National Kidney Foundation's

PRIMER ON KIDNEY DISEASES

SCOTT J. GILBERT, MD
Professor of Medicine, Tufts University School of Medicine
Nephrologist, Tufts Medical Center
Boston, Massachusetts

DANIEL E. WEINER, MD, MS
Associate Professor of Medicine, Tufts University School of Medicine
Nephrologist, Tufts Medical Center
Boston, Massachusetts

Associate Editors
Andrew S. Bomback, MD, MPH
Assistant Professor of Medicine
Department of Medicine, Division of Nephrology
Columbia University College of Physicians and Surgeons
New York, New York

Mark A. Perazella, MD, MS
Professor of Medicine, Section of Nephrology
Medical Director, Yale Physician Associate Program
Department of Medicine, Yale University School of Medicine
Director, Acute Dialysis Services, Yale–New Haven Hospital
New Haven, Connecticut

Marcello Tonelli, MD, SM
Professor of Medicine, University of Alberta
Alberta Kidney Disease Network
Edmonton, Alberta, Canada

Seventh Edition

ELSEVIER

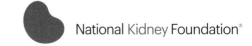

National Kidney Foundation®

ELSEVIER

1600 John F. Kennedy Blvd.
Ste 1800
Philadelphia, PA 19103-2899

NATIONAL KIDNEY FOUNDATION'S PRIMER ON
KIDNEY DISEASES, SEVENTH EDITION

ISBN: 978-0-323-47794-9

Notices

Knowledge and best practice in this field are constantly changing. As new research and experience broaden our understanding, changes in research methods, professional practices, or medical treatment may become necessary.

Practitioners and researchers must always rely on their own experience and knowledge in evaluating and using any information, methods, compounds, or experiments described herein. In using such information or methods they should be mindful of their own safety and the safety of others, including parties for whom they have a professional responsibility.

With respect to any drug or pharmaceutical products identified, readers are advised to check the most current information provided (i) on procedures featured or (ii) by the manufacturer of each product to be administered, to verify the recommended dose or formula, the method and duration of administration, and contraindications. It is the responsibility of practitioners, relying on their own experience and knowledge of their patients, to make diagnoses, to determine dosages and the best treatment for each individual patient, and to take all appropriate safety precautions.

To the fullest extent of the law, neither the Publisher nor the authors, contributors, or editors, assume any liability for any injury and/or damage to persons or property as a matter of products liability, negligence or otherwise, or from any use or operation of any methods, products, instructions, or ideas contained in the material herein.

Previous editions copyrighted 2014, 2009, 2005, 2001, 1998, and 1994 by the National Kidney Foundation.

Library of Congress Cataloging-in-Publication Data

Names: Gilbert, Scott J., editor. | Weiner, Daniel E., editor. | Bomback, Andrew S., editor. | Perazella, Mark A., editor. | Tonelli, Marcello, editor. | National Kidney Foundation, issuing body, publisher.
Title: National Kidney Foundation's primer on kidney diseases / [edited by] Scott J. Gilbert, Daniel E. Weiner ; associate editors, Andrew Bomback, Mark A. Perazella, Marcello Tonelli.
Other titles: Primer on kidney diseases
Description: Seventh edition. | Philadelphia, PA : Elsevier ; [New York City, NY] : National Kidney Foundation, [2018] | Includes bibliographical references and index.
Identifiers: LCCN 2017036332 | ISBN 9780323477949 (pbk. : alk. paper)
Subjects: | MESH: Kidney Diseases | Kidney—pathology
Classification: LCC RC902 | NLM WJ 300 | DDC 616.6/1—dc23 LC record available at https://lccn.loc.gov/2017036332

Content Strategist: Nancy Duffy
Content Development Manager: Lucia Gunzel
Publishing Services Manager: Patricia Tannian
Senior Project Manager: Claire Kramer
Design Direction: Amy Buxton

Printed in China

Last digit is the print number: 9 8 7 6 5 4 3 2 1

Contributors

Ala Abudayyeh, MD
Assistant Professor, Division of Internal Medicine, Section of Nephrology The University of Texas MD Anderson Cancer Center, Houston, Texas
Myeloma, Amyloid, and Other Dysproteinemias

Horacio J. Adrogué, MD
Professor of Medicine, Division of Nephrology, Baylor College of Medicine; the Methodist Hospital; Michael E. DeBakey Veterans Affairs Medical Center, Houston, Texas
Respiratory Acidosis and Alkalosis

Michael Allon, MD
Professor of Medicine, Division of Nephrology, University of Alabama, Birmingham, Alabama
Disorders of Potassium Metabolism

Hina Arif-Tiwari, MD
Assistant Professor, Department of Medical Imaging, Co-Faculty Director, Department of Medical Imaging, South Campus Hospital; Medical Director of Clinical Ultrasound and Research, Department of Medical Imaging, University of Arizona, Banner University Medicine, Tucson, Arizona
Imaging the Kidneys

Jonathan Barratt, PhD, FRCP
The Mayer Professor of Renal Medicine, Infection, Immunity, and Inflammation, University of Leicester; Honorary Consultant Nephrologist, John Walls Renal Unit, University Hospitals of Leicester NHS Trust, Leicester, United Kingdom
Immunoglobulin A Nephropathy and Related Disorders

Jeffrey S. Berns, MD
Professor of Medicine and Pediatrics, Renal, Electrolyte, and Hypertension Division, Perelman School of Medicine at the University of Pennsylvania, Philadelphia, Pennsylvania
Viral Nephropathies: Human Immunodeficiency Virus, Hepatitis C Virus, and Hepatitis B Virus

Petter Bjornstad, MD
Department of Pediatric Endocrinology, University of Colorado School of Medicine, Aurora, Colorado
Pathogenesis, Pathophysiology, and Treatment of Diabetic Nephropathy

Andrew S. Bomback, MD, MPH
Assistant Professor of Medicine, Department of Medicine, Division of Nephrology, Columbia University College of Physicians and Surgeons, New York, New York
Systemic Lupus Erythematosus and the Kidney

C. Barrett Bowling, MD
Assistant Professor of Medicine, Department of Medicine, Duke University School of Medicine, Durham, North Carolina
Kidney Disease in the Elderly

Daniela A. Braun, MD
Division of Nephrology, Boston Children's Hospital, Boston, Massachusetts
Nephronophthisis and Medullary Cystic Kidney Disease

Ursula C. Brewster, MD
Associate Professor of Medicine, Section of Nephrology, Yale School of Medicine, New Haven, Connecticut
Acute Interstitial Nephritis

John M. Carson, MD
Assistant Professor, Department of Medicine, Division of Renal Diseases and Hypertension, University of Colorado, Aurora, Coloado
Hypernatremia

Daniel C. Cattran, MD, FRCP
Professor of Medicine, Department of Medicine, Senior Scientist, Toronto General Research Institute, University Health Network, Toronto, Ontario, Canada
Membranous Nephropathy

Sindhu Chandran, MD
Clinical Associate Professor, Department of Medicine-Nephrology, University of California San Francisco, San Francisco, California
Immunosuppression in Transplantation

Arlene B. Chapman, MD
Professor of Medicine, Chief, Section of Nephrology, University of Chicago, Chicago, Illinois
Polycystic and Other Cystic Kidney Diseases

David Cherney, MD, PhD
Associate Professor, Department of Medicine, Division of Nephrology, University of Toronto, Toronto, Ontario, Canada
Pathogenesis, Pathophysiology, and Treatment of Diabetic Nephropathy

Steven G. Coca, DO, MS
Associate Professor of Medicine, Department of Medicine, Division of Nephrology, Mount Sinai Hospital, New York, New York
Acute Tubular Injury and Acute Tubular Necrosis

Debbie L. Cohen, MD
Professor of Medicine, Clinical Director, Hypertension,
    Co-Director of Neuroendocrine Tumor Program,
    Hospital of the University of Pennsylvania; Department
    of Medicine, Renal Division, University of Pennsylvania,
    Philadelphia, Pennsylvania
Evaluation and Management of Hypertension

Brendan D. Crawford, MD, MS
Fellow, Department of Pediatrics, Division of Nephrology,
    University of Michigan Health System, Ann Arbor,
    Michigan
Genetics and Kidney Disease (APOL1)

Gary C. Curhan, MD, ScD
Physician, Department of Medicine, Renal Division
    and Channing Division of Network Medicine,
    Brigham and Women's Hospital; Professor of
    Medicine, Harvard Medical School; Professor of
    Epidemiology, Harvard School of Public Health,
    Boston, Massachusetts
Nephrolithiasis

Taimur Dad, MD
Nephrologist, Tufts Medical Center; Instructor of
    Medicine, Tufts University School of Medicine, Boston,
    Masssachusetts
Hematuria and Proteinuria

Vivette D. D'Agati, MD
Professor of Pathology, Columbia University College of
    Physicians and Surgeons; Director, Renal Pathology
    Laboratory, Columbia University Medical Center,
    New York, New York
Systemic Lupus Erythematosus and the Kidney

Vimal K. Derebail, MD, MPH, FASN
Assistant Professor of Medicine, University of North
    Carolina Kidney Center, Division of Nephrology and
    Hypertension, University of North Carolina at Chapel
    Hill, Chapel Hill, North Carolina
Sickle Cell Nephropathy

An S. De Vriese, MD, PhD
Division of Nephrology, AZ Sint-Jan Brugge-Oostende AV,
    Brugge, Belgium
Membranous Nephropathy

Dick de Zeeuw, MD, PhD
Professor of Clinical Pharmacology, University of
    Groningen and University Medical School Groningen,
    Groningen, Netherlands
*Pathogenesis, Pathophysiology, and Treatment of Diabetic
Nephropathy*

Thomas D. DuBose, Jr., MD
Professor Emeritus of Medicine, Wake Forest School of
    Medicine, Winston-Salem, North Carolina; Visiting
    Professor, Department of Medicine, University of
    Virginia School of Medicine, Charlottesville,
    Virginia
Metabolic Alkalosis

Michael Emmett, MD
Chief of Internal Medicine, Baylor University Medical
    Center; Professor, Internal Medicine, Texas A&M
    School of Medicine, Dallas, Texas
Approach to Acid-Base Disorders

Pieter Evenepoel, MD, PhD, FERA
Professor of Immunology and Microbiology,
    Nephrology, University Hospitals Leuven, Leuven,
    Belgium
Bone and Mineral Disorders in Chronic Kidney Disease

Todd Fairhead, MD, MSc
Assistant Professor of Medicine, Department of Medicine,
    Division of Nephrology, University of Ottawa and The
    Ottawa Hospital, Ottawa, Ontario, Canda
*Selection of Prospective Kidney Transplant Recipients and
Donors*

Ronald J. Falk, MD
Nan and Hugh Cullman Eminent Professor, Director,
    University of North Carolina Kidney Center; Chair,
    Department of Medicine, University of North Carolina
    School of Medicine, Chapel Hill, North Carolina
Glomerular Clinicopathologic Syndromes
Kidney Involvement in Systemic Vasculitis

Fernando C. Fervenza, MD, PhD
Professor of Medicine, Nephrology and Hypertension,
    Mayo Clinic, Rochester, Minnesota
Membranous Nephropathy

Kevin W. Finkel, MD, FACP, FASN, FCCM
Professor of Medicine and Director, Division of Renal
    Diseases and Hypertension, University of Texas Health
    Science Center at Houston; Professor of Medicine,
    Nephrology Section, University of Texas MD Anderson
    Cancer Center, Houston, Texas
The Kidney in Malignancy

Manuela Födinger, MD
Professor of Laboratory Medicine, Medical Faculty,
    Sigmund-Freud Private University; Institute of Laboratory
    Diagnostics, Kaiser-Franz Josef Spital, Vienna, Austria
Fabry Disease

Rasheed A. Gbadegesin, MD, MBBS
Associate Professor, Department of Pediatrics and
    Nephrology, Duke University Medical Center, Durham,
    North Carolina
Genetics and Kidney Disease (APOL1)

Todd W.B. Gehr, MD
Professor of Medicine, Chairman, Division of Nephrology,
    Virginia Commonwealth University Health System,
    Richmond, Virginia
Edema and the Clinical Use of Diuretics

Scott J. Gilbert, MD
Professor of Medicine, Tufts University School of
    Medicine; Nephrologist, Tufts Medical Center,
    Boston, Massachusetts
Hematuria and Proteinuria

Jagbir S. Gill, MD, MPH
Assistant Professor, Department of Medicine, University of
British Columbia, Vancouver, British Columbia, Canada
Posttransplantation Monitoring and Outcomes

Thomas A. Gonwa, MD
Chair and Professor of Medicine, Department of
Transplantation, Mayo Clinic, Jacksonville, Florida
Hepatorenal Syndrome and Other Liver-Related Kidney Diseases

Arthur Greenberg, MD
Professor of Medicine, Emeritus, Division of Nephrology,
Department of Medicine, Duke University Medical
Center, Durham, North Carolina
Urinalysis and Urine Microscopy

Martin C. Gregory, MD, PhD
Professor of Medicine, Department of Medicine,
University of Utah Health Sciences Center,
Salt Lake City, Utah
Alport Syndrome and Related Disorders

Leal Herlitz, MD
Department of Anatomic Pathology, Cleveland Clinic,
Cleveland, Ohio
Infection-Related Glomerulonephritis

Friedhelm Hildebrandt, MD
William E. Harmon Professor of Pediatrics, Chief, Division
of Nephrology, Boston Children's Hospital, Boston,
Massachusetts
Nephronophthisis and Medullary Cystic Kidney Disease

Gerald A. Hladik, MD
Chief, Doc J. Thurston Distinguished Professor of
Medicine, Division of Nephrology and Hypertension,
University of North Carolina Kidney Center, Chapel
Hill, North Carolina
Overview of Kidney Structure and Function

Michelle A. Hladunewich, MD, MSc
Associate Professor, Division of Nephrology, University of
Toronto, Toronto, Ontario, Canada
The Kidney in Pregnancy

Melanie P. Hoenig, MD
Associate Professor of Medicine, Harvard Medical School;
Renal Division, Beth Israel Deaconess Medical Center,
Boston, Massachusetts
Overview of Kidney Structure and Function

Jonathan Hogan, MD
Assistant Professor of Medicine, Division of Nephrology,
Perelman School of Medicine, University of
Pennsylvania, Philadelphia, Pennsylvania
Minimal Change Nephrotic Syndrome

Andrew A. House, MD, MS, FRCPC, FASN
Professor of Medicine, Chair, Western University Division
of Nephrology, Schulich School of Medicine and
Dentistry, London Health Sciences Centre, University
Hospital, London, Ontario, Canada
Acute Cardiorenal Syndrome

Alastair J. Hutchison, MBChB, MD, FRCP
Professor and Head, Division of Specialist Medicine,
Manchester Institute of Nephrology and
Transplantation, Manchester Royal Infirmary,
Manchester, United Kingdom
Peritoneal Dialysis

T. Alp Ikizler, MD
Catherine McLaughlin-Hakim Professor of Medicine,
Department of Medicine, Vanderbilt University Medical
Center, Nashville, Tennessee
Nutrition and Kidney Disease

Lesley A. Inker, MD, MS
Associate Professor of Medicine, Tufts University School of
Medicine; Nephrologist, Tufts Medical Center, Boston,
Massachusetts
Assessment of Kidney Function in Acute and Chronic Settings
Staging and Management of Chronic Kidney Disease

Michael G. Ison, MD, MS
Professor, Division of Infectious Diseases; Professor, Division
of Organ Transplantation, Northwestern University
Feinberg School of Medicine, Chicago, Illinois
Infectious Complications of Solid Organ Transplantation

Matthew T. James, MD, PhD
Associate Professor, Department of Medicine; Community
Health Sciences, University of Calgary, Calgary, Alberta,
Canada
Management of Acute Kidney Injury

J. Charles Jennette, MD
Kenneth M. Brinkhous Distinguished Professor and Chair,
Department of Pathology and Laboratory Medicine,
University of North Carolina, Chapel Hill,
North Carolina
Glomerular Clinicopathologic Syndromes
Kidney Involvement in Systemic Vasculitis

Renate Kain, MD
Professor of Pathology, Clinical Institute of Pathology,
Medical University of Vienna, Vienna, Austria
Fabry Disease

Jaya Kala, MD
Assistant Professor of Medicine, Division of Renal Diseases
and Hypertension, University of Texas Health Science
Center at Houston, McGovern Medical School,
Houston, Texas
The Kidney in Malignancy

Kamyar Kalantar-Zadeh, MD, MPH, PhD
Professor and Chief, Division of Nephrology, University of
California, Orange, California
Outcomes of Kidney Replacement Therapies

Bobby Kalb, MD
Associate Professor, Director of Magnetic Resonance
Imaging; Chief of Body Section, Vice Chair of Quality
and Safety, Department of Medical Imaging, University
of Arizona, Tucson, Arizona
Imaging the Kidneys

Jeffrey B. Kopp, MD
Branch Chief, Kidney Disease Branch, National Institutes of Diabetes and Digestive and Kidney Disease, National Institutes of Health, Bethesda, Maryland
Focal Segmental Glomerulosclerosis

Greg Knoll, MD, MSc
Professor, Department of Medicine, University of Ottawa; Head, Division of Nephrology, The Ottawa Hospital, Ottawa, Ontario, Canada
Selection of Prospective Kidney Transplant Recipients and Donors

Dhananjay P. Kulkarni, MD
Department of Medicine, Division of Nephrology, Indiana University School of Medicine, Indianapolis, Indianapolis, Indiana
Disorders of Calcium, Phosphorus, and Magnesium Homeostasis

James Lan, MD
Clinical Assistant Professor at the University of British Columbia, Staff Transplant Nephrologist at the Vancouver General Hospital, Vancouver, British Columbia, Canada
Posttransplantation Monitoring and Outcomes

Andrew S. Levey, MD
Professor of Medicine, Dr. Gerald J. and Dorothy R. Friedman Professor of Medicine, Emeritus, Tufts University School of Medicine; Chief, Emeritus, William B. Schwartz Division of Nephrology, Tufts Medical Center, Boston, Massachusetts
Assessment of Kidney Function in Acute and Chronic Settings
Staging and Management of Chronic Kidney Disease

Ed Lewis, MD
Muehrcke Family Professor of Nephrology; Director, Section of Nephrology, Rush University, Medical Center, Chicago, Illinois
Development and Progression of Chronic Kidney Disease

Stuart L. Linas, MD
Professor of Medicine, University of Colorado School of Medicine; Chief of Nephrology, Department of Medicine, Denver Health and Hospital Authority, Denver, Colorado
Hypernatremia

Randy L. Luciano, MD, PhD
Assistant Professor of Medicine, Section of Nephrology, Yale School of Medicine, New Haven, Connecticut
Acute Interstitial Nephritis

Yuliya Lytvyn, PhD
Department of Medicine, Division of Nephrology, University Health Network, University of Toronto, Toronto, Ontario, Canada
Pathogenesis, Pathophysiology, and Treatment of Diabetic Nephropathy

Etienne Macedo, MD, PhD
Assistant Adjunct Professor, Department of Medicine, Division of Nephrology and Hypertension, University of California San Diego, San Diego, California
Clinical Approach to the Diagnosis of Acute Kidney Injury

Nicolaos E. Madias, MD
Maurice S. Segal, MD Professor of Medicine, Tufts University School of Medicine; Physician, Division of Nephrology, St. Elizabeth's Medical Center, Boston, Massachusetts
Respiratory Acidosis and Alkalosis

Diego R. Martin, MD, PhD
Cosden Professor and Chair, Department of Medical Imaging, University of Arizona College of Medicine, Tucson, Arizona
Imaging the Kidneys

Gary R. Matzke, PharmD
Professor and Associate Dean for Clinical Research and Public Policy, Pharmacotherapy and Outcomes Science, School of Pharmacy, Virginia Commonwealth University, Richmond, Virginia
Principles of Drug Therapy in Patients with Reduced Kidney Function

Rajnish Mehrotra, MBBS, MD, MS
Section Head, Division of Nephrology, Harborview Medical Center; Professor of Medicine, University of Washington, Seattle, Washington
Outcomes of Kidney Replacement Therapies

Ankit N. Mehta, MD, FASN
Associate Program Director, Internal Medicine, Baylor University Medical Center; Assistant Professor, Internal Medicine, Texas A & M College of Medicine, Dallas Campus, Dallas, Texas
Approach to Acid-Base Disorders

Ravindra L. Mehta, MBBS, MD, DM
Professor Emeritus, Department of Medicine, Division of Nephrology and Hypertension, University of California San Diego, San Diego, California
Clinical Approach to the Diagnosis of Acute Kidney Injury

Catherine M. Meyers, MD
Director, Office of Clinical and Regulatory Affairs, National Center for Complementary and Alternative Medicine, National Institutes of Health, Bethesda, Maryland
Chronic Tubulointerstitital Disease

Madhukar Misra, MD, FRCP(UK), FACP, FASN
Professor of Medicine, University of Missouri Columbia, Columbia, Missouri
Hemodialysis and Hemofiltration

Sharon M. Moe, MD
Stuart A. Kleit Professor of Medicine and Director, Division of Nephrology, Department of Medicine, Indiana University School of Medicine; Chief of Nephrology, Roudebush Veterans Administration Medical Center, Indianapolis, Indiana
Disorders of Calcium, Phosphorus, and Magnesium Homeostasis

Patrick H. Nachman, MD
Marion Stedman Covington Professor of Medicine, Deputy
    Director, University of North Carolina Kidney Center,
    University of North Carolina, Chapel Hill,
    North Carolina
    Kidney Involvement in Systemic Vasculitis

Lindsay E. Nicolle, MD, FRCPC
Professor Emeritus, Faculty of Health Sciences,
    University of Manitoba, Winnipeg, Manitoba,
    Canada
    Urinary Tract Infection and Pyelonephritis

Thomas D. Nolin, PharmD, PhD
Associate Professor, Department of Pharmacy and
    Therapeutics, University of Pittsburgh School of
    Pharmacy; Department of Medicine, Renal-Electrolyte
    Division, University of Pittsburgh School of Medicine,
    Pittsburgh, Pennsylvania
    *Principles of Drug Therapy in Patients with Reduced Kidney
    Function*

Ann M. O'Hare, MD, MA
Staff Physician, Department of Medicine,
    Department of Veterans Affairs; Professor,
    Division of Nephrology, University of Washington,
    Seattle, Washington
    Kidney Disease in the Elderly

Neesh Pannu, MD, SM
Professor of Medicine, Department of Nephrology and
    Critical Care, University of Alberta, Edmonton, Alberta,
    Canada
    Management of Acute Kidney Injury

Aldo J. Peixoto, MD
Professor of Medicine, Internal Medicine (Nephrology);
    Clinical Chief, Section of Nephrology,
    Yale University School of Medicine, New Haven,
    Connecticut
    Secondary Hypertension

Mark A. Perazella, MD, MS
Professor of Medicine, Section of Nephrology,
    Medical Director, Yale Physician Associate Program,
    Department of Medicine, Yale University Schoool of
    Medicine; Director, Acute Dialysis Services,
    Yale–New Haven Hospital, New Haven,
    Connecticut
    Kidney Disease Caused by Therapeutic Agents
    Chronic Tubulointerstitial Disease

Megan Prochaska, MD
Physician, Renal Division, Brigham and Women's
    Hospital, Harvard Medical School, Boston,
    Massachusetts
    Nephrolithiasis

Laura Ferreira Provenzano, MD
Nephrology and Hypertension Department, Cleveland
    Clinic, Cleveland, Ohio
    Infection-Related Glomerulonephritis

L. Darryl Quarles, MD
UTMG Endowed Professor of Medicine, Department of
    Medicine, University of Tennessee Health Science
    Center, Memphis, Tennessee
    Bone and Mineral Disorders in Chronic Kidney Disease

Jai Radhakrishnan, MD, MS
Professor of Medicine at Columbia University Medical
    Center; Clinical Chief, Division of Nephrology,
    New York Presbyterian Hospital, Columbia Campus,
    New York, New York
    Minimal Change Nephrotic Syndrome

Bharathi Reddy, MD
Assistant Professor of Medicine, Division of Nephrology,
    University of Chicago, Chicago, Illinois
    Polycystic and Other Cystic Kidney Diseases

Dana V. Rizk, MD
Associate Professor of Internal Medicine, Division of
    Nephrology, University of Alabama at Birmingham,
    Birmingham, Alabama
    Polycystic and Other Cystic Kidney Diseases

Claudio Ronco, MD
Director, Department of Nephrology; Director,
    International Renal Research Institute, San Bortolo
    Hospital, Vicenza, Italy
    Acute Cardiorenal Syndrome

Avi Z. Rosenberg, MD, PhD
Assistant Professor of Pathology, Johns Hopkins University
    School of Medicine, Baltimore, Maryland
    Focal Segmental Glomerulosclerosis

Norman D. Rosenblum, MD, FRCPC
Paediatric Nephrologist, Department of Paediatrics; Senior
    Scientist, Program in Developmental and Stem Cell
    Biology, The Hospital for Sick Children; Professor,
    Department of Paediatrics, University of Toronto,
    Toronto, Ontario, Canada
    Kidney Development

Matthew G. Sampson, MD, MSCE
Assistant Professor, Department of Pediatrics and
    Communicable Diseases, Division of Pediatric
    Nephrology, University of Michigan, Ann Arbor,
    Michigan
    Genetics and Kidney Disease (APOL1)

Paul W. Sanders, MD
Professor, Department of Medicine, University of Alabama
    at Birmingham, Birmingham, Alabama
    Myeloma, Amyloid, and Other Dysproteinemias

Mark J. Sarnak, MD, MS
Dr. Gerald J. and Dorothy R. Friedman Professor of
    Medicine, Tufts University School of Medicine; Chief,
    Division of Nephrology, Tufts Medical Center, Boston,
    Massachusetts
    *Cardiac Function and Cardiovascular Disease in Chronic
    Kidney Disesase*

Steven J. Scheinman, MD
President and Dean, Geisinger Commonwealth School of
  Medicine, Scranton, Pennsylvania
  Genetically Based Kidney Transport Disorders

H. William Schnaper, MD
Vice Chair, Academic Affairs, Department of Pediatrics;
  Professor of Pediatrics, Northwestern Medicine,
  Feinberg School of Medicine, Chicago, Illinois
  Focal Segmental Glomerulosclerosis

Sarah Schrauben, MD
University of Pennsylvania Health System, Philadelphia,
  Pennsylvania
  Viral Nephropathies: Human Immunodeficiency Virus,
  Hepatitis C Virus, and Hepatitis B Virus

Richard C. Semelka, MD
Professor and Vice Chair Quality and Safety, Department
  of Radiology, University of North Carolina at Chapel
  Hill, Chapel Hill, North Carolina
  Imaging the Kidneys

Anushree C. Shirali, MD
Assistant Professor of Medicine (Nephrology),
  Department of Internal Medicine, Yale School of
  Medicine, New Haven, Connecticut
  Kidney Disease Caused by Therapeutic Agents

Domenic A. Sica, MD
Professor of Medicine and Pharmacology, Chairman,
  Clinical Pharmacology and Hypertension, Division of
  Nephrology, Virginia Commonwealth University,
  Richmond, Virginia
  Edema and the Clinical Use of Diuretics

Gere Sunder-Plassmann, MD
Division of Nephrology and Dialysis, Department of
  Medicine III, Medical University of Vienna, Vienna,
  Austria
  Fabry Disease

Richard W. Sutherland, MD
Chief, Division of Pediatric Urology, Department of
  Urology, University of North Carolina School of
  Medicine, Chapel Hill, North Carolina
  Obstructive Uropathy

Harold M. Szerlip, MD
Director, Nephrology Division, Director, Nephrology
  Fellowship Program, Baylor University Medical Center;
  Clinical Professor Medicine, Texas A & M College of
  Medicine, Dallas, Texas
  Metabolic Acidosis

Manjula Kurella Tamura, MD, MPH
Professor of Medicine, Department of Medicine/
  Nephrology, Stanford University, Palo Alto,
  California
  Kidney Disease in the Elderly

Jessica Sheehan Tangren, MD
Fellow, Division of Nephrology, Massachusetts General
  Hospital, Boston, Massachusetts
  The Kidney in Pregnancy

Joshua M. Thurman, MD
Professor of Medicine, Division of Renal Diseases and
  Hypertension, University of Colorado Hospital, Aurora,
  Colorado
  Complement-Mediated Glomerulonehpritis and Thrombotic
  Microangiopathy

Marcello Tonelli, MD, SM
Professor of Medicine, University of Alberta, Alberta
  Kidney Disease Network, Edmonton, Alberta,
  Canada

Raymond R. Townsend, MD
Professor of Medicine, Director, Hypertension Program,
  Hospital of the University of Pennsylvania; Department
  of Medicine, Renal Division University of Pennsylvania,
  Philadelphia, Pennsylvania
  Evaluation and Management of Hypertension

Howard Trachtman, MD
Professor of Pediatrics, Director, Division of Nephrology,
  Department of Pediatrics, NYU Langone Medical
  Center, New York, New York
  Minimal Change Nephrotic Syndrome

Jeffrey M. Turner, MD
Assistant Professor of Medicine, Department of Internal
  Medicine, Section of Nephrology, Yale School of
  Medicine, New Haven, Connecticut
  Acute Tubular Injury and Acute Tubular Necrosis

Anand Vardhan, MBBS, MD, DNB, FRCP
Consultant Nephrologist, Manchester Institute of
  Nephrology and Transplantation, Manchester Royal
  Infirmary, Manchester, United Kingdom
  Peritoneal Dialysis

Joseph G. Verbalis, MD
Professor of Medicine and Physiology, Georgetown
  University; Chief, Division of Endocrinology and
  Metabolism, Georgetown University Hospital,
  Washington, District of Columbia
  Hyponatremia and Hypoosmolar Disorders

Flavio G. Vincenti, MD
Professor of Clinical Medicine, Kidney Transplant Service,
  University of California San Francisco, San Francisco,
  California
  Immunosuppression in Transplantation

Marina Vivarelli, MD
Pediatric Nephrology Consultant, Division of Nephrology
  and Dialysis, Ospedale Pediatrico, Bambino Gesù–
  IRCCS, Rome, Italy
  Complement-Mediated Glomerulonephritis and Thrombotic
  Microangiopathy

Raven Voora, MD
Assistant Professor of Medicine, Division of Nephrology and Hypertension, University of North Carolina Kidney Center, University of North Carolina School of Medicine, Chapel Hill, North Carolina
Evaluation and Management of Hypertension

Hani M. Wadei, MD
Associate Professor of Medicine, Department of Transplantation, Mayo Clinic, Jacksonville, Florida
Hepatorenal Syndrome and Other Liver-Related Kidney Diseases

Bradley A. Warady, MD
Professor of Pediatrics, Department of Pediatrics, University of Missouri-Kansas City School of Medicine; Senior Associate Chairman, Chief, Section of Nephrology, Director, Dialysis and Transplantation, Department of Pediatrics, Children's Mercy Hospitals and Clinics, Kansas City, Missouri
Kidney Diseases in Infants and Children

Darcy K. Weidemann, MD, MHS
Assistant Professor of Pediatrics, Department of Pediatrics, University of Missouri-Kansas City School of Medicine; Section of Nephrology, Department of Pediatrics, Children's Mercy Hospital and Clinics, Kansas City, Missouri
Kidney Diseases in Infants and Children

Daniel E. Weiner, MD, MS
Associate Professor of Medicine, Tufts University School of Medicine; Nephrologist, Tufts Medical Center, Boston, Massachusetts
Cardiac Function and Cardiovascular Disease in Chronic Kidney Disease

William L. Whittier, MD, FASN
Associate Professor of Medicine, Department of Internal Medicine, Division of Nephrology, Rush University Medical Center, Chicago, Illinois
Development and Progression of Chronic Kidney Disease

Christopher S. Wilcox, MD, PhD
Chief, Division of Nephrology and Hypertension, George E. Schreiner Chair of Nephrology, Director of the Hypertension Research Center, Georgetown University, Washington, District of Colubmia
Pathogenesis of Hypertension

Jay B. Wish, MD
Professor of Clinical Medicine, Department of Medicine, Indiana University School of Medicine; Medical Director, Dialysis Unit, Indiana University Health University Hospital, Indianapolis, Indiana
Anemia and Other Hematologic Complications of Chronic Kidney Disease

See Cheng Yeo, MBBS, MRCP (UK), MMED (Int Med)
Adjunct Assistant Professor, Consultant and Deputy Head, Department of Renal Medicine, Tan Tock Seng Hospital, Singapore
Immunoglobulin A Nephropathy and Related Disorders

Preface

We are pleased to present the seventh edition of the National Kidney Foundation's *Primer on Kidney Diseases*. The *Primer* has been a key resource for students, residents, fellows, and clinicians ever since publication of the first edition by Arthur Greenberg and his editorial team in 1993. This seventh edition has been extensively revised and updated to address the quickly changing landscape of clinical nephrology while preserving the accessibility and utility that define the *Primer* as the essential resource for clinical challenges in nephrology, electrolyte and acid-base disorders, and hypertensive conditions.

This edition brings change to the *Primer*. Andrew Bomback has joined Mark Perazella and Marcello Tonelli on our editorial team, providing a breadth of expertise and a wealth of clinical experience to this effort. Our group remains committed to the careful selection of content and a diligent editorial process, stressing usability and clinical applicability.

To maintain the *Primer* as a current review of clinical nephrology, we have included new sections that highlight recent advances in nephrology. Our expanding comprehension of the genetic underpinnings of kidney disease is described by Brendan Crawford, Matthew Sampson, and Rasheed Gbadegesin, and a mechanistic approach to complement-mediated kidney diseases and thrombotic microangiopathy is outlined by Joshua Thurman. Advances in onconephrology, diabetic nephropathy, membranous glomerulopathy, focal segmental glomerulosclerosis, hypertension management, and kidney disease in pregnancy are reflected in extensive updates to ensure that the *Primer* remains current, accurate, and practical. Suggested readings have been updated to direct readers to additional material.

We have also expanded the online features with this edition of the *Primer*. Access to Expert Consult is available with the activation code provided on the inside front cover. By visiting www.expertconsult.com, readers are able to access the entire *Primer* electronically in a searchable format, download figures and images, and enjoy additional content. The *Primer* will now fit into your pocket on a smartphone or tablet, delivering the information that you seek when you need it.

We are grateful to the authors and editors who diligently compiled a wealth of information into thorough yet concise reviews, ensuring that the *Primer* maintains its clarity and brevity. We are also grateful to the publisher, designers, and copy editors who strove to create an appealing and highly accessible text with illustrative tables and figures to reinforce key messages. Finally, we would like to dedicate this edition of the *Primer* to Andrew S. Levey, our devoted mentor, committed Chief, and dear friend, who has advanced the approach to clinical nephrology perhaps further than any other in our generation. And yet, his best work lies ahead.

We hope you find the *Primer* to be the same go-to resource clinicians have relied on for the past 25 years.

Scott J. Gilbert, MD
Daniel E. Weiner, MD, MS

Contents

STRUCTURE AND FUNCTION OF THE KIDNEY

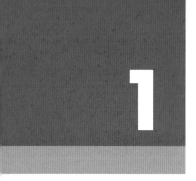

1 Overview of Kidney Structure and Function

Melanie P. Hoenig; Gerald A. Hladik

The kidney plays an essential role in normal homeostasis. The key functions of the kidneys include:

1. *Maintenance of normal body fluid composition.* The kidney plays a primary role in the regulation of both the intracellular and extracellular compartments by retention or excretion of water and electrolytes. The concentration of water, sodium, potassium, calcium, phosphate, and hydrogen are tightly regulated within these body compartments to maintain normal cell size and cellular function.
2. *Excretion of waste products of metabolism and excretion of foreign substances.* The kidney is responsible for excretion of nitrogenous waste that is generated primarily in the liver from normal metabolism. In addition, a wide range of pharmacologic and exogenous toxic compounds are excreted in the urine.
3. *Regulation of blood pressure.* Reduced kidney perfusion or stimulation of the sympathetic nervous system stimulates the release of renin from the juxtaglomerular cells of the kidneys. This enzyme converts angiotensinogen to angiotensin I, which in turn is cleaved to form angiotensin II by angiotensin converting enzyme. Angiotensin II is a potent vasoconstrictive agent. In addition, this peptide hormone can stimulate sodium retention throughout the nephron, but especially in the proximal tubule. Angiotensin II also stimulates the release of aldosterone from the zona glomerulosa of the adrenal gland.
4. *Production of hormones*
   a. *Erythropoietin.* Interstitial fibroblasts produce erythropoietin in response to the hypoxia inducible factor (HIF). Erythropoietin is a glycoprotein hormone that promotes maturation of progenitor erythroid cells into mature red blood cells in the bone marrow.
   b. *Activation of vitamin D.* The final hydroxylation of vitamin D to its active form, 1,25-dihydroxy vitamin D, is achieved by the proximal tubule cells in response to parathyroid hormone. This steroid hormone plays an essential role in calcium and phosphate homeostasis, as well as bone metabolism.

THE KIDNEY AND HOMEOSTASIS

The kidney is the master regulator of homeostasis. Despite substantial variations in intake, environmental conditions, or physical stresses from one individual to another or within the same individual over the course of a few hours, the kidney maintains normal body fluid composition and plasma volume. Important examples include:

- Normal water concentration dictates cell size since water is distributed equally in all body compartments.
- Normal sodium content affects extracellular volume, a key component of which is intravascular volume, organ perfusion, and blood pressure.
- Restriction of potassium primarily to the intracellular space maintains the electrochemical gradient necessary to maintain the negative cell membrane potential required for cells to function normally.
- Normal homeostasis of hydrogen concentration affects protein folding and enzymatic function.
- Since the kidney maintains plasma volume and plays a role in red blood cell production, the kidney also controls the intravascular volume.

MAINTENANCE OF BALANCE

To maintain normal volume and body fluid composition, the kidneys must maintain balance, or "the steady state." Thus intake and production via metabolism must always equal excretion and consumption. Under normal circumstances, excretion can readily match intake. For example, an increase in water intake normally prompts excretion of water as dilute urine. Intake of a diet rich in potassium can stimulate excretion of a large amount of potassium. Similarly, intake of a high-protein diet can prompt excretion of additional nitrogen and acid, but in the setting of volume depletion or reduced kidney function, these prompt responses may be blunted.

BODY FLUID COMPOSITION

The human body is composed primarily of water; in adult men, approximately 60% of the lean body weight is water, with a slightly lower percentage in women and children who tend to have slightly more adipose tissue that contains less water than muscle. Water is distributed among the body compartments such that approximately 2/3 is in the intracellular space and 1/3 in the extracellular space (Fig. 1.1). The extracellular fluid is composed of the interstitium and the vascular fluid. These later compartments are essentially in continuum; fluid in the vasculature is separated from the interstitium only by small differences in oncotic forces generated by plasma proteins and cells. Typical values for the normal electrolytes in plasma and intracellular fluid are shown in Table 1.1.

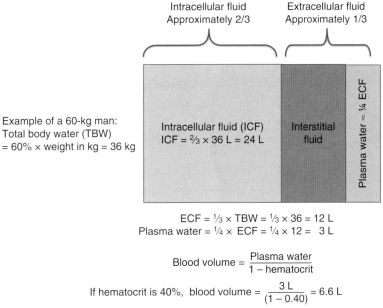

$$\text{Blood volume} = \frac{\text{Plasma water}}{1 - \text{hematocrit}}$$

$$\text{If hematocrit is 40\%, blood volume} = \frac{3 \text{ L}}{(1 - 0.40)} = 6.6 \text{ L}$$

Fig. 1.1 Body fluid compartments, distribution of water, and estimates of compartment volumes.
Total body water (TBW) is distributed in the intracellular fluid (ICF) and extracellular fluid (ECF). Plasma water in the vascular space represents approximately one-fourth of the fluid in the ECF. Using this rubric, body fluid compartment volumes can be estimated.

Table 1.1 Approximate Typical Ion Concentrations, Osmolality, and pH Within the Plasma and Intracellular Fluid

	Plasma (mEq/L)	Intracellular Fluid (mEq/L)
Cations		
Na^+	143	10
K^+	4	138
Ca^{2+} (ionized)	2	<0.0001
Mg^{2+}	1	2
Total Cations	150	150
Anions		
Cl^-	104	4
HCO_3^-	24	10
HPO_4^{2-}, HPO_4^{2-}	2	40
Protein	14	50
Other (organic anions and SO_4^{2-})	6	46
Total Anions	150	150
Osmolality	290 mOsm/L	290 mOsm/L
pH	7.4	7.1

KIDNEY STRUCTURE

The kidneys are positioned along the posterior abdominal wall of the retroperitoneum, each weighing approximately 150 g. Anatomically, the kidneys are divided into two regions: an outer cortex and an inner medulla (Fig. 1.2). The cortex and medulla contain the basic functional units of the kidney, the nephrons, as well as the associated vasculature, nerves, and lymphatic vessels. The nephron consists of the glomerulus, Bowman capsule, and renal tubule (Fig. 1.3). On average, each kidney comprises 1 million nephrons, but this number may vary in individuals from approximately 600,000 to 2 million nephrons per kidney. Distinct functional units form the renal tubule—the proximal tubule, the loop of Henle, the distal convoluted tubule, and the collecting duct. The function and morphology of the tubular epithelium vary in each segment of the nephron (see below). The glomeruli, most of the proximal tubule, and portions of the distal tubule are primarily located in the cortex. The medulla is composed of parallel arrays of the loops of Henle and collecting ducts. On gross inspection, these parallel arrays form the renal pyramids. The rounded apices of the pyramids form the papilla. The urine is maximally concentrated in the renal medulla, and the concentration of solute in the medullary interstitium may exceed that of plasma fourfold.

The process of urine formation begins at the glomerulus. The glomerular filtrate flows into Bowman capsule and enters into the proximal tubule where about two thirds of the filtrate is reabsorbed. Tubular fluid then flows through the thin descending limb of the loop of Henle, and, after a hairpin turn, ascends through the thin ascending limb into the thick ascending limb (TAL) of the loop of Henle. The distal portion of the loop of Henle touches the glomerulus at the juxtaglomerular apparatus (JGA), after which the filtrate flows into the distal convoluted tubule. Fluid in the tubular lumen is maximally dilute at this site. The processed filtrate then flows via the connecting tubule into the cortical and medullary collecting ducts where water is either conserved or excreted. The collecting duct is also the regulatory site of potassium and hydrogen ion secretion. As the filtrate passes through each successive portion of the nephron, a highly orchestrated process of solute reabsorption and secretion

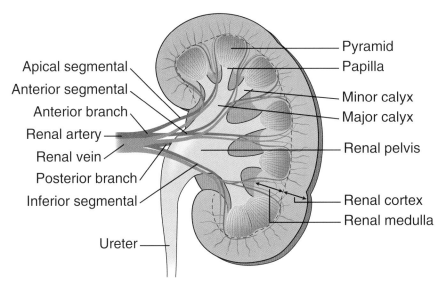

Fig. 1.2 The anatomy of the kidney. The cortex is primarily composed of glomeruli, proximal tubules, and portions of the distal tubule. The medulla contains parallel arrays of the loops of Henle tubules and collecting ducts. The renal arteries of the kidney promptly branch into segmental arteries and then interlobar arteries once within the renal parenchyma (see text for additional details). In contrast to the arterial system, the venous system has extensive collaterals for drainage of the kidney; the venous system maps to the arterial system but there is also a subcapsular venous plexus that drains the kidney (not shown). Nevertheless, if there is obstruction or thrombosis of the renal vein, the kidney will swell.

occurs that results in the excretion of the precise amount water, acid-base equivalents, and electrolytes necessary to maintain homeostasis. Urine subsequently passes from the papillae (the tips of the pyramids) into the minor calyces, which then converge to form two to three major calyces that configure the renal pelvis. The lining of the renal pelvis, the ureter, bladder, and urethra are all epithelial cells that are impermeable to water, known as transitional cells. In the urethra, squamous epithelial cells, which are also impermeable to water, line the lumen.

RENAL CIRCULATION

ANATOMY

The renal circulation is one of the richest vascular beds in the body. The renal arteries originate from the lateral aspect of the aorta and enter the kidneys in the hilum, posterior to the renal veins and anterior to the origin of the ureter. Anatomic variants of the renal arteries and veins are common and can be found in 25% to 40% of patients. During development, blood from transient aortic "sprouts" supplies the kidneys; these degenerate as the kidneys ascend and renal arteries from the lumbar region ultimately perfuse the kidneys. When arteries from earlier in development do not degenerate, there may be residual additional vessels.

The renal arteries enter the kidney in the hilum and then bifurcate first into *segmental arteries* (see Fig. 1.2). The segmental arteries are functional "end arteries" since they serve as the only supply of oxygenated blood to their particular regions of the kidney. The segmental arteries then divide into *interlobar arteries*, and then *arcuate arteries*, which arch around the kidney as they run between the cortex and the outer medulla; the arcuate arteries give rise to the *interlobular arteries* that extend toward the cortex, and en route give rise to an array of arterioles. The *afferent arterioles* divide into the glomerular capillaries and then culminate in another arteriole, the *efferent arteriole*. Thus the glomerular capillary is the only capillary bed in the body flanked by two resistance vessels. Changes in the resistance of the arterioles can affect glomerular pressure and ultimately filtration.

TWO CAPILLARY BEDS IN SERIES

The efferent arterioles then descend toward the medulla and form a second capillary bed; these capillaries are associated with the proximal tubules and are known as the *peritubular capillaries*. The intimate association between this second capillary bed and the tubules creates a relationship such that filtration and reabsorption can be balanced. For example, if filtration is increased, tubular reabsorption is also increased. This is called *glomerulotubular balance*.

MEDULLARY BLOOD SUPPLY

The peritubular capillaries continue straight to the medulla and are called the *vasa recta*. The vasa recta then take a hairpin turn and return to the cortex (see Fig. 1.3). This orientation allows the kidney to return electrolytes and water to the circulation while maintaining the concentration gradient that is created by the loops of Henle. Red blood cells that travel in the vasa recta are subjected to very low oxygen tension and a hyperosmotic environment in the medulla. To withstand the osmotic stress, red blood cells have transporters for urea on the cell surface that allow urea to rapidly enter the cells and help maintain cell size and structure (see below).

GLOMERULUS

The glomerulus is a complex network of capillaries responsible for the selective ultrafiltration of plasma and the clearance of small solutes. The glomerular capillaries are uniquely interposed between two arterioles: the afferent and efferent arterioles. This anatomic configuration allows for the intricate control of glomerular capillary pressure and the glomerular filtration rate (GFR). The glomerular capillaries form the glomerular filtration barrier (Fig. 1.4), which allows for the selective filtration of small solutes such as water, sodium, and urea, while excluding the passage of cells and large proteins such as albumin. The basement membrane, endothelium, and podocytes confer a net negative charge to the filtration barrier. As a result, negatively charged proteins such as albumin are less likely to pass through the filtration

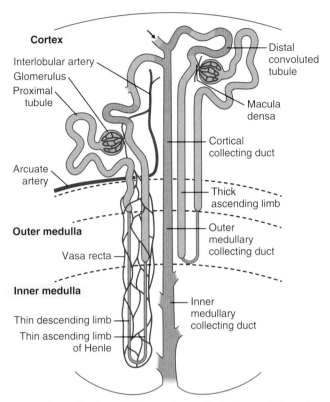

Fig. 1.3 Organization of the nephron. Each human kidney has approximately one million nephrons. Two nephrons are shown here. Each nephron consists of a glomerulus, a proximal convoluted tubule, a thin descending limb and a thin ascending limb of Henle, a thick ascending limb, the macula densa, a distal convoluted tubule, and a connecting tubule. Several nephrons converge and empty into a collecting duct. The collecting duct can be divided into segments based on location: the cortical collecting ducts, the outer medullary collecting duct, and the inner medullary collecting duct. As shown, some glomeruli are deeper and give rise to nephrons with loops of Henle that descend all the way to the papillary tips, whereas more superficial glomeruli have loops of Henle that only reach to the junction of the inner and outer medulla. The interlobular arteries give rise to an array of afferent arterioles, which form the glomerular capillary bundles. Blood exits the glomeruli through the efferent arterioles. These arterioles form a second capillary bed, the peritubular capillaries, which reclaim the fluid and electrolytes reabsorbed in the nephron. In the deeper aspects of the kidney, the peritubular capillaries play a critical role in the maintenance of the osmotic gradient.

barrier. Under normal conditions, only low-molecular-weight proteins and a small amount of albumin are filtered; these are almost completely reabsorbed and catabolized by the proximal tubular epithelial cells. This leads to excretion of 40 to 80 mg of protein per day, primarily composed of uromodulin (previously known as Tamm-Horsfall protein), a mucoprotein secreted by tubular epithelial cells in the thick ascending loop of Henle.

The glomerulus has four major components: the endothelium, the mesangium, the basement membrane, and the podocytes (Fig. 1.5). In addition to important functional roles, the mesangium and podocytes provide a structural scaffold that supports the glomerular capillaries. The glomerular capillaries have an unusually high proportion of *fenestrae*, or clefts, on the endothelial surface (20% to 50%) that facilitate the efficient trafficking of small solutes and water through the filtration barrier. The glycocalyx is a lattice

of negatively charged glycoproteins that overlies the fenestrae that preferentially exclude the passage of negatively charged proteins such as albumin. Aligned between the endothelial cells and the podocytes, is the basement membrane. This structure is composed of a network of extracellular matrix proteins that include type IV collagen, laminin, and heparan sulfate–bound proteoglycans. The basement membrane constrains the filtration of proteins in concert with the endothelium and podocytes, and has an important role in limiting the flux of solutes and fluids. The visceral epithelium is composed of podocytes, specialized cells named for the foot processes that envelop the glomerular capillaries. The foot processes of one podocyte interdigitate with foot processes from neighboring podocytes to form the *slit pore diaphragm.* These specialized intercellular junctions function as a critical barrier to the passage of high-molecular-weight proteins. Podocin and nephrin are two constituent proteins of the slit pore diaphragm essential for the proper structure and function of the filtration barrier. Inactivating mutations of the genes that encode podocin and nephrin lead to severe proteinuric kidney disease.

FACTORS THAT INFLUENCE GLOMERULAR FILTRATION RATE

The GFR is the product of the net filtration pressure along the glomerular capillary (P_{net}) and the surface area of the glomerular capillaries. This relationship can be represented by the following equation:

$$GFR = P_{net} \times Area$$

Transcapillary Starling forces are key determinants of the net filtration pressure. These include the glomerular capillary hydraulic (P_{cap}) and oncotic pressure (π_{cap}), and the interstitial hydraulic (P_{int}) and oncotic pressures (π_{int}). The net filtration pressure can be altered by the permeability of the glomerular capillary (represented by the filtration coefficient, K_f), and the net oncotic pressure may be influenced by the permeability of proteins across the capillary wall, denoted by the reflection coefficient (σ). Quantitatively, these forces are related by the following equation:

$$P_{net} = K_f [(P_{cap} - P_{int}) - \sigma(\pi_{cap} - \pi_{int})]$$

The hydraulic pressure at the origin of the glomerular capillary bed is relatively high at approximately 60 mm Hg and exceeds the capillary oncotic pressure throughout the length of the glomerular capillaries. Together with a very high filtration coefficient, the relatively high glomerular capillary pressure favors the net filtration of fluid from the glomerular capillaries into Bowman space. The capillary oncotic pressure increases along the length of the capillary as filtration of relatively protein-free fluid progresses, resulting in a gradual fall in net filtration pressure as filtration proceeds toward the efferent arteriole. The GFR typically equals about 20% of plasma flow rate. Changes in GFR can result from altered glomerular capillary pressure or permeability or from a change in the surface area of the glomerular capillaries. The relative resistance of the afferent and efferent arterioles affects changes in renal plasma flow, net ultrafiltration pressure, and GFR. A number of physiologic mediators can alter the degree of constriction or dilation of these arterioles.

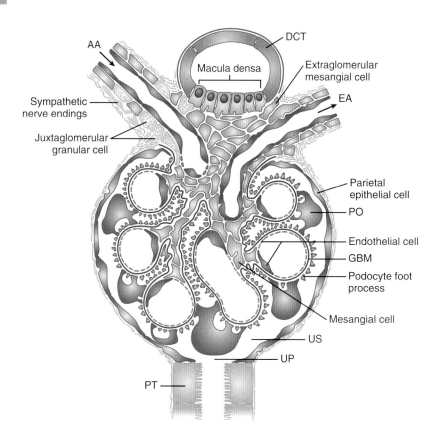

Fig. 1.4 Schematic diagram of a section of a glomerulus and its juxtaglomerular apparatus. *AA*, afferent arteriole; *DCT*, distal convoluted tubule; *EA*, efferent arteriole; *GBM*, glomerular basement membrane; *PT*, proximal tubule; *PO*, epithelial podocyte; *UP*, urinary pole; *US*, urinary space. (Previous edition, Fig. 1.3, Briggs J.)

Angiotensin II, increased activity of the sympathetic nervous system, and circulating catecholamines cause arteriolar vasoconstriction, whereas prostaglandins, nitric oxide, and bradykinin mediate arteriolar vasodilation. During decreases in renal perfusion, prostaglandins tend to maintain or increase glomerular capillary pressure and GFR by causing afferent arteriolar vasodilatation. Correspondingly, in the normal range of autoregulation of GFR (a perfusion pressure of 80 to 180 mm Hg), angiotensin II maintains glomerular capillary pressure and GFR when there is a relative decline in perfusion by inducing vasoconstriction of the efferent arteriole.

MEASUREMENT OF GLOMERULAR FILTRATION RATE

Measurement and estimation of the GFR are extensively reviewed in Chapter 3. The GFR is equal to the total plasma ultrafiltration rate. Normal values are about 120 mL/min per 1.73 m^2 body surface area (BSA) for adult women and 130 mL/min per 1.73 m^2 BSA for adult men, or about 180 L per day. GFR progressively increases with growth during childhood and declines about 1 mL/min per year starting at age 40. GFR can be measured indirectly by determining the clearance of a solute, such as inulin, that is freely filtered by the glomerulus and is neither secreted nor reabsorbed by the renal tubules. In addition, the solute should not be produced or metabolized by the kidney. When these conditions are met, the filtered load is equivalent to the excreted load, allowing for the calculation of GFR.

Creatinine is an endogenous solute commonly used to estimate GFR. Creatinine clearance is less precise than inulin clearance in determining GFR because approximately 10% to 40% of urinary creatinine is derived from the tubular secretion of creatinine in the proximal convoluted tubule.

As a result, creatinine clearance tends to overestimate GFR by about 10% to 15%. The degree of overestimation increases at lower levels of GFR in which the tubular secretion of creatinine is proportionately higher. The serum creatinine level can also be used to assess GFR either alone or through use of estimating equations. As discussed in Chapter 3, the serum creatinine level has limitations for GFR estimation, varying with muscle mass, dietary intake, comorbid illness, age, sex, and volume status. Other filtration markers, like cystatin C, can also be used to estimate GFR. Cystatin C is less influenced by age, sex, and muscle mass compared with serum creatinine and better estimates kidney function at higher levels of GFR.

THE JUXTAGLOMERULAR APPARATUS

The JGA is a specialized conglomeration of cells central to the regulation of GFR, sodium chloride balance, and extracellular fluid volume. It is located at the site where the distal convoluted tubule comes in contact with its own glomerulus and the wall of the afferent arteriole. *Granular cells* are specialized cells in the wall of the afferent arteriole that release renin in response to decreased perfusion or increased sympathetic tone. In addition, decreased uptake of sodium chloride by the kidney-specific Na$^+$/K$^+$/2Cl$^-$ cotransporter (NKCC2) in the macula densa sends a signal to granular cells to release renin.

AUTOREGULATION OF RENAL BLOOD FLOW AND GFR

The JGA plays an important role in the intrarenal regulation of renal blood flow and GFR. Autoregulatory mechanisms

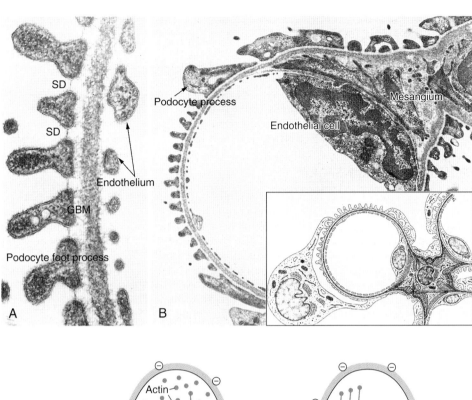

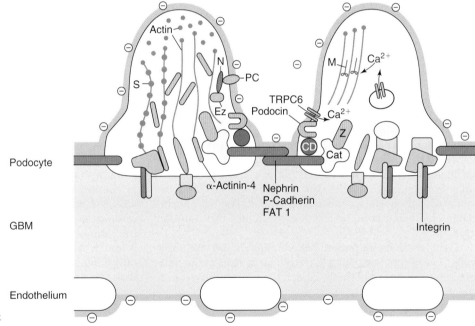

Fig. 1.5 Structure of the glomerular capillary loop and the filtration barrier. (A) The glomerular filtration barrier consists of endothelial cells, the glomerular basement membrane (GBM), and the filtration slit diaphragms (SD) between podocyte foot processes (×34,000). (B) A single capillary loop demonstrates the fenestrated endothelium, the basement membrane, and the foot processes. The mesangium is contiguous with the subendothelial space and provides structural support that permits the cells to withstand the high pressures characteristic of the glomerular capillaries which favor filtration (×13,000). (C) Schematic diagram of the filtration barrier. The porous endothelium is negatively charged. The GBM is composed of type IV collagen and laminin 521, and other components. The filtration SD are created by podocyte foot processes from distinct cells and various molecule. *Cat*, Catenin; *CD*, CD2-associated protein; *EZ*, Ezrin; *FAT 1*, FAT tumor suppressor homolog 1; *M*, myosin; *N*, NERF2; *PC*, podocalyxin; *S*, synaptopodin; *TRPC6*, transient receptor potential-channel 6; *Z*, ZO1. (Previous edition, Fig. 1.5, Briggs J.)

stabilize renal blood flow and GFR during changes in renal perfusion pressure in the range of 80 to 180 mm Hg. Small changes in renal perfusion can influence GFR and potentially cause life-threatening changes in sodium balance. In the absence of significant changes in the effective arterial blood volume (EABV) or underlying kidney disease, two servomechanisms prevent alterations in sodium balance during spontaneous or induced fluctuations in renal perfusion. The first, a rapid myogenic response modulates changes in renal blood flow and GFR after small changes in renal perfusion. Increased hydraulic pressure at the afferent arteriole triggers the intracellular release of calcium that leads to compensatory vasoconstriction. A more delayed mechanism, *tubuloglomerular feedback*, adjusts sodium excretion in response to variations

in renal perfusion in the range of renal autoregulation. An increase in renal perfusion pressure, for example, results in increased NKCC2 activity in the macula densa related to a small but significant increase in single-nephron GFR and the filtered load of sodium chloride. The resultant increase in sodium chloride transport elicits a signal that constricts the afferent arteriole and increases preglomerular vascular resistance. This feedback mechanism counteracts increases in single-nephron GFR arising from increased renal perfusion. Tubuloglomerular feedback is likely altered in chronic kidney disease based on models of chronic nephron loss. Increased tubular sodium chloride levels at the macula densa, for example, result in increased, not decreased, single-nephron GFR in rats after subtotal nephrectomy.

TUBULAR FUNCTION

The volume of the initial glomerular filtrate is approximately 180 L/day in the setting of a normal GFR as derived above, yet most individuals excrete just 1 to 2 L of urine a day. A circuit of tubules, lined with epithelial cells, reabsorbs the majority of the filtrate and assures that the final urine has the appropriate amount of electrolytes, acid, and water.

EPITHELIAL CELL TRANSPORT

Since cells are bound by a lipid bilayer and are impermeable to large molecules, ions, and polar molecules, transport proteins within the epithelial cell membrane help overcome this barrier and facilitate the movement of substances from the filtrate back to the capillaries. The renal tubular cells are polarized cells, characterized by the presence of the Na^+/K^+-ATPase on the basolateral membrane. The Na^+/K^+-ATPase generates an approximately 10-fold higher level of sodium in the extracellular fluid than the intracellular fluid by extruding three intracellular sodium ions in exchange for two extracellular potassium ions with energy derived from the hydrolysis of ATP. This is an example of *primary active transport*. In contrast, transporters on the luminal membrane benefit from the low intracellular concentration of sodium function based on *secondary active transport*. This arrangement allows the kidney to use the concentration gradient created by the low intracellular sodium concentration to reabsorb the majority of sodium in the filtrate.

Movement of sodium into the cell can be achieved with coupled transport of sodium either in the form of cotransport, as with the sodium/glucose cotransporters, or in the form of countertransport as with the Na^+/H^+-exchanger (see below). Facilitated transport using carriers in the membrane can facilitate the movement of molecules such as glucose and urea. Specialized channels favor movement of specific ions along with their electrochemical gradient. The aquaporin water channels permit water to move along the osmotic gradient.

Tight junctions are present between the tubular epithelial cells. These junctions limit paracellular transport so that gradients can be established between the urinary filtrate and the interstitium. These tight junctions are composed of multiple proteins, including claudins, occludins, and cadherins, which permit selective transport of certain ions.

NEPHRON SEGMENTS

The tubular segments vary substantially in both function and morphology. The proximal tubule reabsorbs the bulk of the filtrate, the loop of Henle creates the concentration gradient that is present in the medulla, and the distal nephron sets the final urine composition.

PROXIMAL TUBULE

The proximal tubule is the workhorse of the kidney, and more than 60% of the filtrate is normally reabsorbed in this region. The first portion of the proximal tubule is convoluted and forms a labyrinth within the renal cortex before transitioning to a straight segment that leads to the loop of Henle. To achieve the task of reabsorbing the bulk of the urinary filtrate, the proximal tubule has a lush luminal brush border of microvilli that increases the surface area dramatically (Fig. 1.6). The primary transporter for sodium on the luminal membrane is the Na^+/H^+-exchanger 3 (NHE3). This antiporter also plays a key role in the reclamation of bicarbonate (see below). In addition, NH_4^+ formed in the proximal tubules from glutamine is excreted via the same transporter, as the molar radius of NH_4^+ is similar to H^+. Other important transporters in the proximal tubule include the Na^+/phosphate cotransporters regulated by parathyroid hormone, sodium/glucose transporters, and amino acid transporters. These cells are permeable to water due to the presence of aquaporin 1, and water is reabsorbed in an isosmotic fashion. Tight junctions between proximal tubule cells allow passive reabsorption of water along with paracellular movement of chloride and potassium.

LOOP OF HENLE

At the end of the proximal tubule, the cell type abruptly changes to that of the thin descending limb of Henle (Fig. 1.7). After a hairpin turn, the thin ascending limb of Henle becomes the taller TAL, equipped with the renal-specific NKCC2. NKCC2 requires all four ions for transport. Since the concentration of potassium in the lumen is considerably lower than that of sodium and chloride, additional potassium is supplied by a channel that allows movement of potassium into the lumen, the renal outer medullary potassium channel (ROMK) (Fig. 1.8). NKCC2 plays a critical role in the creation of the medullary concentration gradient. Also of note, the versatile ammonium ion, NH_4^+, can be absorbed by NKCC2 in the K^+ position. The thin limbs are permeable to water, but the TAL cells are not. This differential permeability, along with active transport by the TAL, plays important role in the development of the medullary gradient within the kidney. For this reason, the loop of Henle is considered the *concentrating segment* of the nephron. The net result is that the concentration of the medulla of the kidney is much higher than the rest of the body. This is the only compartment in the body that has a higher osmolality than serum.

When the loop of Henle reaches the cortex, it greets its own glomerulus and forms a unique structure called the *macula densa*. Specialized cells in this structure are equipped with the same NKCC that is used here to provide feedback regarding tubular flow to the parent glomerulus as described above.

DISTAL NEPHRON

DISTAL CONVOLUTED TUBULE

The distal convoluted tubule is the smallest segment of the nephron at only 10 to 12 mm long. Cells in this region are also impermeable to water and include a sodium chloride cotransporter, NCC (Fig. 1.9). Removal of solute without water in this region allows the tubular fluid to become dilute; thus this segment has also been called the *diluting segment*. This segment also has a calcium channel on the luminal membrane, the transient receptor potential channel subfamily V member 5 (TRPV5).

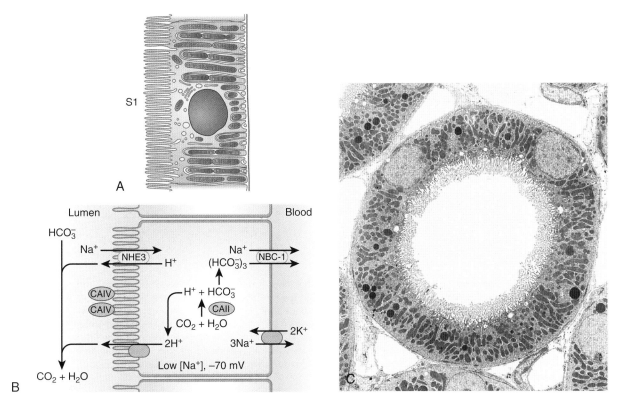

Fig. 1.6 Proximal tubule. (A) Schematic diagram of a typical cell of the proximal convoluted tubule, which is characterized by a prominent luminal brush border that increases the membrane surface area about 40-fold. The basolateral infoldings are lined with mitochondria and interdigitate with the basolateral infoldings of adjacent cells (in the image, infoldings from the neighboring cells are depicted in blue). These adaptations are most prominent in convoluted portion of the proximal tubule, S1. (B) The proximal tubule cell has a variety of transport mechanisms to reabsorb the bulk of the initial urinary filtrate. Primary active transport at the basolateral membrane maintains the low intracellular sodium concentration and returns sodium to the peritubular capillaries. The low intracellular concentration facilitates movement of sodium across the luminal membrane from the filtrate. Sodium is reabsorbed from the Na$^+$/H$^+$-exchanger and other transporters on the luminal membrane. (C) Cross-section of the S1 segment (×3000). *CAII*, carbonic anhydrase II; *CAIV*, carbonic anhydrase IV; *CO$_2$*, carbon dioxide; *H$^+$*, hydrogen ion; *HCO$_3^-$*, bicarbonate; *H$_2$CO$_3$*, carbonic acid; *H$_2$O*, water; *K$^+$*, potassium; *Na$^+$*, sodium; *NBC-1*, electrogenic sodium bicarbonate cotransporter-1; *OH$^-$*, hydroxyl anion. (C from previous edition, Fig. 1.7B, Briggs J.)

COLLECTING DUCT

The collecting duct has two populations of cells: the intercalated cells and the principal cells (Fig. 1.10). These cells are interspersed in the collecting duct and act in concert to create the final urine (Fig. 1.11).

The principal cells have two important roles. First, vasopressin stimulation leads to translocation of aquaporin 2 from intracellular vesicles to the luminal membrane. Then water is reabsorbed along its concentration gradient so that more concentrated urine can be created. Second, under the influence of aldosterone, the epithelial sodium channel (ENaC) facilitates movement of sodium into the cell. This leads to a lumen negative potential, favoring the loss of potassium from the principal cells via ROMK. The neighboring α-intercalated cells are also affected by the luminal negative potential difference as this favors H$^+$ ion secretion via a luminal H$^+$-ATPase. There are also β-intercalated cells that are structurally similar to the α-intercalated cells but with reverse polarity such that the H$^+$-ATPase is on the basolateral membrane and a chloride-bicarbonate exchanger, known as *pendrin*, is on the luminal membrane. These cells play a role in the secretion of bicarbonate in the setting of alkalosis.

Collecting ducts from neighboring nephrons converge in the papilla and empty into the calyces of the renal pelvis.

SALT AND VOLUME REGULATION

THE CELLULAR BASIS FOR TUBULAR SODIUM REABSORPTION

As noted earlier, localization of Na$^+$/K$^+$-ATPase on the basolateral membrane provides energy for reabsorption of solute from the tubular lumen with the help of a series of sodium transporters on the luminal surface of each nephron segment. The key sodium-dependent transporters, many of which are the target of diuretic agents, are listed below.

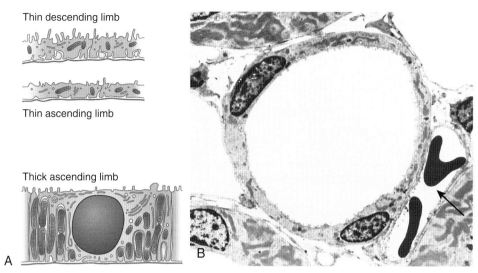

Fig. 1.7 The loop of Henle, composed of the thin descending limb, thin ascending limb, and thick ascending limb, makes a hairpin loop within the medulla. (A) Schematic drawings of the cell morphology. (B) A cross-section through the thin descending limb in the outer medulla. At the lower right aspect of the image, a peritubular capillary is seen with red blood cells *(arrow)*. The thin limbs have shallow epithelia without prominent mitochondria and are permeable to water. The thick ascending limb (TAL), in contrast, is composed of taller epithelial cells with basolateral infoldings and prominent mitochondria. The TAL is impermeable to water; transport in this segment is critical for the generation of interstitial solute gradients (×3000). (Previous edition, Fig. 1.8, Briggs J.)

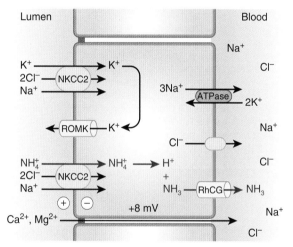

Fig. 1.8 Transport of solutes in the thick ascending limb of Henle. The primary transporter is the sodium-potassium-2 chloride cotransporter (NKCC2) on the luminal membrane, which reabsorbs a significant amount of the filtered load of sodium. In addition, ammonium (NH_4^+), can substitute for potassium (K^+), on the NKCC2. Once in the cell, NH_4^+ dissociates to ammonia (NH_3) because of the higher intracellular pH. NH_3 diffuses into the interstitium through the Rhesus glycoprotein channel (RhCG), where it is then available for secretion into the tubular lumen of a neighboring collecting duct, to act as a buffer for hydrogen ion (H^+). Transport of K^+ into the tubular lumen through ROMK provides K^+ for NKCC2 and generates a lumen positive charge (+8 mV) that drives the paracellular transport of Ca^{2+} and Mg^{2+}. Molecules and ions that are transported out of the tubular epithelial cells on the basolateral membrane enter the surrounding interstitium and the peritubular capillaries that are in close approximation. *Ca^{2+}*, Calcium; *Cl^-*, chloride; *Mg^{2+}*, magnesium; *Na^+*, sodium; *ROMK*, renal outer medullary potassium channel.

1. Proximal tubule: Na^+/H^+-exchanger 3 (NHE3). This transporter is also essential for the return of filtered bicarbonate back into the systemic circulation.
2. Thick ascending limb: $Na^+/K^+/2Cl^-$ (NKCC2). This transporter is responsible for the reabsorption of about 25% of filtered sodium. Its activity is inhibited by the action of loop diuretics, such as furosemide.
3. Distal convoluted tubule: Na^+/Cl^- cotransporter (NCC). This transporter is responsible for about 5% of tubular sodium reabsorption. Thiazide diuretics, like chlorthalidone, inhibit it.
4. Collecting duct: epithelial sodium channel (ENaC). The expression and trafficking of this protein channel to the luminal surface of principal cells is primarily activated by aldosterone, whereas its activity is inhibited by the action of atrial natriuretic peptide. Potassium-sparing diuretics, such as amiloride, inhibit ENaC directly, and mineralocorticoid receptor blockers, such spironolactone, indirectly decrease ENaC expression on the luminal membrane of principal cells.

THE EFFECTIVE ARTERIAL BLOOD VOLUME AND ITS RELATIONSHIP TO THE EXTRACELLULAR FLUID VOLUME

About 85% of plasma circulates in the low-pressure venous side of the circulation, with 15% circulating on the high-pressure arterial side. The EABV is the portion of the circulation, predominantly on the arterial side, that is sensed by baroreceptors that control renal sodium handling and extracellular fluid (ECF) volume. Effective arterial blood volume cannot be measured directly but must be surmised based on the constellation of history, physical examination,

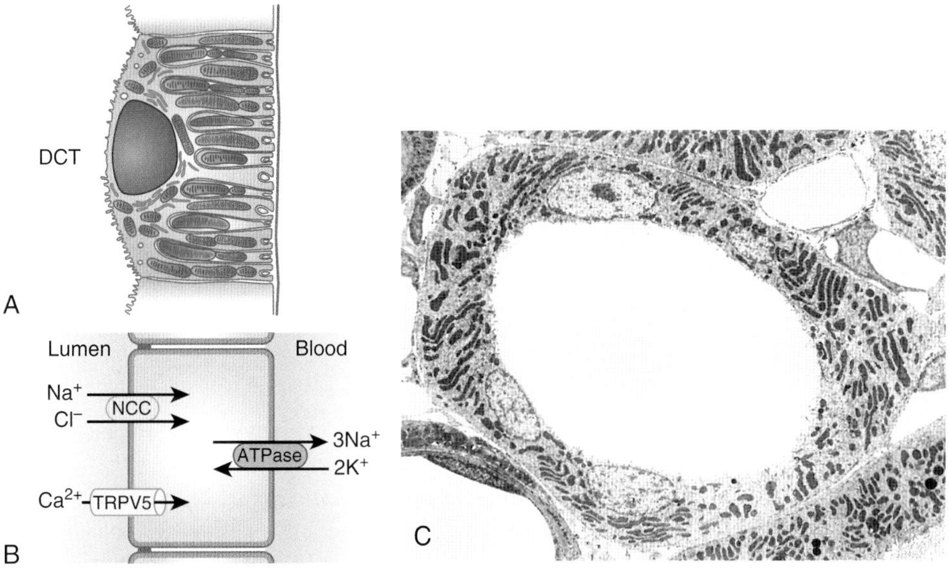

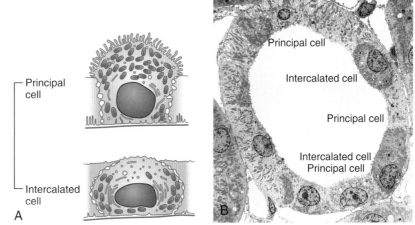

Fig. 1.9 Distal convoluted tubule. The distal convoluted tubule (DCT) is the shortest segment in the nephron. This segment leads to the connecting tubule and features cells similar to the principal cells in the collecting duct. (A) Schematic of the cell morphology of the DCT. (B) A schematic of the major transporters on the DCT, which include the sodium/chloride-cotransporter (NCC) and the calcium transporter, transient receptor potential channel subfamily V member 5 (TRPV5). (C) Cross-section of the DCT (×3000). (C from previous edition, Fig. 1.9, Briggs J.)

Fig. 1.10 The collecting duct is the only segment of the nephron that features two different cell types interspersed: the principal cells (PC) and the intercalated cells (IC). Since these cells are situated next to each other, the electrochemical gradient created by the PCs affects the ICs. (A) Schematic of the cell morphology. (B) Cross section of the collecting duct (×3000). (Previous edition, Fig. 1.10, Briggs J.)

and laboratory findings, including the urinary sodium level. A low urinary sodium level (e.g., <20 mEq/L), for example, usually reflects decreased EABV in the absence of low solute intake or primary polydipsia. The volume of the ECF is largely determined by its content of sodium salts, which in turn is controlled by the excretion or retention of sodium by the kidney. Hence, the kidney plays a pivotal role in regulating ECF volume and maintaining sodium balance.

Normally, the fullness of the EABV parallels that of the ECF volume. However, directional changes in EABV and ECF volume are not always congruent in certain pathologic conditions. For example, the EABV is decreased in congestive heart failure and cirrhosis, diseases often complicated by increased ECF volume and total body sodium. Decreased EABV in these conditions triggers a cascade of events that cause increased tubular reabsorption of sodium to limit further sodium and water losses. These responses are initially corrective and tend to maintain tissue perfusion. With progression of disease,

however, they become maladaptive and result in the formation of edema and excessive activation of the sympathetic nervous system and contribute to increased morbidity and mortality.

THE CLINICAL ASSESSMENT OF ECF VOLUME AND TOTAL BODY SODIUM

A thorough history and physical examination are required for the assessment of ECF volume and total body sodium. The presence of edema or ascites indicates increased ECF volume, whereas postural hypotension suggests decreased ECF volume. In general, the status of ECF volume parallels that of total body sodium content. Two exceptions are pure water loss (dehydration) and the syndrome of inappropriate antidiuretic hormone (SIADH) release. In SIADH, total body sodium is slightly decreased despite increased ECF volume, although the ECF volume expansion is too small to discern by physical examination.

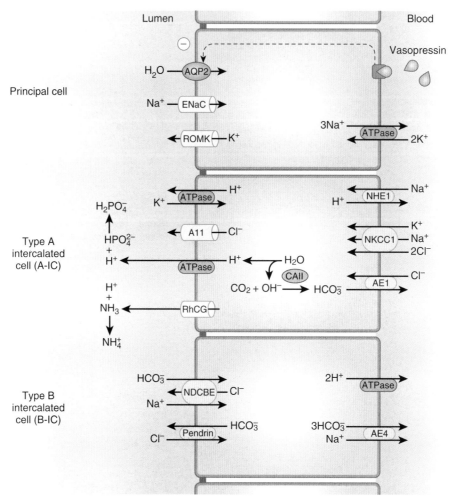

Fig. 1.11 A cartoon of the collecting duct cell types: the principal cell, type A intercalated cell (A-IC), and type B intercalated cell (B-IC). The principal cell (PC) is responsive to vasopressin. When vasopressin binds the V2 receptor, an intracellular cascade leads to phosphorylation of intravesicular aquaporins, which are then targeted to the luminal membrane. PC also expresses ENaC. When ENaC is active, a lumen negative potential favors secretion of potassium from the renal outer medullary potassium channel. The electronegative lumen also promotes H^+ secretion from the type A-IC. This results in the generation of "new bicarbonate," which is extruded from the basolateral membrane by anion exchanger 1 (AE1). The secreted hydrogen can be excreted with titratable acids or ammonia. The type B-I secretes bicarbonate while reabsorbing NaCl.

RENAL TUBULAR HANDLING OF SODIUM

Under normal physiologic conditions, about 67% of the filtered load, or 16,800 mEq of sodium, is reabsorbed in the proximal convoluted tubules; 25% is reabsorbed in the TALs of the loops of Henle; 5% is reabsorbed in distal convoluted tubules; and 3% is reabsorbed in the collecting ducts. Normally, <1% of the filtered load is excreted (50 to 200 mEq per day, depending on dietary sodium intake). The fractional excretion of sodium (FE_{Na}) is the percent of the filtered load of sodium that is excreted in the urine. A simplified equation that is used for calculating the FE_{Na} can be derived as follows:

$$FE_{Na} = \text{Sodium excreted/Filtered load of sodium} \times 100$$

$$\text{Sodium excreted} = U_{Na} \times V$$

$$\text{Filtered load of sodium} = GFR \times P_{Na}$$

Using creatinine clearance as a proxy for GFR,

$$\text{Filtered load of sodium} = (U_{Cr} \times V/P_{Cr}) \times P_{Na}$$

Substituting the equation for the filtered load of sodium into the equation for FE_{Na}:

$$FE_{Na} = \left(\frac{[U_{Na} \times V]}{[GFR \times P_{Na}]} \right) \times 100$$

$$FE_{Na} = U_{Na} \times \frac{V}{[(U_{Cr} \times V/P_{Cr}) \times P_{Na}]} \times 100$$

The volume components cancel out, and the equation can be simplified to:

$$FE_{Na} = \frac{U_{Na}/P_{Na}}{U_{Cr}/P_{Cr}} \times 100\%$$

This equation is useful to decipher the tubular handling of sodium and can be applied to the differential diagnosis of oliguric acute kidney disease. A value of <1% suggests that the kidney is sodium avid and capable of limiting urinary sodium excretion.

CONTROL OF SODIUM EXCRETION

THE PRIMACY OF THE EFFECTIVE ARTERIAL BLOOD VOLUME IN SODIUM HOMEOSTASIS

Under steady-state conditions, urinary sodium excretion matches dietary sodium intake. The slight discrepancy of intake versus urinary excretion stems from extrarenal losses of sodium in the gastrointestinal tract and sweat. The filtered load of sodium is equal to GFR $\times$ P_{Na}, where P_{Na} is equal to the plasma sodium concentration, and is approximately 25,200 mEq/day (180 L/day $\times$ 140 mEq/L). The EABV is the critical component of the circulation that is sensed by baroreceptors and influences renal sodium excretion. An increase in EABV causes increased renal sodium excretion, while decreased EABV causes decreased renal sodium excretion.

THE INTEGRATED COMPENSATORY RESPONSE

Changes in EABV are sensed by low-pressure baroreceptors in the walls of the right atrium and ventricle of the heart, the central veins, and pulmonary vessels, as well as by high-pressure baroreceptors in the afferent arteriole, the carotid sinus, the left ventricle, and the aortic arch. Baroreceptors are mechanoreceptor sensory neurons that constitute the afferent limb of the compensatory response to changes in EABV. Decreased fullness of the EABV induces changes in glomerular and peritubular hemodynamics and activates neurohumoral signals that act in concert to conserve sodium and maintain the EABV. Key regulatory factors that respond to changes in the EABV are the renin-angiotensin-aldosterone system, the sympathetic nervous system, atrial natriuretic peptide, and vasopressin.

THE SYMPATHETIC NERVOUS SYSTEM

A decrease in EABV leads to decreased firing of afferent nerves from baroreceptors, thereby activating the sympathetic nervous system. Increased sympathetic outflow through the renal nerves directly increases sodium reabsorption in the proximal tubule and in other nephron segments. Circulating catecholamines and increased sympathetic renal nerve activity stimulate renin release and liberation of angiotensin II. Severe decrements in EABV eventually cause intense renal arterial vasoconstriction that in turn reduces renal plasma flow and GFR when the renal perfusion pressure is <80 mm Hg. Conversely, decreased sympathetic nerve activation as a consequence of volume expansion is permissive with regard to the excretion of excess sodium.

THE RENIN-ANGIOTENSIN SYSTEM

The renin-angiotensin-aldosterone system regulates both sodium/volume and potassium homeostasis. Angiotensin II and aldosterone have direct effects on the tubular reabsorption of sodium, and angiotensin II has effects on the renal and systemic circulation that tend to maintain or restore the EABV toward normal. Renin is a proteolytic enzyme released from the juxtaglomerular cells of the afferent arterioles in response to three stimuli. These are:

1. Decreased pressure sensed by baroreceptors located within the wall of the afferent arteriole.
2. Signals from the macula densa that sense decreased sodium chloride delivery and transport by NKCC2.
3. Increased sympathetic outflow.

Renin cleaves angiotensinogen, a high-molecular-weight protein that is synthesized predominantly in the liver, to form angiotensin I. Angiotensin I is converted by angiotensin-converting enzyme (produced in the lungs and kidneys) to the biologically active octapeptide angiotensin II. Renin catalyzes the rate-limiting step in angiotensin II formation; therefore plasma levels of renin determine plasma levels of angiotensin II. Angiotensin II directly increases sodium reabsorption in the proximal tubule. In addition, angiotensin II indirectly increases renal sodium reabsorption by altering glomerular hemodynamics and by stimulating the release of aldosterone from the adrenal cortex. Increased systemic levels of angiotensin II also cause intense peripheral vasoconstriction.

ALDOSTERONE

Aldosterone augments sodium reabsorption in the cortical collecting ducts by increasing the activity and expression of ENaCs on the luminal membrane. Aldosterone also plays an important role in stimulating the excretion of potassium (K^+) independent of angiotensin II. The sodium-retaining effects of aldosterone and the effects on K^+ homeostasis are distinct, modulated by the activity of with no lysine (WNK) kinases. This system allows for the independent activation of maximal sodium reabsorption in hypovolemic states or maximal K^+ excretion in hyperkalemic states. The importance of WNK kinases was recognized from genetic studies on patients with a mendelian form of hypertension called type II pseudohypoaldosteronism. WNK4 acts as a switch that enables aldosterone to exert paradoxically different effects during hypovolemia compared to hyperkalemia. With hypovolemia, aldosterone induces changes in WNK4 that enhance NCC activity and inhibit ROMK, analogous to observations seen with type II pseudohypoaldosteronism mutant protein. As a result, both sodium and potassium are conserved. With hyperkalemia, aldosterone triggers increased phosphorylation of WNK4 by decreasing intracellular chloride. Phosphorylation of WNK4 releases its inhibition of ENaC and ROMK, leading to increased distal tubular secretion of K^+.

ATRIAL NATRIURETIC PEPTIDE

Pro-atrial natriuretic peptide (ANP) is released from the atria in response to stretching caused by increased ECF volume. Corin, a trypsin-like serine protease, cleaves pro-ANP to form active ANP. ANP dilates the afferent arteriole and constricts the efferent arteriole, increasing glomerular capillary pressure and GFR. ANP also inhibits sodium uptake in all segments of the nephron but most prominently in the collecting ducts where it inhibits the activity of the ENaC. The sum of these effects is a physiologically appropriate natriuresis during volume expansion that restores the ECF volume toward normal.

VASOPRESSIN (ANTIDIURETIC HORMONE)

Vasopressin is a neurohypophysial hormone released from the posterior pituitary gland in response to increases in extracellular tonicity and decreased fullness of the EABV. Vasopressin stimulates V_1 receptors on the vasculature, thereby promoting vasoconstriction, and has a pivotal role in maintaining water homeostasis (see below). In addition, vasopressin enhances the reabsorption of sodium in the TAL of the loop of Henle and in the collecting duct.

WATER AND OSMOREGULATION

REGULATION OF BLOOD FLUID OSMOLALITY

The serum osmolality is regulated within a narrow window based upon the actions of vasopressin on the kidney. The kidney has the ability to excrete water when there is water excess and limit water loss when there is a deficiency of water (dehydration). Importantly, the kidney does not retain sodium or other solutes when there is excess water to restore osmolality; instead, water excretion is the normal response, provided there are no other stimuli for water retention such as volume depletion.

ROLE OF VASOPRESSIN

Vasopressin, also known as *antidiuretic hormone*, plays a critical role in the regulation of osmolality. An increase in serum osmolality is sensed by specialized cells in the hypothalamus that are equipped with mechanical stretch receptors that depolarize in response to a decrease in cell size in the setting of hyperosmolality. Nonosmotic stimuli for vasopressin release include a decrease in EABV, as noted above, activity of the sympathetic nervous system, pain, nausea, and hypoxia. When vasopressin binds to the V_2 receptors on the basolateral membrane of the principal cells in the kidneys, an intracellular cascade is initiated by cyclic AMP that culminates with the translocation of aquaporin 2 from intracytosolic vesicles to the luminal membrane. The aquaporins on the luminal membrane then permit reclamation of water along the concentration gradient created by the presence of the hypertonic medulla. Vasopressin has a short half-life of just 20 minutes. If the stimulus for vasopressin is removed, the vesicles are targeted for degradation through a complex pathway, and the collecting ducts again become impermeable to water.

MEDULLARY HYPERTONICITY

A hypertonic medulla is necessary to create concentrated urine in the collecting duct. Several mechanisms appear to contribute to the creation of this hypertonic medulla. The NKCC in the TAL promotes the movement of sodium and chloride from the lumen to the interstitial space. In addition, NH_4^+ is also absorbed in this region (see below) where it serves as a pool for subsequent excretion of NH_4^+. A key component of the hypertonic medulla is urea. Although urea has been described as an "ineffective osmole," it is highly polar and, similar to water, crosses cell membranes extremely slowly unless specific transporters are present.

COUNTERCURRENT MECHANISM

The complex architecture of the renal medulla helps create the concentrated medullary interstitium. The parallel arrangement of the tubules equipped with the hairpin turn results in flow of the urinary filtrate in the descending limb opposite to the flow in the ascending limb. This countercurrent flow multiplies the effect of the active transport of NaCl from the TAL into the interstitium to create the concentrated medulla. Important factors that contribute to the concentrated medulla include:

1. There is active transport of NaCl without water in the thick ascending limb of Henle, which leads to an increase in the osmolality of the surrounding interstitium.
2. The descending limb of Henle has high water permeability, such that water moves down its concentration gradient and out of the lumen. This makes the fluid in the lumen more concentrated.
3. The neighboring vascular bundles, the vasa recta, also make a hairpin turn and return to the cortex in the countercurrent configuration. This arrangement assures that blood flow to the medulla does not wash out the gradient; instead, the descending vasa recta lose water and gain urea, whereas the ascending vessels gain water and lose urea.
4. Urea channels in the collecting duct are activated by vasopressin and increase urea absorption from the collecting duct into the interstitium. This serves two purposes: first, an increase in urea in the interstitium increases its osmolality; second, the reabsorption of urea from the filtrate limits the loss of water with urea, which can act as an osmotic diuretic.

TUBULAR OSMOLALITY THROUGHOUT THE NEPHRON

Since the initial filtrate from the glomerulus is generated from plasma, it shares the same osmolality of approximately 290 mOsm/L. As the filtrate moves through the proximal tubule, water is reabsorbed along with solute in an isosmotic fashion so that at the end of the proximal tubule, the luminal fluid still has an osmolality similar to plasma. With the descent into the medulla in the permeable thin descending limb, water leaves the lumen for the hypertonic medulla. By the time the filtrate reaches the hairpin turn of the loop of Henle, the osmolality of the tubular fluid is as high as the surrounding medulla (800 to 1200 mOsm/L). As the fluid ascends in the TAL, which is impermeable to water, solute but not water is removed, so the osmolality decreases. By the time the filtrate reaches the macula densa, it is again similar to plasma. In the distal convoluted tubule, which is also impermeable to water, additional sodium and chloride are removed and the filtrate osmolality can decline to 50 to 100 mOsm/L. In the collecting ducts, if no vasopressin is present, the dilute filtrate created in the distal convoluted tubule is excreted. Depending on the amount of vasopressin present and the osmolality of the medullary interstitium, water leaves the tubular lumen and the final urine becomes more concentrated.

COMPARISON OF VOLUME VERSUS WATER REGULATION

Although osmoregulation and volume regulation have different stimuli, there is considerable overlap. In the setting of volume depletion, the robust and coordinated response by hormones and the sympathetic nervous system prompts reabsorption of both sodium and water regardless of the serum osmolality. In contrast, in the setting of a hyperosmolar state without volume depletion, the sympathetic nervous system and renin-angiotensin-aldosterone axis are not activated, and vasopressin acts alone to facilitate the reabsorption of water without sodium.

REGULATION OF BODY-FLUID ACIDITY AND POTASSIUM

The regulation of body fluid acidity and potassium draws several parallels.

1. The concentrations of potassium (K^+) and hydrogen ion (H^+) are tightly regulated because relatively small perturbations in H^+ and K^+ levels can impair normal cellular function and can result in life-threatening complications.
2. The kidney regulates the excretion of K^+ and H^+ over the course of several hours to days, but immediate extrarenal buffering mechanisms exist to prevent acute life-threatening rises in plasma K^+ and H^+ when there is a surfeit K^+ or H^+.
3. The precise regulation of K^+ and H^+ is coordinated at the same site, the collecting duct. Within the collecting duct, the principal cell is the target of physiologic signals that regulate K^+ secretion, and the α-intercalated cell is the site that mediates H^+ secretion.
4. Both K^+ and H^+ secretion is stimulated by the action of aldosterone.
5. Disturbances of K^+ homeostasis may cause or be associated with acid-base disorders, and acid-base disorders may cause abnormalities in K^+ homeostasis.

SOURCES OF HYDROGEN ION

Oxidation of the cationic amino acids lysine and arginine, as well as the sulfur-containing amino acids cysteine and methionine, generate fixed acid. A typical diet leads to the liberation of approximately 1 mEq/kg body weight, or 50 to 100 mEq, of fixed acid per day. This H^+ is buffered, in part, by consuming extracellular HCO_3^-. In the absence of a mechanism to excrete the daily fixed acid load, the buffer pool would be depleted, leading to metabolic acidosis. Hence, the kidney must excrete fixed acid and generate new bicarbonate to replace the bicarbonate consumed to maintain acid-base homeostasis. Metabolism of carbohydrates and fats also generates H^+, but complete oxidation of these compounds leads to the equimolar removal of H^+. Finally, about 15,000 mmol of volatile acid are produced each day from normal metabolism in the form of carbon dioxide (CO_2), the excretion of which is dependent on adequate ventilation.

REGULATION OF BODY-FLUID ACIDITY

The physiologically appropriate concentration of hydrogen ion (H^+) is 1000-fold less than that of most serum electrolytes, on the order of 37 to 43 nanoequivalents per liter (nEq/L). An increase in the hydrogen ion concentration to >100 nEq/L, or a pH of <7.0, if sustained, is not compatible with life because of altered cellular function. Hence, the concentration of H^+ must be precisely maintained and regulated. The maintenance of the arterial pH at 7.40 relies on buffering by the HCO_3^-/CO_2 system and intracellular molecules, the excretion of fixed acid by the kidney, and effective alveolar ventilation.

THE HCO_3^-/CO_2 SYSTEM

The Henderson-Hasselbalch model of acid-base balance emphasizes the importance of the ratio of HCO_3^- to CO_2 as the major determinant of blood pH. The relationship of arterial pH to HCO_3^-/CO_2 is:

$$pH = 6.1 + \log\left(\frac{[HCO_3^-]}{[0.03 \times P_aCO_2]}\right)$$

Hence, a decrease in $[HCO_3^-]$ or an increase in P_aCO_2 results in a decrease in arterial pH (acidemia), whereas an increase in $[HCO_3^-]$ or a decrease in P_aCO_2 causes an increase in arterial pH (alkalemia). The kidney regulates the concentration of bicarbonate, while the lungs control the level of arterial PCO_2.

ACID-BASE HOMEOSTASIS AND THE KIDNEY

PROXIMAL TUBULAR BICARBONATE REABSORPTION

Proximal tubular reabsorption of bicarbonate does not contribute to fixed acid excretion but is essential for the conservation of filtered bicarbonate. The kidneys filter approximately 4300 mEq of bicarbonate each day. Bicarbonate reabsorption occurs mainly in the proximal tubule, where its transport is governed by the activity of the NHE3 (see Fig. 1.6). H^+ secreted by NHE3 combines with filtered HCO_3^- to form carbonic acid (H_2CO_3), which is then converted to CO_2 and H_2O by carbonic anhydrase IV. CO_2 and H_2O diffuse into the cell through specific channels. Within the cell, water dissociates into OH^- and H^+ while OH^- combines with CO_2 in a reaction catalyzed by carbonic anhydrase II to form HCO_3^-. Intracellular bicarbonate is secreted into the peritubular interstitium by a basolateral sodium/bicarbonate cotransporter 1 (NBC-1, also known as solute carrier family 4 member 4 [SLC4A4]). Intracellular H^+ is then secreted back into the lumen by NHE3 where it again combines with filtered bicarbonate. Proximal secretion of H^+ in exchange for Na^+ results in a minimal fall in the pH of the proximal convoluted tubule because H_2CO_3 rapidly dissociates to CO_2 and H_2O under the influence of abundant carbonic anhydrase present on the luminal surface of the brush border. In total, this mechanism reclaims filtered bicarbonate back into the systemic circulation. Normal bicarbonate reclamation is sufficient to reclaim all of the filtered bicarbonate when the serum bicarbonate is within the normal range. When serum bicarbonate levels exceed normal, the excess bicarbonate overwhelms proximal convoluted tubule reabsorption and is excreted. An exception is in the setting of extracellular volume depletion when angiotensin II activation of NHE3 increases the proximal reabsorption of sodium and with it bicarbonate, regardless of the serum bicarbonate level.

URINARY ACIDIFICATION

The pH of the tubular lumen progressively decreases and reaches its lowest level in the medullary collecting duct. H^+ excretion is predominantly mediated by an H^+-ATPase located on the luminal surface of α-intercalated cells. For every H^+ excreted, an equimolar quantity of HCO_3^- is released into the systemic circulation. The amount of fixed acid that can be excreted as free H^+ is limited by the minimal urine pH of 4.4. The concentration of H^+ at this pH is 0.04 mEq/L. Therefore excretion of an average fixed acid load of about 70 mEq per day as free H^+ cannot be attained at an average daily urine volume of 1.5 L (i.e., it would require a urine volume of about 1750 L). How, then, is the fixed acid load excreted? The answer lies in the activity of two urinary buffers: titratable acid, primarily derived from the buffering capacity of dibasic phosphate (HPO_4^{2-}), and ammonia.

H^+ SECRETION

Water dissociates into H^+ and OH^- in α-intercalated cells (see Fig. 1.11). The H^+ formed is secreted into the tubular lumen by H^+-ATPase, where it is buffered by dibasic phosphate or ammonia and then excreted in the urine. The OH^- combines with intracellular CO_2 to form HCO_3^- in a reaction catalyzed by carbonic anhydrase II. The newly generated HCO_3^- is then transported into the peritubular capillary interstitium by a chloride/bicarbonate exchanger (AE1; band 3 anion transport protein, also known as solute carrier family 4 member 1 [SLC4A1]), where it replenishes the HCO_3^- that was consumed by buffering of fixed acid.

FORMATION AND EXCRETION OF TITRATABLE ACID

Dibasic phosphate (HPO_4^{2-}) is freely filtered at the glomerulus and acts as a buffer for H^+ in both the proximal and distal convoluted tubules. The efficacy of HPO_4^{2-} as an effective buffer is explained by the relationship between urine pH and its pK_a. The pK_a of HPO_4^{2-} is 6.8; therefore about 90% of HPO_4^{2-} buffer capacity occurs above a pH of 5.8. The 30 to 40 mEq of HPO_4^{2-} that is filtered each day accounts for the excretion of approximately one-half of the daily fixed acid load. The buffering activity of HPO_4^{2-} is called titratable acid because it can be measured by titration of the urine with NaOH to a pH of 7.40. The relatively fixed filtered load of HPO_4^{2-} limits the capacity for H^+ excretion as titratable acid. For every H^+ buffered by HPO_4^{2-} and excreted in the urine as ($H_2PO_4^-$), a HCO_3^- is generated and released into the plasma.

FORMATION AND EXCRETION OF AMMONIUM (NH_4^+)

About 30 to 40 mEq of fixed acid per day is excreted in the form of ammonium. During metabolic acidosis, the kidney can increase the generation of ammonium to about 200 mEq per day. Ammonium (NH_4^+) is primarily synthesized in the proximal tubular cells by the deamination of glutamine to glutamate, and further to α-ketoglutarate, yielding two NH_4^+ and two HCO_3^-. Decreased ammoniagenesis occurs when the GFR falls to <45 mL/min per 1.73 m^2 and causes the normal anion gap component of metabolic acidosis in CKD. NH_4^+ is transported into the interstitium in the TAL, substituting for K^+ on the NKCC2 (see Fig. 1.8). Ammonium then dissociates to ammonia (NH_3) in the medullary interstitium because of the relatively higher pH of this compartment. Ammonia is subsequently transported down its concentration gradient into the lumen of the inner medullary collecting duct via the Rhesus (Rh) glycoprotein (RhCG), present on α-intercalated cells. A low concentration of NH_3 is maintained in the tubular lumen because the low luminal pH and the high pK_a of NH_4^+ (pK_a 9) favors generation of NH_4^+. Indeed, the ratio of NH_3 to NH_4^+ is about 1:1000 at a urine pH of 6 and 1:10,000 at a urine pH of 5.0. New HCO_3^- ions are added to the blood pool for every ammonium cation that is trapped in the lumen and then excreted.

ALKALI EXCRETION

Alkalemia is associated with an increase in the number of the bicarbonate-secreting β-intercalated cells relative to α-intercalated cells in the collecting duct. β-intercalated cells function to excrete excess HCO_3^- during metabolic alkalosis.

Increased alkali associated with a diet enriched in fruits and vegetables leads to the liberation of increased citrate and the generation of organic compounds that are bicarbonate equivalents. Increased urinary excretion of citrate occurs after ingestion of a high alkali diet, thereby limiting the degree of alkalosis through the excretion of base equivalents.

REGULATION OF BODY-FLUID POTASSIUM

DISTRIBUTION OF POTASSIUM ION IN THE BODY

Potassium (K^+) plays a critical role in determining the resting cell membrane potential. The transcellular distribution of K^+ is largely determined by the Na^+/K^+-ATPase, which transports Na^+ out of cells in exchange for K^+. As a result, the intracellular concentration of K^+ is maintained at a level of approximately 140 mEq/L, where the normal extracellular concentration of K^+ ranges between 3.5 and 5 mEq/L. Both hypokalemia and hyperkalemia can result in potentially life-threatening cardiac dysrhythmias and paralysis by altering the resting potential of skeletal and cardiac muscle. Therefore, tight regulation of the extracellular potassium concentration is of critical importance for the maintenance of normal cellular function. Total body potassium stores average 50 to 60 mEq/kg, or about 3800 mEq for a 70-kg adult, of which 98% is distributed in the intracellular compartment.

K^+ HOMEOSTASIS AFTER K^+ INTAKE

The rise in the serum K^+ level after ingestion of a K^+ load is attenuated by the intracellular uptake of K^+. A potassium-rich meal stimulates the release of insulin and epinephrine, both of which increase the activity of Na^+/K^+-ATPase to promote the intracellular uptake of K^+, predominantly in skeletal muscle. Increased serum K^+ levels also stimulate the release of aldosterone, which upregulates the excretion of K^+ in the collecting duct.

INFLUENCE OF ACID-BASE STATUS ON K^+ HOMEOSTASIS

Acid-base status must be considered when interpreting the plasma K^+ level because of the influence of the extracellular

H^+ concentration on transcellular potassium flux. Cells buffer increased levels of H^+ in acidemia that results in the shift of K^+ from the intracellular fluid compartment to the extracellular compartment. This occurs to the greatest extent when there is net retention of hydrochloric acid (so-called mineral acidosis). Hence, there is a relative increase in the plasma K^+ level in acidemia. Although there is a relative increase in the serum K^+ level, acidosis does not always cause overt hyperkalemia. Individuals with severe diarrhea, for example, are often K^+ depleted and have hypokalemia despite the presence of acidemia. K^+/H^+ exchange occurs to a lesser extent in organic acidoses, such as lactate acidosis. In organic acidoses, H^+ enters cells along with an accompanying organic acid via an H^+/organic acid transporter, thereby minimizing H^+-K^+ exchange.

Hyperkalemia can cause metabolic acidosis through two mechanisms. First, K^+ entry into cells results in the shift of H^+ into the extracellular compartment. Second, hyperkalemia impairs renal ammonium excretion because the intracellular alkalosis generated from potassium/hydrogen ion exchange inhibits ammoniagenesis. In addition, there is decreased availability of ammonia in the medullary interstitium because increased luminal levels of K^+ result in the preferential transport of K^+ over ammonium by NKCC2 in the TAL of the loop of Henle.

RENAL HANDLING OF K^+

On average, about 50 to 150 mEq of K^+ is excreted in the urine each day, the amount depending on dietary potassium intake. About 90% of filtered K^+ is reabsorbed in the proximal nephron and loop of Henle. Most of the K^+ excreted in the urine is derived from the secretion of K^+ in the cortical collecting duct, the segment of the tubule subject to physiologic regulation. High serum levels of K^+ drive increased K^+ secretion in the collecting duct, whereas K^+ depletion leads to increased reabsorption of K^+ at this site.

K^+ secretion in the cortical collecting duct is influenced by several major factors.

1. Generation of lumen negative charge. Increased electronegativity in the tubular lumen of the collecting duct promotes K^+ excretion by generating a favorable electrochemical gradient for K^+ secretion. Increased delivery of sodium, which is rapidly transported into principal cells through ENaC, leaves behind anions, predominantly chloride, that enhance the generation of lumen electronegativity. Increased delivery of nonabsorbable anions such as keto acids or penicillin metabolites also enhances the lumen negative charge and promotes the secretion of K^+.
2. Aldosterone. Aldosterone enhances lumen electronegativity by increasing the activity and expression of ENaC on the luminal surface of principal cells. The rapid uptake of Na^+ through ENaC exceeds the rate of chloride absorption, thereby generating increased lumen electronegativity. Aldosterone also increases the expression of ROMK on the luminal membrane of principal cells, increasing the permeability to K^+ and amplifying the secretion of K^+. Finally, aldosterone increases the activity of Na^+/K^+-ATPase, thus increasing the intracellular potassium content that drives potassium secretion. In addition to facilitating the excretion of K^+, the resultant lumen negative charge enhances the secretion of H^+ from

α-intercalated cells and the addition of new HCO_3^- into the ECF bicarbonate pool. Hence, increased aldosterone also contributes to the development of metabolic alkalosis.
3. Flow-induced potassium secretion. Increased flow through the aldosterone-sensitive portion of the distal convoluted tubule and the cortical collecting duct increases the secretion of K^+ from principal cells. Increased flow lowers the concentration of K^+ in the tubular lumen, creating a favorable concentration gradient for the secretion of K^+ from principal cells via ROMK. In addition, flow-mediated changes in luminal cilia located on principal cells and α-intercalated cells activate large-conductance calcium, stretch-activated Big Potassium (BK) channels that are expressed on the luminal surface of these cells. Flow-induced K^+ secretion accounts for a significant component of increased urinary K^+ excretion related to volume expansion, diuretic use, and osmotic diuresis.
4. Increased plasma K^+ concentration. Increases in plasma K^+ concentrations raise intracellular K^+ levels, generating a favorable concentration gradient for the excretion of K^+.
5. Metabolic alkalosis. Just as increased concentrations of H^+ in acidemia cause the shift of K^+ out of cells, decreased extracellular H^+ levels in metabolic alkalosis result in increased intracellular levels of K^+ that facilitate the secretion of K^+.

RENAL HANDLING OF GLUCOSE, AMINO ACIDS, ORGANIC ANIONS, AND CATIONS

Glucose and amino acids are freely filtered by the glomerulus and then reabsorbed nearly completely by the end of the proximal tubule. Glucose reabsorption is achieved by the action of sodium/glucose cotransporters (SGLT1 and SGLT2) on the luminal membrane of the proximal tubules. In the early proximal tubule, high-capacity, low-specificity transporters line the luminal membrane and reabsorb the bulk of the filtered glucose. In the late proximal tubule, low-capacity, high-specificity transporters complete this task. Since the glucose concentration in the filtrate is low in comparison to sodium (glucose concentration of 90 mg/dL is equivalent to 5 mmol/L), there is ample sodium available to reabsorb the majority of the filtered load of glucose. Glucose is transported from the cell back to the circulation via the basolateral transporters GLUT1 and GLUT2. The normal glucose absorptive threshold, or tubular transport maximum (Tm), is about 180 mg/dL, but, in the setting of hyperfiltration, glycosuria may develop at lower serum glucose values (Fig. 1.12).

Amino acids are reabsorbed throughout the nephron but primarily in the proximal tubule, with less than 1% of the filtered load of amino acids excreted in the urine. There are a wide array of transporters for amino acids on the luminal and basolateral membranes that have different specificities and different affinities for the neutral, dibasic, and anionic amino acids. Reabsorption of glutamine in the proximal tubule is imporant for the production of ammonium. A dibasic amino acid transporter is responsible for the reabsorption of the amino acid cystine.

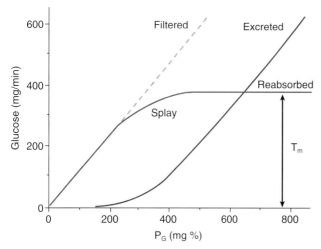

Fig. 1.12 Renal glucose reabsorption is related to the filtered load of glucose. When the filtered load of glucose is low, all of the glucose is reabsorbed and none is excreted. When the plasma glucose concentration (P_G) and the filtered glucose load rise above the maximum tubular (Tm) reabsorptive capacity for the glucose transporters, glucose begins to appear in the urine and is excreted. The "splay" reflects the difference between the theoretical curve and actual observations since there is not a sharp cutoff. As individual nephrons may have different thresholds for glucose reabsorption depending on morphologic features, the Tm reflects the average. (Reprinted from the previous edition, Fig. 1.13.)

The proximal tubule is also the site of secretion of a wide range of organic cations and anions. These include molecules that are too large for filtration and those that are protein bound. This process is facilitated by an array of organic ion transporters on the basolateral and luminal membranes that function in tandem; molecules are first transported from the basolateral surface into the cell and then secreted into the tubular lumen. These transporters from the solute carrier and ATP binding cassette families can facilitate excretion of a host of different molecules. The organic cation transporters secrete medications such as metformin and trimethoprim as well as endogenous substances like creatinine. The organic anion transporters play a role in the secretion of furosemide, tenofovir, and methotrexate, as well as endogenous substances such as urate and exogenous toxins like mercury.

BIBLIOGRAPHY

Carlström M, Wilcox CS, Arendshorst WJ. Renal autoregulation in health and disease. *Physiol Rev.* 2015;95:405-511.

Carrisoza-Gaytan R, Carattino MD, Kleyman TR, Satlin LM. An unexpected journey: conceptual evolution of mechanoregulated potassium transport in the distal nephron. *Am J Physiol Cell Physiol.* 2016;310:C243-C259.

Danziger J, Zeidel ML. Osmotic homeostasis. *Clin J Am Soc Nephrol.* 2015;10:852-862.

Feraille E, Dizin E. Coordinated control of ENaC and Na⁺,K⁺-ATPase in renal collecting duct. *J Am Soc Nephrol.* 2016;27:2554-2563.

Ferenbach DA, Bonventre JV. Kidney tubules: intertubular, vascular, and glomerular cross-talk. *Curr Opin Nephrol Hypertens.* 2016;25: 194-202.

Scott RP, Quaggin SE. Review series: The cell biology of renal filtration. *J Cell Biol.* 2015;209:199-210.

Theilig F, Wu Q. ANP-induced signaling cascade and its implications in renal pathophysiology. *Am J Physiol Renal Physiol.* 2015;308: F1047-F1055.

Weiner ID, Mitch WE, Sands JM. Urea and ammonia metabolism and the control of renal nitrogen excretion. *Clin J Am Soc Nephrol.* 2015;10: 1444-1458.

Weiner ID, Verlander JW. Recent advances in understanding renal ammonia metabolism and transport. *Curr Opin Nephrol Hypertens.* 2016;25:436-443.

Kidney Development

2

Norman D. Rosenblum

DEVELOPMENT OF THE MAMMALIAN KIDNEY

OVERVIEW OF KIDNEY DEVELOPMENT

The permanent mammalian kidney is derived from the metanephros. Establishment of the metanephric kidney is preceded by formation of two other mesenchyme-derived kidney-like structures—the pronephros and the mesonephros. Both are transient kidney-like paired structures that do not contribute to the permanent kidney. The pronephros is the more anterior of these structures and degenerates in mammals. The more posterior structure, the mesonephros, gives rise to male reproductive organs including the rete testis, efferent ducts, epididymis, vas deferens, seminal vesicle, and prostate. In females, the mesonephric portion of the wolffian duct degenerates.

The metanephric kidney is composed of the metanephric mesenchyme and the ureteric bud, both of which are derived from the intermediate mesoderm (Fig. 2.1). Metanephric mesenchyme is the tissue source of all epithelial cell types comprising the mature nephron. The ureteric bud originates as an epithelial outgrowth of the caudal portion of the wolffian duct (also termed the *mesonephric or nephric duct*) (see Fig. 2.1A). Reciprocal inductive interactions between the metanephric mesenchyme and the ureteric bud result in (1) nephrogenesis, defined as formation of the glomerulus and all tubules proximal to the collecting ducts, and (2) branching morphogenesis, defined as growth and branching of the ureteric bud and subsequent formation of the renal collecting system, which is constituted by the cortical and medullary collecting ducts, the renal calyces, and the renal pelvis.

DEVELOPMENT OF THE RENAL COLLECTING SYSTEM

The ureteric bud arises from the wolffian duct in response to signals elaborated by the adjacent metanephric mesenchyme at week 5 of human fetal gestation. Failure to induce ureteric bud outgrowth results in renal agenesis, while outgrowth of more than one ureteric bud can result in kidney malformations including a double collecting system and duplication of the ureter. The position at which the ureteric bud arises from the wolffian duct relative to the metanephric mesenchyme is critical to the nature of the interactions between the ureteric bud and the metanephric mesenchyme. Ectopic positioning of the ureteric bud is associated with renal tissue malformation (dysplasia), which may result from abnormal ureteric bud-metanephric mesenchyme interactions. Ectopic positioning of the ureteric bud is also thought to contribute to the integrity of the ureterovesical junction.

Branching of the ureteric bud occurs immediately following invasion of the metanephric mesenchyme by the ureteric bud. The number of ureteric bud branches is a major determinant of final nephron number, since ureteric bud branch tips induce discrete subsets of metanephric mesenchyme cells to undergo nephrogenesis. Repetitive branching events (see Fig. 2.1C) result in the formation of approximately 15 branch generations. In humans, the first nine branch generations are formed by approximately 15 weeks' gestation. Concomitant with formation of these branches, new nephrons are induced by reciprocal inductive interactions between newly formed ureteric branch tips and surrounding metanephric mesenchyme. By the 20th to 22nd week of gestation, ureteric branching is completed. Thereafter, collecting duct development occurs by extension of peripheral branch segments, and new nephrons form predominantly around the tips of terminal collecting duct branches.

Between the 22nd and 34th week of gestation, the peripheral (cortical) and central (medullary) domains of the developing kidney are established. The renal cortex, which represents 70% of total kidney volume at birth, becomes organized as a relatively compact, circumferential rim of tissue surrounding the periphery of the kidney. The renal medulla, which represents 30% of total kidney volume at birth, has a modified cone shape with a broad base contiguous with cortical tissue. The apex of the cone is formed by convergence of collecting ducts in the inner medulla and is termed the *papilla*. Distinct morphologic differences emerge between collecting ducts located in the medulla and those located in the renal cortex. Medullary collecting ducts are organized into elongated, relatively unbranched linear arrays, which converge centrally in a region devoid of glomeruli. In contrast, collecting ducts located in the renal cortex continue to induce metanephric mesenchyme. The most central segments of the collecting duct system, formed from the first five generations of ureteric bud branching, undergo remodeling by increased growth and dilatation of these tubules to form the pelvis and calyces.

FORMATION OF THE NEPHRON

Nephrons arise from metanephric mesenchyme cells via a process termed *nephrogenesis*. Cells adjacent to the invading ureteric bud are induced to undergo a mesenchymal to epithelial transformation. Initially, mesenchyme cells

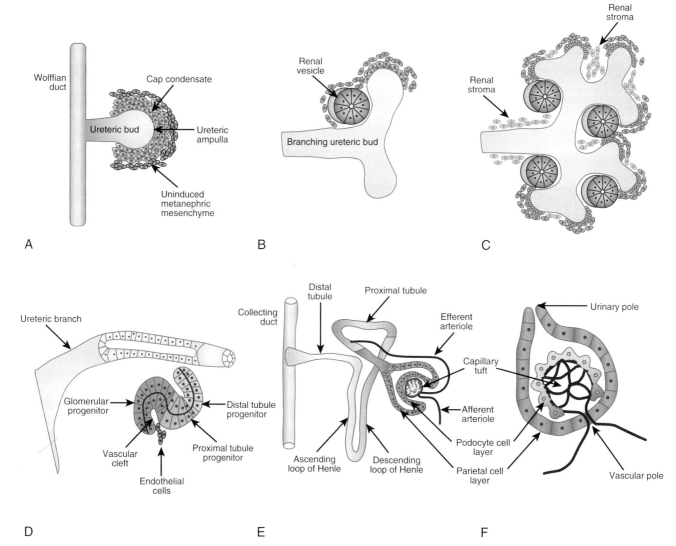

Fig. 2.1 Stages of kidney formation. (A) Induction of the metanephric mesenchyme by the ureteric bud promotes aggregation of mesenchyme cells around the tip of the ureteric bud. (B) Polarized renal vesicles are formed. (C) Stromal cells secrete factors that influence nephrogenesis and branching morphogenesis. (D) Formation of the S-shaped body involves the formation of a proximal cleft that is invaded by angioblasts. (E) The complete nephron is joined to the collecting duct. (F) Glomerulus demonstrating organization of the capillary tuft, podocytes, and parietal epithelial cells.

aggregate to form a four- to five-cell-thick layer, termed a *cap condensate*, around the ampulla of the advancing ureteric bud (see Fig. 2.1A). Near the interface of the ampulla and its adjacent ureteric branch, a cluster of cells separates from the cap condensate and forms an oval mass, called a pretubular aggregate (see Fig. 2.1B). An internal cavity forms within the pretubular aggregate, at which point the structure is called a renal vesicle. Multipotential precursors residing in renal vesicles give rise to all the epithelial cell types of the nephron. Nephron segmentation into glomerular and tubular domains is initiated by the sequential formation of two clefts in the renal vesicle. Creation of a lower cleft, termed the *vascular cleft*, precedes formation of the comma-shaped body. Generation of an upper cleft in the comma-shaped body precedes formation of an S-shaped body, which is characterized by three segments or limbs (see Fig. 2.1D). The middle limb gives rise to the proximal convoluted tubule and the upper limb to the descending and ascending limbs of the loops of Henle and the distal convoluted tubule.

Formation of the glomerulus begins as the vascular cleft broadens and deepens and as the lower limb of the S-shaped body forms a cup-shaped unit (see Fig. 2.1D and F). Epithelial cells lining the inner wall of this cup will comprise the visceral glomerular epithelium, or podocyte layer. Cells lining the outer wall of the cup will form the parietal glomerular epithelium that line the Bowman capsule (see Fig. 2.1F). The glomerular capillary tuft is formed via recruitment and proliferation of endothelial and mesangial cell precursors. Recruitment of angioblasts and mesangial precursors into the vascular cleft results in deformation of the lower S-shaped body limb into a cup-like structure (see Fig. 2.1E). A primitive vascular plexus forms at this capillary loop stage. Podocytes of capillary loop stage glomeruli lose mitotic capacity and begin to form actin-based cytoplasmic extensions, or foot processes, and specialized intercellular junctions, termed *slit diaphragms.* Subsequent development of the glomerular capillary tuft involves extensive branching of capillaries and formation of endothelial fenestrae. Mesangial cells, in turn, populate the core of the tuft and provide structural support to capillary loops through the deposition of extracellular matrix. The full complement of glomeruli in the fetal human kidney is attained by 32 to 34 weeks when nephrogenesis ceases. Subsequent glomerular development involves hypertrophy, and glomeruli reach adult size by 3½ years of age.

RENAL MALFORMATION

DEFINITION AND OVERVIEW

Renal-urinary tract malformations are classified under the overall term, *Congenital Anomalies of the Kidney and Urinary Tract* (CAKUT). These malformations are the most frequently detected abnormalities during intrauterine life (0.1 to 0.7 pregnancies) and are the major cause of childhood kidney failure. In 30% of affected patients, CAKUT occurs in combination with nonrenal malformations as part of a genetic syndrome. Over 200 distinct syndromes feature some type of kidney and urinary tract malformation (Table 2.1).

A classification of kidney and urinary tract malformations follows:

- Aplasia (agenesis): congenital absence of kidney tissue
- Simple hypoplasia: kidney length more than 2 standard deviations below the mean for age, with a reduced nephron number but normal kidney architecture
- Dysplasia ± cysts: malformation of tissue elements
- Isolated dilatation of the renal pelvis ± ureters (collecting system)
- Anomalies of position including the ectopic and fused (horseshoe) kidney

Kidney and urinary tract malformations may be unilateral or bilateral, and, in 50% of affected patients, anomalies of the kidney are associated with structural abnormalities of the lower urinary tract. These structural abnormalities include vesicoureteral reflux (VUR) (25% of cases), ureteropelvic junction obstruction (11% of cases), and ureterovesical junction obstruction (11% of cases). Renal dysplasia is a polymorphic disorder characterized at the microscopic level by abnormal differentiation of mesenchymal and epithelial elements, decreased nephron number, loss of the demarcating zone between the cortex and the medulla, and metaplastic transformation of mesenchyme to cartilage and bone. Dysplastic kidneys range in size from large distended kidneys with multiple large cysts to small kidneys, with or without cysts. A small dysplastic kidney without macroscopic cysts, imaged by ultrasound, is classified as hypoplastic/dysplastic in the absence of a pathologic examination, which distinguishes between simple hypoplasia and dysplasia. The multicystic dysplastic kidney (MCDK) is an extreme form of renal dysplasia.

ETIOLOGY OF HUMAN RENAL-URINARY TRACT MALFORMATION

CAKUT most often occurs in a sporadic manner such that neither a syndrome nor a mendelian pattern of inheritance

Table 2.1   Systemic Syndromes, Chromosomal Abnormalities, and Metabolic Disorders With Kidney or Urinary Tract Malformation

Syndromes

Beckwith-Wiedemann
Cerebro-oculo-renal
CHARGE
DiGeorge
Ectrodactyly, ectodermal dysplasia and cleft/lip palates
Ehlers-Danlos
Fanconi pancytopenia syndrome
Fraser
Fryns
Meckel
Marfan
MURCS association
Oculo-auriculo-vertebral (Goldenhar)
Oculo-facial-digital (OFD)
Pallister-Hall
Renal cyst and diabetes
Simpson-Golabi-Behmel (SGBS)
Tuberous sclerosis
Townes-Brock
VATER
WAGR
Williams-Beuren
Zellweger (cerebrohepatorenal)

Chromosomal Abnormalities

Trisomy 21
Klinefelter
DiGeorge, 22q11
45, X0 (Turner)
(XXY) Klinefelter
Tri 9 mosaic, Tri 13, Tri 18, del 4q, del 18q, dup3q, dup 10q
Triploidy

Metabolic Disorders

Peroxisomal
Glycosylation defect
Mitochondriopathy
Glutaric aciduria type II
Carnitine palmitoyl transferase II deficiency

is obvious. In probands with bilateral renal agenesis or bilateral renal dysgenesis and without evidence of a genetic syndrome or a family history, 9% of first-degree relatives have some type of malformation in the kidney and/or lower urinary tract apparent on ultrasound. An underlying genetic cause may be identified in both sporadic and inherited forms of CAKUT (Table 2.2). In approximately 30% of CAKUT, kidney and/or urinary tract malformation occurs as part of a genetic syndrome, a chromosomal disorder, or an inborn error of metabolism with additional nonkidney manifestations (see Table 2.1).

CAKUT can be caused by prenatal exposure to a variety of prescription and nonprescription drugs (Table 2.3). Angiotensin-converting enzyme inhibitors and angiotensin II receptor blockers cause a particular form of CAKUT termed *renal tubular dysgenesis* (RTD), which is a severe perinatal

Table 2.2 Human Gene Mutations Exhibiting Defects in Renal Morphogenesis

Primary Disease	Gene(s)	Kidney Phenotype
Alagille syndrome	JAGGED1, NOTCH2	Cystic dysplasia
Apert syndrome	FGFR2	Hydronephrosis
Bardet-Biedl syndrome	BBS1	Cystic dysplasia
Beckwith-Wiedemann syndrome	p57^{KIP2}	Medullary dysplasia
Branchio-oto-renal (BOR) syndrome	EYA1, SIX1, SIX5	Unilateral or bilateral agenesis/dysplasia, hypoplasia, collecting system anomalies
Cenani-Lenz syndrome	LRP4	Agenesis, ureteropelvic junction obstruction
Campomelic dysplasia	SOX9	Dysplasia, hydronephrosis
Duane radial ray (Okihiro) syndrome	SALL4	Unilateral agenesis, VUR, malrotation, cross-fused ectopia, pelviectasis
Fraser syndrome	FRAS1, FREM2, GFIP1	Agenesis, dysplasia
Hypoparathyroidism, sensorineural deafness and renal anomalies (HDR) syndrome	GATA3	Dysplasia
Kallmann syndrome	KAL1, FGFR1, PROK2, PROK2R, SEMA3A	Agenesis
Meckel-Gruber syndrome	MKS1, MKS3, NPHP6, NPHP8	Cystic dysplasia
Nephronophthisis	CEP290, GLIS2, RPGRIP1L, NEK8, SDCCAG8, TMEM67, TTC21B	Cystic dysplasia
Okihiro syndrome	SALL4	Unilateral agenesis, VUR, malrotation, ectopia
Pallister-Hall syndrome	GLI3	Dysplasia
Renal-coloboma syndrome	PAX2	Hypoplasia, VUR
Renal dysplasia, isolated	DACH1, BKC1, CDC5L	Dysplasia, VUR
Renal hypoplasia, isolated	BMP4, RET, DSTYK	Hypoplasia
Renal tubular dysgenesis	RAS components	Tubular dysplasia
Renal cysts and diabetes syndrome	HNF1β	Dysplasia, hypoplasia
Rubinstein-Taybi syndrome	CREBBP	Agenesis, hypoplasia
Simpson-Golabi-Behmel syndrome	GPC3	Medullary dysplasia
Smith-Lemli-Opitz syndrome	7-hydroxy-cholesterol reductase	Agenesis, dysplasia
Townes-Brock syndrome	SALL1	Hypoplasia, dysplasia, VUR
VACTERL	TRAP1	VUR, duplex kidney, cystic dysplasia, agenesis
Zellweger syndrome	PEX1	VUR, cystic dysplasia

VUR, Vesicoureteral reflux.

Table 2.3 Clinical Indications to Evaluate for a Renal Anomaly

History of Teratogen Exposure

ACE inhibitors and angiotensin receptor blockers
Alcohol
Alkylating agents
Cocaine
Trimethadione
Vitamin A congeners

Physical Examination Findings

High imperforate anus
Abnormal external genitalia
Supernumerary nipples
Preauricular pits and ear tags, cervical cysts or fistula
Hearing loss
Aniridia
Coloboma or optic disk dysplasia
Hemihypertrophy

ACE, Angiotensin-converting enzyme.

disorder characterized by an absence or paucity of differentiated proximal tubules, early severe oligohydramnios, and perinatal death. The antenatal renal ultrasound in RTD is characteristically normal. RTD may also be caused by mutations in the genes that encode renin, angiotensinogen, angiotensin-converting enzyme, and angiotensin II receptor type 1.

CLINICAL MANAGEMENT OF CONGENITAL ANOMALIES OF THE KIDNEY AND URINARY TRACT

MAJOR CONSIDERATIONS DURING THE ANTENATAL PERIOD

The sensitivity of prenatal ultrasound screening for CAKUT at 23 weeks' gestation is approximately 80%. Assessment of amniotic fluid volume is a key element of the antenatal evaluation. Fetal urine production begins at 9 weeks of gestation and makes a significant contribution to amniotic fluid volume by the onset of the second trimester. By 20 weeks' gestation, 90% of the amniotic fluid volume is determined by fetal urine production. Thus, a decrease in amniotic fluid volume, termed *oligohydramnios*, at or beyond the 20th week of gestation is a surrogate marker of fetal kidney dysfunction. When two kidneys exist, oligohydramnios is observed in bilateral renal agenesis or severe dysgenesis, bilateral ureteric obstruction, or obstruction of the bladder outlet or urethra. When a solitary kidney exists, oligohydramnios is caused by renal dysgenesis or obstruction of urinary outflow. Poor postnatal outcome is highly suggested by the presence of severe oligohydramnios and small, hyperechogenic kidneys.

MANAGEMENT AFTER BIRTH

The clinical presentation of kidney malformations in the postnatal period is dependent on the amount of functioning kidney mass, the presence of bilateral urinary tract obstruction, and the occurrence of urinary tract infection. Bilateral renal agenesis or severe dysplasia is likely to present soon after birth with decreased kidney function. This may be accompanied by oliguria or polyuria. Alternatively, patients may present with a flank mass or an asymptomatic abnormality detected by kidney imaging.

A detailed history and careful physical examination should occur for all infants with antenatally detected CAKUT (see Table 2.3). The physical examination focuses on the pulmonary system, with careful attention to possible pneumothorax associated with pulmonary hypoplasia. Examination of the abdomen may reveal a mass, which represents an MCDK, an obstructed kidney, or an obstructed bladder (e.g., in the posterior urethral valves). A single umbilical artery is associated with CAKUT, particularly VUR. A male infant with prune belly syndrome will have deficient abdominal wall musculature and undescended testes. Physical examination may also reveal abnormalities that occur in multiorgan syndromes associated with CAKUT. Some of the more frequently observed abnormalities include abnormal positioning of the anal orifice, abnormal external genitalia, periauricular pits, and coloboma.

Urine output should be carefully documented. Ultrasound examination of the upper and lower urinary tract should be performed within the first 24 hours of life in newborns with a history of oligohydramnios, progressive antenatal hydronephrosis, a distended bladder on antenatal sonograms, or bilateral severe hydroureteronephrosis. In male infants, a distended bladder and bilateral hydroureteronephrosis may be secondary to posterior urethral valves, a condition that requires immediate kidney imaging and clinical intervention. In general, unilateral anomalies do not require urgent investigation after birth. Kidney ultrasound for unilateral hydronephrosis is not recommended within the first 72 hours of life because urine output gradually increases over the first 24 to 48 hours of life as renal plasma flow and glomerular filtration rate increase. Thus the degree of urinary tract dilatation can be underestimated during this period of transition.

Measurement of serum creatinine should be considered in the postnatal period when there is bilateral kidney disease or an affected solitary kidney. However, measurement should be delayed until after the first 24 hours of life since levels in the first 24 hours reflect maternal serum creatinine. Newborn serum creatinine declines to 0.3 to 0.5 mg/dL (27 to 44 µmol/L) within approximately 1 week in term infants and 2 to 3 weeks in preterm infants.

CLINICAL APPROACH TO SPECIFIC MALFORMATIONS

FETAL ECHOGENIC KIDNEY

Increased echogenicity of one or both kidneys is a frequent presentation of kidney disease in the fetus. Deletions in *TCF2* are the most frequent mutations identified in the fetal echogenic kidney. Other genetic causes include autosomal-dominant and autosomal-recessive forms of polycystic kidney disease. Mutations in *TCF2* are also associated with other renal malformations such as renal hypoplasia and dysplasia, MCDK, renal agenesis, horseshoe kidney, and pelviureteric junction obstruction. Newborns with an antenatal history of hyperechoic kidneys should be studied with a renal ultrasound to further define the phenotype. At this point polycystic kidney disease may be obvious. A genetic metabolic disorder may be indicated by nonrenal findings. In the absence of such findings, a careful physical examination and pelvic ultrasound should be performed to rule out genital abnormalities.

UNILATERAL RENAL AGENESIS

A diagnosis of unilateral renal agenesis requires verification that a second kidney does not exist. Such a "second" kidney may reside in the pelvis or some other ectopic location. A diagnosis of unilateral renal agenesis is supported by compensatory hypertrophy in the normally positioned kidney. Unilateral agenesis is associated with contralateral urinary tract abnormalities including ureteropelvic junction obstruction and VUR in 20% to 40% of cases. Thus imaging of the existing kidney and lower urinary tract is important and should consist of a kidney ultrasound. A voiding cysto-urethrogram (VCUG) may also be indicated in cases that are characterized by hydronephrosis and/or hydroureter. Management of affected patients involves determining the functional status of the existing kidney; if serum creatinine is normal, the long-term prognosis is excellent. However, some studies suggest that some patients ultimately will develop proteinuria and hypertension; accordingly, it is reasonable to propose that individuals with a single functioning kidney should have blood pressure measured, urine tested for protein, periodically continuing into adulthood, and monitoring of comorbidities including body weight.

RENAL DYSPLASIA

The dysplastic kidney is most commonly small for age due to decreased nephrogenesis and may be termed a *hypodysplastic kidney*. However, a large dysplastic kidney may exist in at least two clinical circumstances. First, cystic elements can generate a large kidney, the most extreme example being the MCDK. Second, larger dysplastic kidneys are a feature of somatic overgrowth syndromes including Beckwith-Wiedemann syndrome and Simpson-Golabi-Behmel syndrome. During the antenatal period, a unilateral dysplastic kidney is likely to be discovered as an incidental finding. This may also be the case for bilateral renal dysplasia unless it is associated with oligohydramnios. After birth, bilateral renal dysplasia is associated with a variable degree of decreased kidney function proportional to the severity of the dysplasia. Postnatal ultrasonography of the dysplastic kidney reveals increased echogenicity, loss of corticomedullary differentiation, and cortical cysts. Clinical follow-up involves serial measurement of kidney function. Since renal dysplasia is associated with lower urinary tract abnormalities including VUR, imaging of the lower urinary tract should be considered, particularly if hydronephrosis and/or hydroureter are detected by ultrasound.

MULTICYSTIC DYSPLASTIC KIDNEY

MCDK is a severe form of renal dysplasia that may present as a flank mass. Kidney ultrasound demonstrates a large cystic mass in the renal fossa with a paucity of intervening solid tissue; this appearance is commonly described as a "cluster of grapes." The MCDK is nonfunctional and usually unilateral. If bilateral, it gives rise to Potter syndrome, a syndrome characterized by widely separated eyes with epicanthal folds, a broad nasal bridge, low-set ears, and a receding chin. Complications of MCDK include hypertension and urinary tract infection, but these are rare. Wilms tumor and renal cell carcinoma have also been described in MCDK, but the incidence of malignant complications is not significantly different from the general population. Contralateral urinary tract abnormalities are detected in approximately 25% of cases and include rotational or positional anomalies, renal hypoplasia, VUR, and ureteropelvic junction obstruction.

The natural history of MCDK is gradual reduction in kidney size. By 2 years of life, 60% of kidneys will decrease in size, and 20% to 25% will not be detectable by ultrasound. Increase in the size of the MCDK, a distinctly unusual event, should prompt consideration of removal to rule out malignant transformation. Ultrasound reveals compensatory hypertrophy in the contralateral kidney. Because of the risk of associated anomalies in the contralateral kidney, the possibility of VUR should be considered, particularly in the presence of hydronephrosis/hydroureter, and blood pressure should be measured. Kidney ultrasound is generally recommended at an interval of 3 months for the first year of life and then every 6 months up to involution of the mass, or at least up to 5 years. Nephrectomy should be considered when an MCDK is increasing in size and when hypertension occurs during infancy or early childhood.

RENAL ECTOPIA

Renal ectopia is defined as an abnormally located kidney. Normally, the kidneys lie in the retroperitoneal fossa on either side of the spine in the lumbar region. Rapid caudal growth during embryogenesis results in migration of the developing kidney from the pelvis to the retroperitoneal renal fossa. As the kidney ascends, it rotates 90 degrees such that the renal hilum is directed medially after ascent is complete. Migration and rotation are complete by 8 weeks of gestation.

The most common presentation of an ectopic kidney is a pelvic kidney. Less commonly, the kidney may lie on the contralateral side of the body, a state that is termed *crossed renal ectopia*. Clinical presentation can be asymptomatic or symptomatic. Diagnosis of an ectopic kidney may occur during a routine antenatal ultrasound. Alternatively, a pelvic mass may be palpated on physical examination. Renal ectopia is commonly associated with lower urinary tract anomalies, and VUR is most common, occurring in 20% of crossed renal ectopia, 30% of simple renal ectopia, and 70% of bilateral simple renal ectopia. Other associated urologic abnormalities include contralateral renal dysplasia (4%), cryptorchidism (5%), and hypospadias (5%). Female genital anomalies

such as agenesis of the uterus and vagina or unicornuate uterus have also been associated with ectopic kidneys. Other anomalies described include adrenal, cardiac, and skeletal anomalies.

Identification of an ectopic kidney should prompt a careful physical examination for other anomalies. Serum creatinine should be assessed to track kidney function. In the presence of a dilated collecting system, a VCUG should be performed to rule out VUR, which occurs with a greater incidence in affected patients and which may be associated with urinary tract infection. A 99mTc–dimercaptosuccinic acid (DMSA) scan is also recommended to assess for differential kidney function. A normal-appearing contralateral kidney and no evidence of hydronephrosis in the ectopic kidney suggests that no further evaluation is required, while decreased glomerular filtration rate or an abnormal-appearing contralateral kidney indicates a need for continued follow-up. If the ectopic kidney is severely hydronephrotic and the VCUG examination is normal, then a diuretic renogram with a MAG-3 or diethylenetriaminepentaacetic acid (DTPA) scan should be performed to further assess the degree of obstruction; in mild or moderate hydronephrosis, serial ultrasound is suggested.

RENAL FUSION

Renal fusion is defined as the fusion of two kidneys. The most common fusion anomaly is the horseshoe kidney, in which fusion occurs at one pole of each kidney, usually the lower pole. The fused kidney may lie in the midline (symmetric horseshoe kidney), or the fused part may lie lateral to the midline (asymmetric horseshoe kidney). In a crossed fused ectopic kidney, the kidney from one side has crossed the midline to fuse with the kidney on the other side. Fusion is thought to occur before the kidneys ascend from the pelvis to their normal dorso-lumbar position. As a result, fusion anomalies seldom assume the normal anatomic position. Due to failure of ascent, the renal blood supply may be derived from vessels such as the iliac arteries.

Other associated urologic anomalies include ureteral duplication, ectopic ureter, and retrocaval ureter. Genital anomalies such as bicornuate and/or septate uterus, hypospadias, and undescended testis have also been described. Associated nonkidney anomalies involve the gastrointestinal tract (anorectal malformations such as imperforate anus, malrotation, and Meckel diverticulum), the central nervous system (neural tube defects), and the skeleton (rib defects, clubfoot, or congenital hip dislocation).

Most patients with a horseshoe kidney are asymptomatic and diagnosed incidentally; however, some patients present with pain and/or hematuria due to hydronephrosis with or without obstruction or infection. Causes of hydronephrosis include VUR or obstruction of the collecting system due to renal calculi, ureteropelvic junction obstruction, or external ureteric compression by an aberrant vessel. Infection and calculi likely are due to increased urinary stasis.

Antenatal detection of a horseshoe kidney requires that postnatal ultrasound be performed to confirm the diagnosis and identify any associated urogenital abnormalities. A VCUG is indicated when it is clinically important to rule out VUR. If obstruction is observed, serum creatinine should be measured.

BIBLIOGRAPHY

Abdelhak S, Kalatzis V, Heilig R, et al. A human homologue of the *Drosophila eyes absent* gene underlies Branchio-Oto-Renal (BOR) syndrome and identifies a novel gene family. *Nat Genet.* 1997;15:157-164.

Bamshad M, Lin RC, Law DJ, et al. Mutations in human TBX3 alter limb, apocrine and genital development in ulnar-mammary syndrome. *Nat Genet.* 1997;16(3):311-315.

Barbaux S, Niaudet P, Gubler M-C, et al. Donor splice-site mutations in WT1 are responsible for Frasier syndrome. *Nat Genet.* 1997;17:467-470.

Blake J, Rosenblum ND. Renal branching morphogenesis: morphogenetic and molecular mechanisms. *Semin Cell Dev Biol.* 2014;36C:2-12.

Cain JE, Di Giovanni V, Smeeton J, Rosenblum ND. Genetics of renal hypoplasia: insights into mechanisms controlling nephron endowment. *Pediatr Res.* 2010;68(2):91-98.

Cano-Gauci DF, Song HH, Yang H, et al. Glypican-3-deficient mice exhibit the overgrowth and renal abnormalities typical of the Simpson-Golabi-Behmel syndrome. *J Cell Biol.* 1999;146:255-264.

Cheng HT, Kim M, Valerius MT, et al. Notch2, but not Notch1, is required for proximal fate acquisition in the mammalian nephron. *Development.* 2007;134(4):801-811.

Franco B, Guioli S, Pragliola A, et al. A gene deleted in Kallmann's syndrome shares homology with neural cell adhesion and axonal path-finding molecules. *Nature.* 1991;353:529-536.

Hatada I, Ohashi H, Fukushima Y, et al. An imprinted gene p57KIP2 is mutated in Beckwith Wiedemann syndrome. *Nat Genet.* 1996;14(2):171-173.

Kang S, Graham JM Jr, Olney AH, Biesecker LG. GLI3 frameshift mutations cause autosomal dominant Pallister-Hall syndrome. *Nat Genet.* 1997;15(3):266-268.

Kohlhase J, Wischermann A, Reichenbach H, Froster U, Engel W. Mutations in the SALL1 putative transcription factor gene cause Townes-Brocks syndrome. *Nat Genet.* 1998;18:81-83.

Kreidberg JA. Podocyte differentiation and glomerulogenesis. *J Am Soc Nephrol.* 2003;14(3):806-814.

Li W, Hartwig S, Rosenblum ND. Developmental origins and functions of stromal cells in the normal and diseased mammalian kidney. *Dev Dyn.* 2014;243(7):853-863.

Mackie GG, Stephens FD. Duplex kidneys: a correlation of renal dysplasia with position of the ureteral orifice. *J Urol.* 1975;114:274-280.

McGregor L, Makela V, Darling SM, et al. Fraser syndrome and mouse blebbed phenotype caused by mutations in FRAS1/Fras1 encoding a putative extracellular matrix protein. *Nat Genet.* 2003;34(2):203-208.

Nicolaou N, Pulit SL, Nijman IJ, et al. Prioritization and burden analysis of rare variants in 208 candidate genes suggest they do not play a major role in CAKUT. *Kidney Int.* 2016;89:476-486.

Oda T, Elkahloun AG, Pike BL, et al. Mutations in the human Jagged1 gene are responsible for Alagille syndrome. *Nat Genet.* 1997;16:235-242.

Porteous S, Torban E, Cho N-P, et al. Primary renal hypoplasia in humans and mice with PAX2 mutations: evidence of increased apoptosis in fetal kidneys of Pax2^{1Neu} +/− mutant mice. *Hum Mol Genet.* 2000;9:1-11.

Sakaki-Yumoto M, Kobayashi C, Sato A, et al. The murine homolog of SALL4, a causative gene in Okihiro syndrome, is essential for embryonic stem cell proliferation, and cooperates with Sall1 in anorectal, heart, brain and kidney development. *Development.* 2006;133(15):3005-3013.

Weber S, Moriniere V, Knuppel T, et al. Prevalence of mutations in renal and developmental genes in children with renal hypodysplasia: results of the ESCAPE study. *J Am Soc Nephrol.* 2006;17(10):2864-2870.

3 Assessment of Kidney Function in Acute and Chronic Settings

Lesley A. Inker; Andrew S. Levey

Excretory function of the kidney occurs by glomerular filtration of plasma followed by selective tubular reabsorption or secretion of water and solutes to maintain homeostasis. Because glomerular filtration rate (GFR) is generally considered the best overall assessment of kidney function, this chapter focuses on GFR and its assessment, with other functions of the kidney reviewed elsewhere in the *Primer*.

GLOMERULAR FILTRATION RATE

GFR is the product of the average filtration rate of each single nephron (the filtering unit of the kidneys) multiplied by the number of nephrons in both kidneys. The normal GFR level varies considerably according to age, sex, body size, physical activity, diet, pharmacologic therapy, and physiologic states such as pregnancy. For GFR to be standardized for differences in kidney size (kidney size is proportional to body size), GFR is typically indexed for body surface area, which is computed from height and weight, and then expressed per 1.73 m^2 surface area, which was the mean body surface area of young men and women at the time indexing was first proposed. Normal average GFR values are approximately 130 and 120 mL/min per 1.73 m^2 for young men and women, respectively.

Reductions in GFR can be due to a decline in the nephron number or a decline in the average single-nephron GFR (SNGFR) resulting from physiologic or hemodynamic alterations. However, a rise in SNGFR due to increased filtration pressure (e.g., increased glomerular capillary pressure) or surface area (e.g., glomerular hypertrophy) can compensate for decreases in nephron number; therefore the level of GFR may not reflect the loss of nephrons. As a result, there may be substantial kidney damage before GFR decreases.

Glomerular filtration rate cannot be measured directly in humans; thus "true" GFR cannot be known with certainty. However, GFR can be assessed from clearance measurements (measured GFR [mGFR]) or serum levels of endogenous filtration markers (estimated GFR [eGFR]).

MEASUREMENT OF THE GLOMERULAR FILTRATION RATE

Classically, "measured" GFR is determined from the urinary clearance of an "ideal" filtration marker (inulin). Urinary clearance is calculated as the product of the urinary flow rate (V) and the urinary concentration (U_x) divided by the average plasma concentration (P_x) during the clearance period. Urinary excretion of a substance depends on filtration, tubular secretion, and tubular reabsorption. Substances that are filtered but neither secreted nor reabsorbed by the tubules are ideal filtration markers because their urinary clearance equals GFR. Alternative exogenous filtration markers include iothalamate, iohexol, ethylenediaminetetraacetic acid, and diethylenetriaminepentaacetic acid, which are often chelated to radioisotopes for ease of detection but may differ in their renal handling from inulin. Urinary clearance requires a timed urine collection for measurement of urine volume, and special care must be taken to avoid incomplete urine collections, which will limit the accuracy of the clearance calculation. Plasma clearance is an alternative method to measure GFR and has the advantage of avoiding the need for a timed urine collection but is also affected by extrarenal elimination. All these considerations mean that measured GFR may differ from true GFR.

ESTIMATION OF THE GLOMERULAR FILTRATION RATE

Because of the difficulties in measuring GFR, GFR is often estimated with serum level endogenous filtration markers. For markers that are freely filtered, the plasma level is related to the reciprocal of the level of GFR, but the plasma level of many filtration markers is also influenced by generation, tubular secretion and reabsorption, and extrarenal elimination; these are collectively termed *non-GFR determinants* of the plasma concentration (Fig. 3.1). In the steady state, a constant plasma level is maintained because generation is equal to urinary excretion and extrarenal elimination. Estimating equations incorporate demographic and clinical variables as surrogates for the non-GFR determinants and provide a more accurate estimate of GFR than the reciprocal of the plasma concentration alone. Estimated GFR may differ from measured GFR if it is in the nonsteady state or if there is a discrepancy between the true and average value for the relationship of the surrogate to the non-GFR determinants of the filtration marker. Other sources of error include measurement error in the endogenous filtration marker (including failure to calibrate the assay for the filtration marker to the assay used in the development of the equation) or measurement error in

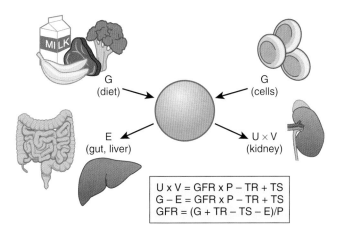

$$U \times V = GFR \times P - TR + TS$$
$$G - E = GFR \times P - TR + TS$$
$$GFR = (G + TR - TS - E)/P$$

Fig. 3.1 Determinants of the serum level of endogenous filtration markers. The serum level (P) of an endogenous filtration marker is determined by its generation (G) from cells and diet, extrarenal elimination (E) by gut and liver, and urinary excretion (U × V) by the kidney. Urinary excretion is the sum of filtered load (glomerular filtration rate [GFR] × P), tubular secretion (TS), minus reabsorption (TR). In the steady state, urinary excretion equals generation and extrarenal elimination. By substitution and rearrangement, GFR can be expressed as the ratio of the non-GFR determinants (G, TS, TR, and E) to the serum level. (Adapted from Stevens LA, Levey AS. Use of measured GFR as a confirmatory test. *J Am Soc Nephrol.* 2009;20: 2305–2313.)

GFR in developing the equation. In principle, the magnitude of all these errors is likely greater at higher measured GFR, although such errors may be more clinically significant at lower measured GFR.

Creatinine is the most commonly used endogenous filtration marker in clinical practice, and cystatin C shows promise. In the past, urea was widely used. The concepts discussed later are relevant for children and adults; however, the specifics of the following discussion focus on estimating GFR in adults. Table 3.1 includes the two most commonly used GFR estimating equations for children.

ENDOGENOUS FILTRATION MARKERS

CREATININE

Metabolism and Excretion

Creatinine, an end product of muscle catabolism, has a molecular mass of 113 Da. It is derived by the metabolism of phosphocreatine in muscle and distributed throughout extracellular fluid. Generation can be increased by creatine intake in meat or dietary supplements. Advantages of creatinine are that it is freely filtered and is easily measured at low cost. The main disadvantage of creatinine is the large number of factors other than GFR that may affect its serum level (termed *non-GFR determinants*), meaning that a given serum creatinine level may correspond to a wide range of true GFRs (see Fig. 3.1 and Table 3.2). The effect of tubular secretion and extrarenal elimination on the serum level of creatinine is greater in patients with reduced GFR. Clinically, it can be difficult to distinguish a rise in serum creatinine due to inhibition of creatinine secretion or extrarenal elimination from a decline in GFR, but these causes should be suspected if the serum level of other filtration markers remains unchanged.

Creatinine Clearance

Creatinine clearance is usually computed from the creatinine excretion in a 24-hour urine collection and a single measurement of serum creatinine in the steady state. There are expected values for creatinine excretion, and deviations from these expected values can provide some indication of errors in timing or completeness of urine collection. Creatinine clearance systematically overestimates GFR because of tubular creatinine secretion. In the nonsteady state (e.g., in acute kidney disease or between dialysis treatments), it is necessary to obtain additional blood samples during the urine collection for more accurate estimation of the average serum concentration.

Equations for Estimating Glomerular Filtration Rate From Serum Creatinine

GFR can be estimated from serum creatinine (eGFRcr) with equations that consider age, sex, race, and body size as surrogates for creatinine generation (see Table 3.1). Despite increasing accuracy of creatinine-based estimating equations over the past several years, all equations are limited by variation in non-GFR determinants of serum creatinine (see Fig. 3.1). In particular, none of these equations will perform well in patients with extreme levels of creatinine generation, such as amputees, very large or small individuals, patients with muscle-wasting conditions, or people with high or low levels of dietary meat intake (see Table 3.2). Because of racial and ethnic differences in diet and body composition, it is unlikely that equations developed in one racial or ethnic group will be accurate in multiethnic populations.

The Kidney Disease Improving Global Outcomes Chronic Kidney Disease (KDIGO CKD) 2013 clinical practice guidelines, as well as other guidelines and commentaries on these guidelines, concur in their recommendation for the use of the Chronic Kidney Disease Epidemiology (CKD-EPI) 2009 creatinine equation, or other equations if they have been shown to be more accurate in specific populations. In particular, this recommendation replaces prior recommendations from the KDOQI CKD 2002 clinical practice guidelines for use of the Cockcroft-Gault formula and Modification of Diet in Renal Disease (MDRD) Study equations. However, the MDRD Study equation is still used by many clinical laboratories, and the Cockcroft-Gault formula is still used by some for drug dosing (see later in this chapter).

The CKD-EPI equation was recently developed with a large database of subjects from research studies and patients from clinical populations with diverse characteristics, including people with and without kidney disease, diabetes, and a history of organ transplantation. The equation includes age, sex, and race (black and white) in addition to creatinine. The CKD-EPI equation was developed with serum creatinine assays standardized to international reference standards and GFR measured by urinary clearance of iothalamate, which overcomes limitations of the Cockcroft-Gault formula. The CKD-EPI equation uses a two-slope "spline" to model the relationship between GFR and serum creatinine, providing more accurate GFR estimates than the MDRD Study equation at higher GFRs (>60 mL/min per 1.73 m²). The CKD-EPI equation is more accurate than the Cockcroft-Gault formula and MDRD Study equation across a wide range of characteristics, including age, sex, race, body mass index, and presence

Table 3.1   Equations for Estimating Glomerular Filtration Rate

Creatinine-Based Equations

Cockcroft-Gault Formula

C_{cr} (mL/min) = (140 – age) × weight/72 × Scr × 0.85 [if female]

MDRD Study Equation for Use With Standardized Serum Creatinine (Four-Variable Equation)

GFR (mL/min per 1.73 m^2) = 175 × $S_{Cr}^{-1.154}$ × age$^{-0.203}$ × 0.742 [if female] × 1.210 [if black]

CKD-EPI Equation for Use With Standardized Serum Creatinine

GFR (mL/min per 1.73 m^2) = 141 × min(Scr/κ, 1)α × max(Scr/κ, 1)$^{1.209}$ × 0.993^{Age} × 1.018 [if female] × 1.157 [if black]
where κ is 0.7 for females and 0.9 for males, α is –0.329 for females and –0.411 for males, min indicates the minimum of Scr/κ or 1,
and max indicates the maximum of Scr/κ or 1.

Female	≤0.7 →	GFR = 144 × (Scr/0.7)$^{-0.329}$		
	>0.7 →	GFR = 144 × (Scr/0.7)$^{-1.209}$		
Male	≤0.9 →	GFR = 141 × (Scr/0.9)$^{-0.411}$	× (0.993)^{Age}	× 1.157 [if black]
	>0.9 →	GFR = 141 × (Scr/0.9)$^{-1.209}$		

Schwartz Formula (Younger Than 18 Years of Age)

GFR = 0.413 × ht/Scr
GFR = 40.7 × [HT/Scr]$^{0.640}$ × [30/BUN]$^{0.202}$

Cystatin C-Based Equations

CKD-EPI Cystatin C Eq. 2012

133 × min(Scys/0.8, 1)$^{-0.499}$ × max(Scys/0.8, 1)$^{-1.328}$ × 0.996^{Age} × 0.932 [if female]
where Scys is serum cystatin C, min indicates the minimum of Scr/κ or 1, and max indicates the maximum of Scr/κ or 1.

Female	≤0.8	GFR = 133 × (Scys/0.8)$^{-0.499}$ × 0.996^{Age} × 0.932
	>0.8	GFR = 133 × (Scys/0.8)$^{-1.328}$ × 0.996^{Age} × 0.932
Male	≤0.8	GFR = 133 × (Scys/0.8)$^{-0.499}$ × 0.996^{Age}
	>0.8	GFR = 133 × (Scys/0.8)$^{-1.328}$ × 0.996^{Age}

Creatinine-Cystatin C-Based Equations

CKD-EPI Creatinine-Cystatin C Eq. 2012

135 × min(Scr/κ, 1)α × max(Scr/κ, 1)$^{-0.601}$ × min(Scys/0.8, 1)$^{-0.375}$ × max(Scys/0.8, 1)$^{-0.711}$ × 0.995^{Age} × 0.969 [if female] × 1.08 [if black]
where Scr is serum creatinine, Scys is serum cystatin C, κ is 0.7 for females and 0.9 for males, α is –0.248 for females and –0.207
for males, min indicates the minimum of Scr/κ or 1, and max indicates the maximum of Scr/κ or 1.

Female	≤0.7	≤0.8	GFR = 130 × (Scr/0.7)$^{-0.248}$ × (Scys/0.8)$^{-0.375}$ × 0.995^{Age} × 1.08 [if black]
		>0.8	GFR = 130 × (Scr/0.7)$^{-0.248}$ × (Scys/0.8)$^{-0.711}$ × 0.995^{Age} × 1.08 [if black]
	>0.7	≤0.8	GFR = 130 × (Scr/0.7)$^{-0.601}$ × (Scys/0.8)$^{-0.375}$ × 0.995^{Age} × 1.08 [if black]
		>0.8	GFR = 130 × (Scr/0.7)$^{-0.601}$ × (Scys/0.8)$^{-0.711}$ × 0.995^{Age} × 1.08 [if black]
Male	≤0.9	≤0.8	GFR = 135 × (Scr/0.9)$^{-0.207}$ × (Scys/0.8)$^{-0.375}$ × 0.995^{Age} × 1.08 [if black]
		>0.8	GFR = 135 × (Scr/0.9)$^{-0.207}$ × (Scys/0.8)$^{-0.711}$ × 0.995^{Age} × 1.08 [if black]
	>0.9	≤0.8	GFR = 135 × (Scr/0.9)$^{-0.601}$ × (Scys/0.8)$^{-0.375}$ × 0.995^{Age} × 1.08 [if black]
		>0.8	GFR = 135 × (Scr/0.9)$^{-0.601}$ × (Scys/0.8)$^{-0.711}$ × 0.995^{Age} × 1.08 [if black]

Schwartz Formula (Less Than 18 Years of Age)

39.1 × (HT/Scr)$^{0.516}$ × (1.8/cysC)$^{0.294}$ × (30/BUN)$^{0.169}$ × (HT/1.4)$^{0.188}$ × 1.099 [if male]

Age in years; weight in kg.
Scr refers to standardized creatinine for all equations except the Cockcroft-Gault formula. For use of the MDRD Study equation without standardized creatinine, use 186 as the intercept.
BUN, Blood urea nitrogren; *Ccr,* creatinine clearance; *CKD-EPI,* Chronic Kidney disease epidemiology corroboration; *GFR,* glomerular filtration
rate; *ht,* height in cm; *HT,* height in m; *MDRD,* Modification in Renal Disease; *Scr,* serum creatinine in mg/dL; *Scys,* cystatin C in mg/L.

or absence of diabetes or history of organ transplantation. With the CKD-EPI equation, it is now reasonable to report eGFR across the entire range of values without substantial bias, and many clinical laboratories have begun to do so.

Since the publication of the CKD-EPI equation, other equations have been developed in selected populations. For example, the Berlin Initiative Study developed an equation in elderly white Germans, and the revised Lund-Malmö equation was developed in Swedish adults. Both equations appear to be equivalent, but not superior, to the CKD-EPI equation. They do not include a race coefficient, though, and so are not useful in blacks.

CYSTATIN C

Metabolism and Excretion

Cystatin C is a 122 amino acid protein with a molecular mass of 13 kDa. Cystatin C is generated by all cells and distributed throughout intravascular fluid. After filtration,

Table 3.2 Primary Use of Estimated Glomerular Filtration Rate Using Creatinine or Cystatin C and Sources of Error in Interpretation

Primary Use	eGFRcr Initial Test for Assessment of GFR	eGFRcys Confirmatory Test for Assessment of GFR
Nonsteady state (AKI)	Change in eGFR lags behind the change in mGFR (eGFR overestimates mGFR when mGFR is declining and underestimates mGFR when mGFR is rising)	Change in eGFR lags behind the change in mGFR (eGFR overestimates mGFR when mGFR is declining and underestimates mGFR when mGFR is rising)
Non-GFR determinants[a]	Directly measured in clinical studies	Hypothesized from clinical observations and epidemiologic studies
Factors affecting generation	Decreased by large muscle mass, high-protein diet, ingestion of cooked meat and creatine supplements Increased by small muscle mass, limb amputation, muscle-wasting diseases	Decreased in hyperthyroidism, glucocorticoid excess, and possibly obesity, inflammation, and smoking Increased in hypothyroidism
Factors affecting tubular reabsorption or secretion	Decreased by drug-induced inhibition of secretion (trimethoprim, cimetidine, fenofibrate)	NA
Factors affecting extrarenal elimination	Decreased by inhibition of gut creatininase by antibiotics Increased by dialysis, large losses of extracellular fluid (drainage of pleural fluid or ascites)	Increased by large losses of extracellular fluid (drainage of pleural fluid or ascites)
Range	Less precise at higher GFR, due to higher biological variability in non-GFR determinants relative to GFR and larger measurement error in Scr and GFR	Less precise at higher GFR, due to higher biological variability in non-GFR determinants relative to GFR, and larger measurement error in Scys and GFR
Interference with assays	Spectral interferences (bilirubin, some drugs) Chemical interferences (glucose, ketones, bilirubin, some drugs)	NA

[a]Errors in eGFRcrcys related to non-GFR determinants of creatinine or cystatin are hypothesized to be less than for eGFRcr and eGFRcys alone. Effects of factors affecting non-GFR determinants refer to effects on eGFR.
AKI, Acute kidney injury; *eGFRcr,* glomerular filtration rate estimates based on serum creatinine; *eGFRcys,* glomerular filtration rate estimates based on cystatin C; *GFR,* glomerular filtration rate; *mGFR,* measured glomerular filtration rate; *Scr,* serum creatinine; *Scys,* serum cystatin C.

approximately 99% of the filtered cystatin C is reabsorbed and catabolized by the proximal tubular cells. There is some evidence for the existence of tubular secretion and extrarenal elimination, which has been estimated at 15% to 21% of renal clearance.

Because cystatin C is not excreted in the urine, it is difficult to study its generation and renal handling. Thus, understanding non-GFR determinants of cystatin C other than GFR relies on epidemiologic associations. Table 3.2 describes some of the key factors thought to be related to cystatin generation. Studies indicate that cystatin C is less affected by muscle metabolism than serum creatinine; thus serum levels of cystatin C are less affected by age, sex, race, and diet than creatinine levels. However, factors other than GFR and muscle mass should be considered when cystatin C levels are interpreted.

Equations for Estimating Glomerular Filtration Rate From Serum Cystatin C

GFR estimates based on cystatin C (eGFRcys) alone are not more accurate than creatinine-based estimating equations (eGFRcr) (see Table 3.1); rather, it is the combination of the two markers (eGFRcr-cys) that generally results in the most accurate estimate in populations with and without CKD.

The CKD-EPI 2012 cystatin C and creatinine-cystatin equations (see Table 3.1) were developed with cystatin C that was measured with assays traceable to the international reference standard in a large database of subjects with diverse characteristics. KDIGO guidelines recommend use of the CKD-EPI 2012 equations if cystatin C is measured. The Berlin Initiative Study (BIS) and Caucasian, Asian, Pediatric, and Adults (CAPA) equations were also developed with standardized cystatin C alone or in combination with creatinine, but thus far they do not seem to have superior performance to the CKD-EPI equations. As standardized cystatin C assays become available for clinical use, the CKD-EPI creatinine-cystatin C equation, or similar or more accurate equations, could be used as a confirmatory test for low eGFRcr.

UREA

The serum urea nitrogen concentration has limited value as an index of GFR because of widely variable non-GFR determinants, primarily urea generation and tubular reabsorption. Urea, an end product of protein catabolism by the liver, has a molecular mass of 60 Da. Reduced kidney perfusion and states of antidiuresis (such as volume depletion or heart failure) are associated with increased urea reabsorption. This leads to a greater decrease in urea clearance than the concomitant decrease in GFR. When measured GFR is less than approximately 20 mL/min per 1.73 m^2, the overestimation of GFR by creatinine clearance due to creatinine secretion is approximately equal to the underestimation of GFR by urea clearance due to urea reabsorption; accordingly, the average of the urea clearance and the creatinine clearance provides a reasonable approximation of the measured GFR. Factors associated with increased generation of urea include protein loading from hyperalimentation or absorption of blood after gastrointestinal hemorrhage. Catabolic states due to infection, corticosteroid administration, or chemotherapy also increase urea generation. Decreased urea generation is seen in severe malnutrition and liver disease.

NOVEL FILTRATION MARKERS

Other markers are under investigation for use instead of or in addition to creatinine and cystatin C to estimate the GFR. Beta-2-microglobulin (B2M) and beta trace protein (BTP) are low-molecular-weight serum proteins that undergo renal handling similar to cystatin C. The CKD-EPI recently published equations with these markers in CKD cohorts. These equations were not more accurate than eGFRcrcys but were less influenced by age, sex, and race than creatinine and less influenced by race than cystatin C. In patients undergoing dialysis, an equation to estimate residual kidney function with a combination of BTP, B2M, and cystatin C was shown to be better than a combination of urea and creatinine.

CLINICAL APPLICATION OF ESTIMATED GLOMERULAR FILTRATION RATE

ROUTINE EVALUATION: INITIAL TESTING WITH eGFRcr WITH CONFIRMATION BY OTHER MEASURES

Creatinine is inexpensive and widely available, and many precise assays exist. The KDIGO CKD 2013 guidelines thus recommended using eGFRcr as an initial test. However, eGFRcr, regardless of the equation, will be less accurate in people with factors affecting serum creatinine other than GFR (see Fig. 3.1). In these situations, confirmation of the eGFRcr is advised (Fig. 3.2). Confirmatory tests could include eGFRcrcys or eGFRcys or a clearance measurement using either an exogenous filtration marker or a timed urine collection for creatinine clearance. Examples of how eGFRcr alone or in combination with confirmatory tests are used in clinical practice are discussed in the following sections.

CHRONIC KIDNEY DISEASE

The level of GFR is used to define and stage CKD. Therefore evaluation of GFR is necessary for the detection, evaluation, and management of CKD. In most circumstances, eGFRcr is sufficient for diagnosis, evaluation, and management. However, there are some circumstances where confirmation of eGFRcr may be helpful (see Fig. 3.2). For example, in some patients,

moderate-to-severe decrease in eGFRcr (45 to 59 mL/min per 1.73 m^2) may be the only indication for the diagnosis of CKD (patients without albuminuria or other markers of kidney disease). In these patients, eGFRcrcys confirms the presence of low GFR and provides prognostic information. Confirmation of the level of GFR may be particularly helpful in deciding whether to avoid agents and medications that are toxic to the kidneys (e.g., iodinated radiocontrast, nonsteroidal antiinflammatory drugs, aminoglycoside antibiotics) or in deciding to initiate dialysis or assess candidacy for kidney donation.

ACUTE KIDNEY DISEASE

Acute kidney injury (AKI) is defined and staged according to the rate of rise in serum creatinine rather than the level of GFR. AKI is one of a number of acute kidney diseases in which GFR may be changing and serum creatinine concentrations are not in the steady state. In the nonsteady state, there is a lag before the rise in the serum marker because of the time required for retention of an endogenous filtration marker, during which eGFR is higher than true GFR (Fig. 3.3). Conversely, following recovery of the GFR, there is a lag before the excretion of the retained marker, during which eGFR is lower than true GFR. During this time, neither the serum level of the marker nor eGFR accurately reflects true GFR. Nonetheless, a change in eGFR in the nonsteady state can be a useful indication of the magnitude and direction of the change in true GFR. If eGFR is falling, the decline in eGFR is less than the decline in true GFR. Conversely, if eGFR is rising, the rise in eGFR is lower than the rise in true GFR. The more rapid the change in estimated GFR, the larger the change in true GFR. Recently, a kinetic equation for change in GFR was developed that allows estimation of the true GFR given the rate of change in eGFR and assumed creatinine generation rate.

Serum cystatin C increases more rapidly than serum creatinine when true GFR declines, likely because of its smaller volume of distribution. More data are required to establish whether eGFRcys is a more sensitive indicator of a rapid GFR decline than eGFRcr.

REDUCED MUSCLE MASS

In certain populations, such as in children, the elderly, and patients with chronic diseases (heart failure, liver failure, organ transplant recipients), neuromuscular diseases, limb amputation, or eating disorders, eGFRcys has been hypothesized to be more accurate than eGFRcr. In patients in whom eGFRcr is likely to be inaccurate because of non-GFR determinants affecting serum creatinine or interference with creatinine assays and in whom there are minimal non-GFR determinants likely affecting cystatin C, it may be preferable to rely on eGFRcys rather than eGFRcr-cys. For example, a recent publication describes better performance of eGFRcys versus eGFRcr or eGFRcrcys in amputees. eGFRcys is less influenced by race and ethnicity than eGFRcr or eGFRcrcys, potentially allowing GFR estimation without specification of race.

DRUG DOSAGE ADJUSTMENT

The Cockcroft-Gault formula has been widely used to assess pharmacokinetic properties of drugs in people with

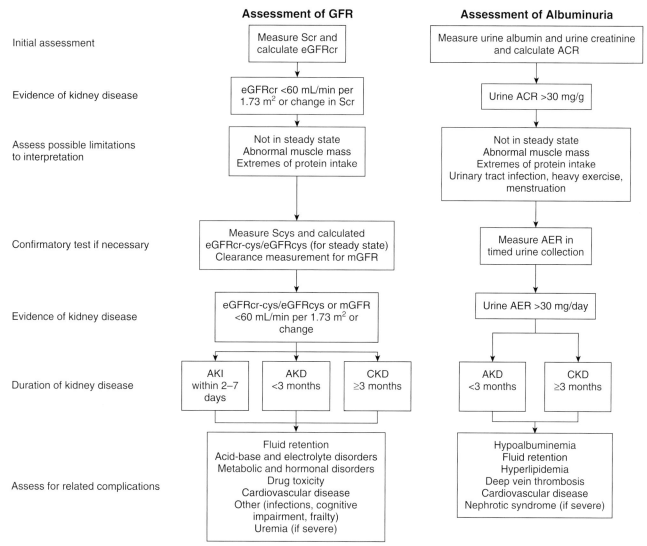

Fig. 3.2 Assessment of glomerular filtration rate (GFR) and albuminuria for detection of acute and chronic kidney disease. The figure illustrates stepwise use of initial and confirmatory tests for GFR and albuminuria for detection of acute and chronic kidney diseases and their association with complications. *ACR,* Albumin-to-creatinine ratio; *AER,* albumin excretion rate; *AKI,* acute kidney injury; *AKD,* acute kidney diseases and disorders; *CKD,* chronic kidney disease; *eGFRcr,* glomerular filtration rate estimates based on serum creatinine; *eGFRcys,* glomerular filtration rate estimates based on cystatin C; *GFR,* glomerular filtration rate; *mGFR,* measured glomerular filtration rate; *Scr,* serum creatinine; *Scys,* serum cystatin C. (Adapted from Levey AS, Becker C, Inker LA. Glomerular filtration rate and albuminuria for detection and staging of acute and chronic kidney disease in adults: a systematic review. *JAMA.* 2015;313(8):837–846.)

impaired kidney function, but its limitations are now widely recognized. The Cockcroft-Gault formula was derived to estimate creatinine clearance, and hence it systematically overestimates GFR because of creatinine secretion. Also, the formula was derived before creatinine standardization (which has led to lower serum values), and therefore it also systematically overestimates creatinine clearance. In addition, inclusion of a term for weight in the numerator leads to systematically overestimating creatinine clearance in patients who are edematous or obese and underestimating it in those who are thin or frail. Finally, the formula systematically underestimates creatinine clearance in the elderly.

In part because of these limitations, the KDIGO 2011 clinical update on drug dosing in patients with acute and chronic kidney diseases recommended using the most accurate method for GFR evaluation for each patient (rather than limiting the evaluation to the Cockcroft-Gault formula) and specifically mentioned consideration of eGFR as it is reported by clinical laboratories (see earlier in this chapter). Because drug dosing is based on body size, it is important to express GFR as milliliter per minute, without indexing for body surface area (BSA), for dosing adjustment based on GFR. Converting eGFR from mL/min per 1.73 m^2 to mL/min requires multiplication by BSA/1.73 m^2. The few

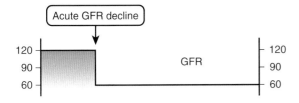

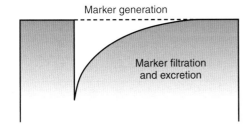

Day	P_marker	eGFR
0	1.0	120
1.5	1.6	79
2.0	1.8	69
2.5	1.9	65
3.0	2.0	60

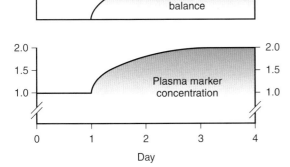

Fig. 3.3 Effect of an acute glomerular filtration rate (GFR) decline on generation, filtration, excretion, balance, and serum level of endogenous filtration markers. After an acute GFR decline, generation of the marker is unchanged, but filtration and excretion are reduced, resulting in retention of the marker (a rising positive balance) and a rising plasma level (nonsteady state). During this time, estimated GFR (eGFR) is greater than true GFR (or measured GFR). Although true GFR remains reduced, the rise in plasma level leads to an increase in filtered load (the product of GFR times the plasma level) until filtration equals generation. At that time, cumulative balance and the plasma level plateau at a new steady state. In the new steady state, eGFR approximates true GFR (or measured GFR). GFR is expressed in units of mL/min per 1.73 m². Tubular secretion, reabsorption, and extrarenal elimination are assumed to be zero. (Adapted from Stevens LA, Levey AS. Use of measured GFR as a confirmatory test. *J Am Soc Nephrol.* 2009;20:2305–2313.)

studies that have compared the efficacy or safety outcomes associated with dosing have suggested superiority or equivalence of GFR-estimating equations to the Cockcroft-Gault formula. For drugs with potential for severe toxicity and for which excretion by the kidney is quantitatively important, it would be prudent to confirm eGFRcr by a clearance measurement.

KEY BIBLIOGRAPHY

CKD-EPI. GFR Calculator—CKD-EPI. N.p., 2016. Web. Retrieved from http://ckdepi.org/equations/gfr-calculator/.

Earley A, Miskulin D, Lamb EJ, Levey AS, Uhlig K. Estimating equations for glomerular filtration rate in the era of creatinine standardization: a systematic review. *Ann Intern Med.* 2012;156:785-795.

Fan L, Inker LA, Rossert J, et al. Glomerular filtration rate estimation using cystatin C alone or combined with creatinine as a confirmatory test. *Nephrol Dial Transplant.* 2014;29:1195-1203.

Fan L, Levey AS, Gudnason V, et al. Comparing GFR estimating equations using cystatin C and creatinine in elderly individuals. *J Am Soc Nephrol.* 2015;26:1982-1989.

Huang N, Foster MC, Lentine KL, et al. Estimated GFR for living kidney donor evaluation. *Am J Transplant.* 2016;16:171-180.

Inker LA, Astor BC, Fox CH, et al. KDOQI US commentary on the 2012 KDIGO clinical practice guideline for the evaluation and management of CKD. *Am J Kidney Dis.* 2014;63:713-735.

Inker LA, Lafayette RA, Upadhyay A, Levey AS. Laboratory evaluation of kidney disease. In: Coffman TM, Falk RJ, eds. *Schrier's Diseases of the Kidney.* Philadelphia: Lippincott Williams and Wilkins; 2012:295-345.

Inker LA, Schmid CH, Tighiouart H, et al. Estimating glomerular filtration rate from serum creatinine and cystatin C. *N Engl J Med.* 2012;367:20-29.

Inker LA, Tighiouart H, Coresh J, et al. GFR estimation using β-trace protein and β2-microglobulin in CKD. *Am J Kidney Dis.* 2016;67:40-48.

Ix JH, Wassel CL, Stevens LA, et al. Equations to estimate creatinine excretion rate: the CKD epidemiology collaboration. *Clin J Am Soc Nephrol.* 2011;6:184-191.

Levey AS, Becker C, Inker LA. Glomerular filtration rate and albuminuria for detection and staging of acute and chronic kidney disease in adults: a systematic review. *JAMA.* 2015;313:837-846.

Levey AS, Inker LA, Coresh J. GFR estimation: from physiology to public health. *Am J Kidney Dis.* 2014;63:820-834.

Levey AS, Stevens LA, Schmid CH, et al. A new equation to estimate glomerular filtration rate. *Ann Intern Med.* 2009;150:604-612.

Liu X, Foster MC, Tighiouart H, et al. Non-GFR determinants of low-molecular-weight serum protein filtration markers in CKD. *Am J Kidney Dis.* 2016;68:892-900.

Matzke GR, Aronoff GR, Atkinson AJ Jr, et al. Drug dosing consideration in patients with acute and chronic kidney disease—a clinical update from Kidney Disease: Improving Global Outcomes (KDIGO). *Kidney Int.* 2011;80:1122-1137.

Rule AD, Teo BW. GFR estimation in Japan and China: what accounts for the difference? *Am J Kidney Dis.* 2009;53:932-935.

Schaeffner ES, Ebert N, Delanaye P, et al. Two novel equations to estimate kidney function in persons aged 70 years or older. *Ann Intern Med.* 2012;157:471-481.

Schwartz GJ, Munoz A, Schneider MF, et al. New equations to estimate GFR in children with CKD. *J Am Soc Nephrol.* 2009;20:629-637.

Stevens LA, Levey AS. Measured GFR as a confirmatory test for estimated GFR. *J Am Soc Nephrol.* 2009;20:2305-2313.

Teo BW, Xu H, Wang D, et al. GFR estimating equations in a multiethnic Asian population. *Am J Kidney Dis.* 2011;58:56-63.

Full bibliography can be found on www.expertconsult.com.

Urinalysis and Urine Microscopy

Arthur Greenberg

The relatively simple chemical tests performed during routine urinalysis rapidly provide important information about a number of primary kidney and systemic disorders. The microscopic examination of the urine sediment is an indispensable part of the evaluation of patients with reduced glomerular filtration, proteinuria, hematuria, urinary tract infection, or nephrolithiasis, and the urine sediment provides valuable clues about the kidney parenchyma.

Urine dipstick tests can be readily automated, and most high-throughput clinical laboratories rely on computerized optical scanning or flow cytometry with automated instruments to perform microscopic urinalyses. Although these give reasonable results for detection of red blood cells (RBCs), white blood cells (WBCs), and squamous epithelial cells, they are unable to reliably identify critical elements such as renal tubular epithelial cells, oval fat bodies, crystals, or casts. Their accuracy for detection even of RBCs and WBCs falls with specimen aging, and sensitivity is reduced within as little as 2 hours after voiding. The interval between collection of a "routine" urine specimen, delivery to the lab, and processing may vary considerably.

When a primary kidney disorder is suspected, the automated urinalysis should be regarded only as a screening test. It does not supplant careful examination under the microscope of a specimen picked up promptly at the bedside, spun down, and examined at once. This task of careful review of the urine under the microscope must not be delegated; it should be performed personally by specialists experienced in examining the urine. Studies show both that a urinalysis performed by a nephrologist is more likely to aid in reaching a correct diagnosis than a urinalysis reported by a clinical chemistry laboratory and that urinalysis performed by physicians without special training is more often inaccurate. The features of a complete urinalysis are listed in Box 4.1.

SPECIMEN COLLECTION AND HANDLING

Urine should be collected with a minimum of contamination. A clean-catch midstream sample is preferred. If this is not feasible, bladder catheterization is appropriate in adults; the risk of inducing a urinary tract infection with a single in-and-out catheterization is negligible. Suprapubic aspiration is used in infants. In the uncooperative male patient, a clean, freshly applied condom catheter and urinary collection bag may be used. Urine in the collection bag of a patient with an indwelling bladder catheter is subject to stasis, but a sample suitable for examination may be collected by withdrawing urine from above a clamp placed on the tube that connects the catheter to the drainage bag.

The chemical composition of the urine changes with standing, and the formed elements within a urine sample degenerate over time. The urine is best examined when fresh, but a brief period of refrigeration is acceptable. Because bacteria multiply at room temperature, bacterial counts from unrefrigerated urine are unreliable. High urine osmolality and low pH favor cellular preservation, and these two characteristics of the first-voided morning urine give it particular value in cases of suspected glomerulonephritis. Some experts favor use of the second morning urine to avoid effects of overnight bladder stasis. However, the most important goal is examination without delay, regardless of what specimen is used.

PHYSICAL AND CHEMICAL PROPERTIES OF THE URINE

APPEARANCE AND ODOR

Normal urine is clear with a faint yellow tinge due to the presence of urochrome. As the urine becomes more concentrated, its color deepens. Bilirubin, other pathologic metabolites, and a variety of drugs may discolor the urine or change its smell. Suspended erythrocytes, leukocytes, or crystals may render the urine turbid. Conditions associated with a change in the appearance or odor of the urine are listed in Table 4.1.

SPECIFIC GRAVITY

The specific gravity of any fluid is the ratio of that fluid's weight to the weight of an equal volume of distilled water. The urine specific gravity is a conveniently determined but inaccurate surrogate for osmolality. Specific gravities of 1.001 to 1.035 correspond to an osmolality range of 50 to 1000 mOsm/kg. A specific gravity near 1.010 connotes isosthenuria, with a urine osmolality matching that of plasma. Relative to osmolality, the specific gravity is elevated when dense solutes, such as protein, glucose, or radiographic contrast agents, are present.

Three methods are available for specific gravity measurement. The hydrometer is the reference standard but requires a sufficient volume of urine to allow flotation of the hydrometer and equilibration of the specimen to the calibrated temperature. The second method is based on the well-characterized relationship between urine specific gravity and refractive index. Refractometers calibrated in specific gravity units are commercially available and require only a drop of urine. Finally, the specific gravity may also be estimated by dipstick.

The specific gravity is used to determine whether the urine is concentrated. During a solute diuresis accompanying hyperglycemia, diuretic therapy, or relief of obstruction, the urine is isosthenuric. In contrast, with a water diuresis caused by overhydration or diabetes insipidus, the specific gravity is typically 1.004 or lower. In the absence of proteinuria, glycosuria, or iodinated contrast administration, a specific gravity of more than 1.018 implies preserved concentrating ability. Iodinated radiographic contrast is very dense, and if the specific gravity is supraphysiologic (i.e., >1.035), one should suspect that contrast is responsible. Measurement of specific gravity is useful in differentiating between prerenal azotemia and acute tubular necrosis (ATN) and in assessing the significance of proteinuria observed in a random voided urine sample. Because the protein indicator strip responds to the concentration of protein, the significance of a borderline reading depends on the overall urine concentration.

ROUTINE DIPSTICK METHODOLOGY

The urine dipstick is a plastic strip to which absorbent tabs impregnated with chemical reagents have been affixed. The reagents in each tab are chromogenic. After timed development, the color is compared with a chart. Some reactions are highly specific. Others are affected by the presence of interfering substances or extremes of pH. Discoloration of the urine with bilirubin or blood may obscure the color changes.

pH

Test pads for pH use indicator dyes that change color with pH. The physiologic urine pH ranges from 4.5 to 8. The determination is most accurate if performed promptly, because growth of urea-splitting bacteria and loss of dissolved carbon dioxide raise the pH. In addition, bacterial metabolism of glucose may produce organic acids that lower pH. These strips are not sufficiently accurate to be used for the diagnosis of renal tubular acidosis. A specimen collected anaerobically under mineral oil should be promptly assayed with a pH electrode when precision is required.

PROTEIN

Protein measurement uses the protein-error-of-indicators principle. The pH at which some indicators change color varies with the protein concentration of the bathing solution. Protein indicator strips are buffered at an acid pH near their

---

Box 4.1 Routine Urinalysis

Appearance and Odor

Specific Gravity

Chemical Tests (Dipstick)

pH
Protein
Glucose
Ketones
Blood
Urobilinogen
Bilirubin
Nitrites
Leukocyte esterase

Microscopic Examination (Formed Elements)

Crystals: urate; calcium phosphate, oxalate, or carbonate; triple phosphate; cystine; drugs
Cells: leukocytes, erythrocytes, renal tubular cells, oval fat bodies, transitional epithelium, squamous cells
Casts: hyaline, granular, red blood cell, white blood cell, tubular cell, degenerating cellular, broad, waxy, lipid laden
Infecting organisms: bacteria, yeast, *Trichomonas,* nematodes
Miscellaneous: spermatozoa, mucous threads, fibers, starch, hair, and other contaminants

---

Table 4.1 Selected Substances That May Alter the Physical Appearance or Odor of the Urine

Color Change	Substances
White	Chyle, pus, calcium phosphate crystals, triple phosphate (struvite) crystals, propofol
Pink/red/brown	Erythrocytes, hemoglobin, myoglobin, porphyrins, beets, blackberries, senna, cascara, levodopa, methyldopa, deferoxamine, phenolphthalein and congeners, food colorings, metronidazole, phenacetin, anthraquinones, doxorubicin, phenothiazines, propofol, triple phosphate (struvite) crystals (salmon colored)
Yellow/orange/brown	Bilirubin, urobilin, phenazopyridine urinary analgesics, senna, cascara, mepacrine, iron compounds, nitrofurantoin, riboflavin, rhubarb, sulfasalazine, rifampin, fluorescein, phenytoin, metronidazole
Brown/black	Methemoglobin, homogentisic acid (alcaptonuria), melanin (melanoma), levodopa, methyldopa
Blue or green, green/brown	Biliverdin, *Pseudomonas* infection, dyes (methylene blue and indigo carmine), triamterene, vitamin B complex, methocarbamol, indican, phenol, chlorophyll, propofol, amitriptyline, triamterene
Purple staining of indwelling plastic urine collection devices	Infection with *Escherichia coli, Pseudomonas, Enterococcus,* others

Odor	Substance or Condition
Sweet or fruity	Ketones
Ammoniac	Urea-splitting bacterial infection
Fetid, pungent	Asparagus (sulfurous breakdown products)
Maple syrup	Maple syrup urine disease
Musty or mousy	Phenylketonuria
"Sweaty feet"	Isovaleric or glutaric acidemia, or excess butyric or hexanoic acid
Rancid	Hypermethioninemia, tyrosinemia

color change point. Wetting them with a protein-containing specimen induces a color change. The protein reaction may be scored from trace to 4+ or by protein concentration. Their equivalence is approximately as follows: trace, 5 to 20 mg/dL; 1+, 30 mg/dL; 2+, 100 mg/dL; 3+, 300 mg/dL; 4+, greater than 2000 mg/dL. Highly alkaline urine, especially after contamination with quaternary ammonium skin cleansers or from patients who abuse sodium bicarbonate, may produce false-positive reactions by overwhelming the pH buffer of the chromogenic tab.

Protein strips are highly sensitive to albumin but less so to globulins, hemoglobin, or light chains. If light chain proteinuria is suspected, more sensitive assays should be used. With acid precipitation tests, an acid that denatures protein (i.e., sulfosalicylic acid) is added to the urine specimen, and the density of the precipitate is related to the protein concentration. Urine that is negative by dipstick but positive by sulfosalicylic acid precipitation is highly suspicious for the presence of light chains. Tolbutamide, high-dose penicillin, sulfonamides, and radiographic contrast agents may yield false-positive turbidimetric reactions. More sensitive and specific tests for light chains, such as immunoelectrophoresis or immunonephelometry, are preferred and necessary for confirmation and more definitive diagnosis.

If the urine is very concentrated, the presence of a modest protein reaction is less likely to correspond to significant proteinuria in a 24-hour collection or when assessed by spot urine protein-to-creatinine ratio. Even so, it is unlikely that a 3+ or 4+ reaction would be seen solely because of a high urine concentration or, conversely, that the urine would be dilute enough to yield a negative reaction despite significant proteinuria. The protein indicator used for routine dipstick analysis is neither sufficiently sensitive nor specific for albuminuria in the moderately increased (30 to 299 mg/g) or high normal range (10 to 29 mg/g).

BLOOD

Reagent strips for blood rely on the peroxidase activity of hemoglobin to catalyze an organic peroxide with subsequent oxidation of an indicator dye. Free hemoglobin produces a homogeneous color. Intact red cells cause punctate staining if present only in small quantity. False-positive reactions occur if the urine is contaminated with other oxidants, such as povidone-iodine, hypochlorite, or bacterial peroxidase. Ascorbate yields false-negative results. Myoglobin is also detected because it has intrinsic peroxidase activity. A urine sample that is positive for blood by dipstick analysis but shows no red cells on microscopic examination is suspect for myoglobinuria or hemoglobinuria. Pink discoloration of serum may occur with hemolysis, but free myoglobin is seldom present in a concentration sufficient to change the color of plasma. A specific assay for urine myoglobin confirms the diagnosis.

SPECIFIC GRAVITY

Specific gravity reagent strips measure ionic strength using indicator dyes with ionic strength-dependent dissociation constants (pKa). They do not detect glucose or nonionic radiographic contrast agents.

GLUCOSE

Dipstick reagent strips are specific for glucose, relying on glucose oxidase to catalyze the formation of hydrogen peroxide, which then reacts with peroxidase and a chromogen to produce a color change. High concentrations of ascorbate or ketoacids reduce test sensitivity; however, the degree of glycosuria occurring in diabetic ketoacidosis is sufficient to prevent false-negative results despite ketonuria.

KETONES

Ketone reagent strips depend on the development of a purple color after acetoacetate reacts with nitroprusside. Some strips can also detect acetone, but none react with β-hydroxybutyrate. False-positive results may occur in patients who are taking levodopa or drugs such as captopril or mesna that contain free sulfhydryl groups.

UROBILINOGEN

Urobilinogen is a colorless pigment produced in the gut from the metabolism of bilirubin. Some is excreted in feces, and the rest is reabsorbed and excreted in the urine. In obstructive jaundice, bilirubin does not reach the bowel, and urinary excretion of urobilinogen is diminished. In other forms of jaundice, urobilinogen is increased. The urobilinogen test is based on the Ehrlich reaction in which diethylaminobenzaldehyde reacts with urobilinogen in acid medium to produce a pink color. Sulfonamides may produce false-positive results, and degradation of urobilinogen to urobilin may yield false-negative results. Better tests are available to diagnose obstructive jaundice.

BILIRUBIN

Bilirubin reagent strips rely on the chromogenic reaction of bilirubin with diazonium salts. Conjugated bilirubin is not normally present in the urine. False-positive results may be observed in patients receiving chlorpromazine or phenazopyridine. False-negative results occur in the presence of ascorbate.

NITRITE

The nitrite screening test for bacteriuria relies on the ability of gram-negative bacteria to convert urinary nitrate to nitrite, which activates a chromogen. False-negative results occur with infection with enterococcus or other organisms that do not produce nitrite, when ascorbate is present, or when urine has not been retained in the bladder long enough (approximately 4 hours) to permit sufficient production of nitrite from nitrate.

LEUKOCYTE ESTERASE

Granulocyte esterases can cleave pyrrole amino acid esters, producing free pyrrole that subsequently reacts with a chromogen. The test threshold is 5 to 15 WBCs per high-power field (WBCs/HPF). False-negative results occur with glycosuria, high specific gravity, cephalexin or tetracycline therapy, or excessive oxalate excretion. Contamination with vaginal material may yield a positive test result without true urinary tract infection.

MICROALBUMIN DIPSTICKS

Albumin-selective dipsticks are available for screening for "microalbuminuria" (moderately increased albuminuria in the range of 30 to 299 mg/g). The most accurate screening occurs when first morning specimens are examined as exercise can increase albumin excretion. One type of dipstick uses colorimetric detection of albumin bound to gold-conjugated antibody. Normally, the urine albumin concentration is less than the 20 μg/L detection threshold for these strips. Unless the urine is very dilute, a patient with no detectable albumin by this method is unlikely to have microalbuminuria. However, because urine concentration varies widely, this assay has the same limitations as any test that only measures concentration. It is useful only as a screening test, and more formal testing is required if albuminuria is detected.

A second type of dipstick has tabs for measurement of both albumin and creatinine concentration, permitting estimation of the albumin-to-creatinine ratio. In contrast to the other dipstick tests described in this chapter, these strips cannot be read by simple visual comparison with a color chart. An instrument is required, but this system is suitable for point-of-care testing. When present on more than one determination, an albumin-to-creatinine ratio of 30 to 300 μg/mg signifies moderately increased albuminuria. Details on the interpretation of urine albumin concentration are provided in Chapters 5 and 26.

MICROSCOPIC EXAMINATION OF THE SPUN URINARY SEDIMENT

SPECIMEN PREPARATION AND VIEWING

The contents of the urine are reported as the number of cells or casts per HPF (×400) after resuspension of the centrifuged pellet in a small volume of urine. The accuracy and reproducibility of this semiquantitative method depend on using the correct volume of urine. Twelve milliliters of urine should be spun in a conical centrifuge tube for 5 minutes at 1500 to 2000 rpm (450 g). After centrifugation, the tube is inverted and drained. The pellet is resuspended in the few drops of urine that remain in the tube after inversion by flicking the base of the tube gently with a finger or with the use of a pipette. Care should be taken to suspend the pellet fully without excessive agitation.

A drop of urine is poured or transferred by pipette onto a microscope slide. The drop should be of sufficient size that a standard 22 × 22 mm coverslip just floats on the urine with a thin rim of urine at the edges. If too little is used, the specimen rapidly dries. If an excess of urine is applied, it will spill onto the microscope objective or stream distractingly under the coverslip. Commercial urine stains or the Papanicolaou stain may be used to enhance detail. Most nephrologists prefer the convenience of viewing unstained urine. Subdued light is necessary. When conventional microscopy is used, the condenser and diaphragm are adjusted to maximize contrast and definition. When the urine is dilute and few formed elements are present, detection of motion of objects suspended in the urine ensures that the focal plane is correct. One should scan the urine at low power (×100) to obtain a general impression of its contents before moving to high power (×400) to look at individual fields. It is useful to scan large areas at low power and then move to high power when an item of interest is located. Cellular elements should be quantitated by counting or estimating the number in at least 10 representative HPFs. Casts may be quantitated by counting

the number per low-power field, although most observers use less specific terms, such as rare, occasional, few, frequent, and numerous.

CELLULAR ELEMENTS

The principal formed elements of the urine are listed (see Box 4.1). The figures in this chapter constitute an atlas of selected formed elements.

ERYTHROCYTES

RBCs (Fig. 4.1A and B) may find their way into the urine from any source between the glomerulus and urethral meatus. The presence of more than two to three erythrocytes per HPF is considered pathologic. Erythrocytes are biconcave disks 7 μm in diameter. They become crenated in hypertonic urine. In hypotonic urine, they swell or burst, leaving ghosts. Erythrocytes originating in the renal parenchyma are dysmorphic, with spicules or blebs (acanthocytes), submembrane cytoplasmic precipitation, membrane folding, and vesicles. Those originating in the collecting system retain their uniform shape. Studies suggest good separation between urologic and intrarenal pathology when phase contrast microscopy is used by experienced observers. In one study, up to 85% of patients with nondysmorphic microscopic hematuria had a urologic disorder, whereas 87.5% of those with dysmorphic hematuria had glomerular disease. Cutoff points for deciding that hematuria is dysmorphic depend on the method used. The number of dysmorphic RBCs as a fraction of total RBCs required to reach the threshold for deciding if hematuria is dysmorphic is lower for conventional than phase contrast microscopy. The presence of proteinuria by dipstick may corroborate the presence of glomerular kidney disease. Of course, many glomerular and tubular disorders do not cause proteinuria.

LEUKOCYTES

Polymorphonuclear leukocytes (PMNs) (see Fig. 4.1C) are approximately 12 μm in diameter and are most readily recognized in a fresh urine sample before their multilobed nuclei or granules have degenerated. Swollen PMNs with prominent granules displaying Brownian motion are termed *glitter* cells. PMNs may indicate urinary tract inflammation, intraparenchymal diseases such as glomerulonephritis or interstitial nephritis, or upper or lower urinary tract infection. Periureteral inflammation, as in regional ileitis or acute appendicitis, may also cause pyuria.

RENAL TUBULAR EPITHELIAL CELLS

Tubular cells (see Fig. 4.1D) are larger than PMNs, ranging from 12 to 20 μm in diameter. Proximal tubular cells are oval or egg shaped and tend to be larger than the cuboidal distal tubular cells. However, because size varies with urine osmolality, these cells cannot be reliably differentiated. In hypotonic urine, it may be difficult to distinguish tubular cells from swollen PMNs. A few tubular cells may be seen in a normal urine sample. More commonly, these cells indicate tubular injury or inflammation from ATN or interstitial nephritis.

OTHER CELLS

Squamous cells (see Fig. 4.1E) of urethral, vaginal, or cutaneous origin are large, flat cells with small nuclei. Transitional

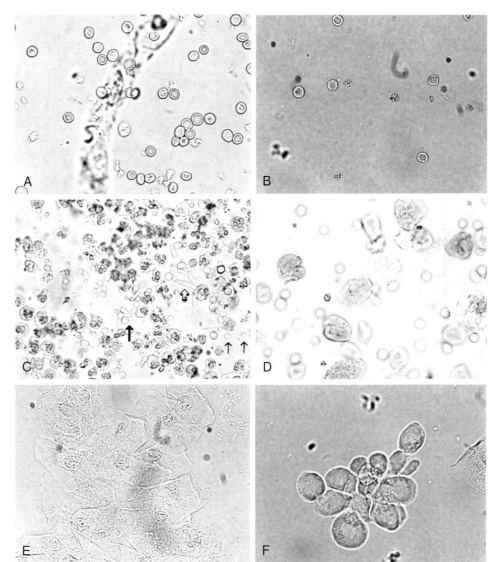

Fig. 4.1 Cellular elements in the urine. In this and subsequent figures, all photographs were made from unstained sediments and were photographed at ×400 original magnification. (A) Nondysmorphic red blood cells (RBCs). They appear as uniform, biconcave disks. (B) Dysmorphic RBCs from a patient with immunoglobulin A nephropathy. Their shape is irregular, with membrane blebs and spicules. (C) Urine obtained from a patient with an indwelling bladder catheter. Innumerable white blood cells as well as individual *(small arrows)*, budding *(single thick arrow)*, and hyphal *(open arrow)* fungal forms are present. (D) Renal tubular epithelial cells. Note the variability of shape. The erythrocytes in the background are much smaller. (E) Squamous epithelial cells. (F) Transitional epithelial cells in a characteristic clump.

epithelial cells (see Fig. 4.1F) line the renal pelvis, ureter, bladder, and proximal urethra. They are rounded cells several times the size of leukocytes and often occur in clumps. In hypotonic urine, they may be confused with swollen tubular epithelial cells.

CASTS AND OTHER FORMED ELEMENTS

Based on their shape and origin, casts are appropriately named. Immunofluorescence studies demonstrate that they consist of a matrix of Tamm-Horsfall urinary glycoprotein (uromodulin) in the shape of the distal tubular or collecting duct segment where they were formed. The matrix has a straight margin that is helpful in differentiating casts from clumps of cells or debris. Use of phase contrast microscopy facilitates identification of casts.

HYALINE CASTS

Hyaline casts (Fig. 4.2A) consist of protein alone. Because their refractive index is close to that of urine, they may be difficult to see with conventional microscopy, requiring

subdued light and careful manipulation of the iris diaphragm to increase diffraction and visual contrast. Hyaline casts are nonspecific. They occur in concentrated urine from healthy individuals, as well as in numerous pathologic conditions.

GRANULAR CASTS

Granular casts (see Fig. 4.2B) consist of finely or coarsely granular material. Immunofluorescence studies show that the fine granules are derived from altered serum proteins. Coarse granules may result from degeneration of embedded cells. Granular casts are nonspecific but usually pathologic. They may be seen after exercise or with simple volume depletion, and as a finding in ATN, glomerulonephritis, or tubulointerstitial disease.

WAXY CASTS

Waxy casts, or broad casts (see Fig. 4.2C), are made of hyaline material with a much greater refractive index than hyaline casts—hence, their description as waxy. They behave as though they are more brittle than hyaline casts, and they frequently

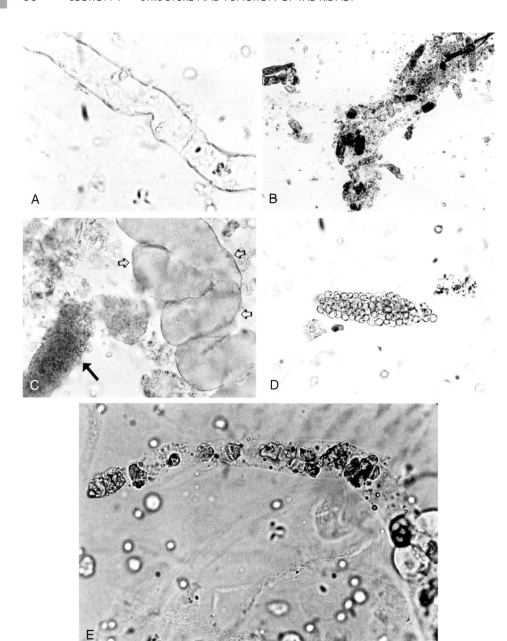

Fig. 4.2 Casts. All images photographed at an original magnification ×100. (A) Hyaline cast. (B) Muddy brown granular casts and amorphous debris from a patient with acute tubular necrosis. (C) Waxy cast *(open arrows)* and granular cast *(solid arrow)* from a patient with lupus nephritis and a telescoped sediment. Note background hematuria. (D) Red blood cell cast. Background hematuria is also present. (E) Tubular cell cast. Note the hyaline cast matrix.

have fissures along their edges. In a systematic review, waxy casts were more common in postinfectious glomerulonephritis, amyloidosis, and individuals with reduced kidney function of either short or long duration. They are rare in membranous nephropathy and focal segmental glomerulopathy. Broad casts form in tubules that have become dilated and atrophic, and from their presence one can infer that the patient has chronic parenchymal disease.

RED BLOOD CELL CASTS

RBC casts indicate intraparenchymal bleeding. The hallmark of glomerulonephritis, they are seen less frequently with tubulointerstitial disease, including allergic interstitial nephritis. RBC casts have been described along with hematuria in healthy individuals after exercise. Fresh RBC casts (see Fig. 4.2D) retain their brown pigment and consist of readily discernible erythrocytes in a tubular cast matrix. Over time, the heme

color is lost, along with the distinct cellular outline. With further degeneration, RBC casts are difficult to distinguish from coarsely granular casts. RBC casts may be diagnosed by the company they keep; they appear in a background of hematuria with dysmorphic red cells, granular casts, and proteinuria. Occasionally, the evidence for intraparenchymal bleeding is a hyaline cast with embedded red cells. These have the same pathophysiologic implication as RBC casts. When only a few RBCs are noted as part of a cast, it is important to focus up and down on the cast to ensure that the RBCs are actually within the cast rather than merely adherent to its surface.

WHITE BLOOD CELL CASTS

WBC casts consist of WBCs in a protein matrix. They are characteristic of pyelonephritis and useful in distinguishing that disorder from lower urinary tract infection. They may also be seen with interstitial nephritis and other tubulointerstitial disorders.

TUBULAR CELL CASTS

Tubular cell casts (see Fig. 4.2E) can consist either of a few tubular cells in a hyaline matrix or a dense agglomeration of sloughed tubular cells. They occur in concentrated urine, but are more characteristically seen with the sloughing of tubular cells that occurs early in the course of ATN.

BACTERIA, YEAST, AND OTHER INFECTIOUS AGENTS

Bacillary or coccal forms of bacteria may be discerned even on an unstained urine sample. Examination of a Gram stain preparation of unspun urine allows estimation of the bacterial count. One organism per HPF of unspun urine corresponds to 20,000 organisms per cubic millimeter. Individual and budding yeasts and hyphal forms occur with *Candida* infection or colonization. *Candida* organisms are similar in size to erythrocytes, but have a greenish hue and are not biconcave disks. When budding forms or hyphae are present, yeast is obvious (see Fig. 4.1C). *Trichomonas* organisms are identified by their teardrop shape and motile flagellum.

LIPIDURIA

In the nephrotic syndrome with lipiduria, tubular cells reabsorb luminal fat. Sloughed tubular cells containing fat droplets are called oval fat bodies. Fatty casts contain lipid-laden tubular cells or free lipid droplets. By light microscopy, lipid droplets appear round and clear with a green tinge. Cholesterol esters are anisotropic, and cholesterol-containing droplets rotate polarized light to produce a "Maltese cross"

appearance. Triglycerides appear similar by light microscopy but are isotropic. Crystals, starch granules, mineral oil, and other urinary contaminants are also anisotropic. Before concluding that anisotropic structures are lipid, the observer must compare polarized and bright-field views of the same object (Fig. 4.3).

CRYSTALS

Crystals may be present spontaneously or may precipitate with refrigeration of a specimen. They can be difficult to type because they have similar shapes; the common urinary crystals are described in Table 4.2. The pH is an important clue to identity because the solubility of many urinary constituents is pH dependent. The three most distinctive crystal forms are cystine, calcium oxalate, and magnesium ammonium (triple) phosphate. Cystine crystals (see Fig. 4.4A) are hexagonal plates that resemble benzene rings. Calcium oxalate crystals (see Fig. 4.4A) are classically described as "envelope shaped" but when viewed as they rotate in the urine under the microscope appear bipyramidal. Coffin lid–shaped triple phosphates (see Fig. 4.4B) are rectangular with beveled ends. Oxalate (see Fig. 4.4C) may also occur as a dumbbell-shaped crystal. Urate may have several forms, including rhomboids (see Fig. 4.4D) or needles (see Fig. 4.4E).

Renally excreted drugs may form crystals, as listed in Table 4.3. Determination of their appearance under polarized light can be informative. Confirmation of the identity of drug crystals requires spectroscopic analysis, which is seldom available clinically. However, review of the patient's drug list combined with a literature search for descriptions of crystals associated with those drugs may be very helpful in determining which drug is responsible for crystalluria, crystal-related acute kidney injury (AKI), or nephrolithiasis.

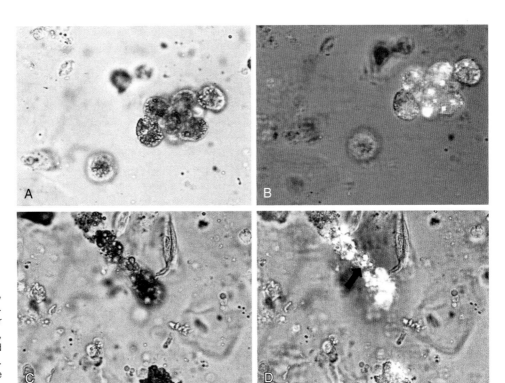

Fig. 4.3 Lipid. (A) Oval fat bodies, as seen by bright-field illumination. (B) Same field as in (A) viewed under polarized light. (C) Lipid-laden cast, bright-field illumination. (D) Same field as in (C) viewed under polarized light. Arrow points to characteristic Maltese cross.

Table 4.2   Common Naturally Occurring Urinary Crystals

Description	Composition	Comment
Crystals Found in Acid Urine		
Amorphous	Uric acid Sodium urate	Cannot be distinguished from amorphous phosphates except by urine pH; may be orange tinted by urochrome
Rhomboid prisms	Uric acid	—
Rosettes	Uric acid	—
Bipyramidal	Calcium oxalate	Also termed "envelope shaped"
Dumbbell shaped	Calcium oxalate	—
Needles	Uric acid	—
Hexagonal plates	Cystine	Presence may be confirmed with nitroprusside test
Crystals Found in Alkaline Urine		
Amorphous	Phosphates	Indistinguishable from urates except by pH
"Coffin lid" (beveled rectangular prisms)	Magnesium ammonium (triple) phosphate	Seen with urea-splitting infection and bacteriuria
Granular masses or dumbbells	Calcium carbonate	Larger than amorphous phosphates
Yellow-brown masses with or without spicules	Ammonium biurate	—

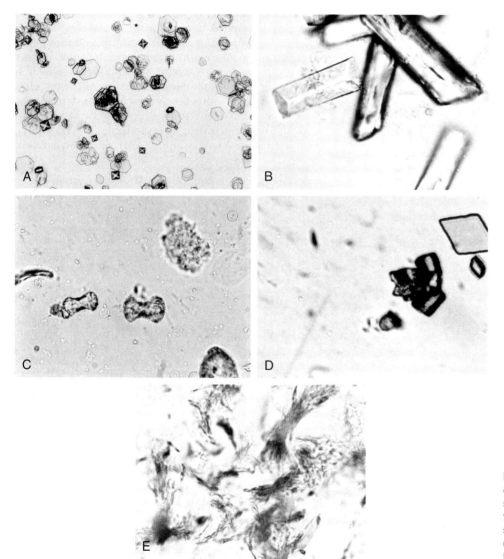

Fig. 4.4 Crystals. (A) Hexagonal cystine and bipyramidal or envelope-shaped oxalate. (B) Coffin lid–shaped triple phosphate. (C) Dumbbell-shaped oxalate. (D) Rhomboid urate. (E) Needle-shaped urate. (A, Courtesy Dr. Thomas O. Pitts.)

Table 4.3   Drug-Induced Crystalluria

Drug	Description	Comment
Amoxicillin	Straw floor broom	—
Ciprofloxacin	Needle or starburst	—
Indinavir	Platelike rectangles, fan shaped, starburst	Causes nephrolithiasis or renal colic. In vitro solubility increased at very low pH. The lowest urine pH achievable in vivo may not actually be acidic enough to lessen crystalluria.
Sulfa drugs	Needles or sheaves of wheat, dumbbell	Reduced solubility at low pH
Radiographic contrast	Needles	Reduced solubility at low pH
Acyclovir, valacyclovir	Needles (birefringent)	—
Methotrexate	Clumped plates	Reduced solubility at low pH
Triamterene	Spherical (birefringent)	Reduced solubility at low pH
Atazanavir	—	More likely at high urine pH
Darunavir	—	—
Orlistat	—	See oxalate, Table 4.2
Ethylene glycol	—	See oxalate, Table 4.2

CHARACTERISTIC URINE SEDIMENTS

The urine sediment is a rich source of diagnostic information. Occasionally a single finding (e.g., cystine crystals) is pathognomonic. More often, the sediment must be considered as a whole and interpreted in conjunction with other clinical and laboratory findings. Several patterns bear emphasis.

In the acute glomerulonephritis, the urine may be pink or pale brown and turbid. Blood and moderate proteinuria are detected by dipstick analysis. The microscopic examination shows dysmorphic RBCs and RBC casts, as well as granular and hyaline casts; WBC casts are rare.

In the nephrotic syndrome, the urine is clear or yellow. Foaminess may be noted because the elevated protein content alters the urine surface tension. In comparison with the sediment of patients with glomerulonephritis, the nephrotic sediment is bland. Hyaline casts and lipiduria with oval fat bodies or lipid-laden casts predominate. Granular casts and a few tubular cells may also be present, along with a few RBCs.

With some forms of chronic glomerulonephritis, a "telescoped" sediment is observed (see Fig. 4.2C). This term refers to the presence of the elements of a glomerulonephritis sediment together with waxy or broad casts, the latter indicative of tubular atrophy. Dipstick findings of heavy proteinuria may be present.

In pyelonephritis, WBC casts and innumerable WBCs are present, along with bacteria. In lower tract infections, WBC casts are absent.

The sediment in ATN (see Fig. 4.2B) characteristically shows tubular cells, tubular cell casts, and muddy brown granular casts. Few diagnoses in medicine have more

immediacy than confirmation of the presence of ATN in a patient with suggestive clinical findings when these elements are noted as the first low-power field to come into focus as the microscope is adjusted. A urine sediment score, derived by totaling points given for the number of renal tubular epithelial cells observed per HPF and the number of granular casts observed per low-power field, has been found in a single-center study to be useful in differentiating ATN from other etiologies of AKI. At least one other similar index has been proposed. This quantitative approach shows promise, but no scoring system has yet been widely validated or gained general acceptance. The use of novel urinary biomarkers to predict onset or severity of AKI has received much ongoing attention. Combining measurement of these markers with suggestive findings on conventional urine microscopy may have additive predictive value, but this also remains a work in progress. The typical urinary findings in individual kidney disorders are discussed in their respective chapters.

BIBLIOGRAPHY

Becker GJ, Garigali G, Fogazzi GB. Advances in urine microscopy. *Am J Kidney Dis.* 2016;67:954-964.

Birch DF, Fairley KF, Becker GJ, et al. *A Color Atlas of Urine Microscopy.* New York: Chapman & Hall; 1994.

Canaris CJ, Flach SD, Tape TG, et al. Can internal medicine residents master microscopic urinalysis? Results of an evaluation and teaching intervention. *Acad Med.* 2003;78:525-529.

Claure-Del Granado R, Macedo E, Mehta RL. Urine microscopy in acute kidney injury: time for a change. *Am J Kidney Dis.* 2011;57:657-660.

Dolscheid-Pommerich RC, Klarmann-Schulz U, Conrad R, Stoffel-Wagner B, Zur B. Evaluation of the appropriate time period between sampling and analyzing for automated urinalysis. *Biochem Med.* 2016;26: 82-89.

Fogazzi GB, Verdesca S, Carigali G. Urinalysis: core curriculum 2008. *Am J Kidney Dis.* 2008;51:1052-1067.

Foot CL, Fraser JF. Uroscopic rainbow: modern matula medicine. *Postgrad Med J.* 2006;82:126-129.

Graff L. *A Handbook of Routine Urinalysis.* Philadelphia: JB Lippincott; 1983.

Kincaid-Smith P. Haematuria and exercise-related haematuria. *Br Med J.* 1982;285:1595-1597.

Lamchiagdhase P, Preechaborisutkul K, Lomsomboon P, Srisuchart P, Tantiniti P, Ra N, Preechaborisutkul B. Urine sediment examination: a comparison between the manual method and the iQ200 automated urine microscopy analyzer. *Clin Chim Acta.* 2005;358:167-174.

Martinez MG, dos Silva S, do Valle AP, Amaro CR, Corrente JE, Martin LC. Comparison of different methods of erythrocyte dysmorphism analysis to determine the origin of hematuria. *Nephron Clin Pract.* 2014;128:88-94.

Perazella MA. Crystal-induced acute renal failure. *Am J Med.* 1999;106: 459-465.

Perazella MA. The urine sediment as a biomarker of kidney disease. *Am J Kidney Dis.* 2015;66:748-755.

Raymond JR, Yarger WE. Abnormal urine color: differential diagnosis. *South Med J.* 1988;81:837-841.

Rutecki GJ, Goldsmith C, Schreiner GE. Characterization of proteins in urinary casts: fluorescent-antibody identification of Tamm-Horsfall mucoprotein in matrix and serum proteins in granules. *N Engl J Med.* 1971;284:1049-1052.

Spinelli D, Consonni D, Garigali G, Fogazzi GB. Waxy casts in the urinary sediment of patients with different types of glomerular diseases: results of a prospective study. *Clin Chim Acta.* 2013;424:47-52.

Stamey TA, Kindrachuk RW. *Urinary Sediment and Urinalysis: A Practical Guide for the Health Professional.* Philadelphia: WB Saunders; 1985.

Tsai JJ, Yeun JY, Kumar VA. Comparison and interpretation of urinalysis performed by a nephrologist versus a hospital-based clinical laboratory. *Am J Kidney Dis.* 2005;46:820-829.

Voswinckel P. A marvel of colors and ingredients: the story of urine test strips. *Kidney Int.* 1994;46(suppl):3-7.

Taimur Dad; Scott J. Gilbert

5 Hematuria and Proteinuria

Kidney disease is recognized as a reduction in the glomerular filtration rate (GFR) or damage to kidney structure or function. This damage is manifested by loss of the integrity of the filtration barrier, impairment of tubular function, or other processes that interfere with normal kidney function. Urinalysis and urine sediment examination are useful tools to detect this damage, and both hematuria and proteinuria are important biomarkers of kidney disease. The appearance of red blood cells (RBCs) in the urine and the presence and type of proteinuria may point to the site of nephron damage and qualify the diagnostic evaluation. For example, blebs on the surface of RBCs in the urine sediment indicate glomerular bleeding as these cells undergo morphologic changes when forced across the glomerular basement membrane (GBM); albuminuria often reflects damage to the filtration barrier with a loss of the charge and size selectivity of the membrane; and low-molecular-weight proteinuria, such as β-2-microglobulin, identifies a failure of proximal tubular protein reabsorption or excessive filtration of pathologic molecules. The persistence of hematuria and the level of proteinuria provide prognostic information as well as an assessment of continued disease activity and response to treatment.

As early kidney damage may occur without clinical correlations, screening for hematuria and proteinuria is encouraged in high-risk populations, such as those with diabetes, hypertension, autoimmune conditions, or a family history of kidney disease. The detection of abnormal levels of these biomarkers warrants a full and complete evaluation by a trained clinician. This chapter explores the significance of hematuria and proteinuria, the mechanisms of their development, the evaluation of these findings, and treatment options.

HEMATURIA

Hematuria is the presence of RBCs in the urine. This can be divided into macroscopic (also known as gross or visible) and microscopic hematuria. Macroscopic hematuria is detected by the naked eye while microscopic hematuria needs either evaluation with a urine dipstick or microscopic urine sediment evaluation. As little as 1 mL of blood in a liter of urine can result in discoloration of the urine. Urine can appear on a spectrum from light pink to dark red/cola colored depending on the concentration of RBCs.

DEFINITION

On microscopic evaluation, the presence of three or more RBCs per high-power field in a centrifuged urine sample is generally considered abnormal. However, there is no absolute cutoff, and lowering this threshold will result in more false-positive results, while increasing this threshold will result in more false-negative results.

ETIOLOGY

The many different causes of hematuria are outlined in Table 5.1. Microscopic hematuria can come from glomerular or nonglomerular sites, with evaluation based on the RBC morphology in the urine sediment and the presence and amount of albuminuria. The most common glomerular causes of asymptomatic hematuria include IgA nephropathy and thin basement membrane disease (TBMD). In about half of affected individuals, immunoglobulin A (IgA) nephropathy can present with gross hematuria following upper respiratory tract infections, although this should be differentiated from postinfectious glomerulonephritis (PIGN). PIGN typically has a longer lag than IgA nephropathy between the infection and the onset of hematuria. TBMD results from genetic defects in type IV collagen that make up the GBM. The inheritance pattern is autosomal dominant, resulting in multiple family members with microscopic hematuria without progressive kidney disease. Glomerular hematuria can be found in healthy individuals after intense exercise, which is benign in nature. Conversely, a family history of hematuria and progressive kidney disease, hearing loss, and ocular abnormalities can indicate Alport syndrome, a genetic condition similar to TBMD in which affected individuals can progress to kidney failure.

Inflammatory diseases of the glomerulus also cause glomerular hematuria. These include lupus nephritis, membranoproliferative glomerulonephritis (MPGN), pauci-immune vasculitis, and antiglomerular basement membrane disease, among others. Direct barotrauma in the setting of hypertensive emergency can result in hematuria. Glomerular diseases that lack significant inflammation but result in increased GBM permeability, such as focal segmental glomerulosclerosis (FSGS), minimal change disease (MCD), and membranous nephropathy, primarily cause proteinuria, but they can also result in hematuria. Hematuria has also been reported as an uncommon finding in diabetic nephropathy.

The presence of pyuria in the setting of hematuria, along with specific symptoms, can point to infection or inflammation being the cause. Numerous bacterial pathogens can cause infectious cystitis. Patients taking immunosuppressant medications can develop infectious cystitis from viruses such as BK polyomavirus. Without infectious symptoms and with sterile cultures, acute or chronic tubulointerstitial disease should be considered, with the latter including analgesic nephropathy.

Table 5.1 Causes of Hematuria

Glomerular

- Pauci-immune (ANCA related) vasculitis/anti-GBM disease
- Alport syndrome
- Thin basement membrane disease
- IgA nephropathy
- Associated with other glomerular diseases (FSGS, MCD, membranous nephropathy)
- Diabetic nephropathy
- Hypertensive emergency
- Exercise induced

Tubular/Interstitial

- Interstitial nephritis
- Papillary necrosis

Urothelial

- Malignancy (involving the kidney, ureters, bladder, or prostate)
- Nephrolithiasis
- Nephrocalcinosis
- Hypercalciuria
- Hyperoxaluria
- Strictures
- Bladder or ureteral polyps

Medications

- Cyclophosphamide/ifosfamide
- Anticoagulation associated[a]

Structural Kidney Diseases

- Acquired or hereditary cystic disease
- Medullary sponge kidney

Other Causes

- Infectious (pyelonephritis, cystitis, urethritis, prostatitis, schistosomiasis, TB, polyoma virus)
- Rejection or trauma in a kidney transplant
- Pelvic radiation
- Sickle cell disease/trait
- Thrombotic microangiopathy
- Post instrumentation of the urinary tract or trauma
- Contamination from menstrual bleeding

Rare Causes

- Analgesic nephropathy
- Renal vein thrombosis
- Renal infarct/necrosis
- Endometriosis of the urinary tract
- Loin pain hematuria syndrome
- Nutcracker syndrome
- Arteriovenous malformations

[a]Also shown to cause glomerular bleeding.
ANCA, Antineutrophil cytoplasmic antibodies; *FSGS,* focal segmental glomerulosclerosis; *GBM,* glomerular basement membrane; *MCD,* minimal change disease; *TB,* tuberculosis.

Table 5.2 Common Medications Causing Urine Discoloration Mimicking Hematuria

Red

- Phenytoin
- Phenazopyridine
- Deferoxamine

Red-Brown

- Metronidazole
- Levodopa

Brown

- Nitrofurantoin
- Chloroquine

Dark Appearing

- Metronidazole
- Methyldopa
- Imipenem-cilastatin

Red-Orange

- Rifampin

malignancy generally increases in older individuals. Other risk factors for urothelial carcinoma include exposure to cigarette smoking, occupational carcinogens, radiation, or medications such as cyclophosphamide. In older men, prostatic hypertrophy can be a cause of hematuria, but caution should be used to exclude malignancy. Hematuria associated with renal colic can be from nephrolithiasis; however, blood clots causing urinary obstruction can cause similar pain. Risk factors for nephrolithiasis, such as hypercalciuria and hyperoxaluria, have also been identified as causes of hematuria. Overanticoagulation can result in hematuria originating in the urothelial tract and has also been implicated, albeit rarely, in glomerular bleeding.

Medications that directly cause hematuria are uncommon, with the exception of a few specific chemotherapeutic agents. Conversely, many medications cause discoloration of urine without actual RBCs or free heme pigment in the urine (Table 5.2). This holds true for certain foods such as beets and for metabolites such as porphyrins, bile pigments, and methemoglobin.

Instrumentation and trauma to the genitourinary tract is commonly associated with hematuria. Similarly, papillary infarction or necrosis (more frequently seen in individuals with sickle cell disease and in a subset of individuals with analgesic nephropathy), kidney infarcts, damage from radiation, or structural kidney disease can all result in hematuria. In addition to causes already mentioned, hematuria in kidney transplant patients can be due to BK polyoma virus infection, rejection, recurrence of original kidney disease (if associated with hematuria), trauma, or structural/anastomotic problems.

DETECTION

Identification of microscopic hematuria is commonly performed with a urine dipstick. The dipstick is performed when there is discoloration of the urine or when there is concern for hematuria. The dipstick relies on the peroxidase activity of the heme molecule, which results in a detectable change in color on an impregnated indicator pad. This sensitive reaction can detect very small amounts of blood in the urine. Positive results can also be present in the setting of free heme pigment from hemoglobin or myoglobin in the urine without intact RBCs (e.g., rhabdomyolysis). False-positive

Although rare in the United States, infections such as tuberculosis or schistosomiasis can cause pyuria and hematuria with sterile bacterial cultures in endemic countries.

Macroscopic hematuria with passage of blood clots in the urine is most often of urothelial origin, and the risk of results can be due to the presence of semen, bacterial peroxidase, highly alkaline urine, or after cleaning the perineum with oxidizing agents. False-negative results can occur in cases of high vitamin C intake.

EVALUATION OF HEMATURIA

The evaluation of hematuria (Fig. 5.1) begins with a careful personal and family history that can provide clues to the possible etiology. Personal history should include prior episodes of hematuria, antecedent travel, upper respiratory tract infection before the onset of hematuria, recent strenuous exercise, history of renal colic or previous nephrolithiasis, passage of blood clots in the urine, pelvic radiation, recent trauma or instrumentation, and initiation of new medications or use of anticoagulants. Hematuria in the setting of menstruation should always be interpreted with caution because of the risk of contamination of the urine sample. Family history should include the presence of hematuria, hearing or ocular disorders, progressive kidney disease, and hematologic abnormalities such as sickle cell

disease/trait or coagulation disorders. Physical examination should explore signs of infection (for pyelonephritis, cystitis, or prostatitis), severe hypertension, edema pointing to possible accompanying hypoalbuminemia from nephrotic syndrome, masses in the setting of kidney or prostatic malignancy, or enlarged kidneys from polycystic kidney disease (PKD).

The next step involves examination of a freshly voided urine sample. Once there is confirmation of heme positivity with a urinary dipstick, the urine should be centrifuged. A dark pellet at the bottom of the tube with clear appearing supernatant indicates the presence of RBCs in the urine. A dark supernatant raises suspicion of free heme pigment, as seen in hemoglobinuria or myoglobinuria, and should prompt evaluation for either intravascular hemolysis or rhabdomyolysis, respectively. This can also be seen if the urine is dilute and has been sitting for a period of time, resulting in osmotic lysis of RBCs. The pellet formed after centrifugation should be re-suspended and evaluated under the microscope. This is generally done with bright field microscopy, although superior evaluation of RBC morphology can be performed

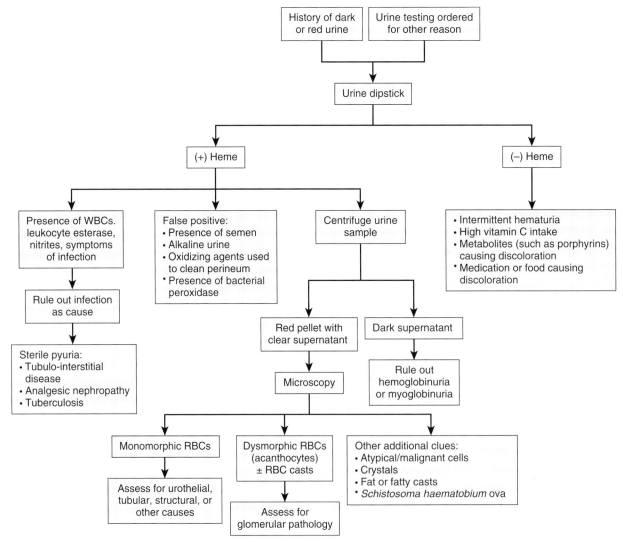

Fig. 5.1 Clinical approach to hematuria. *RBCs*, Red blood cells; *WBCs*, white blood cells.

with phase contrast microscopy. Normal RBC shape results in a biconcave disk appearance. RBCs can appear distorted in the urine for a variety of reasons, resulting in "dysmorphic" RBCs. A specific kind of dysmorphic RBC, called an acanthocyte, has characteristic vesicle-like protrusions and is particularly indicative of glomerular hematuria. Acanthocytes should be distinguished from crenated RBCs, which have spicules after cell shrinkage in concentrated urine (Fig. 5.2). An acanthocyte threshold of greater than 5% can be used for diagnosing glomerular hematuria with high specificity but low sensitivity. The presence of RBC casts and albuminuria further strengthens the diagnosis of glomerular hematuria. Other than RBC morphology, urine microscopy can provide additional clues, such as fat or fatty casts in the setting of accompanying heavy proteinuria, crystals in the setting of nephrolithiasis or hypercalciuria/hyperoxaluria, tubular epithelial cells with intranuclear inclusions (decoy cells) in the presence of BK nephropathy, or atypical appearing cells in the setting of malignancy. The more common test to assess for atypical cells, a stained urine cytology exam by a pathologist, lacks sensitivity.

Laboratory testing should be tailored to the suspected etiology of hematuria. For example, in the setting of a suspected glomerular cause, serum creatinine, electrolytes, and albumin should be checked. Serologic testing can also be performed in the setting of glomerular pathology. Blood counts and coagulation panel can be monitored for the presence of anemia, hemolysis, and coagulation abnormalities.

Imaging plays a vital role in the workup for hematuria. Ultrasound of the kidneys can be used to evaluate kidney structure without exposure to radiation. More sensitive imaging can be performed with computed tomography (CT) scans either with or without intravenous contrast depending on the suspected etiology. Cystoscopy with direct visualization of the urothelial mucosa remains the gold standard for evaluation of the lower urinary tract. Magnetic resonance imaging (MRI) also can be used in the evaluation of hematuria. Finally, kidney biopsy can be performed in the setting of hematuria to achieve a definitive kidney disease diagnosis. Even with the availability of these studies, the etiology of microscopic hematuria may not be identified in a significant proportion

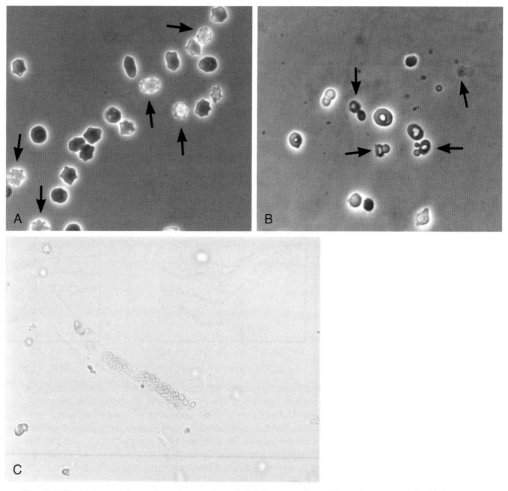

Fig. 5.2 Red blood cells in the urine sediment. (A) Isomorphic erythrocytes, some of which have a crenated appearance *(arrows)*. Phase contrast microscopy, original magnification ×400. (B) Acanthocytes demonstrating membrane blebs *(arrows)*. Phase contrast microscopy, original magnification ×400 (C) Red blood cell cast. Bright field microscopy, original magnification ×100. (A and B, from Fogazzi GB, Verdesca S, Garigali G. Urinalysis: core curriculum 2008. *Am J Kid Dis*. 2008;51:1052–1067.)

of patients. Follow-up evaluation of such patients remains an area of uncertainty.

MANAGEMENT

The management of hematuria depends on the underlying causes, which are discussed elsewhere in the *Primer*. Many of the causes described above may require co-management with urology.

PROTEINURIA

With an intact glomerular filtration barrier and functioning tubules, the amount of protein present in the urine is less than 150 mg/day. Increased levels of proteinuria can indicate kidney damage, and the quantity and type of protein in the urine are important to identify the site and cause of kidney damage. Albuminuria is a marker of damage to the filtration barrier, whereas low-molecular-weight proteins in the urine often indicate tubular injury or overflow proteinuria. Levels of proteinuria in excess of 3.5 g/day

(nephrotic-range) suggest a number of disease processes including FSGS, MCD, membranous nephropathy, and amyloidosis that are distinct from diseases with less than 2 g/day of proteinuria.

The quantification of proteinuria has additional value in assessing prognosis and response to therapy. Higher levels of proteinuria are associated with more rapid GFR decline and higher likelihood of kidney failure in diabetic and nondiabetic kidney disease, and lowering of proteinuria through renin-angiotensin blockade or disease-specific directed therapies is associated with lower rates of progressive GFR loss and kidney failure. Furthermore, the presence of albuminuria, even at low levels of 30 mg/day, is associated with increased all-cause and cardiovascular mortality, left ventricular hypertrophy (LVH), stroke, and vascular calcification, independent of the underlying disease process or the level of kidney function. This was clearly shown in the work of the Chronic Kidney Disease Epidemiology Collaboration (CKD-EPI) consortium (Fig. 5.3). As a result, proteinuria and albuminuria are often monitored as evidence of response to therapy in many primary and secondary kidney diseases, including diabetic nephropathy and hypertensive nephrosclerosis.

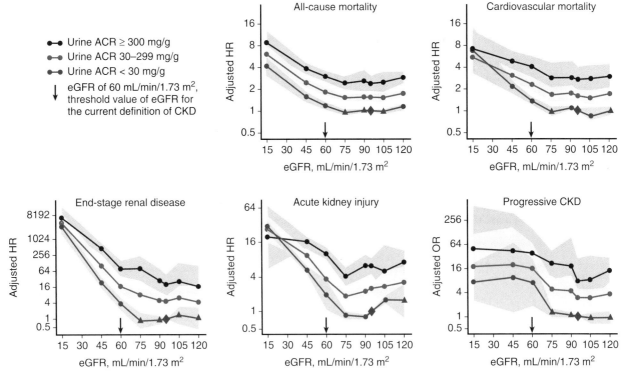

Fig. 5.3 Summary of continuous meta-analysis for general population cohorts with albumin-to-creatinine ratio (ACR). Mortality is reported for general population cohorts assessing albuminuria as urine ACR. Kidney outcomes are reported for general population cohorts assessing albuminuria as either urine ACR or reagent strip. Estimated glomerular filtration rate (eGFR) is expressed as a continuous variable. The three lines represent urine ACR of greater than 30, 30–299, and ≥300 mg/g (<3, 3–29, and ≥30 mg/mmol, respectively) or reagent strip negative and trace, 1+ positive, ≥2+ positive. All results are adjusted for covariates and compared to reference point of eGFR of 95 mL/min per 1.73 m² and ACR of greater than 30 mg/g (<3 mg/mmol) or reagent strip negative (diamond). Each point represents the pooled relative risk (RR) from a meta-analysis. Solid circles indicate statistical significance compared to the reference point (*P* < .05); triangles indicate nonsignificance. Red arrows indicate eGFR of 60 mL/min per 1.73 m², threshold value of eGFR for the current definition of CKD. *CKD*, Chronic kidney disease; *HR*, hazard ratio; *OR*, odds ratio. (From Levey AS, Coresh J. Chronic kidney disease. *Lancet*. 2012;379:165–180.)

DEFINITION

Normal levels of protein in the urine are less than 150 mg/day. This is primarily composed of Tamm-Horsfall protein, with less than 30 mg/day being albumin. Clinical practice guidelines identify levels of albuminuria greater than 30 mg/day that persist for more than 3 months as defining chronic kidney disease (CKD). Urine albumin levels between 30 and 300 mg/day were previously referred to as *microalbuminuria*, whereas levels greater than 300 mg/day were referred to as *macroalbuminuria*. These terms have been replaced by *moderately increased albuminuria* and *severely increased albuminuria*, respectively.

Isolated proteinuria is the condition of greater than 300 mg of protein excretion per day in the absence of abnormalities in the urine sediment, GFR loss, or comorbid conditions (diabetes, hypertension, rheumatologic or infectious diseases). This is often detected incidentally without evidence of edema or nephrotic syndrome.

Proteinuria can also be typed according to its mechanism: *glomerular, tubular, overflow,* and *postrenal.* These are discussed below under Physiology.

Albuminuria greater than 30 mg/day is present in 6.7% of the US general population, with higher prevalence in the elderly and in individuals with comorbidities. The prevalence of albuminuria in individuals with diabetes is 28.8%, and 16% of individuals with hypertension have albuminuria. The prevalence of albuminuria increases after the age of 40, with 3.3% of the adult population with a normal GFR having persistent albuminuria. Albuminuria is 50% more common in women than men (9.7% vs. 6.1%). It is also more common in non-Hispanic black and Mexican American populations when compared to non-Hispanic whites. This likely reflects an increased prevalence of diseases associated with proteinuria in the black community, such as diabetes, hypertension, and primary glomerular diseases, and the risk allele of *APOL1.*

PHYSIOLOGY

Because of the structure of the GBM, small amounts of protein are filtered at the glomerulus by processes of diffusion and convection with the vast majority then reabsorbed through receptor-mediated endocytosis, primary in the proximal convoluted tubule (PCT). A more modest amount of protein, primarily Tamm-Horsfall protein, is secreted by the tubule.

The glomerular filtration barrier is comprised of a fenestrated endothelium, a basement membrane, and an epithelial covering derived from podocyte foot processes and linking slit diaphragms. The endothelial fenestrations are pores of less than 100 nm in diameter coated with glycocalyx that represent the first barrier to protein filtration. The GBM includes a matrix of type IV collagen and laminin comprising a middle lamina densa, with adherent polyanionic proteoglycans like heparan sulfates creating a lamina rara interna (adjacent to the endothelial cells) and lamina rara externa (adjacent to the epithelial cells). The epithelial lining of interdigitating foot processes linked by slit diaphragms of nephrin and podocin provide the final barrier through creation of pores 7 nm in diameter. Together, the intact glomerular filtration barrier provides a size- and charge-specific barrier than allows passage of small (0 to 35 nm)

Table 5.3 Filtration Across the Glomerular Basement Membrane by Size

Substance	Molecular Weight (g/mol)	Filterability
Sodium	23	1.0
Glucose	180	1.0
Inulin	5,500	1.0
Myoglobulin	17,000	0.75
Albumin	69,000	0.005

and uncharged or cationic molecules but reflects molecules of larger size and increasingly anionic charge (Table 5.3).

The primary plasma protein is albumin, a 70-kD molecule with a diameter of 6 nm and an anionic charge (isoelectric point [pI] −4.5). Under normal circumstances, approximately 8 g of albumin is filtered by the glomerulus each day, but nearly all of this is reabsorbed by the PCT through receptor-mediated endocytosis such that less than 20 mg are excreted in the urine. Megalin and cubulin are key factors in this process. An increase in urinary protein excretion occurs with defects in the glomerular filtration barrier, impairment of tubular reabsorption of filtered protein, or an excessive load of filtered proteins that overwhelm the reabsorptive capacity of the tubule.

Glomerular proteinuria is largely albuminuria and other macromolecules, and related to defects in the size- and charge-selective barrier that normally reflect these larger, anionically charged molecules. This can occur with structural changes seen with inflammation, scarring, deposition, or genetic conditions that affect the integral proteins of the filtration barrier (such as nephrin and podocin). Albuminuria typically exceeds 400 mg/day.

Tubular proteinuria is composed of low-molecular-weight proteins (<25 kD), such as β-2-microglobulin, retinol-binding protein, immunoglobulin light chains, and polypeptide fragments, and it is thus unlikely to be identified by the traditional urine dipstick that detects intact albumin. These smaller molecules are normally filtered by the glomerulus and then reabsorbed by the tubule. With tubular pathology seen in tubulointerstitial nephritis, tubular toxicity from heavy-metal poisoning, Dent disease, and Lowe syndrome, the low-molecular-weight proteins are not reabsorbed and appear in the urine. Tubular proteinuria occurs at a level of 200 to 2000 mg/day with albuminuria at less than 400 mg/day, but larger amounts of albuminuria can be seen with coexisting glomerular disease. Urine protein electrophoresis is often used to identify these proteins.

Overflow proteinuria occurs when overproduction and excessive filtration of low-molecular-weight proteins exceeds the reabsorptive capacity of the tubule. This can result in the appearance in the urine of immunoglobulin light chains (with multiple myeloma), lysozyme (with myelomonocytic leukemia), myoglobin (with rhabdomyolysis or inherent muscle disorders), or free hemoglobin (with intravascular hemolysis).

Proteinuria can occur with damage to the collecting system, often referred to as *postrenal proteinuria.* This is seen in conditions including inflammation, irritation, infection, or cancer of the renal pelvis, ureters, bladder, and prostate. The responsible protein is typically nonalbumin (i.e., immunoglobulins), levels are often low, and the duration may be transient.

DETECTION

Proteinuria is most commonly detected with a semi-quantitative urine dipstick and then confirmed with quantitative measures. Repeat testing should be documented on two separate occasions to exclude false positives and transient proteinuria. Two semi-quantitative methods of detecting proteinuria are available.

SEMI-QUANTITATIVE METHODS

The urine dipstick uses pads impregnated with indicator dyes that undergo a colorimetric reaction with albumin in the urine. The common dyes, tetrabromophenol blue and bromocresol green, are very specific but lack sensitivity in the setting of dilute urine or nonalbumin proteins such as immunoglobulin light chains. The reaction on the pad is scored:

Trace	15–30 mg/dL
1+	30–100 mg/dL
2+	100–300 mg/dL
3+	300–1000 mg/dL
4+	>1000 mg/dL

Interpretation must account for urinary concentration (often estimated by the specific gravity). Scores of 2+ and greater are highly suggestive of significant proteinuria, but scores of trace or 1+ are only predictive when the specific gravity is greater than 1.025. In addition to urine concentration, the sensitivity and specificity of the urine dipstick is affected by the presence of other chemicals. False positives are seen with alkaline urine (pH >8) that overwhelms the buffer, drugs (tolbutamide, cephalosporins, chlorhexidine, benzalkonium) that interfere with the reaction, and iodinated radiocontrast agents. As mentioned, false negatives are seen in dilute urine or in the presence of nonalbumin proteins.

A second semi-quantitative method relies on the biuret reaction of urinary proteins with sulfosalicylic acid (SSA). This reaction occurs with all proteins at a sensitivity of 5 to 10 mg/dL. Thus a strongly positive reaction with SSA in the setting of a negative urine dipstick indicates the presence of a nonalbumin protein in the urine, such as immunoglobulin light chains in multiple myeloma. The SSA test is scored:

0	no turbidity (0 mg/dL)
Trace	slight turbidity (1–10 mg/dL)
1+	turbidity through which print can be read (15–30 mg/dL)
2+	white cloud without precipitate through which heavy black lines on a white background can be seen (40–100 mg/dL)
3+	white cloud with fine precipitate through which heavy black lines cannot be seen (150–350 mg/dL)
4+	flocculent precipitate (>500 mg/dL)

False positives with SSA test are seen after iodinated radiocontrast administration.

QUANTITATIVE METHODS

Quantitation of urinary protein excretion is important in individuals with persistent proteinuria to help narrow the spectrum of kidney injury (benign proteinuria vs. nonnephrotic proteinuria vs. nephrotic syndrome) and to monitor progression of disease and response to treatment over time. Two quantitative assessments of proteinuria are available.

The standard for measuring proteinuria is a timed, usually 24-hour, urine collection. These collections are cumbersome to collect, difficult to transport, and often inaccurate because of improper or incomplete collection. Timed collections are particularly challenging for individuals with persistent proteinuria who require frequent measurements. Collections of shorter duration (6 or 12 hours) suffer from wider variability. The completeness of a collection can be assessed by assuming women below the age of 50 excrete 15 to 20 mg creatinine per kilogram lean body mass per day, while men excrete 20 to 25 mg creatinine per kilogram lean body mass. Creatinine excretion declines with advancing age.

An alternative is the measurement in a spot urine collection of the ratio of protein or albumin to creatinine. The urine protein-to-creatinine ratio (UPCR) and urine albumin-to-creatinine ratio (UACR) corrects the protein and albumin measurements (in mg/dL) for urinary concentration or dilution by standardizing for 1 g of daily creatinine excretion. This is expressed in units of mg/g and correlates closely with the daily protein and albumin excretion (Fig. 5.4). Care must be used in interpreting the results in groups that do not meet population norms, such as younger, black and Hispanic, and athletic individuals who excrete more than 1 g of creatinine per day (thus under-estimating protein excretion), or older,

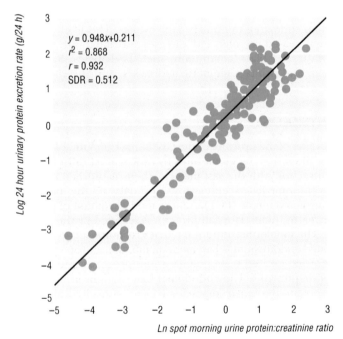

Fig. 5.4 Correlation between ln spot morning urine protein:creatinine ratio and log 24-hour urinary protein in 177 nondiabetic patients with chronic nephropathies and persistent clinical proteinuria, showing regression equation and line. *r,* Correlation coefficient; *r²,* determination coefficient; *SDR,* ln SD of regression line. (From Ruggenenti P, Gaspari F, Perna A, Remuzzi G. Cross sectional longitudinal study of spot morning urine protein:creatinine ratio, 24 hour urine protein excretion rate, glomerular filtration rate, and end stage renal failure in chronic renal disease in patients without diabetes. *BMJ.* 1998;316:504–509.)

white, and more frail individuals who excrete less creatinine (thus overestimating protein excretion). Given diurnal variations in protein excretion, repeat measurements should ideally be performed at the same time each day. Nevertheless, the use of UPCR and UACR are supported by Kidney Disease: Improving Global Outcomes (KDIGO).

EVALUATION OF PROTEINURIA

Once proteinuria has been detected and quantitated, the evaluation requires a careful history, complete physical exam, and directed laboratory testing. The history must include factors associated with kidney disease such as age; race; prior kidney injury; comorbid conditions such as diabetes, hypertension, cancer, and autoimmune diseases; and family history of kidney disease. The physical exam should measure blood pressure, assess for LVH, and evaluate for lymphadenopathy, splenomegaly, edema, arthritis, rash, and sinus disease. A fundoscopic examination is useful for detecting small vessel disease. On laboratory testing, quantification of and typing of proteinuria, examination of the urine sediment for hematuria and casts, estimation of kidney function, measurement of electrolytes, and assessment of serologic markers and infection are performed. Electrocardiogram and echocardiogram are useful in identifying LVH.

Younger individuals are more likely to have benign proteinuria or transient proteinuria. *Transient proteinuria* is a common phenomenon affecting 4% of men and 7% of women. Fever and vigorous exercise are often responsible, and reassessment should occur when the patient is well (free of fever) and after avoidance of vigorous exercise.

Orthostatic proteinuria is seen in children and adolescents (2% to 5%) but is rare in adults over 30 years of age. It can be assessed by doing a split urine collection that includes a supine and an upright collection. The protein content of the upright collection is greater than the supine collection with poor understanding of the mechanism. This is a benign condition with an excellent prognosis and requires no follow-up once identified.

Persistent proteinuria less than 2000 mg/day without features of hematuria, GFR loss, rheumatologic conditions, or abnormal immunologic or serologic tests can often be observed for several months before proceeding with further evaluation. With concerning features, the evaluation is largely driven by findings on the history, physical exam, or other laboratory tests.

The presence of albuminuria in the setting of hematuria is suggestive of glomerular disease and warrants a thorough immunologic and serologic evaluation. Antinuclear antibodies (ANA) and anti-double-stranded DNA (dsDNA) antibodies are typically present in lupus nephritis, and extractable nuclear antigens (Ro, Sm, RNP) can often be identified. Low serum complement levels identify conditions with complement-fixing antigen-antibody complexes, such as lupus nephritis, MPGN, cryoglobulinemic kidney disease, and PIGN. Albuminuria, hematuria, and rapidly declining GFR are worrisome features of a rapidly progressive glomerulonephritis (RPGN), many of which may involve anti-GBM antibodies or antineutrophil cytoplasmic antibodies (ANCAs). ANCA directed against myeloperoxidase (anti-MPO) commonly produces the pathologic injury of microscopic polyangiitis, whereas ANCA against proteinase 3 (anti-PR3) produces

granulomatosis with polyangiitis (previously known as Wegener syndrome). Glomerular proteinuria can also be seen with a number of systemic infections. Hepatitis C (HCV) infection can induce rheumatoid factor and cryoglobulinemic kidney disease. Hepatitis B (HBV) infection has been associated with membranous glomerulopathy, MPGN, and polyarteritis nodosa (PAN). HIV infection is associated with the collapsing variant of FSGS.

Older subjects with an active cancer, a history of cancer, or biomarkers of cancer activity are at risk for membranous nephropathy, MPGN (breast, colon, stomach, lung cancer), or MCD (Hodgkin and non-Hodgkin lymphomas).

Tubular proteinuria is suggested by the presence of nonalbumin protein in the urine. For example, an elevated ratio of β-2-microglobulin-to-albumin in the urine would warrant evaluation for Sjögren syndrome, malignancy, medication toxicity, and heavy metal exposure.

Finally, overflow proteinuria occurs from myoglobinuria after muscle damage from drugs, traumatic injury, or inherited muscle enzyme disorders, hemoglobinuria with intravascular hemolysis or paroxysmal nocturnal hemoglobinuria (PNH), immunoglobulin light chains with multiple myeloma, or lysozyme with myelomonocytic leukemia. These proteins can be measured directly or detected by electrophoresis.

A kidney biopsy is usually reserved for:

- Proteinuria associated with a declining GFR
- Proteinuria in the nephrotic range (greater than 3500 mg/day)
- Proteinuria with features of a glomerular (albuminuria, acanthocytes, RBC casts) or tubular (low-molecular-weight proteins) source
- Persistent proteinuria greater than 500 mg/day in a patient with systemic lupus erythematosus (SLE) or other rheumatologic condition

Patients with diabetes and nephrotic-range proteinuria are not usually biopsied given the frequency of diabetic nephropathy in this population, but dramatic increases in proteinuria that was previously stable may suggest a superimposed condition. Biopsy surveys of diabetic patients identify an alternative etiology in 30% of cases.

MANAGEMENT

Treatment of proteinuria includes disease-specific and general interventions. Disease-specific treatments are discussed elsewhere in the *Primer*, with the objective of targeting the underlying condition to reduce the damage to the kidney and the loss of protein in the urine. General interventions include use of renin-angiotensin blockade that alters glomerular hemodynamics and mediators of fibrosis. The consequences of significant protein loss in the urine, including hyperlipidemia, hypercoagulability, impaired immunologic response, and malnutrition, must not be overlooked.

KEY BIBLIOGRAPHY

Andres A, Praga M, Bello I, Diaz-Rolón JA, et al. Hematuria due to hypercalciuria and hyperuricosuria in adult patients. *Kidney Int.* 1989; 36:96.

Becker GJ, Garigali G, Fogazzi GB. Advances in urine microscopy. *Am J Kidney Dis.* 2015;67:954-964.

Boulware LE, Jaar BG, Tarver-Carr ME, Brancati FL, Powe NR. Screening for proteinuria in US adults: a cost-effectiveness analysis. *JAMA.* 2003;290:3101-3114.

Cohen RA, Brown RS. Microscopic hematuria. *N Engl J Med.* 2003;348: 2330-2338.

Davies R, Jones JS, Barocas DA, Castle EP, et al. Diagnosis, evaluation and follow-up of asymptomatic microhematuria (AMH) in adults: AUA guideline. *J Urol.* 2012;188:2473-2481.

Dickson LE, Wagner MC, Sandoval RM, Molitoris BA. The proximal tubule and albuminuria: really! *J Am Soc Nephrol.* 2014;25:443-453.

Donadio JV, Grande JP. IgA nephrophathy. *N Engl J Med.* 2002;347:738-748.

Fassett RG, Owen JE, Fairley J, Birth DF, Fairley KF. Urinary red-cell morphology during exercise. *Br Med J (Clin Res Ed).* 1982;285:1455-1457.

Fogazzi GB, Verdesca S, Garigali G. Urinalysis: core curriculum 2008. *Am J Kidney Dis.* 2008;51:1052-1067.

Fotheringham J, Campbell MJ, Fogarty DG, El Nahas M, Ellam T. Estimated albumin excretion rate versus urine albumin-creatinine ratio for the estimation of measured albumin excretion rate: derivation and validation of an estimated albumin excretion rate equation. *Am J Kidney Dis.* 2014;63:405-414.

Gaspari F, Perico N, Remuzzi G. Timed urine collections are not needed to measure urine protein excretion in clinical practice. *Am J Kidney Dis.* 2006;47:8-14.

Ginsberg JM, Chang BS, Matarese RA, Garella S. Use of single voided urine samples to estimate quantitative proteinuria. *N Engl J Med.* 1983;309:1543-1546.

Hausmann R, Kuppe C, Egger H, Schweda F, Knecht V, Elger M, Menzel S, Somers D, Braun G, Fuss A, Uhlig S, Kriz W, Tanner G, Floege J, Moeller MJ. Electrical forces determine glomerular permeability. *J Am Soc Nephrol.* 2010;21:2053-2058.

Kashtan C. Alport syndrome. An inherited disorder of renal, ocular, and cochlear basement membranes. *Medicine (Baltimore).* 1999;78:338.

Kelly CJ, Neilson EG. Tubulointerstitial diseases. In: Skorecki K, Chertow GM, Marsden PA, Taal MW, Yu AS, eds. *Brenner & Rector's The Kidney.* 10th ed. Philadelphia: Elsevier; 2016.

Kohler H, Wandel E, Brunck B. Acanthocyturia—a characteristic marker for glomerular bleeding. *Kidney Int.* 1991;40:115-120.

Levey AS, Coresh J. Chronic kidney disease. *Lancet.* 2012;379:165-180.

Ohisa N, Yoshida K, Matsuki R, Suzuki H, et al. A comparison of urinary albumin–total protein ratio to phase-contrast microscopic examination of urine sediment for differentiating glomerular and nonglomerular bleeding. *Am J Kidney Dis.* 2008;52:235-241.

Sharp VJ, Barnes KT, Erickson BA. Assessment of asymptomatic microscopic hematuria in adults. *Am Fam Physician.* 2013;88:747-754.

Tryggvason K, Patrakka J. Thin basement membrane nephropathy. *J Am Soc Nephrol.* 2006;17:813-822.

Full bibliography can be found on www.expertconsult.com.

Imaging the Kidneys

6

Hina Arif-Tiwari; Bobby Kalb; Richard C. Semelka; Diego R. Martin

There has been an impressive evolution and development of diagnostic imaging methods in recent years, expanding the array of techniques that can be used to understand and diagnose kidney diseases. Imaging modalities range from conventional fluoroscopic studies to nuclear medicine techniques to cross-sectional methods based on ultrasound, computed tomography (CT), or magnetic resonance imaging (MRI). Optimal patient care depends on an understanding of potential imaging applications and the benefits and risks related to these techniques. This is a task made more challenging because of continuing and rapid changes in the technology.

IMAGING MODALITIES

ABDOMINAL RADIOGRAPHY AND INTRAVENOUS UROGRAPHY

Historically, plain radiography and intravenous urography (IVU) were the preliminary tools for evaluation of kidney disease; however, these conventional methods provide limited sensitivity and specificity for most important urologic pathologies. Cross-sectional techniques have now superseded plain radiography and IVU to diagnose focal or diffuse kidney parenchymal pathologies and nephrolithiasis.

ULTRASONOGRAPHY

Ultrasonography (US) is a nonionizing technique that produces images in real time. It is a powerful initial kidney imaging modality that is safe, noninvasive, portable, and widely available with a lower initial test cost compared with CT or MRI. In addition, US can be performed in patients with kidney failure as iodinated contrast is not required, and it can readily differentiate between obstructive (surgical) and nonobstructive (medical) causes of kidney failure. However, image quality and detail are limited by a patient's body habitus and the operator's skills.

US can provide information about kidney size, cortical thickness, and echogenicity (Fig. 6.1A–C), and it can easily distinguish between solid and cystic kidney masses; however, characterization and differentiation between complex kidney cysts and cystic kidney tumors are limited by its soft-tissue resolution. In general, focal lesions identified on US require further imaging evaluation with CT or MRI. US is useful in detecting the presence or absence of hydronephrosis. Sensitivity for kidney calculi is generally restricted to calculi greater than 3 to 5 mm located within the renal pelvis, with relative insensitivity to ureteric calculi. Gray-scale ultrasound can be combined with color Doppler duplex imaging to assess patency and flow in kidney vasculature, particularly in the transplant kidney.

COMPUTED TOMOGRAPHY

In the United States, CT is commonly used for imaging the kidneys. CT provides good spatial resolution, with detailed anatomy of the kidney parenchyma, vasculature, and the excretory system. In contrast to other imaging techniques, CT provides the highest sensitivity for detecting fine calcifications within the kidney parenchyma and throughout the collecting system, making unenhanced CT the optimal test for detecting stone disease.

Contrast-enhanced multiphase CT has been used to evaluate kidney masses. Although CT provides high spatial resolution, a relative limitation is soft-tissue contrast. This necessitates more complex diagnostic algorithms for assessing complex cystic kidney lesions that entail the measurement of density units before and after contrast administration. Multiphase CT increases the radiation dose to the patient proportionate to the number of phases used. CT for urologic indications represents the source of greatest diagnostic radiation exposures in our population; three to four CT examinations, or phases within one examination, approximate the radiation exposure determined to cause increased cancer risk in atomic bomb survivors. Contrast allergies are relatively common, and contrast-induced nephropathy (CIN) is a potential risk of iodinated CT contrast. Patients with even moderately impaired kidney function are at risk for CIN, with other risk factors contributing such as advanced age, diabetes, hypertension, heart failure, and volume depletion.

Dual-energy computed tomography (DECT) is a recent advancement in CT hardware that provides information about how substances behave at different energies. The ability to generate virtual unenhanced datasets and improved detection of iodine-containing substances on low-energy images are promising grounds for continued research and development in DECT, targeting the achievement of radiation dose reductions. Potential applications of DECT include distinguishing hyperdense kidney cysts from renal cell carcinoma (RCC), identifying kidney calculi within contrast-filled renal collecting systems, and characterizing the composition of kidney calculi, including the differentiation of uric acid stones from nonuric acid stones. Iterative reconstruction image postprocessing is another recent application in CT that may also lead to significant radiation dose reduction.

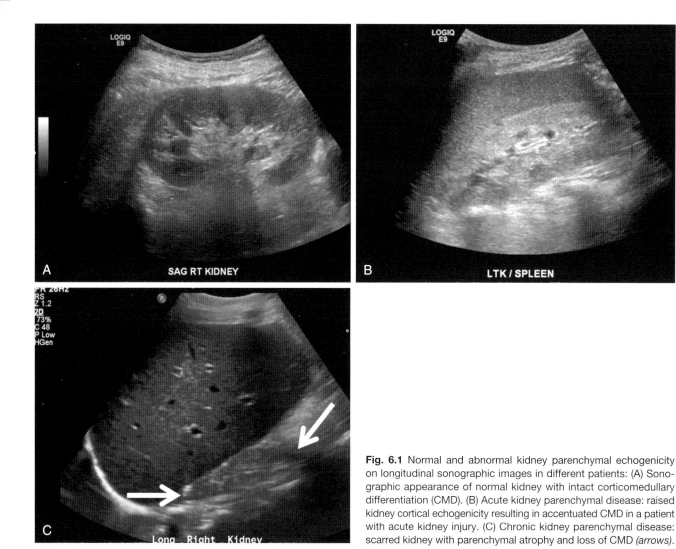

Fig. 6.1 Normal and abnormal kidney parenchymal echogenicity on longitudinal sonographic images in different patients: (A) Sonographic appearance of normal kidney with intact corticomedullary differentiation (CMD). (B) Acute kidney parenchymal disease: raised kidney cortical echogenicity resulting in accentuated CMD in a patient with acute kidney injury. (C) Chronic kidney parenchymal disease: scarred kidney with parenchymal atrophy and loss of CMD *(arrows)*.

KIDNEY SCINTIGRAPHY

Radionuclide studies of the kidney have been used to provide imaging-based qualitative assessment of kidney function. However, these techniques suffer from low spatial resolution and do not provide detailed analysis of both structure and function. The test is based on time-resolved imaging of the kidney after intravenous administration of a radiopharmaceutical that is either filtered (technetium-diethylene triamine pentaacetic acid [Tc-DTPA]) or secreted by the tubule (technetium-mercapto acetyl triglycine [Tc-MAG3]). The use of radioactive tracers, particularly in monitoring applications where the study will be repeated, raises the concern of radiation risk, which is increased in younger patients.

MAGNETIC RESONANCE IMAGING

MRI is evolving as a robust imaging technique for comprehensive evaluation of the kidneys and the collecting system (Fig. 6.2A–C). Excellent intrinsic tissue contrast and high spatial resolution of MRI results in more sensitive detection and specific characterization of focal and diffuse kidney pathologies, including complex cystic lesions considered problematic on CT or US. Because there is no ionizing radiation, MRI is

an ideal imaging technique for assessment of kidney masses, particularly in younger patients or in patients requiring serial studies. In patients with reduced kidney function, gadolinium-chelate-based contrast agents (GBCA) have been associated with nephrogenic systemic fibrosis (NSF), which is discussed separately.

Advantages of MRI include multiplanar imaging, multiphase contrast-enhanced imaging, and acquisition of multiple types of soft-tissue contrast with an array of sequences. This ensures optimal soft tissue contrast for detection and characterization of disease. This array of image contrast may be obtained with the most up-to-date, fast imaging techniques that allow for a total scan time of less than 20 minutes yet without any concern for radiation dose accumulation as with CT.

Multiple sequences that yield specific tissue information can be used. Fluid-sensitive T2W images (half-Fourier acquisition single-shot echo train, HASTE) and T2-like sequences (true free induction with steady-state free precision, TFISP) are helpful in evaluating the collecting system because of the intrinsic high signal intensity of urine. Precontrast and dynamic postcontrast T1W three-dimensional (3D) gradient echo fat-suppressed images in arterial, capillary, venous, and delayed phases demonstrate improved spatial resolution vital

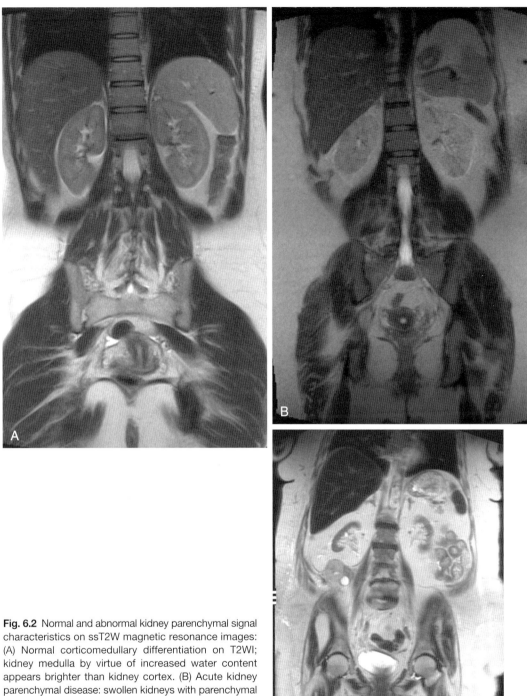

Fig. 6.2 Normal and abnormal kidney parenchymal signal characteristics on ssT2W magnetic resonance images: (A) Normal corticomedullary differentiation on T2WI; kidney medulla by virtue of increased water content appears brighter than kidney cortex. (B) Acute kidney parenchymal disease: swollen kidneys with parenchymal edema demonstrating bright signal and resultant loss of corticomedullary differentiation (CMD) in patient with bilateral pyelonephritis. (C) Chronic kidney parenchymal disease in another patient with parenchymal atrophy and loss of CMD.

for resolving masses and vascular anatomy. Arterial phase can also be optimized for evaluation of renal artery anatomy.

Functional data analysis with magnetic resonance nephro-urography (MRNU) allows for evaluation of kidney physiology in a manner that was not previously possible. Both structural and functional data can be extracted in a single examination, with measurements of renal blood flow (RBF) and glomerular filtration rate (GFR).

STRUCTURAL IMAGING

T2W and steady-state magnetization (TFISP) imaging offers excellent structural evaluation of the kidneys and can display collecting system morphology, even in a nondistended system, because of the bright signal of native urine. Focal lesions, filling defects, and obstructive causes of urinary tract dilation can be identified even in the absence of contrast excretion.

FUNCTIONAL IMAGING

Similar to inulin, gadolinium chelates are freely filtered at the glomerulus and are neither secreted nor absorbed by the renal tubules. Therefore the rate of gadolinium uptake in the kidney is related to the RBF. Accelerated 3D volumetric T1W gradient echo sequence (GRE) facilitates imaging of the gadolinium contrast as it arrives through the feeding renal artery and perfuses the kidney parenchyma. Rapid increase in concentration of gadolinium is seen as it enters the kidney parenchyma equivalent to the blood perfusion through the kidney. Although a portion of the perfused contrast leaves the kidney through the renal vein, another portion remains in the kidney because of glomerular filtration.

Assessments of kidney parenchymal volume, and calculations of kidney perfusion in terms of RBF and GFR, are made by semiautomated methods based on mathematical modeling.

MRNU can identify the cause of obstruction in the renal collecting system, including congenital anomalies such as ureteropelvic junction obstruction (Fig. 6.3A–C) and acquired conditions such as stone disease, transitional cell carcinoma of the upper and lower tract, and extrinsic compression from retroperitoneal fibrosis. Preoperative assessment of kidney function using MRNU in cases of RCC may direct surgical planning toward a potential nephron-sparing procedure. Comprehensive imaging can be obtained for kidney transplant donor and recipient evaluation, and this process is discussed later in this chapter.

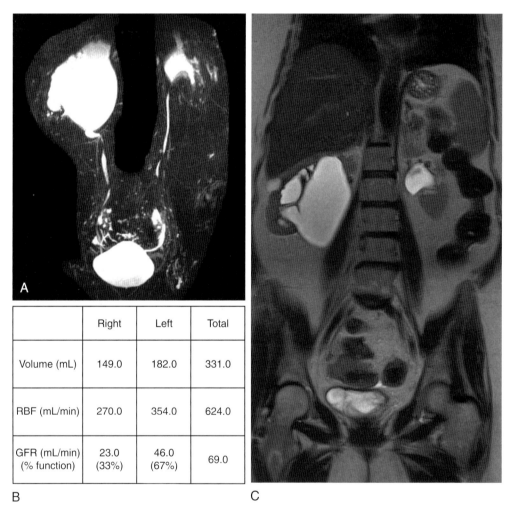

	Right	Left	Total
Volume (mL)	149.0	182.0	331.0
RBF (mL/min)	270.0	354.0	624.0
GFR (mL/min) (% function)	23.0 (33%)	46.0 (67%)	69.0

Fig. 6.3 Sixty-one-year-old woman with right-sided hydronephrosis presenting with persistent right-sided pain and recurrent pyelonephritis. During evaluation for possible surgical intervention, the patient underwent a mercaptoacetyltriglycine scan that demonstrated split kidney function as 45% on the right and 55% on the left, relatively symmetric findings given the extent of right kidney damage from multiple prior bouts of infection. A magnetic resonance imaging was obtained that demonstrated severe right-sided hydronephrosis in the configuration of a uteropelvic junction (UPJ) obstruction on 3D T2W maximum intensity projection (MIP) image (A), with abnormal signal of the right kidney parenchyma on coronal single-shot T2-weighted imaging (B), a finding in keeping with diminished function. Quantitative kidney functional data (C) shows significantly impaired kidney function on the right relative to the left (33% vs. 67%), a finding that was significantly underestimated with nuclear medicine. The patient underwent subsequent robotic pyeloplasty. *GFR,* Glomerular filtration rate; *RBF,* renal blood flow.

RISKS AND BENEFITS OF IMAGING CONTRAST IN KIDNEY DISEASE

In patients with reduced GFR, including those receiving dialysis, the choice of contrast-enhanced CT or MR should be based on the expected diagnostic benefits.

NSF is a systemic fibrotic disorder that occurs in patients with advanced chronic kidney disease (CKD) or severe acute kidney injury who were exposed to one or more doses of certain GBCAs. Delayed excretion and prolonged tissue exposure to circulating free GBCA is likely a key factor in the relationship between reduced GFR and NSF. The largest subset of cases has occurred in dialysis-dependent patients (either hemodialysis or peritoneal dialysis) who had a delay between contrast exposure and dialysis. On average, patients developing NSF have been exposed to multiple GBCA doses or a large single dose, and most documented cases have been associated with gadobenate dimeglumine (Gadodiamide).

Available data from both clinical reports and animal studies support the conclusion that different GBCA formulations have different relative risks of NSF with the risk associated with the relative agent chemical stability. Recommended guidelines to minimize the risk of NSF include use of macrocyclic GBCAs, because of their relatively stable structure, or stable linear GBCAs with higher relaxivity. Relaxivity is a measure of signal generated by the GBCA, with the higher relaxivity of an agent resulting in a lower required dose. Regardless of the GBCA used, the objective is to administer the minimum dose necessary to achieve a diagnostic MRI. Hemodialysis is effective at lowering the serum concentrations of GBCAs and should be performed as soon as possible after GBCA administration. Currently, dialysis is advocated only in patients who are on dialysis before the MRI, as the mortality and morbidity risk of hemodialysis may be greater than the risk of developing NSF following the exposure to stable GBCAs.

Precautions to reduce NSF risk include use of more stable GBCA, use of lowest possible dose, and postprocedure dialysis for patients who are dialysis-dependent. Following the institution of these precautions and more judicious use of GBCA in patients with kidney disease, no new cases of NSF have been described in the United States since 2010, and the risk of NSF with more stable GBCAs appears low. Centers have more recently reported that NSF incidence has diminished after observing these precautions, while continuing to use MRI with selected GBCA enhancement even in patients who are treated with dialysis if warranted.

CIN is defined as an acute decrease in kidney function after exposure to iodinated contrast agents (ICAs) in the absence of another explanation. This is the third most common cause of hospital-acquired acute kidney injury. Multiple risk factors are associated with CIN, including reduced GFR, volume depletion, diabetes, congestive cardiac failure, advanced age, and type and dose of ICA. Evidence suggests that ICA osmolarity and viscosity may relate to CIN risk. For patients receiving dialysis, preservation of residual kidney function is associated with improved outcomes, and ICAs may jeopardize residual kidney function in these patients.

The selection of contrast, specifically GBCAs versus ICAs versus no contrast, should be individualized based on a careful risk-benefit assessment. Consideration of alternative studies, including nonenhanced examination protocols, should always occur. In general, there are more unenhanced options available for the evaluation of soft tissues and blood vessels using MRI than CT. If a contrast-enhanced CT or MRI is warranted, the test most likely to provide a result that will impact management should be performed with a goal of minimizing delayed or missed diagnoses and the need for study repetition.

CYSTIC KIDNEY LESIONS

KIDNEY CYSTS

Kidney cysts represent the most common focal kidney lesion in adults. Cysts in the kidney have been classified and characterized by Bosniak into four categories: *Category I:* Simple benign cysts with negligible likelihood of malignancy; *Category II:* Benign cystic lesions that are minimally complicated; *Category IIF (F for follow-up):* Cysts less complex than category III and likely to be benign but given their complexity require follow-up studies to prove their nature; *Category III:* More complicated cystic lesions that require follow-up imaging and/or surgical excision; *Category IV:* Masses that are clearly malignant cystic carcinomas.

IMAGING FEATURES

US is the preferred method to differentiate cystic from solid lesions because of its ease of performance and lower cost. It is also accurate in differentiating simple kidney cysts (Fig. 6.4A–D) from complex cystic kidney masses. Although CT is widely used for characterization of cystic kidney masses, kidney lesions are best evaluated with triple-phase multidetector row CT (i.e., unenhanced, arterial phase, and nephrographic phase) with increasing radiation risk. Enhancing thick septations, solid components, or change in attenuation between 10 and 15 Hounsfield units (HU) after intravenous administration of contrast material are considered suspicious. Cystic angiomyolipomas (AMLs), oncocytomas, and infections may also show enhancement, whereas hypovascular papillary cancers may demonstrate less enhancement. MR imaging with better soft-tissue contrast resolution is 100% sensitive and 95% specific for distinguishing benign and malignant kidney cysts. Precontrast T1W images can easily identify intracyst hemorrhage in Bosniak Category IIF, which is challenging on CT. Signal intensity changes in dynamic postcontrast 3D T1-weighted GRE can delineate septae, solid elements, and nodules within a fluid-filled cyst or its wall. T2-weighted sequences also complement the 3D T1W GRE sequences for accurate characterization of kidney cysts (see Fig. 6.4A–D).

AUTOSOMAL-DOMINANT POLYCYSTIC KIDNEY DISEASE

Autosomal-dominant polycystic kidney disease (ADPKD) is the most common hereditary kidney cystic disease and the third most common cause of end-stage kidney disease (ESKD). Imaging features of ADPKD may differ according to the severity of the disease. An inverse linear correlation exists between kidney volume and GFR.

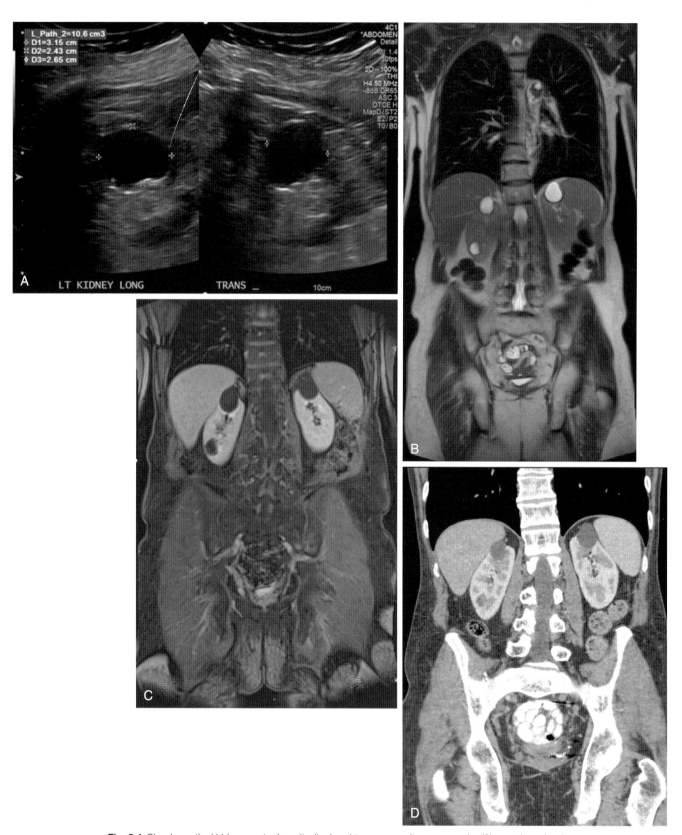

Fig. 6.4 Simple cortical kidney cysts. Longitudinal and transverse ultrasonography (A) reveals a simple, uncomplicated, exophytic cystic lesion consistent with Bosniak Category I cyst. Coronal T2W image (B) in another patient, depicting multiple simple cortical kidney cysts without definable wall that do not show any internal enhancement on post contrast magnetic resonance and computed tomography images (C and D).

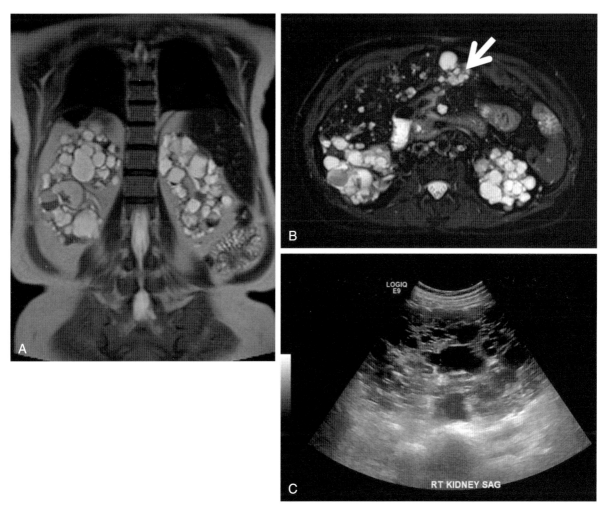

Fig. 6.5 Autosomal-dominant polycystic kidney disease. Coronal (A) and fat-saturated axial (B) ssT2W images. The kidneys are markedly enlarged with numerous cysts. Majority of cysts demonstrate increased T2 signal consistent with simple cyst, but a sizable fraction have varying signal and layering material suggestive of blood products of differing age. Note hepatic cysts *(arrow)*; iron in liver and spleen in reticuloendothelial uptake pattern suggests secondary hemochromatosis. Longitudinal sonogram (C) reveals innumerable cysts of varying sizes replacing the right kidney parenchyma.

IMAGING FEATURES

As ADPKD progresses, both kidneys enlarge massively with architectural distortion and display numerous cysts of varying sizes (Fig. 6.5A–C). Cysts can be seen on US, although because of the large size of the kidneys, the utility of US is severely limited in reproducibility in follow-up examinations. Unenhanced CT can evaluate cyst hemorrhage and calcifications. Extrarenal cysts in the liver and pancreas can be identified by either CT or MRI. The Consortium for Radiologic Imaging Studies of Polycystic Kidney Disease (CRISP) favors MRI-based correlation of kidney and cyst volume measurements that can be used as indicators of disease progression or treatment response. Accurate RBF estimations can be obtained on MR imaging when disease progression parallels the increase in kidney volume and declining GFR. Although there is no increased risk of RCC in ADPKD, MRI remains the preferred method of assessing a solid mass amid multiple cysts.

ACQUIRED CYSTIC DISEASE OF DIALYSIS

Acquired cystic disease of dialysis occurs in patients on maintenance dialysis. Over time, the atrophic kidneys develop multiple small cortical, typically exophytic, cysts. These cysts are at increased risk of hemorrhage and development of RCC.

IMAGING FEATURES

The kidneys appear small and echogenic on US and may demonstrate multiple cysts. US may also be used to screen for potential complications of intracyst hemorrhage and evolution of RCC in asymptomatic patients. Unenhanced CT can detect cyst hemorrhage and kidney or ureteric stones. Multiphase pre- and postcontrast-enhanced CT is required for comprehensive evaluation of cystic kidneys and for the evaluation of possible RCC. MR is well suited for evaluating cystic disease of dialysis (Fig. 6.6A and B). Differentiation between nonenhancing hemorrhagic cysts (bright on precontrast T1W

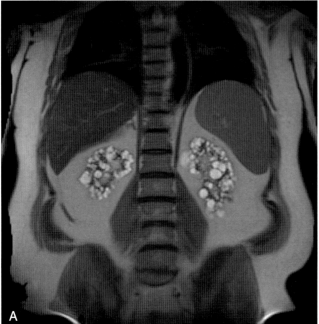
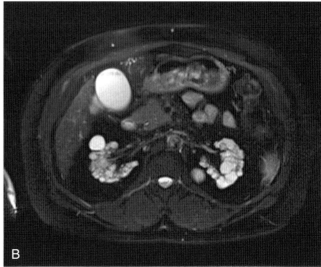

Fig. 6.6 Acquired cystic disease of dialysis. Coronal (A) and fat-saturated axial (B) ssT2W images. Multiple cysts less than 2 cm in diameter are present in both kidneys located predominantly in the kidney cortex. Background kidneys show atrophic parenchymal change.

images) and vascularized renal cell cancer can safely and easily be achieved after administration of a stable and/or high-relaxivity GBCA.

SOLID KIDNEY MASSES

ANGIOMYOLIPOMA

AML is a benign kidney tumor composed of variable amounts of smooth muscle, blood vessels, and mature adipocytes. Diagnosis is usually based on detection of fat. Eighty percent of AMLs are isolated and sporadic, whereas 20% occur in patients with tuberous sclerosis and are often bilateral and multiple. Larger AMLs present the risk of hemorrhage.

IMAGING FEATURES

On US, AML appears as a solid echogenic mass with echodensity comparable to the renal sinuses. CT can identify AML based on an attenuation value of −10 or less HU, predicting the presence of fat. Being vascular lesions, AML may enhance and must be differentiated from RCC by the presence and distribution of fat. This can be depicted on ssT2W sequences and pre- and postcontrast fat-saturated T1W GRE MR images, where areas of signal dropout represent focal macroscopic fat in the lesion, confirming the diagnosis of AML (Fig. 6.7A–C).

RENAL CELL CARCINOMA

Improved imaging of kidney masses by US, CT, and MRI has led to a smaller average size of neoplasm at time of initial detection. Currently, approximately 30% of all RCCs are incidentally identified on imaging studies performed for other reasons.

IMAGING FEATURES

US can delineate kidney masses larger than 25 mm. Sensitivity of US decreases to about 25% for smaller lesions. US is limited in differentiating between benign and malignant solid kidney masses. Extension of RCC into renal vein and inferior vena cava can be evaluated on duplex Doppler imaging. CT can characterize kidney masses larger than 10 mm, and the nephrographic phase of dynamic contrast-enhanced CT is most sensitive for detecting tumors that appear as heterogeneous enhancing solid mass with or without cystic/necrotic changes. Vascular extension and potential metastases can be assessed for treatment planning. The superior soft tissue detail and multiphase and multiplanar capabilities of MRI aid in sensitive detection and staging of RCC (Fig. 6.8A–D), although multiphase CT exposes patients to higher radiation risk. Pre- and postcontrast T1W 3D-GRE images can distinguish cystic and hypovascular RCC from other benign kidney lesions, even when less than 2 cm. Subtraction imaging may further increase sensitivity in hemorrhagic or proteinaceous cystic masses. MRI also helps assess treatment response in patients receiving focal targeted therapy (see Fig. 6.8A–D).

NEPHROLITHIASIS AND OBSTRUCTIVE UROPATHY

Acute flank pain is a frequent clinical presentation in the emergency department (ED). Nearly 22% of all CT examinations performed for the evaluation of acute abdominal pain in the ED are for clinical suspicion of urolithiasis.

IMAGING FEATURES

Plain radiograph KUB (kidney, ureter, and bladder) and IVU are no longer the preferred methods of diagnosis of

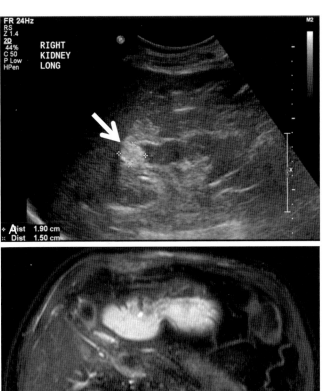

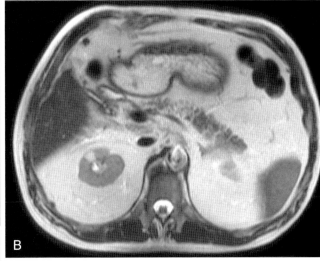

Fig. 6.7 Angiomyolipoma predominantly containing fat. (A) Longitudinal sonogram shows highly echogenic well-marginated kidney mass *(arrow)*. The lesion is high signal intensity on ssT2W images (B) and low signal intensity on fat-suppressed images (C).

kidney stone disease. US is a rapid, safe, and readily available tool for evaluation of renal colic. Although US has limited sensitivity for small kidney stones and ureteric stones, obstructive hydronephrosis can easily be detected. US is useful in young patients, pregnant women, and those requiring multiple follow-up examinations. Unenhanced CT is the most sensitive (95% to 98%) and specific (96% to 98%) test for urolithiasis (Fig. 6.9A–C). Identification of the number, size, and location of calculi and diagnosis of hydronephrosis can be routinely made. The role of MRI is still evolving in the evaluation of acute abdominal pain in the emergency setting. Calcium fails to generate MR signal, thereby limiting the sensitivity of MRI to detect kidney stones; however, MRI can detect perirenal fluid as an indicator of acute kidney obstruction and other abdominal pathologies.

KIDNEY INFECTION

Pyelonephritis and kidney abscess usually result from an ascending infection in the urinary tract. In uncomplicated cases, routine radiologic imaging is not usually required for diagnosis or treatment.

IMAGING FEATURES FOR ACUTE PYELONEPHRITIS

US is not sensitive for diagnosis of acute pyelonephritis, although changes in echogenicity due to edema (hypoechoic), hemorrhage (hyperechoic), and hypoperfusion (visible with duplex Doppler) can sometimes be seen in the kidney parenchyma with associated hydronephrosis (Fig. 6.10A–C). Kidney scintigraphy using radiolabeled white blood cells or gallium can be used to locate kidney infection, because photopenic areas of focal or global reduced uptake are seen with tubular radiotracer agent (Tc DMSA). Infected kidneys show a alternating bands of enhancement (striated nephrogram) and perinephric inflammatory changes in Gerota's fascia on contrast-enhanced CT or MRI (see Fig. 6.10A–C).

IMAGING FEATURES FOR KIDNEY ABSCESS

Kidney abscess on US appears as a hypoechoic mass with through transmission that lacks internal flow on duplex Doppler images, differentiating it from solid masses. A hypoattenuating area with peripheral enhancement is seen on contrast-enhanced CT. Extraparenchymal collections can be identified on either CT or MRI. Mixed signal on T1 and T2W MR images is seen with increased peripheral

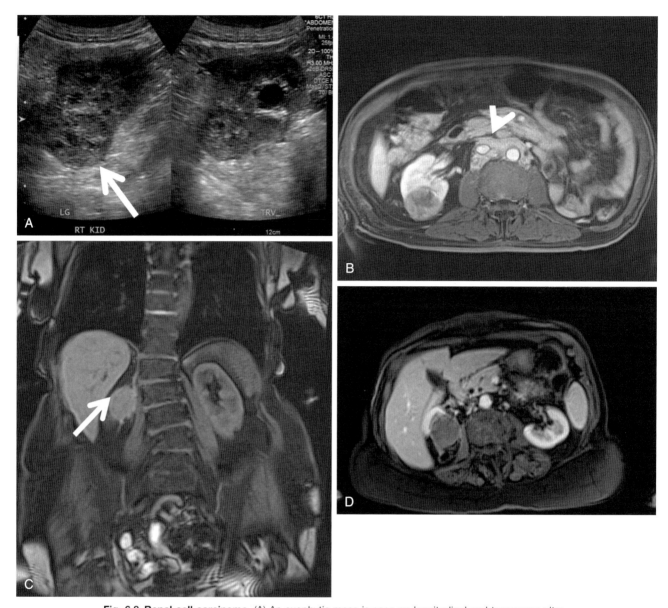

Fig. 6.8 Renal cell carcinoma. (A) An exophytic mass is seen on longitudinal and transverse ultra-sonogram *(arrow)*. (B) Avidly enhancing solid right kidney tumor is shown on early phase T1W fat-suppressed gadolinium-enhanced gradient echo sequence (GRE) image in keeping with renal cell carcinoma–clear cell type. There is metastatic confluent retroperitoneal lymphadenopathy *(arrowhead)*. (C) After image-guided microwave ablation of the tumor (in a different patient with clear cell renal cell carcinoma) increased signal on precontrast coronal T1W fat-suppressed GRE image is seen suggestive of posttherapy hemorrhagic change *(arrow)*. Note the lesion does not show any internal enhancement or viable tissue on axial T1W fat-suppressed gadolinium-enhanced GRE image (D), indicating complete response to local treatment.

inflammatory edema. Postgadolinium T1W images show a nonenhancing central core with perinephric enhancement (see Fig. 6.10A–C).

RENAL ARTERY STENOSIS

Renovascular hypertension is a leading cause of potentially correctable secondary hypertension, and early diagnosis of renal artery stenosis (RAS) may be important for treatment. Renal vascular disease likely is responsible for 1% to 5% of cases of hypertension. At least two-thirds of these cases are caused by atherosclerosis, whereas fibromuscular dysplasia

accounts for most of the remaining cases. Although catheter angiography is the reference standard test for RAS, CT and MR angiography are noninvasive alternative tools that have comparable diagnostic performance using the latest generation technologies.

IMAGING FEATURES

Duplex Doppler is a moderately accurate, cost-effective, operator-dependent technique for initial evaluation of RAS. Peak systolic velocity greater than 100 to 200 cm/sec is considered indicative of RAS. Angiotensin-converting enzyme (ACE) inhibitor scintigraphy may be used to demonstrate impaired

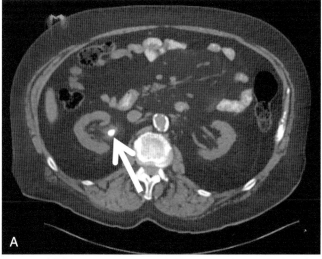

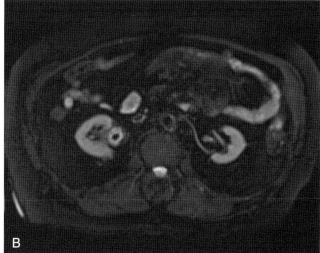

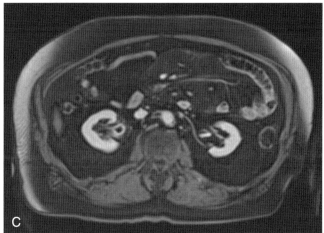

Fig. 6.9 Nephrolithiasis. (A) Unenhanced axial CT image shows right nephrolithiasis with mild urothelial thickening *(arrow)*. Fat-saturated axial (B) ssT2W and delayed phase T1W fat-suppressed gadolinium-enhanced gradient echo sequence (GRE) image (C) shows a signal void in the renal pelvis representing the stone. Note, there is high signal of urine surrounding the nephrolith on the ssT2W fluid-sensitive image (B). Excretion of contrast in both kidney collecting systems is present on the delayed phase T1W fat-suppressed gadolinium-enhanced GRE image; the hyperintense signal of the gadolinium aids identification of the stone.

kidney function in patients with renovascular hypertension; important information regarding kidney size, perfusion, and excretory capacity can be obtained from scintigraphic images and computer-generated time-activity curves. Two major agents have been used: technetium-DTPA, a filtered agent; or MAG-3, a tubular excreted agent. Using these techniques, RAS can be diagnosed based on two criteria: (1) asymmetry of kidney size and function and (2) specific captopril-induced changes in the renogram. However, overall sensitivity and specificity of scintigraphy for RAS-induced renovascular hypertension has been questioned.

CT angiography (CTA) is an excellent examination for obtaining information about the arterial anatomy and for evaluation of stenosis. High spatial resolution CTA is now routinely combined with sophisticated image postprocessing software that can produce 3D volume renderings to provide images that are interpreted more easily. Advancement in MR technology now offers detailed evaluation of vascular anatomy. Additionally, MRI techniques have been developed to provide kidney functional assessment including measures of perfused kidney parenchymal volume, blood flow, and GFR. Renal artery imaging has been routinely obtained using GBCA-enhanced MR angiography. Newer methods using flow-sensitive balanced fast-field echo technique are providing alternatives to GBCA. For detection of greater than 50% narrowing of the renal artery, most studies have shown excellent correlation between conventional angiography and MR angiography (sensitivity >95% and specificity >90%). Earlier reports have indicated that limitations of MR angiography include overestimation of moderate stenosis, but the latest generation MR technologies are significantly improving the capacity to generate higher quality images reliably. Catheter angiography remains the reference standard, but this is an invasive test that requires direct administration of concentrated iodinated contrast into the kidneys, which has been associated with significant acute and long-term kidney dysfunction in at-risk patients.

INTERVENTION

Therapeutic procedures are fundamentally based on techniques including balloon angioplasty and stent placement. Unfortunately, both short-term and long-term results have not been found to correlate with the degree of stenosis, whether unilateral or bilateral. The ability to predict good long-term response to renal angioplasty and stenting remains an active area of investigation.

KIDNEY PARENCHYMAL DISEASE AND KIDNEY TRANSPLANTATION

DIFFUSE KIDNEY PARENCHYMAL DISEASE

Diffuse kidney parenchymal diseases are common medical conditions. A variety of disease processes may involve the parenchyma and be classified into the following broad

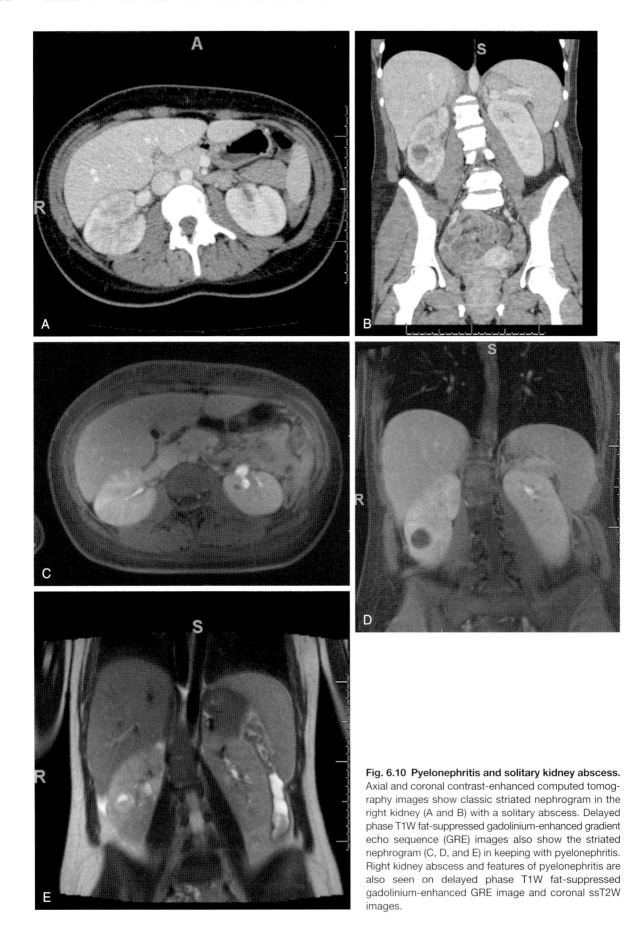

Fig. 6.10 Pyelonephritis and solitary kidney abscess. Axial and coronal contrast-enhanced computed tomography images show classic striated nephrogram in the right kidney (A and B) with a solitary abscess. Delayed phase T1W fat-suppressed gadolinium-enhanced gradient echo sequence (GRE) images also show the striated nephrogram (C, D, and E) in keeping with pyelonephritis. Right kidney abscess and features of pyelonephritis are also seen on delayed phase T1W fat-suppressed gadolinium-enhanced GRE image and coronal ssT2W images.

categories: glomerular disease, acute and chronic tubulointerstitial disease, diabetic nephropathy and nephrosclerosis, other forms of microvascular disease, ischemic nephropathy caused by disease of the main renal arteries, obstructive nephropathy, and infectious kidney disease. Radiologic techniques have limited specificity in the diagnosis of various types of diffuse kidney parenchymal diseases because imaging features are overlapping in these pathologies. Nevertheless, there remains a growing clinical need for accurate, reproducible, and noninvasive measures of kidney function.

IMAGING FEATURES

Obstructive and nonobstructive causes of kidney failure may be differentiated using US as the initial imaging test. Kidney size and parenchymal thickness are useful parameters to assess chronicity. Enlarged kidneys usually indicate an acute parenchymal process, but they can be seen with chronic infiltrative kidney disease, diabetic nephropathy, and HIV-associated nephropathy. Contracted, small kidneys suggest a chronic disease (see Figs. 6.1 and 6.2). Increased kidney cortical echogenicity may be useful in suggesting the presence of kidney parenchymal disease. Kidney failure poses restriction to the use of nephrotoxic iodinated contrast, and noncontrast CT fails to provide additional diagnostic information. Scintigraphic techniques have been the mainstay of kidney function measurements for assessment of GFR. These methods require timed blood sampling and have been shown to have decreased precision with diminished GFR, especially when lower than 30 mL/min. MRI with MRNU can confirm the findings of US in cases of diminished corticomedullary differentiation and can offer detailed anatomic information regarding the kidney parenchyma and collecting system. It also provides quantitative measures of kidney function that may be applied to each kidney.

KIDNEY TRANSPLANTATION

Kidney transplantation has emerged as the treatment of choice for ESKD patients, on average providing improved quality of life and lower healthcare costs compared with dialysis. Given the importance of kidney transplantation and the limitation of available donor kidneys, detailed analysis of factors that affect transplant survival is critical (Fig. 6.11A–E).

IMAGING FEATURES

US is the principal imaging test used in perioperative patients for assessment of complications including perinephric fluid collections, hematomas, and urinoma. In addition, Doppler duplex US is used to evaluate renal vein thrombosis and to measure the renal artery resistive index [RI = (peak systolic velocity − end diastolic velocity)/peak systolic velocity]. An elevated RI (>0.80) in the main renal artery and its branches has been considered predictive of transplant failure. Changes in the renal vascular compliance result in increased in vascular resistance. Elevated RI can also be seen in other causes of transplant dysfunction including acute tubular necrosis (ATN), rejection, and immunosuppression toxicity and graft vascular complications.

Ultrasound lacks ionizing radiation and may be used safely for follow-up longitudinal studies. US is also frequently used for image-guided biopsy of the transplant kidney.

Preoperative CTA of potential donors can depict variant arterial and venous anatomy, vascular disorders, and other unexpected abnormalities. Ionizing radiation remains a limitation in both the donor and recipient, and the added risk of CIN may preclude the use of iodinated contrast in CT imaging in some kidney transplant recipients. Noncontrast CT imaging is limited in its ability to evaluate pelvic soft tissues, the transplanted kidney and collecting system, and the renal vasculature.

Impaired transplant function on radionucleotide study is attributed to either obstruction of urine outflow or to other causes. No additional information can be obtained on nuclear medicine examinations to delineate among the causes of kidney failure.

MAGNETIC RESONANCE NEPHROUROGRAPHY

MRI benefits from excellent soft-tissue details even in the absence of gadolinium, and avoids radiation. It may be used for preoperative imaging evaluation for both potential kidney donors and recipients. Comprehensive pretransplant evaluation of the kidney donor can be performed with assessment of kidney parenchymal, arterial, venous, and ureteric anatomy and measurement of differential kidney function.

In posttransplant recipient evaluation, comprehensive structural and functional analysis can be performed.

- *Anatomic imaging:* T2W HASTE sequences and T2W-like TFISP images offer morphologic details of the collecting system based on the bright signal of urine, allowing identification of causes of obstruction such as stenosis, extrinsic compression, or anastomotic fibrosis of the transplant ureter.
- *Functional imaging:* Postoperative hematomas and proteinaceous debris or hemorrhage in the collecting system can be identified as high signal on precontrast T1W images. Gadolinium perfusion technique can be used to extract kidney functional volume, RBF, and GFR. Dynamic postcontrast 3D GRE T1W images can assist in accurately delineating postoperative complications and causes of transplant failure.

This modality can be useful in the evaluation of a number of posttransplant conditions, including:

1. *Vascular disorders:*
   a. Renal artery thrombosis or stenosis: Narrowing or abrupt cutoff in the main renal artery or its branch is seen in the angiographic phase. Segmental lack of perfusion in a renal artery territory can be depicted by functional imaging.
   b. Renal vein thrombosis: T2W images demonstrate thrombus as loss of patent dark vascular lumen.
2. *Intrinsic kidney disorders:*
   a. ATN: Normal cortical enhancement with markedly delayed medullary perfusion and excretion is shown, similar to the scintigraphic appearance of ATN.
   b. Hyperacute and accelerated acute rejection: Intrinsic graft dysfunction with ischemic microvascular injury manifests as striated nephrogram.
   c. Acute rejection: Blood oxygen level–dependent (BOLD) MRI can detect changes in hemoglobin oxygenation

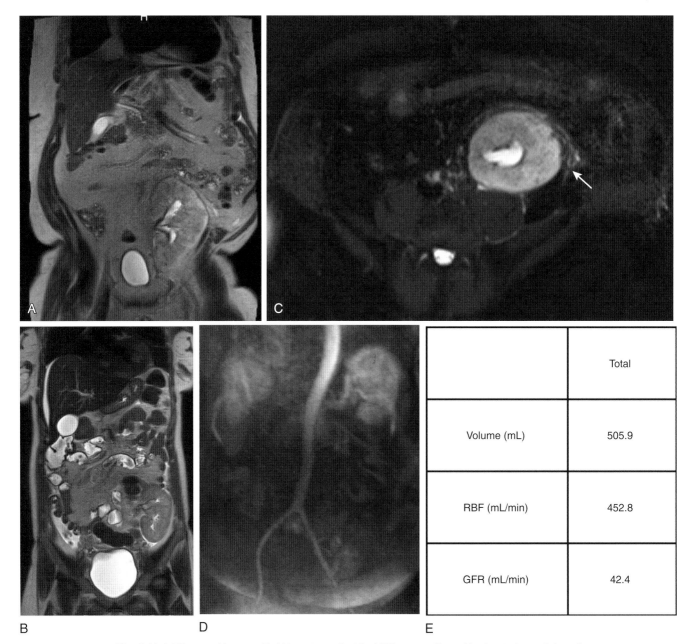

Fig. 6.11 A 53-year-old man with kidney transplant in 1995, presenting with elevated creatinine of uncertain etiology. Magnetic resonance imaging (MRI) demonstrated markedly abnormal signal in the transplant kidney parenchyma on coronal T2W images (A). Compare this appearance with the T2 signal and corticomedullary differentiation of a normal transplant kidney (B). The abnormal graft kidney demonstrated surrounding edema on axial T2W fat-saturated images (C, *arrow*), and dynamic postcontrast functional imaging (D) demonstrated overall reduced perfusion of the transplant kidney. The transplant vasculature was patent, and the overall MRI features maintained an intrinsic etiology for graft dysfunction. The transplant edema and reduction in perfusion is a pattern that has been seen in acute rejection. Quantitative functional analysis (E) showed marked decreased function of the transplant kidney, and subsequent graft biopsy confirmed acute cellular rejection. *GFR*, Glomerular filtration rate; *RBF*, renal blood flow.

and thus assesses kidney tissue oxygenation. It can help differentiate ATN from acute rejection.

d. Chronic rejection: Loss of kidney corticomedullary differentiation on T2 and T1W images is seen. This is a nonspecific finding that depicts impaired kidney function.

SUMMARY

Medical imaging plays a critical role in the diagnosis and management of kidney disease, and this role is continuing to evolve with new advances in diagnostic techniques. US provides a valuable first-line tool for the evaluation of most localized kidney pathologies, including the detection of solid masses, characterization of cystic masses, detection of hydronephrosis, and diagnosis of kidney calculi. CT provides the greatest sensitivity for calcifications within the kidney or urinary tract, including kidney calculi. CT has been used to detect and characterize kidney masses, but cystic lesions require more challenging multiphase contrast-enhanced methodology combined with quantitative density measurements. MRI has developed technically, and currently provides an alternative to ultrasound and CT for better detection and characterization of solid and cystic masses. In addition, MRI techniques are developing to provide qualitative and quantitative assessment of diffuse parenchymal disease and measures of kidney function, including RBF, parenchymal perfusion, and glomerular filtration. Both CT and MRI use contrast agents with potential toxic effects in the setting of impaired kidney function, although these risks can be managed. An understanding of iodinated and gadolinium-chelate-based contrast agents is imperative. Overall, excessive use of CT is increasingly raised as a safety concern because of radiation exposure risks. US and MRI provide alternatives with high levels of safety.

KEY BIBLIOGRAPHY

Craig W, Wagner B, Travis M. Pyelonephritis: radiologic-pathologic review. *Radiographics*. 2008;28:255-276.

Escobar GA, Campbell DN, et al. Randomized trials in angioplasty and stenting of the renal artery: tabular review of the literature and critical analysis of their results. *Ann Vasc Surg*. 2012;26:434-442.

Hartman D, Choyke P, Hartman M. A practical approach to the cystic renal mass. *Radiographics*. 2004;24:S101-S115.

Heinz-Peer G, Schoder M, Rand T, et al. Prevalence of acquired cystic kidney disease and tumors in native kidneys of renal transplant recipients: a prospective US study. *Radiology*. 1995;195:667-671.

Kalb B, Sharma P, Salman K. Acute abdominal Pain—is there a potential role for MRI in the setting of the Emergency Department in a patient with renal calculi? *J Magn Reson Imaging*. 2010;32:1012-1023.

Kalb B, Vatow J, Salman K. Magnetic resonance nephrourography: current and developing techniques. *Radiol Clin North Am*. 2008;46:11-24.

Martin DR. Nephrogenic system fibrosis: a radiologist's practical perspective. *Eur J Radiol*. 2008;66:220-224.

Martin DR, Brown M, Semelka R. *Primer on MR Imaging of the Abdomen and Pelvis*. 1st ed. New York: John Wiley & Sons; 2005.

Martin DR, Kalb B, Salman K, et al. Kidney transplantation: structural and functional evaluation using MR nephro-urography. *J Magn Reson Imaging*. 2008;28:805-822.

Martin DR, Krishnamoorthy S, Kalb B, et al. Decreased incidence of NSF in patients on dialysis after changing gadolinium contrast-enhanced MRI protocols. *J Magn Reson Imaging*. 2010;31:440-446.

Martin DR, Semelka R, Chapman A, et al. Nephrogenic systemic fibrosis versus contrast-induced nephropathy: risks and benefits of contrast-enhanced MR and CT in renally impaired patients. *J Magn Reson Imaging*. 2009;30:1350-1356.

Martin DR, Sharma P, Salman K. Individual kidney blood flow measured by contrast enhanced magnetic resonance first-pass perfusion imaging. *Radiology*. 2008;246:241-248.

Michaely H, Schoenberg S, Oesingmann N. Renal artery stenosis—functional assessment with dynamic MR perfusion measurements—feasibilty study. *Radiology*. 2006;238:586-596.

Mousa AY, Campbell JE, Stone PA. Short- and long-term outcomes of percutaneous transluminal angioplasty/stenting of renal fibromuscular dysplasia over a ten-year period. *J Vasc Surg*. 2012;55:421-427.

Prando A, Prando D, Prando P. Renal cell carcinoma: unusual imaging manifestations. *Radiographics*. 2006;26:233-244.

Radermacher J, Mengel M, Ellis S, et al. The renal arterial resistance index and renal allograft survival. *N Engl J Med*. 2003;349:115-124.

Semelka RC, Shoenut JP, Magro CM, et al. Renal cancer staging: comparison of contrast-enhanced CT and gadolinium-enhanced fat-suppressed spin-echo and gradient-echo MR imaging. *J Magn Reson Imaging*. 1993;3:597-602.

Silva A, Morse B, Hara Robert B, et al. Dual-energy (spectral) CT: applications in abdominal imaging. *Radiographics*. 2011;31:1031-1046.

Soulez G, Pasowicz M, Benea G, et al. Renal artery stenosis evaluation: diagnostic performance of gadobenate dimeglumine–enhanced MR angiography—comparison with DSA. *Radiology*. 2008;247:273-285.

Tublin M, Bude R, Platt JF. The resistive index in renal Doppler sonography: where do we stand? *AJR Am J Roentgenol*. 2003;180:885-892.

Full bibliography can be found on www.expertconsult.com.

ACID-BASE AND ELECTROLYTES

7

Hyponatremia and Hypoosmolar Disorders

Joseph G. Verbalis

The incidence of hyponatremia depends on the patient population screened and the criteria used to define the disorder. Hospital incidences of 15% to 22% are common if hyponatremia is defined as any serum sodium concentration ($[Na^+]$) of less than 135 mmol/L, but in most studies only 1% to 4% of patients have a serum $[Na^+]$ lower than 130 mmol/L, and fewer than 1% have a value lower than 120 mmol/L. Multiple studies have confirmed prevalence ranging from 7% in ambulatory populations up to 38% in acutely hospitalized patients. Older individuals are particularly susceptible to hyponatremia, with reported incidence as high as 53% among institutionalized geriatric patients. Although most cases are mild, hyponatremia is important clinically because (1) acute severe hyponatremia can cause substantial morbidity and mortality; (2) mild hyponatremia can progress to more dangerous levels during management of other disorders; (3) general mortality is higher in hyponatremic patients across a wide range of underlying co-morbidities; and (4) overly rapid correction of chronic hyponatremia can produce severe neurologic complications and death.

DEFINITIONS

Hyponatremia is of clinical significance only when it reflects corresponding plasma hypoosmolality. Plasma osmolality (P_{osm}) can be measured directly by osmometry and is expressed as milliosmoles per kilogram of water (mOsm/kg H_2O). P_{osm} can also be calculated from the serum $[Na^+]$, measured in millimoles per liter (mmol/L), and the glucose and blood urea nitrogen (BUN) levels, both expressed as milligrams per deciliter (mg/dL), as follows:

$$P_{osm} = 2 \times Serum\,[Na^+] + Glucose/18 + BUN/2.8$$

Because the glucose and BUN concentrations are normally dwarfed by the sodium concentration, osmolality can be estimated simply by doubling the serum $[Na^+]$. All three methods produce comparable results under most conditions. However, total osmolality is not always equivalent to *effective osmolality*, which is sometimes referred to as the *tonicity* of the plasma. Solutes that are predominantly compartmentalized in the extracellular fluid (ECF) are effective solutes because they create osmotic gradients across cell membranes and lead to osmotic movement of water from the intracellular fluid (ICF) compartment to the ECF compartment. In contrast, solutes that permeate cell membranes (e.g., urea,

ethanol, methanol) are not effective solutes, because they do not create osmotic gradients across cell membranes, and therefore they are not associated with secondary water shifts. Only the concentration of effective solutes in plasma should be used to determine whether clinically significant hypoosmolality is present. In most cases, these effective solutes include sodium, its associated anions, and glucose (but only in the presence of insulin deficiency, which allows the development of an ECF/ICF glucose gradient); importantly, urea, a solute that penetrates cells, is not an effective solute.

Hyponatremia and hypoosmolality are usually synonymous, with two important exceptions. First, *pseudohyponatremia* can be produced by marked elevation of serum lipids or proteins. In such cases, the concentration of Na^+ per liter of serum water is unchanged, but the concentration of Na^+ per liter of serum is artifactually decreased because of the increased relative proportion occupied by lipid or protein. Although measurement of serum or plasma $[Na^+]$ by ion-specific electrodes, currently used by most clinical laboratories, is less influenced by high concentrations of lipids or proteins than is measurement of serum $[Na^+]$ by flame photometry, such errors nonetheless can still occur when serum samples are diluted before measurement in autoanalyzers. However, because direct measurement of P_{osm} is based on the colligative properties of only the solute particles in solution, increased lipids or proteins will not affect the measured P_{osm}. Second, high concentrations of effective solutes other than Na^+ can cause relative decreases in serum $[Na^+]$ despite an unchanged P_{osm}; this commonly occurs with marked hyperglycemia. Misdiagnosis can be avoided again by direct measurement of P_{osm} or by correcting the serum $[Na^+]$ by 1.6 mmol/L for each 100 mg/dL increase in blood glucose concentration greater than 100 mg/dL (although some studies have suggested that 2.4 mmol/L may be a more accurate correction factor, especially when the glucose is very high).

PATHOGENESIS

The presence of significant hypoosmolality indicates an excess of water relative to solute in the ECF. Because water moves freely between the ICF and ECF, this also indicates an excess of total body water relative to total body solute. Imbalances between water and solute can be generated initially either by *depletion* of body solute more than body water or by *dilution* of body solute because of increases in body water out of proportion to body solute (Box 7.1). However, this distinction represents an oversimplification, because most hypoosmolar states include variable contributions of both solute depletion and water retention. For example, isotonic solute losses occurring during an acute hemorrhage do not produce hypoosmolality until the subsequent retention of water from ingested or infused hypotonic fluids causes a secondary dilution of the remaining ECF solute. Nonetheless, this concept has proved useful because it provides a logical framework for understanding the diagnosis and treatment of hypoosmolar disorders.

DIFFERENTIAL DIAGNOSIS

The diagnostic approach to hypoosmolar disorders should include a careful history (especially concerning medications and diet); physical examination with emphasis on clinical assessment of ECF volume status, including measurement of orthostatic vital signs, and a thorough neurologic evaluation; measurement of serum or plasma electrolytes, glucose, BUN, creatinine, and uric acid; calculated and/or directly measured P_{osm}; and determination of simultaneous urine sodium and osmolality. Although the prevalence varies according to the population being studied, a sequential analysis of hyponatremic patients who were admitted to a large university teaching hospital showed that approximately 20% were hypovolemic, 20% had edema-forming states, 33% were euvolemic, 15% had hyperglycemia-induced hyponatremia, and 10% had kidney failure. Consequently, euvolemic hyponatremia generally constitutes the largest single group of hyponatremic patients found in this setting. A definitive diagnosis is not always possible at the time of presentation, but an initial categorization based on the patient's clinical ECF volume status allows selection of appropriate initial therapy in most cases (Fig. 7.1).

DECREASED EXTRACELLULAR FLUID VOLUME (HYPOVOLEMIA)

Clinically detectable hypovolemia, determined most sensitively by careful measurement of orthostatic changes in blood pressure and pulse rate, usually indicates some degree of solute depletion. Elevations of the BUN and uric acid concentrations are useful laboratory correlates of decreased ECF volume. Even isotonic or hypotonic volume losses can lead to hypoosmolality if water or hypotonic fluids are ingested or infused as replacement. A low urine sodium concentration (U_{Na}) in such cases suggests a nonrenal cause of solute depletion, whereas a high U_{Na} suggests renal causes of solute depletion (see Box 7.1). Diuretic use is the most common cause of hypovolemic hypoosmolality, and thiazides are much more commonly associated with severe hyponatremia than loop diuretics.

Although diuretics represent a prime example of solute depletion, the pathophysiologic mechanisms underlying diuretic-associated hypoosmolality are complex and have multiple components, including sodium depletion with secondary stimulation of arginine vasopressin (AVP) secretion, and impaired diluting ability of the inner medullary collecting duct, both leading to significant degrees of free water retention. Many patients do not manifest clinical evidence of marked hypovolemia, in part because ingested water has been retained in response to nonosmotically stimulated secretion of AVP, as is generally true for all disorders of solute depletion. To complicate diagnosis further, the U_{Na} may be high or low depending on when the last diuretic dose was

---

Box 7.1   Pathogenesis of Hypoosmolar Disorders

Depletion (Primary Decreases in Total Body Solute + Secondary Water Retention)[a]

Renal Solute Loss

Diuretic use
Solute diuresis (glucose, mannitol)
Salt-wasting nephropathy
Mineralocorticoid deficiency

Nonrenal Solute Loss

Gastrointestinal (diarrhea, vomiting, pancreatitis, bowel obstruction)
Cutaneous (sweating, burns)
Blood loss

Dilution (Primary Increases in Total Body Water ± Secondary Solute Depletion)[b]

Impaired Renal Free Water Excretion

Increased proximal reabsorption
    Hypothyroidism
Impaired distal dilution
    SIADH
    Glucocorticoid deficiency
Combined increased proximal reabsorption and impaired distal dilution
    Congestive heart failure
    Cirrhosis
    Nephrotic syndrome
Decreased urinary solute excretion
    Beer potomania
    Low protein/solute diet

Excess Water Intake

Primary polydipsia
Dilute infant formula
Fresh water drowning

[a]Virtually all disorders of solute depletion are accompanied by some degree of secondary retention of water by the kidneys in response to the resulting intravascular hypovolemia; this mechanism can lead to hypoosmolality, even when the solute depletion occurs via hypotonic or isotonic body fluid losses.
[b]Disorders of water retention primarily cause hypoosmolality in the absence of any solute losses, but in some cases of SIADH, secondary solute losses occur in response to the resulting intravascular hypervolemia and can further aggravate the hypoosmolality. (However, this pathophysiology probably does not contribute to the hyponatremia of edema-forming states such as congestive heart failure and cirrhosis, because in these cases, multiple factors favoring sodium retention result in an increased total body sodium load.)
SIADH, Syndrome of inappropriate antidiuretic hormone secretion.
Modified from Verbalis JG. The syndrome of inappropriate antidiuretic hormone secretion and other hypoosmolar disorders. In: Coffman TM, Falk RJ, Molitoris BA, Neilson EG, Schrier RW, eds. *Diseases of the Kidney and Urinary Tract.* 9th ed. Philadelphia: Lippincott Williams and Wilkins; 2013:2012–2054.

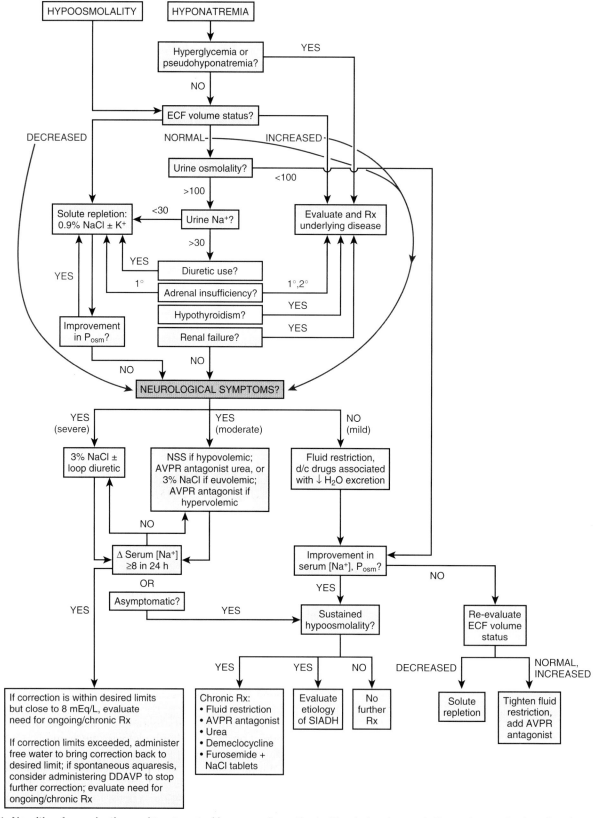

Fig. 7.1 Algorithm for evaluation and treatment of hypoosmolar patients. The dark red arrow in the center emphasizes that the presence of central nervous system dysfunction resulting from hyponatremia should always be assessed immediately, so that appropriate therapy can be started as soon as possible in significantly symptomatic patients, even while the outlined diagnostic evaluation is proceeding. Values for osmolality are in mOsm/kg H_2O, and those referring to serum Na^+ concentration are in mmol/L. Δ, Change (in concentration); *1°*, Primary; *2°*, secondary; *AVPR*, arginine vasopressin receptor; *d/c*, discontinue; *DDAVP*, desmopressin; *ECF*, extracellular fluid volume; P_{osm}, plasma osmolality; *Rx*, treatment; *SIADH*, syndrome of inappropriate antidiuretic hormone secretion. (Modified from Verbalis JG. The syndrome of inappropriate antidiuretic hormone secretion and other hypoosmolar disorders. In: Coffman TM, Falk RJ, Molitoris BA, Neilson EG, Schrier RW, eds. *Diseases of the Kidney and Urinary Tract.* 9th ed. Philadelphia: Lippincott Williams and Wilkins; 2013:2012–2054.)

taken. Consequently, any suspicion of diuretic use mandates careful consideration of this diagnosis. A low serum $[K^+]$ is an important clue to diuretic use, because few other disorders that cause hyponatremia and hypoosmolality also produce appreciable hypokalemia. Whenever the possibility of diuretic use is suspected in the absence of a positive history, a urine screen for diuretics should be performed.

Most other causes of renal or nonrenal solute losses resulting in hypovolemic hypoosmolality will be clinically apparent, although some cases of salt-wasting nephropathies (e.g., chronic interstitial nephropathy, polycystic kidney disease, obstructive uropathy, Bartter syndrome) or mineralocorticoid deficiency (e.g., Addison's disease) can be challenging to diagnose during the early phases of the disease.

NORMAL EXTRACELLULAR FLUID VOLUME (EUVOLEMIA)

Virtually any disorder associated with hypoosmolality can manifest with an ECF volume status that appears normal by standard methods of clinical evaluation. Because clinical assessment of ECF volume status is not very sensitive, normal or low levels of serum BUN and uric acid are helpful laboratory correlates of relatively normal ECF volume.

Conversely, a low U_{Na} suggests a depletional hypoosmolality secondary to ECF losses with subsequent volume replacement by water or other hypotonic fluids; as discussed earlier, such patients may appear euvolemic by all the usual clinical parameters used to assess ECF volume status. Primary dilutional disorders are less likely in the presence of a low U_{Na} (<30 mmol/L), although this pattern can occur in hypothyroidism as well.

A high U_{Na} (≥30 mmol/L) generally suggests a dilutional hypoosmolality such as the *syndrome of inappropriate antidiuretic hormone secretion* (SIADH; see Box 7.1). SIADH is the most common cause of euvolemic hypoosmolality in clinical practice. The criteria necessary for a diagnosis of SIADH remain essentially unchanged since defined by Bartter and Schwartz in 1967 (Box 7.2), but several points deserve emphasis. First, true hypoosmolality must be present, and hyponatremia secondary to pseudohyponatremia or hyperglycemia must be excluded. Second, the urinary osmolality (U_{osm}) must be inappropriate for the low P_{osm}. This does not require that the U_{osm} be greater than P_{osm} but merely that the urine not be maximally dilute (i.e., U_{osm} should not exceed 100 mOsm/kg H_2O in adults, although this may be somewhat higher in older adults). U_{osm} need not be inappropriately elevated at all levels of P_{osm} but simply at some level of P_{osm} less than 275 mOsm/kg H_2O. This is evident in patients with a reset osmostat who suppress AVP secretion at some level of P_{osm}, resulting in maximal urinary dilution and free water excretion at plasma osmolalities falling below this level. Although some consider a reset osmostat to be a separate disorder rather than a variant of SIADH, such cases nonetheless illustrate that some hypoosmolar patients can exhibit an appropriately dilute urine at some, although not all, plasma osmolalities. Third, clinical euvolemia must be present to diagnose SIADH, and this diagnosis cannot be made in a hypovolemic or significantly edematous patient. Importantly, this does not mean that patients with SIADH cannot become hypovolemic for other reasons, but in such cases it is impossible to diagnose the underlying SIADH until the patient is

---

Box 7.2 Criteria for the Diagnosis of Syndrome of Inappropriate Antidiuretic Hormone Secretion

Essential Criteria

1. Decreased effective osmolality of the ECF (P_{osm} less than 275 mOsm/kg H_2O)
2. Inappropriate urinary concentration (U_{osm} greater than 100 mOsm/kg H_2O with normal kidney function) at some level of plasma hypoosmolality
3. Clinical euvolemia, as defined by the absence of signs of hypovolemia (orthostasis, tachycardia, decreased skin turgor, dry mucous membranes) or hypervolemia (subcutaneous edema, ascites)
4. Elevated urinary sodium excretion despite a normal salt and water intake
5. Normal thyroid, adrenal, and kidney function

Supplemental Criteria

1. Abnormal water load test (inability to excrete at least 80% of a 20-mL/kg water load in 4 h and/or failure to dilute U_{osm} to less than 100 mOsm/kg H_2O)
2. Plasma vasopressin (AVP) level inappropriately elevated relative to plasma osmolality
3. No significant correction of serum sodium concentration ($[Na^+]$) with volume expansion but improvement after fluid restriction

AVP, Arginine vasopressin; *ECF,* extracellular fluid; P_{osm}, plasma osmolality; U_{osm}, urinary osmolality.
Modified from Verbalis JG. The syndrome of inappropriate antidiuretic hormone secretion and other hypoosmolar disorders. In: Coffman TM, Falk RJ, Molitoris BA, Neilson EG, Schrier RW, eds. *Diseases of the Kidney and Urinary Tract.* 9th ed. Philadelphia: Lippincott Williams and Wilkins; 2013:2012–2054.

---

rendered euvolemic. The fourth criterion, renal salt wasting, has probably caused the most confusion regarding SIADH. The importance of this criterion lies in its usefulness in differentiating hypoosmolality caused by a decreased effective intravascular volume (in which case renal Na^+ conservation occurs) from dilutional disorders in which urinary Na^+ excretion is normal or increased because of ECF volume expansion. However, U_{Na} can also be high in renal causes of solute depletion, such as diuretic use or Addison's disease, and, conversely, patients with SIADH can have a low urinary Na^+ excretion if they subsequently become hypovolemic or solute depleted, conditions sometimes produced by imposed salt and water restriction. Consequently, although high urinary Na^+ excretion is generally the rule in patients with SIADH, its presence does not necessarily confirm this diagnosis, nor does its absence exclude it. The final criterion emphasizes that SIADH remains a diagnosis of exclusion, and the absence of other potential causes of hypoosmolality must always be verified. Glucocorticoid deficiency and SIADH can be especially difficult to distinguish, because either primary or secondary hypocortisolism can cause elevated plasma AVP levels and, in addition, can have direct renal effects to prevent maximal urinary dilution. Therefore no patient with chronic hyponatremia should be diagnosed as having SIADH without a thorough evaluation of adrenal function, preferably via a rapid adrenocorticotropin (ACTH) stimulation test; acute

Box 7.3   Common Causes of Syndrome of Inappropriate Antidiuretic Hormone Secretion

Tumors

Pulmonary/mediastinal (bronchogenic carcinoma, mesothelioma, thymoma)
Nonchest (duodenal carcinoma, pancreatic carcinoma, ureteral/prostate carcinoma, uterine carcinoma, nasopharyngeal carcinoma, leukemia)

Central Nervous System Disorders

Mass lesions (tumors, brain abscesses, subdural hematoma)
Inflammatory diseases (encephalitis, meningitis, systemic lupus, acute intermittent porphyria, multiple sclerosis)
Degenerative/demyelinative diseases (Guillain-Barré, spinal cord lesions)
Miscellaneous (subarachnoid hemorrhage, head trauma, acute psychosis, delirium tremens, pituitary stalk section, transsphenoidal adenomectomy, hydrocephalus)

Drugs

Stimulated AVP release (nicotine, phenothiazines, tricyclic antidepressants)
Direct renal effects and/or potentiation of AVP antidiuretic effects (desmopressin, oxytocin, prostaglandin synthesis inhibitors)
Mixed or uncertain actions (ACE inhibitors, carbamazepine and oxcarbazepine, chlorpropamide, clofibrate, clozapine, cyclophosphamide, 3,4-methylenedioxy-methamphetamine ["Ecstasy"], omeprazole, serotonin reuptake inhibitors, vincristine)

Pulmonary Diseases

Infections (tuberculosis, acute bacterial or viral pneumonia, aspergillosis, empyema)
Mechanical/ventilatory (acute respiratory failure, COPD, positive-pressure ventilation)

Other

HIV and AIDS
Prolonged strenuous exercise (marathon, triathlon, ultramarathon, hot-weather hiking)
Postoperative state
Senile atrophy
Idiopathic

ACE, Angiotensin-converting enzyme; *AIDS,* acquired immunodeficiency syndrome; *AVP,* arginine vasopressin; *COPD,* chronic obstructive pulmonary disease.
Modified from Verbalis JG. The syndrome of inappropriate antidiuretic hormone secretion and other hypoosmolar disorders. In: Coffman TM, Falk RJ, Molitoris BA, Neilson EG, Schrier RW, eds. *Diseases of the Kidney and Urinary Tract.* 9th ed. Philadelphia: Lippincott Williams and Wilkins; 2013:2012–2054.

hyponatremia of obvious origin, such as that occurring postoperatively or in association with pneumonitis, may be treated without adrenal testing as long as there are no other clinical signs or symptoms suggestive of adrenal dysfunction. Many different disorders have been associated with SIADH, and these can be divided into several major etiologic groups (Box 7.3).

Some cases of euvolemic hyponatremia do not fit particularly well into either a dilutional or a depletional category. Chief among these is the hyponatremia that occurs in patients who ingest large volumes of beer with little food intake for prolonged periods, called *beer potomania.* Even though the volume of fluid ingested may not seem sufficiently excessive to overwhelm renal diluting mechanisms, in these cases free water excretion is limited by very low urinary solute excretion, resulting in water retention and dilutional hyponatremia. However, because such patients have very low sodium intakes as well, it is likely that relative depletion of body Na^+ stores also contributes to the hypoosmolality in some cases. A similar pathophysiology can occur in patients on vegetarian diets with insufficient protein and sodium intake.

INCREASED EXTRACELLULAR FLUID VOLUME (HYPERVOLEMIA)

The presence of hypervolemia, as detected clinically by the presence of significant edema and/or ascites, indicates whole-body sodium excess, and hypoosmolality in these patients suggests a relatively decreased effective intravascular volume or pressure leading to water retention as a result of both elevated plasma AVP levels and decreased distal delivery of glomerular filtrate. Such patients usually have a low U_{Na} because of secondary hyperaldosteronism, but under certain conditions the U_{Na} may be elevated (e.g., glucosuria in diabetics, diuretic therapy). Hyponatremia generally does not occur until fairly advanced stages of diseases such as congestive heart failure, cirrhosis, and nephrotic syndrome, so the diagnosis is usually not difficult. Kidney failure can also cause retention of both sodium and water, but in this case, the factor limiting excretion of excess body fluid is not decreased effective circulating volume but rather decreased glomerular filtration.

It should be remembered that even though many edema-forming states have secondary increases in plasma AVP levels as a result of decreased effective arterial blood volume, they are nonetheless not classified as SIADH because they fail to meet the criterion of clinical euvolemia (see Box 7.2). Although it can be argued that this distinction is semantic, this criterion remains important because it allows segregation of identifiable etiologies of hyponatremia that are associated with different methods of evaluation and therapy.

Several situations can cause hyponatremia because of acute water loading in excess of renal excretory capacity. Primary polydipsia can cause hypoosmolality in a small subset of patients with some degree of underlying SIADH, particularly psychiatric patients with long-standing schizophrenia who are taking neuroleptic drugs or, rarely, patients with normal kidney function in whom the volumes ingested exceed the maximum renal free water excretory rate of approximately 500 to 1000 mL/h.

Endurance exercising, such as marathon or ultramarathon racing, has been associated with sometimes fatal hyponatremia, primarily as a result of ingestion of excessive amounts of hypotonic fluids during the exercise that exceed the water excretory capacity of the kidney. This is called *exercise-associated hyponatremia* (EAH). Many athletes with EAH have met diagnostic criteria for SIADH immediately following prolonged exercise, which serves to decrease further their free water excretory capacity both during and following exercise. Although the stimuli for AVP secretion during endurance excise have not been fully elucidated, potential candidates include baroreceptor activation, nausea, cytokine release from muscle rhabdomyolysis, and exercise itself. Most cases of EAH are associated with weight gain, reflecting the excess water retention, but patients are usually classified as clinically euvolemic, because water retention alone without sodium excess, as observed in these patients, does not generally produce clinical manifestations of hypervolemia such as edema or ascites. Rarely cases of EAH may present as hypovolemic with hypotension and tachycardia as a result of underreplaced sweat sodium losses.

CLINICAL MANIFESTATIONS OF HYPONATREMIA

Hypoosmolality is associated with a broad spectrum of neurologic manifestations, ranging from mild, nonspecific symptoms (e.g., headache, nausea) to more significant deficits (e.g., disorientation, confusion, obtundation, focal neurologic deficits, seizures). In the most severe cases, death can result from respiratory arrest after tentorial herniation with subsequent brainstem compression. This neurologic symptom complex, termed *hyponatremic encephalopathy,* primarily reflects brain edema resulting from osmotic water shifts into the brain caused by the decreased effective P_{osm}. Significant symptoms generally do not occur until the serum $[Na^+]$ falls to less than 125 mmol/L, and the severity of symptoms can be roughly correlated with the degree of hypoosmolality. However, individual variability is marked, and the level of serum $[Na^+]$ at which symptoms will appear cannot be accurately predicted for any individual patient.

Furthermore, several factors other than the severity of hypoosmolality also affect the degree of neurologic dysfunction. Most important is the rate at which hypoosmolality develops. Rapid development of severe hypoosmolality is frequently associated with marked neurologic symptoms, whereas gradual development over several days or weeks is often associated with relatively mild symptomatology despite achievement of an equivalent degree of hypoosmolality. This occurs because the brain can counteract osmotic swelling by secreting intracellular solutes, both electrolytes and organic osmolytes, via a process called *brain volume regulation.* Because this is a time-dependent process, rapid development of hypoosmolality can result in brain edema before adaptation can occur; with slower development of hypoosmolality, brain cells can lose solute sufficiently quickly to prevent the development of brain edema and subsequent neurologic dysfunction.

Underlying neurologic disease also can significantly affect the level of hypoosmolality at which central nervous system symptoms appear. For example, moderate hypoosmolality is usually not of major concern in an otherwise healthy patient, but it can precipitate seizure activity in a patient with underlying epilepsy. Nonneurologic metabolic disorders (e.g., hypoxia, hypercapnia, acidosis, hypercalcemia) similarly can also affect the level of P_{osm} at which central nervous system symptoms occur. Recent studies have suggested that some patients may be susceptible to a vicious cycle in which hypoosmolality-induced brain edema causes noncardiogenic pulmonary edema, and the resulting hypoxia and hypercapnia then further impair the ability of the brain to volume regulate, leading to more brain edema, neurologic deterioration, and death in some

cases. Other clinical studies suggest that menstruating women and young children may be particularly susceptible to the development of neurologic morbidity and mortality during hyponatremia, especially in the acute postoperative setting. The true clinical incidence and underlying pathophysiologic mechanisms responsible for these sometimes catastrophic outcomes remain to be determined.

Finally, the issue of whether mild to moderate hyponatremia is truly "asymptomatic" has been challenged by recent studies showing subtle defects in cognition and gait stability in hyponatremic patients that appear to be reversed by correction of the disorder. The functional significance of the gait instability was illustrated in a study of Belgian patients with hyponatremia who were judged to be "asymptomatic" at the time of presentation to an emergency department (ED). These patients demonstrated a markedly increased incidence of falls, despite being apparently "asymptomatic." The clinical significance of the gait instability and fall data has been further evaluated by multiple independent studies that have shown increased bone fractures in hyponatremic subjects. More recently published studies have shown that hyponatremia is associated with increased bone loss in experimental animals, and a significant increase in odds ratio for osteoporosis and fractures in humans. Thus the major clinical significance of chronic hyponatremia may lie in the increased morbidity and mortality associated with falls and fractures in older populations.

TREATMENT

Although various authors have published recommendations for the treatment of hyponatremia, no standardized treatment algorithms are universally accepted, with many having significant differences of opinion regarding best practices. There is a dearth of evidence-based data on which to base true guidelines, and most of the literature reflects expert opinions. A synthesis of several expert recommendations for treatment of hyponatremia is illustrated in Fig. 7.1. This algorithm is based primarily on the neurologic symptomatology of hyponatremic patients rather than the serum $[Na^+]$ or on the chronicity of the hyponatremia, which is often difficult to ascertain.

If any degree of clinical hypovolemia is present, the patient should be considered to have a solute depletion-induced hypoosmolality and should be treated with isotonic (0.9%) NaCl at a rate appropriate for the estimated volume depletion. If diuretic use is known or suspected, fluid therapy should be supplemented with potassium (30 to 40 mmol/L), even if the serum $[K^+]$ is not low because of the propensity of such patients to have total body potassium depletion. Patients with diuretic-induced hyponatremia usually respond well to isotonic NaCl and do not require 3% NaCl unless they exhibit severe neurologic symptoms. However, such patients often have an electrolyte-free water diuresis after their ECF volume deficit has been corrected, because normalization of the ECF volume removes the hypovolemic stimulus to AVP secretion, resulting in a more rapid correction of the serum $[Na^+]$ than that predicted from the rate of saline infusion.

Most often, the hypoosmolar patient is clinically euvolemic, but several situations dictate a reconsideration of potential solute depletion, even in the patient without clinically apparent hypovolemia. These include low U_{Na} (<20 to 30 mmol/L), any history of recent diuretic use, and any suggestion of primary adrenal insufficiency. Whenever a reasonable likelihood of depletion, rather than dilution, hypoosmolality exists, it is appropriate to treat initially with isotonic NaCl. If the patient has SIADH, no significant harm will have been done with a limited (1 to 2 L) saline infusion, because such patients will excrete excess NaCl without markedly changing their P_{osm}. However, this therapy should be abandoned if the serum [Na⁺] does not improve because longer periods of continued isotonic NaCl infusion can worsen hyponatremia by virtue of cumulative water retention.

Treatment of euvolemic hypoosmolality varies depending on the presentation. If all criteria for SIADH are met, except that the U_{osm} is low, the patient should simply be observed, because this presentation may represent spontaneous reversal of a transient form of SIADH. If there is any suspicion of either primary or secondary adrenal insufficiency, glucocorticoid replacement should be started immediately after completion of a rapid ACTH stimulation test. Prompt water diuresis after initiation of glucocorticoid treatment strongly supports glucocorticoid deficiency, but the absence of a quick response does not exclude this diagnosis, because several days of glucocorticoid therapy may be necessary for normalization of P_{osm}.

Hypervolemic hypoosmolality is usually treated initially with diuretics and other measures directed at the underlying disorder. Such patients rarely require any therapy to increase P_{osm} acutely but often benefit from varying degrees of sodium and water restriction to reduce body fluid retention. However, worsened hyponatremia as a result of aggressive loop diuretic therapy in combination with continued or increased fluid intake and/or ineffectiveness of fluid restriction sometimes necessitates additional treatment of the hyponatremia, particularly via vasopressin receptor antagonists (vaptans), because saline administration can worsen fluid retention.

RATE OF CORRECTION

In any case of significant hyponatremia, one is challenged by how quickly the P_{osm} should be corrected. Although hyponatremia is associated with a broad spectrum of neurologic symptoms, sometimes leading to death in severe cases, too rapid correction of severe hyponatremia can produce the osmotic demyelination syndrome (ODS), a brain demyelinating disease that also can cause substantial neurologic morbidity and mortality. Clinical and experimental results suggest that optimal treatment of hyponatremia must entail balancing the risks of hyponatremia against the risks of correction for each patient. Several factors should be considered: the severity of the hyponatremia, the duration of the hyponatremia, and the patient's symptom burden. Neither sequela from hyponatremia itself nor ODS after therapy is very likely in a patient whose serum [Na⁺] is greater than 125 mmol/L, although in some cases significant symptoms can develop even with serum [Na⁺] greater than 125 mmol/L if the rate of fall of serum [Na⁺] has been rapid. The importance of the duration and symptom burden of hyponatremia relates to how well the brain has volume regulated in response to the hyponatremia, and, consequently, to the degree of risk for demyelination with rapid correction. Cases of acute

hyponatremia (arbitrarily defined as hyponatremia of less than 48-hour duration) are usually symptomatic if the hyponatremia is severe (i.e., <125 mmol/L). These patients are at greatest risk from neurologic complications caused by the hyponatremia itself, and the serum [Na⁺] should be corrected to higher levels promptly, most often with the use of 3% NaCl unless the patient is undergoing a spontaneous aquaresis, in which case the correction will occur without intervention. Conversely, patients with more chronic hyponatremia (greater than 48-hour duration) who have mild to moderate neurologic symptoms are at little immediate risk from complications of hyponatremia itself but can develop demyelination after overly rapid correction. There is no indication to correct the serum [Na⁺] in these patients rapidly, and slower acting therapies, such as fluid restriction or vaptans, which correct serum [Na⁺] over 24 to 48 hours, should be used rather than 3% NaCl.

Although these extreme situations have clear treatment indications, most patients have hyponatremia of indeterminate duration and varying degrees of neurologic impairment. This group presents the most challenging treatment decision because the hyponatremia has been present sufficiently long to allow some degree of brain volume regulation but not long enough to prevent an element of brain edema and neurologic symptoms. Most authors recommend prompt treatment for such patients because of their symptoms but with methods that allow a controlled and limited correction of their hyponatremia. Reasonable correction parameters consist of a rate of correction of serum [Na⁺] in the range of 0.5 to 2 mmol/L per hour, as long as the total magnitude of correction does not exceed 12 mmol/L during the first 24 hours and 18 mmol/L throughout the first 48 hours of correction. However, maximum correction rates should be even lower (no more than 8 mmol/L in 24 hours) if certain risk factors for the development of ODS are present, including alcoholism, liver disease, malnutrition, hypokalemia, and a very low serum [Na⁺] (≤105 mmol/L). Treatments for individual patients should be chosen within these limits, depending on their symptoms. For patients who are only moderately symptomatic, one should proceed at the lower recommended limit of 0.5 mmol/L per hour; in those who manifest more severe neurologic symptoms, initial correction at a rate of 1 to 2 mmol/L per hour is appropriate.

HYPERTONIC SALINE

Controlled corrections of hyponatremia can be accomplished with hypertonic (3%) NaCl solution administered via continuous infusion, because patients with euvolemic hypoosmolality (e.g., SIADH) usually will not respond to isotonic NaCl. An initial infusion rate can be estimated by multiplying the patient's body weight (in kilograms) by the desired rate of increase in serum [Na⁺] in mmol per liter per hour. For example, in a 70-kg patient, increasing serum [Na⁺] by approximately 1 mmol/L per hour will require an infusion of 3% NaCl at 70 mL/h, whereas increasing serum [Na⁺] by approximately 0.5 mmol/L per hour is achieved by infusing 35 mL/h. Furosemide (20 to 40 mg IV) can be used to treat volume overload occurring as a result of 3% NaCl, in some cases anticipatorily, in patients at risk of volume overload as a result of sodium administration.

VAPTANS

Alternatively, vaptans can be used to increase the serum [Na$^+$] by stimulating renal free water excretion, or *aquaresis*, thereby leading to increased serum [Na$^+$] in the majority of patients with hyponatremia resulting from SIADH, congestive heart failure, or cirrhosis. Although the optimal use of AVP receptor antagonists in any setting has not yet been fully determined, the US Food and Drug Administration (FDA) has now approved conivaptan and tolvaptan for the treatment of euvolemic and hypervolemic hyponatremia, and the European Medicines Agency (EMA) has approved tolvaptan for the treatment of SIADH.

Conivaptan is FDA approved for euvolemic and hypervolemic hyponatremia in hospitalized patients. It is available only as an intravenous preparation and is administered as a 20-mg loading dose over 30 minutes, followed by a continuous infusion of 20 or 40 mg/day. In general the 20-mg continuous infusion is used for the first 24 hours to gauge the initial response. If the correction of serum [Na$^+$] is felt to be inadequate (e.g., <5 mmol/L), then the infusion rate can be increased to 40 mg/day. Therapy is limited to a maximum duration of 4 days because of drug interactions with other agents metabolized by the CYP3A4 hepatic isoenzyme. Importantly, for conivaptan and all other vaptans, it is critical that the serum [Na$^+$] concentration is measured frequently during the active phase of correction of the hyponatremia (a minimum of every 6 to 8 hours but more frequently in patients with risk factors for development of ODS). If the correction approaches 12 mmol/L in the first 24 hours, the infusion should be stopped and the patient monitored on a fluid restriction. If the correction exceeds 12 mmol/L, consideration should be given to administering sufficient water, either orally or as intravenous D$_5$W, to bring the overall correction below 12 mmol/L. The maximum correction limit should be reduced to 8 mmol/L during the first 24 hours in patients with risk factors for the development of osmotic demyelination, as described previously. The most common adverse effects include injection-site reactions, which are generally mild and usually do not lead to treatment discontinuation, headache, thirst, and hypokalemia.

Tolvaptan, an oral AVP receptor antagonist, is FDA approved for treatment of dilutional hyponatremias and EMA approved for treatment of SIADH. In contrast to conivaptan, oral administration allows it to be used for both short-term and long-term treatment of hyponatremia. Similar to conivaptan, tolvaptan treatment must be initiated in the hospital so that the rate of correction can be monitored carefully. Patients with a serum [Na$^+$] less than 125 mmol/L are eligible for therapy with tolvaptan as primary therapy; if the serum [Na$^+$] is ≥125 mmol/L, tolvaptan therapy is only indicated if the patient has symptoms that could be attributable to the hyponatremia and the patient is resistant to attempts at fluid restriction. The starting dose of tolvaptan is 15 mg on the first day, and the dose can be titrated to 30 and 60 mg at 24-hour intervals if the serum [Na$^+$] remains less than 135 mmol/L or the increase in serum [Na$^+$] has been <5 mmol/L in the previous 24 hours. As with conivaptan, it is essential that the serum [Na$^+$] concentration be measured frequently during the active phase of correction of the hyponatremia (a minimum of every 6 to 8 hours but more frequently in patients with

risk factors for development of osmotic demyelination). Limits for safe correction of hyponatremia and methods to compensate for overly rapid corrections are the same as described previously for conivaptan. One additional factor that helps to avoid overly rapid correction with tolvaptan is the recommendation that fluid restriction not be used during the active phase of correction, thereby allowing the patient's thirst to compensate for an overly vigorous aquaresis. Side effects include dry mouth, thirst, increased urinary frequency, dizziness, and nausea.

Because inducing increased renal fluid excretion via either a diuresis or an aquaresis can cause or worsen hypotension in patients with hypovolemic hyponatremia, vaptans are contraindicated in this patient population. Clinically significant hypotension was not observed in either the conivaptan or tolvaptan clinical trials in euvolemic and hypervolemic hyponatremic patients, although orthostatic hypotension as a result of the aquaresis has been reported. Although vaptans are not contraindicated with decreased kidney function, these agents generally will not be effective if the serum creatinine is greater than 2.5 mg/dL. Tolvaptan is contraindicated in patients with cirrhosis or liver failure because of some cases of reversible hepatotoxicity using this drug at high doses in clinical trials of polycystic kidney disease.

CLINICAL TARGETS OF ACUTE TREATMENT

Regardless of the method or initial rate of correction chosen, acute treatment should be interrupted after any of three endpoints is reached: (1) the patient's symptoms are abolished, (2) a safe serum [Na$^+$] (typically, 125 mmol/L) has been reached, or (3) a total magnitude of correction of 12 to 18 mmol/L has been achieved. It follows from these recommendations that serum [Na$^+$] levels must be carefully monitored at frequent intervals during the active phases of treatment (every 2 to 4 hours for 3% NaCl administration; every 6 to 8 hours for vaptan administration) to adjust therapy so that the correction stays within accepted guidelines. It cannot be emphasized too strongly that it is necessary to correct the P$_{osm}$ acutely only to a safe range rather than to normal levels. As a practical point, after an acute correction has reached 8 mmol, the need for continued acute therapy should be carefully assessed, because ongoing correction may result in an overcorrection by the time the next serum [Na$^+$] is available (see Fig. 7.1). In some situations, patients may spontaneously correct their hyponatremia via a water diuresis. If the hyponatremia is acute (e.g., psychogenic polydipsia with water intoxication), such patients do not appear at risk for ODS. However, if the hyponatremia has been chronic (e.g., hypocortisolism, diuretic therapy), intervention should be considered to limit the rate and magnitude of correction of serum [Na$^+$], such as administration of desmopressin 1 to 2 µg IV or infusion of hypotonic fluids to match urine output, using the same therapeutic endpoints as for active corrections.

MAINTENANCE HYPONATREMIA TREATMENT

Some patients will benefit from continued treatment of hyponatremia following discharge from the hospital. One important exception is those patients with the reset osmostat syndrome; because the hyponatremia of such patients is not progressive but rather fluctuates around their reset level of serum [Na$^+$], no therapy is generally required. For most other cases of mild to moderate SIADH, fluid restriction represents the least toxic therapy and is the treatment of choice. It should usually be tried as the initial therapy, with pharmacologic intervention reserved for refractory cases in which the degree of fluid restriction required to avoid hypoosmolality is so severe that the patient is unable, or unwilling, to maintain it. In general, the higher the urine solute concentration, as reflected by either U$_{osm}$ or the sum of urine Na$^+$ and K$^+$, the less likely it is that fluid restriction will be successful because of lower renal electrolyte-free water excretion.

If pharmacologic treatment is necessary, the choices include urea, furosemide in combination with NaCl tablets, demeclocycline, and the vasopressin receptor antagonists. Although each of these treatments can be effective in individual circumstances, the only drugs currently approved by the FDA and EMA for treatment of hyponatremia are the vasopressin receptor antagonists. For patients who have responded to either conivaptan or tolvaptan in the hospital, consideration should be given to continuing tolvaptan as an outpatient after discharge. In patients with established chronic hyponatremia, tolvaptan has been shown to be effective at maintaining a normal [Na$^+$] for as long as 4 years on continued daily therapy. However, many patients with hospitalized hyponatremia have a transient form of SIADH without the need for long-term therapy. In the conivaptan open-label study, approximately 70% of patients treated as an inpatient for 4 days had normal serum [Na$^+$] concentrations 7 and 30 days after cessation of the vaptan therapy in the absence of chronic therapy for hyponatremia.

Deciding which patients with hospitalized hyponatremia are candidates for long-term therapy should be based on the etiology of the SIADH, because patients with some causes of SIADH are more likely to experience persistent hyponatremia that may benefit from long-term treatment with tolvaptan following discharge. Nonetheless, for any individual patient this simply represents an estimate of the likelihood of requiring long-term therapy. In all cases, consideration should be given to a trial of stopping the drug at 2 to 4 weeks following discharge to see if hyponatremia recurs. Seven days is a reasonable period of tolvaptan cessation to evaluate the presence of continued SIADH, because this period was sufficient to demonstrate recurrence of hyponatremia in the tolvaptan SALT clinical trials. Serum [Na$^+$] should be monitored every 2 to 3 days following cessation of tolvaptan so that the drug can be resumed as quickly as possible in those patients with recurrent hyponatremia, since the longer the patient is hyponatremic, the greater the risk of subsequent osmotic demyelination with overly rapid correction of the low serum [Na$^+$].

Guidelines for the appropriate treatment of hyponatremia, and particularly the role of vaptans relative to other treatments such as oral urea, are still evolving. Of special interest will be studies to assess whether more effective treatment of hyponatremia can reduce the incidence of falls and fractures in older patients, the use of health care resources for both inpatients and outpatients with hyponatremia, and the markedly increased morbidity and mortality of patients with hyponatremia associated with multiple disease states. Consequently, the indications for treatment of water-retaining disorders in patients without symptomatic hyponatremia must await further studies specifically designed to assess the effects of treatment of hyponatremic patients on clinically relevant outcomes, as well as clinical experience that better delineates efficacies and potential toxicities of all treatments for hyponatremia.

KEY BIBLIOGRAPHY

Adrogué HJ, Madias NE. Diagnosis and treatment of hyponatremia. *Am J Kidney Dis.* 2014;64:681-684.

Berl T. Vasopressin antagonists. *N Engl J Med.* 2015;372:2207-2216.

Berl T, Quittnat-Pelletier F, Verbalis JG, et al. Oral tolvaptan is safe and effective in chronic hyponatremia. *J Am Soc Nephrol.* 2010;21:705-712.

Corona G, Giuliani C, Parenti G, et al. Moderate hyponatremia is associated with increased risk of mortality: evidence from a meta-analysis. *PLoS ONE.* 2013;8:e80451.

Ellison DH, Berl T. Clinical practice. The syndrome of inappropriate antidiuresis. *N Engl J Med.* 2007;356:2064-2072.

Fenske W, Stork S, Koschker AC, et al. Value of fractional uric acid excretion in differential diagnosis of hyponatremic patients on diuretics. *J Clin Endocrinol Metab.* 2008;93:2991-2997.

Greenberg A, Verbalis JG, Amin AN, et al. Current treatment practice and outcomes. Report of the hyponatremia registry. *Kidney Int.* 2015;88:167-177.

Hoorn EJ, Rivadeneira F, van Meurs JB, et al. Mild hyponatremia as a risk factor for fractures: the Rotterdam Study. *J Bone Miner Res.* 2011;26:1822-1828.

Kovesdy CP, Lott EH, Lu JL, et al. Hyponatremia, hypernatremia, and mortality in patients with chronic kidney disease with and without congestive heart failure. *Circulation.* 2012;125:677-684.

Renneboog B, Musch W, Vandemergel X, et al. Mild chronic hyponatremia is associated with falls, unsteadiness, and attention deficits. *Am J Med.* 2006;119:71-78.

Rosner MH, Kirven J. Exercise-associated hyponatremia. *Clin J Am Soc Nephrol.* 2007;2:151-161.

Schrier RW, Gross P, Gheorghiade M, et al. Tolvaptan, a selective oral vasopressin V2-receptor antagonist, for hyponatremia. *N Engl J Med.* 2006;355:2099-2112.

Spasovski G, Vanholder R, Allolio B, et al. Clinical practice guideline on diagnosis and treatment of hyponatraemia. *Nephrol Dial Transplant.* 2014;29(suppl 2):1-139.

Sterns RH. Disorders of plasma sodium. *N Engl J Med.* 2015;372:1267-1269.

Usala RL, Fernandez SJ, Mete M, et al. Hyponatremia is associated with increased osteoporosis and bone fractures in a large U.S. health system population. *J Clin Endocrinol Metab.* 2015;100:3021-3031.

Verbalis JG. Brain volume regulation in response to changes in osmolality. *Neuroscience.* 2010;168:862-870.

Verbalis JG, Barsony J, Sugimura Y, et al. Hyponatremia-induced osteoporosis. *J Bone Miner Res.* 2010;25:554-563.

Verbalis JG, Goldsmith SR, Greenberg A, et al. Diagnosis, evaluation, and treatment of hyponatremia: expert panel recommendations. *Am J Med.* 2013;126(10 suppl 1):S1-S42.

Verbalis JG, Grossman A, Hoybye C, et al. Review and analysis of differing regulatory indications and expert panel guidelines for the treatment of hyponatremia. *Curr Med Res Opin.* 2014;30:1201-1207.

Wald R, Jaber BL, Price LL, et al. Impact of hospital-associated hyponatremia on selected outcomes. *Arch Intern Med.* 2010;170:294-302.

Full bibliography can be found on www.expertconsult.com.

Hypernatremia 8

John M. Carson; Stuart L. Linas

The serum sodium concentration ([Na$^+$]) is the ratio of sodium to water in the extracellular fluid (ECF) compartment. It is determined by the relationship among total body sodium, potassium, and water, the latter of which typically is the main determinant. Dysnatremias, or derangements in serum [Na$^+$], include both hyponatremia and hypernatremia. This chapter focuses on the etiology and management of hypernatremia, a hyperosmolar state defined by serum [Na$^+$] exceeding 145 mEq/L.

Hypernatremia itself is not a disorder but rather a laboratory abnormality caused by an underlying pathologic process. The diagnostic approach to hypernatremia must consider the determinants of the serum [Na$^+$]. Although excesses in total body sodium and, very rarely, excesses in total body potassium can lead to hypernatremia, the majority of cases result from deficits in total body water (TBW).

To simplify the management of hypernatremia, this chapter considers the balance of TBW and sodium separately. This important concept will be illustrated by dividing the water and sodium components of the ECF compartment into separate theoretical beakers (Fig. 8.1). The goal is to determine appropriate, timely therapies for a disorder that is associated with a high degree of morbidity and mortality.

DEFINITIONS

Normal serum [Na$^+$] is 135 to 145 mEq/L. This range is generally maintained despite large individual variations in salt and water intake. Hypernatremia is *always* a water problem and sometimes also a salt problem. There is no predictable relationship between serum [Na$^+$] (a measure of osmolality and tonicity) and total body salt or volume status. More specifically, although hypernatremia confirms the presence of a relative water deficit, the isolated laboratory finding of a serum [Na$^+$] greater than 145 mEq/L does not reveal anything about a person's volume status. As a result, hypernatremia may occur in the setting of hypovolemia, euvolemia, or hypervolemia, as indicated in Fig. 8.1.

DEHYDRATION AND VOLUME DEPLETION

Comparing the terms "dehydration" and "volume depletion" illustrates the distinction between water and sodium balance. Although *dehydration* is commonly used to describe a person's volume status, this use is inaccurate. Dehydration does not equal volume depletion. Rather, *dehydration* is a description of water balance, whereas *volume depletion* refers to a person's sodium balance. Although these two clinical scenarios may coexist, they should not be confused. It is important that

the two terms are not used interchangeably and that a patient's water and sodium balance be considered independently when addressing dysnatremias clinically.

HYPEROSMOLALITY AND HYPERTONICITY

Hypernatremia always reflects a hyperosmolar state, whereas the reverse is not always true. For example, hyperosmolality may also be a consequence of severe hyperglycemia or elevated blood urea nitrogen, as is seen in kidney failure. Furthermore, hyperosmolality does not necessarily mean hypertonicity. For example, uremia is a hyperosmolar but not a hypertonic state. Urea is an ineffective osmole because it can freely cross cell membranes, unlike sodium; therefore urea contributes to osmolality but not to tonicity. In contrast to urea, sodium, which is unable to cross cell membranes freely, is an effective osmole and is the primary cation that affects plasma osmolality (P$_{osm}$). Hypernatremia is a hypertonic state in which water will flow from the intracellular to the extracellular space, resulting in cellular dehydration and shrinkage.

BACKGROUND

Hypernatremia is all about water. A more accurate term for hypernatremia might be "hypoaquaremia" because it literally means a state in which there is too little water in the intravascular space and therefore too little water in the intracellular space. To begin any discussion of hypernatremia (or hyponatremia), it is important to understand that dysnatremias are actually disorders of water homeostasis.

Water distributes throughout all body compartments, with two-thirds in the intracellular and one-third in the extracellular compartment. Three-quarters of the water in the extracellular compartment is located in the interstitial space, and one-quarter is in the intravascular space. Water is lost (or gained) in the same proportions as it is distributed throughout all body compartments. Pure water loss does not affect plasma volume status or hemodynamics significantly until very late because of the normal distribution of water throughout all body compartments. For example, for every 1 L of water deficit, only approximately 80 mL is lost from the intravascular (plasma) compartment.

EPIDEMIOLOGY

The incidence of hypernatremia in all hospitalized patients ranges from less than 1% to approximately 3%. However, in critically ill patients, the overall prevalence of hypernatremia

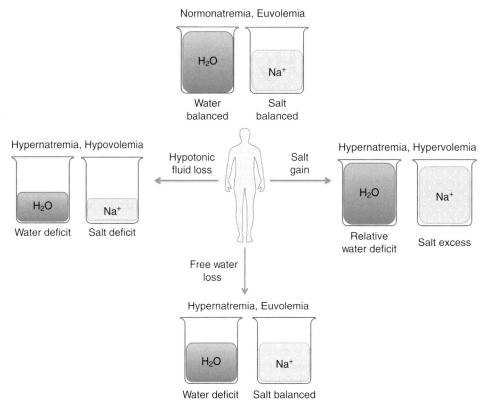

Fig. 8.1 Diagnostic approach to hypernatremia. The pathophysiology of hypernatremia is best understood by separating water and salt balance, done so here by theoretical beakers. Water balance determines the serum sodium, whereas salt balance determines volume status. The beakers at the top of the figure represent normal physiology with water and salt in balance. In the three remaining cases of hypernatremia there is a water deficit with varying degrees of salt balance or volume status. Refer to Table 8.1 for further details regarding the specific causes of hypernatremia for each group of salt balance.

ranges between 9% and 26% and is hospital acquired in approximately 80% of these cases. Hypernatremia present at the time of hospital admission is primarily a disease of older adults and of those with mental illness or impaired sensorium. Most patients with hypernatremia on admission to the hospital have concomitant infections. Hypernatremia that is present on hospital admission is generally treated earlier than hypernatremia that develops during the hospital course, most likely because of increased attention paid to individual laboratory values and volume status on hospital admission.

In contrast, hospital-acquired hypernatremia is typically seen in patients who are younger than those with hypernatremia on admission, with an age distribution similar to that of the general hospitalized population. Hospital-acquired hypernatremia is largely iatrogenic from inadequate and/or inappropriate fluid prescription and therefore is largely preventable. It results from a combination of decreased access to water, disease processes that may increase insensible losses or interfere with the thirst mechanism, and administration of loop diuretics. Approximately half of patients with hospital-acquired hypernatremia are intubated and therefore have no free access to water. Of the remaining 50%, most have altered mental status.

Patients at highest risk for hospital-acquired hypernatremia are those at the extremes of age (infants and older adults),

those with altered mental status, and those without access to water (i.e., intubated or debilitated patients). In addition to the impaired thirst and decreased urinary concentrating ability that accompany advanced age, older patients have a lower baseline TBW content, making smaller changes in water balance more clinically relevant.

CLINICAL MANIFESTATIONS

SYMPTOMS

Clinical symptoms related to hypernatremia can be attributed to cellular dehydration and shrinkage due to the loss of intracellular water. Loss of intracellular water occurs throughout the body, but the primary symptoms are neurologic. The severity of neurologic symptoms is more dependent on the rate of rise in serum $[Na^+]$ than on the absolute value. Polyuria and polydipsia are frequently the presenting symptoms of diabetes insipidus (DI), with or without the presence of hypernatremia.

Neurologic symptoms comprise a continuum that begins with fatigue, lethargy, irritability, and confusion and progresses to seizures and coma. Additional symptoms of hypernatremia include anorexia, nausea, vomiting, and generalized muscle weakness. Altered mental status can be both a cause and an effect of hypernatremia and consequently can be difficult to distinguish clinically. In addition, cellular dehydration and shrinkage can lead to rupture of cerebral veins because of traction, which results in focal intracerebral and subarachnoid hemorrhages; this occurs more often in infants than in adults.

SIGNS

Signs of hypernatremia depend, in part, on its cause and severity. Abnormal subclavicular and forearm skin turgor and altered sensorium are commonly found in patients with hypovolemic or euvolemic hypernatremia, whereas patients with hypervolemic hypernatremia typically have classic signs of volume overload, such as elevated neck veins and edema.

PATHOPHYSIOLOGY

A sound understanding of the normal physiology of water and salt balance is integral to the understanding and management of dysnatremias. The intracellular and extracellular body compartments exist in osmotic equilibrium. The development of hypernatremia is most commonly the result of increased water losses combined with inadequate intake. Rarely does hypernatremia occur as a consequence of excessive sodium intake.

Regulation of plasma [Na^+] is determined by the regulation of P_{osm}, of which plasma [Na^+] is the primary determinant. Normal P_{osm} is between 285 and 295 mOsm/kg. If the P_{osm} varies by 1% to 2% in either direction, physiologic mechanisms are in place to return the P_{osm} to normal. In the case of hypernatremia or hyperosmolality, receptor cells in the hypothalamus detect increases in P_{osm}; in response, they stimulate thirst to increase water intake and simultaneously stimulate antidiuretic hormone (ADH) release to limit renal water losses (by increasing water reabsorption in the collecting duct). Under normal conditions, the body is able to maintain the serum osmolality under tight control. The goal of "normonatremia" is to avoid changes in cellular volume and thereby prevent potential disruptions in cellular structure and function. The body's normal physiologic defense against hypernatremia is twofold: an endogenous thirst stimulus and renal conservation of water.

As with other electrolyte disturbances, the pathophysiology of hypernatremia can be easily categorized into two phases—an initiation phase and a maintenance phase. Simply stated, the initiation, or generation, phase must be caused by a net water loss or, less commonly, a net sodium gain. For hypernatremia to exist as anything more than a transient state, there must be a maintenance phase, defined necessarily by inadequate water intake.

Water metabolism is primarily controlled by arginine vasopressin (AVP) or ADH, as it is commonly termed. ADH is produced in the hypothalamus (supraoptic and paraventricular nuclei) and is stored in and secreted by the posterior pituitary. ADH release can be stimulated by either increases in P_{osm} or decreases in mean arterial pressure or blood volume. In the setting of hypernatremia, the primary stimulus for the release of ADH comes from osmoreceptors located in the hypothalamus. ADH acts on the vasopressin type 2 (V_2)

receptors in the collecting duct to cause increased water reabsorption from the tubular lumen via insertion of aquaporin-2 channels.

The kidney's primary role in hypernatremia is to concentrate the urine maximally, preventing further loss of electrolyte-free fluid. For the kidney to do so, the following must be present: (1) a concentrated medullary interstitium, (2) ADH to insert aquaporin-2 channels into the apical membranes of the collecting duct, and (3) the ability of collecting duct cells to respond to ADH.

In a steady state, water intake must equal water output. Obligatory renal water loss is directly dependent on solute excretion and urinary concentrating ability. If a person has to excrete, for example, 700 mOsm of solute per day (primarily Na^+, K^+, and urea), and the maximum urinary osmolality (U_{osm}) is 100 mOsm/kg, then the minimum urine output requirement will be 7 L. However, if the kidneys are able to concentrate the urine to a U_{osm} of 700 mOsm/kg, urine output would need to be only 1 L.

Thirst, on the other hand, is an ADH-independent mechanism of defense against hypertonicity. Like ADH release, thirst is triggered by osmoreceptors located in the hypothalamus. The intense thirst stimulated by hypernatremia may be impaired or absent in patients with altered mental status or hypothalamic lesions and in older adults. It is important to note that patients with moderate to severe increases in electrolyte-free water losses may maintain eunatremia because of the powerful thirst mechanism. For example, a patient with nephrogenic DI may maintain a normal serum [Na^+] if given unlimited access to water but may develop marked hypernatremia in situations in which access to water is restricted (e.g., altered mental status, mechanical ventilation, nothing by mouth status during hospitalization).

Although ADH activity is a pivotal physiologic defense against hyperosmolality, only an increase in water intake can replace a water deficit. An increase in ADH activity in collecting tubules can only help to decrease ongoing water losses but cannot replace water that has already been lost. Therefore both ADH-dependent and ADH-independent mechanisms are integral to the body's efforts to protect against hypernatremia or hyperosmolality.

The brain has multiple defense mechanisms designed to protect it from the adverse effects of cellular dehydration. As the serum [Na^+] rises, water moves from the intracellular to the extracellular space to return the serum osmolality to the normal range. Almost immediately, there is an increase in the net leak of serum electrolytes (primarily Na^+ and K^+) into the intracellular space, which increases intracellular osmolality. In addition, there is an increased production of cerebrospinal fluid, with movement into the interstitial areas of the brain. Within approximately 24 hours, brain cells generate *osmolytes* or *idiogenic osmoles* (e.g., amino acids, trimethylamines, myoinositol) to increase intracellular osmolality to draw water intracellularly. This process restores intracellular volume over a period of days, thereby decreasing the adverse clinical impact of hypernatremia (i.e., cellular dehydration). The increase in transcellular transport of electrolytes is somewhat transient because over time it interferes with normal cellular function. Idiogenic osmoles clearly serve a protective role, but their removal is also slow (days) when isotonicity has been reestablished. The clinical implication of the slow removal of these idiogenic osmoles is that correction of hypernatremia (hypertonicity) must be gradual to avoid cellular swelling or cerebral edema.

PATHOGENESIS AND DIAGNOSTIC APPROACH

Hypernatremia most commonly results from the combination of increased water loss and decreased water intake. Any clinical condition associated with increased water loss or decreased water intake predisposes to hypernatremia. In general, for hypernatremia to occur, the rate of water excretion must exceed that of water intake. Hypernatremia secondary to sodium loading, which is less common, is an exception to this basic principle.

Water losses occur via the genitourinary and gastrointestinal tracts, as well as via the skin and respiratory tract as insensible losses. DI and osmotic diuresis result in excess urinary loss of water, and excess water is lost via stool in severe diarrhea. Conditions that increase insensible losses include fever, burns, open wounds, and hyperventilation.

Although hypernatremia is due to an imbalance of water homeostasis, there may be a concomitant salt disturbance. After a thorough clinical history is obtained and a complete physical examination performed, the first decision point in the evaluation of any patient with hypernatremia is to determine the patient's sodium balance or volume status (see Fig. 8.1).

Hypernatremia can be seen in patients whose sodium balance is negative (hypovolemic), normal (euvolemic), or positive (hypervolemic), but in all cases a negative water balance is present. Determining the patient's sodium balance is essential to planning the appropriate therapy.

NEGATIVE SODIUM BALANCE

Hypernatremia due to the loss of hypotonic fluids is associated with both a negative sodium balance and a negative water balance (Table 8.1). In such cases, hypernatremia develops because the sustained loss of water exceeds that of sodium. These patients usually manifest typical signs of sodium depletion, or hypovolemia, such as tachycardia and orthostatic hypotension. Determination of the urine sodium concentration ($[U_{Na}]$) can help distinguish between renal losses, such as from diuretics or osmotic diuresis ($[U_{Na}]$ >20 mEq/dL), and extrarenal losses, such as from diarrhea or vomiting ($[U_{Na}]$ <20 mEq/dL).

NORMAL SODIUM BALANCE

Hypernatremia in patients with a normal sodium balance results from the loss of electrolyte-free fluid, or pure water (see Table 8.1). These patients have a normal total body sodium (and are therefore euvolemic) but are TBW depleted. The causes of hypernatremia in patients with a normal sodium

Table 8.1   Causes of Hypernatremia

RENAL CAUSES OF WATER DEFICIT		
Salt Deficit (Urine [Na⁺] >20 mEq/dL)	Salt Balanced (U_{osm}/P_{osm} <1)	Salt Excess
Diuresis	*Diabetes Insipidus (See Box 8.1)*	Mineralocorticoid excess
Medication (loop diuretic)	ADH-dependent	
Post-AKI	Central	
Postobstructive	Nephrogenic	
Osmotic (glucose, urea, mannitol)	Acquired	
	ADH-independent	
	Electrolyte disturbance	
	Drug-induced	
	Chronic kidney disease	
	Malnutrition	
EXTRARENAL CAUSES OF WATER DEFICIT		
Salt Deficit (Urine [Na⁺] <20 mEq/dL)	Salt Balanced (U_{osm}/P_{osm} <1)	Salt Excess
Gastrointestinal	*Increased Insensible Losses*	*Excessive Na⁺ Intake*
Vomiting	Cutaneous (fever, sweating, increased temperature, burns)	Saline
Diarrhea	Respiratory (tachypnea)	Bicarbonate
Nasogastric suction		Salt ingestion
Enterocutaneous fistula	*Decreased Intake*	Hyperalimentation/TPN
	Primary hypodipsia (older adults, hypothalamic, or osmoreceptor dysfunction)	Hypertonic dialysate
Cutaneous	Reset osmostat	
Sweating	Limited access to water (altered mental status, iatrogenic)	
Burns		
	Intracellular Shift	
	Seizures	
	Severe exercise	

ADH, Antidiuretic hormone; *AKI*, acute kidney injury; *[Na⁺]*, sodium ion concentration; *P_{osm}*, plasma osmolality; *U_{osm}*, urine osmolality, *TPN*, total parenteral nutrition.

Box 8.1   Causes of Diabetes Insipidus

ADH Dependent

Central DI (Lack of ADH Release)

Congenital
Trauma
Neurosurgery
Primary or secondary CNS tumor
Infiltrative disorder
    Sarcoidosis, tuberculosis
Hypoxic encephalopathy
    Post cardiac arrest, Sheehan syndrome
Hemorrhage
Infection
    Meningitis, encephalitis
Aneurysm
Idiopathic

Nephrogenic DI (Unresponsive to ADH)

Hereditary
    X-linked recessive
    Defect in V_2 receptor or aquaporin channel
    May be complete or partial

Gestational DI (Degradation of ADH)

Vasopressinase mediated
Occurs in peripheral circulation

ADH Independent

Acquired Nephrogenic DI

Electrolyte disturbances
    Hypercalcemia
    Hypokalemia
Drug induced
    Lithium, demeclocycline, amphotericin B,
    foscarnet, methoxyflurane, vaptans
Chronic interstitial kidney disease
    Medullary cystic disease, sickle cell disease,
    amyloidosis, Sjögren syndrome
Malnutrition
    Decreased medullary gradient

ADH, Antidiuretic hormone; *CNS*, central nervous system; *DI*, diabetes insipidus.

Gestational DI should be evident from the clinical history. The manifestations are similar to those of nephrogenic DI in that there is little or no increase in U_{osm} with exogenous vasopressin; however, gestational DI responds to desmopressin acetate (dDAVP), a synthetic analogue of ADH that is unaffected by vasopressinase.

Nephrogenic DI can be either hereditary (genetic defect of the V_2 receptor gene or aquaporin water channel) or acquired. Acquired nephrogenic DI may be reversible and includes any clinical condition in which the kidney is unable to maximally concentrate the urine. The mechanisms of acquired nephrogenic DI are ADH independent. The most common cause of acquired nephrogenic DI is chronic lithium use. The mechanism of lithium-induced nephrogenic DI includes both a decrease in density of V_2 receptors and decreased expression of aquaporin-2 channels. Hypercalcemia, hypokalemia, and severe malnutrition are other common examples of reversible nephrogenic DI. Hypercalcemia can induce a reversible nephrogenic DI through inhibition of sodium reabsorption in the loop of Henle, which impairs the generation of an adequate medullary gradient and reduces concentrating ability. In addition, dysregulation of the aquaporin-2 channel can be seen with hypercalcemia. Hypokalemia causes nephrogenic DI by decreasing collecting tubule responsiveness to ADH. Decreased protein intake leads to decreased urea production and therefore a decreased medullary gradient with inability to maximally concentrate the urine.

A high U_{osm} suggests extrarenal losses as the cause of euvolemic hypernatremia. To generate a high U_{osm}, the kidney must be able to concentrate the urine, an ability that requires intact ADH-dependent mechanisms. Insensible losses are the primary source of electrolyte-free water loss in this subgroup of patients. Increased insensible losses occur via the skin (burns, sweat), respiratory tract (tachypnea), or both.

Finally, patients with hypodipsia or adipsia may develop euvolemic hyponatremia. Most often, they have normally functioning kidneys but lack adequate water intake. These patients typically have a high U_{osm} and low urine output. Idiopathic hypodipsia occurs, but identification of an impaired thirst mechanism as the primary disorder causing hypernatremia should lead to a more thorough neurologic investigation to rule out the presence of hypothalamic tumors or disorders. An impaired thirst mechanism or limited access to water in the setting of DI can result in severe hypernatremia and can be life threatening.

POSITIVE SODIUM BALANCE

Hypernatremia resulting from total body sodium gain is the least common type of hypernatremia (see Table 8.1). In these cases, total body sodium is uniformly increased, but TBW may be increased or unchanged, depending on the cause. An increase in extracellular volume should be readily identifiable by the presence of hypervolemia on clinical examination. This clinical presentation is usually iatrogenic, resulting from hypertonic fluid administration (saline or bicarbonate), and it reflects a gain of sodium without an appropriate gain of water. Excess mineralocorticoid activity can also result in hypernatremia with a positive sodium balance and, in the absence of typical iatrogenic risk factors, should alert the clinician to evaluate for potential causes of mineralocorticoid excess.

balance may be renal or extrarenal. In these cases, urine osmolality (U_{osm}), which reflects ADH levels and function, is often more helpful than U_{Na}. A low U_{osm} is consistent with renal losses and therefore with low ADH levels or function (DI), whereas a high U_{osm} suggests extrarenal losses of free water and intact secretion of and response to ADH.

Etiologies of DI may be central, nephrogenic, or gestational (Box 8.1). The key diagnostic step in determining a central versus a nephrogenic cause is based on the response to exogenous hormone replacement (i.e., vasopressin). A finding of little or no increase in U_{osm} after administration of exogenous vasopressin is diagnostic of nephrogenic DI. However, it is important to remember that central or nephrogenic DI may be partial: either ADH is present but in insufficient quantity (partial central DI) or there is an incomplete response to ADH in the collecting duct (partial nephrogenic DI).

One rare form of DI is gestational, or pregnancy-related, DI, which is caused by production of placental vasopressinase.

An example of hypernatremia in the setting of positive sodium balance is the hemodynamically stable hypernatremic patient with acute respiratory distress syndrome (ARDS) and an elevated central venous pressure. This relative hypervolemic hypernatremic state reflects an imbalance of both water and salt. Commonly, the physician might be concerned that administration of the free water necessary to correct the serum $[Na^+]$ (e.g., 3 L) would cause the patient to become fluid overloaded. This would be in direct contrast to the goal of a net negative fluid balance for optimal management of ARDS. However, because of the normal distribution of water, less than 10% (i.e., <300 mL for administration of 3 L) of the administered water, either intravenously or enterally, would remain in the vascular space; therefore the fluid administration would not materially impact the patient's volume status. In addition, it is imperative to understand that further diuresis to obtain a net negative sodium balance, in the absence of water administration, will exacerbate the hypernatremia by increasing free water urinary losses.

TREATMENT

Treatment goals of hypernatremia include both replacement of the free water deficit and prevention or reduction of ongoing water loss. The amount, route, and rate of replacement depend on the severity of symptoms, rate of onset, concurrent clinical conditions, and the patient's sodium balance. Correction of the latter in a hemodynamically unstable patient is always a priority, no matter how severe the hypernatremia. In this setting, ECF depletion should always be corrected with 0.9% saline before the water deficit is addressed. After the patient is hemodynamically stable, it is important to focus on the treatment of the water deficit because the complications of hypernatremia frequently result from its inappropriate correction or treatment, not the electrolyte disturbance itself. Management of hypernatremia should include identification of the underlying cause in addition to correction of the hypertonic state. Treatment of hypernatremia can, most often, be broken down into the following seven steps (Box 8.2).

Step 1. Determine Sodium Balance. Evaluation of the patient's sodium balance, or volume status, is a critical first step for both appropriate diagnosis and treatment of hypernatremia. This information should be obtained through a thorough history and physical examination. If the patient is hemodynamically unstable from sodium depletion, this should be addressed first with the administration of normal saline.

Step 2. Calculate Free Water Deficit. Before initiating therapy, it is both prudent and appropriate to quantify the deficit and develop a treatment plan for the individual patient. Calculation of the water deficit represents only a snapshot in time. If it were possible to prevent any further water losses, insensible or otherwise, the calculated water deficit would be the amount that must be administered to normalize the serum $[Na^+]$, as shown in Box 8.3, Formula 1:

$$\text{Water deficit} = TBW \times (\text{plasma } [Na^+]/140 - 1)$$
$$= (0.5 \text{ or } 0.6) \times \text{lean body weight} \times$$
$$(\text{plasma } [Na^+]/140 - 1)$$

where the lean body weight is expressed in kilograms. TBW is generally considered to be 50% of lean body weight in women and 60% in men. In this equation, 140 may be replaced by the target serum $[Na^+]$. For example, if the current $[Na^+]$ is 160 mEq/L and the goal is to reduce the $[Na^+]$ by 10 mEq/L in 24 hours, then 150 mEq/L is substituted for 140 in the equation. This method may be used to calculate the water deficit for any target serum $[Na^+]$.

Step 3. Choose a Replacement Fluid. The choice of fluid for repletion of a free water deficit depends on the clinical assessment of the patient's sodium balance. Specifically, a key determination is whether the deficit is the result of a pure water loss, requiring only water repletion, or a hypotonic fluid loss, which requires both water and salt repletion. In general, patients with a pure water loss should be repleted with the use of enteral free water (oral or nasogastric tube) or by intravenous administration of 5% dextrose in water (D_5W). Patients with a deficit of both salt and water should be repleted with a combination of salt and water. This correction may be accomplished by the administration of 0.2% or 0.45% saline or with the use of separate intravenous solutions, one for water repletion (D_5W) and one for correction of the salt deficit (0.9% saline). The potential advantage of using two separate infusions is the avoidance of continued salt repletion after the volume deficit has been corrected.

The route of repletion must also be determined. As with nutritional repletion, the enteral route for repletion of free water is preferable; however, it is not always an option as patients commonly have altered mental status. Water can be repleted through a nasogastric tube if gut function is not compromised. The enteral route is preferable because it avoids the administration of the dextrose required to provide water intravenously. Dextrose may increase serum osmolality via hyperglycemia, which can lead to an osmotic diuresis and the unwanted renal clearance of additional electrolyte-free

---

Box 8.2 Approach to the Treatment of Hypernatremia

Step 1. Determine sodium balance.
Step 2. Calculate free water deficit.
Step 3. Choose a replacement fluid.
Step 4. Determine rate of repletion.
Step 5. Estimate ongoing "sensible" losses.
Step 6. Estimate ongoing "insensible" losses.
Step 7. Determine underlying cause, if possible.

Box 8.3 Important Water Balance Formulas

Formula 1	$\text{Water deficit} = TBW \times (\text{plasma } [Na^+]/140 - 1)$ $= (0.5 \text{ or } 0.6) \times \text{lean body weight}$ $\times (\text{plasma } [Na^+]/140 - 1)$
Formula 2	$\Delta[Na^+]_s = [Na^+]_{inf} - [Na^+]_s/TBW + 1$
Formula 3	$\text{Urine output} = C_{electrolytes} + C_{electrolyte\text{-}free}$ or $C_{electrolyte\text{-}free} = V \times [1 - \{(U_{Na} + U_K)/P_{Na}\}]$

water. Most commonly, correction of the free water deficit will be done, at least initially, via the intravenous route.

Step 4. Determine Rate of Repletion. The rate of correction of serum $[Na^+]$ is recommended to be approximately 0.5 mEq/L/h, or a decrease of 10 to 12 mEq/L in a 24-hour period. No human studies have been performed to substantiate the appropriateness of this rate. However, based on animal studies, this reflects the observed rate of cerebral de-adaptation, or the rate at which the brain is able to shed electrolytes and idiogenic osmoles acquired in the adaptive response to cellular dehydration. An important exception to this recommended rate of correction occurs in acutely symptomatic patients who have seizures or acute obtundation, potentially requiring intubation for airway protection. In these circumstances, the rate of correction can be 1 to 2 mEq/L/h initially, with the overall rate still not to exceed the recommended 10 to 12 mEq/L in 24 hours. Furthermore, acute symptoms suggest that the hypernatremia developed rapidly, and, consequently, the brain has not had time to adapt. If adaption to hypernatremia has not yet occurred, the risk that cerebral edema will complicate rapid correction is minimal. If the duration of hypernatremia is unknown, the clinician should err on the side of caution and avoid rapid correction. However, if the onset is known to be acute (i.e., developing within the past 24 hours), the serum $[Na^+]$ can be corrected more quickly because brain adaptation does not occur this quickly.

The calculation of water deficit shown in Step 2 (see Formula 1) is particularly useful for hypernatremia caused by pure water losses. However, in multiple observational studies a concomitant sodium deficit is present in more than 50% of hypernatremia cases. For this reason, it is frequently necessary to replace both water and sodium deficits, which may be accomplished with 0.2% or 0.45%. Table 8.2 lists the sodium concentrations of commonly used intravenous fluids. Formula 2 can be clinically useful for predicting the change in serum $[Na^+]$ that will occur with infusion of 1 L of a particular fluid and, accordingly, choosing an appropriate rate of infusion.

$$\Delta[Na^+]_s = [Na^+]_{inf} - [Na^+]_s/TBW + 1$$

where $\Delta[Na^+]_s$ is the change in serum $[Na^+]$ per L of fluid infused, $[Na^+]_{inf}$ is the concentration of sodium in the infusate, $[Na^+]_s$ is the patient's current concentration of sodium, and TBW is 50% of ideal body weight for women, or 60% for men, expressed in liters (L).

Step 5. Estimate Ongoing "Sensible" Losses. The formulas presented for calculation of the water deficit (see Step 2) and estimation of the impact of a particular infusate on serum $[Na^+]$ (see Step 4) both assume a closed system. They do not account for any ongoing renal or extrarenal losses. In patients with DI or an osmotic diuresis due to hyperglycemia or administration of mannitol, ongoing urinary water losses can be significant. Formula 3 is clinically useful in estimating the amount of ongoing renal water losses, based on clearance (C) of the electrolyte and electrolyte-free components of the urinary fluid:

$$Urine\ output = C_{electrolytes} + C_{electrolyte-free}$$

or

$$C_{electrolyte-free} = V \times [1 - \{(U_{Na} + U_K)/P_{Na}\}]$$

where U_{Na} is the urine sodium concentration, U_K is the urine potassium concentration, and P_{Na} is the plasma sodium concentration, all expressed in milliequivalents per liter (mEq/L). Volume (V) may be expressed in any increment of time, with subsequent extrapolation to a 24-hour period.

The following example illustrates the utility of this free water clearance formula. If the random $U_{Na} = 25$ mEq/L, $U_K = 15$ mEq/L, and $P_{Na} = 160$ mEq/L, then 25% of the urine output can be attributed to the clearance of electrolytes, and 75% is electrolyte-free water. In the setting of a serum $[Na^+]$ of 160 mEq/L, urine with 75% electrolyte-free water clearance is inappropriate. The U_{osm} can help to distinguish whether the high free water clearance represents an osmotic diuresis or DI. A high U_{osm} would be consistent with an osmotic diuresis (from glucose, urea, or mannitol), whereas a low U_{osm} would be consistent with DI.

Step 6. Estimate Ongoing "Insensible" Losses. Ongoing insensible losses include urine and stool output, as well as losses from the skin and respiratory tracts. It is reasonable to assume insensible losses of 10 to 15 mL/kg/day for women and 15 to 20 mL/kg/day for men, with factors such as fever, ambient temperature, infection, burns, open wounds, and tachypnea causing an increase in insensible losses.

Step 7. Identify and Treat Underlying Causes. Although the mainstay of treatment of hypernatremia is repletion of the water deficit, attempts to prevent additional losses should be undertaken. In central DI, for example, treatment with a V_2 agonist (i.e., desmopressin) is critical. Nephrogenic DI is considerably more difficult to treat, but treatment can include administration of a thiazide diuretic to create a mildly volume-depleted state and, consequently, decreased water delivery to the collecting ducts. Low-protein and low-sodium diets can also help to decrease the amount of obligatory solute

Table 8.2 Distribution of Commonly Used Fluids[a]

Fluid	Infusate $[Na^+]$ (mEq/L)	% ECF Distribution[a]	% Intravascular Distribution[a]
D_5W	0	33	8
0.225% NaCl in D_5W	38.5	50	12.5
0.45% NaCl	77	62.5	15.5
lactated Ringer solution	130	100	25
0.9% NaCl in water	154	100	25

[a]The distribution of water is assumed to be ⅔ intracellular and ⅓ extracellular, with the extracellular distribution being ¼ intravascular and ¾ interstitial.
D_5W, 5% Dextrose in water; *ECF*, extracellular fluid; *[Na⁺]*, sodium ion concentration; *NaCl*, sodium chloride.

Box 8.4   Special Considerations for Treatment of Hypernatremia

Negative Sodium Balance

Correct water and salt deficit
Treat underlying condition (e.g., hyperglycemia, urinary obstruction)

Normal Sodium Balance

Correct water deficit
CDI: Administer dDAVP and correct underlying disorder
GDI: Administer dDAVP (vasopressinase does not cleave dDAVP)
NDI (reversible): remove offending medication, correct electrolyte abnormality
NDI (irreversible): thiazide diuretic, NSAIDs, decrease salt intake
NDI (lithium-related): amiloride and thiazide diuretic, acetazolamide

Positive Sodium Balance

Correct water deficit and sodium/volume overload
Diuretics
Dialysis if concurrent kidney failure is present

CDI, Central diabetes insipidus; *dDAVP,* desmopressin; *GDI,* gestational diabetes insipidus; *NDI,* nephrogenic diabetes insipidus; *NSAIDs,* nonsteroidal antiinflammatory drugs.

Box 8.5   Hypernatremia Key Points

- Hypernatremia always reflects a hyperosmolar state.
- Hypernatremia is always a water problem and sometimes a salt problem.
- Patients must have a defect in their thirst mechanism or limited access to free water for hypernatremia to persist.
- The sodium concentration itself does not provide any information about total body salt or volume status.
- A calculation of the water deficit represents only a snapshot in time.
- Formulas should be considered an adjunct tool, not a substitute for sound clinical judgment and frequent monitoring of the serum [Na$^+$].
- Failure to consider ongoing sensible and insensible losses is the most common cause of undercorrection.

---

clearance and thereby decrease the urine output. See Box 8.4 for further condition-specific treatment recommendations.

The treatment approach described earlier applies primarily to hypernatremia in the setting of normal or negative sodium balance. Treatment of hypernatremia with a positive sodium balance is quite different and relies primarily on correction of the hypervolemic state with diuretics. An important consideration in this clinical scenario is that, although gain of sodium is the primary disturbance, there is still a relative lack of water. Diuresis in the absence of water repletion will exacerbate the hypernatremia. Loop diuretics interfere with the concentrating mechanism of the kidneys and therefore cause an inappropriate loss of electrolyte-free water in addition to the desired natriuresis. For this reason, it is imperative to replete the free water deficit in these patients and to calculate their ongoing losses using Formula 3 (see Step 5) to achieve adequate repletion. This is of particular concern in those patients who are without free access to water.

Common mistakes encountered in the treatment of hypernatremia include both undercorrection and overcorrection. Undercorrection is most commonly caused by underestimation of ongoing sensible and insensible losses. Formula 3 allows the clinician to obtain a more accurate reflection of ongoing renal electrolyte-free water loss. In addition, it is important to identify and account for insensible losses applicable to the individual patient. Overcorrection, or overly rapid correction, poses the greater danger. Because the formulas described here are only a guide and lack precision for individual patients, it is critical that serum chemistry values be checked frequently to ensure that the expected and actual rates of correction are similar. The clinician can then adjust the treatment decisions as needed and avoid the potentially devastating neurologic complications of overcorrection.

All formulas used to facilitate treatment of hypernatremia have limitations. Specifically, the formulas do not factor in ongoing sensible or insensible losses and use TBW, which is an imprecise term. These formulas should be considered as adjunctive tools but should not replace sound clinical judgment. The isolated use of these formulas to guide therapy could prove deleterious to the patient if used in lieu of appropriate clinical assessment. For these reasons, it is critical that serum [Na$^+$] be measured frequently (typically, every 2 hours initially) to assess whether the patient is responding as predicted. This is particularly important for patients with significant unmeasurable losses (e.g., diarrhea, burns) and for those patients with particularly high ongoing measurable losses (as frequently occurs with DI).

COMPLICATIONS OF HYPERNATREMIA

In several large observational studies, hypernatremia is independently associated with both an increased length of hospital stay and increased mortality. It is unclear whether hypernatremia is simply a marker of illness severity or it contributes directly to an increase in mortality. Acute (≤24 hours) hypernatremia with serum [Na$^+$] levels greater than 160 mEq/L is associated with a 75% mortality rate in adults, whereas chronic hypernatremia is associated with a much lower rate of approximately 10%. Even modest hospital-acquired hypernatremia has been associated with increased mortality in patients with serum [Na$^+$] greater than 150 mEq/L, demonstrating a severity of illness-adjusted relative risk of 2.6 for death. Increased mortality and increased length of stay in patients with hypernatremia have been seen across a broad spectrum of patient populations, including both medical and surgical intensive care patients. A decreased level of consciousness occurring as a complication of hypernatremia is an important prognostic indicator associated with mortality. Although the mechanism of the high mortality is not known, it is clear that a judicious approach to diagnosis and treatment of hypernatremia is imperative (Box 8.5).

As discussed earlier, neurologic sequelae can occur both with hypernatremia and with its correction. Decreased cell volume impairs tissue function, and overly rapid correction can cause cerebral edema if adaptation has occurred. In addition to the adverse central nervous system effects, hypernatremia also inhibits insulin release and increases insulin resistance, thereby predisposing patients to hyperglycemia. Hypernatremia also decreases hepatic gluconeogenesis, lactate clearance, and cardiac function. A patient's level of consciousness, rather than the absolute serum [Na⁺], is a more important prognostic indicator of mortality.

Adverse sequelae associated with hypernatremia are often underappreciated and frequently lead to a delay in treatment. Studies have shown that fewer than 50% of patients with hospital-acquired hypernatremia receive free water replacement within 24 hours of the first identified elevated serum [Na⁺], and the majority take longer than 72 hours to treat. Furthermore, patients whose hypernatremia is corrected within 72 hours have a lower mortality than those whose hypernatremia is not corrected within 72 hours. In light of the significant associations with adverse physiologic sequelae, increased length of stay, and increased mortality seen with hospital-acquired hypernatremia, hypernatremia should not be viewed as an incidental or negligible electrolyte abnormality.

KEY BIBLIOGRAPHY

Adler SM, Verbalis JG. Disorders of body water homeostasis in critical illness. *Endocrinol Metab Clin North Am.* 2006;35:873-894.

Adrogue HA, Madias NE. Aiding fluid prescription for the dysnatremias. *Intensive Care Med.* 1997;23:309-316.

Adrogue HJ, Madias NE. Hypernatremia. *N Engl J Med.* 2000;342: 1493-1499.

Alshayeb HM, Showkat A, Babar F, et al. Severe hypernatremia correction rate and mortality in hospitalized patients. *Am J Med Sci.* 2011;341: 356-360.

Berl T, Robertson G. Pathophysiology of water metabolism. In: Brenner BM, ed. *The Kidney.* 6th ed. Philadelphia: WB Saunders; 2000: 866-893.

Chassagne P, Druesne L, Capet C, et al. Clinical presentation of hypernatremia in elderly patients: a case control study. *J Am Geriatr Soc.* 2006;54:1225-1230.

Darmon M, Timsit J, Francais A, et al. Association between hypernatraemia acquired in the ICU and mortality: a cohort study. *Nephrol Dial Transplant.* 2010;25:2502-2510.

de Groot T, Sinke AP, Kortenoeven MLA, et al. Acetazolamide attenuates lithium-induced nephrogenic diabetes insipidus. *J Am Soc Nephrol.* 2016;27:2082-2091.

Funk G, Lindner G, Druml W, et al. Incidence and prognosis of dysnatremias present on ICU admission. *Intensive Care Med.* 2010;36:304-311.

Hall JB, Schmidt GA, Wood LDH. Electrolyte disorders in critical care. In: Hall JB, Schmidt GA, Wood LDH, eds. *Principles of Critical Care.* 3rd ed. New York: McGraw-Hill; 2005:1161-1166.

Hoorn EJ, Betjes M, Weigel J, et al. Hypernatraemia in critically ill patients: too little water and too much salt. *Nephrol Dial Transplant.* 2008;23:1562-1568.

Liamis G, Kalogirou M, Saugos V, et al. Therapeutic approach in patients with dysnatraemias. *Nephrol Dial Transplant.* 2006;21:1564-1569.

Lien YH, Shapiro JI, Chan L. Effect of hypernatremia on organic brain osmoles. *J Clin Invest.* 1990;85:1427-1435.

Lindner G, Funk G, Lassnigg A, et al. Intensive care-acquired hypernatremia after major cardiothoracic surgery is associated with increased mortality. *Intensive Care Med.* 2010;36:1718-1723.

Lindner G, Funk G, Schwarz C, et al. Hypernatremia in the critically ill is an independent risk factor for mortality. *Am J Kidney Dis.* 2007;50: 952-957.

Nguyen MK, Kurtz I. Analysis of current formulas used for treatment of the dysnatremias. *Clin Exp Nephrol.* 2004;8:12-16.

Palevsky PM. Hypernatremia. *Semin Nephrol.* 1998;18:20-30.

Palevsky PM, Bhagrath R, Greenberg A. Hypernatremia in hospitalized patients. *Ann Intern Med.* 1996;124:197-203.

Polderman K, Schreuder W, van Schijndel R, et al. Hypernatremia in the intensive care unit: an indicator of quality of care? *Crit Care Med.* 1999;27:1105-1108.

Rose BD, Post TW. *Clinical Physiology of Acid-Base and Electrolyte Disorders.* 5th ed. New York: McGraw-Hill; 2001.

Full bibliography can be found on www.expertconsult.com.

9 Edema and the Clinical Use of Diuretics

Domenic A. Sica; Todd W.B. Gehr

Chlorothiazide, which became available in 1958, ushered in the modern era of diuretic therapy, initially for the treatment of edematous states and shortly thereafter for the treatment of essential hypertension. Over the ensuing 60 years, diuretics have emerged as important therapeutic tools. First, they are capable of reducing blood pressure (BP), while simultaneously decreasing the morbidity and mortality that attends the poorly treated hypertensive state. Diuretics are currently considered as one of several first-line therapies suggested by various guideline-promulgating committees. In addition, they remain a necessary treatment tool for volume overload states, such as nephrotic syndrome and heart failure (HF), in that they afford important decongestion benefits. This chapter reviews the various diuretic classes and the physiologic adaptations that ensue from their use and establishes the basis for their use in the treatment of volume overload and various types of hypertension.

INDIVIDUAL CLASSES OF DIURETICS

The predominant nephron sites of action of the various diuretic classes are represented in Fig. 9.1. Inter- and intraclass differences exist for all diuretic groups. The diuretic classes of note include proximal tubular, distal convoluted tubule (DCT) and loop diuretics, potassium (K^+)-sparing agents, and osmotic diuretics.

PROXIMAL TUBULAR DIURETICS

The administration of a carbonic anhydrase (CA) inhibitor ordinarily results in a brisk alkaline diuresis. By inhibiting CA, these compounds decrease the generation of intracellular H^+, which is a prerequisite for the absorption of sodium (Na^+); therein resides their primary diuretic action (see Fig. 9.1). Although CA inhibitors work at the proximal tubule (PT) level where the bulk of Na^+ reabsorption occurs, their final diuretic effect is lessened by reabsorption in more distal nephron segments. Acetazolamide is currently the only CA inhibitor used mainly for its diuretic properties; other CA inhibitors are used topically in the treatment of glaucoma. Acetazolamide is readily absorbed and is eliminated by tubular secretion ($\approx 50\%$). Its use is constrained by its transient action and because prolonged use results in a metabolic acidosis, among other side effects. Alternatively, acetazolamide (250 to 500 mg daily) corrects the metabolic alkalosis that can occur with thiazide or loop diuretic therapy. Acetazolamide should be used cautiously in patients with advanced kidney

failure because it systemically accumulates with repeat dosing with resultant neurologic side effects. In addition, acetazolamide may reduce the glomerular filtration rate (GFR) when given intravenously; however, the dose dependency of this process is poorly understood. The anticonvulsant topiramate inhibits CA and therein can cause metabolic acidosis. Patients with a history of renal calculi or known renal tubular acidosis should receive topiramate with some caution, if at all, unless other treatment options are not available.

DISTAL CONVOLUTED TUBULE DIURETICS

The major site of action of thiazide diuretics is the early DCT where they inhibit the coupled reabsorption of Na^+ and chloride (Cl^-). The water-soluble thiazides such as hydrochlorothiazide (HCTZ) also inhibit CA when given at high doses, and therein further increase Na^+ excretion. Thiazides also inhibit NaCl/fluid reabsorption in the medullary-collecting duct. In addition to these varied effects on Na^+ excretion, thiazide diuretics impair urinary diluting capacity without affecting urinary concentrating mechanisms, reduce calcium (Ca^{++}) and urate excretion, and increase magnesium (Mg^{++}) excretion. The most widely prescribed drug in this class is HCTZ. The onset of diuresis with HCTZ occurs within 2 hours, peaks between 3 and 6 hours, and dose-dependently continues for upward to 12 hours. The half-life ($t_{1/2}$) of HCTZ is prolonged both in decompensated HF and kidney failure. Doses of thiazide diuretics in the 100 to 200 mg/day range are required to initiate a diuresis in patients with chronic kidney disease (CKD), although the overall natriuretic response is arbitrated by the GFR/filtered Na^+ load.

The concept of "class effect" is debated relative to the actions of DCT diuretics, as applied to both BP reduction and cardiovascular (CV) outcomes. Much of the recent debate on diuretic class effect has centered on the differences between chlorthalidone and HCTZ. Although chlorthalidone and HCTZ are structurally similar, they differ pharmacokinetically in that chlorthalidone has a longer $t_{1/2}$ of 40 to 60 hours versus 3.2 to 13.1 hours for HCTZ, as well as a larger volume of distribution by virtue of its extensive partitioning into red blood cells. This latter feature creates a depot that promotes continuous streaming of chlorthalidone (red cell → plasma → tubular secretion). This plasma half-life difference for chlorthalidone correlates with a more extended diuretic effect and is a likely explanation for the observation that chlorthalidone is a better mg-for-mg antihypertensive than HCTZ.

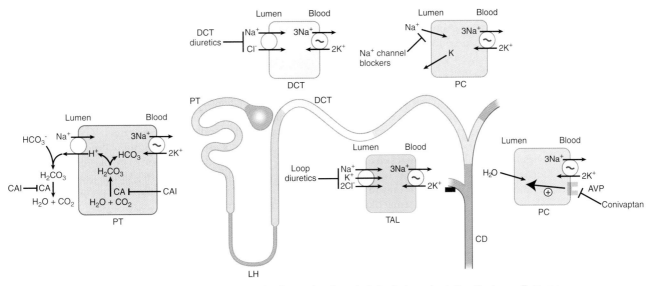

Fig. 9.1 Predominant sites and mechanisms of action of clinically important diuretic drugs. Patterns identify sites of action along the nephron and corresponding cell types affected. The proximal tubule (PT, *purple segment*) is represented by a typical PT cell. The loop of Henle (LH) includes a thick ascending limb (TAL, *green segment*), and a typical TAL cell is shown in green. The distal convoluted tubule (DCT, *blue segment*) is represented by a typical DCT cell in blue. The collecting duct (CD, *yellow and orange segments*) includes principal cells (PC), shown in yellow. Note that, for clarity, two principal cells are shown. Both water and salt pathways exist in the same cells. Both intracellular and luminal actions of carbonic anhydrase (CA) inhibitors in suppressing CA are important in their ability to reduce sodium (Na^+) reabsorption by the renal proximal tubule. Note that Na^+ channel blockers probably act along the last half of the DCT and in the connecting tubule as well as in the CD. Spironolactone and eplerenone (not shown) are competitive mineralocorticoid receptor antagonists and act primarily in the cortical collecting tubule. Aquaretics, such as conivaptan or tolvaptan, inhibit water reabsorption by PC by blocking the action of arginine vasopressin on V_2 receptors. V_2 receptors facilitate insertion of aquaporin 2 water channels in the luminal membrane.

LOOP DIURETICS

Loop diuretics act predominantly at the luminal membrane in the thick ascending limb (TAL) of the loop of Henle where they compete with Cl^- for binding to the $Na^+/K^+/2Cl^-$ cotransporter, thereby inhibiting Na^+ and Cl^- reabsorption. Loop diuretics also have qualitatively minor effects on Na^+ reabsorption within other nephron segments. Other clinically relevant effects of loop diuretics include a decrease in both free water (H_2O) excretion and absorption during H_2O loading and dehydration, respectively, a 30% increase in fractional Ca^{++} excretion, a significant increase in Mg^{++} excretion, as well as a brief increase followed by a more long-lived decrease in uric acid excretion. Loop diuretics also stimulate renal prostaglandin synthesis, particularly that of the vasodilatory prostaglandin E_2 (PGE_2). Angiotensin-II, generated following the administration of intravenous loop diuretics, coupled with an increased synthesis of PGE_2, are the likely reasons for the shift in renal blood flow (RBF) from the inner to the outer renal cortex with these drugs; however, both total RBF and GFR are maintained when loop diuretics are administered to normal subjects.

The available loop diuretics include bumetanide, ethacrynic acid, furosemide, and torsemide. These compounds are highly protein bound, mainly to albumin; therefore to gain access to their tubular site of action they must be secreted as is the case for thiazide diuretics. This process occurs via probenecid-sensitive organic anion transporters localized to the PT. Tubular secretion of loop diuretics may be interfered by elevated levels of endogenous organic acids, as arise in CKD, and by drugs that share the same transporter site, such as salicylates and nonsteroidal antiinflammatory drugs (NSAIDs). Uremic toxins and fatty acids can decrease loop diuretic protein binding and further alter diuretic pharmacokinetics.

Diuretic excretion rates approximate drug delivery to the medullary TAL and correlate with the observed natriuretic response. The relationship between the urinary loop diuretic excretion rate and natriuresis is that of an S-shaped sigmoidal curve. A normal dose-response relationship (as is typically seen in the untreated patient with hypertension) can be shifted (downward and rightward) by a variety of clinical conditions ranging from volume depletion ("braking phenomenon") to HF or nephrotic syndrome (disease-state alterations) to various drug therapies. As an example of the latter, NSAIDs modify this dose-response relationship by inhibiting prostaglandin synthesis and blunting an expected diuretic effect. Finally, the binding of loop diuretics to urinary protein seems not to be the basis for the blunted diuretic effect in the setting of nephrotic syndrome as was suggested early on.

Furosemide is the most widely used diuretic in this class; however, its use is complicated by variable absorption with a bioavailability ranging from 12% to 112%. The coefficient of variation for absorption varies from 25% to 43% for different furosemide products, and exchanging one furosemide formulation for another will not standardize patient absorption and/or response to oral furosemide. Bumetanide and torsemide are better absorbed than is furosemide. The consistency of torsemide's absorption and its longer duration of action are features to consider when loop diuretic therapy is needed in the chronic HF patient. Loop diuretics are commonly used in the patient with CKD, with the renal clearance of these drugs reduced in parallel with the degree of reduction in kidney function. In general, furosemide pharmacokinetics are more significantly changed in CKD than the other loop diuretics, with both its renal metabolism and intact clearance reduced in CKD. Alternatively, bumetanide and torsemide undergo significant hepatic metabolism, which is only marginally impacted by CKD, and in CKD their pharmacokinetic profiles only change as the result of decreased renal clearance of the intact molecules.

DISTAL POTASSIUM-SPARING DIURETICS

There are two classes of K$^+$-sparing diuretics: competitive antagonists of aldosterone, such as spironolactone or eplerenone, and compounds that work independent of aldosterone, such as amiloride and triamterene. Drugs in this class reduce active Na$^+$ absorption in the late DCT/collecting duct (CD). In so doing, basolateral Na$^+$/K$^+$-ATPase activity falls off, intracellular K$^+$ concentration decreases, and the electrochemical gradient for K$^+$ is lowered, thereby reducing K$^+$ secretion. K$^+$-sparing diuretics also reduce Ca^{++} and Mg^{++} excretion, which is a useful feature in the HF patient. Because K$^+$-sparing diuretics are only modestly natriuretic, their clinical utility resides more in their K$^+$-sparing capacity, particularly when more proximally acting diuretics increase distal Na$^+$ delivery or in the instance of either primary or secondary aldosteronism.

Spironolactone is a well-absorbed, highly protein-bound, lipid-soluble K$^+$-sparing diuretic with a 20-hour half-life. The onset of action for spironolactone is characteristically slow, with a peak response at times 48-hours or more after the initial dose. 7α-thiomethylspirolactone and canrenone are the two main metabolites of spironolactone that account for a good portion of its mineralocorticoid receptor blocking activity. Spironolactone, unlike amiloride and triamterene, remains active (as a diuretic and antihypertensive agent) in advanced kidney failure in that its locus of action is basolateral; thus it does not require glomerular filtration or tubular secretion to gain access to its effect site. Eplerenone is a mineralocorticoid receptor antagonist that is highly selective for the aldosterone receptor; accordingly, its much lower affinity for androgen and progesterone receptors results in considerably less gynecomastia than is the case with spironolactone. Typically, eplerenone is at best a very mild diuretic, and its antihypertensive effects originate from nondiuretic aspects of its action.

Amiloride and triamterene are K$^+$-sparing diuretics that block epithelial Na$^+$ channels (ENaC) in the luminal membrane of the CD. They are both actively secreted by cationic transporters that reside in the PT, and each has but a very modest natriuretic effect. The cationic nature of these compounds is such that they interfere with the tubular secretion of creatinine. Both drugs are seldom used in HF for diuresis; rather, they may be used for their K$^+$- and Mg^{++}-sparing properties. Amiloride and triamterene are both

extensively renally cleared and will accumulate with repetitive dosing in the setting of a reduced GFR.

OSMOTIC DIURETICS

Mannitol is a polysaccharide diuretic given intravenously that is freely eliminated by glomerular filtration. Mannitol is poorly reabsorbed along the length of the nephron and thereby exerts a dose-dependent osmotic effect. This osmotic effect traps water and solutes in the tubular fluid, thus increasing Na$^+$, K$^+$, Cl$^-$, and HCO$_3^-$ excretion. The plasma t$_{1/2}$ of mannitol depends on the level of kidney function but usually is between 30 and 60 minutes; thus its diuretic properties are quite transient. Mannitol has been used to reduce the incidence of acute kidney injury (AKI) in patients undergoing cardiopulmonary bypass, having rhabdomyolysis, or following exposure to contrast media. The findings from studies of these circumstances do not support a more widespread use of mannitol to prophylactically forestall development of AKI. Because mannitol also expands extracellular fluid (ECF) volume and can precipitate pulmonary edema in patients with HF, it should be used cautiously, if at all, in these patients. Moreover, excessive mannitol administration, particularly in the setting of a reduced GFR, can cause dilutional hyponatremia, hyperkalemia, and/or AKI. The latter is dose-dependent, relates to afferent arteriolar vasoconstriction, and commonly corrects with the elimination of excess mannitol as may be accomplished with hemodialysis.

ADAPTATION TO DIURETIC THERAPY

Diuretic-induced inhibition of Na$^+$ reabsorption in one nephron segment elicits important adaptations in other nephron segments, which not only limits their antihypertensive and fluid-depleting actions but also contributes to the development of side effects. Although a portion of this resistance to diuretic effect is a normal consequence of diuretic use, disease-state related diuretic resistance is often encountered in patients with clinical disorders such as HF, cirrhosis, and kidney failure states marked by proteinuria.

The initial dose of a diuretic normally produces a brisk diuresis, which is quickly followed by a new equilibrium state in which daily fluid and electrolyte excretion either matches or is less than intake with body weight stabilizing. In nonedematous patients given either a thiazide or a loop diuretic, this adaptation, or *braking phenomenon*, occurs within 1 to 2 days and limits net weight loss to 1 to 2 kg. This braking phenomenon is most evident in normal subjects given a loop diuretic. For example, furosemide administered orally to subjects ingesting a high-Na$^+$ diet (270 mmol/24 hours) produced an initial brisk natriuresis, which resulted in a negative Na$^+$ balance over the ensuing 6 hours. This was followed by an 18-hour period when Na$^+$ excretion was reduced to levels well below the prescribed Na$^+$ intake, resulting in a positive Na$^+$ balance. This postdiuresis Na$^+$ retention matched the initial natriuresis with the result at the end of the day being a neutral Na$^+$ balance state and no weight loss. After 3 successive days of furosemide administration, a similar pattern of Na$^+$ loss and retention was demonstrated each day (Fig. 9.2). This phenomenon is quite reproducible, being evident after even a month of furosemide administration. However,

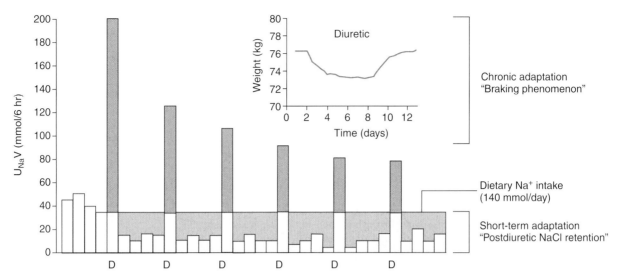

Fig. 9.2 Effect of a loop diuretic on urinary sodium (Na⁺) excretion. Each bar represents a 6-hour time interval. Purple bars indicate periods during which urinary Na⁺ excretion ($U_{Na}V$) exceeds that of dietary intake. Blue areas indicate periods of postdiuretic Na⁺ retention, during which dietary Na⁺ intake exceeds urinary Na⁺ excretion. The horizontal black line indicates dietary Na⁺ intake per 24-hour period. Changes in the magnitude of the natriuretic response over several days are reflective of the "braking phenomenon." Inset shows the effect of diuretics on weight (and extracellular fluid volume) during several days of diuretic administration. (Data redrawn from Wilcox CS, Mitch WE, Kelly RA, et al. Response of the kidney to furosemide: I. Effects of salt intake and renal compensation. *J Lab Clin Med.* 1983;102:450–458.)

if Na⁺ intake is kept very low, balance can remain negative after a single dose of furosemide, even though there is some blunting of the initial natriuretic response.

The mechanistic basis for the braking phenomenon is complex. The relationship between natriuresis and the rate of furosemide excretion is shifted to the right in subjects receiving a low-salt diet, which denotes a blunting of tubular response. The importance of ECF volume depletion in postdiuretic Na⁺ retention has been clearly shown, although there is an ECF volume-independent component to this process as well. The latter appears to be unrelated to aldosterone, as spironolactone therapy has little effect on the Na⁺ retention. Structural hypertrophy in the distal nephron also occurs in rats receiving prolonged infusions of loop diuretics. These structural changes are marked by increased distal nephron Na⁺ and Cl⁻ absorption and K⁺ secretion, phenomena which are aldosterone independent. These structural adaptations may contribute to postdiuretic Na⁺ retention and to diuretic tolerance in humans, and could explain the Na⁺ retention persisting for up to 2 weeks after loop diuretic therapy is discontinued.

NEUROHUMORAL RESPONSE TO DIURETICS

Plasma renin activity (PRA) and plasma aldosterone concentrations rise within minutes of receiving an intravenous diuretic, a process that is independent of volume loss and/or sympathetic nervous system (SNS) activation. This rise in PRA is caused by inhibition of NaCl reabsorption at the macula densa in conjunction with loop-diuretic stimulation of renal prostaglandin release. This first wave of neurohumoral effects, although transient, recognizably increases afterload and for a short period of time may lessen the efficacy of a

loop diuretic. Shortly after this initial rise in PRA, diuretics cause a more sustained increase in PRA and aldosterone arising from an increase in SNS activity (β-agonism) and a fall in ECF volume. The increase in renal prostaglandin production is the likely explanation for the preload reduction and decrease in ventricular filling pressures that occur within 15 minutes of loop diuretic administration.

DIURETIC TREATMENT OF EDEMA

The pathophysiology of Na⁺ and H₂O retention in the patient with edema is typically characterized by a complex interchange of hemodynamic and neurohumoral factors. For example, systemically perceived arterial underfilling sets into motion related Na⁺ and H₂O retention in the patient with HF. The level of neurohormonal activation, the degree of renal vasoconstriction, and the extent to which renal perfusion pressure is reduced moderate this process. In other instances, such as in the patient with a reduced GFR and/or nephrotic syndrome, Na⁺ and H₂O retention derives from a more primary set of renal processes. In each instance, however, efforts should be directed toward correcting the underlying disease state even as diuretic use is being strongly considered.

There are two important considerations that should be brought to bear before and/or concurrent with initiation of diuretic therapy: the need to restrict dietary Na⁺ intake (2 to 4 g Na⁺ day) and dose reduction/elimination of drugs that foster Na⁺ retention, such as NSAIDs, nonspecific vasodilators like hydralazine and minoxidil, and high-dose β-blockers or central α-agonists as used in the treatment of hypertension. Once a decision is made to initiate diuretic therapy, the choice of drug, dosage, and the frequency of dosing can be a subjective process focusing on both the etiology and extent of the volume overload. There is a treatment hierarchy among the thiazide diuretics, and more long-acting compounds, such as chlorthalidone or metolazone, are preferred in the edematous patient. A compound, such as chlorthalidone, can be quite effective in the setting of mild to moderate edema given once or twice daily in the 25- to 50-mg/day range. When the underlying disease state worsens and/or dietary Na^+ restriction cannot be adequately maintained, then conversion to a loop diuretic–based regimen becomes the more practiced approach. Combination diuretic therapy can be considered thereafter, either because the severity of the edema requires "sequential nephron blockade" or because the underlying disease state is particularly sensitive to medications other than loop diuretics, as is the case for spironolactone (50 → 400-mg/day range) use in the patient with advanced cases of cirrhosis and ascites.

Determining the minimally effective dose for a diuretic effect is a necessary clinical exercise, particularly in the patient with a reduced GFR (Fig. 9.3). Gradually increasing a diuretic dose until a response is seen will establish the threshold/effect dose, and thereafter the frequency of dosing can be established based on clinical circumstances. The beginning dose from which dose titration proceeds is influenced by both the level of kidney function and the severity of the edematous state. If kidney function is reduced, the diuretic dose-response curve shifts to the right and the maximal effectiveness, based on absolute Na^+ excretion rate, can be significantly reduced, therein making dietary Na^+ restriction of considerable importance. In a pointedly edematous patient with CKD, furosemide 40 mg, torsemide 10 mg, and bumetanide 1 to 2 mg, with each compound being given twice daily, would be considered adequate starting doses that could then be gradually incremented until the desired effect is achieved. Often, the dose that elicits an increase in urine output can be continued indefinitely unless the underlying disease state worsens and/or dietary Na^+ intake becomes inordinately high. Conversely, a diuretic dose that establishes "euvolemia" can occasionally be lowered and restriction of dietary Na^+ intake given added opportunity to minimize edema redevelopment. Diuretic dose reduction should always be a sought after consideration, as it minimizes loss of K^+, Mg^{++}, and, in the case of loop diuretics, Ca^{++}.

DIURETIC RESISTANCE: CAUSES AND TREATMENT

Volume control in the majority of edematous patients is an attainable goal, albeit one that requires an organized application of the principles of diuretic therapy. The "diuretic-resistant" patient is found in both inpatient and ambulatory settings. In the instance of hospitalized patients, diuretic resistance is linked to the complex nature of the volume-retaining state with multiple organ systems in play, and acuity of illness is the major determinant. In the case of the diuretic-resistant ambulatory patient, an excessive intake of Na^+ is a key factor that can oftentimes go overlooked. Several factors are brought to bear in determining a "dry" or "target" weight in the edematous patient including symptom relief, which incorporates patient input into the treatment equation, the extent of comorbid illnesses, as well as what

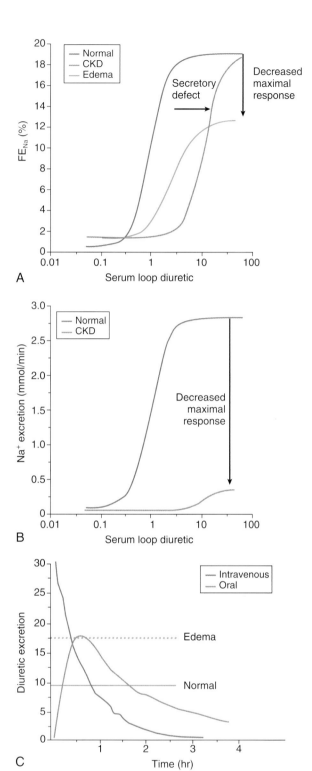

Fig. 9.3 (A) Comparison of effects of chronic kidney disease (CKD) and conditions marked by edema on the loop diuretic dose response, expressed as fractional Na^+ excretion (FE_{Na}). Diuretic delivery via secretion into the lumen is impaired in CKD (pharmacokinetic abnormality), whereas the response to delivered drug is diminished with edema (pharmacodynamic defect). (B) Effect of CKD on the absolute response to a loop diuretic. Compare with panel A. (C) Pharmacokinetics of intravenous and oral loop diuretics. The diuretic thresholds for normal and edematous individuals are shown as horizontal lines; whereas a normal individual responds appropriately to either an intravenous or oral diuretic, some edematous individuals can only reach threshold excretion with intravenous diuretic administration.

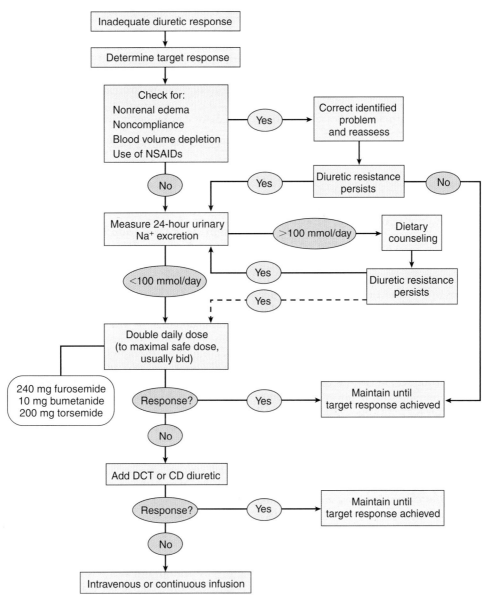

Fig. 9.4 Algorithm for the treatment of the diuretic-resistant patient. Combination diuretic regimens are addressed in the text. Maximal recommended loop diuretic doses given as monotherapy are provided in the yellow box. Note that higher doses are recommended for patients with acute kidney injury. Larger doses may improve the natriuretic response because of a lengthier duration of action; however, this can occur at the cost of increased side effects. *CD*, collecting duct; *DCT*, distal convoluted tubule; *NSAIDs*, nonsteroidal antiinflammatory drugs. (Modified with permission from Wilcox CS. Diuretics. In: Brenner B, ed. *Brenner and Rector's The Kidney*. 5th ed. Philadelphia: WB Saunders; 1996.)

can be realistically accomplished with available therapies. An organized and systematic approach to diuretic therapy can allow for the development of a safe and maximally effective dosing regimen (Fig. 9.4).

As discussed, poorly regulated Na⁺ intake can eliminate the net negative Na⁺ balance that might otherwise occur with a good diuretic regimen. A 24-hour urine Na⁺ excretion greater than 100 mmol/day is a reasonable marker of adequate diuretic action; however, obtaining a complete 24-hour urine collection can prove burdensome. An alternative approach to assessing the adequacy of diuretic action is to obtain an FE_{Na} 1 to 2 hours after ingestion of a well-absorbed loop diuretic, such as torsemide. If this value is greater than 2%, then "true" diuretic resistance is unlikely. The slow rate and

variable extent of diuretic absorption, as is the case with furosemide, can create the impression that diuretic resistance is present when the resistance is more a matter of altered absorptive pharmacokinetics; however, this is a less common issue at higher furosemide doses (>80 to 120 mg/day) based on the surfeit of available drug.

Impairment in the renal clearance of a diuretic may be a factor in attenuating diuretic response. In the setting of CKD, the tubular secretion of a loop diuretic is slowed, requiring that larger doses of drug be given to reach serum levels high enough to exceed the pathologic impediment to luminal drug delivery. Conversion from an intravenous to an orally administered loop diuretic can prove to be an arbitrary process. In the instance of furosemide, which on average is 50% absorbed, twice as much diuretic must be given orally to match what might have been being given intravenously; however, oral furosemide has a wide coefficient of variation for absorption, and this day-to-day variability in absorption can be misconstrued as diuretic resistance.

Nephrotic syndrome often presents as a diuretic-resistant state. Alterations in both the pharmacokinetics and pharmacodynamics of loop diuretics account for this attenuation of diuretic effect. Loop diuretic delivery is impaired in the hypoalbuminemic individual in that the renal secretion of diuretics is strongly dependent on the prevailing plasma albumin concentration. In patients with decompensated nephrotic syndrome, the dose-response relationship for diuretic effect is shifted to the right (higher threshold for effect) and downward (reduction in maximal response or decreased sensitivity). Diuretics can bind to albumin in tubular fluid, which decreases the amount of unbound, active drug available for interaction at its tubular receptor. When urinary albumin concentrations are greater than 4 g/L, as much as 65% of the diuretic reaching the tubular fluid is bound to albumin. Consequently, starting doses 2 to 3 times higher than the normal dose are recommended to ensure delivery of adequate free drug to its site of action. Strategies to reduce the degree of proteinuria with agents that interrupt renin-angiotensin-aldosterone system (RAAS) activity should always be pursued in the patient with nephrotic syndrome. The cornerstone of therapy for nephrotic syndrome-related edema is that of restricting Na^+ intake, an approach that most times needs to be supported by diuretic therapy. However, the inherent "reduced" response often requires more frequent dosing of a loop diuretic. Other therapeutic options to treat the volume overload that marks nephrotic syndrome include two or three diuretic combinations, and the timed but separate administration of albumin and furosemide (see Diuretic Dosing Strategies).

Hemodynamic considerations are common in the patient with diuretic resistance, particularly when reduced ejection fraction forms of HF are in play. Agents, such as dobutamine, that are positive inotropes can favorably influence RBF and diuretic action in the patient with systolic HF. Allowing BP to drift up by holding (or lowering) the dose of RAAS inhibitors can aid in restoring diuretic action in that these drugs often reduce BP below a critical threshold for diuretic effect, particularly when small or large vessel disease is present in the renal vascular bed. In addition, diuretic dosing should not occur close to dosing of RAAS inhibitors, whenever possible, as to the latter's ability to critically lower BP.

There are a number of other approaches to diuretic therapy in the patient with diuretic resistance, including high-dose oral loop diuretic therapy, diuretic rotation, combination diuretic therapy, continuous infusion therapy, admixed albumin/furosemide, and high-dose loop diuretic and hypertonic saline, that can be individually used (see Diuretic Dosing Strategies). These approaches are not mutually exclusive and, for the most part, are empirically used with limited scientific basis for the selection of one over the other. When the aforementioned principles of therapy are applied, most diuretic-resistant patients respond to diuretic therapy, albeit in a variable fashion. A major limiting factor in "diuresing" the volume-overloaded patient, however, is

the ensuing reduction in GFR. Obtaining effective control of ECF volume excess requires a certain artfulness with careful timing of the ongoing diuresis to avoid subsequent response-limiting reductions in GFR and what are often preventable electrolyte complications. As such, when the principles of diuretic therapy are carefully applied to the management of the volume-overloaded patient, more times than not a patient can be safely and effectively diuresed.

SPECIAL DIURETIC DOSING STRATEGIES

Not uncommonly, simple approaches to diuretic resistance fail (see Fig. 9.4). Several strategies can be used to control edema in such patients, including maneuver of increasing the frequency with which a diuretic is administered.

High-Dose Oral Loop Diuretics

Very high doses of loop diuretics have been offered as an alternative for the management of diuretic resistance, although this approach has been used with some hesitation, presumably because of worry about possible ototoxicity. Nevertheless, it has been demonstrated in an outpatient population that the oral administration of furosemide (dosage range 700 to 1000 mg/day) was both a safe and effective decongestion therapy for advanced stage HF. With regard to the supposed toxicity of this approach, when furosemide is given to the patient with HF, absorption is typically both delayed and incomplete, in part relating to gut wall edema that decreases the systemic concentrations attained with such a dosing approach.

Diuretic Rotation

The rotation from one diuretic class to another and, occasionally, rotation within a class may induce diuresis in a patient previously poorly responsive to the diuretic effects of a different compound. This practice has not been critically examined, however, and at best remains hearsay. If response varies among orally administered diuretics within the same class, most times it relates to differences in the rate/extent of absorption and the positive effect gained from a more efficient time course for urinary drug delivery. Also, better hemodynamics may be in play when converting from one diuretic to another, which can be the basis for a differing response.

Combination Diuretic Therapy

The use of diuretic combinations in diuretic-resistant states, such as nephrotic syndrome or HF, is predicated on the ability of diuretics of different classes to effect sequential nephron blockade and thereby produce a summed response. Another consideration in how combination diuretic therapy relates to the capacity of a thiazide diuretic to minimize the development of loop diuretic–related DCT cell hypertrophy that might otherwise increase Na^+ absorption. Although most all combinations of diuretics have been tried, a thiazide together with a loop diuretic with or without a K^+-sparing diuretic are what have been most frequently used in clinical practice. The metolazone-furosemide combination is commonly used when significant volume removal is most essential. The onset of an augmented diuretic response to a loop diuretic and metolazone is often unpredictable owing to the erratic pattern of absorption for metolazone. Achieving adequate systemic concentrations of metolazone to potentiate a loop diuretic may require multiple doses and thus several hours to days of dosing. In the instance of the patient unable to take oral medications, intravenous chlorothiazide (500 to 1000 mg) may be used together with a loop diuretic. Cost considerations make intravenous chlorothiazide add-on therapy less compelling than loop diuretic therapy with metolazone in the patient able to take in oral medications.

In the ambulatory setting when circumstances are typically less pressing, a starting dose of between 2.5 and 5.0 mg of metolazone daily or every other day can be given together with a loop diuretic. With the initiation of combination therapy, the dosage of a loop diuretic is generally kept constant until a response is evident. Once a diuretic response occurs, the frequency of administration of metolazone can be decreased, and oftentimes the loop diuretic dose can be lowered. In all instances, careful monitoring of the achieved diuretic response is warranted to avoid overdiuresis and/or significant electrolyte depletion. If either occurs, both drugs should be discontinued and therapeutic measures instituted in anticipation of a continuing diuresis, as the plasma half-life of metolazone is variably prolonged when kidney function is reduced.

Diuretic Infusions

Pharmacokinetic and pharmacodynamic considerations have suggested hypothetical advantages to the continuous infusion of a loop diuretic compared with bolus therapy in the diuretic-resistant patient; however, the studies addressing any such differences between infusion and bolus therapy generally have been quite heterogeneous and confounded by variables of study size, level of kidney function, prevailing BPs, concomitant vasoactive therapies, and differing primary disease states. Some clarity, however, has been given to this controversy in recent studies in acute decompensated HF comparing bolus to intravenous furosemide wherein those receiving a continuous infusion of furosemide fared no better in terms of global symptom assessment. However, patients who received bolus furosemide therapy had, if anything, worsened kidney function, and the use of loop diuretic infusions became a matter of personal preference.

Albumin and Furosemide Coadministration

In the patient with edema and hypoalbuminemia consideration has been given as how best to administer a loop diuretic such as furosemide. Two options exist: giving albumin and furosemide as separate infusions or *ex vivo* premixing both in a syringe. If separate albumin infusions and intravenous furosemide are considered, then candidates for use should be severely hypoalbuminemic patients in whom aggressively applied traditional approaches have failed to elicit an adequate diuresis. Albumin has been shown to exert maximal effect of intravascular volume expansion within 30 to 60 minutes of administration, and this should be considered if this approach is taken, even with its not having been reproducibly shown to be better than loop diuretic therapy alone. In addition, premixed loop diuretic and albumin in a syringe has been studied in cirrhotic patients with ascites (40 mg of furosemide and 25 g of albumin premixed ex vivo vs. 40 mg of furosemide alone), but the ex vivo admixture approach did not improve the natriuretic response; thus this too is not a worthwhile approach.

Hypertonic Saline and Loop Diuretic Therapy

This combination may seem counterintuitive based on the presence of the already volume-expanded state that typifies diuretic resistance. In point of fact owing to its osmotic effect, the hypertonic saline causes a rapid mobilization of fluids from the third space into the vascular compartment that transiently compensates for disease state–related vascular "underfilling." Ensuing improvement in systemic and renal hemodynamics improves the chance of a response to an administered diuretic as evidenced by an upward and leftward shift in the loop diuretic dose-response curve. As an example, one such regimen used furosemide (250 to 1000 mg/bid i.v.) plus hypertonic saline (150 mL H_2O with NaCl 1.4% to 4.6%) and was shown to be a safe and effective alternative to repeated paracentesis when treating hospitalized patients with cirrhosis and otherwise refractory ascites.

Nesiritide and Loop Diuretic Therapy

Early on in its development, nesiritide had been suggested to enhance the natriuretic effect of loop-diuretic therapy. This premise derives from the generally favorable effect of nesiritide on cardiac hemodynamics, as well as its positive effects on the neurohormonal profile that typifies HF. Recent studies in stable HF patients have shown, however, that nesiritide and furosemide used together afford no incremental benefit for Na^+ excretion compared with furosemide given alone. This may relate to a nesiritide-related fall in BP and therein a reduction in tubular delivery of furosemide to its effect site. Nesiritide should be reserved as a last step in trying to enhance diuretic action in the patient with diuretic resistance. In such patients, however, pretherapy BP should be high enough that any ensuing reduction in BP does not unfavorably influence the varied aspects of diuretic action.

Vasopressin Receptor Antagonists

These drugs increase free H_2O clearance more so than enhancing Na^+ excretion. As a class, these agents have been considered for addition to loop diuretic–based regimens to intensify overall diuretic effect without concern for worsening of neurohumoral status or an adverse effect on RBF or GFR. Agents in this class do not have a well-established role in the outpatient management of the patient with diuretic resistance unless development of hyponatremia is limiting the use of more conventional combination diuretic therapy. Of note, costing considerations can come into play with the outpatient use of these drugs.

SPECIAL CONSIDERATIONS IN EDEMA MANAGEMENT

ISOLATED ULTRAFILTRATION

In certain patients with diuretic-resistant edema, isolated peripheral venovenous ultrafiltration (UF) may be of some use, particularly in the patient with acute/chronic decompensated HF. This approach is now readily available at the bedside with much more simplified technology. Studies suggest that UF, particularly in acute decompensated HF, may allow for more effective fluid removal compared with a high-dose diuretic therapy approach, with improved quality of life, more rapid symptomatic improvement, and longer out-of-hospital stays. Questions of note with this approach include whether the beneficial effects, such as the improvement in volume status and an observed decrease in neurohormonal activation, are enduring phenomena following a several-day course of UF therapy. It also remains open to further investigation as to the degree to which previous diuretic resistance is lessened following a several-day course of UF therapy.

END-STAGE KIDNEY DISEASE

In a subset of end-stage kidney disease (ESKD) patients whose intake between dialysis sessions is inordinately high, the interdialytic weight gain is significant. Such patients are candidates for loop diuretic therapy if sufficient residual kidney function exists to allow for a meaningful diuretic response. If loop diuretic therapy is to be considered in the patient undergoing hemodialysis, then high doses or combination diuretic therapy is generally required if a clinically relevant diuresis is to be achieved. Loop diuretic use may lessen interdialytic weight gain and can make reaching target weight easier. Patients with residual kidney function (urine output greater than 200 cc per day) on diuretic therapy are almost twice as likely to retain residual kidney function after 1 year as are patients not receiving loop diuretics.

DIALYTIC REMOVAL

Because of the typically high plasma protein binding common to all loop diuretics, less than 10% of the total body stores of any of the loop diuretics are eliminated during a routine hemodialysis session. Accordingly, diuretic dosing in the ESKD patient with some residual kidney function can occur without any concern as to meaningful extracorporeal clearance.

DIURETIC-RELATED ADVERSE EVENTS

Diuretic-related side effects can be divided into those with recognizable mechanisms, such as electrolyte and/or metabolic aberrations, and those that are more obscure mechanistically, such as impotence or idiosyncratic drug reactions. Electrolyte changes are the most common side effects with diuretics and ostensibly most noticeable with the more potent loop diuretics, but the strength of a diuretic is likely not as critical as might be its duration of action. For example, thiazide-type diuretics, such as chlorthalidone and metolazone, while less potent than a loop diuretic, can still cause significant hypokalemia and hypomagnesemia owing to their long-lived duration of action.

HYPONATREMIA

Hyponatremia is a potentially serious complication of diuretic therapy. Thiazide diuretics are more apt to cause hyponatremia than loop diuretics in that they increase Na^+ excretion and preclude maximal urine dilution while leaving unimpeded the kidney's inherent concentrating ability. Not all thiazide diuretics are the same in their likelihood to lead to hyponatremia. Those treated with chlorthalidone are 1.7 times more likely to be hospitalized with hyponatremia than those

prescribed HCTZ. Elderly women treated with thiazide diuretics are most frequently affected, and the onset of hyponatremia is usually within the first few weeks of therapy. Withholding diuretics, restricting free H_2O intake, and normalizing serum K^+ values if hypokalemia exists can treat mild asymptomatic hyponatremia. Severe symptomatic hyponatremia complicated by seizures requires emergent correction, although too rapid or overcorrection of the hyponatremia should be avoided as central pontine myelinolysis has occurred in such situations. The optimal rate at which serum Na^+ is corrected in the diuretic-induced hyponatremic patient is still a matter of some debate.

HYPOKALEMIA AND HYPERKALEMIA

Hypokalemia is a common finding in patients treated with loop and/or thiazide diuretics. Mechanisms that contribute to hypokalemia with diuretic use include enhanced flow-dependent K^+ secretion in the distal nephron, a fall in luminal Cl^- concentration in the distal tubule, metabolic alkalosis, and stimulation of aldosterone and/or vasopressin release, both of which promote distal K^+ secretion. It is unusual for serum K^+ values to drop to less than 3.0 mmol/L in diuretic-treated outpatients, apart from there being a very high dietary Na^+ intake, a long-acting diuretic being given as is the case with chlorthalidone or metolazone, or in the presence of hyperaldosteronism. Although diuretic-induced hypokalemia in the range of 3.0 to 3.5 mmol/L can be associated with increased ventricular ectopy and altered glucose homeostasis, the cardiac ramifications of mild diuretic-induced hypokalemia are still debated. Profound degrees of hypokalemia with serum K^+ concentrations less than 2.5 mmol/L, however, can lead to generalized muscle weakness, torsades de pointes, and at the extremes, rhabdomyolysis and accompanying AKI.

Potassium-sparing diuretics, such as triamterene and amiloride, and mineralocorticoid-receptor antagonists, such as spironolactone and eplerenone, reduce urinary K^+ and Mg^{++} excretion when it might otherwise increase with either thiazide or loop diuretic therapy. In certain instances, significant K^+ retention occurs with K^+-sparing diuretics that hyperkalemia ensues. Hyperkalemia with K^+-sparing diuretics is usually encountered in patients with other risk factors including a preexisting reduction in GFR, the occurrence of acute-on-chronic kidney failure, use of K^+ supplements or salt substitutes, treatment with an angiotensin-converting enzyme (ACE) inhibitor or an angiotensin receptor blocker, NSAID use, or in the presence of metabolic acidosis/hyporeninemic hypoaldosteronism. The administration of trimethoprim-sulfamethoxazole (Bactrim) or heparin therapy, inclusive of subcutaneous heparin regimens, can also reduce urinary K^+ excretion and therein lead to the development of hyperkalemia.

ACID-BASE CHANGES

Mild metabolic alkalosis is a not uncommon feature of thiazide diuretic therapy, particularly at higher doses. Severe metabolic alkalosis is more often seen with loop diuretic use. The generation of a metabolic alkalosis with diuretic therapy is largely due to contraction of the ECF space affected by urinary losses of a relatively HCO_3^- free fluid. Diuretic-induced metabolic alkalosis is corrected with administration of K^+

and/or Na^+ Cl^-, although the latter may be unworkable in already volume-expanded patients, such as those with HF. In such circumstances, a K^+-sparing diuretic or a CA inhibitor, such as acetazolamide, may be considered for use. Acetazolamide use under these circumstances is often empiric with limited information as to dose-response relationships. Metabolic alkalosis can also lessen the natriuretic response to a loop diuretic, a factor of some particular relevance to the diuretic-resistant patient. All K^+-sparing diuretics can cause metabolic acidosis, an occurrence of most significance to the elderly and/or CKD patient. It may take several days for acid-base balance to be restored after discontinuation of a K^+-sparing diuretic.

HYPOMAGNESEMIA

Loop diuretics inhibit Mg^{++} reabsorption in the loop of Henle, a site where about 30% of the filtered load of Mg^{++} is reabsorbed. All K^+-sparing diuretics also diminish the heightened Mg^{++} excretion that arises from thiazide or loop diuretic use. Cellular Mg^{++} depletion occurs in 20% to 50% of patients in the course of thiazide therapy, particularly with long-acting thiazide-type diuretics such as chlorthalidone, and can be present notwithstanding an otherwise normal serum Mg^{++}. Hypomagnesemia-related symptoms include depression and muscle weakness, as well as nystagmus, tetany, and positive Chvostek and Trousseau signs. Refractory hypokalemia, as well as hypocalcemia, and an array of atrial/ventricular arrhythmias can occur, with torsades de pointes being a particularly troubling finding. Many of these abnormalities and, in particular, refractory hypokalemia and hypocalcemia correct quickly with small amounts of Mg^{++} replacement.

HYPERURICEMIA

Thiazide diuretic therapy dose dependently increases serum urate concentrations by as much as 35%, an effect related to reduced renal clearance of urate and one that is most conspicuous in those with high pretherapy urate clearance values. Decreased urate clearance may be linked to increased urate reabsorption secondary to diuretic-related ECF volume depletion and/or competition for its tubular secretion because both diuretics and urate undergo tubular secretion by the same organic anion transporter pathway. Hyperuricemia itself has been linked to new-onset hypertension, CV events, and perhaps the development and progression of CKD. It is unclear as to the level of association of these items to hyperuricemia stemming from diuretic therapy. Serum uric acid levels probably should be regularly monitored in diuretic-treated patients as it relates to its implied risk as a marker for CV disease.

HYPERGLYCEMIA

Prolonged thiazide diuretic therapy impairs glucose tolerance and can lead to the development of diabetes mellitus. Hyperglycemia/glucose intolerance has been linked to diuretic-induced hypokalemia, which inhibits insulin secretion by β cells. Diuretic-associated glucose intolerance appears to be dose dependent, less frequent with loop diuretics, and in many cases reversible upon withdrawal of the agent. In the Systolic Hypertension in the Elderly Program, the risk

of new-onset diabetes with the diuretic chlorthalidone was 45% higher for each 0.5-mEq/L drop in serum K^+. Although the data on reversibility in HCTZ-treated patients appear conflicting, long-term thiazide therapy can be looked at as causing only minor changes, if any at all, in fasting serum glucose concentration, an effect that might be reversed with the concurrent use of a K^+-sparing diuretic.

HYPERLIPIDEMIA

Short-term thiazide diuretic therapy can dose dependently elevate serum total cholesterol levels, modestly increase low-density lipoprotein cholesterol, and raise triglyceride levels, while minimally changing high-density lipoprotein cholesterol concentrations. All diuretics, including loop diuretics, cause these lipid changes, with the possible exception of indapamide. The mechanism of diuretic-induced dyslipidemia remains uncertain, but it has been ascribed to insulin resistance and/or reflex activation of the RAAS and SNS consequent to a decrease in plasma volume. Several long-term studies with thiazide diuretics have shown cholesterol levels return to their respective baseline at 1 year.

OTOTOXICITY

Loop diuretics are well established as ototoxic agents. Loop diuretics are direct inhibitors of the $Na^+/K^+/2Cl^-$ cotransport system, which also exists in the marginal and dark cells of the stria vascularis and are responsible for endolymph secretion. The ototoxicity of these agents may be due to variations in the ionic composition and endolymph volume. Loop diuretic-induced ototoxicity usually occurs within 20 minutes of infusion and is typically reversible, although permanent deafness has been reported, particularly with ethacrynic acid. Ototoxicity is clearly related to both the rate of infusion and the peak serum concentrations of a diuretic and appears to be a more likely occurrence with furosemide than bumetanide. In general, ototoxicity can be minimized by slow continuous infusion (<4 mg/min) rather than bolus injection and use of divided oral dose regimens. Furosemide serum concentrations being maintained less than 50 μg/mL reduce the risk of ototoxicity; however, furosemide concentrations are not readily available and can only be interpretatively applied in a retrospective manner in the patient who developed ototoxicity. Patients with kidney failure and those receiving concomitant aminoglycoside therapy are at greatest risk of developing ototoxicity with furosemide.

DRUG ALLERGY

Photosensitivity dermatitis occurs rarely in the course of treatment with furosemide or a thiazide diuretic. HCTZ more commonly causes photosensitivity than do the other thiazides. Acute allergic interstitial nephritis (AIN) with fever, rash, and eosinophilia, although an uncommon complication of diuretics, can cause permanent kidney failure if the drug exposure is sufficiently prolonged. This phenomenon may be abrupt in its development or more insidious, occurring months after therapy is begun with a thiazide diuretic or, less commonly, with furosemide. Not uncommonly, early changes in kidney function in the diuretic-treated patient with AIN can be mistakenly attributed to diuretic-related volume changes and in so doing allow the allergic process to proceed in an unrestrained manner. The chemical structure of ethacrynic acid differs from that of the other loop diuretics and makes it a nontoxic replacement in patients having experienced diuretic-related allergic complications.

ADVERSE DRUG INTERACTIONS

Loop diuretics can increase the likelihood of aminoglycoside nephrotoxicity. By causing hypokalemia and/or hypomagnesemia, diuretics in general increase digitalis toxicity. Plasma lithium (Li$^+$) concentrations can increase with diuretic therapy if significant volume contraction occurs; however, this is a variable and somewhat unpredictable phenomenon. Li$^+$ levels should be carefully monitored in those patients receiving Li$^+$ in conjunction with diuretics. NSAIDs can dose dependently antagonize the effects of diuretics and predispose diuretic-treated patients to a generally reversible form of AKI that is nonproteinuric in nature. The combination of indomethacin and triamterene may be particularly hazardous in that a prolonged form of AKI can occur. Triamterene can also induce crystal formations that are brown, spherical, and assume a Maltese cross appearance under polarized light with crystal formation prevented with alkalization of urine to a pH of ≥7.5. Kidney stone formation is less common with triamterene use than is crystalluria. This phenomenon is unique to triamterene among K$^+$-sparing diuretics. A typically reversible form of kidney failure may also develop in RAAS-inhibitor-treated patients who are excessively diuresed.

BIBLIOGRAPHY

Brater DC. Diuretic therapy. *N Engl J Med.* 1998;339:387-395.

Chalasani N, Gorski JC, Horlander JC, Craven R, Hoen H, Maya J, Brater DC. Effects of albumin/furosemide mixtures on responses to furosemide in hypoalbuminemic patients. *J Am Soc Nephrol.* 2001;12:1010-1016.

Costanzo MR, Ronco C. Isolated ultrafiltration in heart failure patients. *Curr Cardiol Rep.* 2012;14:254-264.

Felker GM, Lee KL, Bull DA, Redfield MM, Stevenson LW, Goldsmith SR, LeWinter MM, Deswal A, Rouleau JL, Ofili EO, Anstrom KJ, Hernandez AF, McNulty SE, Velazquez EJ, Kfoury AG, Chen HH, Givertz MM, Semigran MJ, Bart BA, Mascette AM, Braunwald E, O'Connor CM, NHLBI Heart Failure Clinical Research Network. Diuretic strategies in patients with acute decompensated heart failure. *N Engl J Med.* 2011;364:797-805.

Fliser D, Schröter M, Neubeck M, Ritz E. Co-administration of thiazides increases the efficacy of loop diuretics even in patients with advanced renal failure. *Kidney Int.* 1994;46:482-488.

Freda BJ, Slawsky M, Mallidi J, Braden GL. Decongestive treatment of acute decompensated heart failure: cardiorenal implications of ultrafiltration and diuretics. *Am J Kidney Dis.* 2011;58:1005-1017.

Goldsmith SR, Gilbertson DT, Mackedanz SA, Swan SK. Renal effects of conivaptan, furosemide, and the combination in patients with chronic heart failure. *J Card Fail.* 2011;17:982-989.

Hari P, Bagga A. Co-administration of albumin and furosemide in patients with the nephrotic syndrome. *Saudi J Kidney Dis Transpl.* 2012;23:371-372.

Hix JK, Silver S, Sterns RH. Diuretic-associated hyponatremia. *Semin Nephrol.* 2011;31:553-566.

Karadsheh F, Weir MR. Thiazide and thiazide-like diuretics: an opportunity to reduce blood pressure in patients with advanced kidney disease. *Curr Hypertens Rep.* 2012;14:416-420.

Kassamali R, Sica D. Acetazolamide—a forgotten diuretic agent. *Cardiol Rev.* 2011;19:276-278.

Rosner MH, Gupta R, Ellison D, Okusa MD. Management of cirrhotic ascites: physiological basis of diuretic action. *Eur J Intern Med.* 2006;17:8-19.

Shankar SS, Brater DC. Loop diuretics: from the Na-K-2Cl transporter to clinical use. *Am J Physiol Renal Physiol.* 2003;284:F11-F21.

Sica DA. Metolazone and its role in edema management. *Congest Heart Fail.* 2003;9:100-105.

Sica DA. Diuretic use in chronic kidney disease. *Nat Rev Nephrol.* 2011;8:100-109.

Sica DA, Gehr TW. Diuretic combinations in refractory oedema states: pharmacokinetic-pharmacodynamic relationships. *Clin Pharmacokinet.* 1996;30:229-249.

Sica DA, Gehr TW. Diuretic use in stage five chronic kidney disease and end-stage renal disease. *Curr Opin Nephrol Hypertens.* 2003;12:483-490.

Tuttolomondo A, Pinto A, Parrinello G, Licata G. Intravenous high-dose furosemide and hypertonic saline solutions for refractory heart failure and ascites. *Semin Nephrol.* 2011;31:513-522.

Wilcox CS. New insights into diuretic use in the patient with chronic renal disease. *J Am Soc Nephrol.* 2002;13:798-805.

Zillich AJ, Garg J, Basu S, Bakris GL, Carter BL. Thiazide diuretics, potassium, and the development of diabetes: a quantitative review. *Hypertension.* 2006;48:219-224.

Disorders of Potassium Metabolism

10

Michael Allon

MECHANISMS OF POTASSIUM HOMEOSTASIS

Total body potassium is about 3500 mmol. Approximately 98% of this total is intracellular, primarily in skeletal muscle, and to a lesser extent in the liver. The remaining 2% (about 70 mmol) is in the extracellular fluid. Two homeostatic systems help maintain potassium homeostasis. The first system regulates potassium excretion from the kidney and gut. The second regulates potassium shifts between the extracellular and intracellular fluid compartments.

EXTERNAL POTASSIUM BALANCE

The average American diet contains about 100 mmol (4 g) of potassium per day. Dietary potassium intake may vary widely from day to day. To stay in potassium balance, it is necessary to increase potassium excretion when dietary potassium increases and decrease potassium excretion when dietary potassium decreases. Normally the kidneys excrete 90% to 95% of dietary potassium, with the remaining 5% to 10% excreted by the gut. Potassium excretion by the kidney is a relatively slow process, taking 6 to 12 hours to eliminate an acute load.

RENAL HANDLING OF POTASSIUM

To understand the physiologic factors that determine renal excretion of potassium, it is critical to review the main features of tubular potassium handling. Plasma potassium is freely filtered across the glomerular capillary into the proximal tubule. It is subsequently completely reabsorbed by the proximal tubule and loop of Henle. In the distal tubule and the collecting duct, potassium is secreted into the tubular lumen. For practical purposes, urinary excretion of potassium reflects potassium secretion into the lumen of the distal tubule and collecting duct. Thus any factor that stimulates potassium secretion increases urinary potassium excretion; conversely, any factor that inhibits potassium secretion decreases urinary potassium excretion.

PHYSIOLOGIC REGULATION OF RENAL POTASSIUM EXCRETION

Five major physiologic factors stimulate distal potassium secretion (i.e., increase excretion): aldosterone, high distal sodium delivery, high urine flow rate, high [K^+] in tubular cell, and metabolic alkalosis (Table 10.1). Aldosterone directly increases the activity of Na^+/K^+-adenosine triphosphatase (ATPase) in the collecting duct cells, thereby stimulating secretion of potassium into the tubular lumen. Medical conditions that impair aldosterone production or secretion (e.g., diabetic nephropathy, chronic interstitial nephritis) or drugs that inhibit aldosterone production or action (e.g., nonsteroidal antiinflammatory drugs [NSAIDs], angiotensin converting enzyme [ACE] inhibitors, angiotensin receptor blockers [ARBs], heparin, spironolactone) decrease potassium secretion by the kidney. Conversely, medical conditions associated with increased aldosterone levels (primary hyperaldosteronism, secondary hyperaldosteronism due to diuretics or vomiting) increase potassium loss in the urine. Although there is profound secondary hyperaldosteronism in congestive heart failure and cirrhosis, each of these conditions may be associated with hyperkalemia because of decreased delivery of sodium to the distal nephron. Many diuretics increase renal potassium excretion by a number of mechanisms, including high distal sodium delivery, high urine flow rate, metabolic alkalosis, and hyperaldosteronism due to volume depletion. Poorly controlled diabetes commonly increases urinary potassium excretion due to osmotic diuresis with high urinary flow rate and high distal delivery of sodium.

Reabsorption of sodium in the collecting duct occurs through selective sodium channels. This creates an electronegative charge within the tubular lumen relative to the tubular epithelial cell. This in turn promotes secretion of cations (K^+ and H^+) into the lumen. Therefore drugs that block the sodium channel in the collecting duct decrease potassium secretion. Conversely, in Liddle syndrome, a rare genetic disorder in which the sodium channel is constitutively open, avid sodium reabsorption results in excessive potassium secretion.

ADAPTATION IN CHRONIC KIDNEY DISEASE

In patients with chronic kidney disease (CKD), three major mechanisms protect against hyperkalemia: (1) increased renal potassium excretion mediated by aldosterone, (2) increased intestinal potassium excretion, and (3) increased potassium excretion per nephron. The kidney compensates for reduced nephron number in CKD by increasing the efficiency of potassium excretion. Clearly there is a limit to kidney compensation, and a significant loss of kidney function impairs the ability to excrete potassium, thereby predisposing to a positive potassium balance and a tendency toward hyperkalemia. In most patients with CKD, overt hyperkalemia

Table 10.1   Physiologic Factors Increasing Renal Potassium Excretion

Factor	Mechanism	Medical Conditions Affecting It	Drugs Affecting It
Aldosterone	Increase Na$^+$/K$^+$-ATPase activity in collecting duct	Diabetic nephropathy Interstitial nephritis Primary hyperaldosteronism Secondary hyperaldosteronism	NSAIDs ACE inhibitors ARB Heparin Spironolactone
Distal Na$^+$ delivery	Create electrochemical gradient	Uncontrolled diabetes	Loop diuretics Thiazide diuretics
Urine flow	Increase concentration gradient	Uncontrolled diabetes	Loop diuretics Thiazide diuretics
Tubular [K$^+$]	Increase concentration gradient	Hyperkalemia	—
Metabolic alkalosis	Decreased proximal Na$^+$ reabsorption	Primary hyperaldosteronism	Loop diuretics Thiazide diuretics

ACE, Angiotensin converting enzyme; *ARB*, angiotensin receptor blocker; *NSAIDs*, nonsteroidal antiinflammatory drugs.

does not occur until the glomerular filtration rate (GFR) falls below 10 mL/min. Serum aldosterone levels are elevated in many patients with CKD. Aldosterone stimulates the activity of both Na$^+$/K$^+$-ATPase and H$^+$/K$^+$-ATPase, thereby promoting secretion of potassium in the collecting duct and defending against hyperkalemia. These adaptive mechanisms are less effective in patients with acute kidney injury (AKI) as compared with CKD. Moreover, patients with AKI are often hypotensive, resulting in hypoperfusion and release of potassium from ischemic tissues. For these reasons, severe hyperkalemia occurs more frequently in patients with AKI as compared with those with CKD.

A subset of patients with CKD fail to increase aldosterone levels appreciably; as a result, they develop hyperkalemia at moderate levels of GFR loss (<50 mL/min), typically in association with nonanion gap metabolic acidosis (type IV renal tubular acidosis). This condition is most commonly encountered with diabetic nephropathy and chronic interstitial nephritis. Moreover, administration of drugs that inhibit aldosterone production or secretion (e.g., ACE inhibitors, ARBs, NSAIDs, heparin) may provoke hyperkalemia in patients with mild to moderate CKD.

INTESTINAL POTASSIUM EXCRETION

Like the renal collecting duct, the small intestine and colon secrete potassium in response to aldosterone. In normal individuals, intestinal potassium excretion plays a minor role in potassium homeostasis, accounting for about 10% of total potassium excretion. However, in patients with significant GFR loss, intestinal potassium secretion is increased three- to fourfold with a significant contribution to potassium homeostasis. This adaptation is limited and is inadequate to compensate for the loss of excretory function in patients with advanced kidney failure.

INTERNAL POTASSIUM BALANCE

Extracellular fluid [K$^+$] is approximately 4 mEq/L, whereas the intracellular [K$^+$] is approximately 150 mEq/L. Because of the uneven distribution of potassium between the fluid compartments, a relatively small net shift of potassium from the intracellular to the extracellular fluid compartment produces marked increases in plasma potassium. Conversely,

a relatively small net shift from the extracellular to the intracellular fluid compartment produces a marked decrease in plasma potassium. Unlike renal excretion of potassium that requires several hours, potassium shift between the extracellular and intracellular fluid compartment (also referred to as extrarenal potassium disposal) is extremely rapid, occurring within minutes.

Clearly, in patients with advanced kidney failure whose capacity to excrete potassium is marginal, extrarenal potassium disposal plays a critical role in the prevention of life-threatening hyperkalemia following potassium-rich meals. The following example will illustrate this important principle. Suppose that a 70-kg anephric patient with a serum potassium of 4.5 mmol/L eats 1 cup of pinto beans, which contains 35 mmol of potassium. Initially, the dietary potassium is absorbed into the extracellular fluid compartment (20% × 70 kg = 14 L). This amount of dietary potassium will increase the serum potassium by 2.5 mmol/L (35 mmol/14 L). In the absence of extrarenal potassium disposal, the patient's serum potassium would rise acutely to 7.0 mmol/L, a level frequently associated with serious ventricular arrhythmias. In practice, the increase in serum potassium is much smaller because of efficient physiologic mechanisms that promote potassium shifts into the intracellular fluid compartment.

EFFECTS OF INSULIN AND CATECHOLAMINES ON EXTRARENAL POTASSIUM DISPOSAL

The two major physiologic factors that stimulate transfer of potassium from the extracellular to the intracellular fluid compartments are insulin and epinephrine. The stimulation of extrarenal potassium disposal by insulin and beta-2 adrenergic agonists is mediated by stimulation of the Na$^+$/K$^+$-ATPase activity, primarily in skeletal muscle cells. Interference with these two physiologic mechanisms (insulin deficiency or beta-2 adrenergic blockade, respectively) predisposes to hyperkalemia. On the other hand, excessive insulin or epinephrine levels predispose to hypokalemia.

The potassium-lowering effect of insulin is dose-related within the physiologic range of plasma insulin, and is independent of its effect on plasma glucose. Even the low physiologic levels of insulin present during fasting promote extrarenal potassium disposal. In nondiabetic individuals, hyperglycemia stimulates endogenous insulin secretion, thereby decreasing the serum potassium. In insulin-dependent diabetics, endogenous insulin production is limited, and significant hyperglycemia may occur. Hyperglycemia results in plasma hypertonicity, which promotes potassium shifts out of the cells and produces paradoxic hyperkalemia.

The potassium-lowering action of epinephrine is mediated by beta-2 adrenergic stimulation and is blocked by nonselective beta-blockers but not by selective beta-1 adrenergic blockers. Alpha-adrenergic stimulation promotes shifts of potassium *out of cells* into the extracellular fluid compartment, leading to an increase in serum potassium. Epinephrine is a mixed alpha-adrenergic and beta-adrenergic agonist, such that its net effect on serum potassium reflects the balance between its beta-adrenergic (potassium-lowering) and alpha-adrenergic (potassium-raising) effects. In normal individuals, the beta-adrenergic effect of epinephrine predominates over the alpha-adrenergic effect, such that the serum potassium decreases. In contrast, the alpha-adrenergic effect of epinephrine on potassium shifts is much more prominent in patients with severe kidney failure; as a result, patients undergoing dialysis are refractory to the potassium-lowering effect of epinephrine.

EFFECT OF ACID-BASE DISORDERS ON EXTRARENAL POTASSIUM DISPOSAL

Acid-base disorders produce internal potassium shifts in a less predictable manner. As a general rule, metabolic alkalosis shifts potassium into cells, whereas metabolic acidosis shifts potassium out of cells. However, the nature of the metabolic acidosis determines its effect on serum potassium. Cells are relatively impermeable to chloride. With mineral acidoses, the entry of protons (but not chloride) into cells results in a reciprocal release of potassium from cells to maintain electroneutrality. In contrast, cells are highly permeable to organic anions. The addition of an organic acid to the extracellular fluid results in parallel shifts of protons and organic anions into the cells, with no net change in the electric balance; as a result, potassium is not released from cells. Thus mineral acidoses (i.e., hyperchloremic, normal anion gap metabolic acidosis) typically result in hyperkalemia, whereas organic metabolic acidoses (e.g., lactic acidosis) do not affect the serum potassium. Bicarbonate administration to individuals with normal kidney function decreases serum potassium, but this effect is largely due to enhanced urinary excretion of potassium. In contrast, bicarbonate administration to patients undergoing dialysis (in whom the capacity for urinary potassium excretion is negligible) does not lower plasma potassium acutely. Moreover, bicarbonate administration does not potentiate the potassium-lowering effects of insulin or albuterol in patients undergoing dialysis.

LABORATORY TESTS TO EVALUATE POTASSIUM DISORDERS

DIFFERENTIAL DIAGNOSIS OF HYPOKALEMIA AND HYPERKALEMIA

The clinical history, medication review, family history, and physical examination are sufficient to create a rapid differential diagnosis of most potassium disorders. In selected patients, the etiology of hypokalemia or hyperkalemia is not apparent, and additional specialized laboratory tests may be useful. Measurement of the fractional excretion of potassium (FE_K) may help distinguish between renal and nonrenal etiologies of hyperkalemia and hypokalemia. The general principle underlying this test is that the kidney compensates for hyperkalemia by increasing potassium excretion and compensates for hypokalemia by decreasing potassium excretion. In contrast, when potassium excretion is inappropriate for the serum potassium, this suggests a renal etiology. The optimal use of FE_K to inform the differential diagnosis requires that this value be obtained before the potassium abnormality (hyperkalemia or hypokalemia) is corrected.

FRACTIONAL EXCRETION OF POTASSIUM

FE_K is the percent of potassium filtered into the proximal tubule that appears in the urine. It represents potassium clearance corrected for GFR, or Cl_K/Cl_{Cr}. Since the clearance of any substance can be calculated from UV/P, this ratio can be algebraically transformed to:

$$[(U_K V/P_K)/(U_{Cr} V/P_{Cr})] \times 100\%$$

The V in the numerator and denominator cancel out, giving a simplified formula:

$$[(U_K/P_K)/(U_{Cr}/P_{Cr})] \times 100\%$$

where U_K and U_{Cr} are the concentrations of potassium and creatinine in the urine, respectively, and P_K and P_{Cr} are the corresponding serum concentrations. For an individual with normal kidney function on a typical dietary potassium intake, the FE_K is approximately 10%. When hypokalemia is a result of extrarenal causes (low potassium diet, gastrointestinal losses, potassium shifts into cells), the kidney conserves potassium and the FE_K is low. In contrast, hypokalemia due to renal potassium losses is associated with an increased FE_K. Similarly, in the setting of hyperkalemia, a high FE_K suggests an extrarenal etiology, whereas a low FE_K is consistent with a renal etiology. If a urine creatinine measurement is not available, one can often use U_K alone to differentiate between renal and extrarenal causes of hyperkalemia. Specifically, in a hypokalemic patient, $U_K > 20$ mEq/L suggests a renal etiology, whereas $U_K < 20$ mEq/L suggests an extrarenal etiology.

Several factors limit the utility of the FE_K in the differential diagnosis of potassium disorders. The FE_K is increased when dietary potassium is increased, and it is decreased when dietary potassium is decreased. Furthermore, in patients with CKD, there is an adaptive increase in potassium excretion per functioning nephron, such that FE_K increases. This means that the "normal" value for a given individual can vary substantially, making it difficult to determine the significance of a high or low FE_K.

HYPOKALEMIA

HYPOKALEMIA VERSUS POTASSIUM DEFICIENCY

It is important to distinguish between potassium deficiency and hypokalemia. Potassium deficiency is the state resulting from a persistent negative potassium balance (i.e., potassium excretion exceeding potassium intake). Hypokalemia refers to a low plasma potassium concentration. Hypokalemia can be due to either potassium deficiency (inadequate potassium intake or excessive potassium losses) or net potassium shifts from the extracellular to the intracellular fluid compartment. A patient may have severe potassium deficiency without manifesting hypokalemia. An important example is a patient presenting with diabetic ketoacidosis. Such patients have typically had severe hyperglycemia with osmotic diuresis for several days, leading to high levels of renal potassium excretion and potassium deficiency. However, as a result of insulin deficiency and hyperglycemia-induced hyperosmolality, there is a concomitant shift of potassium out of the cells into the extracellular fluid compartment. At presentation to the hospital, such patients are frequently normokalemic or even hyperkalemic. Once they are treated with exogenous insulin, there is a rapid shift of potassium back into the cells, and within a few hours the patients develop significant hypokalemia. Conversely, patients hospitalized with an acute myocardial infarction commonly have hypokalemia due to stress-induced catecholamine release and enhanced extrarenal potassium disposal, even though they have a normal external potassium balance.

CLINICAL DISORDERS ASSOCIATED WITH HYPOKALEMIA

Table 10.2 provides a list of the most common causes of hypokalemia. The kidney can avidly conserve potassium, such that hypokalemia due to inadequate potassium intake is a rare event requiring prolonged starvation ("tea and toast diet"). Therefore hypokalemia is usually due to excessive potassium losses from the gut or the kidney or to potassium shifts from the extracellular to the intracellular fluid compartments. Prolonged vomiting causes potassium losses, in part due to potassium present in gastric secretions (~10 mEq/L) but primarily due to renal losses because of secondary hyperaldosteronism from volume depletion. Severe diarrhea, either due to disease or laxative abuse, results in significant potassium excretion in the stool.

Hypokalemia due to excessive renal potassium losses is seen with a number of clinical syndromes. Conceptually, it is useful to classify hypokalemia as associated with hypertension or with normal blood pressure (Fig. 10.1). When hypokalemia

is associated with hypertension, measurements of plasma renin and aldosterone may be helpful in the differential diagnosis. Several physiologic observations are relevant in this regard. First, aldosterone, a mineralocorticoid, stimulates sodium reabsorption and potassium secretion in the collecting duct. Second, the physiologic stimulus for aldosterone secretion is activation of the renin-angiotensin axis. Moreover, aldosterone-induced sodium retention suppresses the renin-angiotensin axis by negative feedback. Third, glucocorticoids at high concentrations bind to mineralocorticoid receptors and mimic their physiologic actions. And fourth, glucocorticoids are stimulated by adrenocorticotropic

Table 10.2 Causes of Hypokalemia

Inadequate potassium intake (severe malnutrition)
Extrarenal potassium losses
- Vomiting
- Diarrhea
Hypokalemia due to urinary potassium losses
- Diuretics (loop diuretics, thiazides, acetazolamide)
- Osmotic diuresis (e.g., hyperglycemia)
- Hypokalemia with hypertension
  - Primary hyperaldosteronism
  - Glucocorticoid-remediable hypertension
  - Malignant hypertension
  - Renovascular hypertension
  - Renin-secreting tumor
  - Essential hypertension with excessive diuretics
  - Liddle syndrome
  - 11β hydroxysteroid dehydrogenase deficiency
    - Genetic
    - Drug induced (chewing tobacco, licorice, some French wines)
  - Congenital adrenal hyperplasia
- Hypokalemia with a normal blood pressure
  - Distal renal tubular acidosis (type I)
  - Proximal renal tubular acidosis (type II)
  - Bartter syndrome
  - Gitelman syndrome
  - Hypomagnesemia (cis-platinum, alcoholism, diuretics)
Hypokalemia due to potassium shifts
- Insulin administration
- Catecholamine excess (acute stress)
- Familial periodic hypokalemic paralysis
- Thyrotoxic hypokalemic paralysis

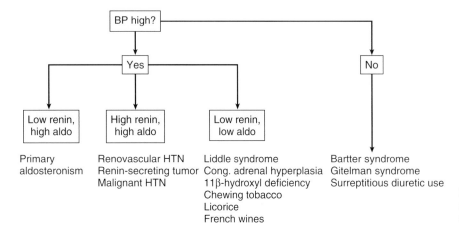

Fig. 10.1 Differential diagnosis of hypokalemia, using blood pressure (BP) and plasma renin and aldosterone (aldo). *HTN,* Hypertension.

hormone (ACTH) and suppress ACTH production by negative feedback.

Primary hyperaldosteronism is due to autonomous (non-renin-mediated) secretion of aldosterone by the adrenal cortex. This results in avid sodium retention and potassium secretion by the distal nephron. Patients present with volume-dependent hypertension, hypokalemia, and metabolic alkalosis. Biochemical evaluation reveals a *high serum aldosterone level and suppressed plasma renin*. An abdominal computed tomography (CT) scan reveals either a unilateral adrenal adenoma or bilateral adrenal hyperplasia. The former is treated surgically, and the latter with aldosterone antagonism. *Glucocorticoid-remediable hyperaldosteronism* (GRA) is a rare, autosomal dominant condition in which there is fusion of the 11β-hydroxylase and aldosterone synthase genes. As a result, aldosterone secretion is stimulated by ACTH; abnormally high levels of aldosterone result from physiologic levels of ACTH but can be suppressed by dexamethasone. Patients with GRA have a very similar clinical presentation to those with primary hyperaldosteronism (volume-dependent hypertension, hypokalemia, high serum aldosterone, and low serum renin), except that they are younger and have a family history of hypertension.

Patients with *renovascular hypertension, renin-secreting tumors,* and severe *malignant hypertension* may also present with severe hypertension and hypokalemia. In contrast to patients with primary hyperaldosteronism, these patients have secondary hyperaldosteronism (i.e., *high serum renin and aldosterone levels*). Of course, patients with essential hypertension may also have hypokalemia and high plasma renin and aldosterone levels if they are treated with loop or thiazide diuretics.

Patients with *11β-hydroxysteroid dehydrogenase deficiency,* a rare genetic disorder, have a defect in the conversion of cortisol to cortisone in the peripheral tissues. This results in high tissue cortisol levels that activate the mineralocorticoid receptors, producing hypokalemia and hypertension. Such patients have *low serum renin and aldosterone levels.* Chewing tobacco, certain brands of licorice, and some French red wines contain *glycyrrhizic acid,* which inhibits 11β-hydroxysteroid dehydrogenase. Ingestion of these foods may produce hypokalemia, volume-dependent hypertension, and low serum renin and aldosterone levels, similar to the clinical presentation of congenital 11β-hydroxysteroid dehydrogenase deficiency.

Patients with *congenital adrenal hyperplasia* have a deficiency of 11β-hydroxylase, an enzyme required in the common pathways for mineralocorticoids and glucocorticoids. These patients have low serum renin and aldosterone levels, high levels of DOCA (deoxycorticosterone acetate, a mineralocorticoid), and high levels of androgen. Boys exhibit early puberty, and girls exhibit virilization with hirsutism and clitoromegaly. This condition improves with exogenous corticosteroids to suppress ACTH.

Liddle syndrome is a rare autosomal dominant disorder caused by a defect of the sodium channel, such that there is increased sodium absorption and potassium secretion in the collecting duct. Patients present with hypokalemia, hypertension, and volume overload. Their biochemical profile reveals a *low serum renin and aldosterone.* The patients' blood pressure and serum potassium improve dramatically after inhibiting the sodium channel with amiloride.

Hypokalemia due to excessive renal potassium excretion is also seen in a number of clinical conditions in which hypertension is infrequent. Both distal (type I) and proximal (type II) renal tubular acidoses (RTA) are associated with kaliuresis and hypokalemia; both conditions present with a normal anion gap metabolic acidosis. *Distal RTAs* are frequently associated with hypercalciuria and calcium oxalate kidney stones. *Proximal RTAs* are rare in adults and often associated with a generalized defect in proximal tubular function (Fanconi syndrome), manifesting with glycosuria (with a normal serum glucose), hypophosphatemia with phosphaturia, and a low serum uric acid with uricosuria.

Bartter syndrome is a rare familial disease characterized by hypokalemia, metabolic alkalosis, hypercalciuria, normal blood pressure, and high plasma renin and aldosterone levels. Serum magnesium is usually normal. It has been associated with a number of mutations that inhibit active sodium reabsorption in the thick ascending limb of the loop of Henle, including mutations in the $Na^+/K^+/2Cl^-$-cotransporter, ClC-Kb, and ROMK (see Chapter 38). These patients act as if they are chronically ingesting loop diuretics; for this reason, they are difficult to distinguish clinically from patients with surreptitious diuretic ingestion. Patients with *Gitelman syndrome* differ in that they have hypocalciuria and hypomagnesemia. Gitelman syndrome has been linked to a mutation in the renal thiazide-sensitive Na^+/K^+-cotransporter. These patients act as if they are chronically ingesting thiazide diuretics.

Familial hypokalemic periodic paralysis is a rare, autosomal dominant disorder in which affected individuals develop periodic episodes of severe muscle weakness in association with profound hypokalemia, due to rapid shifts of potassium from the extracellular to the intracellular fluid compartment. Interestingly, even when the patient has complete paralysis, the diaphragm and bulbar muscles are spared, such that the patient is able to breathe, swallow, talk, and blink. The paralysis resolves within hours of potassium ingestion. The patients are asymptomatic with normal serum potassium levels in between the acute episodes. *Thyrotoxic hypokalemic paralysis* is an unusual manifestation of hyperthyroidism, seen primarily in Asian patients. The clinical presentation is similar to that of hypokalemic periodic paralysis, except that the paralytic episodes cease when the hyperthyroidism is corrected.

DRUG-INDUCED HYPOKALEMIA

A number of drugs have the potential to cause hypokalemia, either by stimulating renal potassium excretion or by blocking extrarenal disposal. Exogenous mineralocorticoids mimic the effects of aldosterone, thereby stimulating distal potassium secretion. High doses of glucocorticoids possess some mineralocorticoid activity and have a similar effect. Most *diuretics,* including loop diuretics, thiazide diuretics, and acetazolamide, increase renal potassium excretion. A number of drugs, including *alcohol, diuretics,* and cis-*platinum,* cause renal magnesium wasting and hypomagnesemia. For reasons that are not well understood, hypomagnesemia impairs renal potassium conservation. Thus these patients may have associated hypokalemia that is refractory to potassium supplementation until the magnesium deficit is corrected.

Drugs that promote extrarenal potassium disposal may also result in hypokalemia. This phenomenon can be seen after the administration of an acute dose of *insulin.* Similarly, *beta-2 agonists* (either intravenous or nebulized), including albuterol and terbutaline, frequently result in acute hypokalemia.

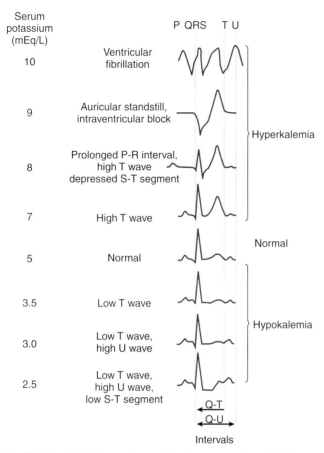

Fig. 10.2 Typical electrocardiographic changes associated with hypokalemia and hyperkalemia.

CLINICAL MANIFESTATIONS OF HYPOKALEMIA

Hypokalemia may produce electrocardiographic abnormalities, including a flattened T wave and a U wave (Fig. 10.2). Hypokalemia also appears to increase the risk of ventricular arrhythmias in patients with ischemic heart disease or patients taking digoxin. Severe hypokalemia is associated with variable degrees of skeletal muscle weakness, even to the point of paralysis. Rarely, diaphragmatic paralysis from hypokalemia can lead to respiratory arrest. There may also be decreased motility of smooth muscle, manifesting with ileus or urinary retention. Severe hypokalemia may occasionally produce rhabdomyolysis.

Severe hypokalemia also interferes with the urinary concentrating mechanism in the distal nephron, resulting in nephrogenic diabetes insipidus. Such patients have a low urine osmolality in the face of high serum osmolality and are refractory to vasopressin.

TREATMENT OF HYPOKALEMIA

The acute treatment of hypokalemia requires potassium supplementation, either intravenously or orally. The correlation between serum potassium and total potassium deficit in hypokalemic patients is quite poor. A given patient's serum potassium is a reflection of both external potassium balance and transcellular potassium shifts. The percent of administered exogenous potassium that remains in the extracellular fluid

compartment is variable. Thus it is difficult to predict how much potassium replacement will be required for a particular patient. If the patient is hypokalemic in the setting of potassium deficiency, a large amount of potassium replacement is needed. In contrast, hypokalemia that is primarily due to transcellular potassium shifts requires relatively little potassium repletion. Without adequate monitoring, it is possible to give too much potassium and make the patient hyperkalemic. Therefore one should give multiple small doses of potassium, with frequent checks of serum potassium values.

Oral potassium administration is safer than the intravenous route and less likely to produce an overshoot in the serum potassium. Each oral dose should not exceed 20 to 40 mEq of potassium. Intravenous potassium chloride should be reserved for severe, symptomatic hypokalemia (<3.0 mEq/L) or for patients who cannot ingest oral potassium. Intravenous potassium chloride should not be given any faster than 10 mmol/hour in the absence of continuous EKG monitoring. The serum potassium should be rechecked every 2 to 3 hours to confirm a clinical response and avoid an overshoot.

Correction of the underlying medical condition may prevent recurrence of hypokalemia after its correction. If the patient has a chronic condition associated with persistent urinary potassium losses, such that hypokalemia is likely to recur, the patient should be encouraged to increase the intake of foods high in potassium (especially fresh fruits, nuts, and legumes). In some patients, chronic oral potassium supplementation may be necessary.

HYPERKALEMIA

Pseudohyperkalemia is a factitious elevation of the serum potassium caused by in vitro release of potassium from blood cells or platelets. It may be seen with in vitro hemolysis, thrombocytosis, or severe leukocytosis. Pseudohyperkalemia due to hemolysis is readily apparent because the serum is pink. Pseudohyperkalemia due to severe thrombocytosis or leukocytosis can be confirmed by drawing simultaneous blood samples in tubes with and without anticoagulant; if potassium in the latter (serum) is higher than in the former (plasma), the diagnosis is confirmed.

True hyperkalemia is caused by a positive potassium balance (increased potassium intake or decreased potassium excretion) or an increase in net potassium shift from the intracellular to the extracellular fluid compartment. Table 10.3 provides a list of the most common causes of hyperkalemia. In practice, most patients who develop severe hyperkalemia have multiple contributory factors. For example, a patient with CKD due to diabetic nephropathy may be medicated with an ACE inhibitor and have mild hyperkalemia. However, when he is started on indomethacin for acute gouty arthritis, the patient rapidly develops severe hyperkalemia.

DRUG-INDUCED HYPERKALEMIA

A large number of drugs have the potential to cause hyperkalemia, either by inhibiting renal potassium excretion or by blocking extrarenal disposal (Table 10.4). Most individuals taking these drugs will not develop hyperkalemia. Patients with advanced CKD are at the highest risk, especially if they have a high dietary potassium intake or are taking additional

Table 10.3   Causes of Hyperkalemia

Pseudohyperkalemia
- Hemolysis
- Thrombocytosis
- Severe leukocytosis
- Fist clenching

Decreased renal excretion
- Acute or chronic kidney disease
- Aldosterone deficiency (e.g., type IV renal tubular acidosis) Frequently associated with diabetic nephropathy, chronic interstitial nephritis, or obstructive nephropathy
- Adrenal insufficiency (Addison disease)
- Drugs that inhibit potassium excretion
- Kidney diseases that impair distal tubule function
  - Sickle cell anemia
  - Systemic lupus erythematosus

Abnormal potassium distribution
- Insulin deficiency
- Beta-blockers
- Metabolic or respiratory acidosis
- Familial hyperkalemic periodic paralysis

Abnormal potassium release from cells
- Rhabdomyolysis
- Tumor lysis syndrome

Table 10.4   Mechanisms for Drug-Induced Hyperkalemia

Decrease renal potassium excretion
    Block sodium channel in the distal nephron
- Potassium-sparing diuretics: amiloride, triamterene
- Antibiotics: trimethoprim, pentamidine

    Block aldosterone production
- ACE inhibitors (e.g., captopril, enalapril, lisinopril, benazepril)
- Angiotensin receptor blockers
- NSAIDs and COX-2 inhibitors
- Heparin
- Tacrolimus

    Block aldosterone receptors
- Spironolactone
- Eplerenone

    Block Na^+/K^+-ATPase activity in the distal nephron
- Cyclosporine

Inhibit extrarenal potassium disposal
- Block beta-2 adrenergic–mediated extrarenal potassium disposal: nonselective beta-blockers (e.g., propranolol, nadolol, timolol)
- Block Na^+/K^+-ATPase activity in skeletal muscles: digoxin overdose (not therapeutic doses)
- Inhibit insulin release (e.g., somatostatin)

Potassium release from injured cells
- Drug-induced rhabdomyolysis (e.g., lovastatin, cocaine)
- Drug-induced tumor lysis syndrome (chemotherapy agents in acute leukemias and high-grade lymphomas)
- Depolarizing paralytic agents (e.g., succinylcholine)

Drug-induced acute kidney injury

ACE, Angiotensin converting enzyme; *NSAIDs,* nonsteroidal antiinflammatory drugs.

medication that predisposes to hyperkalemia. Most *diuretics* (loop diuretics, thiazide diuretics, acetazolamide) increase urinary potassium excretion and tend to cause hypokalemia. However, potassium-sparing diuretics inhibit urinary potassium excretion and predispose to hyperkalemia by one of two mechanisms. *Spironolactone* and *eplerenone* are competitive inhibitors of aldosterone; they bind to the aldosterone receptors in the collecting duct, thereby inhibiting Na^+/K^+-ATPase activity, and indirectly limiting potassium secretion. The immunosuppressive drug, *cyclosporine,* also blocks Na^+/K^+-ATPase activity in the distal nephron. Two other potassium-sparing diuretics, *amiloride* and *triamterene,* bind to the sodium channel in the collecting duct. This inhibits sodium reabsorption in the distal nephron and thereby limits the establishment of an electrochemical gradient required for potassium secretion. Interestingly, two antibiotics, *trimethoprim* (one of the components of Bactrim) and *pentamidine,* have also been shown to block the sodium channel in the collecting duct and therefore predispose patients to hyperkalemia. In addition, trimethoprim has been shown to inhibit the collecting tubule H^+/K^+-ATPase.

Because aldosterone plays an important role in enhancing renal potassium excretion in patients with kidney failure, drugs that inhibit aldosterone production (either directly or indirectly) predispose such patients to hyperkalemia. Angiotensin II is a potent stimulator of aldosterone production in the adrenal cortex. ACE inhibitors inhibit the production of angiotensin II, thereby decreasing aldosterone levels. Similarly, angiotensin II receptor blockers also inhibit aldosterone production. Prostaglandins stimulate renin production, and prostaglandin inhibitors (NSAIDs) inhibit the production of renin, thereby indirectly decreasing aldosterone production. This effect is seen even with "renal-sparing NSAIDs," such as sulindac (a nonselective COX-1 and COX-2 inhibitor). Hyperkalemia may also be caused by selective COX-2 inhibitors. Heparin has been shown to directly inhibit the production of aldosterone in the renal cortex, primarily by decreasing the number and affinity of angiotensin II receptors in the zona glomerulosa. This effect occurs even with the low doses of subcutaneous heparin or enoxaparin used for prophylaxis of venous thrombosis in hospitalized patients (e.g., 5000 units q12h). Tacrolimus, an immunosuppressant drug, may also cause hyperkalemia by inhibiting aldosterone synthesis. Oral contraceptives containing drospirenone (a progestin) inhibit renal potassium excretion and may provoke hyperkalemia in women with CKD.

Given the stimulation of extrarenal potassium disposal by beta-adrenergic agonists, it is not surprising that beta-2 antagonists can predispose to hyperkalemia. This effect is seen primarily with nonselective beta-blockers (e.g., propranolol, nadolol, carvedilol), rather than beta-selective blockers (e.g., atenolol, metoprolol). There is significant systemic absorption of topical beta-blockers, and severe hyperkalemia may rarely be provoked by timolol eye drops. Drugs inhibiting endogenous insulin release, such as *somatostatin,* have been rarely implicated as a cause of hyperkalemia in patients with kidney failure. Presumably, long-acting somatostatin analogs, such as octreotide, would have a similar effect on serum potassium. *Digoxin overdose* causes inhibition of Na^+/K^+-ATPase activity in skeletal muscle cells and may manifest with hyperkalemia. This effect is rarely seen at therapeutic doses of the drug. Depolarizing paralytic agents used for general anesthesia, such as *succinylcholine*, can occasionally produce hyperkalemia by causing potassium to leak out of the cells.

Finally, drugs can also induce hyperkalemia indirectly by causing release of intracellular potassium from injured cells (e.g., rhabdomyolysis with *statins* and *cocaine*, or tumor lysis syndrome when chemotherapy is administered in patients with acute leukemia or high-grade lymphoma). Moreover, drug-induced AKI may be associated with secondary hyperkalemia.

A common clinical dilemma occurs when patients with CKD develop hyperkalemia after being started on an ACE inhibitor or ARB. One would like to continue this drug due to its renoprotective benefit. Therapeutic options for this scenario include reducing the dose of ACE inhibitor or ARB, starting or increasing the dose of a loop or thiazide diuretic, discontinuing other medications that promote hyperkalemia, and reinforcing dietary potassium restriction. Fludrocortisone (0.1 to 0.2 mg daily) can be tried in refractory cases, although it may promote peripheral edema and hypertension resulting from avid sodium retention. Finally, the patient should be questioned about constipation, as the addition of laxatives may promote fecal potassium excretion.

FASTING HYPERKALEMIA IN PATIENTS UNDERGOING DIALYSIS

Prolonged fasting decreases plasma insulin concentrations, thereby promoting potassium shifts from the intracellular to the extracellular fluid compartments. In normal individuals, the excess potassium is excreted in the urine such that the plasma potassium remains constant. In kidney failure, the potassium entering the extracellular fluid compartment during fasting cannot be excreted, thereby resulting in progressive hyperkalemia. The phenomenon of fasting hyperkalemia may be clinically significant in patients undergoing dialysis who fast longer than 8 to 12 hours before a surgical or radiologic procedure. Occasionally, such patients develop life-threatening hyperkalemia during a prolonged fast. The hyperkalemia can be prevented by the administration of intravenous dextrose (to stimulated endogenous insulin secretion) for the duration of the fast. If the patient is diabetic, insulin must be added to the dextrose infusion to prevent paradoxic hyperkalemia.

CLINICAL MANIFESTATIONS OF HYPERKALEMIA

Hyperkalemia may produce progressive electrocardiographic abnormalities, including peaked T waves, flattening or absence of P waves, widened QRS complexes, and sine waves (see Fig. 10.2). The major risk of severe hyperkalemia is the development of life-threatening ventricular arrhythmias.

Severe hyperkalemia, like severe hypokalemia, can cause skeletal muscle weakness, even to the point of paralysis and respiratory failure. Hyperkalemia impairs urinary acidification by decreasing collecting tubule apical H^+/K^+-ATPase, which may result in a renal tubular acidosis (type IV RTA). Hyperkalemia stimulates endogenous aldosterone secretion but not insulin secretion.

TREATMENT OF HYPERKALEMIA

Severe hyperkalemia associated with electrocardiographic changes is a life-threatening state requiring emergent

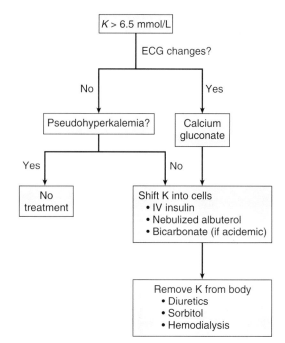

Fig. 10.3 Approach to treatment of hyperkalemia. (Reproduced from Shingarev R, Allon M. A physiologic approach to the treatment of acute hyperkalemia. *Am J Kidney Dis.* 2010;56:578–584.)

intervention (Fig. 10.3). If the patient's EKG is suspicious for hyperkalemia, one should initiate therapy without waiting for laboratory confirmation. If the patient has kidney failure, urgent dialysis is required for removal of potassium from the body. Because of the inevitable delay in initiating dialysis, the following temporizing measures must be initiated promptly:

1. *The first step is to stabilize the myocardium.* Acute administration of intravenous calcium gluconate does not change plasma potassium but does transiently improve the EKG. The effect of 10 mL of 10% calcium gluconate solution over 1 minute is almost immediate. If there is no improvement in the EKG appearance within 3 to 5 minutes, the dose should be repeated. Although calcium chloride has more elemental calcium per ampule than calcium gluconate, it is generally avoided in patients with a peripheral venous access as it may cause skin necrosis if it infiltrates.
2. *The second step is to shift potassium* from the extracellular to the intracellular fluid so as to rapidly decrease the serum potassium. This involves administration of insulin and/ or a beta-2 agonist.
   a. *Intravenous insulin* is the fastest way to lower the serum potassium. The plasma potassium starts to decrease within 15 minutes. Intravenous glucose is given concurrently to prevent hypoglycemia. Regular insulin is administered as 10 units along with a 50-mL bolus of 50% dextrose (1 ampule of D_{50}), followed by a continuous infusion of 5% dextrose at 100 mL/hour to prevent late hypoglycemia. In patients with diabetes, the serum glucose should be ascertained with a glucometer; if it is >300 mg/dL, one can administer the intravenous insulin without concomitant 50% dextrose. One should never give dextrose without insulin for the acute

treatment of hyperkalemia; in patients with inadequate endogenous insulin production, the resulting hyperglycemia can produce a paradoxical increase in serum potassium.

b. *Beta-agonists.* One should give 20 mg of albuterol (a beta$_2$-agonist) by inhalation over 10 minutes. The onset of action is 30 minutes; the concentrated form of albuterol (5 mg/mL) should be used to minimize the inhalation volume. The dose required to lower plasma potassium is considerably higher than that used to treat asthma, because only a small fraction of nebulized albuterol is absorbed systemically. Thus 0.5 mg of intravenous albuterol (available in Europe but not in the United States) produces a comparable change in plasma potassium to that seen after 20 mg of nebulized albuterol. The potassium-lowering effect of albuterol is additive to that of insulin.

c. *Sodium bicarbonate* administration can lower serum potassium by enhancing renal potassium excretion in patients with CKD who are not yet on dialysis. However, bicarbonate administration is of dubious value for treatment of hyperkalemia in patients without residual kidney function. It takes at least 3 to 4 hours for the serum potassium to start to decrease after bicarbonate administration to patients undergoing dialysis, so this modality is not useful for the acute management of hyperkalemia. Moreover, bicarbonate administration does not enhance the potassium-lowering effects of insulin or albuterol. Bicarbonate administration is still indicated if the patient has severe metabolic acidosis (serum bicarbonate <10 mmol/L).

3. Once the previous temporizing measures have been performed, further interventions are done to *remove potassium from the body*.

a. *Diuretics.* Loop and thiazide diuretics work if the patient has adequate kidney function.

b. Sodium polystyrene sulfate (SPS, *Kayexalate*) is a resin exchanger that moves potassium from the blood into the gut, in exchange for an equal amount of sodium. It is relatively slow acting, requiring 1 to 2 hours before plasma potassium decreases. Each gram of SPS removes 0.5 to 1.0 mmol of potassium. It is administered as 50 g in 30 mL sorbitol by mouth or 50 g in a retention enema. The rectal route is faster and more reliable. The studies documenting the efficacy of SPS for treatment of hyperkalemia are generally small and of relatively low quality. A recent randomized, double-blinded clinical trial of 31 patients with CKD and mild hyperkalemia allocated patients to receive SPS or placebo for 7 days. Those treated with SPS had a mean decrease in serum potassium of about 1.0 mmol/L. A recent study suggested that a single standard oral dose of SPS may not be efficacious in decreasing the serum potassium within 4 hours in normokalemic hemodialysis patients, despite a documented increase in potassium excretion by the gut. Whether this modality is effective in hyperkalemic dialysis patients, or when given in multiple doses, remains to be determined. However, given this uncertainty, frequent monitoring of plasma potassium in patients treated with SPS is warranted. The use of SPS has been associated with colonic necrosis in rare cases, particularly when combined with sorbitol, leading to a "black box" warning by the FDA.

c. Several new colonic potassium binders are becoming available.

   i. *Patiromer* is a polymer that binds potassium in exchange for calcium in the gut that has recently received FDA approval. It has been compared to placebo in two randomized, double-blinded clinical trials of patients with CKD and hyperkalemia, many of whom had diabetes or heart failure and were receiving concomitant ACE inhibitor or ARB treatment. Both the short-term study (28 days) and the long-term study (1 year) demonstrated a significant (~1 mmol/L) and sustained reduction in serum potassium in patients receiving patiromer. The safety profile was excellent, with the exception of mild hypomagnesemia in a minority of patients. The starting dose of patiromer is 4.2 to 12.6 g twice daily. Concern exists about the binding of patiromer to other oral medication, and dosing should be spaced by 6 hours from other medications.

   ii. *Zirconium cyclosilicate* is a cation (sodium-potassium) exchanger that has a ninefold higher potassium binding capacity (per gram) than SPS. An initial short-term (28 days) trial in CKD patients with hyperkalemia demonstrated that 98% of patients normalized their serum potassium within 48 hours. Many of the patients had diabetes or congestive heart failure and were receiving concomitant ACE inhibitor or ARB treatment. A larger study of 753 patients demonstrated a dose-dependent decrease in serum potassium during zirconium administration, with the greatest decrease observed when the patients received 5 to 10 g thrice daily. The side-effect profile was quite favorable. Zirconium is not yet approved by the FDA. Although there are no head-to-head comparisons between Kayexalate, patiromer, and zirconium, the newer agents appear to lower serum potassium more consistently and have fewer side effects.

d. *Hemodialysis* is the definitive treatment for patients with advanced kidney failure and severe hyperkalemia.

For patients with moderate hyperkalemia, not associated with electrocardiographic changes, it is frequently sufficient to discontinue the drugs predisposing to hyperkalemia.

To prevent a recurrence of hyperkalemia once the acute treatment has been provided, the following measures are useful:

1. Counsel the patient on dietary potassium restriction of 40 to 60 mEq (1 to 1.5 g) per day (Table 10.5).
2. Avoid medications that interfere with renal excretion of potassium (Table 10.3). ACE inhibitors and ARB play a major role in slowing the progression of CKD. For this reason, when patients on these medications develop hyperkalemia, one should first attempt to decrease dietary potassium intake, treat constipation if present to maximize gastrointestinal excretion of potassium, stop other drugs contributing to hyperkalemia, add a diuretic, reduce the dose of ACE inhibitor or ARB, or add Kayexalate or patiromer. Only if all other measures fail to control the hyperkalemia should the ACE inhibitor or ARB be discontinued.
3. Avoid drugs that interfere with potassium shifts from the extracellular to the intracellular compartments (e.g., nonselective beta-blockers).

Table 10.5   Potassium Content of Selected Foods

Food	Potassium (mg)	Potassium (mEq)
Pinto beans (1 cup)	1370	35
Raisins (1 cup)	1106	28
Honeydew (1/2 melon)	939	24
Nuts (1 cup)	688	18
Black-eyed peas (1 cup)	625	16
Collard greens (1 cup)	498	13
Banana (1 medium)	440	11
Tomato (1 medium)	366	9
Orange (1 large)	333	9
Milk (1 cup)	351	9
Potato chips (10)	226	6

4. When patients undergoing hemodialysis are fasted in preparation for surgery or a radiologic procedure, administer intravenous 10% dextrose at 50 mL/hour to prevent hyperkalemia. If the patient is diabetic, 10 units of regular insulin should be added to each liter of 10% dextrose.

5. In selected patients, chronic medication with loop diuretics can be used to stimulate urinary potassium excretion.

6. Specific therapy may be indicated for the underlying etiology, when available. For example, patients with *adrenal insufficiency* require replacement with exogenous glucocorticoids and mineralocorticoids. In patients with *hyperkalemic periodic paralysis* (a rare, autosomal dominant disorder in which affected individuals develop periodic episodes of severe muscle weakness in association with profound hyperkalemia), prophylactic aerosolized albuterol can prevent both exercise-induced hyperkalemia and muscle weakness.

BIBLIOGRAPHY

Bakris GL, Pitt B, Weir MR. Effect of patiromer on serum potassium level in in patients with hyperkalemia and diabetic kidney disease: the amethyst-DN randomized clinical trial. *JAMA.* 2015;314:151-161.

Epstein M, Lifschitz MD. Potassium homeostasis and dyskalemias: the respective roles of renal, extrarenal and gut sensors in potassium handling. *Kidney Int Suppl.* 2016;6:7-15.

Gruy-Kapral C, Emmett M, Santa Ana CA, Porter JL, Fordtran JS, Fine KD. Effect of single dose resin-cathartic therapy on serum potassium concentration in patients with end-stage renal disease. *J Am Soc Nephrol.* 1998;9:1924-1930.

Kosiborod M, Rasmussen HS, Lavin P. Effect of sodium zirconium cyclosilicate on potassium lowering for 28 days among outpatients with hyperkalemia: the harmonize randomized clinical trial. *JAMA.* 2014;312:2223-2233.

Krishna GG, Steigerwalt SP, Pikus R, Kaul R, Narins RG, Raymond KH, Kunau RT. Hypokalemic states. In: Narins RG, ed. *Clinical Disorders of Fluid and Electrolyte Metabolism.* New York: McGraw-Hill; 1994:659-696.

Kurtz I. Molecular pathogenesis of Bartter's and Gitelman's syndromes. *Kidney Int.* 1998;54:1396-1410.

Lepage L, Dufour AC, Doiron J, et al. Randomized clinical trial of sodium polystyrene sulfonate for the treatment of mild hyperkalemia in CKD. *Clin J Am Soc Nephrol.* 2015;10:2136-2142.

Lifton RP, Dluhy RG, Powers M, et al. A chimaeric 11 beta-hydroxylase/aldosterone synthase gene causes glucocorticoid-remediable aldosteronism and human hypertension. *Nature.* 1992;355:262-265.

Packham DK, Rasmussen HS, Lavin PT. Sodium zirconium cyclosilicate in hyperkalemia. *N Engl J Med.* 2015;372:222-231.

Putcha N, Allon M. Management of hyperkalemia in dialysis patients. *Semin Dial.* 2007;20:431-439.

Salem MM, Rosa RM, Batlle DC. Extrarenal potassium tolerance in chronic renal failure: implications for the treatment of acute hyperkalemia. *Am J Kidney Dis.* 1991;18:421-440.

Shimkets RA, Warnock DG, Bositis CM, et al. Liddle's syndrome: heritable human hypertension caused by mutations in the beta subunit of the epithelial sodium channel. *Cell.* 1994;79:407-414.

Shingarev R, Allon M. A physiologic approach to the treatment of acute hyperkalemia. *Am J Kidney Dis.* 2010;56:578-584.

Weir MR, Bakris GL, Bushinsky DA. Patiromer in patients with kidney disease and hyperkalemia receiving RAAS inhibitors. *N Engl J Med.* 2015;372:211-221.

Disorders of Calcium, Phosphorus, and Magnesium Homeostasis

11

Sharon M. Moe; Dhananjay P. Kulkarni

Disorders of mineral metabolism (calcium, phosphorus, magnesium) are common, especially in hospitalized patients. The extracellular concentrations of these ions are less than 1% of total body stores, and the principal site of storage is bone. Thus serum levels may not always reflect underlying pathology. Knowledge of the complex homeostasis of these ions is critical in formulating the differential diagnosis of these disorders affecting these ions and in the appropriate treatment of these disorders. This regulation occurs in four major target organs (intestine, kidney, parathyroid glands, and bone) via the complex integration of four hormones (parathyroid hormone [PTH], vitamin D and its derivatives, fibroblast growth factor 23 [FGF23], and alpha-klotho [α-klotho, hereafter called klotho]). An understanding of normal physiology is necessary to accurately diagnose and treat disorders of calcium, phosphorus, and magnesium.

NORMAL PHYSIOLOGY

PARATHYROID HORMONE

PTH is released in response to hypocalcemia (Fig. 11.1) and maintains calcium homeostasis by three mechanisms: (1) increasing bone mineral dissolution, thus releasing calcium and phosphorus; (2) increasing renal reabsorption of calcium and excretion of phosphorus; and (3) enhancing the gastrointestinal absorption of both calcium and phosphorus indirectly through its effects on the synthesis of $1,25(OH)_2$-vitamin D. In healthy individuals, the increase in serum PTH level in response to hypocalcemia effectively restores serum calcium levels while maintaining normal serum phosphorus levels.

PTH enhances the conversion of 25(OH)-vitamin D [calcidiol] to $1,25(OH)_2$-vitamin D [calcitriol], with the latter decreasing PTH secretion at the level of the parathyroid glands and completing a typical endocrine feedback loop. In primary hyperparathyroidism, PTH is secreted autonomously from adenomatous glands without regard to physiologic stimuli. In contrast, in secondary hyperparathyroidism, the glands initially respond appropriately; however, after a prolonged period of chronic kidney disease (CKD) and secondary hyperparathyroidism, the hyperplastic glands become adenomatous and therefore unresponsive to stimuli that would normally suppress PTH secretion (sometimes called tertiary hyperparathyroidism). After entering the circulation, PTH binds to PTH receptors that are located throughout the body. Therefore disorders of PTH excess or insufficiency not only affect serum levels of calcium and phosphorus but also lead to bone, cardiac, skin, neurologic, and other manifestations.

PTH is cleaved from a precursor preprohormone to an 84-amino-acid protein in the parathyroid gland, where it is stored with other PTH-protein fragments in secretory granules for release. After release, the circulating 1- to 84-amino-acid protein has a half-life of 2 to 4 minutes. It is then further cleaved into N-terminal, C-terminal, and midregion fragments of PTH, which are finally metabolized in the liver and kidneys. PTH secretion can be triggered by hypocalcemia, hyperphosphatemia, or calcitriol deficiency, whereas profound hypomagnesemia can reduce PTH release. The extracellular concentration of ionized calcium is the most important determinant of minute-to-minute PTH levels. Active secretion of PTH from stored granules in response to hypocalcemia is controlled by the calcium-sensing receptor (CaSR), and mutations of the CaSR gene can lead to syndromes of hypercalcemia or hypocalcemia through dysregulated PTH release. The CaSR is expressed in thyroid C-cells and in the kidney, where it controls renal excretion of calcium in the thick ascending limb of the loop of Henle in response to changes in serum calcium concentration.

Through the years, a succession of increasingly sensitive assays has been developed to measure PTH. A major difficulty in measuring PTH accurately is cross-reactivity with inactive, circulating PTH-protein fragments that may accumulate in CKD. Early assays targeted the C-terminus but were inaccurate in patients with kidney disease because of accumulation of these fragments. Subsequent N-terminus assays resulted in similar problems. Accuracy was improved by the development of a two-site antibody test (commonly called the "INTACT" assay) to detect full-length (1–84, or active) PTH molecules. In this assay, a capture antibody binds to the N-terminus, and a second antibody binds to the C-terminus. However, because the N-terminal antibody is at amino acid 7 instead of amino acid 1, this intact assay still detects some retained C-terminal fragments (although less than the older assays). These fragments accumulate in CKD, leading to falsely elevated values in assays of intact PTH such that values above the normal range are associated with complications of hypoparathyroidism at the level of bone. In addition, there are normal minute-to-minute oscillations in PTH secretion that account for some of the variability in measurements in patients. Finally, there is no common reference standard used in the available intact

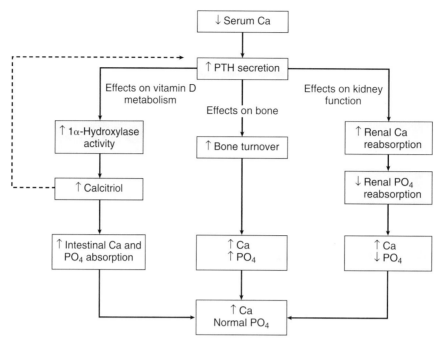

Fig. 11.1 Normal homeostatic response to hypocalcemia. In the presence of hypocalcemia, secretion of parathyroid hormone (PTH) is increased. PTH acts on three target organs. PTH works at the intestine indirectly by first increasing the 1α-hydroxylase activity in the kidney; this enzyme converts calcidiol to calcitriol, which increases intestinal absorption of both calcium and phosphorus. Calcitriol then negatively feeds back on the parathyroid glands to suppress PTH release *(dotted line)*. In bone, PTH increases bone turnover, resulting in a release of calcium and phosphorus. Last, PTH works directly on the kidney to increase renal calcium reabsorption and to decrease renal phosphorus reabsorption. The net effect is a rise in serum calcium but no net change in serum phosphorus. The blue boxes indicate homeostatic steps in the kidney that are abnormal in people with chronic kidney disease. Because of diminished kidney mass, conversion of calcidiol to calcitriol and phosphorus excretion are impaired.

PTH assays. This means that there can be considerable differences between various manufacturers' assays, which may be mitigated by using the same lab for all PTH assays and evaluating trends in PTH levels rather than isolated values.

VITAMIN D

Vitamin D is called a "vitamin" because it is an essential nutrient that must come from an exogenous source if it cannot be manufactured in humans in sufficient quantity; however, this is a misnomer, because vitamin D is a hormone that can be synthesized in the skin. Vitamin D_2 (ergocalciferol) from plants and vitamin D_3 (cholecalciferol) primarily from oily fish are the main exogenous sources in a Western diet outside of supplementation in food products. In the skin, 7-dehydrocholesterol is converted to vitamin D_3 in response to sunlight, which is inhibited by sunscreen of skin protection factor (SPF) 8 or greater. After entering the blood, vitamins D_2 and D_3 from diet or skin bind to vitamin D–binding protein and are carried to the liver, where they are hydroxylated to yield 25(OH)D, often called calcidiol; accordingly, blood calcidiol levels are a direct assessment of the nutritional (dietary) intake and skin conversion of vitamin D. Some clinical assays measure hydroxylated forms of both D_2 and D_3, whereas others measure the total level of 25(OH)D (D_2 + D_3). 25(OH)D (calcidiol) is then converted in the kidney to 1,25(OH)$_2$D (calcitriol) by the action of 1α-hydroxylase

(the CYP27B1 isoenzyme of the cytochrome P-450 system). In the kidney, CYP27B1 activity is affected by almost every hormone involved in calcium homeostasis. Its activity is stimulated by PTH, estrogen, calcitonin, prolactin, growth hormone, low serum calcium, and low serum phosphorus, and inhibited by calcitriol and FGF23 providing feedback loops of regulation. FGF23 also stimulates CYP24, leading to accelerated degradation of both calcidiol and calcitriol, and thus contributing to the known vitamin D deficiency of CKD.

Calcitriol circulates in the bloodstream bound to vitamin D–binding protein. The free form of 1,25(OH)$_2$D enters the target cell, where it interacts with its nuclear vitamin D receptor (VDR). This complex then combines with the retinoic acid X receptor to form a heterodimer, which in turn interacts with the vitamin D response element (VDRE) on the target gene. The major functions of 1,25(OH)$_2$D are carried out in three target organs: (1) the small intestine, where it regulates the intestinal absorption of calcium and, to a lesser degree, phosphorus and possibly magnesium; (2) the parathyroid gland, where it inhibits PTH synthesis at the level of messenger RNA transcription; and (3) the osteoblast/osteocytes in bone, where it directly stimulates the secretion of FGF23. Importantly, the kidney CYP27B1 is essential for the feedback loops between calcitriol and both PTH and FGF23.

In addition to the role of vitamin D in mineral metabolism, the VDR is expressed in multiple organs, and 1α-hydroxylase activity can be detected in extrarenal tissues including immune cells, muscle cells, and myocardiocytes. Both 25(OH)D and 1,25(OH)$_2$D can be taken up by extrarenal cells, with the former then converted intracellularly to 1,25(OH)$_2$D. These features may mediate autocrine or paracrine effects of vitamin D outside its classic target tissues, especially effects on cell differentiation and proliferation and immune function. Recent studies in both normal and CKD patients have demonstrated widespread vitamin D (calcidiol) insufficiency and deficiency. Low levels of this precursor to calcitriol are associated with hyperparathyroidism, falls, fractures, cardiovascular disease, mortality, and cancers in the general population. However, repletion has not yet been shown to improve clinical outcomes in CKD.

FIBROBLAST GROWTH FACTOR 23

FGF23 is a phosphatonin, which is a group of proteins that were identified from the study of genetic disorders characterized by hypophosphatemia due to urinary phosphate wasting, and from cases of tumor-induced osteomalacia associated with urinary phosphate wasting. FGF23 is made by osteocytes, a subgroup of osteoblasts that are interconnected through a series of canaliculi within cancellous (trabecular) bone. FGF23 directly inhibits the conversion of 25(OH)D to 1,25(OH)$_2$D through downregulation of the CP27B1 in the kidney and increases the catabolism of both forms of vitamin D through stimulation of CYP24. FGF23 also inhibits PTH, while 1,25(OH)D and PTH stimulate FGF23, completing a feedback loop (Fig. 11.2). Thus FGF23 provides the key PTH-bone link and kidney-bone link. Levels of FGF23 are elevated as early as CKD stage 2 and are associated with left ventricular hypertrophy and increased mortality. In the kidney, FGF23 acts through the FGF receptor and its coreceptor klotho; however, in cardiomyocytes, FGF23 acts independently of klotho. In addition to FGF23, there are other phosphatonins, such as matrix extracellular phosphoglycoprotein (MEPE), that may provide an intestine-kidney link.

KLOTHO

Alpha-klotho null mice have apparent premature aging: early demise, infertility, arteriosclerosis and arterial calcification, osteoporosis, hyperphosphatemia, emphysema, and skin atrophy, paralleling observations of FGF23 null mice. It was thus named klotho after the Greek goddess who spins the thread of life. Alpha-klotho is a 130-kDa transmembrane protein that is predominantly expressed in the distal tubule of the kidney but also in multiple other tissues. The extracellular domain is also cleaved by proteases including a disintegrin and metalloproteinase (ADAM10 and ADAM17) and secreted into the blood, urine, and cerebrospinal fluid where it functions as a hormone. Thus there is both tissue klotho and secreted (soluble or circulating) klotho. In the kidney, tissue klotho serves as a coreceptor for FGF23, and receptor activation leads to increased urinary excretion of phosphorus. Klotho also stimulates calcium reabsorption in the distal tubule by preventing endocytosis (stabilizing) of the major calcium channels, TRPV5 and TRPV6. Therefore klotho may work with FGF23 to increase urinary phosphorus content but also ensures that the urine with high phosphorus does not also have high calcium (and thus prevents supersaturation of the urine). Both FGF23 (from bone) and klotho (in the kidney) are stimulated by 1,25(OH)$_2$D, and both FGF23 and klotho stimulate renal 1-alpha hydroxylase (CYP27B1) to complete the endocrine feedback loop. In addition, cleaved/soluble klotho stimulates FGF23 secretion from bone and can affect kidney phosphate homeostasis even in the absence of membrane klotho. Thus klotho joins FGF23,

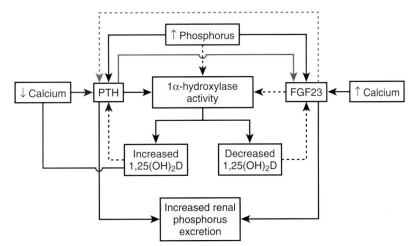

Fig. 11.2 Hormonal control of phosphorus. In the setting of increased phosphorus intake or hyperphosphatemia, both parathyroid hormone (PTH) and fibroblast growth factor 23 (FGF23) are stimulated and induce renal phosphorus excretion. However, PTH and FGF23 have opposing effects on the CYP27B1 (1α-hydroxylase) to increase and decrease 1,25(OH)$_2$D (calcitriol) production, respectively. The increased calcitriol then feeds back to inhibit PTH, and the decreased calcitriol then feeds back to inhibit FGF23 (as calcitriol normally stimulates FGF23). Hypocalcemia also stimulates PTH, and recent data suggests hypercalcemia stimulates FGF23. The solid lines represent an increase in levels; the dotted lines represent a decrease or inhibition of levels. (Adapted from Moe SM, Sprague SM. Chronic kidney disease–mineral bone disorder. In: Taal MW, Chertow GM, Marsden PA, Skorecki K, Yu ASL, Brenner BM, eds. *Brenner and Rector's the Kidney.* 9th ed. Philadelphia: Elsevier Saunders; 2012:2023.)

PTH, and calcitriol in a series of feedback loops that ensure optimal concentrations of calcium and phosphorus in bone and blood.

CALCIUM

Serum calcium levels are tightly controlled within a narrow range, usually 8.5 to 10.5 mg/dL (2.1 to 2.6 mmol/L). However, the serum calcium level is a poor reflection of overall total body calcium, because the intravascular space contains only 0.1% to 0.2% of extracellular calcium, which in turn represents only 1% of total body calcium, with nearly all total body calcium stored in bone. Only ionized calcium, approximately 50% of total serum calcium, is physiologically active, with the remaining 50% of total serum calcium bound to albumin or anions such as citrate, bicarbonate, and phosphorus (Fig. 11.3).

Calcium absorption across the intestinal epithelium occurs via a vitamin D–dependent, saturable (transcellular) and independent, nonsaturable (paracellular) pathway. In states of adequate dietary calcium, the paracellular mechanism prevails, but the vitamin D–dependent pathways are critical in calcium-deficient states. Usually the dietary intake of calcium is about 600 to 1000 mg/day in healthy adults. Out of every 1 g of ingested calcium, 600 mg is excreted in feces and 200 mg via the urine, thus leading to a net absorption of approximately 200 mg/day. The duodenum is the major site of calcium absorption, although the other segments of the small intestine and the colon also contribute to net calcium absorption. In addition, there is an obligatory secretion of calcium into the gut. Individuals on a calcium-free diet will have a net loss of calcium from the body in stool resulting in a negative calcium balance.

In the intestine and in the kidney, transcellular absorption occurs via three steps: (1) the entry of calcium from the lumen into the cells via transient receptor potential vanilloid (TRPV) channels, (2) the intracellular calcium then associates with calbindin to be "ferried" to the basolateral membrane, and (3) calcium is removed from the enterocytes predominantly via the calcium-ATPase, with the Na/Ca exchanger (NCX) playing a minor role. All of the key regulatory components of active calcium transport, TRPV, calbindin, Ca-ATPase, and NCX, are upregulated by calcitriol. At the level of the kidney, vitamin D and PTH work together to control calcium reabsorption and excretion.

In the kidney, the majority (60% to 70%) of calcium is reabsorbed passively in the proximal tubule, driven by a gradient that is generated by reabsorption of sodium and water. In the thick ascending limb, another 20% to 30% of calcium is reabsorbed via paracellular transport driven by the lumen positive net charge. The remaining 10% of calcium reabsorption occurs in the distal convoluted tubule, the connecting tubule, and the initial portion of the cortical collecting duct. The final regulation of urinary calcium excretion is carried out in these distal segments.

PHOSPHORUS

Inorganic phosphorus is critical for numerous normal physiologic functions, including skeletal development, cell membrane phospholipid content and function, cell signaling, platelet aggregation, and energy transfer through mitochondrial metabolism. Normal homeostasis maintains serum concentrations between 2.5 and 4.5 mg/dL (0.81 to 1.45 mmol/L). The terms *phosphorus* and *phosphate* are often used interchangeably, but, strictly speaking, "phosphate" refers to the inorganic form that is in equilibrium (pK 6.8) between HPO_4^{2-} and $H_2PO_4^-$ at physiologic pH in a ratio of about 4:1. For that reason, phosphorus is usually expressed in millimoles (mmol) rather than milliequivalents (mEq) per liter (L); however, as most laboratories report this inorganic component as "phosphorus," we will use this term in the remainder of this chapter. Levels are highest in infants and decrease throughout growth, reaching adult levels in the late teenage years.

Total adult body stores of phosphorus are approximately 700 g, of which 85% is contained in bone. Of the remainder, 14% is intracellular and only 1% is extracellular. Of this extracellular phosphorus, 70% is organic and contained within phospholipids, and 30% is inorganic. Of the latter, 15% is protein bound, and the remaining 85% is either complexed with sodium, magnesium, or calcium or is circulating as the free monohydrogen or dihydrogen forms. Accordingly, only 0.15% of total body phosphorus (15% of extracellular phosphorus) is freely circulating, and this is the portion that is measured. Therefore, as with calcium, serum measurements reflect only a small fraction of total body phosphorus and do not accurately indicate total body stores in the setting of abnormal homeostasis (e.g., CKD).

The average American diet contains approximately 1000 to 1400 mg of phosphorus per day, and the recommended daily allowance (RDA) is 800 mg/day. Approximately two thirds of the ingested phosphorus is excreted in the urine and the remaining third in stool. In general, high-protein foods and dairy products contain the most phosphorus, whereas fruits and vegetables contain the least. In addition, grain-based (e.g., soy) protein contains phosphorus bound with phytate, making it less bioavailable. Many prepackaged and fast foods

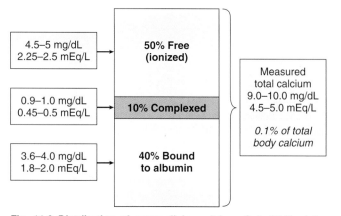

Fig. 11.3 Distribution of extracellular calcium. Only 0.1% of the total body calcium is in the extracellular space; the other 99.9% is localized in bone. The serum calcium concentration reported by the clinical laboratory is total serum calcium. However, only approximately 50% of this total calcium is the physiologically active ionized component. The other 50% of serum calcium is composed of the 10% of the total calcium that is complexed to anions such as bicarbonate, phosphate, and citrate and the 40% that is bound to albumin.

contain extra phosphorus as a preservative, which may not be identified on food labels and vary from lot to lot. Therefore it is difficult to predict accurately the dietary intake based on food type alone. Between 60% and 70% of dietary phosphorus is absorbed by the gut, in all intestinal segments. Medications that bind dietary phosphorus can decrease the net amount of phosphorus absorbed by decreasing the amount of free phosphorus available for absorption. In patients with CKD, such phosphate binders are used to compensate for the loss of renal phosphorus excretion.

Passive enteric absorption (which is dependent on the luminal phosphorus concentration) occurs via the epithelial brush border sodium-phosphate cotransporter (NPT2b), driven by the sodium gradient created by the energy-using basolateral Na^+/K^+-ATPase transporter. The NPT2b sits in the terminal web, just below the brush border in "ready-to-use" vesicles that traffic to the brush border in response to acute and chronic changes in phosphorus concentration. Calcitriol can upregulate the NPT2b and thereby actively increase phosphorus absorption.

Most inorganic phosphorus is freely filtered by the glomerulus. Approximately 70% to 80% of the filtered load is reabsorbed in the proximal tubule, the primary site of regulated phosphorus reabsorption in the kidney, with the remaining 20% to 30% reabsorbed in the distal tubule. Hypophosphatemia stimulates CYP27B1, thereby increasing conversion of calcidiol to calcitriol, which in turn increases intestinal phosphorus absorption. Calcitriol also stimulates renal tubular phosphorus reabsorption, leading to a reduction in urinary phosphorus excretion. In the presence of hyperphosphatemia, there is a rapid increase in urinary excretion of phosphorus, mediated by the levels of serum phosphorus, PTH, and FGF23. Although the effects are more minor, renal phosphorus excretion is also increased by volume expansion, metabolic acidosis, glucocorticoids, and calcitonin and is decreased by growth hormone and thyroid hormone. Because of the capacity of the kidney to increase urinary phosphorus excretion, sustained hyperphosphatemia is not seen clinically without impairment of kidney function.

MAGNESIUM

Magnesium plays an important role in neuromuscular function, control of cardiac excitability and vasomotor tone, mitochondrial function and energy metabolism, and DNA and protein synthesis. Magnesium is also a cofactor for many transporters involved in the regulation of sodium, potassium, and calcium. Normal magnesium levels are 0.7 to 1.1 mmol/L (1.4 to 2.2 mEq/L). Magnesium is the fourth most abundant mineral in the body, and many individuals are deficient because of a reduction in soil magnesium content (and thus fruit and vegetable content) over the past few decades. Similar to calcium and phosphorus, a minority (1%) of total body magnesium is located in the extracellular space, approximately 20% in the intracellular space bound to ribosomes and other cellular organelles, and the remaining content in soft tissue. Approximately 60% of total body magnesium is stored in bone as a component of hydroxyapatite from which it freely disassociates and enters the blood. Another 30% of intracellular stores are in skeletal muscle. As a consequence (and similar to calcium and phosphorus), the serum magnesium level is a poor indicator of the total body stores. Magnesium acts as an antagonist to intracellular calcium, and the ratio of intracellular magnesium to calcium is important in the regulation of calcium transport proteins.

At this time, there are no known hormones that specifically regulate magnesium homeostasis or balance. Approximately 30% of the dietary magnesium is absorbed, mostly in the small intestine via paracellular pathways with a smaller contribution in the colon. In the colon, absorption from the lumen is predominantly active via transient receptor potential melastatin type 6 channel (TRPM6) and TRPM7, the activity of which is downregulated by increased intracellular magnesium and is independent of vitamin D. Extrusion of magnesium from the basolateral side may be through the Na^+/Mg^{++} exchanger CNNM4 based on data from rodent models. However, humans with VNNM4 mutations do not have hypomagnesemia.

About 10% to 20% of filtered magnesium is reabsorbed in the proximal convoluted tubule, and reabsorption decreases with extracellular volume expansion in parallel with that of sodium and calcium. Unlike other divalent ions, most (75%) magnesium is reabsorbed passively through paracellular pathways in the thick ascending limb of the loop of Henle, driven by a lumen-positive voltage in a specific cation-permeable channel formed by the tight junction proteins Claudin-16 (formerly called paracellin), Claudin-14, and Claudin-19. Mutations of the latter proteins have a role in the development of familial hypomagnesemia with hypercalciuria and nephrocalcinosis. About 5% to 10% of magnesium is reabsorbed in the distal convoluted tubule, driven primarily by the luminal membrane potential established by the voltage-gated potassium channel and facilitated by TRMP6, which is located at the luminal membrane of the distal convoluted tubule. Estrogen, insulin, magnesium, and pH may alter expression or function of this transporter.

BONE

The majority of the total body stores of calcium and phosphorus are located in bone in the form of hydroxyapatite $[Ca_{10}(PO_4)_6(OH)_2]$. Trabecular (cancellous) bone comprises 15% to 20% of bone. Trabecular bone is located predominantly in the epiphyses of the long bones and serves a metabolic function. There is a relatively rapid exchange of calcium between trabecular bone and plasma (days to weeks), as evidenced by a short turnover rate of the radioisotope ^{45}calcium. In contrast, cortical (compact) bone is located in the shafts of long bones and comprises 80% to 90% of bone. This bone serves primarily a protective and mechanical function, and it has a calcium turnover rate of months. The nonmineral component of bone consists principally (90%) of highly organized cross-linked fibers of type I collagen; the remainder consists of proteoglycans and "noncollagen" proteins such as osteopontin, osteocalcin, osteonectin, and alkaline phosphatase. The predominant cell types involved in bone turnover are osteoclasts, the bone-resorbing cells derived from circulating hematopoietic cells, and osteoblasts, the bone-forming cells derived from the marrow. These cells are important in bone remodeling, which occurs in response to hormones, cytokines, and changes in mechanical forces and can in turn affect calcium and phosphorus homeostasis.

DISORDERS OF MINERAL METABOLISM

HYPERCALCEMIA

Ionized calcium represents the biologically active fraction of total serum calcium. In the presence of hypoalbuminemia, there is a proportionate increase in ionized calcium relative to total calcium, so that measurements of total serum calcium in patients with hypoalbuminemia may underestimate the amount of physiologically active (ionized) calcium. A commonly used formula to estimate ionized calcium from total serum calcium is to add 0.8 mg/dL to the total calcium value for every 1-mg/dL decrease in serum albumin below 4 mg/dL. In certain circumstances, such as the presence of increased concentrations of proteins capable of binding calcium (e.g., phosphate and citrate), paraproteinemias, or abnormally high or low blood pH, direct measurement of serum ionized calcium is essential, especially if intravenous (IV) calcium infusion is contemplated. In patients with advanced CKD on dialysis, this estimating formula is not very accurate.

DISORDERS OF MINERAL METABOLISM

CLINICAL MANIFESTATIONS OF HYPERCALCEMIA

The severity of symptoms caused by hypercalcemia depends on the degree and rate of rise in serum calcium. Gastrointestinal symptoms such as nausea, vomiting, constipation, abdominal pain, and, rarely, peptic ulcer disease may occur. Neuromuscular involvement includes altered mentation, impaired concentration, fatigue, lethargy, and muscle weakness. Hypercalcemia can impair renal water handling by inducing nephrogenic diabetes insipidus and sodium wasting. The resulting diuresis worsens the hypercalcemia, because volume depletion limits the protective hypercalciuria and exacerbates the volume-dependent proximal tubule reabsorption of calcium. In addition, volume depletion may lead to acute kidney injury, which further limits calcium excretion and favors an additional increase in serum calcium. The hypercalciuria associated with prolonged hypercalcemia can rarely lead to nephrolithiasis and nephrocalcinosis. Cardiovascular effects include hypertension and shortening of the QT interval on the electrocardiogram (ECG). Although cardiac arrhythmias are uncommon, hypercalcemia can trigger digitalis toxicity.

DIFFERENTIAL DIAGNOSIS OF HYPERCALCEMIA

The most common causes of hypercalcemia are malignancy and hyperparathyroidism; in most series, these two diagnoses account for more than 80% of cases. The remaining causes are listed in Box 11.1, with key causes discussed in more detail in the following paragraphs.

Malignancy

Malignancy is the most common cause of hypercalcemia in hospitalized patients, and the presence of hypercalcemia in cancer patients confers a poor prognosis. Hypercalcemia can result from direct invasion of bone by metastatic disease (local osteolytic hypercalcemia [LOH]). In LOH, tumor cells within the bone marrow space produce a variety of inflammatory cytokines, collectively termed osteoclast-activating

---

Box 11.1　Causes of Hypercalcemia

Malignancy
　Local osteolytic hypercalcemia
　Humoral hypercalcemia of malignancy (PTHrp)
　Hematologic malignancies such as lymphoma where
　　there is ectopic calcitriol synthesis
Hyperparathyroidism
Thyrotoxicosis
Granulomatous diseases (sarcoidosis, histoplasmosis,
　tuberculosis)
Drug-induced
　Vitamin D
　Thiazide diuretics
　Estrogens and antiestrogens
　Androgens (breast cancer therapy)
　Vitamin A
　Lithium
Immobilization
Total parenteral nutrition
Impaired kidney function (AKI or CKD), usually in the setting
　of medications such as calcium-containing phosphate
　binders or calcitriol or its analogues

AKI, Acute kidney injury; *CKD,* chronic kidney disease; *PTHrp,* parathyroid hormone–related peptide.

---

factors, which lead to net bone resorption and hypercalcemia. PTH levels are suppressed in response to the hypercalcemia. This mechanism is common with hypercalcemia resulting from breast cancer or multiple myeloma. Hypercalcemia can also result from the production of circulating factors that stimulate osteoclastic resorption of bone. Humoral hypercalcemia of malignancy is caused by secretion of parathyroid hormone–related peptide (PTHrp) by tumor cells. PTHrp bears similarity to PTH only in the initial 8-amino-acid sequence, but this homology permits binding to the PTH receptor, leading to increased bone turnover and hypercalcemia. Specific assays are available to distinguish circulating PTHrp from PTH. Finally, hypercalcemia in malignancy can result from increased production of calcitriol, which stimulates gastrointestinal absorption of calcium. Various lymphoid tumors, most notably Hodgkin lymphoma, have been shown to synthesize large quantities of calcitriol.

Hyperparathyroidism

The incidence of *primary hyperparathyroidism* has declined during the past 30 years, but it is still the second most common cause of hypercalcemia. In most cases, primary hyperparathyroidism is caused by a benign adenoma of a single parathyroid gland that autonomously secretes PTH. The disorder may be sporadic, familial, or inherited as a component of the constellation of multiple endocrine neoplasia (MEN). The elevation in PTH results in increased intestinal absorption of calcium through stimulation of calcitriol production, increased osteoclastic bone resorption, and increased renal tubular reabsorption of calcium. However, because of the elevation in serum calcium, the filtered load of calcium exceeds the ability of the kidney to reabsorb calcium, leading to hypercalciuria and potentially to nephrolithiasis. *Secondary hyperparathyroidism* is caused by diffuse hyperplasia of all four glands in response to ongoing stimuli such as hypocalcemia or hyperphosphatemia. Iatrogenic hypercalcemia may occur in patients with secondary hyperparathyroidism treated with calcium-based phosphate binders or calcitriol and its derivatives. Secondary hyperparathyroidism can also cause hypercalcemia via increased bone resorption when the glands become adenomatous and no longer respond to the change in calcium—a stage often called *tertiary hyperparathyroidism*.

Lithium may interfere with the CaSR, leading to a "resetting" of the parathyroid gland sensitivity such that higher levels of calcium are needed to decrease PTH. Clinically, these patients may appear to have hyperparathyroidism, but hypercalcemia resolves when lithium is stopped.

Vitamin D Excess

Hypercalcemia from excessive exogenous intake of native vitamin D supplements (ergocalciferol and cholecalciferol) is rare, because 1α-hydroxylase (CYP27B1) activity is tightly regulated by calcium levels. In contrast, the excessive administration of calcitriol or of other active vitamin D analogues, such as paricalcitol or doxercalciferol, which bypass this regulatory step at the level of the kidney, can lead to hypercalcemia. These drugs are commonly used in the treatment of secondary hyperparathyroidism in CKD. An endogenous source of excess calcitriol is production by nonkidney tissue. Lymphomas and granulomatous diseases such as sarcoidosis, tuberculosis, and leprosy likely cause hypercalcemia via increased production of calcitriol by monocytes and macrophages that possess 1α-hydroxylase activity.

Familial Hypocalciuric Hypercalcemia

Inactivating mutations of the CaSR cause familial hypocalciuric hypercalcemia (FHH), a rare hereditary disease with autosomal-dominant transmission. Calcium is unable to activate the mutant receptor in the kidney, leading to increased renal reabsorption of calcium into the blood from the tubular fluid and hypocalciuria, usually with urine calcium excretion less than 100 mg/day. Because this mutation may also affect the receptor at the level of the parathyroid gland, PTH may be slightly elevated out of proportion to the degree of hypercalcemia. Other clues pointing to this diagnosis include a family history of asymptomatic hypercalcemia. Probands are often discovered after parathyroidectomy fails to correct hypercalcemia.

APPROACH TO THE PATIENT WITH HYPERCALCEMIA

Clinicians may approach patients with hypercalcemia by reviewing the list in Box 11.1. An alternative approach is to formulate a differential diagnosis based on the physiology of calcium homeostasis (Fig. 11.4) and tailoring diagnostic studies to the suspected pathophysiology.

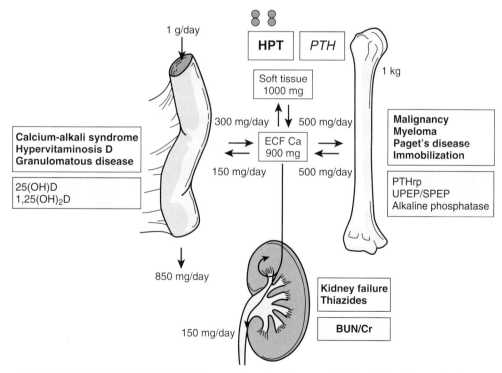

Fig. 11.4 Approach to a patient with hypercalcemia. The normal daily calcium balance is shown, demonstrating the fluxes between the serum compartment and intestine and bone as well as the excretion of calcium. The patient with hypercalcemia must have an abnormality at the parathyroid glands *(top)*, intestine *(left)*, bone *(right)*, or kidney *(bottom)*. The yellow boxes represent causes of hypercalcemia that are associated with abnormalities at each of these target organs. The blue boxes indicate diagnostic tests that may be abnormal in these disorders. *BUN*, Blood urea nitrogen; *Cr*, creatinine; *ECF*, extracellular fluid; *HPT*, hyperparathyroidism; *PTH*, parathyroid hormone; *PTHrp*, parathyroid hormone–related peptide; *SPEP*, serum protein electrophoresis; *UPEP*, urine protein electrophoresis.

Parathyroid Glands

The normal response to hypercalcemia is suppression of PTH secretion. Interpretation of a PTH level (normal: 10 to 65 pg/mL) must always be performed in conjunction with a simultaneously measured calcium level. For example, if the serum calcium level is 11.5 mg/dL and the PTH is 50 pg/mL, the circulating level of PTH is inappropriately high, suggesting hyperparathyroidism. Conversely, if the calcium is 8.5 mg/dL and the PTH is 70 pg/mL, then the elevated PTH is appropriate. Because PTH increases urinary phosphorus excretion, a normal or high-normal PTH level with hypercalcemia and a low or low-normal phosphorus level are essentially diagnostic of primary hyperparathyroidism but only when kidney function is normal. Radionuclide sestamibi imaging may be helpful in localizing an adenomatous gland; however, there is a high risk of false-negative scans, and an experienced parathyroid surgeon can usually locate the enlarged gland. Rarely, glands are found in the mediastinum. Parathyroid cancers secrete excess PTH, leading to severe hyperparathyroidism, and marked hypercalcemia may be present.

Bone

Hypercalcemia of bony origin occurs either because of enhanced bone turnover (osteoclast activity greater than osteoblast activity or net bone resorption greater than bone formation) caused by local tumor invasion or increased secretion of hormonal factors by tumor cells (PTHrp, calcitriol, and PTH). Alternatively, immobilization may lead to the release of calcium from the bone, especially in the setting of excess turnover. Diagnostic studies for bone-induced hypercalcemia include PTH, PTHrp, urine and serum protein electrophoresis and immunofixation (to diagnose myeloma), and alkaline phosphatase. The latter is markedly elevated in Paget disease and other high bone turnover states.

Intestine

Enhanced intestinal absorption of calcium can occur in conditions that result in elevated circulating levels of calcidiol or calcitriol. This can occur because of vitamin D toxicity with very high calcidiol levels, calcitriol therapy in patients with secondary hyperparathyroidism, calcitriol-producing granulomatous diseases and lymphomas, and hyperparathyroidism, which in turn increases calcitriol synthesis. In addition, excess calcium ingestion, especially with alkali, can lead to hypercalcemia. This is now referred to as *calcium-alkali syndrome* and was previously called *milk-alkali syndrome*, named for the combination of therapies used to treat peptic ulcer disease (sodium bicarbonate and milk) before the advent of proton pump blockers. To detect vitamin D toxicity, levels of both 25(OH)vitD (calcidiol) and 1,25(OH)$_2$vitD (calcitriol) should be measured. This is particularly important as many patients are taking large quantities of cholecalciferol in supplements and vitamins. In the setting of exogenous vitamin D intake, calcidiol levels will be high and calcitriol levels normal to high. In the setting of granulomatous production of calcitriol, calcitriol levels will be high; calcidiol levels are nondiagnostic but will usually be at the lower end of normal to low.

Kidneys

With volume depletion, serum calcium levels rise, and mild hypercalcemia can result. Thiazide diuretics, by blocking distal tubular sodium reabsorption, enhance the NCX. This results in a reduction in urinary calcium excretion and hypercalcemia. These effects are used to advantage in the treatment of hypercalciuria in patients with nephrolithiasis. In most cases, the rise in serum calcium in response to thiazide diuretics does not result in clinical hypercalcemia, and any rise is rapidly reversible. When thiazides induce hypercalcemia and the patient is not clinically volume depleted, there may be underlying hyperparathyroidism. PTH acts at the kidney to increase tubular reabsorption of calcium. Even so, patients with hypercalcemia from hyperparathyroidism tend to have an elevated urine calcium excretion, because the filtered load of calcium is so high. In primary hyperparathyroidism, the urinary calcium/creatinine ratio is usually greater than 0.2 (mg/mg), whereas, in patients with FHH, the urinary calcium/creatinine ratio is less than 0.01 mg/mg. Ideally, a 24-hour urine collection should be measured, but a spot collection may differentiate primary hyperparathyroidism from FHH.

TREATMENT OF HYPERCALCEMIA

The ultimate goal of therapy is to remedy the underlying cause of hypercalcemia; however, patients who present with acute symptoms of hypercalcemia require immediate treatment to reduce the serum levels. The safest and most effective treatment in patients with normal cardiac and kidney function is IV volume expansion with normal saline, which reduces proximal tubular reabsorption of sodium, water, and calcium. Most patients with symptomatic hypercalcemia are volume depleted at presentation because of the polyuria and natriuresis induced by hypercalcemia. In severe cases, very aggressive volume resuscitation may be required, with close attention to the patient's cardiopulmonary status to avoid volume overload. After volume expansion is achieved, calcium reabsorption can be further reduced with IV loop diuretics, such as furosemide, that blocks the Na$^+$-K$^+$-2Cl$^-$ cotransporter in the thick ascending limb, thereby disrupting the favorable electrochemical gradient for passive (paracellular) calcium reabsorption. As patients must be adequately hydrated before the diuretic is administered to avoid worsening hypovolemia and hypercalcemia, accurate assessment of intake and output is critical to optimize this treatment approach.

If these conservative treatments fail to restore normocalcemia, other pharmacologic options should be used (Table 11.1). Because the response to these agents is not immediate, their use in patients with severe symptoms of hypercalcemia may be appropriate early in the course of management. In the United States, the bisphosphonates pamidronate and zoledronic acid are approved for the treatment of malignancy-associated hypercalcemia. These agents block osteoclast-mediated bone resorption by inducing osteoclast apoptosis. Typically, a clinical response is seen within 2 to 4 days, with a nadir in serum calcium within 4 to 7 days. Caution is required, because acute kidney injury has been reported with rapid administration of bisphosphonates or in settings of volume depletion. Calcitonin has the advantage of a rapid reduction of serum calcium, but its use is limited by a short duration of action and tachyphylaxis. Glucocorticoids are effective first-line agents, along with saline diuresis, when the hypercalcemia is mediated by elevated circulating levels of calcitriol due to granulomatous disorders or lymphoma.

Table 11.1   Treatments for Hypercalcemia

Agent	Mode of Action	Dose
IV saline	Increases tubular flow and excretion of calcium	Based on patient's cardiovascular status and level of kidney function; 200–500 mL/hour
IV furosemide or loop diuretics	Block NKCC2 channel in loop of Henle, thus reducing positive electrochemical gradient for passive calcium reabsorption	20–40 mg intravenously after volume resuscitation; dose may need to be adjusted based on level of kidney function
IV bisphosphonates	Inhibit osteoclastic activity	Pamidronate, 60–90 mg over 4 hours Zoledronate, 4–8 mg over 15 min
Calcitonin	Inhibits bone resorption and enhances calcium excretion	4–12 IU/kg IM/SQ every 12 hours
Glucocorticoids	Inhibit conversion of 25(OH)D to 1,25(OH)$_2$D	Hydrocortisone, 200 mg/day IV for 3 days Prednisone, 60 mg/day PO for 10 days
Cinacalcet	Allosteric activator of CaSR, mimicking increased calcium to reduce PTH	30 mg daily to twice daily, to a maximum dose of 90 mg twice daily; give with food to reduce nausea

CaSR, Calcium-sensing receptor; *IV*, intravenous; *NKCC2*, Na^{2+}/K$^+$/2Cl$^2-$–cotransporter; *PTH*, parathyroid hormone.

Mild hypercalcemia is usually not symptomatic and may not require aggressive therapy.

The approach to patients with hyperparathyroidism is more controversial. In primary hyperparathyroidism, asymptomatic hyperparathyroidism may be identified after work-up of hypercalcemia noted on a routine lab screen. A National Institutes of Health consensus conference recommended that asymptomatic patients undergo surgical removal of the enlarged parathyroid gland if the serum calcium is 1.0 mg/dL greater than the laboratory upper limit of normal together with dual-energy X-ray absorptiometry (DEXA) T-score of −2.5 present at any major site or the patient is older than 50 years. An alternative to surgical parathyroidectomy is the use of cinacalcet, a calcimimetic. This agent is an allosteric activator of the CaSR that "mimics" higher levels of calcium, thereby decreasing PTH secretion and serum calcium. For primary hyperparathyroidism, the dose is usually 30 mg twice daily, titrating up to 90 mg twice daily.

HYPOCALCEMIA

With true hypocalcemia, the ionized calcium concentration is low; however, in patients with hypoalbuminemia, there is a decrease in total calcium but not necessarily a decrease in ionized calcium. In patients with excess citrate (from blood transfusions) or acute administration of bicarbonate, the percentage of calcium that is bound to these negatively charged ions increases; this reduces the free ionized calcium, usually with only a minimal change in total calcium. Acute respiratory alkalosis also lowers the ionized calcium as a decrease in the hydrogen ion concentration leads to protons dissociating from binding sites on other proteins. This increases protein binding of ionized calcium, thereby decreasing ionized calcium. Because the actual magnitude of any change in these circumstances may be hard to predict, the ionized calcium concentration is best measured directly.

CLINICAL MANIFESTATIONS OF HYPOCALCEMIA

Symptoms only occur with changes in the free ionized calcium, and most patients with mild hypocalcemia exhibit very few

symptoms. Large or abrupt changes in ionized calcium may lead to symptoms including perioral numbness and spasms of the hands and feet. In some patients, progression to tetany or seizures occurs. This increased neuromuscular reactivity can be demonstrated by eliciting the Chvostek sign or Trousseau sign. The Chvostek sign is tested by tapping on the facial nerve near the temporal mandibular joint and watching for grimacing caused by spasm of the facial muscles. The Trousseau sign is tested by inflating a blood pressure cuff to a pressure greater than the systolic blood pressure for 3 minutes and watching for spasm of the outstretched hand. Of these two signs, Trousseau is more specific. If these clinical signs are positive, hypocalcemia should be confirmed by measurement of ionized calcium.

DIFFERENTIAL DIAGNOSIS OF HYPOCALCEMIA

The causes of hypocalcemia are best organized mechanistically.

Vitamin D Deficiency

Vitamin D, once activated to calcitriol, is the primary determinant of intestinal calcium absorption. Individuals may be deficient in vitamin D because of poor absorption from dietary sources (e.g., malabsorption, short bowel, poor nutrition); lack of sun exposure; abnormal conversion of D2/D3 to calcidiol in the liver (cirrhosis, some drugs); or decreased renal conversion of calcidiol to calcitriol (CKD). These patients have low levels of vitamin D and an increase in PTH.

Hypoparathyroidism

Deficiency or inactivity of PTH results in hypocalcemia. This may be caused by inadvertent removal of the parathyroid glands during thyroid surgery or by radiation therapy, congenital defects, or autoimmune disease. These patients have an inappropriately low PTH for their low calcium levels. In the absence of PTH, the only mechanism to increase serum calcium is via intestinal absorption stimulated by the administration of vitamin D (usually in the active form, calcitriol) and oral calcium. Hypomagnesemia may also cause resistance to PTH as well as suppression of PTH release.

Pseudohypoparathyroidism

The term *pseudohypoparathyroidism* describes a group of disorders that are characterized by hypocalcemia and hypophosphatemia, elevated PTH levels, and lack of tissue responsiveness to PTH. The magnesium and calcidiol levels are normal. A PTH infusion test can confirm the tissue resistance. IV administration of PTH normally results in increased urinary cyclic adenosine monophosphate (cAMP) and phosphorus excretion, but patients with pseudohypoparathyroidism lack this response. The most common form of pseudohypoparathyroidism is type Ia, Albright hereditary osteodystrophy, which is also associated with short stature, round facies, obesity, brachydactyly, and other defects.

Tissue Consumption of Calcium

Hypocalcemia may result from the precipitation of calcium into extraskeletal tissue, such as occurs in pancreatitis. In addition, excess bone formation in some malignancies with osteoblastic bone metastases may cause the bone to take up excess calcium acutely. After parathyroidectomy, there is an acute drop in serum calcium and phosphorus because of the "hungry bone syndrome," wherein calcium and phosphorus are rapidly taken up because of the sudden reduction in PTH. This phenomenon is more severe and more protracted in patients with kidney failure who are undergoing parathyroidectomy as a treatment for severe secondary hyperparathyroidism. In acute hyperphosphatemia caused by rhabdomyolysis or tumor lysis syndrome, phosphorus binds to calcium, leading to a fall in ionized calcium. Similarly, the infusion of citrate, a preservative in blood and plasma transfusions, can reduce ionized calcium as discussed earlier. Last, sepsis is also associated with hypocalcemia, although the mechanism is not clear.

TREATMENT OF HYPOCALCEMIA

IV calcium infusions are indicated only in the setting of symptomatic hypocalcemia, and they should not be administered to patients with severe hyperphosphatemia because of the risk of ectopic precipitation of calcium phosphate. IV calcium comes in two forms: calcium gluconate (10-mL vial = 94 mg elemental calcium) and calcium chloride (10-mL vial = 273 mg elemental calcium). Calcium chloride is typically used only during cardiopulmonary resuscitation because its infusion is painful and can cause vein sclerosis. Importantly, patients who are not symptomatic should be repleted with oral, not IV, calcium. The most common oral supplement is calcium carbonate, starting with 1 to 2 g of elemental calcium 3 times daily (1250 mg calcium carbonate = 500 mg elemental calcium), given away from meals. The amount of calcium absorbed will be increased if calcitriol (0.25 μg twice daily to start) is coadministered. Any hypomagnesemia should be treated concomitantly, and, if appropriate, patients may be changed from loop to thiazide diuretics to decrease urinary calcium excretion.

HYPERPHOSPHATEMIA

Hyperphosphatemia can result from increased intestinal absorption, from cellular release or rapid shifts of phosphorus from the intracellular to the extracellular compartment, or from decreased kidney excretion. Persistent hyperphosphatemia (>12 hours) occurs almost exclusively in the setting of impaired kidney function. Increased intestinal absorption is usually caused either by the use of phosphate-containing oral purgatives or enemas, or by vitamin D overdoses. Increased tissue release of phosphorus is commonly seen in acute tumor lysis syndrome, rhabdomyolysis, hemolysis, hyperthermia, profound catabolic stress, or acute leukemia. These disorders can also lead to acute kidney injury, limiting renal phosphate excretion and further exacerbating the hyperphosphatemia. Rarely, thyrotoxicosis or acromegaly leads to hyperphosphatemia. Acute hyperphosphatemia usually does not cause symptoms unless there is a significant reciprocal reduction of serum calcium. The treatment of acute hyperphosphatemia includes volume expansion, dialysis, and administration of phosphate binders. In the setting of normal kidney function, or even mild to moderate kidney disease, hyperphosphatemia is usually self-limited because of the capacity of the kidney to excrete a phosphorus load. Sequelae and treatment of hyperphosphatemia related to CKD, including bone disease and cardiovascular disease, are discussed in detail in Chapter 54.

HYPOPHOSPHATEMIA

Hypophosphatemia can occur with decreased phosphorus intake (decreased intestinal absorption or increased gastrointestinal losses) or with excess renal wasting because of renal tubular defects or hyperparathyroidism. In addition, low serum phosphorus levels may also occur in the setting of extracellular-to-intracellular shifts. In the case of cellular shifts, total body phosphorus may not be depleted. By convention, hypophosphatemia is often graded as mild (<3.5 mg/dL), moderate (<2.5 mg/dL), or severe (<1.0 mg/dL). Moderate and severe hypophosphatemia usually occur only if there are multiple causes (Box 11.2).

CLINICAL MANIFESTATIONS OF HYPOPHOSPHATEMIA

Hypophosphatemia is fairly common, observed in approximately 3% of all hospitalized patients, 10% of hospitalized alcoholic patients, and 70% of mechanically ventilated patients. Symptoms, including muscle weakness (and difficulty weaning from the ventilator), hemolysis, impaired platelet and white blood cell function, rhabdomyolysis, and, in moderate to severe cases, neurologic disorders. Hypophosphatemia is probably overtreated in the intensive care unit, where the "difficult to wean" patient may be given phosphorus when the low phosphorus levels are actually caused by cellular shifts due to respiratory alkalosis. A careful review of the trend in serum phosphorus with arterial blood pH can help discern which patients need to be treated.

DIFFERENTIAL DIAGNOSIS OF HYPOPHOSPHATEMIA

The differential diagnosis and treatment approach are based on the cause and site of phosphate loss. The cause is usually clinically apparent, but if it is not, the simplest test is measurement of the 24-hour urine phosphorus excretion. The expected kidney response to hypophosphatemia is avid reabsorption. If the urinary excretion is less than 100 mg/24 hours, then the kidney is responding appropriately to hypophosphatemia, and the cause must be impaired intake, gastrointestinal losses, or extracellular-to-intracellular shifts.

Box 11.2   Causes of Hypophosphatemia

Decreased Intestinal Absorption

Antacid abuse or excessive calcium supplement use
Malabsorption and chronic diarrhea
Vitamin D deficiency
Starvation or anorexia
Alcoholism

Increased Urinary Losses

Primary hyperparathyroidism
Following kidney transplantation
Extracellular volume expansion
Glucosuria (after treatment of DKA)
Postobstructive or resolving ATN diuresis
Acetazolamide
Fanconi syndrome
X-linked and vitamin D–dependent rickets
Oncogenic osteomalacia

Redistribution

Respiratory alkalosis
Alcohol withdrawal
Severe burns
Postfeeding syndrome
Leukemic blast crisis
Treatment of hyperglycemia

ATN, Acute tubular necrosis; *DKA*, diabetic ketoacidosis.

Decreased Oral Intake

The average American diet contains excessive amounts of phosphorus. All proteins and dairy products contain phosphorus, and phosphorus is used as a preservative in most processed foods. Decreased intake of phosphorus is usually seen only with generalized poor oral intake, gastrointestinal losses from diarrhea and malabsorption, or alcoholism. Occasionally, patients abuse antacids or take excessive calcium supplements, both of which bind phosphorus.

Redistribution

Approximately 15% of the extraskeletal phosphorus is intracellular, and hypophosphatemia may result from a shift to intracellular stores. In most situations, this shift is not clinically detectable; however, if there is underlying phosphate depletion, more profound hypophosphatemia may be observed. The most common clinical cause of this form of hypophosphatemia is hyperglycemia with or without ketoacidosis. The glucose-induced osmotic diuresis results in a net deficit of phosphorus, whereas cellular glucose uptake stimulated by insulin during treatment further causes a shift of the extracellular phosphorus into cells as glycogen stores are repleted. In this setting, hypophosphatemia is usually transient and, in general, should not be treated. In patients who are malnourished, sudden "refeeding" may shift phosphorus into cells, which can be lethal in severe starvation or anorexia nervosa. Respiratory, but not metabolic, alkalosis also increases the intracellular flux of phosphorus. Even in normal subjects, severe hyperventilation (to a carbon dioxide tension [PCO_2] of <20 mm Hg) may lower serum phosphorus concentrations to less than 1.0 mg/dL. Therefore, in ventilated patients,

arterial blood gases may be helpful in differentiating shifts resulting from true phosphorus depletion. Last, in hungry bone syndrome after parathyroidectomy (described earlier), there is increased bone uptake of phosphorus and resultant hypophosphatemia.

Increased Urinary Losses

Phosphorus clearance by the kidney is primarily determined by the phosphorus concentration, urinary flow, PTH, and FGF23 and other phosphatonins. Patients who are overly volume-expanded exhibit less proximal tubular reabsorption of phosphorus in parallel with reduced proximal sodium and water reabsorption. Similarly, patients with glucosuria and postobstructive diuresis experience increased urinary flow and phosphorus losses. In primary hyperparathyroidism, there is increased urinary phosphorus excretion caused by elevated PTH levels. Both congenital and acquired Fanconi syndrome are characterized by increased urinary phosphorus excretion because of defects in proximal tubule reabsorption, together with renal glucosuria, hypouricemia, aminoaciduria, and, potentially, proximal (type 2) renal tubular acidosis. Acquired forms of Fanconi syndrome may be seen in multiple myeloma and after administration of some chemotherapy agents (cisplatin, ifosfamide, and 6-mercaptopurine), outdated tetracycline, or the antiretroviral agent tenofovir.

Rickets and Osteomalacia

Hypophosphatemia can lead to impaired bone mineralization. Several genetic disorders are associated with hypophosphatemia and rickets in children. Autosomal-dominant hypophosphatemic rickets (ADHR) is rare and associated with a mutation that limits normal degradation of FGF23. Autosomal recessive hypophosphatemic rickets (ARHR), also rare, is caused by a mutation in the gene encoding dentine matrix protein (DMP), a locally produced inhibitor of FGF23. X-linked hypophosphatemic rickets (XLH), the most common form of rickets, is due to a mutation called PHEX (phosphate regulating gene with homologies to endopeptidases located on the X chromosome), which normally degrades FGF23. Mutations in PHEX therefore lead to inappropriate levels of FGF23. Thus what previously was thought to be multiple disorders are now all linked back to abnormalities in FGF23. In tumor-induced osteomalacia, tumors of mesenchymal origin secrete phosphatonins such as FGF23, MEPE, or FRP4, which upregulate the renal sodium phosphate cotransporter with resultant renal phosphate wasting.

TREATMENT OF HYPOPHOSPHATEMIA

Treatment is usually necessary for patients with moderate to severe hypophosphatemia. Increasing oral phosphorus intake is the preferred treatment because IV administration of phosphate complexes with calcium and can lead to extraskeletal calcifications. Oral supplementation can be given with skim milk (1000 mg/quart), whole milk (850 mg/quart), Neutra-Phos K capsules (250 mg/capsule; maximum dose, 3 tabs every 6 hours), or Neutra-Phos solution (128 mg/mL). Oral phosphorus may induce or exacerbate diarrhea. Milk is much better tolerated, is a source of protein, and is cheaper. The concomitant administration of vitamin D may enhance its absorption. If necessary, phosphorus may be replaced intravenously as potassium phosphate

(3 mmol/mL of phosphorus, 4.4 mEq/mL of potassium) or sodium phosphate (3 mmol/mL of phosphorus, 4.0 mEq/mL of sodium) in a single administration, usually mixed in 50 mL of normal saline.

HYPERMAGNESEMIA

Hypermagnesemia is present when the serum level is greater than 2.9 mg/dL (1.2 mmol/L), although clinical manifestations typically do not occur until serum levels are greater than 4 mg/dL (1.6 mmol/L). Signs and symptoms include hyporeflexia (usually the first sign) and weakness that may progress to paralysis and can involve the diaphragm. Cardiac findings are bradycardia, hypotension, and cardiac arrest. ECG findings include prolonged PR, QRS, and QT intervals, and complete heart block may occur when the levels are as high as 15 mg/dL (6.2 mmol/L). Of note, moderate hypermagnesemia can inhibit the secretion of PTH, which may lead to hypocalcemia and subsequent prolonged QT interval.

DIFFERENTIAL DIAGNOSIS OF HYPERMAGNESEMIA

Because hypermagnesemia appears to stimulate renal excretion, it is "self-regulating," and prolonged hypermagnesemia generally occurs only when there is reduced kidney function. Hypermagnesemia is usually iatrogenic from laxatives, antacids, or intravenous magnesium administration. Levels will be purposefully elevated in the treatment of eclampsia, but they resolve quickly with cessation of therapy because of renal excretion. Other causes of a mild elevation of magnesium include theophylline intoxication, tumor lysis syndrome, acromegaly, FHH, and adrenal insufficiency.

TREATMENT OF HYPERMAGNESEMIA

Treatment begins with avoiding magnesium-containing medications, including some laxatives and antacids, in patients with reduced kidney function. In the presence of normal kidney function, asymptomatic hypermagnesemia will resolve and no treatment is indicated. If hypermagnesemia is symptomatic, IV administration of calcium gluconate (~90 to 180 mg of elemental calcium) over 10 to 20 minutes will help antagonize the effect of the excessive magnesium. Supportive therapy may include mechanical ventilation and the placement of a temporary pacemaker. With adequate kidney function, volume expansion with IV saline facilitates renal excretion of magnesium. In the case of kidney failure, dialysis is required.

HYPOMAGNESEMIA

Serum magnesium less than 1.3 mg/dL (0.53 mmol/L) defines hypomagnesemia. Similar to calcium and phosphorus, a minority of magnesium is in the extracellular space; however, unlike calcium there is no "ionized" magnesium measurement available. Therefore, when blood magnesium levels are normal, this does not exclude magnesium deficiency. On the other hand, when there is severe magnesium deficiency, there is almost always hypomagnesemia. In patients with normal magnesium levels but clinical suspicion of hypomagnesemia, urine magnesium should be checked. If low, this confirms magnesium depletion.

Renal wasting of magnesium can be diagnosed in the presence of hypomagnesemia if there is more than 24 mg of

magnesium in the 24-hour urine collection or if the fractional excretion of magnesium is greater than 2%. The fractional excretion of magnesium is calculated as follows:

$$FEM_g = \frac{U_{Mg} \times P_{Cr}}{P_{Mg} \times U_{Cr} \times 0.7} \times 100$$

where U and P are urinary and plasma concentrations of magnesium (Mg) and creatinine (Cr).

CLINICAL MANIFESTATIONS OF HYPOMAGNESEMIA

Hypomagnesemia is seen in 10% of hospitalized patients and 20% of patients in the ICU. Forty percent of patients with hypomagnesemia will have hypokalemia, and 20% will have hypocalcemia, hypophosphatemia, or hyponatremia. Notably, hypokalemia may appear refractory to potassium replacement until the magnesium is repleted, believed to be secondary to intracellular magnesium changes that alter renal outer medullary potassium channel (ROMK) potassium reabsorption, although this may not be the only mechanism. Thus magnesium levels should be evaluated in hypokalemia. Patients with severe hypomagnesemia may have clinical neurologic or cardiovascular abnormalities. Symptoms include muscle cramps, generalized fatigue, and ileus. With more severe depletion, confusion, ataxia, nystagmus, tremor, hyperreflexia, fasciculations, tetany, and seizures may occur. Cardiac arrhythmia may occur, particularly with patients on digoxin, with ECG changes including prolonged PR and QT intervals with a widened QRS complex. Torsades de pointes is the other classic finding. Magnesium levels are not generally included on routine blood chemistry panels, and thus patients at risk (malnutrition, chronic diarrhea, alcoholism, use of diuretics or digoxin) should be specifically tested for hypomagnesemia.

DIFFERENTIAL DIAGNOSIS OF HYPOMAGNESEMIA

Hypomagnesemia may be caused by (1) decreased intake, as in chronic alcoholism and malabsorption syndromes; (2) increased gastrointestinal losses; (3) increased renal losses; or (4) intravascular chelation and extravascular deposition, as seen with hypocalcemia (Box 11.3). The latter can occur when substances that complex with magnesium become available, such as fatty acids released in acute pancreatitis and citrate. It also occurs in the hungry bone syndrome following parathyroidectomy. Renal losses occur in the presence of hypercalcemia (where calcium competes with magnesium to be reabsorbed in the thick ascending limb), osmotic diuresis, volume expansion (because of the decreased magnesium reabsorption associated with the increased tubular flow), and genetic disorders or drugs that lead to defects in tubular magnesium transport. Culprit drugs include diuretics, aminoglycosides, amphotericin B, cisplatin, and calcineurin inhibitors such as cyclosporine and tacrolimus, making it important to monitor magnesium blood levels when these drugs are used. Similar to calcium and phosphorus, shifts from the extracellular to intracellular space can occur, particularly with treatment of diabetic ketoacidosis and alcohol withdrawal. In contrast to the rapid shifts of calcium and phosphorus from bone to maintain serum levels, this potential compensatory mechanism for magnesium may take weeks and thus is not a factor in acute homeostasis of blood levels.

Box 11.3   Causes of Hypomagnesemia

Decreased Intake

Prolonged fasting
Chronic alcoholism
Protein-calorie malnutrition
Inadequate parenteral nutrition

Gastrointestinal Losses

Chronic diarrhea
Laxative abuse
Malabsorption syndromes
Massive resection of the small intestine
Neonatal hypomagnesemia

Kidney Losses

Drugs
    Diuretics
    Amphotericin B
    Aminoglycosides
    Cisplatin
    Pentamidine
    Proton pump inhibitors
    Cyclosporine
    Tacrolimus
    Foscarnet
    Cetuximab
High urinary output states
    Postobstructive diuresis
    Diuretic phase of acute tubular necrosis
    Posttransplantation polyuria
Inherited hypomagnesemia
    Gitelman syndrome
    Bartter syndrome
    Other genetic transient receptor potential abnormalities
Primary hyperaldosteronism
Hypercalcemic states
Phosphate depletion
Chronic metabolic acidosis
Idiopathic renal wasting

Miscellaneous

Acute pancreatitis
Hungry bone syndrome
Diabetic ketoacidosis
Acute intermittent porphyria

Table 11.2   Examples of Magnesium Supplementation

Source	Mass of Elemental Magnesium[a]
Mag-Ox 400 PO (Mg oxide)	240 mg per tablet = 20 mEq per tablet
Uro-Mag 140 PO (Mg oxide)	85 Mg = 7 mEq
Magnesium gluconate 500 (tablet or liquid)	27 Mg = 2.3 mEq
Slow-Mag PO (Mg chloride)	64 Mg = 5.3 mEq
MagTab SR (84 Mg elemental mg per tab)	84 Mg tablet = 7 mEq
Magnesium sulfate 1 g IV	96 Mg = 8 mEq

[a]Mg of magnesium per tablet = mEq magnesium per tablet.
IV, Intravenous.

gastrointestinal symptoms including diarrhea. In some cases, amiloride may be effective in reducing renal wasting. In severe symptomatic hypomagnesemia, 1 to 2 g of IV magnesium sulfate may be administered over 15 to 30 minutes, followed by an infusion of 5 to 6 g over 24 hours, with levels checked daily (but as far away from the last infusion as possible) to avoid overrepletion. As only a portion of intravenously administered magnesium is retained, repeat magnesium levels several days later are needed to determine the efficacy of repletion. Dosing for IV and oral administration of magnesium is presented in Table 11.2.

BIBLIOGRAPHY

de Baaij JH, Hoenderop JG, Bindels RJ. Magnesium in man: implications for health and disease. *Physiol Rev.* 2015;95:1-46.

Glendenning P, Chew GT. Controversies and consensus regarding vitamin D deficiency in 2015: whom to test and whom to treat? *Med J Aust.* 2015;202:470-471.

Grober U, Schmidt J, Kisters K. Magnesium in prevention and therapy. *nutrients.* 2015;7:8199-8226.

Hansen KE, Johnson MG. An update on vitamin D for clinicians. *Curr Opin Endocrinol Diabetes Obes.* 2016;23:440-444.

Hu MC, Kuro-o M, Moe OW. Renal and extrarenal actions of Klotho. *Semin Nephrol.* 2013;33:118-129.

Huang CL, Kuo E. Mechanism of hypokalemia in magnesium deficiency. *J Am Soc Nephrol.* 2007;18:2649-2652.

Kelly A, Levine MA. Hypocalcemia in the critically ill patient. *J Intensive Care Med.* 2013;28:166-177.

Marcocci C, Cetani F. Clinical practice. Primary hyperparathyroidism. *N Engl J Med.* 2011;365:2389-2397.

Moe SM. Calcium homeostasis in health and in kidney disease. *Compr Physiol.* 2016;6:1781-1800.

Olauson H, Larsson TE. FGF23 and Klotho in chronic kidney disease. *Curr Opin Nephrol Hypertens.* 2013;22:397-404.

TREATMENT OF HYPOMAGNESEMIA

Magnesium should be administered cautiously in the presence of kidney dysfunction. In asymptomatic hypomagnesemia, up to 720 mg of oral elemental magnesium can be given per day, although oral magnesium salts are associated with

12 Approach to Acid-Base Disorders

Ankit N. Mehta; Michael Emmett

Acid-base disorders can have major clinical and diagnostic implications. If they generate extreme acidemia or alkalemia, the abnormal pH itself may result in pathophysiologic consequences. For example, the tertiary structure of proteins is altered by extreme pH conditions, potentially affecting the activity of enzymes and ion transport systems. Consequently, every metabolic pathway may be impacted by acidemia or alkalemia. In addition, extreme acidemia can depress cardiac function, impair the vascular response to catecholamines, and cause arteriolar vasodilation and venoconstriction, with resultant systemic hypotension and pulmonary edema. Insulin resistance, reduced hepatic lactate uptake, and accelerated protein catabolism are other effects of acidemia. Alkalemia can generate cardiac arrhythmias, produce neuromuscular irritability, and contribute to tissue hypoxemia. In alkalemic patients, cerebral and myocardial blood flow falls, and respiratory depression occurs. Potassium disorders, a common accompaniment of acid-base perturbations, also contribute to the morbidity.

Although mild and moderate acid-base disorders may not directly affect physiologic function, the identification of such disorders may be an important diagnostic clue to the existence of serious medical conditions. Whenever an acid-base disorder is identified, the underlying cause should be sought. This diagnostic imperative often overrides the importance of any therapeutic intervention directed at the pH itself. The situation is analogous to the discovery of fever or hypothermia. Although very high or very low temperatures can themselves be dangerous and require aggressive therapy directed at restoration of a more normal temperature, often more important is the effort to identify and treat the underlying cause of the abnormal temperature. Similarly, the recognition of an acid-base disorder must generate a search for its clinical cause or causes, and recognition of a mixed acid-base disorder should trigger an investigation to determine the etiology of each component.

The acid-base status of the extracellular fluid (ECF) is carefully regulated to maintain the arterial pH in a narrow range between 7.36 and 7.44 (hydrogen ion concentration $[H^+]$ 44 to 36 nEq/L). The pH is stabilized by multiple buffer systems in the ECF, cells, and bone. The CO_2 tension (pCO_2), primarily under neurorespiratory control, and the serum bicarbonate concentration ($[HCO_3^-]$), primarily under renal/metabolic regulation, are the most important variables in this complex system of buffers.

Currently three different methodologic approaches are widely used to describe normal acid-base status and simple and mixed acid-base disorders.

1. The *physiologic method* uses measurements of arterial pH, pCO_2, and $[HCO_3^-]$, together with an analysis of the anion gap (AG) and a set of compensation rules.
2. The *base excess (BE) method* uses measurements of arterial pH and pCO_2, and calculation of the BE and the AG.
3. The *physicochemical method* uses measurements of arterial pH and pCO_2 together with the calculated apparent (SIDa) and effective (SIDe) "Strong Ion Difference," the "Strong Ion Gap" (SIG = SIDa − SIDe), and the total concentration of plasma weak acids (Atot).

Each of these approaches can be effectively used to characterize acid-base disorders, each has its vocal proponents and detractors, and each has certain unique characteristics that may be particularly helpful under certain conditions. We believe the physiologic method is the most straightforward and the easiest model to understand and use. It is generally acceptable in most clinical circumstances and will be the method we use in this chapter.

The physiologic method to the elucidation of acid-base disorders uses the following information:

1. Recognition of diagnostic clues provided by the patient's history and physical examination
2. Analysis of the serum $[HCO_3^-]$, arterial pH, and pCO_2 (Although a blood gas analysis is not always necessary to make a diagnosis, it is generally required for complicated cases.)
3. Knowledge of the predicted compensatory response to simple acid-base disorders
4. Calculation of the AG, with consideration of the expected "baseline" AG for each patient
5. Analysis of the degree of change (Δ) in AG and the degree of Δ in $[HCO_3^-]$ to see if the magnitude of these respective changes is reciprocal. This has been dubbed the Delta/Delta or $\Delta[AG]/\Delta[HCO_3^-]$.

ACIDEMIA, ALKALEMIA, ACIDOSIS, AND ALKALOSIS

The normal arterial blood pH range is between 7.36 and 7.44 ($[H^+]$ between 44 and 36 nEq/L). Acidemia is defined as an arterial pH <7.36 ($[H^+]$ >44 nEq/L) and may result from a primary elevation in pCO_2, a fall in $[HCO_3^-]$, or both. Alkalemia is defined as an arterial pH >7.44 ($[H^+]$ <36 nEq/L). Alkalemia may result from a primary increase in $[HCO_3^-]$, a fall in pCO_2, or both.

The relationship among pH, pCO_2, and HCO_3^- concentrations is described by the familiar Henderson-Hasselbalch equation:

$$pH = 6.1 + \log([HCO_3^-]/(0.03 \times pCO_2)).$$

Acidosis and alkalosis are pathophysiologic processes that, if unopposed by therapy or complicating disorders, would cause acidemia or alkalemia, respectively.

SIMPLE (SINGLE) ACID-BASE DISTURBANCES AND COMPENSATION

The simple acid-base disorders are divided into primary metabolic and primary respiratory disturbances. Each of these simple, or single, acid-base disorders generates a compensatory response that acts to return the blood pH back toward the normal range. By convention, the physiologic approach to acid-base analysis considers the compensatory response to a simple acid-base disorder to be an integral component of that disorder. Hence there are four primary simple acid-base disturbances (six if each respiratory disorder is divided into an acute and chronic phase):

- *Metabolic acidosis:* The underlying pathophysiology tends to reduce the serum bicarbonate concentration $[HCO_3^-]$. Although we refer to serum bicarbonate here, it is often directly measured as total CO_2, which includes bicarbonate (HCO_3^-), carbonic acid (H_2CO_3), and dissolved CO_2. The latter two components account for a very small fraction of the total (roughly 1.2 mEq/L at normal pCO_2). Therefore, for clinical purposes, total CO_2 is equated to serum bicarbonate concentration. Causes include excess generation of metabolic acids, excessive exogenous acid intake, reduced kidney excretion of acid, or excessive exogenous loss of HCO_3^- (usually in stool or urine). Metabolic acidosis reduces the arterial plasma pH and generates a hyperventilatory compensatory response, which reduces the arterial pCO_2 and blunts the degree of acidemia.
- *Metabolic alkalosis:* The underlying pathophysiology tends to increase the $[HCO_3^-]$. Causes include exogenous intake of HCO_3^- salts (or salts that can be converted to HCO_3^-) and/or endogenous generation of HCO_3^-. Regardless of the origin of the HCO_3^-, the pathology must also include reduced or impaired renal HCO_3^- excretion. Metabolic alkalosis increases the arterial plasma pH and generates a hypoventilatory compensatory response, which increases the arterial pCO_2 and blunts the degree of alkalemia.
- *Respiratory acidosis:* The underlying pathophysiology tends to increase the arterial pCO_2. The compensatory response is an increase of the plasma $[HCO_3^-]$ due to rapid generation from buffers and, over a period of days, renal HCO_3^- generation and retention.
- *Respiratory alkalosis:* The underlying pathophysiology tends to decrease the arterial pCO_2. The compensatory response reduces the plasma $[HCO_3^-]$. This occurs acutely as H^+ is released from buffers and chronically, over a period of days, as the kidneys excrete HCO_3^- and/or retain acid.

The magnitude of each compensatory response is proportional to the severity of the primary disturbance. Generally, respiratory responses to primary metabolic acid-base disorders

occur rapidly (within an hour) and are fully developed within 12 to 36 hours. In contrast, the compensatory metabolic alterations triggered by the primary respiratory disorders are divided into two phases. A chemical buffering response occurs within minutes (acute), whereas the quantitatively more significant kidney response takes several days (chronic) to develop fully. Hence each primary respiratory disorder is subdivided into an acute and a chronic disorder to differentiate the expected compensatory response.

The expected degree of compensation for each simple disorder has been determined by studying patients with isolated simple disorders and normal subjects with experimentally induced acid-base disorders. These data have been used to create various graphic acid-base nomograms, simple mathematical relationships, and a number of mnemonic methods for predicting expected compensation ranges. Fig. 12.1 and Table 12.1 provide some of these "compensation rules." Appropriate compensation should generally be present in all patients with an acid-base disorder, and when it is not identified, a complex, or mixed, acid-base disorder must be considered.

In general, with one exception, compensatory responses return the pH toward the normal range but do not completely normalize the pH. The exception is chronic respiratory alkalosis, wherein compensation results in a pH that is normal. With all other disorders, some degree of acidemia or alkalemia remains, even after full compensation. Compensatory responses result in the pCO_2 moving in the same direction as the primary $[HCO_3^-]$ change in case of metabolic acid-base disorder and the $[HCO_3^-]$ moving in the same direction as the primary pCO_2 change in case of respiratory acid-base disorder (see Table 12.1). If the pCO_2 and $[HCO_3^-]$ are deranged in the opposite directions (i.e., the pCO_2 or $[HCO_3^-]$ is increased and the other variable is decreased), then a mixed disturbance must exist.

ANION GAP

The ion profile of normal serum is depicted in Fig. 12.2A. In any solution, the total cation charge concentration must be equal to the total anion charge concentration (all measured in units of electrical charge concentration; i.e., mEq/L). Now consider only the three serum electrolytes that are at the highest concentration—namely, Na^+, Cl^-, and HCO_3^-. The cation charge concentration $[Na^+]$ normally exceeds the sum of the anion charge concentrations $[Cl^-]$ and $[HCO_3^-]$. If the sum of the two anions is subtracted from [Na], an "AG" is noted (see Fig. 12.2B):

$$AG = [Na^+] - ([Cl^-] + [HCO_3^-])$$

This AG is of course a function of the decision to consider only the three major serum electrolytes and not other ions that normally exist in serum. Nevertheless, the AG, as defined in this fashion, is a very useful diagnostic tool.

The normal value of the AG varies among laboratories as a result of the wide variety of analyte measurement technologies and unique normal ranges for each instrument. Typically, the normal AG range is considered to be 8 to 12 mEq/L. The normal AG is primarily composed of anionic albumin and, to a lesser degree, other proteins, sulfate, phosphate, urate, and various organic acid anions such as lactate. In

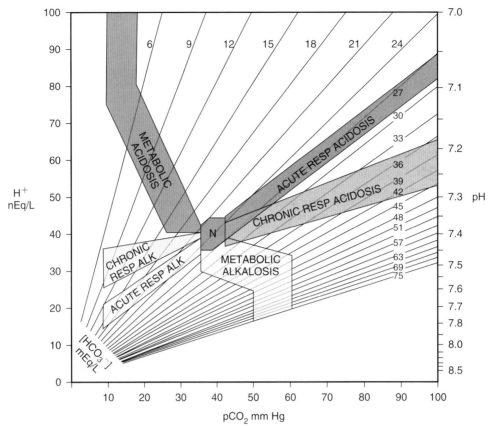

Fig. 12.1 The acid-base map. Shaded areas represent the 95% confidence limits for zones of compensation for the simple acid-base disorders. Numbered diagonal lines represent isopleths of plasma bicarbonate concentration ([HCO$_3^-$]). Laboratory values that fall within a colored zone are consistent with the simple acid-base disorder as shown. If the values fall outside a colored zone, a mixed acid-base disorder is likely. *ALK*, Alkalosis; *N*, normal range; *RESP*, respiratory. (Modified and updated from Goldberg M, Green SB, Moss ML, Marhacli MS, Garfinkel D. Computer-based instruction and diagnosis of acid-base disorders. *JAMA*. 1973;223:269–275.)

Table 12.1   Acid-Base Rules: Changes in pH, pCO$_2$, and [HCO$_3^-$] and Expected Compensatory Responses in Simple Disturbances

Primary Disorder	pH	Initial Chemical Change	Compensatory Response	Expected Compensation
Metabolic acidosis	Low	↓ [HCO$_3^-$]	↓ pCO$_2$	$pCO_2 = (1.5 \times [HCO_3^-]) + 8 \pm 2$ $pCO_2 = [HCO_3^-] + 15$ $pCO_2 = $ decimal digits of pH
Metabolic alkalosis[a]	High	↑ [HCO$_3^-$]	↑ pCO$_2$	pCO$_2$ variably increased $pCO_2 = (0.9 \times [HCO_3^-]) + 9$
Respiratory Acidosis				$\boldsymbol{pCO_2 = (0.7 \times [HCO_3^-]) + 20}$
Acute	Low	↑ pCO$_2$	↑ [HCO$_3^-$]	[HCO$_3^-$] increases 1 mEq/L for every 10 mm Hg increase in pCO$_2$
Chronic	Low	↑ pCO$_2$	Further ↑ [HCO$_3^-$]	[HCO$_3^-$] increases 3 to 4 mEq/L for every 10 mm Hg increase in pCO$_2$
Respiratory Alkalosis				
Acute	High	↓ pCO$_2$	↓ [HCO$_3^-$]	[HCO$_3^-$] decreases 2 mEq/L for every 10 mm Hg decrease in pCO$_2$
Chronic	High	↓ pCO$_2$	Further ↓ [HCO$_3^-$]	[HCO$_3^-$] decreases 5 mEq/L for every 10 mm Hg decrease in pCO$_2$

[a]Compensation formulas for metabolic alkalosis have wide confidence limits because the pCO$_2$ of individuals with this disorder varies greatly at any given [HCO$_3^-$].
[HCO$_3^-$], Serum bicarbonate concentration; *pCO$_2$*, arterial partial pressure of carbon dioxide.

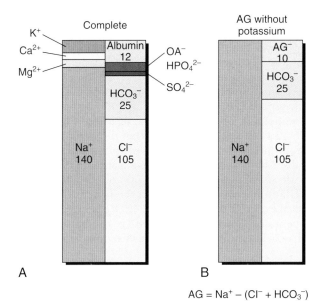

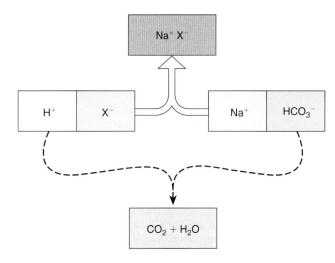

$$AG = Na^+ - (Cl^- + HCO_3^-)$$

Fig. 12.2 The ionic anatomy of plasma. All units are milliequivalents per liter (mEq/L). (A) Ion profile of normal serum. (B) Calculation of the anion gap *(AG)* using the concentrations of sodium, chloride, and bicarbonate concentrations only. *OA,* Organic acid.

		METABOLIC ACIDOSIS	
	Normal	Hyperchloremic	High AG
Na^+	140	140	140
Cl^-	105	115	105
HCO_3^-	25	15	15
AG	10	10	20
ΔHCO_3^-	0	−10	−10
ΔAG	0	0	+10
Lactate	1	1	11

Fig. 12.3 Pathogenesis of a metabolic acidosis. If any relatively strong acid, HX (where X– is an anion), is added to a solution containing $NaHCO_3$, there is decomposition of some HCO_3^- and an equivalent increase of the X^- concentration. If HX is HCl, then a hyperchloremic, or normal anion-gap, acidosis develops. If HX is any acid other than HCl, such as lactic acid or a keto acid, then a high anion-gap acidosis develops.

general, if the concentration of these "unmeasured" anions increases, the AG increases. Conversely, the AG falls when the concentration of unmeasured anions is reduced. For example, hypoalbuminemia is a common cause of a reduced AG, with the AG falling about 2.5 mEq/L for each 1 g/dl reduction of albumin below the normal range.

The disorders that produce metabolic acidosis can be subdivided on the basis of an increased or normal AG. An examination of the AG equation reveals that the only way the $[HCO_3^-]$ can fall while the AG remains normal is for the $[Cl^-]$ to increase relative to the $[Na^+]$. Consequently, all "non-AG" metabolic acidoses must be hyperchloremic metabolic acidoses. This is shown graphically in Fig. 12.3.

Most often, an elevated AG indicates the presence of a metabolic acidosis. Several mnemonics have been published as guides to the most common clinically relevant etiologies of high AG metabolic acidosis. We suggest the mnemonic "GOLDMARK" for this purpose (Glycols [ethylene, propylene, and diethylene], Oxoproline [acetaminophen], L-Lactate, D-Lactate, Methanol, Aspirin, Renal failure, Ketoacidosis). However, a high AG can sometimes occur in the absence of metabolic acidosis. Exceptions include:

- Dehydration, as the loss of water in excess of salts, increases the concentration of all electrolytes, including albumin and other unmeasured ions, thereby increasing the AG.
- Rapid infusion, and transient accumulation, of metabolizable sodium salts such as lactate, acetate, citrate, and so on. To the extent these salts are metabolized, they generate $NaHCO_3$, and the AG does not increase; if metabolic conversion is delayed, the AG increases.
- Infusion of nonmetabolizable sodium salts, other than sodium chloride or bicarbonate. For example, anionic antibiotics such as carbenicillin and penicillin G may be infused as sodium (or potassium) salts and, to the extent that they accumulate, increase the AG.

- Metabolic alkalosis causes a small increase in AG (usually less than 3 to 4 mEq/L) as a result of (1) increased concentrations of the anions of organic acids (mainly lactate), which accumulate because of metabolic stimulation of production, and (2) increased concentration of albumin, due to ECF volume contraction.
- Laboratory error, or measurement artifact, of one or more analytes.

MIXED ACID-BASE DISTURBANCES

A mixed acid-base disturbance is the simultaneous occurrence of two or more simple acid-base disturbances. Mixed acid-base disorders may develop concurrently or sequentially. The disorders may be additive, with each process having a similar directional effect on pH. Alternatively, they may oppose each other, having offsetting effects on pH. Sometimes three simultaneous acid-base disorders, or a triple acid-base disturbance, can be identified.

Recognition of mixed acid-base disorders is important for several reasons. First, when these disorders are additive (i.e., concurrent metabolic and respiratory acidoses or concurrent metabolic and respiratory alkaloses), the pH excursions may become severe, with toxic consequences. When offsetting disorders coexist, the pH may be normal or near normal. Nonetheless, their identification serves as an important diagnostic clue to the underlying pathophysiology. Mixed disorders often suggest specific clinical derangements. For example, concurrent high AG metabolic acidosis and respiratory alkalosis are typical of salicylate poisoning, whereas patients with diabetic ketoacidosis often vomit and may present with concurrent high AG metabolic acidosis and metabolic alkalosis.

INADEQUATE OR "EXCESSIVE" COMPENSATION

The expected compensatory responses shown in the acid-base nomogram (see Fig. 12.1) and described in Table 12.1 are used to determine whether respiratory compensation for a metabolic disorder, or metabolic compensation for a respiratory disorder, is quantitatively appropriate, inadequate, or excessive. The arterial pH, pCO_2, and [HCO_3^-] values are required for this determination; therefore, a blood gas analysis

is necessary for complete characterization of the acid-base disturbance. If a patient with a metabolic acidosis has a pCO_2 that is lower than the expected compensatory response, a respiratory alkalosis also exists; conversely, a pCO_2 that is too high indicates a complicating respiratory acidosis. Analogously, if a primary respiratory acid-base disorder is identified, then the measured [HCO_3^-] should be in the range predicted by the nomogram or compensation rules (see Fig. 12.1 and Table 12.1). It should be noted that the determination of the appropriate compensation range for any primary respiratory disorder also requires the classification of that disorder as acute (from minutes to 1 to 2 days) or chronic (>2 days), a decision that is usually based on the patient's history and physical exam. If the measured [HCO_3^-] is higher than the compensatory range expected with a respiratory acidosis, then a coexistent metabolic alkalosis should be considered;

Table 12.2   Mixed Metabolic Acidosis and Respiratory Acidosis (Clinical Example 1)

Analyte	Normal Concentration	High AG Metabolic Acidosis With Appropriate Compensation	MIXED HIGH AG METABOLIC ACIDOSIS AND RESPIRATORY ACIDOSIS	
			Mixed High AG Metabolic Acidosis and Mild Respiratory Acidosis	Mixed High AG Metabolic Acidosis and Severe Respiratory Acidosis
Na^+	140	140	140	140
K^+	4.0	5.0	5.0	5.0
Cl^-	105	105	105	105
HCO_3^-	25	15	15	15
AG	10	20	20	20
pCO_2	40	30	40	50
pH	7.42	7.32	7.20	7.10

AG, Anion gap; *pCO_2,* arterial carbon dioxide tension.

Table 12.3   Mixed Metabolic Alkalosis and Chronic Respiratory Acidosis (Clinical Example 2)

Analyte	Normal Concentration	Chronic Respiratory Acidosis With Appropriate Compensation	Metabolic Alkalosis With Appropriate Compensation	Mixed Chronic Respiratory Acidosis and Metabolic Alkalosis
Na^+	140	140	140	140
K^+	4.0	5.0	3.4	3.5
Cl^-	105	98	98	90
HCO_3^-	25	32	31	37
AG	10	10	12	13
pCO_2	40	60	43	60
pH	7.42	7.35	7.47	7.41

Table 12.4   Mixed Metabolic Acidosis and Respiratory Alkalosis (Clinical Example 3)

Analyte	Normal Concentration	High AG Metabolic Acidosis With Appropriate Compensation	MIXED METABOLIC ACIDOSIS AND RESPIRATORY ALKALOSIS	
			Mild Respiratory Alkalosis	Severe Respiratory Alkalosis
Na^+	140	140	140	140
K^+	4.0	5.0	5.0	5.0
Cl^-	105	105	105	105
HCO_3^-	25	15	15	15
AG	10	20	20	20
pCO_2	40	30	25	20
pH	7.42	7.32	7.4	7.5

AG, Anion gap; *pCO_2,* arterial carbon dioxide tension.

Table 12.5 Simple and Mixed Metabolic and Respiratory Alkalosis (Clinical Example 4)

| Analyte | Normal Concentration | SIMPLE ALKALOSIS | | MIXED METABOLIC AND CHRONIC RESPIRATORY ALKALOSIS | |
		Metabolic Alkalosis With Appropriate Compensation	Chronic Respiratory Alkalosis With Appropriate Compensation	Mild Metabolic Alkalosis	Severe Metabolic Alkalosis
Na^+	140	140	140	140	140
K^+	4.0	3.2	3.4	3.1	2.9
Cl^-	105	96	108	103	96
HCO_3^-	25	32	19	23[a]	29
AG	10	12	12	14	15
PCO_2	40	44	30	30	30
pH	7.42	7.48	7.42	7.51	7.61

[a]Note that a lack of metabolic compensation—the serum $[HCO_3^-]$ has not decreased—in the presence of chronic respiratory alkalosis is consistent with coexisting metabolic alkalosis. This pattern could also exist in simple *acute* respiratory alkalosis.
AG, Anion gap; *PCO₂*, arterial carbon dioxide tension.

Table 12.6 Mixed Metabolic Acidosis and Metabolic Alkalosis (Clinical Example 5)

| Analyte | Normal Concentration | High AG Metabolic Acidosis With Appropriate Compensation | Normal AG Metabolic Acidosis With Appropriate Compensation | MIXED METABOLIC ALKALOSIS AND METABOLIC ACIDOSIS | |
				High AG Metabolic Acidosis and Metabolic Alkalosis	Normal AG Metabolic Acidosis and Metabolic Alkalosis
Na^+	140	140	140	140	140
K^+	4.0	5.0	3.8	4.0	4.0
Cl^-	105	105	115	95	105
HCO_3^-	25	15	15	25	25
AG	10	20	10	20	10
PCO_2	40	30	30	40	40
pH	7.42	7.32	7.32	7.42	7.42

AG, Anion gap; *PCO₂*, arterial carbon dioxide tension.

conversely, if the $[HCO_3^-]$ is too low, a coexistent metabolic acidosis should be considered. Examples of such mixed acid-base disorders are provided in Tables 12.2–12.5, and they are discussed later in this chapter (see the "Clinical Examples" section).

THE DELTA/DELTA ($\Delta AG/\Delta HCO_3^-$)

Whenever an AG metabolic acidosis exists as a single acid-base disorder, the magnitude of the increase in AG should be quantitatively similar to the magnitude of reduction in $[HCO_3^-]$. If the AG increases by 10 mEq/L as a result of an accumulation of keto acids that have titrated the serum bicarbonate, then the $[HCO_3^-]$ should also decrease by about 10 mEq/L (see Fig. 12.3). The absolute value of each change should be equivalent, such that $\Delta[AG] = \Delta[HCO_3^-]$.

If the increase in AG above its baseline (the ΔAG) exceeds the fall in $[HCO_3^-]$ from its baseline of 24 mEq/L (the ΔHCO_3^-), then the presence of an additional acid-base disorder that has elevated the $[HCO_3^-]$ is suggested. Two situations usually cause this discrepancy. Most often, it is the result of a coexistent metabolic alkalosis (Table 12.6 and clinical example 5). Another possibility is a coexistent chronic respiratory

acidosis for which compensation has increased the $[HCO_3^-]$ to a value greater than the normal range (Fig. 12.4). The resulting arterial pH and pCO_2 should allow the clinician to readily distinguish between these possibilities.

Conversely, if the increase of the AG is smaller than the fall in $[HCO_3^-]$ from a normal baseline of about 24 mEq/L (i.e., $\Delta AG < \Delta HCO_3^-$), the $[Cl^-]$ must be increased relative to $[Na^+]$. The presence of relative hyperchloremia usually indicates the existence of a hyperchloremic metabolic acidosis, or compensation for chronic respiratory alkalosis. Again, the resulting arterial pH and pCO_2 should allow one to readily distinguish between these possibilities.

These $\Delta AG/\Delta HCO_3^-$ comparisons usually assume that the AG has started in the normal range. If the initial AG is abnormally low to begin with (e.g., if the patient has a very low albumin concentration), then the excursion (or Δ) must begin from this lower baseline.

CLINICAL EXAMPLES

CLINICAL EXAMPLE 1

A patient becomes septic and develops lactic acidosis. If that same patient also develops acute respiratory distress syndrome

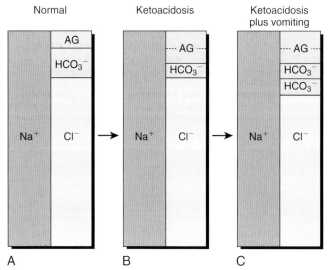

Fig. 12.4 The effect of ketoacidosis plus vomiting on the ionic profile of blood. (A) The normal electrolyte pattern. (B) The development of a typical anion gap *(AG)* metabolic acidosis. (C) The superimposed effect of vomiting, which causes proton loss without the loss of any organic acid anions. This results in a decrease in the serum chloride concentration and an increase in the bicarbonate concentration. The latter normalizes the [HCO$_3^-$], but the AG remains large because the keto acid concentration is unchanged by the vomiting.

(ARDS), then mild or severe respiratory acidosis may occur as well (see Table 12.2).

CLINICAL EXAMPLE 2

A patient with chronic obstructive pulmonary disease (COPD) may show a pattern of chronic respiratory acidosis, as depicted in the first chronic respiratory acidosis column of Table 12.3, whereas a patient receiving loop diuretic therapy may develop metabolic alkalosis, as shown in the next column of Table 12.3. If a patient with COPD is treated with a loop diuretic, the pattern in the last column of the table may develop. Note that a chronic pCO$_2$ of 55 mm Hg should raise the [HCO$_3^-$] to about 31 mEq/L, so the [HCO$_3^-$] of 34 mEq/L is too high. Also, note that this has resulted in a pH of 7.41, which is too high. Patients with chronic respiratory acidosis should not have a pH in the mid- to normal range; their pH should remain slightly acidic, even after full compensation.

CLINICAL EXAMPLE 3

Patients with uncomplicated AG metabolic acidosis will have a reduced [HCO$_3^-$], an appropriately reduced pCO$_2$, and an acidic pH. Superimposed respiratory alkalosis will further reduce the pCO$_2$ and raise the pH toward normal or even enough to generate alkalemia (see Table 12.4). Patients with aspirin overdose will often present with this mixed acid-base pattern. Inhibition of normal oxidative metabolic reactions causes an accumulation of multiple organic acidoses and hence the AG metabolic acidosis. Acetylsalicylic acid also directly contributes to the large AG. Simultaneously, the toxic levels of salicylate stimulate central hyperventilation. The pattern in the last column of Table 12.4 is typically seen in adults with this disorder. Infants with salicylate poisoning more typically present with less marked respiratory alkalosis, so their arterial pH is generally acidic.

CLINICAL EXAMPLE 4

Metabolic alkalosis occurs with elevation of the [HCO$_3^-$], and compensation should increase the pCO$_2$. Respiratory alkalosis is seen with a reduced pCO$_2$, and compensation should decrease the [HCO$_3^-$]. Hence, in simple alkaloses, both components should deviate in the same direction. If the [HCO$_3^-$] is increased and the pCO$_2$ is decreased, then metabolic alkalosis and respiratory alkalosis coexist (see Table 12.5). This mixed acid-base disorder is often seen in patients with severe liver disease. Chronic respiratory alkalosis is extremely common as a result of diaphragmatic elevation, A-V shunting, and a deranged hormonal milieu that stimulates ventilation. Nausea and vomiting occur frequently, and nasogastric suction is often employed. These disorders and treatments generate metabolic alkalosis, which complicates the chronic respiratory alkalosis. Combined, these disorders can generate extreme alkalemia.

CLINICAL EXAMPLE 5

The combination of mixed metabolic acidosis with high AG and metabolic alkalosis can develop in different ways.

1. A large AG metabolic acidosis may develop in a patient with preexisting metabolic alkalosis. In this situation, the [HCO$_3^-$] falls from a supranormal level as the AG develops (see Table 12.6).
2. Metabolic alkalosis may develop in a patient with a large AG metabolic acidosis. The metabolic alkalosis raises the [HCO$_3^-$], while the AG remains large.
3. AG metabolic acidosis and metabolic alkalosis can develop simultaneously.

In each of these scenarios, the elevated AG remains as a residual marker of the metabolic acidosis. However, the magnitude of increase of the AG is greater than the [HCO$_3^-$] fall from its baseline. This relationship can be expressed as the Delta/Delta or Δ[AG]/Δ[HCO$_3^-$], which will be increased above 1 (the Δ[AG] > Δ[HCO$_3^-$]).

Patients with diabetic ketoacidosis have metabolic acidosis with a large AG. If nausea and vomiting occur, they generate a simultaneous or sequential metabolic alkalosis through loss of acidic gastric fluids. Although the final arterial pH is typically acid, it may sometimes become normal or even alkaline if the alkalosis is more severe than the acidosis. Regardless of the resultant pH and [HCO$_3^-$], the large AG remains a major chemical clue to the presence of a metabolic acidosis. A similar pattern is seen when uremic patients develop nausea and vomiting.

OTHER MIXED ACID-BASE DISORDERS

The combination of a hyperchloremic metabolic acidosis and metabolic alkalosis may be more difficult to diagnose. In these patients, there is no residual AG increase to indicate that an underlying metabolic acidosis exists. Instead, the hyperchloremic acidosis reduces the [HCO$_3^-$] and increases the [Cl$^-$], whereas the metabolic alkalosis increases the [HCO$_3^-$] and decreases the [Cl$^-$] (see Table 12.6). If the two disorders are of similar intensity, the final [HCO$_3^-$] and [Cl$^-$] may be restored to their normal ranges with a normal AG. This mixed disorder can be suspected on the basis of the history,

Table 12.7   Metabolic Acidosis, Metabolic Alkalosis, and Respiratory Alkalosis: A Triple Acid-Base Disturbance

Analyte	Normal Concentrations	Case 1: Metabolic Alkalosis With Appropriate Compensation	Case 2: High AG Metabolic Acidosis With Appropriate Compensation	Case 3: Mixed Metabolic Acidosis and Metabolic Alkalosis	Case 4: Mixed Metabolic Acidosis, Metabolic Alkalosis, and Respiratory Alkalosis
Na^+	140	140	140	140	140
K^+	4.0	3.4	4.5	4.5	4.5
Cl^-	105	89	105	92	92
HCO_3^-	25	38	12	25	25
AG	10	13	23	23	23
PCO_2	40	46	26	40	30
pH	7.42	7.54	7.29	7.42	7.54

AG, Anion gap; *PCO₂*, arterial carbon dioxide tension.

clinical setting, and physical exam. For example, a patient with gastroenteritis who has a history of both watery diarrhea and vomiting may have this mixed acid-base disorder, despite a normal pH, pCO₂, [HCO₃⁻], AG, and [Cl⁻]. Marked hypokalemia may be present. If the vomiting improves but the diarrhea continues, overt hyperchloremic metabolic acidosis and acidemia may be revealed.

Other forms of mixed acid-base disorders are combinations of different metabolic acidosis disorders or, much less commonly, metabolic alkalosis disorders. For example, it is not uncommon for ketoacidosis to coexist with lactic acidosis; similarly, hyperchloremic acidosis caused by diarrhea or renal tubular acidosis may present in conjunction with lactic acidosis or uremic acidosis. Some patients with nausea and vomiting may medicate themselves with baking soda. The vomiting generates HCO₃⁻, and the baking soda is a form of exogenous alkali (sodium bicarbonate).

Mixed respiratory acid-base disorders can also develop, and they are usually suspected on the basis of the history and clinical setting rather than any specific laboratory results. The patient with chronic obstructive lung disease who presents with recent pulmonary deterioration, caused by a mucus plug or pneumonia, may have chronic respiratory acidosis and a superimposed acute respiratory acidosis. A pregnant woman with underlying hyperventilation who ingests an overdose of sedating drugs and develops respiratory depression will have chronic respiratory alkalosis and a superimposed acute respiratory alkalosis.

TRIPLE ACID-BASE DISTURBANCES

A relatively common and the most readily diagnosed type of triple acid-base disturbance is due to the combination of an elevated AG metabolic acidosis, metabolic alkalosis, and either respiratory acidosis or respiratory alkalosis. The offsetting

effects of the coexistent metabolic acidosis and alkalosis result in a low, normal, or elevated [HCO₃⁻]. Regardless of the [HCO₃⁻], there is a large ΔAG, which exceeds the Δ[HCO₃⁻]. This is the clue to the double disorder of metabolic acidosis and metabolic alkalosis. The final [HCO₃⁻] that results from these two disorders is the parameter that should determine the degree of respiratory compensation and pCO₂. If the pCO₂ is lower than expected, a third disorder, respiratory alkalosis, exists. If the pCO₂ is higher than expected, the third disorder is respiratory acidosis.

A clinical example is shown in Table 12.7. Case 1 is a patient who vomits and develops metabolic alkalosis. The [HCO₃⁻] increases to 38 mEq/L, the pCO₂ increases to 46 mm Hg, and the AG increases slightly. Case 2 illustrates the findings expected with high AG metabolic acidosis, such as lactic acidosis. The [HCO₃⁻] has fallen by 13 mEq/L, and the AG has increased by the same amount. If the patient represented by Case 1 develops severe ECF volume depletion, then lactic acidosis may ensue (Case 3). Accordingly, the [HCO₃⁻] falls, in this example from 38 to 25 mEq/L (a ΔHCO₃⁻ of 13 mEq/L), and the AG also increases by a Δ of 23 mEq/L. The chemistries in Case 3 show a normal [HCO₃⁻], despite an AG of 23 mEq/L. The discrepancy between the normal [HCO₃⁻] and the large AG is the major clue to this mixed acid-base disorder. The normal [HCO₃⁻], which is the result of equally severe degrees of metabolic acidosis and metabolic alkalosis, should be associated with a normal pCO₂. The last column (Case 4) shows an example of a pCO₂ that is too low, indicating that a third disorder, respiratory alkalosis, is also present. If the pCO₂ had been 50 mm Hg, then respiratory acidosis, metabolic alkalosis, and metabolic acidosis would be the triple disturbance.

The flow charts in Figs. 12.5 and 12.6 show one general approach to the diagnostic workup of a patient with either acidemia or alkalemia.

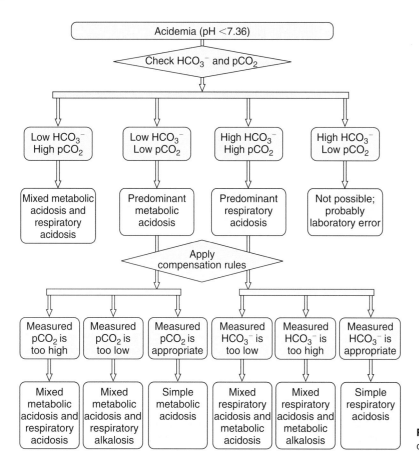

Fig. 12.5 A flowchart showing one approach to the diagnostic workup of a patient with acidemia.

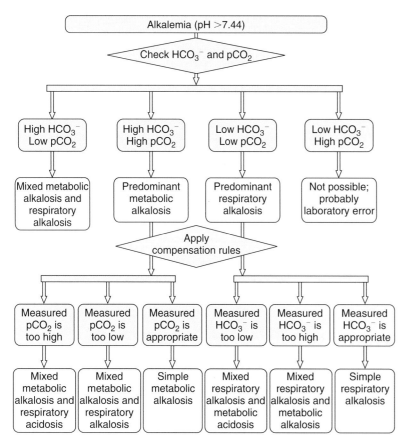

Fig. 12.6 A flowchart showing one approach to the diagnostic workup of a patient with alkalemia.

BIBLIOGRAPHY

Adrogué HJ, Gennari FJ, Galla JH. Assessing acid-base disorders. *Kidney Int.* 2009;76:1239-1247.

Emmett M, Narins R. Clinical use of the AG. *Medicine (Baltimore).* 1977;56:38-54.

Emmett M, Seldin DW. Evaluation of acid-base disorders from plasma composition. In: Seldin DW, Giebisch G, eds. *The Regulation of Acid-Base Balance.* New York: Raven Press; 1989:213-263.

Gabow PA, Kaehny WD, Fennessey PV. Diagnostic importance of an increased serum anion gap. *N Engl J Med.* 1980;303:854-858.

Madias NE. Renal acidification responses to respiratory acid-base disorders. *J Nephrol.* 2010;23(suppl 16):S85-S91.

Madias NE, Adrogué HJ. Respiratory alkalosis and acidosis. In: Seldin DW, Giebisch G, eds. *The Kidney: Physiology and Pathophysiology.* 3rd ed. Philadelphia: Lippincott/Williams & Wilkins; 2000:2131-2166.

Mehta AN, Emmett JB, Emmett M. GOLD MARK: an AG mnemonic for the 21st century. *Lancet.* 2008;372:892.

Narins RG, Emmett M. Simple and mixed acid-base disorders: a practical approach. *Medicine (Baltimore).* 1980;59:161-187.

Palmer BF, Alpern RJ. Metabolic alkalosis. *J Am Soc Nephrol.* 1997;8:1462-1469.

Rastegar A. Use of the DeltaAG/DeltaHCO3– ratio in the diagnosis of mixed acid-base disorders. *J Am Soc Nephrol.* 2007;18:2429-2431.

13 Metabolic Acidosis

Harold M. Szerlip

Metabolic acidosis describes a process in which nonvolatile acids accumulate in the body. For practical purposes, this can result from either the addition of protons or the loss of base. The consequence of this process is a decline in the major extracellular buffer, bicarbonate, and, if unopposed, a decrease in extracellular pH. Depending on the existence and the magnitude of other acid-base disturbances, however, the extracellular pH may be low, normal, or even high. Normal blood pH is between 7.36 and 7.44, corresponding to a hydrogen ion concentration of 44 to 36 nmol/L.

Because the body tightly defends against changes in pH, a decreased pH sensitizes both peripheral and central chemoreceptors, which triggers an increase in minute ventilation. This compensatory respiratory alkalosis helps offset a marked fall in pH. Because increased ventilation is a compensatory mechanism stimulated by the acidemia, it never returns the pH to normal. The expected partial pressure of carbon dioxide (pCO_2) for any given degree of metabolic acidosis can be estimated by adding 15 back to the bicarbonate,

$$pCO_2 = 15 + HCO_3$$

or by using Winters' formula: $pCO_2 = (1.5 \times [HCO_3]) + 8 \pm 2$.

OVERVIEW OF ACID-BASE BALANCE

To maintain extracellular pH within the normal range, the daily production of acid must be excreted from the body (Fig. 13.1). The vast majority of acid production results from the metabolism of dietary carbohydrates and fats. Complete oxidation of these metabolic substrates produces CO_2 and water. The 15,000 mmoles of CO_2 produced daily are efficiently exhaled by the lungs and are therefore known as "volatile acid." As long as ventilatory function remains normal, this volatile acid does not contribute to changes in acid-base balance. Nonvolatile or fixed acids are produced by the metabolism of sulfate-containing and phosphate-containing amino acids. In addition, incomplete oxidation of fats and carbohydrates results in the production of small quantities of lactate and other organic anions, which when excreted in the urine represent a loss of base. Individuals consuming a typical meat-based diet produce approximately 1 mmol/kg/day of hydrogen ions. Fecal excretion of a small amount of base also contributes to total daily acid production.

The kidney is responsible not only for the excretion of the daily production of fixed acid but also for the reclamation of the filtered bicarbonate. Bicarbonate reclamation occurs predominantly in the proximal tubule, mainly through the Na^+-H^+ exchanger. Active transporters in the distal tubule secrete hydrogen ion against a concentration gradient. Although urinary pH can fall to as low as 4.5, if there were no urinary buffers, this would account for very little acid excretion. For example, to excrete 100 mmoles of H^+ into unbuffered urine at a minimum urine pH of 4.5 ([H^+] = 32 mmol/L) would require a daily urine volume of 3000 L. Fortunately, urinary phosphate and creatinine help buffer these protons, allowing the kidney to excrete approximately 40% to 50% of the daily fixed acid load as titratable acid (TA), so called because they are quantitated by titrating the urine pH back to that of plasma, 7.4. In addition to TA, renal excretion of acid is supported by ammoniagenesis. NH_3 is generated in the proximal tubule by the deamidation of glutamine to glutamate, which is subsequently deaminated to yield α-ketoglutarate. The enzymes responsible for these reactions are upregulated by acidosis and hypokalemia. Hyperkalemia, on the other hand, reduces ammoniagenesis. NH_3 builds up in the renal interstitium and passively diffuses into the tubule lumen along the length of the collecting duct, where it is trapped by H^+ as ammonium (NH_4^+).

Under conditions of increased acid production, the normal kidney can increase acid excretion primarily by augmenting NH_3 production. Renal acid excretion varies directly with the rate of acid production. Net renal acid excretion (NAE) is equal to the sum of TA and NH_4^+, minus any secreted HCO_3^- [NAE = (TA + NH_4^+) − HCO_3^+]. Thus the etiology of a metabolic acidosis can be divided into four broad categories: (1) overproduction of fixed acids, (2) increased extrarenal loss of base, (3) decrease in the kidney's ability to secrete hydrogen ions, and (4) inability of the kidney to reclaim the filtered bicarbonate (Fig. 13.2).

EVALUATION OF URINARY ACIDIFICATION

The cause of metabolic acidosis often is evident from the clinical situation. However, because the kidney is responsible for both the reclamation of filtered HCO_3^- and the excretion of the daily production of fixed acid, to evaluate a metabolic acidosis it may be necessary to assess whether the kidney is appropriately able to reabsorb HCO_3^-, secrete H^+ against a gradient, and excrete NH_4^+ (Table 13.1). The simplest test is to measure the urine pH. Although urine pH can be measured using a dipstick, the lack of precision of this

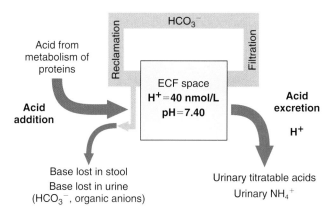

Fig. 13.1 Maintenance of acid-base homeostasis requires that the addition of acid to the body is balanced by excretion of acid. Production of fixed nonvolatile acid occurs mainly through the metabolism of proteins. A small quantity of base also is lost in the stool and urine. Acid excretion occurs in the kidney through the secretion of H^+ buffered by titratable acids and NH_3. Bicarbonate filtration and reclamation by the kidney are normally a neutral process.

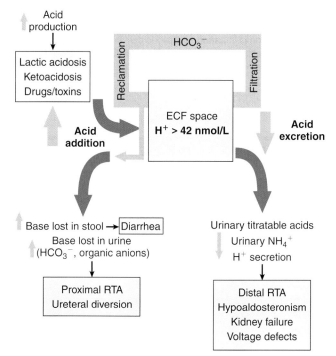

Fig. 13.2 Metabolic acidosis can result from increased acid production, increased loss of base in stool or urine, or decreased H^+ secretion in the distal tubule. The causes of these processes are shown. *RTA*, Renal tubular acidosis.

Table 13.1   Tests of Renal Acid Excretion

Urine pH (enhanced by furosemide)
NH_4^+ excretion
- Urine NH_4^+
- Urine anion gap
- Urine osmolal gap

Urine pCO$_2$ with bicarbonate loading
Fractional excretion of HCO_3^-

---

technique prevents it from being useful in making clinical decisions. Although it has been suggested that urine be collected under oil and the pH measured, using a pH electrode to prevent the loss of CO_2, in fact when the urine pH is less than 6.0, the amount of dissolved CO_2 is minimal and the use of oil is unnecessary. Under conditions of acid loading, urine pH should be below 5.5. A pH of higher than 5.5 usually reflects impaired distal hydrogen ion secretion. Measuring the pH after challenging the patient with the loop diuretic furosemide will increase the sensitivity of this test by providing Na^+ to the distal tubule for reabsorption. The reabsorption of Na^+ creates a negative electrical potential in the lumen and enhances H^+ secretion. It is important, however, to rule out urinary infections with urea-splitting organisms, which will increase pH. An elevated urine pH may also be misleading in conditions associated with volume depletion and hypokalemia, as can occur in diarrhea. In contradistinction to furosemide, volume depletion with decreased sodium delivery to the distal tubule impairs distal H^+ secretion. Furthermore, hypokalemia, by enhancing ammoniagenesis, raises the urine pH.

Because renal excretion of NH_4^+ accounts for the majority of acid excretion, measurement of urine NH_4^+ provides important information. Urinary NH_4^+ excretion can be decreased by a variety of mechanisms, including a primary decrease in ammoniagenesis by the proximal tubule, as seen in chronic kidney disease (CKD), or decreased trapping in the distal tubule either secondary to decreased H^+ secretion or an increased delivery of HCO_3^-, which will preferentially buffer H^+, making it unavailable to form NH_4^+. Although direct measurement of NH_4^+ is becoming more readily available in clinical laboratories and is the gold standard, many laboratories still do not perform this assay. An estimate of NH_4^+ excretion, however, is easily obtained by calculating the urine anion gap (UAG) or urine osmole gap. If, as is usual, the anion balancing the charge of the NH_4^+ is Cl^-, the UAG $[(Na^+ + K^+) - Cl^-]$ should be negative because the chloride is greater than the sum of Na^+ and K^+ (Fig. 13.3). Although the measurement of the UAG in conditions of acid loading is often reflective of NH_4^+ excretion, the presence of anions other than Cl^- (such as keto anions or hippurate) makes it a less reliable assessment of NH_4^+ than the urine osmole gap (see Fig. 13.3). The urine osmole gap is calculated as follows: [measured urine osmolality − calculated urine osmolality], where calculated urine osmolality is $[2(Na^+ + K^+) + (urea\ nitrogen/2.8) + (glucose/18)]$. The osmole gap is made up primarily of NH_4^+ salts. Thus half of the gap represents NH_4^+. An osmole gap of greater than 100 mmol/L signifies normal NH_4^+ excretion.

Another test of distal H^+ ion secretory ability is measurement of urine pCO_2 during bicarbonate loading. Distal delivery of HCO_3^- in the presence of normal H^+ secretory capacity results in elevated pCO_2 in the urine. When there is a secretory defect, urine pCO_2 does not increase. In this case, accurate measurement of urine pCO_2 requires that the urine be collected under oil to prevent the loss of CO_2 into the air.

COMPLICATIONS OF ACIDOSIS

Although it has been accepted that a decrease in extracellular pH has detrimental effects on numerous physiologic

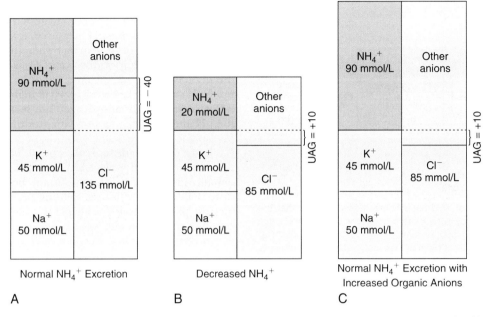

Fig. 13.3 In the presence of acidemia, the kidney increases NH_4^+ excretion. The urine anion gap *(UAG)* is an indirect method for estimating urine NH_4^+. (A) If the accompanying anion is chloride, the UAG ($Na^+ + K^+ - Cl^-$) will be negative, reflecting the large quantity of NH_4^+ in the urine. (B) A decrease in NH_4^+ secretion occurs when ammoniagenesis is diminished, H^+ secretion is impaired, or there is delivery of HCO_3^- to the distal tubule. In these cases, the UAG will be inappropriately positive. (C) If anions other than Cl are excreted (e.g., ketones, hippurate), the UAG will be positive despite increased NH_4^+ excretion, because these anions are not used in calculation of the gap.

parameters and should be aggressively treated, this dogma has been challenged. The proponents of treatment argue that acidemia depresses cardiac contractility, blocks activation of adrenergic receptors, and inhibits the action of key enzymes. Uncontrolled clinical studies are not easy to interpret because of the difficulties in separating the effects of the acidosis from the effects of the underlying illness. Most controlled studies investigating the role of acidosis on cellular processes have been done in isolated cells or organs; therefore the effects of acidemia on whole-body physiology and their applicability to humans are unclear.

The effect of pH on cardiac function has been strongly debated. Cardiac output is determined by multiple components, and it is the sum of the effects on these individual components that determines the net effect of acidemia on cardiac function. Myocardial contractile strength and changes in vascular tone determine cardiovascular performance, and the relative contributions of each in the context of acidemia remain to be clarified. Because of differing effects of acidemia on contractile force, vascular tone, and sympathetic discharge, it is difficult to predict what happens to cardiac output from studies using isolated myocytes or perfused hearts.

During continuous infusion of lactic acid, it has been shown that cardiac output and the rate of development of left ventricular force increase. In addition, fractional shortening of the left ventricle as assessed by transthoracic echocardiography appears to be normal, even in cases of severe acidemia. The pH at which cardiac output and blood pressure fall remains unclear.

APPROACH TO ACID-BASE DISORDERS

Complete evaluation of acid-base status requires a routine electrolyte panel, measurement of serum albumin, and arterial blood gas analysis (see Chapter 12). The traditional approach to metabolic acidosis relies on the calculation of the anion gap (AG) and the subsequent separation of metabolic acidosis into those with an elevated AG and those in which the AG is normal, or so-called hyperchloremic metabolic acidosis (HCMA; Fig. 13.4). The AG is defined as the difference between the concentration of sodium, the major cation, and the sum of the concentrations of chloride and bicarbonate, the major anions: $Na^+ - [Cl^- - HCO_3^-]$. Because the concentration of potassium changes minimally, its contribution is ignored for convenience. Obviously, electrical neutrality must exist, and the sum of the anions must equal the sum of the cations. The gap results because the unmeasured anions, such as sulfate, phosphate, organic anions, and especially the weak acid proteins, are greater than the unmeasured cations (i.e., magnesium). Thus it would seem upon examination of a basic chemistry panel that cations exceed anions, creating an AG. The normal AG is 10 ± 2 mEq/L. Any increase in the AG, even in the face of a normal or frankly alkalemic pH, represents the accumulation of acids and the presence of an acidosis. In many cases, the anions that make up the gap are not easily identifiable.

The one caveat in using the AG is to recognize that the normal gap is predominantly composed of the negative charge on albumin. When hypoalbuminemia is present, the AG must be corrected for the serum albumin. For each 1-g/dL decrease

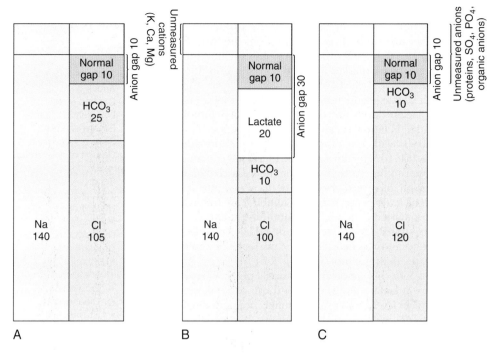

Fig. 13.4 The anion gap (AG) is equal to $[Na^+] + ([Cl^-] + [HCO_3^-])$, which is equal to the unmeasured anions minus the unmeasured cations. (A) The normal anion gap is 10 ± 2. (B) In an AG acidosis there is a decrease in $[HCO_3^-]$ and an increase in organic anions (e.g., lactate), which results in an elevated anion gap. (C) In a hyperchloremic acidosis, there is a decrease in $[HCO_3^-]$ and an increase in [Cl], with no change in anion gap.

in the serum albumin, the calculated AG should be increased by 2.5 mEq/L. Thus the corrected AG can be estimated as AGc = AG + 2.5 (4 − serum albumin). If the AG is not corrected, the presence of a metabolic acidosis may be masked. This is especially true in critically ill patients, who typically have decreased serum albumin.

ANION GAP ACIDOSIS

As previously described, an increased AG represents the accumulation of nonchloride acids. The mnemonic GOLD-MARK is a useful tool that helps identify the causes of an AG acidosis (Fig. 13.5). AG acidosis can be divided into four major categories (Table 13.2): (1) lactic acidosis, (2) keto-acidosis, (3) toxin/drugs, and (4) severe kidney failure. In all but kidney failure, the accumulation of acids is caused by their overproduction. These acids dissociate into protons, which are quickly buffered by HCO_3^-, and into their respective conjugate bases, the unmeasured anions. As long as these anions are retained in the body and not excreted, they contribute to the elevation in the AG.

LACTIC ACIDOSIS

Lactic acidosis is a common AG acidosis and by far the most serious of all high-AG acidoses. Anaerobic metabolism of glucose (glycolysis) occurs in the extramitochondrial cytoplasm and produces pyruvate as an intermediary. If this were the end of the glycolytic process, there would be a net production of two protons and a metabolically unsatisfactory reduction of NAD to NADH. Fortunately, pyruvate rapidly undergoes one of two metabolic fates: (1) under anaerobic conditions, because of the high NADH/NAD ratio, pyruvate is quickly reduced by lactate dehydrogenase to lactate, releasing energy, consuming a proton, and decreasing the NADH/NAD ratio, thus allowing for continued glycolysis; or (2) in the presence

- Glycols
- Oxoproline (pyroglutamic acid – acetaminophen)
- L-lactate
- D-lactate

- Methanol
- Aspirin
- Renal failure
- Ketoacidosis

Fig. 13.5 GOLDMARK is a useful mnemonic to remember the common causes of an anion gap metabolic acidosis.

Table 13.2   Causes of Anion Gap Acidosis

Lactic acidosis
- Type A
- Type B
- D-Lactic acidosis

Ketoacidosis
- Diabetic ketoacidosis
- Alcoholic ketoacidosis
- Starvation ketosis

Toxins/drugs
- Methanol
- Ethylene glycol
- Acetaminophen
- Salicylate

Kidney failure (with severe reductions in glomerular filtration rate)

of oxygen, pyruvate diffuses into the mitochondria and, after oxidation by the pyruvate dehydrogenase (PDH) complex, enters the tricarboxylic acid cycle, where it is completely oxidized to CO_2 and water. Neither of these pathways results in the production of H^+. During glycolysis, glucose metabolism produces two molecules of lactate and two molecules of adenosine triphosphate (ATP). It is the hydrolysis of ATP

(ATP = ADP + H$^+$ + Pi) that releases protons. Therefore the acidosis does not occur because of the production of lactate but because under hypoxic conditions the hydrolysis of ATP is greater than ATP production. Thus the buildup of lactate is a surrogate marker for ATP consumption during hypoxic states.

Although lactate production averages about 1300 mmol/day, serum lactate levels are typically less than 1 mmol/L because lactate is either reoxidized to pyruvate and enters the tricarboxylic acid cycle or is used by the liver and kidney via the Cori cycle for gluconeogenesis. Increased concentration of lactate can therefore result from decreased oxidative phosphorylation, increased glycolysis, or decreased gluconeogenesis. Lactate levels between 2 and 3 mmol/L are frequently found in hospitalized patients. Some of these patients will go on to develop frank acidosis, but others will have no adverse events. Lactic acidosis is defined as the presence of a lactate level of greater than 5 mmol/L.

There is a poor correlation among arterial pH, uncorrected AG, and serum lactate levels, even in those patients with a serum lactic acid level greater than 5 mmol/L. Approximately 25% of patients with serum lactate levels between 5 and 9.9 mmol/L have a pH greater than 7.35, and as many as half have AGs of less than 12.

Lactic acidosis has been traditionally divided into types A and B (Table 13.3). Type A, or hypoxic lactic acidosis, results from an imbalance between oxygen supply and oxygen demand. In type B lactic acidosis, oxygen delivery is normal, but oxidative phosphorylation is impaired. This is seen in patients who have inborn errors of metabolism or who have ingested drugs or toxins. It has become increasingly clear, however, that lactic acidosis is often caused by the simultaneous existence of both hypoxic and nonhypoxic factors, and in many cases it is difficult to separate one from the other. For example, hereditary partial defects in mitochondrial metabolism, as well as age-related declines in cytochrome IV complex activity, may result in lactic acidosis with a lesser degree of hypoxia than in patients without such defects. Even in cases of shock, in which tissue oxygen delivery is obviously inadequate, decreased portal blood flow and reduced hepatic clearance of lactate contribute to the acidosis. Similarly, in sepsis there is a decrease in both tissue perfusion and in the ability to use oxygen. Therefore this division based solely on cause is largely of historic and conceptual interest.

The presence of lactic acidosis is considered a poor prognostic sign. Studies have found that, as lactate levels increase above 4 mmol/L, the probability of survival decreases precipitously; however, it is unclear whether the blood lactate level is an independent contributor to mortality or whether it represents an epiphenomenon confounded by the severity of the patient's illness. Just as important to prognosis is the body's ability to metabolize lactate after the restoration of tissue perfusion. Patients able to reduce their lactate by half within 18 hours of resuscitation have a significantly greater chance of survival. In all likelihood, the inability to metabolize lactate is a surrogate marker for organ dysfunction.

TYPE A LACTIC ACIDOSIS

Lactic acidosis is commonly observed in conditions in which oxygen delivery is inadequate, such as low cardiac output, hypotension, severe anemia, and carbon monoxide poisoning. States of hypoperfusion are more prone to the accumulation

Table 13.3   Lactic Acidosis

Type A
- Generalized seizure
- Extreme exercise
- Shock
- Cardiac arrest
- Low cardiac output
- Severe anemia
- Severe hypoxemia
- Carbon monoxide poisoning

Type B
- Sepsis
- Thiamine deficiency
- Uncontrolled diabetes mellitus
- Malignancy
- Hypoglycemia
- Drugs/toxins
  - Ethanol
  - Metformin
  - Zidovudine
  - Didanosine
  - Stavudine
  - Lamivudine
  - Zalcitabine
  - Salicylate
- Linezolid
  - Propofol
  - Niacin
  - Isoniazid
  - Nitroprusside
  - Cyanide
  - Catecholamines
  - Cocaine
  - Acetaminophen
  - Streptozotocin
  - Pheochromocytoma
  - Sorbitol/fructose
  - Malaria
- Inborn errors of metabolism

Other
- Hepatic failure
- Respiratory or metabolic alkalosis
- Propylene glycol
- D-Lactic acidosis

of lactate than hypoxemic states. In the latter, tissue oxygenation is often preserved due to compensatory mechanisms such as increased cardiac output, augmented red blood cell production, and a reduced affinity of hemoglobin for oxygen. In all cases of type A lactic acidosis, oxygen is unavailable to the mitochondria, and pyruvate, unable to enter the tricarboxylic acid cycle, is reduced to lactate.

TYPE B LACTIC ACIDOSIS

Sepsis

Although sepsis is frequently associated with hypotension and thus type A lactic acidosis, lactic acidosis also may develop during sepsis, even when oxygen delivery and tissue perfusion appear to be unimpeded. In fact, in the right clinical setting, a lactate level greater than 4 mmol/L has become a surrogate marker for severe sepsis independent of hypotension—so-called compensated shock. It has been postulated that in sepsis there is both an overproduction of pyruvate and an inhibition of PDH activity (the rate-limiting state in oxidative phosphorylation). Because of the increased NADH/NAD ratio, pyruvate is rapidly reduced to lactate. In septic patients with lactic acidosis, dichloroacetate, an activator of the PDH complex, lowers lactate levels significantly, suggesting that tissue oxygenation is adequate to support oxidative phosphorylation and therefore not the limiting factor.

Drugs

Numerous drugs and toxins can cause lactic acidosis. The biguanide derivatives phenformin and metformin are recognized causes of lactic acidosis. Phenformin was withdrawn from the US market in 1976 because of the high frequency of lactic acidosis in association with its use. Both of these agents bind to complex 1 of the mitochondrial respiratory chain, inhibiting its activity. Metformin, a newer biguanide, has a markedly lower incidence of lactic acidosis than phenformin, possibly because it is less lipid soluble and thus has limited ability to cross the mitochondrial membrane and bind to the mitochondrial complex. Almost all reported cases of metformin-associated lactic acidosis have occurred in patients with underlying CKD. It has been suggested that the present incidence of lactic acidosis in diabetics is no greater than the incidence of lactic acidosis before the introduction of metformin, and thus the association of metformin with lactic acidosis is more "guilt by association." A causative role, however, is suggested by the observations that in isolated mitochondria, metformin inhibits the respiratory chain and that the incidence of lactic acidosis approaches zero when the drug is prescribed according to recommendations.

Lactic acidosis is being increasingly recognized in patients with human immunodeficiency virus infection who are taking nucleoside reverse-transcriptase inhibitors. These agents, particularly stavudine, but also zidovudine, didanosine, and lamivudine, have been associated with severe lactic acidosis, often with concomitant hepatic steatosis. Nucleoside analogues inhibit mitochondrial DNA polymerase-γ. This causes mitochondrial toxicity and a decrease in oxidative phosphorylation, resulting in lipid accumulation within the liver and in decreased oxidation of pyruvate. Of note, hyperlactatemia without frank lactic acidosis is often present in patients on these medications. What converts these mild elevations in lactate levels into frank lactic acidosis is not known.

Salicylate intoxication often produces lactic acidosis. This occurs both because the salicylate-induced respiratory alkalosis stimulates lactate production and because of the inhibitory effects of salicylates on oxidative metabolism. Ethanol ingestion may cause mild elevations in lactate levels, secondary to impaired hepatic conversion of lactate to glucose. In addition, the metabolism of ethanol increases the NADH/NAD ratio, favoring the conversion of pyruvate to lactate. Concomitant thiamine deficiency, as is often seen in alcohol abusers, may exacerbate the acidosis.

Linezolid, an oxazolidinone antibiotic approved for use in methicillin- and vancomycin-resistant gram-positive organisms, has been reported to be associated with lactic acidosis. The presumed mechanism is mitochondrial toxicity. Infusions of high-dose propofol have also been associated with lactic acidosis.

Vitamin Deficiencies

Deficiency of thiamine, a cofactor for PDH, can also result in lactic acidosis. Patients requiring total parenteral nutrition may develop thiamine deficiency if not supplemented with this vitamin. During a national shortage of parenteral vitamin preparations, numerous cases of lactic acidosis were reported from inadequate thiamine supplementation.

Systemic Disease

Diabetes is often associated with lactic acidosis. Even under basal conditions, patients with diabetes have mildly elevated lactate levels. This is thought to be secondary to decreased PDH activity caused by free fatty acid oxidation by liver and muscle. Lactate increases even more during diabetic ketoacidosis (DKA), possibly secondary to decreased hepatic clearance. This accumulation of lactate contributes to the elevated AG present in ketoacidosis.

Malignancy

Lactic acidosis has been detected in patients with acute rapidly progressive hematologic malignancies, such as leukemia or lymphoma. Lactate levels usually parallel disease activity. Rapidly proliferating cells have a high rate of anaerobic glycolysis (so-called Warburg effect) producing excessive amounts of lactate. In addition, the increased blood viscosity and microvascular aggregates that are frequently found in acute leukemia cause regional hypoperfusion. Overproduction of lactate may also result from a large tumor burden and rapid cell lysis.

Alternate Sugars

The use of sorbitol or fructose as irrigants during prostate surgery or in tube feedings can cause lactic acidosis. The metabolism of these sugars consumes ATP, inhibiting gluconeogenesis and stimulating glycolysis, leading to the accumulation of excess lactate.

Propylene Glycol

Propylene glycol is a common vehicle for many drugs, including topical silver sulfadiazine and intravenous preparations of nitroglycerin, diazepam, lorazepam, phenytoin, etomidate, and trimethoprim-sulfamethoxazole, among others. In addition, because of its better safety profile, newer formulations of antifreeze also contain propylene glycol. Although it is considered relatively safe, many case reports indicate toxicity. Approximately 40% to 50% of administered propylene glycol is oxidized by alcohol dehydrogenase to both D-lactic acid and L-lactic acid. Toxic patients commonly develop an unexplained AG acidosis with increased serum osmolality. Considering that patients receiving many of the medications solubilized with propylene glycol frequently have other possible causes for their acidosis, it is important to be aware of this iatrogenic cause for the acidosis. Correction of the metabolic abnormalities quickly occurs following discontinuation of the medication.

D-LACTIC ACIDOSIS

This unusual form of AG acidosis is the result of the accumulation of the D-isomer of lactate. Unlike the lactate produced by glycolysis in animals, which is the L-isomer, colonic bacteria produce both the L-isomer and the D-isomer. Overproduction of D-lactate occurs in patients with short-bowel syndrome and is usually precipitated by a high carbohydrate intake. Increased delivery of carbohydrates due to the shortened bowel and an overgrowth of bacteria is responsible for this overproduction. Mammalian clearance of D-lactate is far less efficient than that of L-lactate, and, with increased production within the gut, D-lactate accumulates within the blood. Because D-lactate is not detected on the routine assay, which measures only L-lactate, diagnosis requires a high clinical suspicion. Patients typically present with mental status changes, ataxia, and nystagmus. Treatment consists of an oral fast with intravenous nutrition and restoration of gut flora to normal through the administration of oral antibiotics. In severe cases, hemodialysis can decrease the concentration of D-lactate.

TREATMENT OF LACTIC ACIDOSIS

The treatment of lactic acidosis is fraught with controversy. The most important step is treatment of the underlying cause. In sepsis, restoring oxygenation with mechanical ventilation and perfusion with pressors or inotropes are of paramount importance, although these interventions do not always improve the lactic acidosis. In some patients with medication-induced lactic acidosis, withdrawal of the offending agent may be sufficient. There are anecdotal case reports of successful use of riboflavin or L-carnitine to treat lactic acidosis associated with nucleoside analogues.

Often these measures fail, and clinicians are faced with the decision of whether to give sodium bicarbonate in an effort to increase serum pH. There are several potential problems with this approach. First, as previously discussed, it is not clear to what extent acidosis is deleterious and therefore whether normalizing pH is of any benefit. Also, increasing pH may actually increase lactic acid production. Sodium bicarbonate is often given as a hypertonic solution, which can lead to hypernatremia and cellular dehydration. Perhaps most important is the possibility that the administration of HCO_3^- can cause a paradoxic decrease in intracellular pH despite an increase in extracellular pH. Bicarbonate combines with hydrogen, forming carbonic acid, which is then converted to CO_2 and water. pCO_2 increases with the titration of acid by bicarbonate and rapidly diffuses into cells, causing acidification, while bicarbonate remains extracellular. Thus it is difficult to recommend the use of bicarbonate for the treatment of a low serum pH alone. If the serum pH is less than 7.1, however, many clinicians, despite the lack of supporting data, opt for treatment because a further small decline in serum bicarbonate can have a profound effect on serum pH.

Other buffers may be better tolerated insofar as they buffer hydrogen ions without increasing CO_2. One such buffer is tris-hydroxymethyl aminomethane (THAM), a biologically inert amino acid that can buffer both CO_2 and protons. It does not lead to production of CO_2 and thus works well in a closed system. The protonated molecule is excreted by the kidney and should be used cautiously in patients with kidney failure. Potential side effects include hyperkalemia, hypoglycemia, ventilatory depression, and hepatic necrosis in neonates. Despite THAM being available for many years, there are no studies demonstrating improved outcomes with the use of THAM. The acute dose in milliliters of 0.3 mol/L solution can be derived using the following formula: dose in milliliters = lean body weight (kg) × decrease in HCO_3^-

from normal (mmol/L). The first 25% to 50% of the dose is given over 5 minutes and the rest over 1 hour. Alternatively, a steady infusion of no more than 3.5 L/day can be given for several days.

Dichloroacetate has also been used in the treatment of lactic acidosis. This agent stimulates the activity of PDH, increasing the rate of pyruvate oxidation and thereby decreasing lactate levels. A large multicenter trial in humans showed a reduction in serum lactate, an increase in pH, and an increase in the number of patients able to resolve their hyperlactatemia. Despite these favorable changes, no improvement in hemodynamic parameters or mortality was found.

Various modes of kidney replacement therapy have been used in the treatment of lactic acidosis. Standard bicarbonate hemodialysis treats acidosis primarily by diffusion of bicarbonate from the bath into the blood and is thus another form of bicarbonate administration, albeit with several advantages. Hypernatremia and volume overload are not a concern with bicarbonate administered via hemodialysis. Also, hemodialysis removes lactate. Although the removal of lactate does not increase serum pH, there is some evidence that the lactate ion itself is harmful. Unfortunately, there are no randomized, prospective trials demonstrating the benefit of dialysis in lactic acidosis, and its use in the absence of other indications cannot be routinely recommended.

Several studies have shown that high-volume hemofiltration using either lactate or bicarbonate buffered replacement fluid can rapidly correct metabolic acidosis. These studies have been small, and the degree and type of acidosis have been poorly characterized. In addition, other treatment measures have usually been instituted, making it difficult to draw conclusions about the effectiveness of this treatment. Nevertheless, hemofiltration remains a potential therapeutic option.

Peritoneal dialysis has also been used in the treatment of metabolic acidosis. Although there are case reports of success using this modality, a randomized study comparing lactate-buffered peritoneal dialysis with continuous hemofiltration showed that hemofiltration corrected acidosis more quickly and more effectively than peritoneal dialysis. Whether newer bicarbonate-buffered peritoneal dialysis solution will be more efficacious remains unknown.

DIABETIC KETOACIDOSIS

DKA is another common cause of an AG acidosis. Although DKA may be the initial presentation of diabetes mellitus, more commonly patients have a known diagnosis of diabetes and either have been noncompliant with their insulin regimen or have a precipitating factor such as infection. Patients are generally polyuric and polydipsic, but if volume depletion becomes severe enough, polyuria may not be seen. Although DKA is classically seen in type 1 diabetes, it can also occur in patients with type 2 diabetes. DKA results from insulin deficiency and concomitant increase in counterregulatory hormones such as glucagon, epinephrine, and cortisol. This hormonal milieu leads to an inability of cells to use glucose, causing them to oxidize fatty acids as fuel, producing large amounts of keto acids. A diagnosis of DKA requires a pH less than 7.35, elevated AG, positive serum ketones of at least 1:2 dilutions, and decreased serum bicarbonate. However, not all patients with DKA meet these criteria. If kidney perfusion and glomerular filtration rate (GFR) are well maintained, ketones (anions) are rapidly excreted by the kidney in place of chloride. With the loss of these anions in the urine, the AG acidosis may be replaced by a mixed AG/hyperchloremic acidosis or even a pure hyperchloremic acidosis. Furthermore, an increase in the NADH/NAD ratio, which frequently occurs during DKA, causes ketones to shift from acetoacetate to β-hydroxybutyrate, which is not detected on the standard nitroprusside test used to identify serum and urinary ketones. If this occurs, serum ketones may appear to be negative or only trace positive. Finally, vomiting may result in a metabolic alkalosis, which would raise the serum bicarbonate toward the normal range. In this case, the serum AG would almost certainly be elevated, and the astute clinician will not be fooled.

TREATMENT

The treatment of DKA consists of three parts: fluid resuscitation, insulin administration, and correction of potassium deficits. Patients with DKA often have profound deficits of both sodium and free water. Hypovolemia, as demonstrated by hemodynamic compromise, should always be treated first. Patients should rapidly receive 1 to 2 L of 0.9% saline until their blood pressure is stabilized. Thereafter, hypotonic fluids in the form of 0.45% saline should be administered to correct free water deficits while continuing to provide volume. Insulin should be administered only after fluid resuscitation is well under way. If insulin is given precipitously, the rapid uptake of glucose by the cells will cause water to follow because of the fall in extracellular osmolality, potentially resulting in cardiovascular collapse. A continuous regular insulin infusion of 0.1 units/kg/h is given; use of an initial bolus of 0.1 unit/kg is controversial. If the glucose does not decline by 50 to 100 mg/dL/h, the infusion should be increased by 50%. As tissue perfusion improves, β-hydroxybutyrate is converted to acetoacetate, and serum ketones paradoxically increase but then should decrease. Serum glucose usually approaches normal before ketosis is resolved. When glucose is less than 250 mg/dL, intravenous fluids should be changed to 5% dextrose to avoid hypoglycemia while awaiting resolution of ketosis. The insulin infusion should be continued until the AG closes, the HCO_3^- rises above 14 mmol/L, and the patient is taking food orally. Although the ADA recommends continuing the insulin infusion until the HCO_3^- is greater than 18 mmol/L, regeneration of HCO_3^- may take up to 24 hours after the termination of ketogenesis, and this is not hastened by insulin. A subcutaneous insulin dose should be given at least 1 hour before stopping the drip to avoid rebound ketosis.

Most patients with DKA have total-body potassium depletion. Nevertheless, their serum potassium may be normal to high because of a shift out of the cells caused by the hyperglycemia-induced hyperosmolality and the insulinopenia. When insulin is restored, extracellular potassium is rapidly taken up by cells, and severe hypokalemia may ensue. Therefore the addition of potassium to the intravenous fluids is recommended at a concentration of 10 to 20 mEq/L as soon as serum potassium falls below 4.5 mEq/L. Needless to say, this management algorithm requires frequent laboratory tests.

Although bicarbonate therapy has been used in severe DKA, this use is not supported by the literature. In fact, bicarbonate administration, even in patients with pH less than 7.0, has not been shown to be advantageous. In almost all cases, the acidosis rapidly improves with appropriate management without the use of bicarbonate. Thus the administration of sodium bicarbonate to patients with DKA cannot be routinely recommended. It is important, however, that these patients be monitored in a setting where they can be closely observed and where frequent analyses of their arterial blood gases and electrolytes can be obtained.

ALCOHOLIC KETOACIDOSIS

Alcoholic ketoacidosis (AKA) usually presents with an AG acidosis and ketonemia but without significant hyperglycemia. The classic presentation is that of a patient who has been on an alcohol binge, develops nausea and vomiting, and stops eating. The patient typically presents 24 to 48 hours after the cessation of oral intake and may complain of abdominal pain and shortness of breath. Alcohol levels are low or even unmeasurable by the time AKA develops. AKA is similar to DKA in that it is a state of insulinopenia and increased counterregulatory hormones; in fact, the levels of these hormones are similar in both disorders. In AKA, normoglycemia to hypoglycemia is usually observed, despite a hormonal milieu favoring hyperglycemia, because decreased NAD curtails hepatic gluconeogenesis, and starvation depletes glycogen stores. Patients with AKA, however, can occasionally present with hyperglycemia, and distinguishing it from DKA in those cases can be difficult. AKA almost always presents with an AG, but acidemia is less universal. Patients often have concurrent metabolic alkalosis from vomiting or respiratory alkalosis from liver disease. Thus patients with AKA may not be acidemic and rarely do they have a simple metabolic acidosis. Because of the increased NADH/NAD ratio, the primary keto acid present is β-hydroxybutyrate; therefore serum ketones may be reported as negative. This ratio also favors the formation of lactic acid. Finally, electrolyte disorders, including hypokalemia, hypophosphatemia, and hypomagnesemia, are common.

TREATMENT

Therapy of AKA is straightforward and consists of volume repletion, provision of glucose (except in those patients with hyperglycemia), and correction of any electrolyte abnormalities. Patients are often volume depleted from vomiting combined with poor oral intake. Thiamine must be provided before or concurrently with glucose to avoid precipitating Wernicke encephalopathy. Acidosis resolves as insulin increases, and counterregulatory hormones are turned off in response to glucose infusion. The clinician must maintain a high degree of suspicion for AKA, as the acid-base disturbance may be subtle on routine laboratory analyses, with patients often demonstrating an elevated AG as the only abnormality. Chronic alcoholics often have hypoalbuminemia, which can further obscure the interpretation of the AG. Any patient with nausea and vomiting with a recent history of alcohol abuse should probably be treated for presumptive AKA until the diagnosis is clearly ruled out.

STARVATION KETOSIS

During prolonged fasting, insulin levels are suppressed, whereas glucagon, epinephrine, growth hormone, and cortisol levels are increased. This hormonal milieu results in increased lipolysis, with release of free fatty acids into the blood and stimulation of hepatic ketogenesis. The concentrations of both β-hydroxybutyrate and acetoacetate increase over the course of several weeks, resulting in a mild AG metabolic acidosis.

TOXINS AND DRUGS

ETHYLENE GLYCOL

Ingestion of various toxins can cause severe metabolic acidosis with an increased AG and should always be suspected in these cases. Ethylene glycol is a sweet liquid often found in antifreeze. Ingestion of 100 mL or more can be fatal. Ethylene glycol is metabolized by alcohol dehydrogenase into glycolic acid and subsequently oxalic acid. This generates NADH, which encourages the formation of lactic acid. The AG acidosis results from the accumulation of the various acid metabolites of ethylene glycol as well as lactic acidosis. Diagnosis can be difficult because ethylene glycol is not detected on routine toxicology assays. It should be suspected in anyone who presents with intoxication, a low blood alcohol, and a markedly increased AG metabolic acidosis without ketonemia. The serum osmolar gap may help detect ethylene glycol. Serum osmolar gap is the difference between the calculated serum osmolarity $[([Na^+] \times 2) + (glucose/18) + (BUN/2.8)]$ and the actual serum osmolality as measured by the laboratory. A difference greater than about 10 to 15 mOsm/kg suggests the presence of an unmeasured, osmotically active substance, which in the right clinical setting could be a toxin. However, it is important to understand the limitations of this approach. Some laboratories measure serum osmolality using the vapor pressure methodology rather than the freezing point depression, and volatile substances such as alcohols may not be detected. As the osmotically active alcohol is metabolized into the various acids, the osmolar gap disappears. Thus, early after ingestion, the osmolar gap is elevated without a significant increase in the AG. As the alcohol is metabolized, the osmolar gap decreases while the AG increases. Examination of the urine may reveal calcium oxalate crystals, a finding that can be considered pathognomonic. However, the absence of these crystals does not rule out the ingestion of ethylene glycol. Precipitation of calcium oxalate may occasionally cause hypocalcemia. Because fluorescein is added as a colorant to antifreeze, the urine of a patient with antifreeze ingestion may fluoresce under a Wood lamp.

METHANOL

Methanol is an alcohol often found in solvents or as an adulterant in alcoholic beverages. Toxicity is usually caused by ingestion of as little as 30 mL but has also been reported after inhalation. Methanol is metabolized by alcohol dehydrogenase to formaldehyde and then to formic acid, resulting in an elevated AG acidosis. As with ingestions of other alcohols, NAD depletion favors the production of lactate. Methanol is less intoxicating than either ethanol or ethylene glycol. The most characteristic symptom of methanol toxicity is blurry vision. Blindness may occur due to optic nerve involvement, and pancreatitis may be seen in up to two-thirds of patients. As described previously, early after ingestion an osmolar gap may be found. The diagnosis of both ethylene glycol and methanol poisoning can be confirmed by specific toxicologic assays, but treatment should never be delayed while awaiting these results.

TREATMENT OF TOXIC ALCOHOL INGESTIONS

Treatment of both ethylene glycol and methanol toxicity is based on the fact that it is the metabolites of these alcohols that are actually harmful. Both substances are metabolized by alcohol dehydrogenase. Blocking the activity of this enzyme will prevent the metabolic acidosis and allow the alcohol to be excreted by the kidneys or removed by dialysis. Because alcohol dehydrogenase has a much higher affinity for ethanol than for either ethylene glycol or methanol, use of ethanol as a competitive inhibitor was the traditional treatment. Ethanol is supplied as a 10% solution in 5% dextrose in water (D5W). A loading dose of 0.8 to 1.0 g/kg body weight followed by an infusion of 100 mg/kg/h should be sufficient to maintain a blood alcohol level of 100 to 150 mg/dL. However, in some patients with marked ethanol tolerance, this rate will need to be doubled. Fomepizole (4-methylpyrazole), a competitive inhibitor of alcohol dehydrogenase, has replaced ethanol as the treatment of choice. Fomepizole is a more potent inhibitor of alcohol dehydrogenase than ethanol and does not lead to central nervous system (CNS) depression. An initial loading dose of 15 mg/kg body weight is followed 12 hours later by 10 mg/kg every 12 hours for four doses, and then 15 mg/kg every 12 hours for four more doses. Although fomepizole, because of its potency, has begun to call into question the need for dialysis, until more studies are available, it is recommended that dialysis be instituted in all patients with suspected ingestions of ethylene glycol or methanol who have end organ damage (kidney failure or visual impairment) and whose pH is less than 7.2. Both compounds can be rapidly removed by hemodialysis. Hemodialysis can also help improve the acidosis by providing a source of bicarbonate. It is important to double the rate of any ethanol infusion or increase the dose of fomepizole while a patient is receiving hemodialysis. For either ingestion, gastric lavage with charcoal should be performed when ingestion has occurred within the preceding 2 to 3 hours.

SALICYLATE TOXICITY

The ingestion of salicylates is an important cause of mixed acid-base disturbances, producing both a respiratory alkalosis (salicylate is a direct respiratory stimulant) and a metabolic acidosis. Metabolic acidosis results from the accumulation of both lactic and keto acids. Salicylic acid, by itself, accounts for only a small quantity of the acid load. The common presenting sign of salicylate toxicity is tachypnea. The patient may also complain of tinnitus with serum concentrations of salicylic acid of 20 to 45 mg/dL or higher. Other CNS manifestations are agitation, seizures, and even coma. Both noncardiogenic pulmonary edema and upper gastrointestinal bleeding may occur. Hypoglycemia occurs in children but is rare in adults. Other symptoms include nausea, vomiting, and hyperpyrexia.

In the setting of salicylate overdose, peak serum concentrations are achieved 4 to 6 hours after ingestion. The severity of the ingestion can be predicted by the Done nomogram, which plots the toxic salicylate level at varying time points following ingestion. This nomogram cannot be used with chronic ingestions or with the ingestion of enteric-coated aspirin. The treatment of salicylate toxicity consists of supportive care, removal of unabsorbed compounds using charcoal lavage, administration of bicarbonate, and, if necessary, hemodialysis. Because the dissociation constant (pK) of salicylic acid is 3.0, alkalinization keeps the drug in its polar dissociated form, preventing diffusion into the CNS. In addition, because tissue salicylic acid is in equilibrium with the nondissociated compound in the plasma, alkalinization also decreases tissue levels. Concurrent alkalinization of the urine traps salicylate in the tubule, promoting its excretion. Hemodialysis is indicated in all patients with altered mental status, kidney failure that causes a decrease in renal excretion, volume overload that prevents the administration of bicarbonate, or salicylate levels greater than 100 mg/dL.

PYROGLUTAMIC ACIDOSIS

It is increasingly recognized that glutathione depletion can cause an AG acidosis. This underreported acidosis occurs in patients who often have underlying infections and are treated with acetaminophen, even at therapeutic doses. Glutathione depletion decreases the negative feedback inhibition on γ-glutamylcysteine synthetase, resulting in an increase in pyroglutamic acid (5-oxoproline). Measurement of urine 5-oxoproline levels will confirm the diagnosis.

KIDNEY FAILURE

Kidney failure is a well-recognized cause of metabolic acidosis. With the reduction in nephron mass that occurs in CKD, there is decreased ammoniagenesis in the proximal tubule. Many patients with diminished kidney function may also have specific acidification defects in the form of a renal tubular acidosis (RTA). As the GFR declines, the kidney is unable to secrete the daily production of fixed acid. Serum bicarbonate may begin to decline when the GFR falls below 40 mL/min/1.73 m^2.

The acidosis of kidney failure is associated with either a normal AG or an elevated AG. With mild to moderate reductions in GFR, the anions that comprise the gap are excreted normally, and the acidosis reflects decreased ammoniagenesis and is therefore hyperchloremic. As kidney failure worsens, the kidney loses its ability to excrete various anions, and the accumulation of sulfate, phosphate, and other anions produces an elevated AG. With better control of phosphorus and more intensive dietary modifications, many patients initiating kidney replacement therapy may not manifest an AG.

Despite daily net positive acid balance, it is unusual for HCO_3^- to fall below 15 mmol/L. Why the acidosis of CKD is rarely severe is unclear. Whether this lack of severity is secondary to buffering of the retained protons in bone or retention of organic anions usually lost in the urine that are instead subsequently converted to HCO_3^- is controversial. The buffering of protons by bone results in the loss of calcium and negative calcium balance. In addition, chronic acidosis causes protein breakdown, muscle wasting, and negative nitrogen balance. Maintaining acid-base balance close to normal may prevent these consequences.

The metabolic acidosis commonly found in patients with CKD can easily be corrected with oral bicarbonate. Usually two 650-mg (7.8 mEq) tablets 3 times a day will keep the serum bicarbonate in the normal range. It is rare that hemodialysis has to be initiated solely for the purpose of correcting acidosis.

HYPERCHLOREMIC METABOLIC ACIDOSIS

Acidosis associated with a normal AG, HCMA, has a limited number of causes (Fig. 13.6). HCMA can occur in CKD when reduced ammoniagenesis impairs the kidney's ability to excrete the daily acid load. In individuals with normal or near-normal kidney function, it can be divided into cases caused by the kidney's failure to reabsorb HCO_3^- or secrete the daily fixed load of H$^+$, commonly known as RTA, and cases in which renal acid-base handling is normal. In contrast to AG acidosis, most cases of HCMA are easily treated with supplemental base.

KIDNEY CAUSES OF HYPERCHLOREMIC METABOLIC ACIDOSIS

RTAs represent a heterogeneous cause of HCMA in which the kidney is unable to maintain acid-base balance, despite normal or near-normal GFR. There is often confusion regarding the RTAs because no standard nomenclature exists, numerous diverse transport defects have been identified, and the literature often presents contradictory information. A grasp of the underlying pathophysiology makes the approach to these disorders more comprehensible. The RTAs can be divided into four major categories: (1) primary defects in ammoniagenesis, (2) hypoaldosteronism, (3) disorders of the proximal tubule, and (4) disorders of the distal tubule (Fig. 13.6). The distal tubule defects can be further divided into those with hypokalemia and those with hyperkalemia (Fig. 13.7).

DEFECTIVE AMMONIAGENESIS

One of the most common causes of an HCMA is the inability of the kidney to generate ammonia because of CKD. By definition, RTA refers to a specific acid excretory defect occurring despite the presence of normal or near-normal kidney function. Thus it bears emphasis that the HCMA of CKD is not classified as an RTA. As the number of nephrons decreases with CKD, there is a proportional decrease in the production of ammonia. As mentioned previously, when GFR falls below 40 mL/min/1.73 m^2, the kidney is less able to excrete the daily acid load, and HCO_3^- begins to decline with a concomitant increase in the serum Cl$^-$, producing HCMA. Only when the GFR falls below 15 to 20 mL/min/1.73 m^2 does the kidney lose the ability to secrete anions, thus converting this HCMA into an AG acidosis. It must be stressed that the acidosis in kidney failure, whether manifested by hyperchloremia or an AG, is primarily caused by defective ammoniagenesis. As such, the UAG will be positive because of the decrease in ammonia excretion, while urine pH will be less than 5.5.

HYPOALDOSTERONISM

Primary and secondary hypoaldosteronism are common disorders causing hyperkalemia and metabolic acidosis (Table 13.4). Hyporeninemic hypoaldosteronism (type IV RTA) is the most frequently encountered variety of this disorder. This disorder is usually seen in patients with diabetes and mild CKD. The precise cause of hyporeninemia has not been clearly defined. The finding that hypertension is frequently present and that the disorder may be partly reversed with

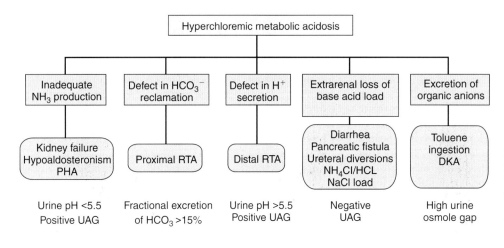

Fig. 13.6 The etiology of hyperchloremic metabolic acidosis. Shown at the bottom are useful diagnostic tools. *DKA,* Diabetic ketoacidosis; *PHA,* pseudohypoaldosteronism; *RTA,* renal tubular acidosis; *UAG,* urine anion gap.

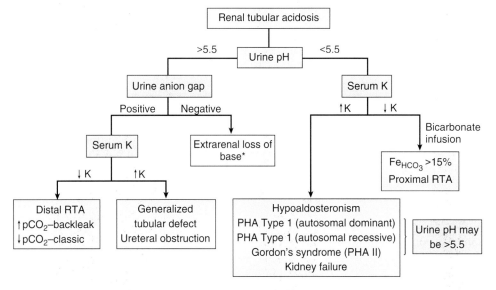

Fig. 13.7 Evaluation of renal tubular acidosis. FE_{HCO_3}, Fractional excretion of bicarbonate; *PHA,* pseudohypoaldosteronism; *RTA,* renal tubular acidosis. Note that extrarenal loss of base is not a form of renal tubular acidosis.

Table 13.4 Hypoaldosteronism

Primary
- Addison disease
- Congenital enzyme defects
- Drugs
  - Heparin
  - Angiotensin converting enzyme inhibitors
  - Angiotensin receptor blockers

Hyporeninemic hypoaldosteronism (type IV RTA)

Pseudohypoaldosteronism I (autosomal dominant)—mineralocorticoid resistance

---

chronic furosemide use suggests that renin suppression may be secondary to chronic volume overload. The cause of the hypoaldosteronism also has not been fully explained. Renin suppression alone should not cause hypoaldosteronism, because hyperkalemia is a potent stimulus of aldosterone secretion, and anephric individuals still secrete aldosterone. The acidosis is primarily caused by decreased ammoniagenesis as a result of the associated hyperkalemia induced by the aldosterone deficiency. Hypoaldosteronism, by diminishing distal sodium reabsorption, also results in a less negative lumen potential, thus decreasing the rate of H^+ secretion

but not the electromotive force of the pump. Because the hydrogen pump is not defective, urine pH is usually less than 5.5.

Patients with type IV RTA are usually asymptomatic, with only minor laboratory abnormalities (mild hyperkalemia and decreased HCO_3^-). However, when renal potassium handling is further perturbed by various stressors (including sodium depletion, which decreases the delivery of sodium to the distal tubule; a high-potassium diet; and potassium-sparing diuretics or medications that further decrease renin and aldosterone levels, such as angiotensin-converting enzyme inhibitors, angiotensin receptor blockers, nonsteroidal antiinflammatory drugs, or heparin), marked hyperkalemia ensues with a decline in ammoniagenesis. Most patients can be treated by removing the insult to potassium homeostasis, restricting potassium intake, and providing supplemental bicarbonate. Proving that type IV RTA is present requires the demonstration of low renin and aldosterone levels after sodium depletion. Because of practical considerations, these tests are rarely ordered, and most patients will be treated empirically.

Autosomal-dominant pseudohypoaldosteronism (PHA) type I is an uncommon disorder caused by a mutation in the renal mineralocorticoid receptor, resulting in decreased affinity for aldosterone. This genetic disorder presents in childhood with hyperaldosteronism, hyperkalemia, metabolic acidosis, salt wasting, and hypotension. Autosomal dominant PHA type I becomes less severe with age. Carbenoxolone and glycyrrhizic acid (found in true licorice) both inhibit 11-β-hydroxysteroid dehydrogenase, the enzyme in the kidney that converts cortisol, which binds the mineralocorticoid receptor to cortisone, which does not bind. They can be used to treat this disorder by increasing the intrarenal supply of mineralocorticoid.

PROXIMAL RENAL TUBULAR ACIDOSIS

Proximal RTA, often called type II RTA (because it was the second type described), is a defect in the ability of the proximal tubule to reclaim filtered HCO_3^- (Table 13.5). In type II RTA, the proximal tubule has a diminished threshold (approximately 15 mmol/L instead of the normal 24 mmol/L) for HCO_3^- reabsorption. When plasma HCO_3^- falls below this threshold, complete reabsorption occurs. Proximal RTA can be congenital or acquired and may exist as an isolated defect in HCO_3^- reabsorption or as part of a more generalized transport defect known as Fanconi syndrome, in which there is diminished reabsorption of other solutes across the proximal tubule. Patients with proximal RTA and Fanconi syndrome, in addition to the loss of HCO_3^-, inappropriately excrete amino acids, glucose, phosphorus, and uric acid in their urine.

As would be expected, mutations in the Na^+-H^+ exchanger on the luminal membrane, the Na^+-HCO_3^- cotransporter on the basolateral membrane, and cytosolic carbonic anhydrase have all been implicated in the isolated hereditary and sporadic forms of proximal RTA. Several drugs that block carbonic anhydrase, including the diuretic acetazolamide and the anticonvulsant topiramate, also cause isolated HCO_3^- wasting. Proximal RTA with Fanconi syndrome is frequently found in patients with cystinosis, Wilson disease, Lowe syndrome, multiple myeloma, and light chain disease, among others. A decrease in ATP production, which reduces basolateral Na^+/K^+-ATPase activity, is the presumed etiology of this global transport defect. Drugs, particularly the cyclophosphamide analogue ifosfamide, and cidofovir, used in the treatment of cytomegalovirus retinitis, are associated with a generalized proximal tubulopathy.

Because distal H^+ excretion is normal, urine pH during steady state, when the HCO_3^- is below the lowered threshold and bicarbonaturia is absent, will be less than 5.5. At this time, the serum HCO_3^- will be between 15 and 18 mEq/L. It is important to recognize that whenever the HCO_3^- increases above the reabsorptive threshold, HCO_3^- will appear in the urine and the pH will be greater than 6.5. Although ammoniagenesis is preserved in proximal RTA, direct or indirect measurement of urine NH_4^+ may reveal an inappropriately low excretion. This can occur because HCO_3^-, which escapes proximal reabsorption, serves as a buffer sink for secreted H^+, thus reducing the trapping of NH_4^+. The diagnosis of proximal RTA is established by demonstrating a fractional excretion of HCO_3^- greater than 15%, while supplemental bicarbonate is administered in an attempt to increase the serum bicarbonate to normal.

Treatment of proximal RTA is difficult because the administered base is rapidly excreted in the urine. Extremely large amounts of base (10 to 15 mmol/kg/day) are frequently needed, and therefore compliance is limited. The increased delivery of HCO_3^- to the distal nephron induces or exacerbates hypokalemia. It is recommended that frequent doses of a mixture of Na^+ and K^+ salts of bicarbonate and citrate be used.

DISTAL RENAL TUBULAR ACIDOSIS

Classic Distal Renal Tubular Acidosis With Hypokalemia

Distal RTA, also known as type I RTA, represents the inability of the distal tubule to acidify the urine (Table 13.6). As with proximal RTA, the distal variety can be congenital or acquired. Abnormalities have been identified in both the luminal H^+-ATPase and the basolateral Cl^--HCO_3^- exchanger. The acquired form is associated with autoimmune diseases, especially systemic lupus and Sjögren syndrome; dysproteinemia; and kidney transplant rejection. Immunocytochemical

---

Table 13.5 Causes of Proximal Renal Tubular Acidosis

Isolated defects in HCO_3 reabsorption
- Carbonic anhydrase inhibitors
- Acetazolamide
- Topiramate
- Sulfamylon
- Carbonic anhydrase deficiency

Generalized defects in proximal tubular transport
- Cystinosis
- Wilson disease
- Lowe syndrome
- Galactosemia
- Multiple myeloma
- Light chain disease
- Amyloidosis
- Vitamin D deficiency
- Ifosfamide
- Cidofovir
- Lead
- Aminoglycosides

Table 13.6 Causes of Distal Renal Tubular Acidosis With Hypokalemia

Familial
- Defective HCO_3^--Cl^- exchanger (autosomal dominant)
- Defective H^+-ATPase (autosomal recessive)

Endemic
- Thai endemic distal renal tubular acidosis

Drugs
- Amphotericin
- Toluene
- Lithium
- Ifosfamide
- Foscarnet
- Vanadium
- Systemic disorder
- Sjögren syndrome
- Cryoglobulinemia
- Systemic lupus erythematosus
- Kidney transplant rejection

studies have revealed decreased staining of the H^+-ATPase and Cl^--HCO_3^- exchanger in patients with the acquired form of distal RTA. Ifosfamide, which is also associated with a proximal RTA, can cause a distal defect. Amphotericin, which creates pores in membranes forming ion channels, causes a distal RTA by allowing the back leak of protons across the luminal membrane. The classic finding in type I RTA is an inappropriately high urine pH (greater than 5.5).

Because H^+ secretion is defective in distal RTA, less NH_4^+ can be trapped in the lumen of the tubule, and the UAG will be positive, reflecting this decrease in NH_4^+ excretion. Besides having an inappropriately high urine pH and a positive UAG, distal RTA can be further characterized by measuring urine pCO_2 during an HCO_3^- infusion. Distal delivery of HCO_3^- in the presence of a normal H^+ secretory capacity results in elevated pCO_2 in the urine. When there is a H^+ secretory defect, urine pCO_2 will not increase. As would be expected, in amphotericin-induced RTA when H^+ ion secretion is unaffected, urine pCO_2 increases normally. Occasionally, it may be difficult to distinguish HCMA induced by diarrhea from a distal RTA. Diarrhea results in HCMA and hypokalemia. Because the hypokalemia increases renal ammoniagenesis, urine pH may be inappropriately elevated. Thus, on the surface, both forms of acidosis appear similar. Measurement of the UAG will easily distinguish the markedly elevated urine NH_4^+ with its negative AG found in diarrheal illness from the low NH_4^+ excretion and positive AG found with distal RTA. The one caveat is that sodium must be delivered to the distal tubule, as shown by urine Na^+ above 20 mmol/L.

Classic distal RTA is associated with hypokalemia (due to augmented distal K^+ secretion in lieu of H^+ secretion in exchange for Na^+ reabsorption), hypocitraturia (from augmented proximal tubule cell reabsorption), hypercalciuria (from the buffering of H^+ in bone and loss of calcium), and nephrocalcinosis. The treatment of distal RTA is simply to supply enough base (2 to 3 mmol/kg/day) to counter the daily fixed production of acid. This can be administered as a mixture of sodium and potassium salts of either bicarbonate or citrate.

Distal Renal Tubular Acidosis With Hyperkalemia

Although many textbooks place distal RTA with hyperkalemia under the rubric of type 4 RTA (hyporenin-hypoaldosteronism), it is more appropriate to call it distal RTA with hyperkalemia, because it has a pathophysiology that differs from type 4 RTA. This disorder can be further divided into two broad general categories: (1) a generalized defect of both distal tubular H^+ and K^+ secretion or (2) a primary defect in Na^+ transport often called a "voltage defect" (Table 13.7).

Generalized Distal Tubule Defect. Unlike classic distal RTA, a more generalized distal tubule defect can occur, in which both H^+ and K^+ secretion is impaired. This has been best identified in cases of ureteral obstruction and in patients with interstitial kidney disease resulting from sickle cell anemia or systemic lupus erythematosus. In animals with ureteral obstruction, immunocytochemical staining has revealed loss of the apical H^+-ATPase. Why hyperkalemia occurs is less clear. Because K^+ excretion cannot be augmented by diuretics, a primary defect in K^+ transport is likely. Similar to classic distal RTA, urine pH is greater than 5.5.

Table 13.7   Causes of Distal Renal Tubular Acidosis With Hyperkalemia

Lupus nephritis
Obstructive nephropathy
Sickle cell anemia
Voltage defects
Familial
- Pseudohypoaldosteronism type I (autosomal recessive)
- Pseudohypoaldosteronism type II (autosomal recessive)— Gordon syndrome

Drugs
- Amiloride
- Triamterene
- Trimethoprim
- Pentamidine

Distal Sodium Transport Defects. Several disorders have been characterized by defective sodium transport in the distal tubule. The reabsorption of Na^+ by the distal tubule generates a lumen-negative potential. This electrical negativity helps promote the secretion of K^+ and H^+. Any drug or disorder that interferes with this lumen-negative potential will diminish both K^+ and H^+ secretion. These are commonly classified as voltage defects. Autosomal-recessive PHA type I is a syndrome in which there is loss of function of the epithelial sodium channel (ENaC) in the distal tubule. Numerous mutations have been described in various subunits of this channel. This disease manifests in childhood with marked hyperkalemia, metabolic acidosis, hyperaldosteronism, and salt wasting. Because the ENaC also exists in other tissue, including lung, colon, and sweat glands, patients with this disorder often have symptoms related to these organs. Treatment consists of providing a high salt intake. Drugs that block ENaC produce a similar metabolic picture. These include the potassium-sparing diuretics amiloride and triamterene, as well as trimethoprim and pentamidine.

Another well-recognized disorder of distal transport is PHA type II, also known as Gordon syndrome (see Chapters 38 and 66). Individuals with this condition have mild volume overload with suppressed renin and aldosterone, hypertension, hyperkalemia, and metabolic acidosis. Mutations in two members of a family of serine-threonine kinases, WNK1 and WNK4 (*With No K* [K = lysine]), cause this syndrome. These kinases appear to have an important role in the regulation of Cl^- transport in numerous different tissues. It appears that defects in these kinases result in an increase in the number of neutral NaCl transporters (NCCT) and thus increase NaCl transport across the distal convoluted tubule. Less sodium is delivered to the more distal tubule segments for reabsorption, which curtails the generation of the lumen-negative potential. This results in decreased H^+ and K^+ secretion. Supporting this hypothesis is the fact that Gordon syndrome can be treated with thiazide diuretics, which block the NCCT.

The acidosis in all of these sodium transport disorders is secondary to decreased H^+ secretion caused by an unfavorable electrical gradient in the distal tubule and the decreased ammoniagenesis caused by the hyperkalemia. Whether the urine pH is less than 5.5 depends on how severely H^+ secretion is affected.

COMBINED PROXIMAL AND DISTAL RENAL TUBULAR ACIDOSIS

This is an extremely uncommon disorder, previously called type 3 RTA. As would be expected, both proximal HCO_3^- reabsorption and distal H^+ secretion are impaired. Mutations in the gene for cytosolic carbonic anhydrase can cause such a defect. As already discussed, ifosfamide can also cause a combined defect.

INCOMPLETE DISTAL RENAL TUBULAR ACIDOSIS

Patients with incomplete distal RTA will come to medical attention because of calcium stone disease and nephrocalcinosis. Serum HCO_3^- is normal, but urine pH never falls below 5.5, even after acid loading with NH_4Cl or $CaCl_2$. This disorder likely represents a milder form of distal RTA. Frank metabolic acidosis may become evident when patients are stressed by diarrhea or other conditions that require compensation by augmented renal proton secretion.

EXTRARENAL CAUSES OF HYPERCHLOREMIC METABOLIC ACIDOSIS

EXTRARENAL BICARBONATE LOSS

The loss of base during episodes of diarrhea or with the overzealous use of laxatives is associated with HCMA. Loss of HCO_3^- can also occur with pancreatic fistulae or with pancreas transplants if drainage of the pancreatic duct is into the bladder. Ureteral diversions using an isolated sigmoid loop were frequently associated with bicarbonate loss because of Cl-HCO_3^- exchange across bowel mucosa. These ureteral-sigmoidostomies have largely been replaced with ureteral diversions using ileal conduits, which have less surface area and contact time for loss of HCO_3^- to occur. If these become obstructed, however, HCMA can still develop.

ACID LOAD

An obvious cause of an HCMA is ingestion or infusion of a chloride salt of an acid. Both NH_4Cl and $CaCl_2$ can result in a metabolic acidosis and can be used as a provocative test to assess urinary acidification. In addition, total parenteral nutrition using hydrochloric acid salts of various amino acids can produce a metabolic acidosis if an insufficient quantity of base (usually acetate) is added to the infusion mixture. Another form of acid load is NaCl. Volume resuscitation with 0.9% NaCl will often produce an HCMA. This occurs because of "dilution" of the plasma HCO_3^- by the more acidic saline solution (pH 7.0) and because volume expansion diminishes proximal HCO_3^- reabsorption.

URINARY LOSS OF ANIONS

As previously discussed, if organic anions are excreted in the urine, they represent a source of base lost from the body. Although involving the kidney, this cannot be viewed as being caused by an intrinsic kidney defect. Because of the low renal threshold for the excretion of keto acids, patients with DKA, if able to maintain their intravascular volume or if volume resuscitated, will excrete these anions in place of Cl^-, resulting in HCMA. A similar metabolic disturbance exists after toluene exposure. Toluene is a common solvent found in paint products and glues. Exposure is generally by inhalation, either accidental or intentional. Toluene is rapidly absorbed through the skin and mucous membranes and metabolized to hippuric acid. Hippurate is quickly excreted by the kidney, leaving behind an HCMA. Although hippurate is not a base, its rapid excretion into the urine conceals the AG origins of this disturbance. Both of these disorders are usually easily discovered after taking an adequate history.

KEY BIBLIOGRAPHY

Alper SL. Genetic diseases of acid-base transporters. *Annu Rev Physiol.* 2002;64:899-923.

Adrogue HJ, Madias NE. Management of life-threatening acid-base disorders. *N Engl J Med.* 1998;338:26-34, 107–111.

Bonny O, Rossier B. Disturbances of Na/K balance: pseudohypoaldosteronism revisited. *J Am Soc Nephrol.* 2002;13:2399-2414.

Brent J, McMartin K, Phillips S, et al. Fomepizole for the treatment of methanol poisoning. *N Engl J Med.* 2001;344:424-429.

Carlisle EJ, Donnelly SM, Vasuvattakul S, et al. Glue-sniffing and distal renal tubular acidosis: sticking to the facts. *J Am Soc Nephrol.* 1991;1:1019-1027.

Chang CT, Chen YC, Fang JT, Huang CC. Metformin-associated lactic acidosis: case reports and literature review. *J Nephrol.* 2002;15:398-402.

Claessens YE, Cariou A, Monchi M, et al. Detecting life-threatening lactic acidosis related to nucleoside-analog treatment of human immunodeficiency virus-infected patients, and treatment with l-carnitine. *Crit Care Med.* 2003;31:1042-1047.

Dargan PI, Wallace CI, Jones AL. An evidence based flowchart to guide the management of acute salicylate (aspirin) overdose. *Emerg Med J.* 2002;19:206-209.

DuBose TD Jr, Mcdonald GA. Renal tubular acidosis. In: Dubose TD, Hamm LL Jr, eds. *Acid-Base and Electrolyte Disorders: A Companion to Brenner and Rector's The Kidney.* Philadelphia: WB Saunders; 2002:189-206.

Figge J, Jabor A, Kazda A. Anion gap and hypoalbuminemia. *Crit Care Med.* 1998;26:1807-1810.

Fraser AD. Clinical toxicologic implications of ethylene glycol and glycolic acid poisoning. *Ther Drug Monit.* 2002;24:232-238.

Han J, Kim G-H, Kim J, et al. Secretory-defect distal renal tubular acidosis is associated with transporter defect in H+-ATPase and anion exchanger-1. *J Am Soc Nephrol.* 2002;13:1425-1432.

Hood VL, Tannen RL. Protection of acid-base balance by pH regulation of acid production. *N Engl J Med.* 1998;339:819-826.

Igarashi T, Sekine T, Inatomi J, Seki G. Unraveling the molecular pathogenesis of isolated proximal renal tubular acidosis. *J Am Soc Nephrol.* 2002;13:2171-2177.

Ishihara K, Szerlip HM. Anion gap acidosis. *Semin Nephrol.* 1998;18:83-89.

Izzedine H, Launay-Vacher V, Isnard-Bagnis C, Derray G. Drug-induced Fanconi's syndrome. *Am J Kid Dis.* 2003;41:292-309.

Karet FE. Inherited distal renal tubular acidosis. *J Am Soc Nephrol.* 2002;13:2178-2184.

Kirschbaum B, Sica D, Anderson F. Urine electrolytes and the urine anion and osmolar gaps. *J Lab Clin Med.* 1999;133:597-604.

Lemann J Jr, Bushinsky DA, Hamm LL. Bone buffering of acid and base in humans. *Am J Physiol Renal Physiol.* 2003;285:F811-F832.

Levraut J, Grimaud D. Treatment of metabolic acidosis. *Curr Opin Crit Care.* 2003;9:260-265.

Full bibliography can be found on www.expertconsult.com.

Metabolic Alkalosis

Thomas D. DuBose, Jr.

Metabolic alkalosis represents the inability of the kidney to excrete an excessive amount of bicarbonate present in extracellular fluid (ECF) due to factors that generate the net gain of bicarbonate and secondary factors that maintain the alkalosis. Disorders that generate metabolic alkalosis include vomiting, diuretics, chloride and volume depletion, hypokalemia, and primary or secondary hyperaldosteronism. Differentiation of these diverse etiologies requires a careful assessment of ECF volume status, blood pressure, and potassium stores. Although uncommon, excessive exogenous alkali loads may also cause metabolic alkalosis under certain circumstances. This chapter summarizes the diverse clinical causes of metabolic alkalosis and the pathophysiologic basis of each disorder. Special attention is devoted to the diagnosis of each entity, and, from this perspective, an approach to the therapy and ultimate correction of this acid-base disorder is outlined in detail.

PATHOGENESIS

The pathogenesis of metabolic alkalosis requires two processes: (1) generation and (2) maintenance. Generation occurs by net gain of bicarbonate ions [HCO_3^-] or net loss of nonvolatile acid (usually HCl by vomiting) from the extracellular fluid. Although the kidneys have an impressive capacity to excrete HCO_3^- under normal circumstances, in the maintenance stage of metabolic alkalosis, the kidneys fail to excrete HCO_3^-, with HCO_3^- retained because of volume contraction, a low glomerular filtration rate (GFR), or depletion of chloride (Cl^-) or potassium (K^+). Maintenance of metabolic alkalosis, therefore, represents a failure of the kidneys to eliminate HCO_3^- in the usual manner. Retention, rather than excretion, of excess alkali by the kidney is promoted when (1) volume depletion, Cl^-, and K^+ deficiency exist in combination with a reduced GFR, or (2) hypokalemia prevails because of autonomous hyperaldosteronism. In the first example, alkalosis is typically corrected by administration of NaCl and KCl, whereas, in the latter example, it is necessary to address the alkalosis by pharmacologic or surgical intervention rather than saline administration.

In assessing a patient with metabolic alkalosis, two questions should be considered: First, what is the source of alkali gain (or acid loss) that generated the alkalosis? Second, what mechanisms are operating to prevent excretion of excess HCO_3^-, thereby maintaining, rather than correcting, the alkalosis?

DIFFERENTIAL DIAGNOSIS

To establish the cause of metabolic alkalosis (Box 14.1), it is necessary to assess the extracellular fluid volume (ECV) status, the recumbent and upright blood pressure, and the serum potassium concentration ([K^+]). In hypertensive patients with chronic hypokalemia, it is also helpful to evaluate the renin-angiotensin system. For example, the presence of chronic hypertension and chronic hypokalemia in an alkalemic patient suggests either mineralocorticoid excess or a hypertensive patient receiving diuretics. Low plasma renin activity and urine [Na^+] and [Cl^-] values greater than 20 mEq/L in a hypertensive patient not taking diuretics are consistent with primary mineralocorticoid excess.

The combination of hypokalemia and alkalosis in a nonedematous patient with a low or normal BP can pose a challenging diagnostic problem. Possible causes include Bartter or Gitelman syndromes, magnesium deficiency, vomiting, exogenous alkali, and diuretic ingestion. Determination of urine electrolytes (especially [Cl^-]) and screening of the urine for diuretics may be helpful. When the urine chloride concentration is measured (Table 14.1), it should be considered in context with assessment of the ECV status of the patient. A low urine [Cl^-] (i.e., <10 mEq/L) indicates avid Cl^- retention by the kidney and denotes ECV depletion, even if the urine Na^+ is high (i.e., >20 mEq/L), whereas a high urine [Cl^-] in the absence of concurrent diuretic use suggests inappropriate chloride loss resulting from a renal tubular defect or mineralocorticoid excess. If the urine is alkaline with an elevated urine [Na^+] and [K^+], but the urine [Cl^-] is lower than 10 mEq/L, the diagnosis is usually either vomiting (overt or surreptitious) or alkali ingestion. If the urine is relatively acidic and has low concentrations of Na^+, K^+, and Cl^-, the most likely possibilities are previous vomiting, the posthypercapnic state, or previous diuretic ingestion. If, on the other hand, neither the urine [Na^+], [K^+], nor [Cl^-] is depressed, magnesium deficiency, Bartter or Gitelman syndromes, or active diuretic use should be considered. Gitelman syndrome is distinguished from Bartter syndrome by the presence of hypocalciuria. In addition, hypomagnesemia may be present in both but is more common in Gitelman syndrome.

Box 14.1 Causes of Metabolic Alkalosis

Exogenous HCO₃⁻ Loads

Acute alkali administration
Milk-alkali syndrome
Use of NaOH in "freebasing" of crack cocaine
Street cocaine "cut" with baking soda
Baking soda pica in pregnancy
Bicarbonate precursors (citrate, acetate) in chronic or acute kidney disease
Alkali NG tube feedings, particularly in settings of low GFR

Effective ECV Contraction, Normotension, K⁺ Deficiency, and Secondary Hyperreninemic Hyperaldosteronism

Gastrointestinal origin
  Vomiting
  Gastric aspiration
  Congenital chloridorrhea
  Villous adenoma
  Combined administration of sodium polystyrene sulfonate (Kayexalate) and aluminum hydroxide
  Cystic fibrosis and volume depletion
  Gastrocystoplasty
  Chronic laxative abuse
  Cl⁻-deficient infant formula
Kidney origin
  Diuretics (remote use of thiazides or loop diuretics)
  Edematous states
  Posthypercapnic state
  Hypercalcemia–hypoparathyroidism
  Recovery from lactic acidosis or ketoacidosis
  Nonreabsorbable anions (e.g., intravenous penicillin derivatives such as carbenicillin or ticarcillin)
  Mg²⁺ deficiency
  K⁺ depletion
  Bartter syndrome
  Gitelman syndrome
  Carbohydrate refeeding after starvation
  Pendred syndrome (during thiazide diuretic use or intercurrent illness)

ECV Expansion, Hypertension, K⁺ Deficiency, and Hypermineralocorticoidism

Associated with high renin
  Renal artery stenosis
  Accelerated hypertension
  Renin-secreting tumor
  Estrogen therapy
Associated with low renin
  Primary aldosteronism
    • Adenoma
    • Hyperplasia
    • Carcinoma
    • Glucocorticoid suppressible
  Adrenal enzymatic defects
    • 11β-Hydroxylase deficiency
    • 17α-Hydroxylase deficiency
  Cushing syndrome or disease
    • Ectopic corticotropin
    • Adrenal carcinoma
    • Adrenal adenoma
    • Primary pituitary
  Other
    • Licorice
    • Carbenoxolone
    • Chewing tobacco (containing glycyrrhizinic acid)
    • Lydia Pinkham tablets

Gain-of-Function Mutation of ENaC With ECV Expansion, Hypertension, K⁺ Deficiency, and Hyporeninemic Hypoaldosteronism

Liddle syndrome

ECV, Extracellular fluid volume; *ENaC*, epithelial sodium channel; *GFR*, glomerular filtration rate.

Table 14.1 Diagnosis of Metabolic Alkalosis

Low Urinary [Cl⁻] (<10 mEq/L)	High or Normal Urinary [Cl⁻] (>15–20 mEq/L)
Normotension	**Hypertension**
Vomiting, nasogastric Aspiration	Primary aldosteronism
Diuretics	Cushing syndrome
Posthypercapnia	Renal artery stenosis
Bicarbonate treatment of organic acidosis	Renal failure plus alkali therapy
K⁺ deficiency	**Normotension or Hypotension**
Hypertension	Mg²⁺ deficiency
Liddle syndrome	Severe K⁺ deficiency
	Bartter syndrome
	Gitelman syndrome
	Diuretics

METABOLIC ALKALOSIS DUE TO EXOGENOUS BICARBONATE LOADS

ALKALI ADMINISTRATION

Administration of base to individuals with normal kidney function rarely causes alkalosis since the normal kidney has a high capacity for HCO₃⁻ excretion. Nevertheless, in patients with coexistent hemodynamic disturbances, alkalosis may develop because the normal capacity to excrete HCO₃⁻ has been exceeded. Examples include patients receiving oral or intravenous HCO₃⁻, acetate loads (parenteral hyperalimentation solutions), citrate loads (transfusions, continuous renal replacement therapy, or infant formula), or antacids in conjunction with cation-exchange resins (aluminum hydroxide and sodium polystyrene sulfonate). Moreover, metabolic alkalosis may develop when there is a coexisting problem that results in enhanced reabsorption of HCO₃⁻, such as volume depletion, a reduction in GFR, potassium depletion, or hypercapnia.

In patients with acute kidney injury or advanced chronic kidney disease, overt alkalosis can develop after alkali administration because the capacity to excrete HCO_3^- is exceeded or coexistent hemodynamic disturbances have caused enhanced HCO_3^- reabsorption. In this regard, baking soda ingestion should be considered in CKD patients, especially when baking soda is used as a home remedy for dyspepsia. The use of tube feedings in elderly patients in long-term care facilities has been associated with metabolic alkalosis, as tube feeding preparations in the elderly are a common and underappreciated source of alkali loads. Plasma electrolytes should be monitored more frequently in these patients. Other examples of acute metabolic alkalosis resulting from alkali ingestion include the association of pica for baking soda in pregnancy. Additionally, the use of crack cocaine has been described as a cause of severe alkalosis in patients undergoing hemodialysis as "freebasing" involves the addition of alkali (NaOH, a component of household drain cleaner) to cocaine hydrochloride.

MILK-ALKALI SYNDROME

A long-standing history of excessive ingestion of milk and antacids, termed milk-alkali syndrome, is a historically important cause of metabolic alkalosis. There has been a resurgence of this syndrome since the 1990s following increased use of calcium carbonate and vitamin D for osteoporosis. The majority of patients with this form of milk-alkali syndrome are asymptomatic women with incidental hypercalcemia, previously unappreciated CKD, and hypophosphatemia. Older women on diuretics and ACE inhibitors appear to be at higher risk. Both hypercalcemia and excess vitamin D increase renal tubular HCO_3^- reabsorption. A critical component of this syndrome is reduced GFR. Patients with this disorder are prone to developing nephrocalcinosis, progressive CKD, and metabolic alkalosis. Discontinuation of alkali ingestion is usually sufficient to correct the alkalosis, but the kidney disease may be irreversible if nephrocalcinosis is advanced.

CITRATE-BASED CONTINUOUS RENAL REPLACEMENT THERAPY

If citrate is used for regional anticoagulation in continuous renal replacement therapy, metabolic alkalosis can be expected. The metabolism of citrate by the liver and skeletal muscle results in a net gain of HCO_3^-. Strategies have been advanced to reduce the complications of regional trisodium citrate anticoagulation (hypocalcemia, metabolic alkalosis, use of 0.1 N HCl, and subsequent hyponatremia) by using anticoagulant citrate dextrose formula A.

METABOLIC ALKALOSIS ASSOCIATED WITH EFFECTIVE INTRAVASCULAR VOLUME CONTRACTION AND SECONDARY HYPERRENINEMIC HYPERALDOSTERONISM

GASTROINTESTINAL ORIGIN

Gastrointestinal loss of H^+, Cl^-, Na^+, and K^+ from vomitus or gastric aspiration results in retention of HCO_3^-. The loss of fluid and electrolytes results in contraction of the ECV and stimulation of the renin-angiotensin system. Volume contraction causes a reduction in GFR and an enhanced capacity of the renal tubule to reabsorb HCO_3^-. Excess angiotensin II stimulates Na^+/H^+ exchange in the proximal tubule. During active vomiting, there is continued addition of HCO_3^- to plasma in exchange for Cl^-, and the plasma $[HCO_3^-]$ exceeds the reabsorptive capacity of the proximal tubule. Aldosterone and endothelin also stimulate the proton-transporting adenosine triphosphatase (H^+-ATPase) in the distal nephron, resulting in enhanced capacity for distal nephron HCO_3^- absorption and, paradoxically, aciduria. When the excess $NaHCO_3$ reaches the distal tubule, potassium secretion is enhanced by aldosterone and the delivery of the poorly reabsorbed anion, HCO_3^-. Thus the predominant cause of hypokalemia is urinary loss of K^+ and not gastrointestinal potassium wasting.

Hypokalemia has selective effects on renal tubular bicarbonate absorption and ammonium production that are counterproductive to metabolic alkalosis. Hypokalemia dramatically increases the activity of the proton pump (H^+/K^+-ATPase) in the cortical and medullary collecting tubule for reabsorbing K^+, but this occurs at the expense of both enhanced net acid excretion and HCO_3^- absorption. Hypokalemia also increases ammonium production independently of acid-base status, which, in the face of enhanced H^+ secretion, results in increased ammonium production and excretion; this in turn adds new bicarbonate to the systemic circulation (increase in net acid excretion). Therefore hypokalemia plays an important role in the seemingly maladaptive response of the kidney to maintain the alkalosis. Because of contraction of the ECV and hypochloremia, Cl^- is avidly conserved by the kidney. This can be recognized clinically by a low urinary chloride concentration (see Table 14.1). Correction of the contracted ECV with isotonic NaCl and repletion of the K^+ deficit correct the acid-base disorder, because such therapy restores the ability of the kidney to excrete excess bicarbonate.

CONGENITAL CHLORIDORRHEA

Congenital chloridorrhea, a rare autosomal-recessive disorder, causes metabolic alkalosis by an extrarenal mechanism of severe diarrhea, fecal acid loss, and HCO_3^- retention. The disease is the result of mutations in the *SLC26A3* gene that disrupt the ileal and colonic HCO_3^-/Cl^- anion exchange mechanism so that Cl^- cannot be reabsorbed in the gut. The parallel Na^+/H^+ ion exchanger remains functional, allowing Na^+ to be reabsorbed and H^+ to be secreted. Therefore the stool has high concentrations of H^+ and Cl^-, causing Na^+ and HCO_3^- retention in the extracellular fluid. The alkalosis is sustained by concomitant ECV contraction, hyperaldosteronism, and K^+ deficiency. Delivery of Cl^- to the distal nephron is low because of volume contraction. As in cystic fibrosis, this low delivery of Cl^- results in impaired HCO_3^- secretion by the β-intercalated cell. Therapy consists of oral supplementation of sodium and potassium chloride. Administration of proton pump inhibitors may reduce chloride secretion by the parietal cells and improve the diarrhea. The long-term outcome is good with daily supplementation of NaCl and KCl.

VILLOUS ADENOMA

Metabolic alkalosis has been described in cases of villous adenoma. K^+ depletion probably induces the alkalosis since colonic secretion is alkaline.

GASTROCYSTOPLASTY

Augmentation of the bladder by gastrocystoplasty, although uncommon, has been used as an alternative to enterocystoplasty. Implantation of a segment of vascularized stomach into the bladder in children with reduced bladder capacity has been associated with hypokalemia, hypochloremia, and metabolic alkalosis. Gastrointestinal complications have also been reported. Oral potassium chloride should be administered chronically.

RENAL ORIGIN

The generation of metabolic alkalosis through renal mechanisms involves three processes for increasing distal nephron H$^+$ secretion and enhancing net acid excretion (ammonium) excretion: (1) high delivery of Na$^+$ salts to the distal nephron, (2) excessive elaboration of mineralocorticoids, and (3) K$^+$ deficiency (Fig. 14.1).

DIURETICS

Drugs that induce distal delivery of sodium salts, such as thiazide and loop diuretics, diminish ECV without altering total body bicarbonate content. Consequently the serum [HCO$_3^-$] increases. The chronic administration of diuretics generates a metabolic alkalosis by increasing distal salt delivery, thereby enhancing K$^+$ and H$^+$ secretion by the collecting tubule. The alkalosis is maintained by persistent contraction of the ECV, secondary hyperaldosteronism, K$^+$ deficiency, and activation of the H$^+$/K$^+$-ATPase, as long as diuretic administration continues. Hypokalemia also enhances ammonium production and excretion. Repair of the alkalosis is achieved by withholding the diuretic, providing isotonic saline to correct the ECV deficit, and repleting potassium.

BARTTER SYNDROME

Both classic Bartter syndrome and the antenatal type are inherited as autosomal-recessive disorders that impair salt absorption in the thick ascending limb (TAL) of the loop of Henle; this results in salt wasting, volume depletion, and activation of the renin-angiotensin system. These manifestations are the result of loss-of-function mutations of one of the genes that encode three transporters involved in NaCl absorption in the TAL. The most prevalent disorder is a mutation of the gene *NKCC2*, which encodes the Na$^+$/K$^+$/2Cl$^-$ cotransporter on the apical membrane. A second mutation has been discovered in the gene *KCNJ1*, which encodes the ATP-sensitive apical K$^+$ conductance channel (ROMK) that operates in parallel with the Na$^+$/K$^+$/2Cl$^-$ cotransporter to recycle K$^+$. Both defects can be associated with antenatal Bartter syndrome or with classic Bartter syndrome. A mutation of the *CLCNKb* gene encoding the voltage-gated basolateral chloride channel (ClC-Kb) is associated only with classic Bartter syndrome, is milder, and is rarely associated with nephrocalcinosis. All three defects have the same net effect: loss of Cl$^-$ transport in the TAL, causing enhanced delivery of NaCl that stimulates K$^+$ and H$^+$ secretion by the collecting tubule, causing hypokalemia and metabolic alkalosis.

Antenatal Bartter syndrome has been observed in consanguineous families in association with sensorineural deafness, a syndrome linked to chromosome 1p31. The responsible gene, *BSND*, encodes a subunit, barttin, that co-localizes with the ClC-Kb channel in the TAL and K$^+$-secreting epithelial

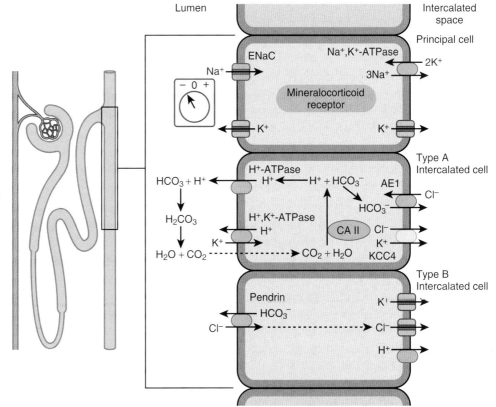

Fig. 14.1 Contribution of the distal nephron to the maintenance of metabolic alkalosis. Extracellular volume depletion maintains metabolic alkalosis by increasing the activity of the epithelial sodium channel in principal cells (*top cell,* labeled ENaC) through enhanced elaboration of mineralocorticoid (secondary hyperaldosteronism). This further aggravates potassium wasting by increasing the negative transepithelial potential. Similarly, secondary hyperaldosteronism enhances H$^+$ secretion in Type A intercalated cells that inappropriately enhance absorption of HCO$_3^-$, rather than its excretion. Correction of metabolic alkalosis with volume depletion requires correction of ECF and potassium deficits. When accomplished, the kidney can excrete HCO$_3^-$ efficiently.

cells in the inner ear. Barttin appears to be necessary for the function of the voltage-gated chloride channel. Expression of ClC-Kb is lost when co-expressed with mutant barttins. Therefore mutations in *BSND* define a fourth category of patients with Bartter syndrome.

Such defects predictably lead to ECV contraction, hyperreninemic hyperaldosteronism, and increased delivery of NaCl to the distal nephron, with consequent alkalosis, urinary K^+ wasting, and hypokalemia. Secondary overproduction of prostaglandins, juxtaglomerular apparatus hypertrophy, and vascular pressor unresponsiveness ensue. Most patients have hypercalciuria and normal serum magnesium levels, distinguishing this disorder from Gitelman syndrome.

Bartter syndrome is inherited as an autosomal-recessive defect. Most patients are homozygotes or compound heterozygotes for different mutations in one of these four genes, whereas a few patients with the clinical syndrome have no discernible mutation in any of these genes. Plausible explanations include unrecognized mutations in other genes, a dominant-negative effect of a heterozygous mutation, or other mechanisms. In addition, activating mutations in the calcium-sensing receptor, CaSR, on the basolateral cell surface of the TAL inhibits the function of ROMK, recapitulating the phenotype of inherited Bartter syndrome.

For diagnosis, Bartter syndrome must be distinguished from surreptitious vomiting, diuretic administration, and laxative abuse. The finding of a low urinary Cl^- concentration is helpful in identifying the vomiting patient (see Table 14.1). The urinary Cl^- concentration in a patient with Bartter syndrome would be expected to be normal or increased rather than depressed.

The therapy for Bartter syndrome focuses on repair of the hypokalemia through inhibition of the renin-angiotensin-aldosterone system or the prostaglandin-kinin system, using propranolol, amiloride, spironolactone, prostaglandin inhibitors, and angiotensin-converting enzyme inhibitors, as well as direct repletion of the deficits of potassium and magnesium.

GITELMAN SYNDROME

Patients with Gitelman syndrome resemble the Bartter syndrome phenotype in that an autosomal-recessive metabolic alkalosis is associated with hypokalemia, normal to low blood pressure, volume depletion with secondary hyperreninemic hyperaldosteronism, and juxtaglomerular hyperplasia. However, the consistent presence of hypocalciuria and the frequent presence of hypomagnesemia are useful in distinguishing Gitelman syndrome from Bartter syndrome on clinical grounds. These unique features mimic the effects of chronic thiazide diuretic administration. Missense mutations of the gene *SLC12A3*, which encodes the thiazide-sensitive sodium chloride cotransporter in the distal convoluted tubule (NCC), account for the clinical features, including the classic finding of hypocalciuria. However, it is not clear why these patients have pronounced hypomagnesemia. A study demonstrated that peripheral blood mononuclear cells from patients with Gitelman syndrome express mutated NCC messenger RNA (mRNA). In a large consanguineous Bedouin family, missense mutations were noted in *CLCNKb*, but the clinical features overlapped between Gitelman and Bartter syndromes.

Compared with Bartter syndrome, Gitelman syndrome becomes symptomatic later in life and is associated with milder salt wasting. A large study of adults with proven Gitelman syndrome and NCC mutations showed that salt craving, nocturia, cramps, and fatigue were more common than in sex-matched and age-matched controls. Women experience exacerbation of symptoms during menses, and they may experience complicated pregnancies.

Treatment of Gitelman syndrome consists of a diet high in potassium and potassium salts, typically with the addition of magnesium supplementation. Amiloride is often more helpful than spironolactone or eplerenone, with dose escalation to as much as 10 mg twice daily. Amiloride may be used in combination with spironolactone or eplerenone. Importantly, almost all patients with Gitelman syndrome exhibit some degree of salt craving, some of which may be extreme. To the extent possible, offending foods high in salt should be identified and avoided, because salt loading increases distal delivery of NaCl and greatly amplifies K^+ secretion by the cortical collecting tubule. Careful questioning of dietary practices is necessary to expose unusual salt appetites. Angiotensin-converting enzyme inhibitors have been suggested in selected patients for which frank hypotension is not a complication.

PENDRED SYNDROME

Pendred syndrome consists of sensorineural deafness and goiter caused by impaired iodide uptake, and it is ascribed to a defect in the pendrin co-transporter (encoded by *SLC26A4*). Pendrin is expressed on the apical membrane of type B intercalated cells of the collecting tubule. Although these patients typically do not have acid-base disorders, two recent reports of severe metabolic alkalosis with hypokalemia (one was a patient prescribed a thiazide diuretic, and another case occurred with alcoholism and severe vomiting after a cochlear implant) suggest that these patients are susceptible because of the inability of type B intercalated cells to secrete bicarbonate. These reports also underscore the importance of bicarbonate secretion during alkalotic challenges. Diuretics should not be prescribed to patients with Pendred syndrome, and clinicians should be aware that protracted vomiting may lead to severe metabolic alkalosis.

NONREABSORBABLE ANIONS AND MAGNESIUM DEFICIENCY

Administration of large quantities of nonreabsorbable anions, such as with penicillin derivatives like carbenicillin, can enhance distal acidification and K^+ secretion by increasing the negative transepithelial potential difference. Mg^{2+} deficiency frequently accompanies hypokalemia, and both electrolyte abnormalities must be corrected to ameliorate the metabolic alkalosis.

POTASSIUM DEPLETION

Pure K^+ depletion causes metabolic alkalosis although usually of only modest severity. Hypokalemia independently enhances renal ammoniagenesis, which increases net acid excretion and thereby the return of "new" bicarbonate to the systemic circulation. When access to salt and K^+ is restricted, more severe alkalosis develops. Activation of the H^+/K^+-ATPase in the collecting duct by chronic hypokalemia probably plays a major role in maintenance of the alkalosis. Specifically, chronic hypokalemia has been shown to markedly increase the abundance of the colonic H^+/K^+-ATPase mRNA and protein in the outer medullary collecting duct. Alkalosis associated with severe K^+ depletion is resistant to salt administration, with repair of the K^+ deficiency necessary to correct the alkalosis.

POSTLACTIC ACIDOSIS OR KETOACIDOSIS

When an underlying stimulus for the endogenous generation of lactic acid or ketoacid is removed rapidly, as with the repair of circulatory insufficiency or administration of insulin therapy, the lactate or ketones are metabolized to yield an equivalent amount of HCO_3^-. Other sources of new HCO_3^- are additive to the original alkali generated by organic anion metabolism to create a surfeit of HCO_3^-. Such sources include new HCO_3^- added to the blood by the kidneys as a result of enhanced acid excretion during the preexisting period of acidosis, and exogenous alkali administered during the treatment phase of the acidosis. Acidosis-induced contraction of the ECV acts to sustain the alkalosis.

POSTHYPERCAPNIA

Prolonged CO_2 retention with chronic respiratory acidosis enhances tubular HCO_3^- absorption and the generation of new HCO_3^- (increased net acid excretion). If the partial pressure of carbon dioxide in arterial blood ($PaCO_2$) is returned to normal by mechanical ventilation or other means, metabolic alkalosis results from the persistently elevated [HCO_3^-]. Associated ECV contraction does not allow complete repair of the alkalosis by correction of the $PaCO_2$ alone, and alkalosis persists until isotonic saline is infused.

METABOLIC ALKALOSIS ASSOCIATED WITH HYPERALDOSTERONISM AND HYPERTENSION

ASSOCIATED WITH HIGH RENIN

Hyperreninemia promotes conversion of angiotensin I to angiotensin II, causing severe vasoconstriction and aldosterone release. The clinical features of functional renal artery stenosis are related primarily to activation of the renin-angiotensin-aldosterone system, causing renovascular hypertension (contralateral kidney) and ischemic nephropathy (affected kidney). Patients typically present with resistant hypertension that may be unresponsive to high doses of multiple antihypertensive agents. In addition, approximately 16% of adult patients also exhibit hypokalemia and metabolic alkalosis. Additional examples of metabolic alkalosis, hypokalemia, and hypertension can also occur with renin-secreting tumors of the kidney, accelerated hypertension, and estrogen therapy (see Box 14.1).

ASSOCIATED WITH LOW RENIN

PRIMARY HYPERALDOSTERONISM

Increased aldosterone levels may result from autonomous adrenal overproduction or secondary aldosterone release caused by the overproduction of renin by the kidneys. In both situations, the normal feedback of ECV on aldosterone production is disrupted, and hypertension is the result of ECF volume expansion. Excessive production of aldosterone also increases net acid excretion and may result in metabolic alkalosis, which is worsened by associated K^+ deficiency. ECV expansion from salt retention causes hypertension, and urinary acidification is enhanced by aldosterone and K^+ deficiency through an increase in the activity of the H^+-ATPase and H^+/K^+-ATPase, respectively. The kaliuresis worsens K^+ depletion, resulting in a urinary concentrating defect, polyuria, and polydipsia.

LIDDLE SYNDROME

Liddle syndrome is associated with severe hypertension presenting in childhood, accompanied by hypokalemia and metabolic alkalosis. These features resemble those of primary hyperaldosteronism, but renin and aldosterone levels are suppressed (pseudohyperaldosteronism). Liddle originally described patients with low renin and low aldosterone levels that did not respond to spironolactone. The defect is inherited as an autosomal-dominant form of monogenic hypertension and is attributed to an abnormality in the gene that encodes the β or the γ subunit of the renal epithelial Na^+ channel (ENaC) on the apical membrane of principal cells in the cortical collecting duct. This defect leads to constitutive activation of this channel. Either mutation results in deletion of the cytoplasmic tail (C-terminus) of the affected subunit. The C-termini contain a PY amino acid motif that is highly conserved, and essentially all mutations in Liddle syndrome patients involve disruption or deletion of this motif. Such PY motifs are important in regulating the number of sodium channels in the luminal membrane by binding to the WW domains of the Nedd4-like family of ubiquitin protein ligases. Disruption of the PY motif dramatically increases the surface localization of the ENaC complex by failing to internalize or degrade (Nedd4 pathway) the channels from the cell surface. Ultimately, persistent Na^+ absorption results in volume expansion, hypertension, hypokalemia, and metabolic alkalosis.

GLUCOCORTICOID-REMEDIABLE HYPERALDOSTERONISM

Glucocorticoid-remediable hyperaldosteronism is an autosomal-dominant form of hypertension, the features of which resemble primary aldosteronism (hypokalemic metabolic alkalosis and volume-dependent hypertension). However, in this disorder glucocorticoid administration corrects the hypertension as well as the excessive excretion of 18-hydroxysteroid in the urine. This disorder occurs from an unequal crossover between two genes located in close proximity on chromosome 8, resulting in the glucocorticoid-responsive promoter region of the gene encoding the 11β-hydroxylase (*CYP11B1*), attaching to the structural portion of the *CYP11B2* gene encoding aldosterone synthase. The chimeric gene produces excess amounts of aldosterone synthase unresponsive to serum potassium or renin levels; however, production can be suppressed by glucocorticoid administration. Although this syndrome is a rare cause of primary aldosteronism, it is important to diagnose since the treatment is unique and the syndrome can be associated with severe hypertension and stroke, especially during pregnancy.

CUSHING SYNDROME

Abnormally high glucocorticoid production as a result of adrenal adenoma, carcinoma, or ectopic corticotropin production causes metabolic alkalosis. The alkalosis may be ascribed to coexisting mineralocorticoid (deoxycorticosterone and corticosterone) hypersecretion. Alternatively, glucocorticoids may have the capability of enhancing net acid secretion and NH_4^+ production through cross-reactivity with mineralocorticoid receptors.

MISCELLANEOUS CONDITIONS

Ingestion of licorice or licorice-containing chewing tobacco can cause a typical pattern of mineralocorticoid excess. Glycyrrhizinic acid contained in authentic licorice inhibits 11β-hydroxysteroid dehydrogenase. This enzyme is responsible for converting cortisol to cortisone, an essential step in protecting the mineralocorticoid receptor from cortisol. When the enzyme is inactivated, cortisol can occupy type I mineralocorticoid receptors, mimicking aldosterone. Genetic apparent mineralocorticoid excess (AME) resembles excessive ingestion of licorice, with volume expansion, low renin and aldosterone levels, and a salt-sensitive form of hypertension that may include metabolic alkalosis and hypokalemia. In genetic AME, 11β-hydroxysteroid dehydrogenase is defective, and monogenic hypertension develops. Hypertension responds to thiazides and spironolactone but without abnormal steroid products in the urine.

SYMPTOMS OF METABOLIC ALKALOSIS

Patients with metabolic alkalosis experience changes in central and peripheral nervous system function similar to those of hypocalcemia. This results from the binding of free calcium to anionic protein sites exposed in alkalemia, lowering the ionized calcium concentration. Symptoms may include confusion, obtundation, and a predisposition to seizures, paresthesia, muscular cramping, tetany, aggravation of arrhythmias, and hypoxemia in chronic obstructive pulmonary disease. Related electrolyte abnormalities include hypokalemia and hypophosphatemia.

TREATMENT OF METABOLIC ALKALOSIS

The maintenance phase of metabolic alkalosis represents a failure of the kidney to excrete bicarbonate efficiently because of chloride or potassium deficiency, continuous mineralocorticoid elaboration, or both. Treatment depends on the cause of the metabolic alkalosis, and it is primarily directed at correcting the underlying stimulus for HCO_3^- generation and restoring the ability of the kidney to excrete the excess HCO_3^-. A history of vomiting, diuretic use, or alkali therapy and assessment of the urine chloride concentration, arterial blood pressure, and volume status (particularly the presence or absence of orthostasis; see Box 14.1) all help guide diagnosis and treatment.

A high urine chloride level and hypertension suggest that primary mineralocorticoid excess is present. If primary aldosteronism is diagnosed, correction of the underlying cause (adenoma, bilateral hyperplasia, Cushing syndrome) will reverse the alkalosis. Patients with bilateral adrenal hyperplasia may respond to spironolactone. Normotensive patients with a high urine chloride level may have Bartter or Gitelman syndrome if diuretic use or vomiting can be excluded. A low urine chloride level and relative hypotension suggest a chloride-responsive metabolic alkalosis such as vomiting or nasogastric suction. Loss of $[H^+]$ by the stomach or kidneys can be mitigated by the use of proton pump inhibitors or the discontinuation of diuretics. The second aspect of treatment is to remove the factors that sustain HCO_3^- reabsorption, such as ECV contraction or K^+ deficiency. Although K^+ deficits should be repleted, NaCl therapy is usually sufficient to reverse the alkalosis if ECV contraction is present, as indicated by a low urine $[Cl^-]$.

Patients with congestive heart failure or unexplained volume expansion represent special challenges in the critical care setting. Patients with a low urine chloride concentration, usually indicative of a "chloride-responsive" form of metabolic alkalosis, may not tolerate normal saline infusion. Renal HCO_3^- loss can be accelerated by administration of the carbonic anhydrase inhibitor acetazolamide (125–250 mg intravenously) if associated conditions preclude infusion of saline (i.e., clinical evidence of congestive heart failure). Acetazolamide is usually effective in patients with adequate kidney function but can exacerbate urinary K^+ losses and cause hypokalemia. Dilute hydrochloric acid (0.1 N HCl) infused into a central vein is sometimes recommended. Several potentially serious complications, such as hemolysis, venous sclerosis, and imprecise dosing, result in a very high risk-to-benefit ratio. It is not recommended except in extreme metabolic alkalosis (pH >7.6) in patients unresponsive to or intolerant of isotonic saline infusion, acetazolamide, or ammonium chloride administration. Oral NH_4Cl is preferable to intravenous 0.1 N HCl, except in patients with liver disease.

KEY BIBLIOGRAPHY

Birkenhager R, Otto E, Schurmann MJ, et al. Mutation of BSND causes Bartter syndrome with sensorineural deafness and kidney failure. *Nat Genet.* 2001;29:310-314.

Conn JW, Rovner DR, Cohen EL. Licorice-induced pseudoaldosteronism: hypertension, hypokalemia, aldosteronopenia, and suppressed plasma renin activity. *JAMA.* 1968;205:492.

Cruz DN, Shaer AJ, Bia MJ, et al. Gitelman's syndrome revisited: an evaluation of symptoms and health-related quality of life. *Kidney Int.* 2001;59:717-719.

Diskin CJ, Stokes TJ, Dansby M, et al. Recurrent metabolic alkalosis and elevated troponins after crack cocaine use in a hemodialysis patient. *Clin Exp Nephrol.* 2006;10:156-158.

DuBose TD Jr. Disorders of acid-base balance. In: Skorecki K, Chertow GM, Marsden PA, Taal MW, Yu SL, eds. *Brenner and Rector's The Kidney.* 10th ed. Philadelphia: Elsevier; 2016:511-558.

Felsenfeld AJ, Levine BS. Milk alkali syndrome and the dynamics of calcium homeostasis. *Clin J Am Soc Nephrol.* 2006;4:641-654.

Fitzgibbons LJ, Snoey ER. Severe metabolic alkalosis due to baking soda ingestion: case reports of two patients with unsuspected antacid overdose. *J Emerg Med.* 1999;17:57-61.

Gennari FJ. Pathophysiology of metabolic alkalosis: a new classification based on the centrality of stimulated collecting duct ion transport. *Am J Kidney Dis.* 2011;58:626-636.

Grotegut CA, Dandolu V, Katari S, et al. Baking soda pica: a case of hypokalemic metabolic alkalosis and rhabdomyolysis in pregnancy. *Obstet Gynecol.* 2006;107:484-486.

Hebert SC, Gullans SR. The molecular basis of inherited hypokalemic alkalosis: Bartter's and Gitelman's syndromes. *Am J Physiol.* 1996;271: F957-F959.

Hernandez R, Schambelan M, Cogan MG, et al. Dietary NaCl determines severity of potassium depletion-induced metabolic alkalosis. *Kidney Int.* 1987;31:1356.

Hihnala S, Kujala M, Toppari J, et al. Expression of SLC26A3, CFTR and NHE3 in the human male reproductive tract: role in male subfertility caused by congenital chloride diarrhea. *Mol Hum Reprod.* 2006;12: 107-111.

Jamison RL, Ross JC, Kempson RL, et al. Surreptitious diuretic ingestion and pseudo-Bartter's syndrome. *Am J Med.* 1982;73:142.

Kamynina E, Staub O. Concerted action of ENaC, Nedd4-2, and Sgk1 in transepithelial Na+ transport. *Am J Physiol Renal Physiol.* 2002;283: F377.

Lifton RP, Dluhy RG, Powers M, et al. Hereditary hypertension caused by chimaeric gene duplications and ectopic expression of aldosterone synthase. *Nat Genet.* 1992;2:66-74.

Morgera S, Haase M, Ruckert M, et al. Regional citrate anticoagulation in continuous hemodialysis: acid-base and electrolyte balance at an increased dose of dialysis. *Nephron Clin Pract.* 2005;101:c211-c219.

Sanei-Moghaddam A, Wilson T, Kumar S, et al. An unfortunate case of Pendred syndrome. *J Laryngol Otol.* 2011;125:965-967.

Schroeder ET. Alkalosis resulting from combined administration of a "nonsystemic" antacid and a cation-exchange resin. *Gastroenterology.* 1969;56:868-874.

Shimkets RA, Warnock DG, Bositis CM, et al. Liddle's syndrome: heritable human hypertension caused by mutations in the beta subunit of the epithelial sodium channel. *Cell.* 1994;79:407.

Yi JH, Han SW, Song JS, et al. Metabolic alkalosis from unsuspected ingestion: use of urine pH and anion gap. *Am J Kidney Dis.* 2012;59:577-581.

Full bibliography can be found on www.expertconsult.com.

15 Respiratory Acidosis and Alkalosis

Nicolaos E. Madias; Horacio J. Adrogué

RESPIRATORY ACIDOSIS

Respiratory acidosis, or primary hypercapnia, is the acid-base disturbance initiated by an increase in the carbon dioxide tension of body fluids and in whole-body CO_2 stores. Hypercapnia acidifies body fluids and elicits an adaptive increment in the plasma bicarbonate concentration $[HCO_3^-]$ that should be viewed as an integral part of the respiratory acidosis. Arterial CO_2 tension (Pco_2), measured at rest and at sea level, is greater than 45 mm Hg in simple respiratory acidosis. Lower values of Pco_2 might still signify the presence of primary hypercapnia in the setting of mixed acid-base disorders (e.g., eucapnia, rather than the expected hypocapnia, in the presence of metabolic acidosis). Another special case of respiratory acidosis is the presence of arterial eucapnia, or even hypocapnia, in association with venous hypercapnia in patients who have an acute severe reduction in cardiac output but relative preservation of respiratory function (i.e., pseudo-respiratory alkalosis).

PATHOPHYSIOLOGY

The ventilatory system is responsible for maintaining Pco_2 within normal limits by adjusting minute ventilation ($\dot{V}_E$) to match the rate of CO_2 production. $\dot{V}_E$ consists of two components: ventilation distributed in the gas-exchange units of the lungs (alveolar ventilation, $\dot{V}_A$) and ventilation wasted in dead space ($\dot{V}_D$). Hypercapnia can result from increased CO_2 production, decreased $\dot{V}_A$, or both. Decreased $\dot{V}_A$ can occur from a reduction in $\dot{V}_E$, an increase in $\dot{V}_D$, or a combination of the two.

The main elements of the ventilatory system are the respiratory pump, which generates a pressure gradient responsible for airflow, and the loads that oppose such action. The respiratory pump comprises the cerebrum, brainstem, spinal cord, phrenic and intercostal nerves, and the muscles of respiration. The respiratory loads include the ventilatory requirement (CO_2 production, O_2 consumption), airway resistance, lung elastic recoil, and chest wall/abdominal resistance. Most frequently, primary hypercapnia develops from an imbalance between the strength of the respiratory pump and the weight of the respiratory loads, thereby resulting in a decreased $\dot{V}_A$. Impairment of the respiratory pump can occur because of depressed central drive, abnormal neuromuscular transmission, or muscle dysfunction. Causes of augmented respiratory loads include ventilation/perfusion mismatch (increased $\dot{V}_D$), augmented airway flow resistance, lung/pleural/chest wall stiffness, impaired diaphragmatic function, and increased ventilatory demand. An increased $\dot{V}_D$ occurs in many clinical conditions, including emphysema, cystic fibrosis, asthma, and other intrinsic lung diseases, as well as chest wall disorders. A less frequent cause of primary hypercapnia is failure of CO_2 transport caused by decreases in pulmonary perfusion, a condition that occurs in cardiac arrest, circulatory collapse, and pulmonary embolism (thrombus, fat, air).

Overproduction of CO_2 is usually matched by increased excretion so that hypercapnia is prevented. However, patients with marked limitation in pulmonary reserve and those receiving constant mechanical ventilation might experience respiratory acidosis due to increased CO_2 production caused by increased muscle activity (agitation, myoclonus, shivering, seizures), sepsis, fever, or hyperthyroidism. Increments in CO_2 production might also be imposed by the administration of large carbohydrate loads (>2000 kcal/day) to nutritionally bereft, critically ill patients or during the decomposition of bicarbonate infused in the course of treating metabolic acidosis.

The major threat to life from CO_2 retention in patients who are breathing room air is the associated obligatory hypoxemia (in accordance with the alveolar gas equation). When the arterial oxygen tension (Po_2) falls to less than 40 to 50 mm Hg, harmful effects can occur, especially if the fall is rapid. In the absence of supplemental oxygen, patients in respiratory arrest develop critical hypoxemia within a few minutes, long before extreme hypercapnia ensues. Because of the constraints of the alveolar gas equation, it is not possible for Pco_2 to reach values much higher than 80 mm Hg while the level of Po_2 is still compatible with life. Extreme hypercapnia with Pco_2 values exceeding 100 mm Hg is occasionally seen in patients receiving oxygen therapy, and in fact, it is often the result of uncontrolled oxygen administration.

SECONDARY PHYSIOLOGIC RESPONSE

An immediate rise in plasma $[HCO_3^-]$ owing to titration of nonbicarbonate body buffers occurs in response to acute hypercapnia. This adaptation is complete within 5 to 10 minutes after the increase in Pco_2. On average, plasma $[HCO_3^-]$ increases by about 0.1 mEq/L for each 1 mm Hg acute increment in Pco_2; as a result, the plasma hydrogen ion concentration $[H^+]$ increases by about 0.75 nEq/L for each 1 mm Hg acute increment in Pco_2. Therefore the overall limit of adaptation of plasma $[HCO_3^-]$ in acute respiratory acidosis is quite small; even when Pco_2 increases to levels of 80 to 90 mm Hg, the increment in plasma $[HCO_3^-]$ does not exceed 3 to 4 mEq/L. Moderate hypoxemia does not alter the adaptive response to acute respiratory acidosis. On the other hand, preexisting hypobicarbonatemia (from metabolic acidosis or chronic respiratory alkalosis) enhances the magnitude of the bicarbonate response to acute hypercapnia, whereas this response is diminished in hyperbicarbonatemic states (from metabolic alkalosis or chronic respiratory acidosis). Other electrolyte changes observed in acute respiratory acidosis include mild increases in plasma sodium (1 to 4 mEq/L), potassium (0.1 mEq/L for each 0.1 unit decrease in pH), and phosphorus, as well as small decreases in plasma chloride and lactate concentrations (the latter effect originating from inhibition of the activity of 6-phosphofructokinase and, consequently, glycolysis by intracellular acidosis).

A small reduction in the plasma anion gap is also observed, reflecting the decline in plasma lactate and the acidic titration of plasma proteins. Acute respiratory acidosis induces glucose intolerance and insulin resistance that are not prevented by adrenergic blockade. These changes are likely mediated by direct effects of the low tissue pH on skeletal muscle.

The adaptive increase in plasma $[HCO_3^-]$ observed in the acute phase of hypercapnia is amplified markedly during chronic hypercapnia as a result of the generation of new bicarbonate by the kidneys. Both proximal and distal acidification mechanisms contribute to this adaptation, which requires 3 to 5 days for completion. The renal response to chronic hypercapnia includes chloruresis and the generation of hypochloremia. On average, plasma $[HCO_3^-]$ increases by about 0.35 mEq/L for each 1 mm Hg chronic increment in P_{CO_2}; as a result, the plasma $[H^+]$ increases by about 0.3 nEq/L for each 1 mm Hg chronic increase in P_{CO_2}. More recently, a substantially steeper slope for the change in plasma $[HCO_3^-]$ was reported (0.51 mEq/L for each 1 mm Hg chronic increase in P_{CO_2}), but the small number of blood gas measurements, one for each of 18 patients, calls into question the validity of this conclusion. Empiric observations indicate a limit of adaptation of plasma $[HCO_3^-]$ on the order of 45 mEq/L.

The renal response to chronic hypercapnia is not altered appreciably by dietary sodium or chloride restriction, moderate potassium depletion, alkali loading, or moderate hypoxemia. The extent to which chronic kidney disease of variable severity limits the renal response to chronic hypercapnia remains unknown. Obviously patients with end-stage kidney disease cannot mount a renal response to chronic hypercapnia (i.e., generation of new bicarbonate by the kidneys), making them subject to severe acidemia. The degree of acidemia is more pronounced in patients who are receiving hemodialysis rather than peritoneal dialysis because the former treatment maintains, on average, lower plasma $[HCO_3^-]$. Recovery from chronic hypercapnia is crippled by a chloride-deficient diet. In this circumstance, despite correction of the level of P_{CO_2}, plasma $[HCO_3^-]$ remains elevated as long as the state of chloride deprivation persists, thus creating the entity of "posthypercapnic metabolic alkalosis." Chronic hypercapnia is not associated with appreciable changes in the anion gap or in plasma concentrations of sodium, potassium, or phosphorus.

ETIOLOGY

Respiratory acidosis can develop in patients who have normal or abnormal airways and lungs. Tables 15.1 and 15.2 present, respectively, causes of acute and chronic respiratory acidosis. Some conditions can cause both types of the disorder. This classification accounts for the usual mode of onset and duration of the various causes, and it emphasizes the biphasic time course that characterizes the secondary physiologic response to hypercapnia. Primary hypercapnia can result from disease or malfunction within any element of the regulatory system that controls respiration, including the central and peripheral nervous system, respiratory muscles, thoracic cage, pleural space, airways, and lung parenchyma. Not infrequently, more than one cause contributes to the development of respiratory acidosis in a given patient. A vital capacity less than 1 L in patients with myasthenic crisis predicts impending acute respiratory failure with CO_2 retention. Chronic obstructive pulmonary disease (COPD), including emphysema, chronic bronchitis, and small-airway disease, is the most common cause of chronic hypercapnia. Importantly, certain causes of chronic respiratory acidosis (e.g., COPD) can superimpose an element of acute respiratory acidosis during periods of decompensation (e.g., pneumonia, major surgery, heart failure).

CLINICAL MANIFESTATIONS

Because hypercapnia almost always occurs with some degree of hypoxemia, it is often difficult to determine whether a specific manifestation is the consequence of the elevated P_{CO_2} or the reduced P_{O_2}. Clinical manifestations of respiratory acidosis arising from the central nervous system, collectively known as hypercapnic encephalopathy, include irritability, inability to concentrate, headache, anorexia, mental cloudiness, apathy, confusion, incoherence, combativeness, hallucinations, delirium, and transient psychosis. Progressive narcosis or coma might develop in patients receiving oxygen therapy, especially those with an acute exacerbation of chronic respiratory insufficiency, in whom P_{CO_2} levels of 100 mm Hg or even higher can occur. In addition, frank papilledema (pseudotumor cerebri) and motor disturbances, including myoclonic jerks, flapping tremor identical to that observed in liver failure, sustained myoclonus, and seizures may develop. Focal neurologic signs (e.g., muscle paresis, abnormal reflexes) might be observed. The neurologic symptom burden depends on the magnitude of hypercapnia, the rapidity with which it develops, the severity of acidemia, and the degree of accompanying hypoxemia. Severe hypercapnia can be misdiagnosed as a cerebral vascular accident or an intracranial tumor.

The hemodynamic consequences of respiratory acidosis include a direct depressing effect on myocardial contractility. An associated sympathetic surge, sometimes intense, leads to increases in plasma catecholamines; however, during severe acidemia (blood pH lower than approximately 7.20), receptor responsiveness to catecholamines is markedly blunted. Hypercapnia results in systemic vasodilatation via a direct action on vascular smooth muscle; this effect is most obvious in the cerebral circulation, where blood flow increases in direct relation to the level of P_{CO_2}. By contrast, CO_2 retention can produce vasoconstriction in the pulmonary circulation resulting in pulmonary hypertension and right-sided heart failure (cor pulmonale). Similarly, CO_2 retention can lead to vasoconstriction in the renal circulation that may be the result at least in part of an enhanced sympathetic activity.

Table 15.1   Causes of Acute Respiratory Acidosis

Normal Airways and Lungs	Abnormal Airways and Lungs
Central Nervous System Depression	***Upper Airway Obstruction***
General anesthesia	Coma-induced hypopharyngeal obstruction
Sedative overdose (opiates, benzodiazepines, tricyclic antidepressants, barbiturates)	Aspiration of foreign body or vomitus
Head trauma	Laryngospasm
Cerebrovascular accident	Angioedema
Central sleep apnea	Epiglottitis
Cerebral edema	Obstructive sleep apnea
Brain tumor	Inadequate laryngeal intubation
Encephalitis	Laryngeal obstruction post intubation
Hypothyroidism	
Hypothermia	***Lower Airway Obstruction***
Starvation	Generalized bronchospasm
	Acute severe asthma
Neuromuscular Impairment	Bronchiolitis of infancy and adult
Cervical spine injury or disease (trauma, syringomyelia)	Disorders involving pulmonary alveoli
Transverse myelitis (multiple sclerosis)	Severe bilateral pneumonia
Guillain-Barré syndrome	Acute respiratory distress syndrome
Acute intermittent porphyria	Severe pulmonary edema
Tick paralysis	
Status epilepticus	***Pulmonary Perfusion Defect***
Botulism, tetanus	Cardiac arrest[a]
Crisis in myasthenia gravis	Severe circulatory failure[a]
Electrolyte abnormalities (hyperkalemia, hypokalemia, hypophosphatemia, hypercalcemia, hypermagnesemia)	Massive pulmonary thromboembolism
	Fat or air embolus
Eaton-Lambert syndrome	
Hyperthyroidism	
Drugs or toxic agents (e.g., curare, succinylcholine, aminoglycosides, organophosphates, shellfish poisoning, ciguatera poisoning, procainamide myopathy)	
Ventilatory Restriction	
Rib fractures with flail chest	
Pneumothorax	
Hemothorax	
Impaired diaphragmatic function (e.g., peritoneal dialysis, ascites)	
Iatrogenic Events	
Misplacement or displacement of airway cannula during anesthesia or mechanical ventilation	
Bronchoscopy-associated hypoventilation or respiratory arrest	
Increased CO_2 production with constant mechanical ventilation (e.g., due to high-carbohydrate diet or sorbent-regenerative hemodialysis)	

[a]May produce "pseudorespiratory alkalosis."
Modified from Madias NE, Adrogué HJ. Respiratory alkalosis and acidosis. In: Alpern RJ, Moe OW, Kaplan M (eds). *Seldin and Giebisch's The Kidney: Physiology and Pathophysiology*. London: Academic Press; 2013: 2113–2138.

Mild to moderate hypercapnia is usually associated with an increased cardiac output, normal or increased blood pressure, warm skin, a bounding pulse, and diaphoresis. However, if hypercapnia is severe or considerable hypoxemia is present, decreases in both cardiac output and blood pressure may be observed.

Concomitant therapy with vasoactive medications (e.g., β-adrenergic receptor blockers) or the presence of congestive heart failure may further impair the hemodynamic response. Cardiac arrhythmias, particularly supraventricular tachyarrhythmias not associated with major hemodynamic compromise, are common, especially in patients receiving digitalis. They do not result primarily from the hypercapnia but rather reflect the associated hypoxemia and sympathetic discharge, concomitant medication, other electrolyte abnormalities, and

underlying cardiac disease. Cardiac arrhythmias are also observed after initiation of mechanical ventilation and likely result from sudden correction of acidemia. Retention of salt and water is commonly observed in sustained hypercapnia, especially in the presence of cor pulmonale. In addition to the effects of heart failure on the kidney, multiple other factors may be involved, including the prevailing stimulation of the sympathetic nervous system and the renin-angiotensin-aldosterone axis, increased renal vascular resistance, and elevated levels of antidiuretic hormone and cortisol.

DIAGNOSIS

Whenever CO_2 retention is suspected, arterial blood gases should be obtained. Venous blood sampling can be effectively

Table 15.2 Causes of Chronic Respiratory Acidosis

Normal Airways and Lungs	Abnormal Airways and Lungs
Central Nervous System Depression	***Upper Airway Obstruction***
Sedative overdose (narcotics, benzodiazepines, tricyclic antidepressants)	Tonsillar and peritonsillar hypertrophy
Primary alveolar hypoventilation (Ondine's curse)	Retropharyngeal disorders
Obesity-hypoventilation syndrome (Pickwickian syndrome)	Paralysis of vocal cords
Brain tumor	Severe laryngeal or tracheal disorders (stenosis, tumors, angioedema, tracheomalacia)
Brainstem disease	Obstructive goiter
Bulbar poliomyelitis	Airway stenosis after prolonged intubation
Hypothyroidism	Thymoma, aortic aneurysm
Hypothermia	
Starvation	***Lower Airway Obstruction***
	Chronic obstructive lung disease (bronchitis, bronchiolitis, bronchiectasis, emphysema)
Neuromuscular Impairment	
Poliomyelitis	***Disorders Involving Pulmonary Alveoli***
Multiple sclerosis	Severe chronic pneumonitis
Muscular dystrophy	Diffuse infiltrative disease (e.g., alveolar proteinosis)
Amyotrophic lateral sclerosis	End-stage interstitial lung disease
Diaphragmatic paralysis	Severe pulmonary vascular disease
Myxedema	
Myopathic disease	
Hyperthyroidism	
Eaton-Lambert syndrome	
Glycogen storage and mitochondrial diseases	
Ventilatory Restriction	
Kyphoscoliosis, spinal arthritis	
Morbid obesity	
Pectus excavatum	
Thoracoplasty	
Ankylosing spondylitis	
Fibrothorax	
Hydrothorax	
Impaired diaphragmatic function	

Modified from Madias NE, Adrogué HJ. Respiratory alkalosis and acidosis. In: Alpern RJ, Moe OW, Kaplan M (eds). *Seldin and Giebisch's The Kidney: Physiology and Pathophysiology*. London: Academic Press; 2013: 2113–2138.

used to assess acid-base status and obtain information about the oxygenation of the tissues. If the acid-base profile of the patient reveals hypercapnia in association with acidemia, at least an element of respiratory acidosis must be present. However, hypercapnia can be associated with a normal or an alkaline pH because of the simultaneous presence of additional acid-base disorders (see Chapter 12). Information from the patient's history, physical examination, and ancillary laboratory data should be used for an accurate assessment of the acid-base status.

THERAPEUTIC PRINCIPLES

Treatment of acute respiratory acidosis should focus on four critical steps: (1) ensuring a patent airway, (2) restoring adequate oxygenation by delivering an oxygen-rich inspired mixture, (3) securing adequate ventilation to repair the abnormal blood gas composition, and (4) reversing or treating the underlying cause, if possible. Patients with suspected opiate or benzodiazepine overdose should receive antidote treatment (naloxone or flumazenil, respectively). Indications for endotracheal intubation/mechanical ventilation include

protection of the airway, relief of respiratory distress, improvement of pulmonary gas exchange, assistance with airway and lung healing, and application of appropriate sedation and neuromuscular blockade. As noted, acute respiratory acidosis poses its major threat to survival not because of hypercapnia or acidemia but because of the associated hypoxemia. The goal of oxygen therapy is to maintain a Po_2 of at least 60 mm Hg but not higher than 100 mm Hg and peripheral oxygen saturation of $\geq 90\%$; yet a Po_2 of 50 to 55 mm Hg might help prevent respiratory depression in patients with hypercapnia and chronic hypoxemia. Supplemental oxygen can be administered to spontaneously breathing patients via nasal cannulas, Venturi masks, or non-rebreathing masks. Oxygen flow rates ≤ 5 L/min can be used with nasal cannulas, each increment of 1 L/min increasing the Fio_2 by approximately 4%. Venturi masks, calibrated to deliver Fio_2 between 24% and 50%, are most useful in patients with COPD, as they allow the Po_2 to be titrated, thus minimizing the risk of CO_2 retention. Respiratory depression resulting from oxygen administration may be prevented by maintaining a peripheral saturation between 90% and 93%. Patients expected to require low levels of supplemental oxygen may be started at 1 to 2 L/min via nasal cannula or 24% to 28% Fio_2 via Venturi mask with gradual increases of 1 L/min or 4% to 7% Fio_2.

If the target Po_2 is not achieved with these measures and the patient is conscious, cooperative, hemodynamically stable, and able to protect the lower airway, a method of noninvasive ventilation through a mask can be used (e.g., bilevel positive airway pressure [BiPAP]). With BiPAP, the inspiratory-pressure support decreases the patient's work of breathing, and the expiratory-pressure support improves gas exchange by preventing alveolar collapse.

Endotracheal intubation with mechanical ventilatory support should be initiated if adequate oxygenation cannot be secured by noninvasive measures, if progressive hypercapnia or obtundation develops, or if the patient is unable to cough and clear secretions. Large tidal volumes during mechanical ventilation often lead to alveolar overdistention, which results in hypotension and barotrauma, two life-threatening complications. To overcome these complications, prescription of tidal volumes of 6 mL/kg body weight (instead of the conventional level of 12 mL/kg body weight), to achieve plateau airway pressures of <30 cm H_2O, has been proposed. Because an increase in Pco_2 develops (but rarely exceeds 80 mm Hg), this approach is termed *permissive hypercapnia* or *controlled mechanical hypoventilation*. If the resultant hypercapnia reduces the blood pH to less than 7.20, many physicians would prescribe bicarbonate; however, this strategy is controversial, and others would intervene only for pH values on the order of 7.00. Several studies indicate that permissive hypercapnia affords improved clinical outcomes. Heavy sedation and neuromuscular blockade are frequently needed with this therapy. After discontinuation of neuromuscular blockade, some patients develop prolonged weakness or paralysis. Contraindications to permissive hypercapnia include cerebrovascular disease, brain edema, increased intracranial pressure, and convulsions; depressed cardiac function and arrhythmias; and severe pulmonary hypertension. Notably, most of these entities can develop as adverse effects of permissive hypercapnia itself, especially in the presence of substantial acidemia.

Cardiopulmonary bypass represents a form of mechanical cardiopulmonary support that is often applied intraoperatively to facilitate cardiac surgery. A more prolonged type of extracorporeal life support, known as extracorporeal membrane oxygenation (ECMO), can be used in the intensive care unit in neonates, children, and adults. Application of ECMO involves either a venoarterial (VA) or venovenous (VV) vascular access. Both types provide respiratory support, but only VA ECMO provides hemodynamic support.

The presence of a concurrent *metabolic* acidosis is the primary indication for alkali therapy in patients with acute respiratory acidosis. Administration of sodium bicarbonate to the spontaneously breathing patient with simple respiratory acidosis is not only of questionable efficacy but also involves considerable risk. Concerns include pH-mediated depression of ventilation, enhanced CO_2 production because of bicarbonate decomposition, and volume expansion; however, alkali therapy may have a role in patients with severe bronchospasm by restoring the responsiveness of the bronchial musculature to β-adrenergic agonists. Successful management of intractable asthma in patients with blood pH lower than 7.00 by administering sufficient sodium bicarbonate to raise blood pH to greater than 7.20 has been reported.

Patients with chronic respiratory acidosis frequently develop episodes of acute decompensation that can be serious or life threatening. Common culprits include pulmonary infections, use of narcotics, and uncontrolled oxygen therapy. In contrast to acute hypercapnia, injudicious use of oxygen therapy in patients with chronic respiratory acidosis can produce further reductions in alveolar ventilation. Respiratory decompensation superimposes an acute element of CO_2 retention and acidemia on the chronic baseline. Only rarely can one remove the underlying cause of chronic respiratory acidosis, but maximizing alveolar ventilation with relatively simple maneuvers is often successful in the management of respiratory decompensation. Such maneuvers include treatment with antibiotics, bronchodilators, or diuretics; avoidance of irritant inhalants, tranquilizers, and sedatives; elimination of retained secretions; and gradual reduction of supplemental oxygen, targeting a Po_2 of about 50 to 55 mm Hg. Administration of adequate quantities of chloride (usually as the potassium salt) prevents or corrects a complicating element of metabolic alkalosis (commonly diuretic-induced) that can further dampen the ventilatory drive. Acetazolamide may be used as an adjunctive measure, but care must be taken to avoid potassium depletion. Potassium and phosphate depletion should be corrected, as they can contribute to the development or maintenance of respiratory failure by impairing the function of skeletal muscles. Restoration of the Pco_2 of the patient to near its chronic baseline should proceed gradually, over a period of many hours to a few days. Overly rapid reduction in Pco_2 in such patients risks the development of sudden, posthypercapnic alkalemia with potentially serious consequences, including reduction in cardiac output and cerebral blood flow, cardiac arrhythmias (including predisposition to digitalis intoxication), and generalized seizures. In the absence of a complicating element of metabolic acidosis, and with the possible exception of the severely acidemic patient with intense generalized bronchoconstriction who is undergoing mechanical ventilation, there is no role for alkali administration in chronic respiratory acidosis.

RESPIRATORY ALKALOSIS

Respiratory alkalosis, or primary hypocapnia, is the acid-base disturbance initiated by a reduction in carbon dioxide tension of body fluids and in whole-body CO_2 stores. Hypocapnia alkalinizes body fluids and elicits an adaptive decrement in plasma [HCO_3^-] that should be viewed as an integral part of the respiratory alkalosis. The level of Pco_2 measured at rest and at sea level is lower than 35 mm Hg in simple respiratory alkalosis. Higher values of Pco_2 may still indicate the presence of an element of primary hypocapnia in the setting of mixed acid-base disorders (e.g., eucapnia, rather than the anticipated hypercapnia, in the presence of metabolic alkalosis).

PATHOPHYSIOLOGY

Primary hypocapnia most commonly reflects pulmonary hyperventilation caused by increased ventilatory drive. The latter results from signals arising from the lung, from the peripheral (carotid and aortic) or brainstem chemoreceptors, or from influences originating in other centers of the brain. Hypoxemia is a major stimulus of alveolar ventilation, but Po_2 values lower than 60 mm Hg are required to elicit this effect consistently. Additional mechanisms for the generation of primary hypocapnia include maladjusted mechanical ventilators, extrapulmonary elimination of CO_2 by a dialysis device or ECMO, and decreased CO_2 production (e.g., sedation, skeletal muscle paralysis, hypothermia, hypothyroidism) in patients receiving constant mechanical ventilation.

A condition termed *pseudorespiratory alkalosis* occurs in patients who have profound depression of cardiac function and pulmonary perfusion but have relative preservation of alveolar ventilation, including patients with advanced circulatory failure and those undergoing cardiopulmonary resuscitation. In such patients, venous (and tissue) hypercapnia is present because of the severely reduced pulmonary blood flow that limits the amount of CO_2 delivered to the lungs for excretion. On the other hand, arterial blood reveals hypocapnia because of the increased ventilation-to-perfusion ratio ($\dot{V}_A/\dot{Q}$), which causes a larger than normal removal of CO_2 per unit of blood traversing the pulmonary circulation. However, absolute CO_2 excretion is decreased, and the body CO_2 balance is positive. Therefore respiratory acidosis, rather than respiratory alkalosis, is present. Such patients may have severe venous acidemia (often resulting from mixed respiratory and metabolic acidosis) accompanied by an arterial pH that ranges from mild acidemia to frank alkalemia. In addition, arterial blood may show normoxemia or hyperoxemia, despite the presence of severe hypoxemia in venous blood. Therefore both arterial and mixed (or central) venous blood sampling is needed to assess the acid-base status and oxygenation of patients with critical hemodynamic compromise.

SECONDARY PHYSIOLOGIC RESPONSE

Adaptation to acute hypocapnia is characterized by an immediate drop in plasma $[HCO_3^-]$, principally as a result of titration of nonbicarbonate body buffers. This adaptation is completed within 5 to 10 minutes after the onset of hypocapnia. Plasma $[HCO_3^-]$ declines, on average, by approximately 0.2 mEq/L for each 1 mm Hg acute decrement in Pco_2; consequently the plasma $[H^+]$ decreases by about 0.75 nEq/L for each 1 mm Hg acute reduction in Pco_2. The limit of this adaptation of plasma $[HCO_3^-]$ is on the order of 17 to 18 mEq/L. Concomitant small increases in plasma chloride, lactate, and other unmeasured anions balance the decline in plasma $[HCO_3^-]$; each of these components accounts for about one-third of the bicarbonate decrement. Small decreases in plasma sodium (1 to 3 mEq/L) and potassium (0.2 mEq/L for each 0.1 unit increase in pH) may be observed. Severe hypophosphatemia can occur in acute hypocapnia because of the translocation of phosphorus into the cells.

A larger decrement in plasma $[HCO_3^-]$ occurs in chronic hypocapnia as a result of renal adaptation to the disorder, which involves suppression of both proximal and distal acidification mechanisms. Completion of this adaptation requires 2 to 3 days. Plasma $[HCO_3^-]$ decreases, on average, by about 0.4 mEq/L for each 1 mm Hg chronic decrement in Pco_2; as a consequence, plasma $[H^+]$ decreases by approximately 0.4 nEq/L for each 1 mm Hg chronic reduction in Pco_2. The

limit of this adaptation of plasma $[HCO_3^-]$ is on the order of 12 to 15 mEq/L. About two-thirds of the decline in plasma $[HCO_3^-]$ is balanced by an increase in plasma chloride concentration, and the remainder reflects an increase in plasma unmeasured anions; part of the remainder results from the alkaline titration of plasma proteins, but most remains undefined. Plasma lactate does not increase in chronic hypocapnia, even in the presence of moderate hypoxemia. Similarly, no appreciable change in the plasma concentration of sodium occurs. In sharp contrast with acute hypocapnia, the plasma concentration of phosphorus remains essentially unchanged in chronic hypocapnia. Although plasma potassium is in the normal range in patients with chronic hypocapnia at sea level, hypokalemia and renal potassium wasting have been described in subjects in whom sustained hypocapnia was induced by exposure to high altitude. Patients with end-stage kidney disease maintained on chronic replacement therapy are obviously at risk for development of severe alkalemia in response to chronic hypocapnia, because the damaged kidneys cannot generate a secondary decrease in plasma $[HCO_3^-]$. For example, this situation arises when such a patient develops marked hyperventilation because of severe pneumonia. This risk is somewhat higher in patients undergoing peritoneal dialysis rather than hemodialysis because the former treatment maintains, on average, higher plasma $[HCO_3^-]$.

ETIOLOGY

Primary hypocapnia is the most frequent acid-base disturbance encountered; it occurs in normal pregnancy and with high-altitude residence. Table 15.3 lists the major causes of respiratory alkalosis. Most are associated with the abrupt appearance of hypocapnia, but in many instances the process is sufficiently prolonged to permit full chronic adaptation. Consequently, no attempt has been made to separate these conditions into acute and chronic categories. Some of the major causes of respiratory alkalosis are benign, whereas others are life threatening. The hyperventilation syndrome refers to a condition characterized by episodes of acute hyperventilation associated with fear, anxiety, and sense of impending doom in the absence of significant cardiopulmonary disease. Primary hypocapnia is particularly common among the critically ill, occurring either as the simple disorder or as a component of mixed disturbances. Its presence constitutes an ominous prognostic sign, with mortality increasing in direct proportion to the severity of the hypocapnia.

CLINICAL MANIFESTATIONS

Rapid decrements in Pco_2 to half the normal values or lower are typically accompanied by paresthesias of the extremities, chest discomfort (especially in patients manifesting increased airway resistance), circumoral numbness, lightheadedness, confusion, and, rarely, tetany or generalized seizures. These manifestations are common in patients with the hyperventilation syndrome. These patients also report dyspnea at rest; they need to sigh frequently, and minimal exertion may result in significant dyspnea. These manifestations are seldom present in the chronic phase. Episodes of acute hyperventilation may occasionally lead to posthyperventilation apnea caused by the depletion of CO_2 stores; the resulting hypoxemia can have serious consequences.

Table 15.3 Causes of Respiratory Alkalosis

Hypoxemia or Tissue Hypoxia	Subarachnoid hemorrhage
Decreased inspired O$_2$ tension	Cerebrovascular accident
High altitude	Meningoencephalitis
Bacterial or viral pneumonia	Tumor
Aspiration of food, foreign body, or vomitus	Trauma
Laryngospasm, Angioedema	***Drugs or Hormones***
Drowning	Nikethamide, ethamivan
Cyanotic heart disease	Doxapram
Severe anemia	Xanthines
Left shift deviation of the HbO$_2$ curve	Salicylates
Hypotension[a]	Catecholamines
Severe circulatory failure[a]	Angiotensin II
Pulmonary edema	Vasopressor agents
	Progesterone
Stimulation of Chest Receptors	Medroxyprogesterone
	Dinitrophenol
Pneumonia	Nicotine
Acute asthma	
Pneumothorax	***Miscellaneous***
Hemothorax	Exercise
Flail chest	Pregnancy
Acute respiratory distress syndrome	Hyperthyroidism
	Sepsis
Cardiac failure	Chronic liver disease
Noncardiogenic pulmonary edema	Mechanical hyperventilation
	Heat exposure
Pulmonary embolism	Heart-lung machine
Interstitial lung disease	ECMO
	Heat exposure
Central Nervous System Stimulation	Recovery from metabolic acidosis
Voluntary	
Pain	
Anxiety, Hyperventilation syndrome	
Psychosis	
Fever	

[a]May produce "pseudorespiratory alkalosis."
ECMO, Extracorporeal membrane oxygenation; *HbO$_2$*, oxyhemoglobin.
Modified from Madias NE, Adrogué HJ. Respiratory alkalosis and acidosis. In: Alpern RJ, Moe OW, Kaplan M (eds). *Seldin and Giebisch's The Kidney: Physiology and Pathophysiology*. London: Academic Press; 2013: 2113–2138.

Acute hypocapnia decreases cerebral blood flow, which in severe cases may reach values less than 50% of normal, resulting in cerebral hypoxia. This hypoperfusion has been implicated in the pathogenesis of the neurologic manifestations of acute respiratory alkalosis along with other factors, including hypocapnia per se, alkalemia, pH-induced shift of the oxyhemoglobin dissociation curve, and decrements in the levels of ionized calcium and potassium. Some evidence indicates that cerebral blood flow returns to normal in chronic respiratory alkalosis.

Patients who are actively hyperventilating manifest no appreciable changes in cardiac output or systemic blood pressure. By contrast, acute hypocapnia in the course of passive hyperventilation, as typically observed during mechanical ventilation in patients with a depressed central nervous system or receiving general anesthesia, frequently results in a major reduction in cardiac output and systemic blood pressure, increased peripheral vascular resistance, and substantial hyperlactatemia. This discrepant response probably reflects the decline in venous return caused by mechanical ventilation in passive hyperventilation. Although acute hypocapnia does not lead to cardiac arrhythmias in normal volunteers, it appears that it contributes to the generation of both atrial and ventricular tachyarrhythmias in patients with ischemic heart disease. Chest pain and ischemic ST-T wave changes have been observed in acutely hyperventilating subjects with or without coronary artery disease. Coronary vasospasm and Prinzmetal angina can be precipitated by acute hypocapnia in susceptible subjects. The pathogenesis of these manifestations has been attributed to the same factors that are incriminated in the neurologic manifestations of acute hypocapnia.

DIAGNOSIS

Careful observation can detect abnormal patterns of breathing in some patients, yet marked hypocapnia may be present without a clinically evident increase in respiratory effort. Therefore an arterial blood gas analysis should be obtained whenever hyperventilation is suspected. In fact, the diagnosis of respiratory alkalosis, especially the chronic form, is frequently missed; physicians often misinterpret the electrolyte pattern of hyperchloremic hypobicarbonatemia as indicative of a normal anion gap metabolic acidosis. If the acid-base profile of the patient reveals hypocapnia in association with alkalemia, at least an element of respiratory alkalosis must be present. Primary hypocapnia, however, may be associated with a normal or an acidic pH as a result of the concomitant presence of other acid-base disorders. Notably, mild degrees of chronic hypocapnia commonly leave blood pH within the high-normal range. As always, proper evaluation of the acid-base status of the patient requires careful assessment of the history, physical examination, and ancillary laboratory data (see Chapter 12). After the diagnosis of respiratory alkalosis has been made, a search for its cause should ensue. The diagnosis of respiratory alkalosis can have important clinical implications, often providing a clue to the presence of an unrecognized, serious disorder (e.g., sepsis) or indicating the severity of a known underlying disease.

THERAPEUTIC PRINCIPLES

Management of respiratory alkalosis must be directed whenever possible toward correction of the underlying cause. Respiratory alkalosis resulting from severe hypoxemia requires oxygen therapy. The widely held view that hypocapnia, even if severe, poses little risk to health is inaccurate. In fact, transient or permanent damage to the brain, heart, and lungs can result from substantial hypocapnia. In addition, rapid correction of severe hypocapnia can lead to reperfusion injury in the brain and lung. Therefore severe hypocapnia in hospitalized patients must be prevented whenever possible, and if it is present, a slow correction is most appropriate.

The long-term management of the hyperventilation syndrome centers on education regarding the nature of the underlying condition and cognitive-behavioral therapy. Other measures may include breathing retraining, β-blockers, benzodiazepines, and serotonin reuptake inhibitors. Rebreathing into a closed system (e.g., a paper bag) is not recommended, because of the potential of hypoxemia in patients with underlying respiratory or cardiovascular disease. Administration of 250 to 500 mg acetazolamide can be beneficial in the management of signs and symptoms of high-altitude sickness, a syndrome characterized by hypoxemia and respiratory alkalosis. Considering the risks of severe alkalemia, sedation or, in rare cases, skeletal muscle paralysis and mechanical ventilation may be required temporarily to correct marked respiratory alkalosis. Patients maintained on chronic hemodialysis who develop an acute illness resulting in marked hyperventilation may require dialysis against a low-bicarbonate bath. Management of pseudorespiratory alkalosis must be directed at optimizing systemic hemodynamics.

KEY BIBLIOGRAPHY

Adrogué HJ, Chap Z, Okuda Y, et al. Acidosis-induced glucose intolerance is not prevented by adrenergic blockade. *Am J Physiol.* 1988;255: E812-E823.

Adrogué HJ, Madias NE. Management of life-threatening acid-base disorders. *N Engl J Med.* 1998;338:26-34, 107-111.

Adrogué HJ, Madias NE. Respiratory acidosis. In: Gennari FJ, Adrogué HJ, Galla JH, Madias NE, eds. *Acid-Base Disorders and Their Treatment.* Boca Raton: Taylor & Francis Group; 2005:597-639.

Adrogué HJ, Madias NE. Secondary responses to altered acid-base status: the rules of engagement. *J Am Soc Nephrol.* 2010;21:920-923.

Adrogué HJ, Rashad MN, Gorin AB, et al. Assessing acid-base status in circulatory failure. Differences between arterial and central venous blood. *N Engl J Med.* 1989;320:1312-1316.

Arbus GS, Hebert LA, Levesque PR, et al. Characterization and clinical application of the "significance band" for acute respiratory alkalosis. *N Engl J Med.* 1969;280:117-123.

Boulding R, Stacey R, Niven R, Fowler SJ. Dysfunctional breathing: a review of the literature and proposal for classification. *Eur Respir Rev.* 2016;25:287-294.

Brackett NC Jr, Cohen JJ, Schwartz WB. Carbon dioxide titration curve of normal man: Effect of increasing degrees of acute hypercapnia on acid-base equilibrium. *N Engl J Med.* 1965;272:6-12.

Brackett NC Jr, Wingo CF, Muren O, Solano JT. Acid-base response to chronic hypercapnia in man. *N Engl J Med.* 1969;280:124-130.

Davidson AC, Banham S, Elliott M, et al. BTS/ICS guidelines for the ventilator management of acute hypercapnic respiratory failure in adults. *Thorax.* 2016;71:1-35.

Girardis M, Busani S, Damiani E, et al. Effect of conservative vs conventional oxygen therapy on mortality among patients in an intensive care unit. The oxygen-ICU randomized clinical trial. *JAMA.* 2016;316: 1583-1589.

Global Strategy for the Diagnosis, Management and Prevention of COPD, Global Initiative for Chronic Obstructive Lung Disease (GOLD); 2016. http://www.goldcopd.org/; Accessed 30 November 2016.

Grocott MPW, Martin DS, Levett DZH, et al. Arterial blood gases and oxygen content in climbers on Mount Everest. *N Engl J Med.* 2009;360: 140-149.

Kollef M. Respiratory failure. In: Dale DC, Federman DD, eds. *ACP Medicine.* New York: WebMD; 2006:2791-2804.

Krapf R, Beeler I, Hertner D, Hulter HN. Chronic respiratory alkalosis: The effect of sustained hyperventilation on renal regulation of acid-base equilibrium. *N Engl J Med.* 1991;324:1394-1401.

Madias NE, Adrogué HJ. Respiratory alkalosis and acidosis. In: Alpern RJ, Moe OW, Kaplan M, eds. *Seldin and Giebisch's The Kidney: Physiology and Pathophysiology.* 5th ed. London: Academic Press; 2013: 2113-2138.

Madias NE, Wolf CJ, Cohen JJ. Regulation of acid-base equilibrium in chronic hypercapnia. *Kidney Int.* 1985;27:538-543.

Malhotra A. Low-tidal-volume ventilation in the acute respiratory distress syndrome. *N Engl J Med.* 2007;357:1113-1120.

Martinu T, Menzies D, Dial S. Re-evaluation of acid-base prediction rules in patients with chronic respiratory acidosis. *Can Respir J.* 2003;10:311-315.

Palmer BF. Evaluation and treatment of respiratory alkalosis. *Am J Kidney Dis.* 2012;60:834-838.

Full bibliography can be found on www.expertconsult.com.

GLOMERULAR DISEASES

16 Glomerular Clinicopathologic Syndromes

J. Charles Jennette; Ronald J. Falk

Glomerular injury results in multiple signs and symptoms, including proteinuria caused by altered permeability of capillary walls, hematuria caused by rupture of capillary walls, azotemia caused by impaired filtration of nitrogenous wastes, oliguria or anuria caused by reduced urine production, edema caused by salt and water retention, and hypertension caused by fluid retention and other factors. The nature and severity of disease in a given patient are dictated by the nature and severity of glomerular injury.

Glomerular syndromes include asymptomatic hematuria or proteinuria, nephrotic syndrome, nephritic (glomerulonephritic) syndrome, rapidly progressive glomerulonephritis, and syndromes with concurrent glomerular and extrarenal features, such as pulmonary-renal syndrome and dermal-renal syndrome. Specific glomerular diseases tend to produce characteristic syndromes of kidney dysfunction (Table 16.1). The diagnosis of a glomerular disease requires recognition of one of these syndromes followed by collection of data to determine which specific glomerular disease is present. Alternatively, if reaching a specific diagnosis is not possible or not necessary, the physician should at least narrow the differential diagnosis to a likely candidate glomerular disease.

Evaluation for pathogenic processes, often by serology, as well as identification of patterns of injury in a kidney biopsy specimen, is required for a definitive diagnosis. Table 16.2 illustrates parameters that are used to categorize glomerulonephritis. Fig. 16.1 shows the relative frequencies that major categories of glomerular disease are identified in kidney biopsy specimens. These frequencies are different from the overall prevalence of these diseases in patients with these syndromes, because some categories of disease have presentations that are more likely to prompt biopsy (e.g., rapidly progressive glomerulonephritis) than other diseases (e.g., steroid-responsive childhood nephrotic syndrome). Fig. 16.2 depicts some of the clinical and pathologic features used to resolve the differential diagnosis in patients with antibody-mediated glomerulonephritis, Figs. 16.3 through 16.6 illustrate the distinctive ultrastructural features of some of the major categories of glomerular disease, Fig. 16.7 illustrates some of the major patterns of immune deposition identified by immunofluorescence microscopy, and Fig. 16.8 illustrates common patterns of injury of focal segmental glomerulosclerosis (FSGS).

HEMATURIA

Hematuria is usually defined as greater than three red blood cells per high-power field observed by microscopic examination in a centrifuged urine sediment (see Chapters 4 and 5). Asymptomatic hematuria is defined as hematuria in the absence of clinical manifestations, such as nephritis or nephrotic syndrome. Most hematuria is not of glomerular origin, and glomerular diseases are associated with fewer than 10% of cases of hematuria in patients who do not have proteinuria; almost 80% of cases of hematuria are caused by bladder, prostate, or urethral disease. Hypercalciuria and hyperuricosuria also can cause asymptomatic hematuria, especially in children.

Microscopic examination of the urine can help determine whether hematuria is of glomerular or nonglomerular origin. Chemical (e.g., osmotic) and physical damage to red blood cells as they pass through the nephron causes structural changes that are not present in red blood cells that have passed directly into the urine from a gross parenchymal injury in the kidney (e.g., a neoplasm or infection) or from a lesion in the urinary tract. Dysmorphic red blood cells have transited the urinary tract from the glomeruli; these cells usually have lost their biconcave configuration and hemoglobin, resulting in cells with multiple membrane blebs and sometimes producing acanthocytes and "Mickey Mouse" cells with surface projections resembling mouse ears. The presence of red blood cell casts and substantial proteinuria further supports a glomerular origin for hematuria.

Published kidney biopsy series conducted in patients with asymptomatic hematuria show differences in the frequencies of identified underlying glomerular lesions. Differences in the nature of the population analyzed (e.g., military recruits vs. patients undergoing routine physical examination) and differences in pathologic analysis (e.g., failure of earlier studies to recognize thin basement membrane nephropathy) account for many of the observed disparities. The data presented in Table 16.3 are derived from patients with hematuria who underwent diagnostic kidney biopsy. The data in the first column equate with asymptomatic hematuria and are similar to findings in other published series. In patients with hematuria, less than 1 g per day of proteinuria, and serum creatinine less than 1.5 mg/dL, the three major biopsy findings were no pathologic abnormality (30%), thin basement membrane nephropathy (26%), and immunoglobulin A (IgA) nephropathy (28%). While thin basement membrane nephropathy virtually always manifests as asymptomatic hematuria or recurrent gross hematuria, IgA nephropathy can manifest as any of the glomerular disease syndromes, because it can cause a variety of glomerular lesions that result in different clinical manifestations (Fig. 16.9).

Alport syndrome is a hereditary disease caused by a defect in the genes that code for basement membrane type IV

Table 16.1 Tendencies of Glomerular Diseases to Manifest Nephrotic and Nephritic Features

Disease	Nephrotic Features	Nephritic Features
Minimal change disease	++++	—
Membranous nephropathy	++++	+
Diabetic glomerulosclerosis	++++	+
Amyloidosis	++++	+
FSGS	+++	++
Fibrillary glomerulonephritis	+++	++
Mesangioproliferative glomerulopathy[a]	++	++
Membranoproliferative glomerulonephritis[b]	++	+++
Proliferative glomerulonephritis[a]	++	+++
Acute postinfectious glomerulonephritis[c]	+	++++
Crescentic glomerulonephritis[d]	+	++++

Most diseases can manifest both nephrotic and nephritic features, but there is usually a tendency for one to predominate. Number of plus signs indicates strength of tendency.

[a]Mesangioproliferative and proliferative glomerulonephritis (focal or diffuse) are structural manifestations (patterns of injury) caused by a number of glomerulonephritides, such as immunoglobulin A nephropathy, C3 glomerulopathy, and lupus nephritis.

[b]Membranoproliferative glomerulonephritis is a pattern of injury with multiple causes, such as immune complex disease (infectious, autoimmune, and monoclonal) and C3 glomerulopathy.

[c]Often a structural manifestation of acute poststreptococcal glomerulonephritis.

[d]Can be immune complex glomerulonephritis (GN), C3 glomerulopathy, antiglomerular basement membrane antibody GN, or associated with antineutrophil cytoplasmic antibodies (ANCA GN). *FSGS*, Focal segmental glomerulosclerosis; *MPGN*, membranoproliferative glomerulonephritis.

collagen (see Chapter 42). In affected men, Alport syndrome initially manifests as asymptomatic microscopic hematuria, sometimes with superimposed episodes of gross hematuria. Although similar within a given kindred, the onset of symptoms varies from childhood to adulthood and typically begins with asymptomatic hematuria. Progressively worsening proteinuria and, eventually, kidney failure may develop, although the rate of progression is variable. Affected women, who are almost always heterozygous, often have intermittent microscopic hematuria but may have no other manifestations of kidney disease.

Kidney biopsy may not be performed to evaluate asymptomatic glomerular hematuria, as the diagnosis may not affect treatment; however, kidney biopsy may provide helpful information and help avoid other unnecessary diagnostic procedures. Many patients with asymptomatic hematuria are subjected to repeated invasive urologic evaluations until a definitive diagnosis can be determined. In these patients, additional urologic evaluation can be avoided if kidney biopsy provides a diagnosis. For example, the presence of mesangial immune deposits with a dominance or codominance of immunohistologic staining for IgA1 is diagnostic for IgA nephropathy (see Fig. 16.7).

Kidney biopsy in a patient with asymptomatic hematuria may reveal unexpected Alport syndrome, which could be helpful for prognostication and family counseling. Females with heterozygous X-linked disease may present with asymptomatic hematuria. Biopsy reveals thin basement membrane lesions as the electron microscopic manifestation of Alport syndrome, whereas men usually have lamina densa laminations. In Alport syndrome, the kidney and skin also have diagnostically useful abnormalities in immunohistologic staining for the alpha chains of type IV collagen.

Table 16.2 Nomenclature of Glomerulonephritis, Composed of Pathogenic Type, Specific Disease Category, and Pathologic Pattern of Injury

Glomerulonephritis Pathogenic Type	Specific Disease Entity Examples	Pattern of Injury: Focal or Diffuse
Immune-complex glomerulonephritis	IgA nephropathy, IgA vasculitis, lupus nephritis, infection-related GN, fibrillary GN with polyclonal Ig deposits	Mesangial, endocapillary, exudative, membranoproliferative, necrotizing, crescentic, sclerosing, or multiple
Pauci-immune glomerulonephritis	MPO-ANCA GN, PR3-ANCA GN, ANCA-negative GN	Necrotizing, crescentic, sclerosing, or mixed
Anti-GBM glomerulonephritis	Anti-GBM GN	Necrotizing, crescentic, sclerosing, or mixed
Monoclonal immunoglobulin (Ig) glomerulonephritis	Monoclonal Ig deposition disease, proliferative GN with monoclonal Ig deposits, immunotactoid glomerulopathy, fibrillary GN with monoclonal Ig deposits	Mesangial, endocapillary, exudative, membranoproliferative, necrotizing, crescentic, sclerosing, or multiple
C3 glomerulopathy	C3 GN, dense deposit disease	Mesangial, endocapillary, exudative, membranoproliferative, necrotizing, crescentic, sclerosing, or multiple

The diagnosis of a glomerular disease should include the pathogenic type or specific disease designation paired with the pattern of injury observed (e.g., anti-GBM glomerulonephritis with diffuse necrotizing and crescentic glomerulonephritis).
ANCA, Antineutrophil cytoplasmic antibody; *GBM*, glomerular basement membrane; *GN*, glomerulonephritis; *IgA*, immunoglobulin A; *MPO*, myeloperoxidase; *PR3*, proteinase 3.
Modified from Sethi S, Haas M, Markowitz GS, et al. Mayo Clinic/Renal Pathology Society Consensus report on pathologic classification, diagnosis, and reporting of GN. *J Am Soc Nephrol*. 2016;27:1278–1287, with permission.

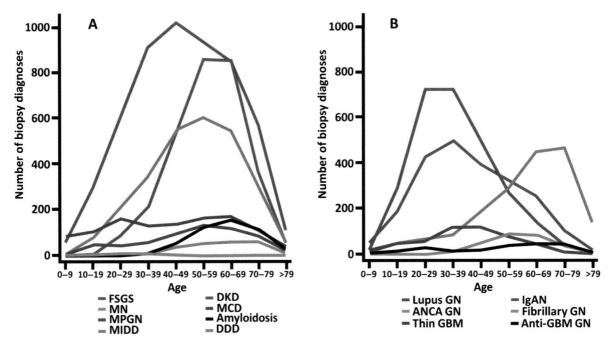

Fig. 16.1 Frequencies of kidney biopsy diagnoses versus age from 1986 to 2015 in the University of North Carolina (UNC) Nephropathology Laboratory. The diagnoses are separated into those that usually cause a glomerulonephritic presentation and those that usually cause the nephrotic syndrome. Approximately one-third of the patients in this kidney biopsy population from UNC were blacks, which influences the high frequency of lupus glomerulonephritis and FSGS. (A) Causes of glomerulonephritis. (B) Causes of nephrotic syndrome. *ANCA,* Antineutrophil cytoplasmic antibody; *DDD,* dense deposit disease; *DKD,* diabetic kidney disease; *FSGS,* focal segmental glomerulosclerosis; *GBM,* glomerular basement membrane; *GN,* glomerulonephritis; *IgA,* immunoglobulin A; *MN,* membranous nephropathy; *MIDD,* monoclonal Immunoglobulin deposition disease; *MCD,* minimal change disease; *MPGN,* membranoproliferative glomerulonephritis; *Lupus,* systemic lupus erythematosus. (From O'Shaughnessy MM, Hogan SL, Poulton CJ, et al. Temporal and demographic trends in glomerular disease epidemiology in the Southeastern United States, 1986–2015. *Clin J Am Soc Nephrol.* 2017;12:614–623.)

ACUTE GLOMERULONEPHRITIS AND RAPIDLY PROGRESSIVE GLOMERULONEPHRITIS

Patients with acute glomerulonephritis or rapidly progressive glomerulonephritis often present with acute onset of nephritis with azotemia, oliguria, edema, hypertension, proteinuria, and hematuria along with an "active" urine sediment that often contains red blood cell casts, pigmented casts, and cellular debris. Rapidly progressive glomerulonephritis is defined clinically by a 50% or greater loss of kidney function within weeks to months and may present with kidney failure.

The pathologic processes that most often associate with acute or rapidly progressive glomerulonephritis are inflammatory glomerular lesions. Lupus glomerulonephritis and IgA nephropathy are the most common causes in children and young adults, whereas antineutrophil cytoplasmic antibody (ANCA) glomerulonephritis is the most common cause in older adults (see Table 16.4 and Fig. 16.1). The nature and severity of glomerular inflammation correlate with the clinical features of the glomerulonephritis (see Fig. 16.9). Note in Fig. 16.9 that the pattern of injury caused by glomerular inflammation can change as time passes; this is

reflected by changes in the clinical manifestations of the glomerulonephritis.

The least severe pattern of injury that can be discerned by light microscopy is mesangial hyperplasia alone, which usually is associated with asymptomatic proteinuria or hematuria, or very mild nephritis. Proliferative glomerulonephritis, which may be focal (affecting less than 50% of glomeruli) or diffuse (affecting more than 50% of glomeruli), is characterized histologically not only by the proliferation of glomerular cells (e.g., mesangial cells, endothelial cells, epithelial cells) but also by the influx of leukocytes, especially neutrophils, monocytes, and macrophages. Necrosis may be present, especially in disease caused by ANCAs or antiglomerular basement membrane (anti-GBM) antibodies. Chronic changes such as glomerular sclerosis, interstitial fibrosis, and tubular atrophy begin to develop within 1 week after the onset of destructive glomerular inflammation and become the dominant features in chronic glomerulonephritis.

Lupus glomerulonephritis (see Chapter 25) provides a model of the interrelationships among pathogenic mechanisms, pathologic patterns of injury, and clinical manifestations of immune complex glomerular disease (see Fig. 16.5). The mildest expressions of lupus nephritis (International Society of Nephrology/Renal Pathology Society [ISN/RPS] class I

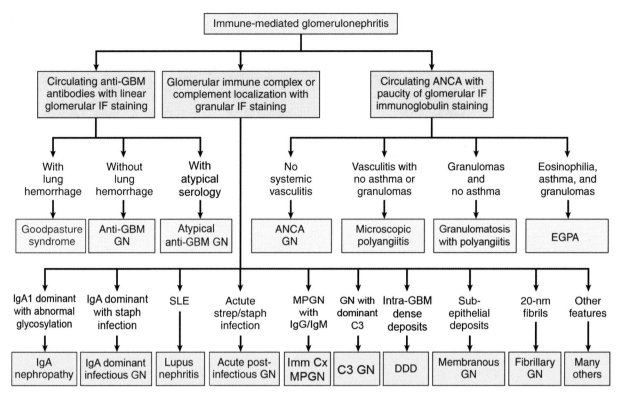

Fig. 16.2 Features that distinguish among different immunopathologic categories of immune-mediated glomerulonephritis. *ANCA,* Antineutrophil cytoplasmic antibody; *DDD,* dense deposit disease (which is a C3 glomerulopathy and not an immune complex disease); *EGPA,* eosinophilic granulomatosis with polyangiitis; *GBM,* glomerular basement membrane; *GN,* glomerulonephritis; *IF,* immunofluorescence microscopy; *IgA,* immunoglobulin A; *Imm Cx,* immune complex; *MPGN,* membranoproliferative glomerulonephritis; *SLE,* systemic lupus erythematosus.

minimal mesangial and class II mesangioproliferative lupus glomerulonephritis) are induced by predominantly mesangial localization of immune complexes, which usually causes only mild nephritis or asymptomatic hematuria and proteinuria. Localization of substantial amounts of nephritogenic immune complexes in the subendothelial zones of glomerular capillaries, where they are adjacent to the inflammatory mediator systems in the blood, induces overt glomerular inflammation (focal or diffuse proliferative lupus glomerulonephritis, class III or IV lupus nephritis) and usually causes severe clinical manifestations of nephritis. Qualitative and quantitative characteristics of the pathogenic immune complexes that result in localization, predominantly in subepithelial zones where they are not in contact with the inflammatory mediator systems in the blood, induce membranous lupus glomerulonephritis (class V lupus glomerulonephritis). This variant usually causes the nephrotic syndrome rather than nephritis. As the nephritogenic immune response in a given patient changes with time, sometimes modified by treatment, transitions may occur among the various lupus nephritis phenotypes.

The structurally most severe form of active glomerulonephritis is crescentic glomerulonephritis, which usually manifests clinically as rapidly progressive glomerulonephritis. In patients with new-onset kidney disease who have a nephritic sediment and serum creatinine greater than 3 mg/dL, glomerulonephritis with crescents is the most common finding in kidney biopsy specimens (see Table 16.3). Crescents are

proliferations of cells within Bowman capsule that include both macrophages and glomerular epithelial cells. Crescent formation is a response to glomerular capillary rupture and therefore is a marker of severe glomerular injury. Crescents, however, do not indicate the cause of glomerular injury, because many different pathogenic mechanisms can cause crescent formation. There is no consensus on how many glomeruli should have crescents to use the term *crescentic glomerulonephritis* in the diagnosis. Most pathologists use the term if more than 50% of glomeruli include crescents, but the percentage of glomeruli with crescents should be specified in the diagnosis even if it is less than 50% (e.g., IgA nephropathy with focal proliferative glomerulonephritis and 25% crescents). Within a specific pathogenic category of glomerulonephritis (e.g., anti-GBM disease, ANCA disease, lupus glomerulonephritis, IgA nephropathy, poststreptococcal glomerulonephritis), the higher the fraction of glomeruli with crescents, the worse the prognosis; however, among pathogenetically different forms of glomerulonephritis, the pathogenic category may be more important in predicting outcome than the presence of crescents. For example, a patient with poststreptococcal glomerulonephritis with 50% crescents has a much better prognosis for kidney survival, even without immunosuppressive treatment, than a patient with anti-GBM glomerulonephritis or ANCA glomerulonephritis with 25% crescents.

The importance of pathogenic category in predicting the natural history of glomerulonephritis indicates that

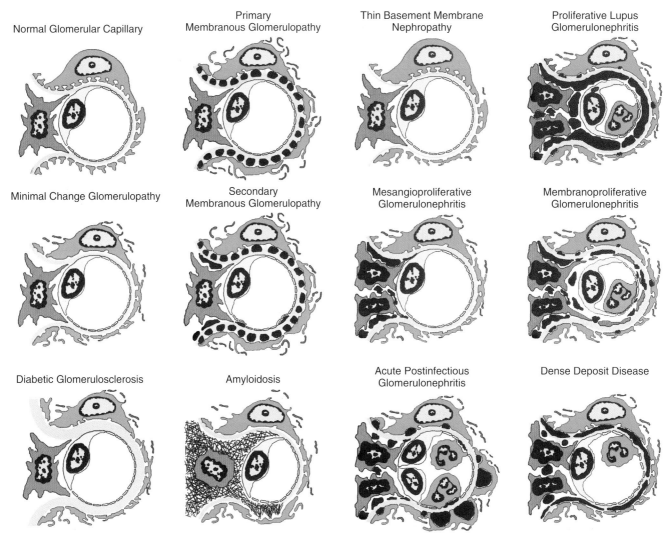

Fig. 16.3 Ultrastructural changes in glomerular capillaries caused by glomerular diseases that typically result in the nephrotic syndrome. In the normal glomerular capillary, note the visceral epithelial cell with intact foot processes *(green)*, endothelial cell with fenestrations *(tan)*, mesangial cell *(brown)* with adjacent mesangial matrix *(light gray)*, and basement membrane with lamina densa *(light blue)* that does not completely surround the capillary lumen but splays out as the paramesangial basement membrane. In minimal change disease, note the effacement of foot processes and microvillus transformation. In diabetic glomerulosclerosis, note the thickening of the lamina densa and expansion of mesangial matrix. In idiopathic membranous glomerulopathy, note the subepithelial dense deposits with adjacent projections of basement membrane (see also Fig. 16.6). In secondary membranous glomerulopathy, note the mesangial and small subendothelial deposits in addition to the requisite subepithelial deposits. In amyloidosis, note the fibrils within the mesangium and capillary wall. (Courtesy J. Charles Jennette, MD.)

Fig. 16.4 Ultrastructural changes in glomerular capillaries caused by glomerular diseases that typically result in hematuria and the nephritic syndrome. In thin basement membrane nephropathy, note the thin lamina densa of the basement membrane (compare to the normal glomerular capillary in Fig. 16.3). In mesangioproliferative glomerulonephritis (e.g., mild lupus nephritis, immunoglobulin A nephropathy), note the mesangial dense deposits and mesangial hypercellularity. In acute diffuse proliferative glomerulonephritis (e.g., poststreptococcal glomerulonephritis), note the endocapillary hypercellularity contributed to by leukocytes, endothelial cells, and mesangial cells and the dense deposits, which include not only conspicuous subepithelial "humps" but also inconspicuous subendothelial and mesangial deposits. In proliferative lupus glomerulonephritis, note the extensive subendothelial and mesangial dense deposits. In membranoproliferative glomerulonephritis (mesangiocapillary glomerulonephritis), note the subendothelial deposits with associated subendothelial interposition of mesangial cytoplasm and deposition of new matrix material resulting in basement membrane replication. In dense deposit disease, note the intramembranous and mesangial dense deposits. (Courtesy J. Charles Jennette, MD.)

the pathologic classification of glomerulonephritis by light microscopy into the morphologic categories based on the pattern of injury as listed in Table 16.2 and shown in Fig. 16.9 is not adequate for optimal management. In addition to determining the pattern and severity of glomerular inflammation, the pathogenic or immunopathologic category of disease must be determined (see Table 16.2 and Fig. 16.2).

If a kidney biopsy is performed, this determination is by immunohistology and electron microscopy (see Figs. 16.2 through 16.7). Immunohistology shows the presence or absence of immunoglobulins and complement components. The distribution (e.g., capillary wall, mesangium), pattern

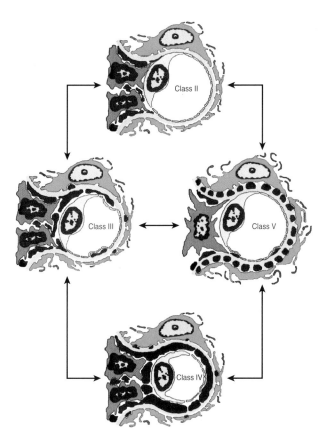

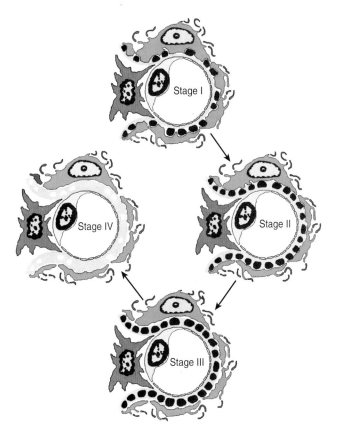

Fig. 16.5 Ultrastructural features of the major classes of lupus nephritis. The sequestration of immune deposits within the mesangium in class II (mesangioproliferative) lupus glomerulonephritis causes only mesangial hyperplasia and mild renal dysfunction. Substantial amounts of subendothelial immune deposits, which are adjacent to the inflammatory mediator systems of the blood, cause focal (class III) or diffuse (class IV) proliferative lupus glomerulonephritis with overt nephritic signs and symptoms. Localization of immune deposits predominantly in the subepithelial zone causes membranous (class V) lupus glomerulonephritis, which usually manifests predominantly as the nephrotic syndrome. (Courtesy J. Charles Jennette, MD.)

Fig. 16.6 Ultrastructural stages in the progression of membranous glomerulopathy. Stage I has subepithelial electron-dense immune complex deposits without adjacent projections of basement membrane material. Stage II has adjacent glomerular basement membrane (GBM) projections that eventually surround the electron-dense immune deposits in stage III. Stage IV has a markedly thickened GBM with electron-lucent zones replacing the electron-dense deposits. (Courtesy J. Charles Jennette, MD.)

(e.g., granular, linear), and composition (e.g., IgA-dominant, IgG-dominant, IgM-dominant, C3-dominant, monoclonal) of immunoglobulin and complement are useful for determining specific types of glomerulonephritis; this is discussed in detail in later chapters that address specific types of glomerular disease. Table 16.4 shows the frequencies of the major pathologic categories of glomerulonephritis in patients with 50% or more crescents who have undergone kidney biopsy. The immune complex category comprises a variety of diseases, including lupus nephritis, IgA nephropathy, immune complex membranoproliferative glomerulonephritis (MPGN), and infection-related glomerulonephritis. Note that most patients with greater than 50% crescents have little or no immunohistologic evidence for immune complex or anti-GBM antibody localization within glomeruli; that is, they have pauci-immune glomerulonephritis. More than 90% of these patients with pauci-immune crescentic glomerulonephritis have circulating ANCAs. Therefore ANCA glomerulonephritis is the most common form of crescentic glomerulonephritis, especially in older adults.

Because both the structural severity (such as the patterns of injury shown in Fig. 16.9) and the immunopathologic and ultrastructural category of disease (such as the categories presented in Figs. 16.2 through 16.7) are important for predicting the course of disease in a patient with glomerulonephritis, the most useful diagnostic terms should include information about both the pattern of injury and etiology and pathogenic causes of the injury (see Table 16.2). Examples are "IgA nephropathy with focal proliferative glomerulonephritis," "diffuse proliferative lupus glomerulonephritis," and "anti-GBM crescentic glomerulonephritis."

Many types of glomerulonephritis are immune-mediated inflammatory diseases and are treated with corticosteroids, cytotoxic drugs, or other antiinflammatory and immunosuppressive agents. The aggressiveness of the treatment should match the aggressiveness of the disease. For example, active class IV lupus nephritis warrants aggressive immunosuppressive treatment, whereas class I or class II lupus nephritis does not. The two most aggressive forms of glomerulonephritis are anti-GBM crescentic glomerulonephritis and ANCA crescentic glomerulonephritis, and the most important factor in improving kidney outcomes is early diagnosis and treatment.

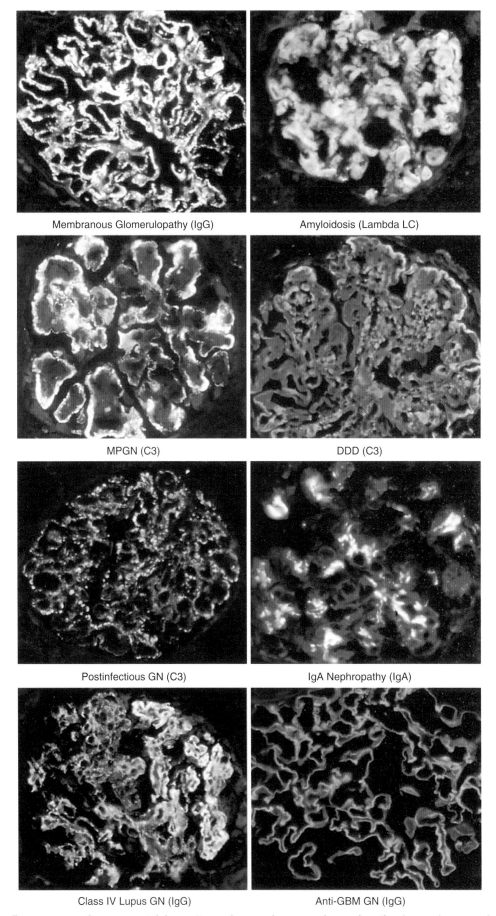

Membranous Glomerulopathy (IgG)

Amyloidosis (Lambda LC)

MPGN (C3)

DDD (C3)

Postinfectious GN (C3)

IgA Nephropathy (IgA)

Class IV Lupus GN (IgG)

Anti-GBM GN (IgG)

Fig. 16.7 Immunofluorescence microscopy staining patterns for membranous glomerulopathy. In membranous glomerulopathy, note the global granular capillary wall staining for IgG. In AL amyloidosis, note the irregular fluffy staining for lambda light chains. In MPGN, note the peripheral granular to bandlike staining for C3. In DDD, note the bandlike capillary wall and coarsely granular mesangial staining for C3. In acute postinfectious GN, note the coarsely granular capillary wall staining for C3. In IgA nephropathy, note the mesangial staining for IgA. In class IV lupus GN, note the segmentally variable capillary wall and mesangial staining for IgG. In anti-GBM GN, note the linear GBM staining for IgG. *anti-GBM,* Antiglomerular basement membrane; *DDD,* dense deposit disease; *GN,* glomerulonephritis; *IgG,* immunoglobulin G; *LC,* light chain; *MPGN,* membranoproliferative glomerulonephritis.

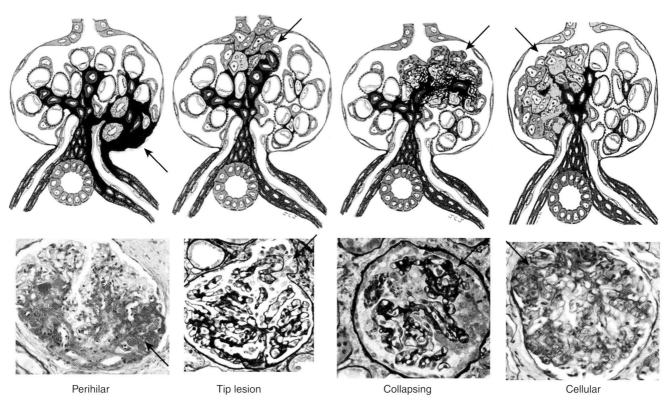

Perihilar   Tip lesion   Collapsing   Cellular

Fig. 16.8 Pathologic variants of focal segmental glomerulosclerosis. Podocytes showing parietal epithelial cells and tubular epithelial cells *(green)*, endothelial cells *(pale yellow)*, mesangial and arteriolar smooth muscle cells *(red)*, macrophages *(light tan)*, and collagenous matrix *(black)*. The photomicrographs of perihilar and cellular focal segmental glomerulosclerosis (FSGS) include periodic acid–Schiff staining, and the images of tip lesion and collapsing FSGS include Jones silver staining. Perihilar FSGS has perihilar sclerosis and adhesion. Tip lesion FSGS has consolidation of the tuft contiguous with the origin of the proximal tubule. Collapsing FSGS has collapse of capillaries with hypertrophy and hyperplasia of overlying epithelial cells. Cellular FSGS has endocapillary hypercellularity with foam cells.

Table 16.3   Kidney Diseases in Patients With Hematuria Undergoing Kidney Biopsy

Disease	Prot <1 g/24 h, Cr <1.5 mg/dL	Prot 1–3 g/24 h	Cr 1.5–3.0 mg/dL	Cr >3 mg/dL
No abnormality	30%	2%	1%	0%
Thin BM nephropathy	26%	4%	3%	0%
IgA nephropathy	28%	24%	14%	8%
GN without crescents[a]	9%	26%	37%	23%
GN with crescents[a]	2%	24%	21%	44%
Other kidney disease[b]	5%	20%	24%	25%
Total	100% (*n* = 43)	100% (*n* = 123)	100% (*n* = 179)	100% (*n* = 255)

An analysis of kidney biopsy specimens evaluated by the University of North Carolina nephropathology laboratory in 1990. Patients with systemic lupus erythematosus were excluded from the analysis. All specimens were evaluated by light, immunofluorescence, and electron microscopy. Columns 1 and 2 are mutually exclusive with regard to proteinuria while columns 1, 3, and 4 are mutually exclusive with regard to serum creatinine.
[a]Proliferative or necrotizing glomerulonephritis other than immunoglobulin A nephropathy or lupus nephritis.
[b]Includes causes for the nephrotic syndrome, such as membranous glomerulopathy and focal segmental glomerulosclerosis.
BM, Basement membrane; *Cr*, serum creatinine; *GN*, glomerulonephritis; *IgA*, immunoglobulin A; *Prot*, proteinuria.
Adapted from Caldas MLR, Jennette JC, Falk RJ, Wilkman AS. NC Glomerular Disease Collaborative Network: what is found by renal biopsy in patients with hematuria? *Lab Invest*. 1990;62:15A.

Light Microscopic Morphology

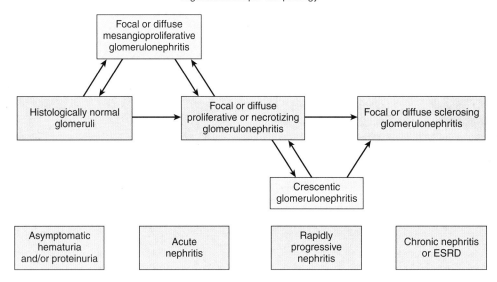

Clinical Manifestations

Fig. 16.9 Morphologic patterns of injury of glomerulonephritis *(top)* **aligned with the usual clinical manifestations** *(bottom).* Certain glomerular diseases, such as antiglomerular basement membrane and antineutrophil cytoplasmic antibody glomerulonephritis, usually exhibit crescentic glomerulonephritis with rapid decline in kidney function if not promptly treated. Others, such as lupus nephritis, have a predilection for causing focal or diffuse proliferative glomerulonephritis with variable rates of progression depending on the activity of the glomerular lesions. Immunoglobulin A nephropathy tends to begin as mild mesangioproliferative lesions but may progress to more severe proliferative lesions. Post-streptococcal glomerulonephritis typically develops an active acute proliferative glomerulonephritis initially but then resolves through a mesangioproliferative phase to normal. *ESRD,* End-stage renal disease. (From Jennette JC, Mandal AK. Syndrome of glomerulonephritis. In: Mandal AK, Jennette JC, eds. *Diagnosis and Management of Renal Disease and Hypertension.* 2nd ed. Durham, NC: Carolina Academic Press; 1994, with permission.)

Table 16.4   Frequency of Pathologic Categories of Crescentic Glomerulonephritis in Consecutive Native Kidney Biopsy Specimens, by Age of Patient

Age (years)	Pauci-Immune	Immune Complex	Anti-GBM	Other[a]
All (*n* = 632)	60%	24%	15%	1%
1–20 (*n* = 73)	42%	45%	12%	0%
21–60 (*n* = 303)	48%	35%	15%	3%
61–100 (*n* = 256)	79%	6%	15%	0%

Crescentic glomerulonephritis defined as glomerular disease with 50% or more crescents.
[a]The "other" category includes all other glomerular diseases, such as thrombotic microangiopathy, diabetic glomerulosclerosis, and monoclonal immunoglobulin deposition disease.
Anti-GBM, Antiglomerular basement membrane.
Modified from Jennette JC. Rapidly progressive and crescentic glomerulonephritis. *Kidney Int.* 2003;63:1164–1172.

ANTIGLOMERULAR BASEMENT MEMBRANE DISEASE

In anti-GBM disease, autoantibodies develop to a specific component of the glomerular basement membrane. More than 90% of patients with glomerulonephritis and linear GBM staining for IgG have identifiable circulating autoantibodies to cryptic, conformational epitopes in the noncollagenous domain of the alpha 3 chain of type IV collagen. Those who do not are called atypical anti-GBM disease, although the nature of the immunoglobulin in the GBMs is not yet well defined and may not be anti-GBM autoantibodies in some patients. Of note, approximately a quarter of patients with anti-GBM glomerulonephritis also are ANCA positive.

After extensive sclerosis of glomeruli and advanced chronic tubulointerstitial injury have developed, significant response to treatment is less likely. Both anti-GBM disease and ANCA-associated GN are treated with immunosuppressive regimens, such as pulse methylprednisolone and cyclophosphamide or rituximab. Plasmapheresis is added to the regimen for anti-GBM disease and for ANCA disease with pulmonary hemorrhage or severe kidney failure. Immunosuppressive treatment usually can be terminated after 3 to 5 months in patients with anti-GBM glomerulonephritis with little risk for recurrence (see Chapter 24).

ANTINEUTROPHIL CYTOPLASMIC ANTIBODY GLOMERULONEPHRITIS

ANCA GN is discussed in Chapter 24. ANCAs are specific for proteins within the granules of neutrophils and the peroxidase-positive lysosomes of monocytes. Two patterns of neutrophil staining discriminate between the major ANCA subtypes: cytoplasmic-staining (C-ANCA) and perinuclear-staining (P-ANCA). Most C-ANCAs are specific for a neutrophil and monocyte proteinase called proteinase 3 (PR3-ANCA), and most P-ANCAs are specific for myeloperoxidase (MPO-ANCA). The initial induction of remission for ANCA glomerulonephritis often is performed for 6 to 12 months, and even then there is risk for recurrence that will require additional immunosuppression. In addition to the clinical and pathologic severity, ANCA specificity influences likelihood of remission, with PR3-ANCA associated with better response to treatment. Thus a fully actionable diagnosis of ANCA glomerulonephritis should include the antigen specificity as well as designations for the clinical and pathologic manifestations—for example, MPO-ANCA microscopic polyangiitis (MPA) and crescentic glomerulonephritis.

GLOMERULONEPHRITIS ASSOCIATED WITH SYSTEMIC DISEASES

Some patients with acute or rapidly progressive glomerulonephritis have a pathogenetically related systemic disease. These forms of glomerulonephritis, with known systemic disease causes, may be referred to as *secondary glomerulonephritides*. Immune complex–mediated glomerulonephritis that is induced by infection may involve an antecedent infection, such as streptococcal pharyngitis or pyoderma, preceding acute poststreptococcal glomerulonephritis. Persistent infections also can cause concurrent glomerulonephritis, such as hepatitis C infection causing immune complex (cryoglobulinemic) MPGN. Membranoproliferative pattern glomerulonephritis can be caused not only by immune complex deposition but also by C3-dominant deposits resulting from alternative complement pathway dysregulation (C3 glomerulopathy) and by monoclonal immunoglobulin deposits that can activate complement (see Table 16.2). Staphylococcal infection, especially methicillin-resistant staph infection, can cause an IgA-dominant immune complex glomerulonephritis that resembles IgA nephropathy. As noted earlier, glomerulonephritis with any of the morphologic expressions shown in Fig. 16.9, as well as membranous glomerulopathy, can be caused by systemic lupus erythematosus (see Fig. 16.6).

Because glomeruli are vessels, glomerulonephritis is a frequent manifestation of systemic small-vessel vasculitides, such as IgA vasculitis (Henoch-Schönlein purpura), cryoglobulinemic vasculitis, MPA, granulomatosis with polyangiitis (GPA, formerly Wegener granulomatosis), or eosinophilic granulomatosis with polyangiitis (EGPA, formerly Churg-Strauss syndrome) (see Chapter 24). IgA vasculitis is caused by vascular localization of IgA-dominant immune complexes,

including deposits and inflammation that are indistinguishable from glomerular lesions of IgA nephropathy. Cryoglobulinemic vasculitis is caused by cryoglobulin deposition in vessels and often is associated with hepatitis C infection. In glomeruli, cryoglobulinemia usually causes an MPGN pattern of injury, but other patterns of proliferative and even membranous glomerulonephritis may develop. In MPA, GPA, and EGPA, there is typically a paucity of immune deposits in vessel walls, usually, but not always, accompanied by circulating ANCAs. Glomerulonephritis associated with and probably caused by ANCAs is characterized pathologically by fibrinoid necrosis and crescent formation and often manifests as a rapidly progressive decline in kidney function. Patients with vasculitis-associated glomerulonephritis typically exhibit clinical manifestations of vascular inflammation in multiple organs, such as skin purpura caused by dermal venulitis, hemoptysis caused by alveolar capillary hemorrhage, abdominal pain caused by gut vasculitis, and peripheral neuropathy (mononeuritis multiplex) caused by vasculitis in the small epineural arteries of peripheral nerves.

A distinctive and severe clinical presentation for glomerulonephritis is pulmonary-renal vasculitic syndrome, in which rapidly progressive glomerulonephritis is combined with pulmonary hemorrhage. ANCA disease is the most common cause for pulmonary-renal vasculitic syndrome, followed by anti-GBM disease. Histologic and immunohistologic examination of involved vessels, including glomeruli in kidney biopsy specimens, is useful in making a definitive diagnosis (see Fig. 16.2). Serologic analysis for anti-GBM antibodies and ANCA and markers for immune complex disease (e.g., antinuclear antibodies, cryoglobulins, antihepatitis C and B antibodies, complement levels) also may indicate the appropriate diagnosis (see Fig. 16.2).

PROTEINURIA

When proteinuria is severe, it causes the nephrotic syndrome, whereas less severe proteinuria, or severe proteinuria of short duration, may be asymptomatic. The nephrotic syndrome is characterized by massive proteinuria (greater than 3 g/24 h per 1.73 m^2), hypoproteinemia (especially hypoalbuminemia), edema, hyperlipidemia, and lipiduria. The most specific microscopic urinalysis finding is the presence of oval fat bodies (see Chapters 4 and 5). These are sloughed tubular epithelial cells that have absorbed excess lipids and lipoproteins in the urine.

Severe nephrotic syndrome predisposes to thrombosis secondary to loss of hemostasis control proteins (e.g., antithrombin III, protein S, protein C), infection secondary to loss of immunoglobulins, and accelerated atherosclerosis caused by hyperlipidemia. Volume depletion and inactivity may further increase the risk for venous thrombosis in nephrotic patients.

Any type of glomerular disease can cause proteinuria. In fact, although proteinuria is a sensitive indicator of glomerular damage, not all proteinuria is of glomerular origin. For example, tubular damage can cause proteinuria but rarely of more than 2 g/24 h. As noted in Table 16.1, some glomerular diseases are more likely to manifest as nephrotic syndrome than others, although virtually any form of glomerular disease may cause nephrotic range proteinuria. The primary kidney diseases that most often manifest as nephrotic syndrome are minimal change disease, FSGS, and membranous glomerulopathy; the secondary forms of kidney disease that often manifest as nephrotic syndrome are diabetic glomerulosclerosis and amyloidosis.

Age and race may predispose to certain causes of nephrotic syndrome. Among children younger than 10 years, about 80% of nephrotic syndrome is caused by minimal change disease, whereas, throughout adulthood, minimal change disease accounts for only about 10% to 15% of primary nephrotic syndrome. In white adults, membranous glomerulopathy is the most common cause for primary nephrotic syndrome, accounting for approximately 40% of cases, whereas FSGS is the most common cause for primary nephrotic syndrome in blacks, accounting for more than 50% of cases. Fig. 16.1 shows the frequencies of different glomerular disease identified by kidney biopsy specimens across a wide age range. Notably, these biopsy data do not correlate directly with the frequencies of these diseases in all nephrotic patients, because all causes of nephrotic syndrome are not biopsied at the same rate. For example, diagnoses of minimal change disease in children and diabetic glomerulosclerosis in adults are often made without biopsy.

Membranous glomerulopathy (see Chapter 19) is the most frequent cause of primary nephrotic syndrome in white people during the fifth and sixth decades of life. It is characterized pathologically by numerous subepithelial immune complex deposits (see Figs. 16.3, 16.6, and 16.7). The glomerular lesion evolves through time, with progressive accumulation of basement membrane material around the capillary wall immune complexes (see Fig. 16.6) and eventual development of chronic tubulointerstitial injury in those patients with progressive disease. Most membranous glomerulopathy is caused by autoantibodies specific for an antigen on visceral epithelial cells, M-type phospholipase A2 receptor (anti-PLA2R). This results in immune complex formation in the subepithelial zone but not in the subendothelial zone of glomeruli. Primary membranous glomerulopathy also can be caused by autoantibodies specific for other proteins—for example, neutral endopeptidase and thrombospondin type I domain-containing 7A (THSD7A).

Patients with membranous glomerulopathy who do not have circulating anti-PLA2R antibodies or PLA2R antigen in glomerular immune complexes are more likely to have membranous glomerulopathy secondary to systemic disease. Membranous glomerulopathy secondary to immune complexes composed of antigens and antibodies in the systemic circulation often have immune complex deposits in the mesangium and may have small subendothelial deposits (see Fig. 16.3). Therefore the ultrastructural identification of mesangial or subendothelial deposits should raise the level of suspicion for secondary membranous glomerulopathy, such as membranous glomerulopathy caused by a systemic autoimmune disease (e.g., lupus, mixed connective tissue disease, autoimmune thyroiditis), infection (e.g., hepatitis B or C, syphilis), or neoplasm (e.g., lung or gut carcinoma). In very young and very old patients, the likelihood of secondary membranous glomerulopathy is greater, although still uncommon. Membranous glomerulopathy occurring in young patients raises the possibility of systemic lupus erythematosus or hepatitis B infection, while in the elderly it raises the possibility of occult carcinoma.

Glomerulonephritis with a membranoproliferative pattern often manifests with mixed nephrotic and nephritic features, sometimes accompanied by hypocomplementemia, especially if it is caused by a C3 glomerulopathy secondary to dysregulation of the alternative complement pathway. MPGN has glomerular capillary wall thickening and hypercellularity by light microscopy. The most common form of MPGN, caused by immune complex disease or C3 glomerulonephritis, is characterized ultrastructurally by subendothelial immune complex deposits that stimulate subendothelial mesangial interposition and replication of basement membrane material. A less common pattern of C3 glomerulopathy that can cause an MPGN pattern of injury is dense deposit disease (DDD) that has intramembranous dense deposits (see Fig. 16.4). This pathognomonic feature, intramembranous dense deposits, is not always accompanied by an MPGN pattern by light microscopy but rather may have a proliferative or mesangioproliferative pattern. Patients with an MPGN pattern by light microscopy may have immune complex disease with substantial immunoglobulin and complement deposits or C3 glomerulopathy with exclusively or predominantly complement deposits with prominent C3 and little or no immunoglobulin (see Fig. 16.7). MPGN with extensive immunoglobulin deposition is an immune complex disease that may be secondary to cryoglobulinemia, neoplasms, or chronic infections (e.g., hepatitis C or B; infected prostheses, such as a ventriculoatrial shunt; chronic bacterial endocarditis; chronic mastoiditis). MPGN with complement deposition but no immunoglobulin, as well as DDD, are not immune complex diseases but rather are secondary to abnormal activation of the alternative complement pathway by a variety of inherited and acquired abnormalities in complement regulation.

In addition to the categories of glomerular disease that usually are associated with nephrotic syndrome, the various forms of proliferative glomerulonephritis account for a substantial proportion of patients who have nephrotic-range proteinuria. Patients with proliferative glomerulonephritis and marked proteinuria usually also have features of nephritis, especially hematuria. Included in this group are patients with lupus nephritis and IgA nephropathy who have nephrotic-range proteinuria. In the United States, approximately 15% of adults with nephrotic-range proteinuria are found to have IgA nephropathy by kidney biopsy.

FSGS is the most common cause for the nephrotic syndrome in blacks, but it affects all races. FSGS is not a specific disease but rather a pattern of injury that can be caused by multiple etiologies and pathogenic mechanisms. Clinical presentations include asymptomatic proteinuria, indolent nephrotic syndrome, rapid-onset nephrotic syndrome, and nephrotic syndrome with rapidly progressive kidney failure. Some forms of FSGS may recur in transplant recipients, suggesting a pathogenic role for a circulating factor. The Columbia classification system recognizes five morphologic variants of FSGS with different patterns of injury: tip lesion, collapsing, cellular, perihilar, and not otherwise specified (NOS) (see Fig. 16.8). NOS is most common and usually presents as asymptomatic proteinuria or indolent nephrotic syndrome. Although the other variants can have any type of proteinuric presentation, tip lesion FSGS usually presents with rapid-onset severe proteinuria resembling minimal change disease, collapsing FSGS with severe proteinuria and often rapidly progressing kidney failure, and perihilar FSGS with subnephrotic proteinuria. FSGS occurs as a primary (idiopathic) disease or secondary to recognized causes. For example, FSGS NOS may be secondary to mutations in podocyte genes, collapsing FSGS secondary to human immunodeficiency virus infection, and perihilar FSGS secondary to obesity or reduced functional nephrons.

Amyloidosis as a cause for the nephrotic syndrome is most frequently seen in older adults. Overall, approximately 10% of adults with unexplained nephrotic syndrome have amyloidosis that appears on kidney biopsy. Currently in the United States, amyloid causing the nephrotic syndrome is approximately 75% AL (amyloid L), and approximately 75% of AL amyloid is composed of λ rather than κ light chains. Patients with κ light chain paraproteins and the nephrotic syndrome are more likely to develop light chain deposition disease (i.e., nodular sclerosis without amyloid fibrils) rather than AL amyloidosis (see Chapter 28). Amyloid composition can be determined by immunofluorescence microscopy (see Fig. 16.7) or mass spectroscopy. In less developed areas of the world where chronic infections are more prevalent, AA amyloidosis (composed of amyloid A protein) is more frequent than AL amyloidosis. In North America, amyloidosis derived from leukocyte cell–derived chemotaxin 2 is most frequent in Latinos and Native Americans. Hereditary forms of amyloidosis are rare—for example, amyloid composed of fibrinogen A, transthyretin, gelsolin, lysozyme, and apolipoprotein A.

CHRONIC GLOMERULONEPHRITIS AND KIDNEY FAILURE

Most glomerular disease, with the possible exceptions of uncomplicated minimal change disease, can progress to chronic glomerular sclerosis with progressively declining kidney function. Chronic glomerular disease is the third leading cause of end-stage renal disease (ESRD) in the United States, after diabetic and hypertensive kidney disease. Clinicopathologic studies of glomerular diseases have shown marked differences in their natural histories. Some diseases, such as anti-GBM and ANCA crescentic glomerulonephritis, result in a high risk for rapid progression to ESRD unless treated. Other diseases, such as IgA nephropathy and FSGS, have more indolent but persistent courses, with ESRD eventually ensuing in a significant number of patients. Some forms of glomerulonephritis, such as acute poststreptococcal glomerulonephritis, may initially manifest with severe nephritis but usually resolve completely with little risk for progression to ESRD, whereas other diseases are unpredictable, such as membranous glomerulopathy, which may remit spontaneously, produce persistent nephrotic syndrome for decades without a decline in kidney function, or progress during several years to ESRD.

Chronic glomerulonephritis is characterized pathologically by varying degrees of glomerular scarring that is always accompanied by cortical tubular atrophy, interstitial fibrosis, interstitial infiltration by chronic inflammatory cells, and arteriosclerosis. As the glomerular, interstitial, and vascular sclerosis worsen, they eventually reach a point at which histologic evaluation of the kidney tissue cannot show the initial cause for the kidney injury, and a pathologic diagnosis of ESRD is all that can be concluded.

KIDNEY BIOPSY

Kidney biopsy is indicated in a patient with kidney disease when all three of the following conditions are met: (1) the cause cannot be determined or adequately predicted by less invasive diagnostic procedures; (2) the signs and symptoms suggest parenchymal disease that can be diagnosed by pathologic evaluation; and (3) the differential diagnosis includes diseases that have different treatments, different prognoses, or both.

Situations in which a kidney biopsy serves an important diagnostic function include nephrotic syndrome in adults, steroid-resistant nephrotic syndrome in children, glomerulonephritis in adults other than clear-cut acute poststreptococcal glomerulonephritis, and acute and chronic kidney injury of unknown cause. In some kidney diseases for which the diagnosis is relatively certain based on clinical data, a kidney biopsy may be of value not only for confirming the diagnosis but also for assessing the activity, chronicity, and severity of injury (e.g., in patients with suspected lupus glomerulonephritis). Although the diagnosis is strongly supported by positive serologic results in patients with anti-GBM and ANCA glomerulonephritis, the extremely toxic treatment that is used for these diseases warrants the additional level of confirmation that a kidney biopsy provides, as well as information about disease severity, potential reversibility of the glomerular damage, and likelihood of kidney failure. Fig. 16.1 demonstrates the types of native kidney diseases that have prompted kidney biopsy among the nephrologists who refer specimens to the University of North Carolina nephropathology laboratory. Nephrologists in community practice performed approximately 80% of these biopsies. Diseases that typically cause nephrotic syndrome (e.g., membranous glomerulopathy, FSGS) were the conditions most often shown by biopsy, followed by diseases that cause nephritis (e.g., lupus nephritis, IgA nephropathy).

Relative or absolute contraindications to percutaneous kidney biopsy include an uncooperative patient, solitary native kidney, hemorrhagic diathesis, uncontrolled severe hypertension, severe anemia, cystic kidney, hydronephrosis, multiple renal arterial aneurysms, acute pyelonephritis, or perinephric abscess and ESRD. Some advocate transjugular kidney biopsy and open kidney biopsy as safer procedures in patients with these risk factors.

Clinically significant complications of kidney biopsy are relatively infrequent but must be kept in mind when determining the risk/benefit ratio of the procedure. Small perirenal hematomas that can be seen on imaging studies (e.g., ultrasonography) are relatively common if observed carefully. With real-time ultrasound or computed tomography guidance, gross hematuria occurs in fewer than 5% of patients, arteriovenous fistula in less than 1%, hemorrhage requiring surgery in less than 1%, and death in less than 0.1%. The rate of arteriovenous fistula formation may be higher with transjugular biopsy.

Light microscopy alone is inadequate for the diagnosis of native kidney diseases, although it may be adequate for assessing kidney allografts, particularly in the immediate posttransplant period. All native kidney biopsy samples should be processed for at least light microscopy and immunofluorescence microscopy. Most renal pathologists advocate performing electron microscopy on all native kidney biopsy specimens; however, some fix tissue for electron microscopy but perform the procedure only if the other microscopic findings suggest that it will be useful.

BIBLIOGRAPHY

Barbour TD, Ruseva MM, Pickering MC. Update on C3 glomerulopathy. *Nephrol Dial Transplant.* 2016;31:717-725.

Beck LH Jr, Salant DJ. Membranous nephropathy: from models to man. *J Clin Invest.* 2014;124:2307-2314.

Bomback AS. Anti-glomerular basement membrane nephritis: why we still "need" the kidney biopsy. *Clin Kidney J.* 2012;5:496-497.

Bose B, Cattran D, Toronto Glomerulonephritis Registry. Glomerular diseases: FSGS. *Clin J Am Soc Nephrol.* 2014;9:626-632.

D'Agati VD, Alster JM, Jennette JC, et al. Association of histologic variants in FSGS clinical trial with presenting features and outcomes. *Clin J Am Soc Nephrol.* 2013;8:399-406.

D'Agati VD, Fogo AB, Bruijn JA, et al. Pathologic classification of focal segmental glomerulosclerosis: a working proposal. *Am J Kidney Dis.* 2004;43:368-382.

Glassock RJ. The pathogenesis of membranous nephropathy: evolution and revolution. *Curr Opin Nephrol Hypertens.* 2012;21:235-242.

Jennette JC. Rapidly progressive crescentic glomerulonephritis. *Kidney Int.* 2003;63:1164-1177.

Jennette JC, Falk RJ, Bacon PA, et al. 2012 revised International Chapel Hill Consensus Conference Nomenclature of Vasculitides. *Arthritis Rheum.* 2013;65:1-11.

Jennette JC, Falk RJ, McGregor JG. Renal and systematic vasculitis. In: Johnson RJ, Feehally J, Floege J, eds. *Comprehensive Clinical Nephrology.* 5th ed. Philadelphia: Elsevier; 2015:287-302.

Jennette JC, Olson JL, Silva FG, et al. Primer on the pathologic diagnosis of renal disease. In: Jennette JC, Olson JL, Silva FG, D'Agati V, eds. *Heptinstall's Pathology of the Kidney.* 7th ed. Philadelphia: Wolters Kluwer; 2015:91-118.

O'Shaughnessy M, Hogan S, Poulton CJ, et al. Temporal and demographic trends in glomerular disease epidemiology in the southeastern United States, 1986–2015. *Clin J Am Soc Nephrol.* 2017;12:614-623.

Said SM, Sethi S, Valeri AM, et al. Renal amyloidosis: origin and clinicopathologic correlations of 474 recent cases. *Clin J Am Soc Nephrol.* 2013;8:1515-1523.

Satoskar AA, Suleiman S, Ayoub I, et al. *Staphylococcus* infection-associated GN—spectrum of IgA staining and prevalence of ANCA in a single-center cohort. *Clin J Am Soc Nephrol.* 2017;12:39-49.

Sethi S, Haas M, Markowitz GS, et al. Mayo Clinic/Renal Pathology Society Consensus report on pathologic classification, diagnosis, and reporting of GN. *J Am Soc Nephrol.* 2016;27:1278-1287.

Sethi S, Nester CM, Smith RJ. Membranoproliferative glomerulonephritis and C3 glomerulopathy: resolving the confusion. *Kidney Int.* 2012;81:434-441.

Suzuki H, Kiryluk K, Novak J, et al. The pathophysiology of IgA nephropathy. *J Am Soc Nephrol.* 2011;22:1795-1803.

Thomas DB, Franceschini N, Hogan SL, et al. Clinical and pathologic characteristics of focal segmental glomerulosclerosis pathologic variants. *Kidney Int.* 2006;69:920-926.

Troxell ML, Houghton DC. Atypical anti-glomerular basement membrane disease. *Clin Kidney J.* 2016;9:211-221.

Weening JJ, D'Agati VD, Schwartz MM, et al. The classification of glomerulonephritis in systemic lupus erythematosus revisited. *Kidney Int.* 2004;65:521-530.

Minimal Change Nephrotic Syndrome

17

Howard Trachtman; Jonathan Hogan; Jai Radhakrishnan

TERMINOLOGY AND HISTOPATHOLOGY

Minimal change disease (MCD) is a common cause of nephrotic syndrome (NS). Also known as lipoid nephrosis, nil disease, and minimal change nephropathy, kidney histology on light microscopy in MCD is relatively normal, lacking the significant glomerular cell proliferation, infiltration by circulating immunoeffector cells, immune deposits, tubulointerstitial changes, or alterations in the glomerular basement membrane (GBM) that characterize other glomerular diseases. The defining feature of MCD is diffuse effacement and fusion of the majority of podocyte foot processes without electron-dense deposits on electron microscopy. There are variants of MCD that are characterized by diffuse mesangial hypercellularity. Immunofluorescence is typically negative or may show low-level focal staining for C3 and IgM.

MCD can also be diagnosed clinically by exhibiting responsiveness to corticosteroid treatment. In children, because MCD is the cause of 90% of cases of idiopathic NS, a kidney biopsy is only warranted if clinical and laboratory evidence, including disease onset before 6 to 9 months of age or following adolescence, unexpected systemic manifestations, or a low serum C3 level, suggest an alternative diagnosis. Children who do not exhibit these characteristics will typically have MCD and will consequently respond to steroids. The nomenclature *steroid-sensitive nephrotic syndrome* (SSNS) is also used to describe such children. Steroid responsiveness is a marker of a favorable long-term prognosis. In contrast, children with steroid-resistant nephrotic syndrome (SRNS) are more likely on subsequent kidney biopsies to show focal segmental glomerulosclerosis (FSGS), a disease that is associated with a worse prognosis. The causes of the NS in adults are more varied, including a higher percentage of cases with other histologies such as membranous nephropathy (MN), FSGS, and membranoproliferative glomerulonephritis (MPGN). Because MCD only accounts for approximately 10% to 15% of adult NS cases, a kidney biopsy is usually warranted in adults to establish the etiology of NS and guide management.

MCD can be the cause of significant short-term morbidity and can manifest with a chronic relapsing course with long-term adverse consequences well into adulthood. Both first-line treatment and secondary therapeutic options for more difficult cases can lead to serious toxicity. Therefore, although the long-term prognosis is excellent, optimal management of MCD requires clinical acumen to balance the risks of untreated disease activity against the potential irreversible hazards of available pharmacologic choices.

PATHOPHYSIOLOGY

The effacement of podocyte foot processes that is a hallmark of MCD may be mediated by various intracellular signaling pathways. For example, markers of focal adhesion complex–mediated Crk-dependent signaling are enhanced in MCD but not FSGS. Moreover, increased production of proteins such as CD80 and angiopoietin-like protein 4 by podocytes in MCD models supports the central role of podocyte damage in the pathogenesis of MCD. It is thought that proteinuria occurs solely because of a defect in glomerular permselectivity, although alterations in tubular reabsorption may contribute.

MCD is unique in that it predominantly reflects a decrease in the negative charge present in endothelial cells, the GBM, and podocytes, thereby causing selective proteinuria. The reduction in negative charge appears to be a diffuse abnormality that manifests in capillaries throughout the body, with leakage of albumin in the peripheral circulation and accumulation of interstitial fluid. The cause of the diminished negative charge density probably results from immune-mediated defects that inhibit sulfate incorporation into the GBM, rather than a genetic mutation in a podocyte protein.

In addition, immunoeffector cells may elaborate soluble molecules, such as vascular endothelial growth factor, that directly increase GBM permeability to protein. It is likely that the molecular identity of circulating permeability factors that cause proteinuria will differ in patients with MCD and FSGS. A link between abnormal T-cell function and MCD was initially proposed more than 30 years ago by Shalhoub, and many studies since then have documented altered subtype distribution and activity of lymphocytes in children with MCD. The pivotal role of the immune system in MCD pathogenesis is underscored by a study in which albuminuria and podocyte foot process effacement was induced by injection of CD34+ stem cells isolated from patients with MCD or FSGS into immunodeficient NOD/SCID mice. This role is also supported by the finding of a higher Th17/Treg cell ratio in children with MCD. Finally, the genetic linkage between HLA-DQA1 and PLCG2 supports a role for adaptive and autoimmunity in the pathogenesis of MCD.

Although MCD can occur in familial clusters with both vertical (parent-child) and horizontal (sibling) patterns of inheritance, it has not been linked to mutations in any of the well-recognized proteins associated with FSGS, such as Wilms tumor-1, TRPC6, or α-actinin-4. Interestingly, there have been observations linking frequently relapsing childhood MCD to allelic heterogeneity in the gene for nephrin, a key component of the slit diaphragm and a major genetic locus

Box 17.1   Secondary Causes of Minimal Change Disease

Malignancy

Hematologic Tumors
    Hodgkin lymphoma
    Non-Hodgkin lymphoma
    Leukemia
Solid Tumors
    Thymoma
    Renal cell carcinoma
    Lung carcinoma
    Mesothelioma

Infection

Syphilis
Mycoplasma
Ehrlichiosis/Anaplasmosis
Strongyloidiasis
Echinococcus
Tuberculosis
HIV
Hepatitis C virus

Drugs

NSAIDs, including COX-2 inhibitors
Antimicrobials (ampicillin, rifampicin, cephalosporins)
Lithium
D-penicillamine
Bisphosphonates (pamidronate)
Sulfasalazines (mesalazine and salazopyrine)
Trimethadione
Immunizations
Interferon-γ

Other Kidney and Systemic Diseases

SLE
Fabry disease
Polycystic kidney disease
IPEX syndrome

HIV, Human immunodeficiency virus; *IPEX*, immune dysregulation polyendocrinopathy, enteropathy, X-linked; *NSAIDs*, nonsteroidal antiinflammatory drugs; *SLE*, systemic lupus erythematosus.

for congenital NS. In addition, in a study of 214 Chinese patients with MCD, variants in the podocin gene were more common than in healthy controls and correlated with proteinuria. Alterations in histone H3 lysine 4 trimethylation in children with MCD raise the possibility that epigenetic changes may contribute to the occurrence of MCD. Polymorphisms in the multidrug resistance-1 gene may influence responsiveness to steroids in patients with MCD.

MCD also is associated with various secondary causes (Box 17.1), including medications, infections, toxins, and malignancies. The pathophysiologic link between these secondary causes and the resulting MCD is not understood.

INCIDENCE

The overall incidence of primary or idiopathic NS, which includes MCD (and its variants), FSGS, MN, and MPGN, is approximately three to five cases/100,000 population/year in children and adults. This rate is fairly constant throughout the world and in most racial and ethnic groups. Recent data suggest that the incidence of MCD is rising in India and Southeast Asia, while FSGS may be increasingly prevalent throughout the world. The contribution of MCD to this general category varies tremendously with the age of the patient. Thus in prepubertal patients more than 6 months of age, MCD accounts for nearly 90% of all cases of idiopathic NS, whereas in adults the percentage of cases attributable to MCD falls to 10% to 15%. Adolescence represents the transition period between the two ends of the spectrum. In a study of 1523 consecutive Chinese patients who underwent biopsy performed during the evaluation of NS, in those aged 14 to 24 years, MCD was documented in 33% of the subgroup. Similarly, in a report of biopsy findings in 538 pediatric patients in Pakistan, among whom 365 were younger children (mean age 7.3 years) and 173 were adolescents (mean age 15.1 years), approximately one-third of the older group had FSGS and only one-fourth had MCD. MN and MPGN also were significantly more common in the older group. These findings suggest that adolescents correspond more closely to adults than they do to younger children.

CLINICAL PRESENTATION

MCD causes NS, manifesting with nephrotic range proteinuria, edema, hypoalbuminemia, and hypercholesterolemia. Edema is the most common presenting symptom of MCD, and the onset may be acute. The onset of MCD may be associated with an antecedent infection, typically respiratory. Infections may also trigger subsequent relapses of MCD. The rapidity of the appearance of edema is characteristic of MCD compared with other etiologies of NS. In children, edema can occur anywhere in the body, including the periorbital region, scrotum, or abdomen. The pathogenesis of edema in NS is complex and represents an interplay between underfill and overfill mechanisms. Less frequent presenting complaints include infections, such as cellulitis secondary to localized accumulation of fluid and skin breakdown, or bacterial peritonitis in patients with ascites. Hypercholesterolemia arises from alterations in lipoprotein lipase activity, and recent data support an important role for derangements in PCSK9 activity in mediating hypercholesterolemia in MCD. The incidence of thromboembolic events, including renal vein thrombosis and pulmonary emboli, is tenfold higher in adults than in children, and typically these events occur in patients with severe hypoalbuminemia.

Urinalysis reveals microscopic hematuria in 10% to 30% of adults and children with MCD, but gross hematuria is rare. Microscopic examination of the urine may also show waxy casts and oval fat bodies. In one series, acute kidney injury (AKI) occurred in 18% of adult patients who presented with NS and were subsequently diagnosed with MCD. These patients tended to be older, male, and hypertensive and had more severe proteinuria and hypoalbuminemia than patients who did not develop AKI. Kidney biopsies of these patients showed a variety of histologic patterns of injury, including tubular atrophy, interstitial inflammation and fibrosis, and atherosclerotic disease. The cause of the AKI is not entirely clear and may reflect primary changes in glomerular permeability, the reason for which is not entirely clear. Serologic tests are usually negative or normal.

INITIAL TREATMENT

Corticosteroids are the time-honored initial therapy for presumed and biopsy-confirmed MCD, and the sensitivity of MCD to steroid treatment prompts many physicians to empirically treat nephrotic patients with glucocorticoids without a kidney biopsy, particularly children. Prednisone is the usual agent prescribed, and the standard dose in pediatric patients is 60 mg/m^2 or 2 mg/kg daily for 4 to 6 weeks, followed by 40 mg/m^2 or 1.5 mg/kg every other day for 4 to 6 weeks. In children, 70% will achieve remission after 10 to 14 days of treatment, and the vast majority will no longer have proteinuria after 4 weeks of therapy. There are conflicting data in the literature as to whether lengthening the course of the initial treatment from 8 to 12 weeks delays the time to first relapse and reduces overall exposure to steroids. Two recent controlled clinical trials indicated that a longer initial course of steroids had no beneficial impact on the development of a frequently relapsing course (discussed later) compared with a standard 8-week course. Efficacy may vary depending on the patient population, and the precise treatment should be guided by the experience at each center.

Adults are treated with oral prednisone 1 mg/kg/day (maxmium, 80 mg/dose) or alternate-day prednisone at 2 mg/kg/day (maximum, 120 mg/dose). However, unlike children, responses in adults may take up to 24 weeks before the patient is designated "steroid responsive" or "steroid resistant." In adults, up to 20% of patients with an initial diagnosis of MCD may be refractory to steroids at the end of 16 weeks.

Treatment of relapse involves similar corticosteroid doses, but usually for a shorter period of time. Various modifications in corticosteroid dosing such as extended tapering schedules, avoidance of every other day administration, and prolonged low-dose hydrocortisone to prevent adrenal insufficiency have been prescribed to prevent relapses and to minimize side effects. Different formulations of steroids such as deflazacort have also been tried with mixed results. Adults do not tolerate relapsing disease as well as children as a consequence of the intrinsic morbidity of MCD and the toxicity related to repeated exposures to corticosteroids. Therefore these patients are often candidates for earlier implementation of second-line immunosuppressive therapy.

SHORT-TERM COURSE

MCD is usually a chronic relapsing disease (Fig. 17.1). Less than 10% of cases will remain completely free of relapses after the initial episode. The remaining patients can be divided into three categories based on clinical course. One-third will have infrequent relapses that are easily managed by intermittent administration of courses of corticosteroids. Another third will have frequent relapses defined by two or more relapses in a 6-month period; however, they too are successfully managed with intermittent administration of courses of corticosteroids. The remaining third are frequently relapsing patients or those with steroid dependence, defined as relapse occurring on alternate-day steroid treatment or within 2 weeks of discontinuing corticosteroids. It has proved difficult to predict short-term prognosis in individual patients (defined as within 2 years after disease onset). Children who go into remission during the first week of corticosteroid treatment and who have no hematuria are more likely to be infrequent relapsers. The presence of small involuted glomeruli, which can be distinguished from other causes of global glomerulosclerosis by the presence of vital podocytes and parietal epithelial cells, may be a marker of frequently relapsing MCD in children.

Patients who experience frequent relapses/steroid dependence usually experience steroid toxicity, and they are candidates for second-line treatments. Key steroid-induced side effects in children are impaired linear growth, obesity, behavioral changes, and cosmetic changes. In addition to these clinical effects, children with MCD also experience altered quality of life and psychosocial adjustment related both to illness-related variables and to alterations in the family

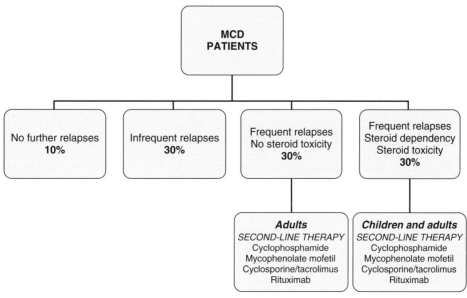

Fig. 17.1 Minimal change disease (MCD): short-term natural history.

climate. In adults, additional evidence of steroid toxicity includes cataracts and altered bone density. Hypertension and hyperlipidemia occur across the age spectrum.

LONG-TERM TREATMENT

IMMUNOSUPPRESSIVE THERAPY

Second-line therapy is used in patients with frequently relapsing, steroid-dependent, or steroid-resistant MCD, as well as those who experience severe steroid side effects (Table 17.1). The first drugs used in this setting were alkylating agents such as cyclophosphamide and chlorambucil. A prolonged remission of at least 1 year was achieved in 70% of patients. With cyclophosphamide, most patients require at least 12 weeks of therapy, and they should be monitored carefully for side effects, including leukopenia, infection, hemorrhagic cystitis, gonadal toxicity, and malignancy. Notably, more than 25% of patients with MCD treated with cyclophosphamide were not in sustained remission after puberty, and they required prolonged immunosuppressive treatment. Thus, because of the serious toxicity associated with alkylating agents, the reluctance to prescribe a second course, and the guarded long-term effect, there has been greater reliance on alternative medications for frequently relapsing or steroid-dependent patients with MCD.

Antimetabolites such as azathioprine and mycophenolate mofetil can reduce the relapse rate by approximately 50%, although they are not as effective as alkylating agents in inducing a permanent remission. They are useful because they have a more favorable side-effect profile, can be administered for an extended period, and require less intensive monitoring.

A third option is calcineurin inhibitors such as cyclosporine and tacrolimus. These agents induce a prolonged remission in nearly 80% to 90% of patients while the patient is taking the drug; however, relapses frequently occur shortly after stopping the drug. In addition, calcineurin inhibitors can cause undesirable cosmetic changes (hair growth and gingival hyperplasia with cyclosporine, alopecia with tacrolimus), hepatoxicity, hypertension, and nephrotoxicity. Therefore patients taking calcineurin inhibitors may require periodic blood tests to monitor drug levels and kidney damage.

Adrenocorticotropic hormone (ACTH), which was widely used in the past, has been reintroduced for the management of MCD. This hormone may act in part as a steroid substitute. In addition, it may act directly on the podocyte to restore functional integrity and normalize proteinuria. More studies are needed to determine the role of ACTH in the current management of MCD.

The newest agent used to treat children with frequently relapsing or steroid-dependent MCD and clinical evidence of steroid-induced side effects is rituximab. Administration of this anti-CD20 monoclonal antibody on B cells results in remission in up to 80% of steroid-sensitive cases when used in combination with calcineurin inhibitors. This was confirmed in a study of 54 children (mean age 11 years) in which open-label administration of rituximab plus low-dose steroids and tacrolimus was as effective as treatment with standard doses of the latter two drugs. The efficacy of rituximab has been confirmed in several small randomized clinical trials. Drawbacks include high cost and uncertain long-term risks.

The decision to recommend a second-line agent in an effort to alleviate the adverse consequences of steroids must be weighed on an individual basis and must take into account the patient's age, sex, and likely compliance with treatment. Consideration should be given to the side-effect profile, the likelihood of reversal of the complication, and the odds that the MCD will spontaneously resolve. Although a number of other immunomodulatory agents have been tried in the past in patients with MCD, data have been collected in relatively

Table 17.1 Second-Line Treatments of Minimal Change Disease

Drug	Dose	Efficacy	Side Effects
Cyclophosphamide	*Children and adults:* 2–2.5 mg/kg/day × 8–12 wk[a]	Prolonged remission (>1 year) in 70%	Leukopenia, hemorrhagic cystitis, alopecia, seizures, gonadal toxicity, malignancy
Chlorambucil	*Children and adults:* 0.15 mg/kg/day × 8–12 wk[a]		
Mycophenolate mofetil	*Children:* 24–36 mg/kg/day or 600 mg/m² /dose BID *Adults:* 1–1.5 g BID	50% reduction in overall relapse rate	Gastrointestinal complaints, leukopenia, elevated liver enzymes
Cyclosporine	*Children and adults:* 4–5 mg/kg/day in divided doses[b]	70%–80% of patients achieve complete remission on treatment	Gingival hyperplasia, tremor, elevated liver enzymes, nephrotoxicity
Tacrolimus	*Children and adults:* 0.05–0.3 mg/kg/day in divided doses[b]	70%–80%	Tremor, nephrotoxicity, alopecia
Rituximab	Children and adults: 375 mg/m² weekly × 4 weeks[c]	80% in steroid responsive MCD	Infection

[a]It is recommended that the duration of therapy be extended to 12 weeks in patients with steroid-dependent disease.
[b]Target trough levels for cyclosporine and tacrolimus are 100–200 ng/mL and 4–8 ng/mL, respectively. Children may require more frequent dosing to maintain a therapeutic drug level. After achieving remission, reduce doses to the lowest dose compatible with staying in remission.
[c]Alternate regimen used in adults is a 1000-mg fixed dose with two administrations 14 days apart.
BID, Twice daily; *MCD*, minimal change disease; *SSNS*, steroid-sensitive nephrotic syndrome.

small studies that hinder broad generalizations about efficacy. In addition, drugs such as levamisole are generally not available in the United States for use in patients with MCD. This underscores the need to develop newer agents that can be used to control proteinuria in patients with MCD, especially in children with steroid toxicity and adults with relapsing disease.

SUPPORTIVE CARE

After the initial diagnosis, patients with MCD are usually monitored with daily dipstick testing for proteinuria. In most patients, relapses are detected by the onset of proteinuria 3 to 4 days before edema ensues. In patients who develop edema before a relapse is recognized or who respond slowly to prednisone, edema can be controlled by prescribing a low-salt (2 g sodium) diet and oral diuretics. Options include loop diuretics, such as furosemide 1 to 2 mg/kg administered once or twice daily, or a thiazide diuretic. In patients who are refractory to standard diuretics, the addition of metolazone, an agent that acts primarily in the cortical collecting duct and to a lesser extent in the proximal tubule, may improve urine output. However, close monitoring is warranted to ensure that the patients do not develop severe hypokalemia, metabolic alkalosis, or intravascular volume contraction. The duration of action of diuretic agents may be diminished secondary to hypoalbuminemia and enhanced renal clearance, but this is rarely clinically significant because the medications are only needed for 1 to 2 weeks until treatment response occurs and proteinuria resolves.

Children who have frequent relapses and persistent edema are at risk for bacterial peritonitis and can be given prophylactic antibiotics. Immunization with the pneumococcal vaccine is also helpful under these circumstances. If feasible, the timing of vaccine administration should be delayed for at least 2 weeks after administration of prednisone to ensure maximal immunologic response.

LONG-TERM PROGNOSIS

The prognosis for children with MCD is excellent, and after a few relapses (which do occur in the majority of childhood MCD), many children eventually go into permanent remission. However, this presumed benign course is based on scarce data of patients followed into adulthood. A recent study of 42 adult patients, median age 28 years, who were monitored for a median of 22 years after the diagnosis of MCD, demonstrated that 33% were still relapsing in adulthood. Children who had a relapsing course and/or required immunosuppressive medications were more likely to have persistent disease in adulthood. Moreover, although final height was normal, nearly half of adult patients with relapsing MCD have excess weight gain, hypertension, cataracts, osteoporosis, and sperm abnormalities. Whether MCD has any long term effect on the incidence or age at onset of cardiovascular disease in adults remains unclear. Clinical outcomes in patients enrolled in large health maintenance organizations indicate that persistent NS is associated with an increased incidence of atherosclerotic disease, and the relative risk in patients with MCD versus more refractory forms of idiopathic NS requires further study. Based on the persistence beyond childhood

of relapsing disease and the development of serious side effects, transition from a pediatric to an adult nephrologist is warranted in patients with relapsing MCD or a history of prolonged steroid or immunosuppressive drug use for MCD as they reach adulthood.

The overwhelming majority of children with MCD have no evidence of progressive chronic kidney disease. Recognizing that the diagnosis of FSGS can be difficult to establish if a kidney biopsy specimen does not include the few abnormal glomeruli at the corticomedullary junction, it is conceivable that the rare cases of presumed MCD with a poor outcome and progressive GFR loss may represent unidentified FSGS.

CONCLUSION

Although MCD is not a common illness, it causes short-term morbidity related to edema and infection. Initial treatment with corticosteroids results in remission of proteinuria in nearly all patients; however, 90% of patients will manifest a frequently relapsing or steroid-dependent course with steroid toxicity. These patients are candidates for treatment with second-line agents such as cyclophosphamide, mycophenolate mofetil, or calcineurin inhibitors. The choice of drug will vary from center to center and reflect local experience and preferences of the individual physician. The disease can persist into adulthood and can lead to chronic sequelae such as bone demineralization, atherosclerosis, and obesity. Therefore long-term follow-up is warranted, particularly in patients who continue to relapse and require immunosuppressive medication. Further research is needed to define better the cause of MCD—specifically, the immunologic basis and/or role of podocyte protein abnormalities—so as to develop more effective treatments that can promote long-term remission without the side effects associated with current therapeutic options.

KEY BIBLIOGRAPHY

Clement LC, Avila-Casado C, Macé C, et al. Podocyte-secreted angiopoietin-like-4 mediates proteinuria in glucocorticoid-sensitive nephrotic syndrome. *Nat Med.* 2011;17:117-122.

Fakhouri F, Bocqueret N, Taupin P, et al. Children with steroid-sensitive nephrotic syndrome come of age: long-term outcome. *J Pediatr.* 2005; 147:202-207.

Garin EH, Diaz LN, Mu W, et al. Urinary CD80 excretion increases in idiopathic minimal-change disease. *J Am Soc Nephrol.* 2009;20: 260-266.

Gbadegesin RA, Adeyemo A, Webb NJ, et al. HLA-DQA1 and PLCG2 are candidate risk loci for childhood-onset steroid-sensitive nephrotic syndrome. *J Am Soc Nephrol.* 2015;26:1701-1710.

George B, Verma R, Soofi AA, et al. Crk1/2-dependent signaling is necessary for podocyte foot process spreading in mouse models of glomerular disease. *J Clin Invest.* 2012;122:674-692.

Gulati A, Sinha A, Jordan SC, et al. Efficacy and safety of treatment with rituximab for difficult steroid-resistant and -dependent nephrotic syndrome: multicentric report. *Clin J Am Soc Nephrol.* 2010;5:2207-2212.

Kisner T, Burst V, Teschner S, et al. Rituximab treatment for adults with refractory nephrotic syndrome: a single-center experience and review of the literature. *Nephron Clin Pract.* 2012;120:c79-c85.

Kitamura A, Tsukaguchi H, Hiramoto R, et al. A familial childhood-onset relapsing nephrotic syndrome. *Kidney Int.* 2007;71:946-951.

Kyriels HA, Levtchenko EN, Wetzels JF. Long-term outcome after cyclophosphamide treatment in children with steroid-dependent and frequently relapsing minimal change nephrotic syndrome. *Am J Kidney Dis.* 2007;49:592-597.

McCarthy ET, Sharma M, Savin VJ. Factors in idiopathic nephrotic syndrome and focal segmental glomerulosclerosis. *Clin J Am Soc Nephrol.* 2010;5:2115-2121.

Mubarak M, Kazi JI, Lanewala A, et al. Pathology of idiopathic nephrotic syndrome in children: are the adolescents different from young children? *Nephrol Dial Transplant.* 2012;27:722-726.

Nachman PH, Jennette JC, Falk RJ. Primary glomerular diseases. In: Brenner BM, ed. The Kidney. 8th ed. Philadelphia: W.B. Saunders Company; 2012:987-1279.

Palmer SC, Nand K, Strippoli GF. Interventions for minimal change disease in adults with nephrotic syndrome. *Cochrane Database Syst Rev.* 2008;(1):CD001537.

Sellier-Leclerc AL, Macher MA, Loirat C, et al. Rituximab efficiency in children with steroid-dependent nephrotic syndrome. *Pediatr Nephrol.* 2010;25:1109-1115.

van Husen M, Kemper MJ. New therapies in steroid-sensitive and steroid-resistant idiopathic nephrotic syndrome. *Pediatr Nephrol.* 2011;26:881-892.

Waldman M, Crew RJ, Valeri A, et al. Adult minimal-change disease: clinical characteristics, treatment, and outcomes. *Clin J Am Soc Nephrol.* 2007;2:445-453.

Wei C, El Hindi S, Li J, et al. Circulating urokinase receptor as a cause of focal segmental glomerulosclerosis. *Nat Med.* 2011;17:952-960.

Zhang L, Dai Y, Peng W, et al. Genome-wide analysis of histone H3 lysine 4 trimethylation in peripheral blood mononuclear cells of minimal change nephrotic syndrome patients. *Am J Nephrol.* 2009;30:505-513.

Zhou FD, Chen M. The renal histopathological spectrum of patients with nephrotic syndrome: an analysis of 1523 patients in a single Chinese center. *Nephrol Dial Transplant.* 2011;26:3993-3997.

Zhu L, Yu L, Wang CD, et al. Genetic effect of the NPHS2 gene variants on proteinuria in minimal change disease and immunoglobulin A nephropathy. *Nephrology (Carlton).* 2009;14:728-734.

Full bibliography can be found on www.expertconsult.com.

Focal Segmental Glomerulosclerosis

18

Jeffrey B. Kopp; Avi Z. Rosenberg; H. William Schnaper

Focal segmental glomerulosclerosis (FSGS) is neither a disease nor a syndrome, but rather a set of clinicopathologic syndromes. The shared histopathologic findings include segmental glomerular scars, often with global glomerular tubulointerstitial scarring, no or nonspecific staining by immunofluorescence (usually for immunoglobulin M [IgM] and C3), and no or minimal inflammatory cells in glomeruli or blood vessels. FSGS accounts for approximately 20% of cases of idiopathic nephrotic syndrome in children and as many as 35% of cases in adults. FSGS can present as nephrotic syndrome, nephrotic range proteinuria without other features of nephrotic syndrome, and subnephrotic proteinuria. FSGS is the most common histopathologic pattern of injury in idiopathic nephrotic syndrome among blacks and, in some published series, the most common pattern among all races. Studies in North America have documented increasing prevalence of FSGS in biopsy series over the past several decades. Spontaneous remission of FSGS is rare, and both untreated and treatment-resistant FSGS frequently progress to kidney failure.

CLINICAL FEATURES AND DIAGNOSIS

Proteinuria in FSGS is typically nonselective, consisting of both small and large proteins, including albumin. Edema, hypoalbuminemia, and hyperlipidemia are typically present in primary FSGS while less common in other forms. Hypertension is common, and decreased glomerular filtration rate (GFR) is noted in approximately one-third of patients at presentation. Microscopic hematuria may be present.

Various nosologies of FSGS have been presented over the years; all are somewhat arbitrary and depend on the judgments about where to split or combine categories. We have suggested that FSGS can be usefully classified into six forms and that making these distinctions can have clinical relevance (Table 18.1). These forms are primary, adaptive, APOL1-associated, high-penetrance genetic, virus-associated, and medication-associated FSGS. Not listed here are cases that show a pattern of focal and segmental glomerular scarring that can result from a variety of inflammatory, proliferative, thrombotic, and hereditary conditions. There are situations where the proper diagnostic approach is unclear, including the case of an individual with diabetes with both classic changes of diabetic nephropathy and focal and segmental glomerular scars. We avoid the term secondary in this chapter, as it serves chiefly to distinguish primary disease (unknown cause) from other forms with known cause, although we recognize the term may have utility. Upon receiving a diagnosis of FSGS based on kidney biopsy findings, we believe that it is essential for the clinician to determine which form of FSGS his or her patient might have and to carry out additional diagnostic testing for this purpose.

THE SIX FOCAL SEGMENTAL GLOMERULOSCLEROSIS CLINICAL SYNDROMES

Three FSGS syndromes are most common, with each of these accounting for approximately one third of FSGS in the United States; the distribution will differ in other countries. Distinction among these forms involves collecting clinical history and laboratory data and evaluating kidney biopsy findings (Table 18.2).

Primary FSGS is the form that is least well understood. Many patients have nephrotic proteinuria, often as part of nephrotic syndrome. Primary FSGS is believed to be due to circulating factor(s), with evidence that it may recur following kidney transplant. The causative factor remains elusive, with candidates that include soluble plasminogen activator urokinase-type receptor (suPAR) and cardiotrophin-like cytokine 1.

Adaptive FSGS (perhaps more correctly termed postadaptive FSGS or maladaptive FSGS) arises from an imbalance between glomerular load (i.e., increased glomerular blood flow, arising from diverse factors) and glomerular capacity (i.e., the maximal effective glomerular capillary surface area), resulting in increased glomerular capillary pressures and thus placing podocytes under mechanical stress. Such maladaptive glomerular hemodynamic alterations can arise through (1) a reduction in the number of functioning nephrons (such as after unilateral renal agenesis, surgical ablation, oligomeganephronia, or any advanced primary kidney disease) or (2) mechanisms that place hemodynamic stress on an initially normal nephron population (as in morbid obesity, cyanotic congenital heart disease, and sickle cell anemia). In adaptive FSGS, proteinuria may be nephrotic range or subnephrotic. Plasma albumin concentration may be normal, even in the presence of nephrotic range proteinuria. Renin-angiotensin-aldosterone system antagonism, particularly when coupled with a diuretic and dietary sodium restriction, may have a particularly dramatic effect in reducing proteinuria in adaptive FSGS, and such a response may help confirm the diagnosis.

APOL1 FSGS is due to coding-region variants in the apolipoprotein L1 gene. These variants are termed G1 and G2 and are seen exclusively in individuals of sub-Saharan African descent. While some have advocated calling this entity APOL1-associated FSGS, recent work adds important

Table 18.1   Six Forms of Focal Segmental Glomerulosclerosis

	Mechanism	Setting	Therapy
Primary FSGS	Presumed circulating molecule	Particularly children and young adults	Immunosuppression
Adaptive FSGS	Mismatch between glomerular load and capacity	Premature birth, small for gestational age obesity	RAAS antagonism
APOL1 FSGS	APOL1 alleles	Sub-Saharan African descent	Depends on phenotype
High-penetrance genetic SGS	>40 genes, nuclear and mitochondrial DNA		Most forms: RAAS antagonism
Virus-associated FSGS	HIV, possibly EBV, parvovirus B19		Antiviral therapy or reduced immunosuppression
Medication–associated FSGS	Interferon (APOL1), bisphosphonate, androgens, lithium		Stop the offending agent

EBV, Epstein-Barr virus; *FSGS,* focal segmental glomerulosclerosis; *HIV,* human immunodeficiency virus; *RAAS,* renin-angiotensin, aldosterone system; *SGS,* Schinzel-Giedion syndrome.

Table 18.2   Data Relevant in Evaluating a Patient With the Histologic Diagnosis of Focal Segmental Glomerulosclerosis

Relevant Clinical History	Laboratory Data	Renal Biopsy Findings
Family history of kidney disease	Serum albumin before therapy	FSGS histologic variant
Birth weight	Urine PCR	Glomerular size (glomerulomegaly)
Gestational age at birth	Percent change in urine PCR following maximal renin-angiotensin-aldosterone therapy and dietary sodium restriction	Electron microscopy: Extent of foot process effacement; podocyte microvillus transformation
Congenital cyanotic heart disease		
Sickle cell disease		
History consistent with reflux nephropathy or reduced renal mass	Change in urine PCR following immunosuppressive therapy	Electron microscopy: tubuloreticular inclusions in glomerular endothelial cells (interferon effect)
Peak and present body mass index: obesity, extreme muscular development		
Viral infection: HIV, parvovirus B19, Epstein-Barr virus		
Medication, past or present: interferon, lithium, bisphosphonate, androgen abuse, chronic use of nephrotoxic drugs		

FSGS, Focal segmental glomerulosclerosis; *HIV,* human immunodeficiency virus; *PCR,* protein to creatinine ratio.
Table adapted from Rosenberg A, Kopp J. Focal segmental glomerulosclerosis. *Clin J Am Soc Nephrol.* 2017;12:502–517.

evidence that the APOL1 kidney risk variants cause glomerular injury. The clinical picture of APOL1 FSGS is diverse and can mimic that of other forms of FSGS, which provides the rationale for having its own category. APOL1 FSGS is a specific form of genetic FSGS; APOL1 FSGS subjects often have a family history of FSGS, but given the requirement for an additional provocative factor for kidney disease to manifest, the inheritance pattern of clinical disease is highly variable and complex among families. Further, the high frequency of APOL1 FSGS (APOL1 is the cause of 72% of FSGS in African descent individuals in the United States and South Africa) sets it apart from other forms of genetic FSGS.

The clinical picture of APOL1 FSGS can mimic that of primary FSGS or adaptive FSGS, and it appears likely that the provocative factors that drive each of these two forms can also elicit perhaps accelerated glomerular scarring in individuals with two *APOL1* risk alleles. APOL1 FSGS is also seen with virus-associated FSGS, augmenting risk for FSGS in this setting. Human immunodeficiency (HIV) infection is the most powerful interactor with APOL1 risk alleles,

and carriage of a single *APOL1* risk allele can associate with risk for FSGS, as shown by data from South Africa. APOL1 FSGS can present as a form of medication-associated FSGS, as interferon increases *APOL1* gene expression and induces FSGS in genetically susceptible individuals. Finally, APOL1 FSGS can present in the setting of glomerulonephritides such as in lupus nephritis with collapsing glomerulopathy. At present, therapy for APOL1 FSGS should be based on whether the clinical presentation mimics primary FSGS, adaptive FSGS, virus-associated FSGS, or medication-associated FSGS. For this reason, *APOL1* genetic testing is not clinically indicated at this time. In the future, that recommendation may change when precision therapies are developed that target cellular pathways activated by the *APOL1* risk alleles.

Three other forms of FSGS are less common. High-penetrance genetic variants, with mendelian or mitochondrial inheritance patterns, manifest FSGS, often with a clinical picture that is neither classic for primary nor adaptive FSGS. There are now over 40 genetic loci implicated in FSGS, and more are identified annually. Several viruses cause FSGS.

Uncontrolled HIV infection is associated with HIV-associated nephropathy, a form of collapsing FSGS. Infection with cytomegalovirus is a probable cause of FSGS, and parvovirus B19 and Epstein-Barr virus are possible causes. Certain medications also cause FSGS, including interferons (as mentioned above), anabolic androgenic steroids (likely a form of adaptive FSGS), bisphosphonates, and lithium.

SHARED PATHWAYS OF GLOMERULAR INJURY

In health, the glomerular filtration barrier functions as a highly organized, semipermeable membrane preventing the passage of large proteins into the urine (Chapter 1). This barrier is composed of the glomerular basement membrane, the podocyte with its slit diaphragm connecting adjacent podocyte foot processes (Fig. 18.1). Tubular function assists with the recycling of the small amount of proteins that cross the glomerular barrier, maintaining the normal urine protein excretion <0.2 g daily. In FSGS, particularly primary FSGS, podocytes may lose their normal cytoarchitecture and, ultrastructurally show foot process fusion, the degree of which is reported in routine kidney biopsy reports. This is relevant as the extent of podocyte injury varies across the various forms of FSGS along a spectrum from limited to essentially complete foot process effacement.

With progressive glomerular injury, podocytes are lost from the glomerulus and excreted in the urine. The degree of podocyte depletion appears to correlate with glomerular sclerosis. When a loss of less than 40% is observed in animal models, limited scarring and mild proteinuria are observed; however, loss of more than 40% of podocytes is often associated with severe proteinuria and significant progressive kidney parenchymal scarring. In addition, initial podocyte injuries may be followed by a propagation of the injury to adjacent podocytes, augmenting frank podocyte loss, to cumulatively exceed these critical podocyte-loss thresholds.

The pathogenesis of the glomerular sclerosing lesions in FSGS is not completely understood, but, in recent years, the complexity of the podocyte and slit diaphragm has been partially elucidated, and specific imperfections in the podocyte architectural and functional components have been identified in children and adults with defined genetic polymorphisms. Several podocyte-associated genetic polymorphisms affecting the components of the slit diaphragm, actin cytoskeleton, cell membrane, nucleus, lysosome, mitochondria, and cytosol have been identified (see Fig. 18.1). The frequency of these polymorphisms varies by phenotype and by ancestry.

Another major potential contributor to glomerular disease is the role of the normal circulating factors in plasma that directly or indirectly influences glomerular function in health and disease. In FSGS, the presence of a circulating factor that results in podocyte effacement and disruption of the glomerular filtration barrier has been suggested for decades. Evidence supporting the presence of a circulating factor is derived from clinical cases that have reported virtual immediate recurrence of massive proteinuria following kidney transplantation as well as from studies with animal models that have demonstrated that plasma from patients with FSGS can increase glomerular permeability to albumin. Using an in vitro assay, Savin and colleagues were the first to demonstrate significantly increased albumin permeability of isolated glomeruli when exposed to plasma from patients with FSGS,

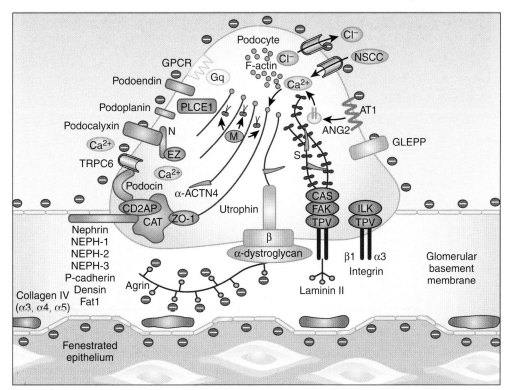

Fig. 18.1 Podocyte cytoarchitecture. (Reprinted with permission from Winn MP. 2007 Young Investigator Award: TRP'ing into a new era for glomerular disease. *J Am Soc Nephrol.* 2008;19:1071–1075.)

yet the specific molecular characteristics and mechanism of action of this permeability factor remained elusive. suPAR has been proposed as a recurrent FSGS factor, but other groups have challenged this finding; if suPAR does contribute to FSGS recurrence, its role is more complicated than initially believed, and recent studies are providing a better picture of the role for suPAR in FSGS.

A single circulating permeability factor may be inadequate to disrupt the filtration barrier. Accordingly, others have hypothesized that a large number of circulating proteins have pro- or antiproteinuric effects on normal glomeruli and that changes in the relative ratio of these circulating proteins may be the major determinant of proteinuria in disease states. In fact, it may be more unlikely that any single protein would cause any specific disease. It is more likely that some particular glomerular diseases have characteristic circulating proteomes that influence the pathogenesis. Other potential soluble proteins implicated in glomerular disease include cardiotrophin-like cytokine, angiopoietin-like-4, vascular endothelial growth factor, and hemopexin.

PATHOLOGY

The kidney biopsy may provide additional pathologic clues that allow for differentiation of primary FSGS from other forms. Fundamentally, FSGS is a segmental solidification of the glomerular tuft with loss of capillary lumina in the sclerosed segment. Early in the disease process, the pattern of glomerular sclerosis is *focal*, involving a subset of glomeruli, and *segmental*, involving a portion of the glomerular tuft, so it may be missed in superficial samples. A more diffuse and global pattern of scarring is usually seen as the disease progresses, which can make it difficult to label the underlying process as FSGS. The actual histologic spectrum of FSGS, however, is diverse. The ultrastructural finding is of importance as well. In FSGS there is glomerular podocyte damage and foot process effacement, which may be patchy in nonprimary forms of FSGS to diffuse in primary processes. It is likely that the podocyte injury pattern of FSGS represents a common pathway for the various forms of FSGS. Because areas of segmental scarring can be observed in a variety of other primary glomerulonephritides, assessing the biopsy for an absence of immune complexes in glomeruli and correlation with systemic findings is critical. In primary FSGS, effacement of the podocytes is typically diffuse and extensive. In HIV-associated nephropathy and other forms of viral FSGS, there is often a collapsing variant of glomerulosclerosis with global rather than segmental involvement along with tubuloreticular inclusions noted on electron microscopy. In patients with remnant kidneys or other forms of adaptive FSGS, glomerular enlargement, perihilar location of segmental scars, arteriolar hyalinosis, and incomplete effacement of the foot processes are often noted (Fig. 18.2).

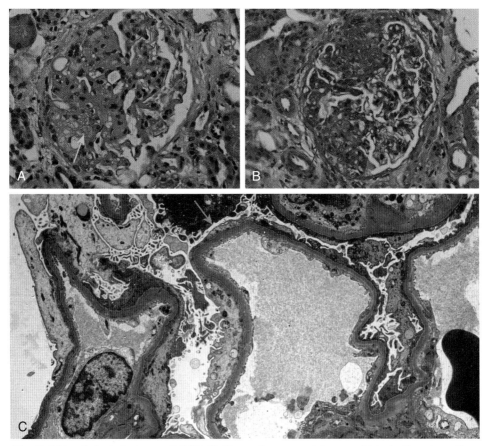

Fig. 18.2 Morphologic features of FSGS. (A) Glomerulus segmentally consolidated with endocapillary foam cells (*blue arrow,* H&E). (B) Hypertrophied podocytes cap segmental consolidated area (*red arrow,* PAS). (C) Podocyte foot processes are fused *(orange arrow)*, and there is focal microvillous transformation (*green arrow,* electron microscopy).

In an effort to classify the histologic spectrum of glomerular lesions associated with FSGS, the Columbia classification for FSGS was put forth. The five discrete histologic patterns of FSGS include the perihilar variant, cellular variant, glomerular tip lesion, collapsing variant, and not otherwise specified (NOS) if none of the features of the other four is present. Several of these patterns may occur in the same biopsy; the pattern with the most adverse prognosis is considered the principal diagnosis as will be discussed shortly. Although the appearance of the glomerular tuft differs in these forms, all share the common feature of podocyte alterations at the ultrastructural level. New insights point toward the conclusion that these morphologic variants may reflect pathogenetic differences and, to some degree, different causes of podocyte injury.

The morphologic classification of FSGS variants may provide prognostic information (Box 18.1). For example, collapsing FSGS exhibits a more aggressive clinical course, with fewer remissions, more frequent kidney failure, and recurrence in the allograft following kidney transplantation, whereas the tip lesion identifies a subset of FSGS that usually responds to steroids and rarely progresses to kidney failure. The cellular lesion is the least common variant of FSGS, identified in only 3% of cases of adult idiopathic FSGS, and the condition is similarly rare in children. This variant is a challenging histopathologic diagnosis to render, and the prognostic significance of cellular FSGS remains unclear. The cellular, collapsing, and tip lesions all share clinical presenting features of heavier proteinuria and more frequent nephrotic syndrome compared with FSGS NOS, suggesting that these three morphologic variants may reflect acute glomerular injury, or possibly a response to heavy proteinuria. However, the prognostic value of morphologic classification of FSGS is not universally acknowledged, reflecting the inherent difficulty of accurately classifying focal patterns of injury based on pathologic examination of limited biopsy tissue and the potential for different types of lesions to coexist in individual biopsy samples.

CLINICAL COURSE

Spontaneous remissions are rare in patients with primary FSGS, occurring in fewer than 5% of patients; if untreated and/or unresponsive, the disease course is typically one of progressive proteinuria and loss of kidney function. Primary and APOL1 FSGS often progress to end-stage kidney disease over a period of 5 to 10 years in perhaps 50% of patients; prognosis appears similar among children and adults. Furthermore, these forms of FSGS may recur after transplantation, contributing significantly to loss of graft function. A rapidly progressive course to kidney failure in the native kidneys predicts a greater risk for recurrence following kidney transplant. The presence of high-penetrance genetic polymorphisms is associated with a lower risk for posttransplant recurrence compared with primary FSGS but is also suggestive of a reduced opportunity for response to immunomodulating therapy. However, partial responses to immunosuppression have been described in children and adults with FSGS-associated genetic polymorphisms. Furthermore, particular forms of genetic FSGS are amenable to targeted therapy, such as coenzyme Q10 supplementation for mitochondrial disorders.

Several clinical and histologic features can be informative with respect to predicting disease course. Female sex appears to be protective and is associated with both slower progression as well as a higher likelihood of a partial or complete remission as compared with men. In contrast, APOL1 FSGS often has an aggressive course, sometimes despite an apparent response to therapy as demonstrated by a reduction in proteinuria. Severe nephrotic-range proteinuria (>10 g/24 hours), impaired kidney function, and increased tubulointerstitial damage on kidney biopsy at the time of presentation all portend a poor prognosis. The collapsing variant is also associated with more rapid progression, whereas the tip lesion, which tends to be responsive to immunosuppression, has a better prognosis. During the course of treatment of FSGS, absence of any response to immunosuppressive therapy is the strongest predictor of a poor prognosis, whereas complete remission of the nephrotic syndrome with normalization of urine protein excretion confers the best prognosis. However, even a partial response to treatment is associated with a significant delay in kidney disease progression and is therefore an acceptable treatment goal. Relapse is common (>50%) and is subsequently associated with more rapid progression and poor kidney survival.

Box 18.1 Morphologic Classification of Focal Segmental Glomerulosclerosis

Perihilar Variant

Perihilar sclerosis and hyalinosis in more than 50% of segmentally sclerotic glomeruli

Tip Lesion

At least one segmental, either cellular or sclerosing, lesion involving the outer 25% of the glomerulus next to the origin of the proximal tubule

Collapsing Variant

At least one glomerulus with segmental or global collapse and overlying podocyte hyperplasia

Cellular Variant

At least one glomerulus with segmental endocapillary hypercellularity occluding lumina with or without foam cells and karyorrhexis

Not Otherwise Specified

At least one glomerulus with segmental increase in matrix obliterating capillary lumina (excludes other variants)

Modified from D'Agati VD, Fogo AB, Bruijn AJ, Jennette JC. Pathologic classification of focal segmental glomerulosclerosis: a working proposal. *Am J Kidney Dis*. 2004;43:368–382.

THERAPY

The treatment of primary FSGS is controversial because of the paucity of randomized, controlled trials and the lack of effective, well-tolerated treatment options (Table 18.3). In

Table 18.3 Overview of Treatment Options for Focal Segmental Glomerulosclerosis

Setting	Therapy	Comment
Nephrotic forms of primary FSGS,* APOL1 FSGS, certain steroid-sensitive FSGS	Prednisone, initially daily or alternate day*	Alternate for patients at high risk for steroid complications include calcineurin inhibitors, mycophenolate mofetil
Steroid-resistant FSGS with nephrotic syndrome*	Calcineurin inhibitor* (cyclosporine and possibly tacrolimus)	—
Refractory FSGS with nephrotic syndrome*	Mycophenolate mofetil ± high-dose dexamethasone*	—
All forms of FSGS with subnephrotic proteinuria	ACE inhibitor or angiotensin receptor blocker, possibly combined with adolsterone antagonist, dietary sodium restriction	Thiazide diuretic may potentiate the antiproteinuric of RAAS antagonism

Recommendations from the Kidney Disease Improving Outcomes Global Initiatives for idiopathic FSGS with nephrotic syndrome are marked with asterisks (*) and are extended here to other forms of FSGS as shown. Cyclosporine has been shown effective in randomized controlled trials of FSGS, while tacrolimus has not. These recommendations would apply, when nephrotic syndrome is present, to primary FSGS, APOL1 FSGS, and certain rare forms of genetic FSGS that may be steroid sensitive.
FSGS, Focal segmental glomerulosclerosis; *RAAS,* renin-angiotensin-aldosterone system.
Table adapted from Rosenberg A, Kopp J. Focal segmental glomerulosclerosis. *Clin J Am Soc Nephrol.* 2017;12:502–517.

patients with nephrotic syndrome, immunosuppression may improve proteinuria and slow progression to kidney failure, but side effects associated with current treatment options, including high doses and prolonged courses of glucocorticoids, cytotoxic agents, and calcineurin inhibitors, are significant, and treatment failure and relapses are common. Immunosuppression typically is not used in primary FSGS with subnephrotic-range proteinuria or in FSGS with a suspected secondary cause; conservative management principles, which target symptoms, are preferred.

Prednisone is the first line of therapy in children and many adults, largely based on data from observational cohorts. The optimal dose and duration of therapy remain uncertain and therefore vary widely across clinical centers. Daily steroid regimens as well as alternate-day regimens have been used. On average, a response is seen within 3 to 4 months, although adults can take longer to respond. Thus, although the minimum requirement of glucocorticoid exposure to define lack of response and resistance remains unclear, many practitioners would define steroid resistance as at least 8 to 16 weeks of therapy without significant improvement in urine protein.

Among children, 20% to 25% experience a complete remission with glucocorticoids. Response rates in adults are lower, and intolerance to steroid therapy tends to be more significant, especially in the presence of advanced age and comorbid conditions such as obesity and diabetes. Steroid resistance, even with prolonged treatment, occurs in more than 50% of adult patients. Prolonged courses of high-dose steroids can result in significant side effects including, but not limited to, cataracts, skin thinning, acne, diabetes, osteoporosis/osteonecrosis, and weight gain, regardless of age.

Cytotoxic agents such as cyclophosphamide have been used with success in children with relapsing and remitting disease and in adults who have demonstrated at least a partial response to prednisone therapy; however, these agents carry significant immediate and long-term risks including infection, propensity to late-onset malignancy, and infertility. Thus in patients with steroid resistance or intolerance, calcineurin

inhibitors are generally second-line therapy and first-line therapy for subjects with primary FSGS who are at increased risk for steroid-associated adverse events. In one randomized controlled trial in steroid-resistant FSGS, patients were randomized to continue on low-dose prednisone either alone or in combination with cyclosporine. The therapy was continued for 26 weeks and then tapered over 4 weeks. The response rate in the cyclosporine-treated patients exceeded 70%, but relapses after discontinuation of therapy were common, exceeding 50%. In a larger randomized trial conducted over 12 months, only 46% of participants experienced a combined complete and partial remission in response to cyclosporine, and 33% relapsed following discontinuation of cyclosporine. In smaller studies, similar rates of complete and partial remission in patients with steroid-resistant or steroid-dependent nephrotic syndrome are seen for tacrolimus and cyclosporine; accordingly, tacrolimus can be considered an alternative calcineurin inhibitor. Calcineurin inhibitors should be used with caution in patients with significant vascular or interstitial disease noted on kidney biopsy and in patients who have an estimated GFR of less than 40 mL/min per 1.73 m² because of the greater potential to cause nephrotoxicity, hyperkalemia, and hypertension in this population.

Other therapeutic options include mycophenolate mofetil (MMF) or rituximab. A randomized controlled trial of children and adults with steroid-resistant FSGS showed that the combination of a 12-month course of MMF with high-dose dexamethasone induced a 33% combined partial and complete remission. Following discontinuation of MMF and dexamethasone, 18% relapsed, demonstrating only a modest improvement with prolonged dexamethasone exposure and MMF. In two randomized controlled trials involving Italian children, rituximab reduced proteinuria in treatment-dependent nephrotic syndrome but did not reduce proteinuria in children with treatment-resistant nephrotic syndrome. A randomized trial involving Indian adults compared prednisolone versus MMF plus low-dose prednisolone and found the latter reach remission faster, with reduced glucocorticoid dose. In kidney allografts, plasma exchange has been successful in treating some patients with recurrent FSGS.

The cornerstone of treatment for adaptive and genetic FSGS is renin-angiotensin-aldosterone system (RAAS) antagonism, which reduces intraglomerular capillary hydrostatic pressure by reducing tone in the efferent glomerular arteriole; this approach should benefit all forms of FSGS (see Table 18.3). The ACE Inhibition in Progressive Renal Disease analysis examined prior studies of proteinuria, excluding studies of diabetes, and showed a benefit to slow progression. In the Effect of Strict Blood Pressure Control and ACE Inhibition on the Progression of CRF in Pediatric Patients (ESCAPE) trial involving children with proteinuric kidney disease, use of an angiotensin converting enzyme inhibitor (ACEi) was associated with slowed progression of GFR loss, and the effect was greatest in those with hypertension, reduced GFR, proteinuria.

A single RAAS agent may be sufficient. Dual blockage with ACEi and an angiotensin receptor blocker (ARB) has been associated with inferior outcomes in older patients with vascular disease or diabetes in the ONTARGET (Ongoing Telmisartan Alone and in conjunction with Ramipril Global Endpoint trial) study, but these results may be irrelevant for the child or young adult with FSGS. Another approach would be to combine an ACEi or ARB with an aldosterone antagonist (spironolactone or eplerenone), together with a thiazide diuretic and dietary sodium restriction to potentiate the antiproteinuric effects, although there are no published data to support this regimen in FSGS. For those with obesity, weight loss may be beneficial.

There are no studies in FSGS addressing blood pressure target. Blood pressure targets for adults with chronic kidney disease (CKD) are below 140/90 mm Hg according to JNC8 recommendations. Data from the African American Study of Kidney Disease and Hypertension (AASK) study suggest a target of 130/70 mm Hg, although this result is suggested based on a subgroup analysis of AASK participants with proteinuria. The recent Systolic Blood Pressure Intervention Trial (SPRINT trial), enrolling hypertensive adults with additional cardiovascular risk factors, found cardiovascular benefit from a systolic blood pressure target of 120 mm Hg but excluded patients with heavy proteinuria. For children with CKD, blood pressure reduction to the 50th percentile for age is associated with slower disease progression.

Control of dyslipidemia with diet and pharmacologic therapy is recommended, and fluid retention and edema may be improved with salt restriction and diuretics. Although the risk of venous thromboembolism is highest in patients with membranous nephropathy, patients with FSGS are also at an increased risk of venous thromboembolism; risk factors include higher hematocrit and relapse of nephrotic syndrome.

ACKNOWLEDGMENT

This work was supported in part by the NIDDK Intramural Research Program, NIH, Bethesda, MD (JBK) and NCATS grant TL1 TR001423 (HWS).

BIBLIOGRAPHY

Brown EJ, Pollak MR, Barua M. Genetic testing for nephrotic syndrome and FSGS in the era of next-generation sequencing. *Kidney Int.* 2014;85:1030-1038.

Cattran DC, Appel GB, Hebert LA, et al. A randomized trial of cyclosporine in patients with steroid-resistant focal segmental glomerulosclerosis. North America Nephrotic syndrome study group. *Kidney Int.* 1999;56:2220-2226.

Chandra P, Kopp JB. Viruses and collapsing glomerulopathy: a brief critical review. *Clin Kidney J.* 2013;6:1-5.

Cravedi P, Kopp JB, Remuzzi G. Recent progress in the pathophysiology and treatment of FSGS recurrence. *Am J Transplant.* 2013;13:266-274.

D'Agati VD. Pathobiology of focal segmental glomerulosclerosis: new developments. *Curr Opin Nephrol Hypertens.* 2012;21:243-250.

D'Agati VD, Kaskel FJ, Falk RJ. Focal segmental glomerulosclerosis. *N Engl J Med.* 2011;365:2398-2411.

Fogo AB. Causes and pathogenesis of focal segmental glomerulosclerosis. *Nat Rev Nephrol.* 2015;11:76-87.

Gipson DS, Trachtman H, Kaskel FJ, et al. Clinical trial of focal segmental glomerulosclerosis in children and young adults. *Kidney Int.* 2011;80:868-878.

Kashgary A, Sontrop JM, Li L, Al-Jaishi AA, Habibullah ZN, Alsolaimani R, Clark WF. The role of plasma exchange in treating post-transplant focal segmental glomerulosclerosis: a systematic review and meta-analysis of 77 case-reports and case-series. *BMC Nephrol.* 2016;17:104.

Konigshausen E, Sellin L. Circulating permeability factors in primary focal segmental glomerulosclerosis: a review of proposed candidates. *Biomed Res Int.* 2016;2016:3765608.

Kopp JB, Nelson GW, Sampath K, et al. APOL1 genetic variants in focal segmental glomerulosclerosis and HIV-associated nephropathy. *J Am Soc Nephrol.* 2011;22:2129-2137.

Lovric S, Ashraf S, Tan W, Hildebrandt F. Genetic testing in steroid-resistant nephrotic syndrome: when and how? *Nephrol Dial Transplant.* 2016;31:1802-1813.

Meyrier A. Focal and segmental glomerulosclerosis: multiple pathways are involved. *Semin Nephrol.* 2011;31:326-332.

Mondini A, Messa P, Rastaldi MP. The sclerosing glomerulus in mice and man: novel insights. *Curr Opin Nephrol Hypertens.* 2014;23:239-244.

Rosenberg A, Kopp J. Focal segmental glomerulosclerosis. *Clin J Am Soc Nephrol.* 2017;12:502-517.

Rosenberg AZ, Naicker S, Winkler CA, Kopp JB. HIV-associated nephropathies: epidemiology, pathology, mechanisms and treatment. *Nat Rev Nephrol.* 2015;11:150-160.

Schell C, Huber TB. New players in the pathogenesis of focal segmental glomerulosclerosis. *Nephrol Dial Transplant.* 2012;27:3406-3412.

Sethna CB, Gipson DS. Treatment of FSGS in children. *Adv Chronic Kidney Dis.* 2014;21:194-199.

Thomas DB, Franceschini N, Hogan SL, et al. Clinical and pathologic characteristics of focal segmental glomerulosclerosis pathologic variants. *Kidney Int.* 2006;69:920-926.

Troyanov S, Wall CA, Miller JA, et al. Focal and segmental glomerulosclerosis: definition and relevance of a partial remission. *J Am Soc Nephrol.* 2005;16:1061-1068.

19

Membranous Nephropathy

Daniel C. Cattran; An S. De Vriese; Fernando C. Fervenza

Membranous nephropathy (MN) is the most common cause of adult-onset nephrotic syndrome in the white population. It is characterized by deposition of immune complexes and complement components in the glomerular capillary wall and attendant new basement membrane synthesis. This histologic pattern is more properly called nephropathy than nephritis, because there is rarely any inflammatory response in the glomeruli or interstitium.

Previously, most cases were termed idiopathic; however, we now know that antibodies to the M-type phospholipase A2 receptor (PLA2R) are present in approximately 70% of patients with MN. More recently, antibodies against another podocyte antigen, the thrombospondin type-1 domain containing 7A (THSD7A), have been described in a minority of patients with MN that are negative for anti-PLA2R antibodies. Taken together, autoantibodies to podocyte-specific antigens account for approximately 80% of the patients with MN, and these cases should be called primary MN. In the remaining 20%, the disease is secondary to a variety of disorders (Table 19.1). The idiopathic designation is made by exclusion and should be reserved for patients who are anti-PLA2R/THSD7A negative and for whom a causative agent cannot be determined. The list of known secondary causes of MN in Table 19.1 is not complete but provides an indication of the wide array of conditions associated with this histologic pattern. In some, such as hepatitis B or thyroiditis, the specific antigen has been identified as part of the immune complex within the deposits in the glomeruli. In others, the association is less well defined, but the designation remains, because treatment of the underlying condition or removal of the putative agent results in resolution of the clinical and histologic features of the disease. In older patients, neoplasms are the most common cause of secondary MN. Recent studies show an association between the presence of anti-THSD7A antibodies and malignancy-associated MN. In the largest cohort of 25 patients with positive anti-THSD7A antibodies, 7 were found to have a malignant tumor. As such, patients with anti-THSD7A–associated MN should be carefully screened for malignancy.

The clinical manifestations of both primary and secondary MN are similar. Hence a careful history, laboratory evaluation, and review of histologic features must be pursued to rule out potential secondary causes. Ongoing vigilance is also necessary, because the causative agent may not be obvious for months or even years after presentation. For example, in about 45% of malignancy-associated MN, kidney disease antedates the diagnosis of malignancy; in 40%, there is a simultaneous presentation; and in the remaining 10%, MN appears after the diagnosis of malignancy.

Primary MN is rare in children. In pediatric MN cases, a careful screening for other types of immunologically mediated disorders, especially systemic lupus erythematosus (SLE), is necessary. In very young children, the diagnosis of MN should raise the possibility of bovine serum albumin (BSA)–induced MN.

There are also marked geographic differences in etiology. The prevalence of anti-PLA2R antibodies in primary MN is lower in Japanese patients (<50%). Other factors impacting geographic variation include malaria in Africa and hepatitis B in East Asia. Universal hepatitis B vaccination has greatly reduced childhood MN associated with hepatitis B.

CLINICAL FEATURES

MN presents in 60% to 70% of cases with features associated with the nephrotic syndrome, such as edema, proteinuria greater than 3.5 g/day, hypoalbuminemia, and hyperlipidemia. The other 30% to 40% of cases present with asymptomatic proteinuria, usually in the subnephrotic range (≤3.5 g/day). The majority of patients present with normal glomerular filtration rate (GFR), but about 10% have diminished kidney function. The urine sediment is often bland, although microscopic hematuria is common. Hypertension is uncommon at presentation, occurring in only 10% to 20% of cases. The clinical features associated with nephrotic range proteinuria in MN can be severe; patients with MN almost always have ankle swelling, and ascites, pleural, and rarely pericardial effusions may also be present. This pattern is particularly common in the elderly, and, unless a urinalysis is performed, these symptoms may be incorrectly labeled as signs of primary cardiac failure. Complications of MN include thromboembolic events and cardiovascular events. A recent study showed that clinically apparent venous thromboembolic events affect about 8% of MN patients, with renal vein thrombosis accounting for 30% of the thromboembolic events. This frequency is substantially lower than that previously reported in studies that used systematic screening for thromboembolic events. Secondary hyperlipidemia is common and characterized by an increase in total and low-density lipoprotein (LDL) cholesterol and often a decrease in high-density lipoproteins (HDLs), a profile associated with increased atherogenic risk.

PATHOLOGY

In early MN, glomeruli appear normal by light microscopy. Increasing the size and number of immune complexes in

Table 19.1 Secondary Causes of Membranous Nephropathy

Etiology	Examples
Neoplasm	Carcinomas, especially solid organ (tumors of the lung, colon, breast, and kidney), leukemia, and non-Hodgkin lymphoma
Infections	Malaria, hepatitis B and C, secondary or congenital syphilis, leprosy
Drugs	Penicillamine, gold
Immunologic	Systemic lupus erythematosus, mixed connective tissue disease, thyroiditis, dermatitis herpetiformis, sarcoidosis
Post kidney transplant	Recurrent disease, de novo membranous nephropathy
Miscellaneous	Sickle cell anemia
Bovine serum albumin	In children

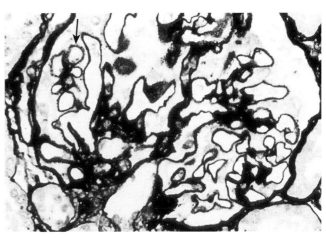

Fig. 19.2 Classic spike pattern along glomerular basement membrane as it grows around deposits (*arrow*; periodic acid–Schiff, original magnification ×400).

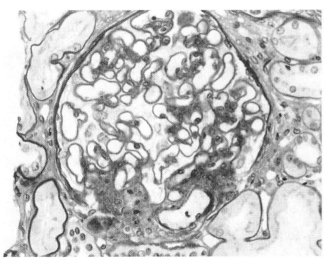

Fig. 19.1 Glomerulus from a patient with membranous nephropathy. Capillary walls are diffusely thickened, and there is no increase in mesangial cells or matrix (periodic acid–Schiff, original magnification ×250).

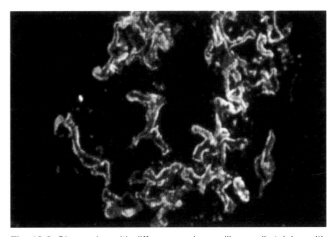

Fig. 19.3 Glomerulus with diffuse granular capillary wall staining with antiimmunoglobulin G antibody (immunofluorescence microscopy, original magnification ×250).

the subepithelial space produces a thickening as well as a rigid appearance of the normally lacy-looking glomerular basement membrane (GBM) on light microscopy (Fig. 19.1). Over time, new basement membrane is formed around the immune complexes (deposits do not stain), producing the spikes along the epithelial side of the basement membrane, which are particularly well visualized when using the silver methenamine stains (Fig. 19.2). In contrast, on immunofluorescence microscopy, these immune complexes do stain, most commonly with antihuman immunoglobulin G (IgG) and complement C3 (Fig. 19.3). This produces a beaded appearance along the GBM (capillary wall), a pattern that is pathognomonic of MN on immunofluorescence. In the most extreme cases, this beading can become so dense that careful examination is required to distinguish it from a linear pattern. On electron microscopy, the majority of cases show extensive podocyte foot process effacement, even at the early stages (Fig. 19.4).

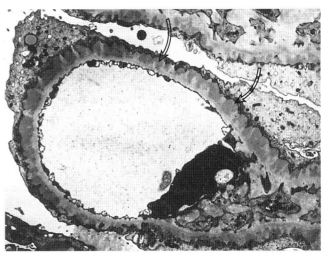

Fig. 19.4 Electron photomicrograph of capillary loop with multiple electron-dense deposits along the subepithelial side of the glomerular basement membrane (*arrows*; original magnification ×7500).

Immune complex deposits are initially formed in the subepithelial space, which explains why a proliferative response, as in a glomerulonephritis, does not occur in MN. A classification system has been developed based on their specific location on electron microscopic examination. In stage I, deposits are located only on the surface of the GBM in the subepithelial location, without evidence of new basement membrane formation; in stage II, deposits are partially surrounded by new basement membranes; in stage III, they are surrounded and incorporated into the basement membrane; and in stage IV, the capillary walls are diffusely thickened, but rarefaction (lucent) zones are seen in intramembranous areas previously occupied by the deposits. Unfortunately, the clinical and laboratory correlations with these stages are poor. In some individual cases of MN, the electron microscopic pattern appears as if there had been waves of complex deposition, with all of the preceding stages present in the same glomerulus. In others cases, deposits appear as if there had been a continuous production of complexes with growth in size over time, producing lesions that are all at a similar stage and that can extend from the surface of the subepithelial space and penetrate all the way through the basement membrane.

Features that favor a secondary cause of MN, in particular an autoimmune disease, include (1) proliferative features (mesangial or endocapillary); (2) full-house pattern of Ig staining (G, M, and A), including staining for C1q on immunofluorescence microscopy; (3) electron dense deposits in the subendothelial location of the capillary wall and mesangium or along the tubular basement membrane and vessel walls; and (4) endothelial tubuloreticular inclusions on electron microscopy. Electron microscopy showing only few superficial scattered subepithelial deposits may suggest a drug-induced secondary MN. Additional diagnostic value may be obtained by staining kidney biopsies for IgG subclasses. IgG1, IgG2, and IgG3 tend to be expressed in lupus MN. IgG4 tends to be more commonly expressed in primary MN and absent in MN secondary to malignancy.

PATHOGENESIS

Over the past decade, major advances have occurred in our understanding of the autoimmune processes involved in the development of human MN.

ANTINEUTRAL ENDOPEPTIDASE ANTIBODIES

The first breakthrough involved a case report of a patient with neonatal MN caused by transplacental transfer of circulating antineutral endopeptidase antibodies. Neutral endopeptidase (NEP) is a membrane-bound enzyme that is able to digest biologically active peptides and is expressed on the surface of human podocytes, syncytiotrophoblastic cells, lymphoid progenitors, and many other epithelial cells, as well as polymorphonuclear leukocytes. Mothers with truncating mutations of the metallomembrane endopeptidase (MME) gene fail to express NEP on cell membranes. NEP-deficient mothers, who were immunized during pregnancy, were able to transplacentally transfer nephritogenic antibodies against NEP to their children, causing MN in the newborns. Rabbits injected with the maternal IgG from

these mothers also developed MN, providing additional proof that the disease is related to circulating anti-NEP antibodies.

ANTIBOVINE SERUM ALBUMIN ANTIBODIES

High levels of circulating anti-BSA antibodies of both IgG1 and IgG4 subclasses have been reported as a cause of secondary MN in children and adults. BSA immunopurified from the serum of children migrated in the basic range of pH, whereas the BSA from adult patients migrated in the neutral region as native BSA. BSA staining colocalized with IgG immune deposits only in four children with circulating cationic BSA but in none of the adults with MN for whom biopsy specimens were available, implying that only cationic BSA can induce MN.

ANTI–M-TYPE PHOSPHOLIPASE A2 RECEPTOR ANTIBODIES

The M (muscle)-type phospholipase A2 receptor (PLA2R) is a member of the mannose receptor family and is composed of an N-terminal cysteine-rich (ricin B) domain, a fibronectin-like II domain, eight C-type lectin-like domains (CTLD), a transmembrane region, and a short cytoplasmic tail containing motifs used in endocytic recycling. Anti-PLA2R antibodies are present in 50% to 80% of adult patients with primary MN and a lesser proportion of affected children. These antibodies are not present in the serum of healthy controls or in patients with other kidney or systemic diseases, yielding a 100% specificity for the lesion of MN. In some studies, small numbers of patients with various forms of secondary MN tested positive for anti-PLA2R antibodies. Whether these cases represent true secondary MN, or rather PLA2R-associated MN with coincident secondary disease, requires further investigation.

A growing body of evidence has documented that PLA2R Ab titer tightly correlates with disease activity in MN, although the majority of the studies to date are retrospective. In one study, 75% of patients with active disease were positive for anti-PLA2R antibodies. This contrasted with positivity in only 37% of patients in partial remission and 10% of patients in complete remission. Remission is reported to occur in 50% of patients with low titers but in only 30% of patients with high titers of anti-PLA2R antibodies at the time of diagnosis. High titers of anti-PLA2R antibody have also been associated with lower response rates and longer time to remission. Antibody titers at the time of clinical remission also correlate with the rate of relapse: patients who become anti-PLA2R negative after immunosuppressive treatment have lower relapse rates than patients who remain positive at the end of treatment. Anti-PLA2R levels may indicate which patients presenting with subnephrotic range proteinuria are likely to progress to full nephrotic syndrome. Moreover, high anti-PLA2R antibodies levels are associated with a high risk of kidney failure over time. In one study, more than 50% of patients with high anti-PLA2R levels had a doubling of serum creatinine over 5-year follow-up. Stratification of patients by antibody levels as low (20 to 86 RU/mL by a commercial enzyme-linked immunosorbent assay [ELISA]), medium (87 to 201 RU/mL), or high (≥202 RU/mL) revealed that after a median follow-up time of 27 months, the clinical end point, defined as an increase of serum creatinine by ≥25% and serum creatinine ≥1.3 mg/dL, was reached in 69% of patients in the high anti-PLA2R antibody levels group, versus in 25% of patients with low antibody levels. Patients with high antibody levels also reached this study end point faster (17.7 months) than patients with low titers (30.9 months). The evolution of PLA2R antibody levels in response to immunosuppression reliably predicts outcome. A decline in levels consistently precedes a decline in proteinuria. Generally, antibody levels decrease rapidly in the first 3 months of treatment and disappear over 6 to 9 months, followed by a remission of proteinuria over 12 to 24 months (or longer, as discussed later), independently of the type of immunosuppressive agent used.

Taken together, these observations strongly suggest that serial quantification of anti-PLA2R antibody levels can help in monitoring disease activity and response to immunosuppressive therapy. When taken in concert with follow-up of proteinuria, antibody testing may allow early intervention and earlier stopping of potent immunosuppressive agents.

Immunofluorescence staining for PLA2R can now be performed on kidney biopsy material. Positive staining mirroring the distribution of immune deposits that are detected on electron microscopy (EM) examination strongly favors primary MN over a secondary form of disease. Some patients may be negative in terms of circulating anti-PLA2R autoantibody at the time of kidney biopsy but still exhibit positive glomerular PLA2R staining. This state could represent completely different phases of the disease, either indicating that PLA2R-associated MN has gone into an immune remission while leaving footprints of the previous immunologic activity or indicating that early disease is present, with the very high affinity between anti-PLA2R autoantibodies and the podocyte antigen, leading to such a rapid depletion of antibodies from the circulation and deposition in the kidney that antibody is not measurable despite active disease.

GENETIC ASSOCIATIONS

Single-nucleotide polymorphisms (SNPs) in the genes encoding M-type PLA2R and HLA complex class II HLA-DQ alpha chain 1 (HLA-DQA1) have been reported in white and Asian populations with MN. The risk for primary MN was significantly higher when both the HLA-DQ1 allele and the PLA2R1 allele were present. Patients carrying one or two alleles for HLA DQA1*05:01 or for DQB1*02:01 have higher anti-PLA2R titers than those with neither of these HLA alleles. A theory has been proposed that the rare confluence of several relatively common factors triggers the development of MN: a particular isoform of HLA-DQA1 that confers increased susceptibility to autoimmunity, polymorphisms in PLA2R1 that alter expression and/or create a unique conformation identified by HLA class II on antigen-presenting cells, and other environmental factors.

ANTITHROMBOSPONDIN TYPE-1 DOMAIN-CONTAINING 7A ANTIBODIES

THSD7A is a transmembrane protein initially described in human endothelial vein cells but also expressed in many organs, including the kidney. The function of THSD7A may relate to binding to extracellular matrix, especially to glycosaminoglycan chains present on matrix proteoglycans.

Immunogold EM has localized the protein within podocytes to the foot process near the slit diaphragm and in endosomal structures. Antibodies against THSD7A, predominantly of the IgG4 subclass, are reported in ~10% of patients with MN that are negative for PLA2R antibodies. So far, anti-THSD7A antibodies have not been detected in healthy controls or in patients with other kidney and systemic diseases, yielding 100% specificity for MN. Limited evidence suggests that, as in the case of PLA2R antibodies, circulating anti-THSD7A antibodies correlate with disease activity and may be used to monitor disease activity in patients with THSD7A-associated disease in the future. A genetic link to the THSD7A locus has not yet been established, possibly because of the small number of cases identified so far. Initially it appeared that anti-PLA2R and anti-THSD7A autoantibodies were mutually exclusive, but several cases of dual antibody positivity have been described. Tissue staining for the THSD7A antigen in kidney biopsies is technically more difficult than the "on or off" pattern described for the PLA2R antigen because a linear staining pattern for THSD7A is seen in normal biopsies and other types of glomerular disease.

DIAGNOSIS

MN is a diagnosis based on histology. Primary/idiopathic and secondary forms have similar clinical presentations. As such, secondary MN should be ruled out by careful history, physical, and laboratory examinations, aided by features on pathology. Investigations should include a complement profile, assays for antinuclear antibodies, rheumatoid factor, hepatitis B surface antigen and hepatitis C antibody, thyroid antibodies, and cryoglobulins. The presence of circulating anti-PLA2R antibodies and/or the detection of PLA2R on kidney biopsies indicates PLA2R-associated MN. Predominance of IgG4 staining strongly suggests primary MN. The assay for anti-THSD7A antibodies is presently not yet commercially available.

Malignancy is associated with MN in approximately 20% of cases in people above 60 years old. More recent epidemiologic data suggest that the standardized incidence ratio of malignancy in MN is in the range of 2 to 3 in all age groups; however, because the absolute incidence of malignancies in younger people is lower, extensive testing for malignancy is not usually performed unless there are clinical clues. In contrast, older patients who present with MN should receive a history and physical examination focused on possible evidence of occult malignancy, especially if they are anti-THSD7A antibody positive. The role of malignancy in anti-PLA2R antibody positive patients is controversial. Positive anti-PLA2R testing has been reported in a minority of patients with MN associated with solid tumors, but oncologic treatment was not accompanied by remission of proteinuria, suggesting that the two processes were not causally related but rather coincidental. The evaluation should consist of most age-appropriate screening tests, including colon cancer screening, mammography, a prostate-specific antigen assay in men, and a chest radiograph (or in high-risk patients, a chest computed tomography). The cost-benefit ratio of this additional screening in the absence of symptoms remains unknown, but, given the dramatic difference in management and outcome, it seems prudent to perform these investigations.

PROGNOSIS OF PRIMARY MEMBRANOUS NEPHROPATHY

NATURAL HISTORY

The natural history of primary MN must be understood before considering specific treatment. Spontaneous complete remissions, defined as a reduction in proteinuria to less than 0.3 g/day, occur in 20% to 30% of patients with primary MN, whereas progressive kidney failure develops in 20% to 40% of cases after more than 5 to 15 years of observation. In the remaining patients, mild to moderate proteinuria persists. A summary review of 11 large studies demonstrated a 10-year kidney survival rate of 65% to 85%, whereas a more recently pooled analysis of 32 reports indicated a 15-year kidney survival rate of 60%. Complicating the understanding of the natural history is the fact that primary MN often follows a spontaneous remitting and relapsing course. Spontaneous complete remission rates have been reported in 20% to 30% of long-term (>10 years) follow-up studies, with 20% to 50% of these cases exhibiting at least one relapse. A complete remission and a lower relapse rate are more common in patients with persistent low-grade (subnephrotic) proteinuria and in women. In contrast, male gender, age greater than 50 years, high levels of proteinuria (more than 6 g/day), abnormal kidney function at presentation, tubulointerstitial disease, and focal and segmental lesions on biopsy are all associated with poorer kidney survival rates.

PREDICTING OUTCOME

Until now, predicting patient outcome has been based on a semiquantitative method that considers the initial creatinine clearance (CrCl), the slope of the CrCl, and the lowest level of proteinuria during a 6-month observation period. The predictive value of the risk score was much greater than that of presence of nephrotic range proteinuria at presentation alone when proteinuria values during 6-month time frames were monitored. When proteinuria was consistently ≥4 g/day, its overall accuracy was 71%; when ≥6 g/day, 79%; and when ≥8 g/day, 84% (Box 19.1). The advantages of the algorithm are that it only requires assessing kidney function and proteinuria, and the risk can be calculated repeatedly during the period of follow-up. Age, sex, degree of nephrosclerosis, and presence of hypertension are relevant but do not add to the predictive ability of this model.

Importantly, proteinuria and serum creatinine may not accurately reflect disease activity. Proteinuria and serum creatinine do not discriminate between immunologically active disease and irreversible structural damage to podocytes and the basement membrane, and a change in proteinuria typically lags behind a change in anti-PLA2R levels by several months. Patients may be judged to be at high risk and exposed to potentially toxic immunosuppressive therapy but could still develop a spontaneous remission. In addition, the observation period required to assess the risk of progression may delay treatment, resulting in significant residual kidney damage. As discussed earlier, the ability for monitoring for PLA2R antibodies has added a new marker that can be used to predict clinical outcomes. Patients with low levels of anti-PLA2R antibodies are more likely to undergo spontaneous

---

Box 19.1   Risk for Progression Based on Proteinuria

Low Risk

Patients with normal serum creatinine/creatinine clearance and proteinuria consistently ≤4 g/24 hours over a 6-month observation period have an excellent long-term renal prognosis.

Medium Risk

Patients with normal and stable kidney function and with proteinuria >4 g but <8 g/24 hours during 6 months of observation have a 55% probability of developing ESRD within 10 years.

High Risk

Patients with persistent proteinuria >8 g/24 hours, independent of the degree of kidney function impairment, have a 66%–80% probability of progression to ESRD within 10 years.

ESRD, End-stage renal disease.

---

remission, suggesting that immunosuppressive treatment may be withheld. On the other hand, persistently elevated or increasing levels of anti-PLA2R antibodies are associated with lower rates of spontaneous remission and an increased risk of progressive loss of kidney function, such that earlier initiation of immunosuppressive treatment should be considered. A serology-based assessment of prognosis for patients with PLA2R-associated MN, that takes into consideration the degree of proteinuria, has been recently been proposed (Fig. 19.5). The hope is that such an approach will improve diagnostic and prognostic accuracy and provide for an individualized treatment of patients with PLA2R-associated MN that will limit unnecessary exposure to immunosuppression. A randomized controlled trial (RCT) comparing the serology-based versus the traditional prognostic approach is needed.

Management of patients with primary MN who are antibody negative is uncertain. Considering that a high proportion of PLA2R and THSD7A-negative patients develop a spontaneous remission, maximizing conservative therapy (discussed later) may be a reasonable initial approach. Studies that have included both anti-PLA2R positive and negative cases seem to indicate a similar natural history and response to treatment for both groups.

RESPONSE GOALS

The treatment target in MN has been debated for some time. Obviously, the best target would be a permanent state of complete remission (<0.3 g/day of proteinuria), but this presently occurs in only 30% to 50% of cases, even when combining spontaneous and drug-induced remissions. However, there is now good evidence that partial remission (<3.5 g/day and a 50% reduction from peak proteinuria) is an appropriate and valid target. Achieving a partial remission is associated with a significant slowing of the decline in kidney function at 10 years when compared with patients who do not experience remission. Most patients experience partial remission, suggesting that the process of remodeling of the GBM may take years to complete and not necessarily reflects

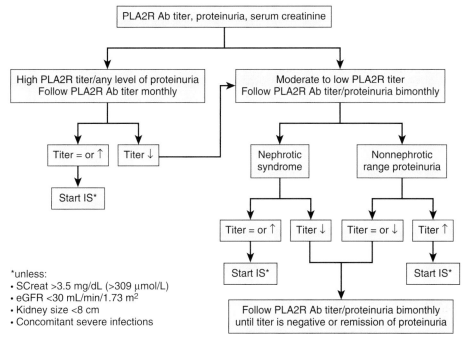

Fig. 19.5 A proposal for a serologic approach to the treatment of antibody positive membranous nephropathy. *eGFR,* Estimated glomerular filtration rate; *IS,* immunosuppression; *PLA2R,* phospholipase A2 receptor; *SCreat,* serum creatinine.

immunologic activity. Repeat biopsy studies in patients who have been successfully treated with rituximab in recurrent MN post kidney transplant showed persistence of deposits containing IgG and complement components for a significant amount of time despite disappearance of circulating anti-PLA2R antibodies. In patients with a history of positive anti-PLA2R or anti-THSD7A antibodies, monitoring these antibodies may help reveal if proteinuria reflects residual damage to the GBM or persistent immunologic disease.

TREATMENT

NONSPECIFIC NONIMMUNOSUPPRESSIVE THERAPY

Nonspecific nonimmunosuppressive treatment involves restricting dietary sodium to less than 2 g/day, restricting protein intake, and controlling blood pressure, hyperlipidemia, and edema; this treatment is applicable to all patients with MN. Blood pressure reduction has been shown to reduce proteinuria and should be part of the management from the time of diagnosis. Angiotensin-converting enzyme (ACE) inhibitors yield improvement in proteinuria beyond that expected by their antihypertensive action alone and, unless there is a specific contraindication, should be a first-line therapy in all cases, even when the blood pressure is not significantly elevated. Angiotensin receptor blockers (ARBs) likely have similar results and should be considered if problems arise with the use of ACE inhibitors. Importantly, evidence that such therapy is beneficial in patients with MN is weak, and the antiproteinuric effect of angiotensin-converting enzyme inhibitors (ACEIs) and ARBs in these patients is modest (<30% decrease from baseline). Although dietary protein restriction has never been associated with a complete

remission of the nephrotic syndrome, it does result in lower levels of proteinuria; however, this needs to be balanced with the risk of malnutrition. Sodium restriction is much more critical, as poor adherence can lead to both an increase in proteinuria and escape from the benefits of renin angiotensin aldosterone system (RAAS) blockade.

TREATMENT FOCUSED ON THE SECONDARY EFFECTS OF MEMBRANOUS NEPHROPATHY

Patients with nephrotic syndrome have elevated total cholesterol and triglycerides, normal or low HDL, and increased LDL. This dyslipidemia probably plays a role in the increased risk for cardiovascular disease in patients with prolonged high-grade proteinuria. Although no trial has been conducted to determine if cholesterol lowering reduces the risk for cardiovascular disease in such patients, most clinicians apply evidence from patients without kidney disease to promote the use of statins in patients with primary MN and persistent high-grade proteinuria. A recent meta-analysis showed a small benefit on proteinuria reduction but no beneficial effect on GFR with statins in these proteinuric conditions.

Studies of the risk for thrombotic disease in primary MN demonstrated a wide variation in prevalence. This is partly related to the rigor of screening (all patients vs. the selection of high-risk patients) and partly to the detection methods used. A study showed that clinically apparent venous thromboembolic events occurred in approximately 7% of patients with primary MN. In this study, a serum albumin level below 2.8 g/dL was the most significant independent predictor of venous thromboembolism. No consensus has emerged as to whether prophylactic anticoagulation should be used in this disease, although a treatment algorithm that assessed risk benefit showed a substantial advantage to prophylactic anticoagulants under these conditions, particularly within the first 2 years of presentation when thromboembolism risk seems highest and if bleeding risk is low. A majority of physicians use anticoagulation as primary prevention only in high-risk cases or reserve its use until after documentation of a thromboembolic event. A proteinuria greater than 10 g/day, positive family history, previous thrombotic event before the patient was known to have MN, prolonged serum albumin levels less than 2 g/dL, bedridden status, or obesity should prompt consideration for the earlier use of prophylactic anticoagulation. The precise mechanism of the hypercoagulable state observed in MN is unclear, although a variety of factors do converge that heighten the thrombotic risk, including a local decrease in perfusion pressure in the renal vein from the lowered oncotic pressure, loss of clotting factors in the urine, increased hepatic production of clotting factors, and perhaps even a genetic predisposition to clot.

IMMUNOSUPPRESSION

As discussed previously, a serology-based approach that takes into consideration anti-PLA2R levels together with the degree of proteinuria will likely be the best way to define prognosis in patients with PLA2R-associated MN. This approach will probably also be applicable to patients with anti-THSD7A–associated MN. Because the majority of the studies regarding the use of immunosuppression in MN were conducted at a time when no antibody testing was available, the evidence presented as follows is based solely on the use of sustained proteinuria as a risk marker for disease progression, although given the commonness of anti-PLA2R positive cases, the treatment benefits are unlikely to be dramatically different.

LOW RISK FOR PROGRESSION

The prognosis for patients with proteinuria ≤4 g/day and with normal kidney function is excellent. In a series of more than 300 cases from three distinct geographic regions followed for more than 5 years, fewer than 8% developed a measurable decrease in kidney function. Normalization of blood pressure and reduction of protein excretion with ACE inhibitors or ARBs should be implemented. Because some patients do progress, long-term follow-up should include regular measurements of blood pressure, kidney function, and proteinuria and should now include monitoring for anti-PLA2R antibodies. Immunosuppression is not recommended, as long as the patient remains in the low risk for progression category. Approximately 50% of patients who present with nonnephrotic proteinuria in MN will eventually progress to nephrotic range proteinuria—most likely those that have high anti-PLA2R levels at presentation. In the majority of cases (70%), this will occur within the first year after diagnosis.

MEDIUM RISK FOR PROGRESSION

Corticosteroid monotherapy appears ineffective in inducing remission of proteinuria in all controlled trials conducted to date and in preventing progression in all but one study.

Although the follow-up periods were limited to less than 4 years, and the dose and duration of corticosteroid treatment varied, it is generally held that steroid monotherapy should not be used in primary MN.

There is evidence for a treatment benefit when corticosteroids are combined with a cytotoxic agent. In a series of RCTs in Italy, a significant increase in both partial and complete remission of proteinuria and preserved kidney function at 10 years was seen after an initial 6-month course of corticosteroids and the alkylating agent, chlorambucil (Ponticelli protocol). Therapy consisted of 1 g of intravenous methylprednisolone on the first 3 days of months 1, 3, and 5, followed by 27 days of oral methylprednisolone at 0.4 mg/kg, alternating in months 2, 4, and 6 with chlorambucil at 0.2 mg/kg per day. This therapeutic regimen was found to be superior to either no treatment or methylprednisolone monotherapy, although in the latter study, the benefit was not significant after 4 years of follow-up. The original regimen was remarkably safe, and all adverse events were reversed after stopping the drugs. When 2.5 mg/kg per day oral cyclophosphamide was substituted for chlorambucil and compared with the original regimen, similar complete and partial remission rates of proteinuria were seen. However, a substantial relapse rate of approximately 30% was seen within 2 years in both groups, regardless of whether they were treated with chlorambucil or cyclophosphamide. Fewer patients had to discontinue cyclophosphamide (5%) compared with chlorambucil (14%). Using this regimen versus conservative therapy, similar long-term results were reported in a trial from India. Regimens using longer term (1 year) cyclophosphamide and lower dose prednisone have also demonstrated an improved outcome, but in these studies the patients were compared with historical controls, and the total cumulative dose of cyclophosphamide far exceeded the total dose used in the Ponticelli protocol.

Initial results of combined use of mycophenolate mofetil (MMF) with high-dose corticosteroids have been similar to cyclophosphamide therapy but with a significantly higher relapse rate after corticosteroids were discontinued (>70% by 3 years posttreatment). Monotherapy with MMF appears ineffective in primary MN.

Cyclosporine has shown results similar to the cytotoxic/steroid regimen in terms of improving proteinuria in the medium risk for progression group. MN patients who remained nephrotic after a minimum of 6 months of observation, and who were unresponsive to a course of high-dose prednisone, were given 6 months of cyclosporine (3 to 5 mg/kg per day) plus low-dose prednisone (maximum 10 mg/day) and were compared with a prednisone-alone/placebo group. Complete or partial remission in proteinuria was seen in 70% of the cyclosporine group compared with 24% of the control group. The relapse rate (40% to 50% within 2 years of discontinuing the drug) was higher than that seen in the Italian trials. A study using a longer duration of cyclosporine treatment at a dose of 2 to 4 mg/kg per day for 12 months, followed by a reduction in the cyclosporine therapy in the range of 1.5 mg/kg per day, showed a much lower relapse rate of approximately 20% within the 2-year period. More recently, a 12-month RCT using tacrolimus monotherapy confirmed the benefit of the calcineurin inhibitors, achieving a partial or complete remission in proteinuria in 75% to 80% of the treated group, as well as a significant slowing of kidney disease progression compared with a control group;

however, nephrotic syndrome reappeared in almost half the patients after tacrolimus withdrawal.

Newer therapeutic options include yearlong injections of synthetic adrenocorticotrophic hormone (ACTH). There have been two small RCTs with this agent showing short-term benefits similar to the results seen with the cytotoxic/steroid regimen, with quite variable adverse effects. A retrospective case series of 11 patients with nephrotic syndrome resistant to previous immunosuppression treated with a natural highly purified ACTH gel formulation (H.P. Acthar Gel), currently approved in the United States for remission of proteinuria in the nephrotic syndrome, reported similar encouraging results. Most patients were treated for a minimum of 6 months, with the longest treatment period being 14 months. Nine of the 11 patients achieved a complete or partial remission. In a more recent study, 20 patients with MN were randomly treated with Acthar Gel, either 40 or 80 IU twice weekly for 120 days. ACTH therapy resulted in a significant reduction in median proteinuria from 9.0 ± 3.3 g/day at baseline to 3.7 ± 4.2 g/day at 12 months. A clear dose-response relationship was also reported, with 80 IU units twice weekly for at least 4 months appearing necessary for maximal effect. The reduction in anti-PLA2R antibodies and the decline in proteinuria correlated in some but not all patients, suggesting a possible direct effect on the podocyte. No serious adverse effects were reported. Although promising, evidence for the efficacy of ACTH in improving long-term kidney outcomes in patients with MN is lacking. It has been suggested that ACTH mediates its effects via melanocortin receptor 1 on podocytes, and this unique interaction may explain why patients who are resistant to previous immunosuppressive therapies respond to ACTH.

Another potential alternative agent is rituximab, a chimeric monoclonal antibody to B cells carrying the CD 20 epitope. Several prospective but nonrandomized pilot studies using rituximab monotherapy have demonstrated complete or partial remission in proteinuria in 60% to 80% of patients by the end of the trial. The great majority of these patients remained in remission long term. A recent study reported that only 18 of the 65 patients treated with rituximab (the majority treated with one single dose) that achieved complete or partial remission had a relapse of proteinuria from 7 to 116 months (median 42 months) after treatment. Lower antibody levels at baseline and full antibody depletion at 6 months after rituximab treatment were strong predictors of remission. In all of the 25 patients that achieved complete remission, it was preceded by complete anti-PLA2R antibody depletion. Reemergence of circulating antibodies predicted disease relapse. A B-cell titrated protocol using a single dose of 375 mg/m^2 rituximab has been proposed to be as effective as the four-dose protocol, at a lower cost. However, recent reports have challenged the success of the single-dose approach. The response to rituximab is independent of patients receiving it as first- or second-line therapy. Rituximab may also allow successful withdrawal of previously calcineurin-inhibitor–dependent patients. Taken in sum, these results suggest that rituximab is effective for inducing remission of proteinuria in a large number of patients with MN, either as initial treatment or for patients refractory to previous therapeutic attempts. The short-term favorable side-effect profile and compliance issues related to this selective therapy seem preferable to the currently used immunosuppressive regimens. There are still some concerns about the long-term effects of rare and fatal complications, including reports of progressive multifocal leukoencephalitis potentially related to B-cell depletion, although to the best of our knowledge, no such case has been reported in patients treated with rituximab monotherapy. A recent RCT of rituximab versus conservative therapy showed no significant difference in remission rate at 6 months, but by 17 months the remission rate in the rituximab group was twice that of the controls. Similar AE rates were reported in both arms and changes in PLA2R titer paralleled proteinuria responsiveness. An RCT testing the efficacy of rituximab versus cyclosporine in the maintenance of remission in MN (MENTOR; ClinicalTrials.gov NCT01180036) is currently under way.

HIGH RISK FOR PROGRESSION

Until recently, this group included patients with worsening kidney function and/or persistent high-grade proteinuria. Given the recent evidence, patients with persistently high anti-PLA2R levels (in the upper tertile) should also be considered high risk. The proportion of patients with primary MN in this category is small, and RCTs focusing on this subgroup are lacking. When an improvement in proteinuria with conservative therapy is not seen within the first 3 months, an earlier start to immunosuppressive therapy is warranted in the majority of cases. Cyclosporine was studied in high-risk MN patients in a small RCT where only 17 of 64 patients in the conservative, pretreatment phase of the study fulfilled the entry criterion of an absolute reduction in kidney function of 10 mL/min in CrCl. These patients were then randomized to either cyclosporine or placebo for 1 year. The patients treated with cyclosporine showed a substantial improvement in proteinuria compared with placebo, which was sustained for ≤2 years in 50% of cases. The rate of progression, as measured by the slope of CrCl, was significantly slowed (by >60%) during cyclosporine treatment, with no improvement in the placebo group. This drug has substantial nephrotoxic potential, and monitoring for nephrotoxicity and other adverse events must be part of any treatment routine that includes this class of agent.

An RCT comparing chlorambucil in conjunction with steroids, cyclosporine, and placebo in patients with MN who had a greater than 20% decline in GFR within 3 to 24 months of study entry found a lower rate of progression in the chlorambucil/steroid group than in both other groups. Significantly more serious adverse events (particularly hematologic issues) were reported in the chlorambucil group. It should be noted that the starting dose of 5 mg/kg/day of cyclosporine used in this study is higher than currently recommended, particularly in patients who already have renal compromise and might have prompted a sudden decrease in estimated glomerular filtration rate (eGFR), which was considered as failure of therapy. The study might thus have underestimated the efficacy of cyclosporine, and in the absence of data on hard kidney end points, no definite conclusions can be made.

Although the algorithm for the management of the high-risk patient (Fig. 19.6) lists the option of switching to a cytotoxic agent plus prednisone regimen if there is a failure to respond to cyclosporine, it must be realized that both options include powerful immunosuppressive agents and carry significant risks. In addition, when GFR is below

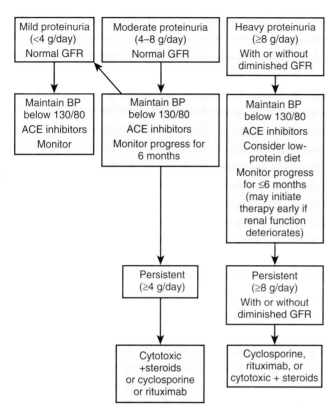

Fig. 19.6 Guideline for the treatment of antibody negative primary membranous nephropathy. Patients may change from one category to another during the course of follow-up. *ACE,* Angiotensin-converting enzyme; *BP,* blood pressure; *GFR,* glomerular filtration rate.

30 mL/min, the dose of cyclophosphamide must be adjusted downward to avoid the risk of significant bone marrow toxicity. Similarly, if the GFR is low (below 30 mL/min per 1.73 m^2) or deteriorating rapidly and/or if the biopsy shows extensive tubular interstitial disease and/or severe vascular changes, calcineurin inhibitors should either be avoided or given with great caution.

Overall, the decision to treat this group of patients is not to be undertaken without carefully weighing the risks and benefits, and often a second opinion is warranted. A repeat biopsy to confirm viable tissue and new subepithelial deposits on EM may help in this difficult situation to consider further treatment.

PROPHYLAXIS OF COMPLICATIONS OF THERAPY

Many large studies in the kidney transplantation field and in postmenopausal women have indicated that agents such as bisphosphonates or supplemental oral calcium and vitamin D reduce bone loss during long-term use of corticosteroids. The use of such agents in primary MN should be considered when a course of therapy includes prolonged prednisone treatment. Trimethoprim-sulfamethoxazole has reduced the incidence of *Pneumocystis jiroveci* infection in patients on prolonged immunosuppressive therapy in both the transplantation field and in certain autoimmune diseases. Its use when the patients with primary MN are exposed to prolonged glucocorticoid treatment, cytotoxic agents, calcineurin inhibitors, or rituximab seems prudent.

MANAGEMENT PLAN FOR PRIMARY MEMBRANOUS NEPHROPATHY

Fig. 19.6 shows a treatment framework for patients with primary MN. In addition, the following general rules should be applied:

1. Establish whether the disease is primary (anti-PLA2R or anti-THSD7A–associated MN) or secondary MN.
2. Patients who are seronegative for anti-PLA2R, kidney biopsy negative for PLA2R antigen, and seronegative for anti-THSD7A may have MN due to still unidentified autoantibodies (idiopathic MN) or may have secondary MN.
3. Antibodies against PLA2R, and possibly antibodies against THSD7A, closely correlate with disease activity. Low baseline and decreasing anti-PLA2R antibody levels strongly predict spontaneous remission, thus favoring conservative therapy.
4. High baseline or increasing anti-PLA2R antibody levels are associated with nephrotic syndrome, lower probability of spontaneous remission, and progressive loss of kidney function, thereby encouraging early initiation of immunosuppressive therapy.
5. Changes in serum anti-PLA2R antibody levels reliably predict response to therapy, and levels at completion of therapy may forecast long-term outcome.
6. Re-emergence of or increase in anti-PLA2R antibody levels predicts clinical relapse, but the timing of these increases is currently largely unknown.
7. For patients who have anti-PLA2R–associated MN, we suggest monitoring proteinuria and antibody levels to guide immunosuppressive therapy (see Fig. 19.5).
8. For patients who are anti-PLA2R negative, we recommend monitoring kidney function during a 6-month period (3 months for the high-risk category patient), establish a risk-for-progression score based on the traditional Toronto proteinuria and kidney function algorithm, and tailor therapy accordingly.
9. Treatment of secondary MN depends on the underlying cause.
10. The first choice specific therapy for patients with a medium risk for progression is cyclophosphamide cycling monthly, with prednisone for 6 months or cyclosporine combined with low-dose prednisone for 6 to 12 months (Kidney Disease: Improving Global Outcomes [KDIGO] guidelines).
11. The first choice specific therapy for high-risk patients defined by high-grade proteinuria but preserved kidney function is cyclosporine for 6 to 12 months. If this fails or if proteinuria is accompanied by low GFR or deteriorating kidney function, a course of cyclophosphamide combined with ≤6 months of prednisone may be considered (KDIGO guidelines).
12. Since the publication of the KDIGO guidelines, there has been considerable evidence for the use of rituximab as equally effective and with lower toxicity than cyclic or calcineurin-based regimes, and this could be considered as alternative initial therapy.
13. ACTH can be considered if all of the above have failed or created intolerable side effects.

14. A significant proportion of the patients who achieved either a partial or complete remission will relapse, especially if they remain anti-PLA2R positive at the time immunosuppression is discontinued. Retreatment with the previously successful regimen (or with one of the other proven regimens if toxicity is a major concern) should be undertaken, but cumulative cyclophosphamide dose should not exceed 36 g (~2 courses of the Poncicelli protocol). This should replace labeling the patient as a treatment failure, because even a partial remission is associated with significantly improved kidney survival.

TREATMENT OF SECONDARY MEMBRANOUS NEPHROPATHY

In the secondary types of MN, attention should be focused on removing the putative agent or treating the underlying cause. If this can be done successfully, both the histopathology and the clinical manifestations typically resolve with time.

KEY BIBLIOGRAPHY

Bech AP, Hofstra JM, Brenchley PE, et al. Association of anti-PLA$_2$R antibodies with outcomes after immunosuppressive therapy in idiopathic membranous nephropathy. *Clin J Am Soc Nephrol.* 2014;9:1386-1392.

Beck LH Jr, Bonegio RG, Lambeau G, et al. M-type phospholipase A2 receptor as target antigen in idiopathic membranous nephropathy. *N Engl J Med.* 2009;361:11-21.

Beck LH Jr, Fervenza FC, Beck DM, et al. Rituximab-induced depletion of anti-PLA2R autoantibodies predicts response in membranous nephropathy. *J Am Soc Nephrol.* 2011;22:1543-1550.

Branten AJ, du Buf-Vereijken PW, Vervloet M, et al. Mycophenolate mofetil in idiopathic membranous nephropathy: a clinical trial with comparison to a historical control group treated with cyclophosphamide. *Am J Kidney Dis.* 2007;50:248-256.

Cattran DC, Appel GB, Hebert LA, et al. Cyclosporine in patients with steroid resistant membranous nephropathy: a randomized trial. *Kidney Int.* 2001;59:1484-1490.

Cattran DC, Greenwood C, Ritchie S, et al. A controlled trial of cyclosporine in patients with progressive membranous nephropathy. Canadian Glomerulonephritis Study Group. *Kidney Int.* 1995;47:1130-1135.

Cravedi P, Ruggenenti P, Sghirlanzoni MC, et al. Titrating rituximab to circulating B cells to optimize lymphocytolytic therapy in idiopathic membranous nephropathy. *Clin J Am Soc Nephrol.* 2007;2:932-937.

Dahan K, Debiec H, Plaisier E, et al. Rituximab for severe membranous nephropathy: a 6-month trial with extended follow-up. *J Am Soc Nephrol.* 2017;28:348-358.

Debiec H, Guigonis V, Mougenot B, et al. Antenatal membranous glomerulonephritis due to anti-neutral endopeptidase antibodies. *N Engl J Med.* 2002;346:2053-2060.

Debiec H, Lefeu F, Kemper MJ, et al. Early-childhood membranous nephropathy due to cationic bovine serum albumin. *N Engl J Med.* 2011;364:2101-2110.

De Vriese AS, Glassock RJ, Nath KA, Sethi S, Fervenza FC. A proposal for a serology-based approach to membranous nephropathy. *J Am Soc Nephrol.* 2017;28:421-430.

Hladunewich MA, Cattran D, Beck LH, Odutayo A, Sethi S, Ayalon R, Leung N, Reich H, Fervenza FC. A pilot study to determine the dose and effectiveness of adrenocorticotrophic hormone (H.P. Acthar® Gel) in nephrotic syndrome due to idiopathic membranous nephropathy. *Nephrol Dial Transplant.* 2014;8:1570-1577.

Hofstra JM, Fervenza FC, Wetzels JF. Treatment of idiopathic membranous nephropathy. *Nat Rev Nephrol.* 2013;9:443-458.

Hoxha E, Thiele I, Zahner G, et al. Phospholipase A2 receptor autoantibodies and clinical outcome in patients with primary membranous nephropathy. *J Am Soc Nephrol.* 2014;25:1357-1366.

Kanigicherla D, Gummadova J, McKenzie EA, et al. Anti-PLA2R antibodies measured by ELISA predict long-term outcome in a prevalent population of patients with idiopathic membranous nephropathy. *Kidney Int.* 2013;83:940-948.

Ponticelli C, Zucchelli P, Passerini P, et al. A 10-year follow-up of a randomized study with methylprednisolone and chlorambucil in membranous nephropathy. *Kidney Int.* 1995;48:1600-1604.

Ruggenenti P, Debiec H, Ruggiero B, et al. Anti-phospholipase A2 receptor antibody titer predicts post-rituximab outcome of membranous nephropathy. *J Am Soc Nephrol.* 2015;26:2545-2558.

Ruggenenti P, Fervenza FC, Remuzzi G. Treatment of membranous nephropathy: time for a paradigm shift. *Nat Rev Nephrol.* 2017 Jul 3;doi:10.1038/nrneph.2017.92.

Seitz-Polski B, Dolla G, Payre C, et al. Epitope spreading of autoantibody response to PLA2R associates with poor prognosis in membranous nephropathy. *J Am Soc Nephrol.* 2016;27:1517-1533.

Stanescu HC, Arcos-Burgos M, Medlar A, et al. Risk HLA-DQA1 and PLA(2)R1 alleles in idiopathic membranous nephropathy. *N Engl J Med.* 2011;364:616-626.

Tomas NM, Hoxha E, Reinicke AT, et al. Autoantibodies against thrombospondin type 1 domain-containing 7A induce membranous nephropathy. *J Clin Invest.* 2016;126:2519-2532.

Full bibliography can be found on www.expertconsult.com.

20

Immunoglobulin A Nephropathy and Related Disorders

See Cheng Yeo; Jonathan Barratt

Immunoglobulin A nephropathy (IgAN) was first described in 1968 by the Parisian pathologist Jean Berger, and at one time it was known as Berger disease. It is the most common pattern of glomerulonephritis (GN) identified in areas of the world where kidney biopsy is widely practiced. IgAN is defined by mesangial IgA deposition accompanied by a mesangial proliferative GN, and it is an important cause of kidney failure. Recurrent visible hematuria is the hallmark of the disease. Closely related to IgAN is Henoch-Schönlein purpura, now referred to as IgA vasculitis (IgAV), and this less common disease is more frequently found in children. IgAV is a small vessel systemic vasculitis characterized by IgA deposition in affected blood vessels, with kidney biopsy findings usually indistinguishable from IgAN.

EPIDEMIOLOGY

IgAN is most common in Caucasian and Asian populations and is relatively rare in people of African descent. The highest worldwide incidence is in Southeast Asia, but this may reflect different approaches to evaluation of kidney disease and different thresholds for kidney biopsy. Peak incidence of IgAN is in the second and third decades of life, and there is a 2 : 1 male to female predominance in North American and Western European populations that is not seen in Asian populations. Subclinical IgAN is estimated to occur in up to 16% of the general population according to postmortem studies. IgAN is occasionally familial, but the majority of cases are sporadic.

CLINICAL PRESENTATION

EPISODIC VISIBLE HEMATURIA

Episodic visible hematuria most frequently occurs in the second or third decades of life and is the presenting complaint in 40% to 50% of patients. The urine is usually brown rather than red and will often be described by the patient as looking like "tea without milk" or "cola-colored." The passage of clots is very unusual. There may be bilateral loin pain accompanying these episodes, which may be due to renal capsular swelling. Hematuria usually follows intercurrent mucosal infection, most commonly in the upper respiratory tract, but it is occasionally seen following gastrointestinal infection and may be provoked by heavy physical exercise. Spontaneous episodes occur as well. The time course is characteristic, with hematuria appearing within 24 hours of the onset of the symptoms of

infection. This differentiates it from the 2- to 3-week delay between infection and subsequent hematuria characteristic of poststreptococcal GN. Visible hematuria resolves spontaneously over a few days in nearly all cases, but nonvisible (microscopic) hematuria may persist between attacks. Most patients only experience a few episodes of visible hematuria, and such episodes typically recur for a few years at most. These episodes are infrequently associated with acute kidney injury (AKI).

ASYMPTOMATIC NONVISIBLE HEMATURIA

Asymptomatic nonvisible hematuria is usually detected during routine health screening and identifies 30% to 40% of patients with IgAN in most series. Hematuria may occur alone or with proteinuria. It is rare for proteinuria to occur without microscopic hematuria in IgAN.

NEPHROTIC SYNDROME

Nephrotic syndrome is uncommon, occurring in only 5% of all patients with IgAN, but it is more common in children and adolescents. Nephrotic-range proteinuria is principally seen in patients with advanced glomerulosclerosis. In those children and adults presenting with concurrent nephrotic syndrome, microscopic hematuria, and mesangial IgA deposition, one should always consider the possibility of the coincidence of the two most common glomerular diseases of young adults: minimal change disease and IgAN. A number of case series have reported patients who, on kidney biopsy, have normal light microscopy, foot process effacement on electron microscopy, and electron-dense mesangial IgA deposits and in whom proteinuria resolved completely in response to corticosteroid therapy. Typically in these cases, following resolution of proteinuria, both nonvisible hematuria and IgA deposits persist.

ACUTE KIDNEY INJURY

AKI is uncommon in IgAN (less than 5% of all cases) and develops by two distinct mechanisms. The first is an acute, severe immune and inflammatory injury resulting in crescent formation, called crescentic IgAN. This may be the first presentation of the disease or can occur superimposed on known mild IgAN. Alternatively, AKI can occur with mild glomerular injury when heavy glomerular hematuria leads to tubular occlusion by red cell casts. This is a reversible phenomenon, and recovery of kidney function occurs with supportive measures.

OTHER PRESENTATIONS

Other presentations of IgAN include hypertension and chronic kidney disease (CKD) where the patient is identified coincidentally.

SECONDARY IMMUNOGLOBULIN A NEPHROPATHY

Mesangial IgA deposition may occur in a number of other diseases, and the kidney biopsy appearances are often indistinguishable from primary IgAN. Although some associations are well established, other anecdotal observations based on single-case reports should be interpreted with caution as IgAN is a common disease. The most common form of secondary IgAN is associated with chronic liver disease, particularly with alcoholic cirrhosis. It is usually thought to be a consequence of impaired hepatic clearance of IgA. Mesangial IgA is a common autopsy finding in patients with chronic liver disease; however, few patients have clinical manifestations of kidney disease other than nonvisible hematuria. IgAN is also reported in association with HIV infection and AIDS. The polyclonal increase in serum IgA, which is a feature of AIDS, has been cited as a predisposing factor for the disease. The closeness of this association has been controversial, as autopsy studies have indicated a prevalence of IgAN between zero and 8%. Treatment of secondary IgAN should be targeted toward the primary disease.

PATHOLOGY

Elevated serum IgA levels are found in 30% to 50% of adult patients with IgAN. Serum IgA levels do not correlate with disease activity or severity. Likewise, measurement of poorly galactosylated IgA1 O-glycoform levels is neither sensitive nor specific enough to be used as a diagnostic test in IgAN, although there is emerging evidence that high levels of poorly galactosylated IgA1 O-glycoforms may correlate with a worse prognosis. The diagnosis of IgAN requires a kidney biopsy.

LIGHT MICROSCOPY

Light microscopic abnormalities may be minimal, but the most common appearance is mesangial hypercellularity (Fig. 20.1). This is most commonly diffuse and global, but focal segmental hypercellularity is also seen. Focal segmental glomerulosclerosis is also described, and crescentic change may be superimposed on diffuse mesangial proliferation with or without associated segmental necrosis. Crescents are a common finding in biopsies performed during episodes of visible hematuria with reduced glomerular filtration rate (GFR).

Tubulointerstitial changes do not differ from those seen in other forms of progressive GN, reflecting the final common pathway of renal parenchymal disease. Mononuclear cell infiltration is associated with tubular atrophy and interstitial fibrosis, ultimately leading to a widening of the cortical interstitium. This finding correlates with a poor prognosis.

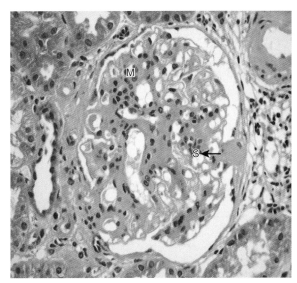

Fig. 20.1 Kidney biopsy showing mesangial proliferation *(M)* and expansion of the mesangial extracellular matrix *(S)* in a patient with IgA nephropathy. A capsular adhesion can also be seen *(arrow)*.

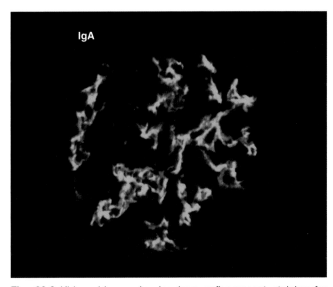

Fig. 20.2 Kidney biopsy showing immunofluorescent staining for mesangial immunoglobulin A *(IgA)*.

IMMUNOHISTOLOGY

The presence of dominant or codominant IgA deposits in the mesangium is the defining feature of IgAN. This is detected in kidney biopsy specimens by immunofluorescence or immunohistochemistry (Fig. 20.2). IgA deposition is diffuse and global. In 15% of cases, IgA is the only deposited immunoglobulin. Other immunoglobulins are also frequently detectable (immunoglobulin [Ig]G in 50% to 70%, IgM in 31% to 66%), but their presence does not appear to correlate with clinical outcome. The complement component C3 is also commonly present.

ELECTRON MICROSCOPY

Electron microscopy shows mesangial and paramesangial electron-dense deposits corresponding to IgA immune

Table 20.1   Oxford Classification of Immunoglobulin A Nephropathy

Histologic Variable	Definition	Score
Mesangial hypercellularity	Mesangial hypercellularity score defined by the proportion of glomeruli with mesangial hypercellularity	M0 ≤0.5 M1 >0.5
Endocapillary hypercellularity	Hypercellularity because of increased number of cells within glomerular capillary lumina, causing narrowing of the lumina	E0 absent E1 present
Segmental glomerulosclerosis	Any amount of the tuft involved in sclerosis but not involving the whole tuft or the presence of an adhesion	S0 absent S1 present
Tubular atrophy/interstitial fibrosis	Percentage of cortical area involved by the tubular atrophy or interstitial fibrosis, whichever is greater	T0 0%–25% T1 26%–50% T2 >50%

Note: Scoring should be assessed on period acid-Schiff-stained sections.

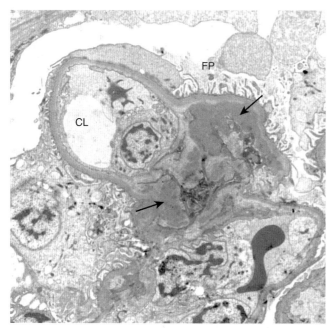

Fig. 20.3 Electron micrograph showing immunoglobulin A immune complex deposition within the mesangium and paramesangium *(arrows)*. *CL,* Capillary loops; *FP,* normal podocyte foot processes.

complexes (Fig. 20.3). The size, shape, quantity, and density of the deposits vary between glomeruli. Glomerular capillary wall deposits may also be seen in the subepithelial or, more commonly, subendothelial space. Capillary loop deposits are associated with disease that is more severe. Glomerular basement membrane abnormalities are seen in 15% to 40% of cases and are associated with heavy proteinuria, more severe glomerular changes, and crescent formation. A group of patients experience thinning of the glomerular basement membrane indistinguishable from thin membrane disease. It remains unclear whether the clinical course of these patients is different.

THE OXFORD CLASSIFICATION OF IMMUNOGLOBULIN A NEPHROPATHY

The Oxford Classification of IgAN, published in 2009, is an international scoring system for evaluating pathologic features on kidney biopsy. Four variables were identified that correlated most strongly with clinical outcome, independent of known clinical risk factors at the time of diagnosis, including the presence of hypertension, reduced GFR, and degree of proteinuria and proteinuria and blood pressure at follow-up: these included the presence of mesangial hypercellularity (M), segmental glomerulosclerosis (S) and tubular atrophy/ interstitial fibrosis (T), and endocapillary hypercellularity (E) (Table 20.1). The first three of these (M, S, and T) were independent predictors of rate of GFR decline and the composite of kidney failure or a 50% decline in GFR. A similar association was seen with endocapillary hypercellularity (E) in patients who had not received immunosuppression; this difference was not observed in patients who received immunosuppression, suggesting that endocapillary lesions are responsive to immunosuppressive treatment. The presence of multiple pathologic features (M, E, S, and/or T) in combination results in additive risk of kidney disease progression. Among the four predictors, studies have consistently demonstrated that the degree of interstitial fibrosis/tubular atrophy is the strongest predictor of kidney survival. The predictive value of these biopsy features was similar in both adults and children. Since its publication, the Oxford Classification of IgAN has been validated in different patient populations from North America, Europe, and Asia, and it is now widely accepted as the histopathologic scoring system of choice for IgAN.

In the original Oxford classification, the presence of crescents did not independently predict clinical outcome in IgAN. However, the Oxford study excluded patients with advanced CKD at presentation or rapid progression to kidney failure. A working subgroup of the IgAN Classification Working Group subsequently demonstrated that crescents were independent predictors of kidney outcomes in a pooled cohort of 3096 patients, leading to the 2017 addition to the Oxford Classification of crescent scores (MEST-C): C0 (no crescents), C1 (crescents in less than one-fourth of glomeruli), and C2 (crescents in over one-fourth of glomeruli). A score of C1 identifies a group of patients with significantly higher risk of poor kidney outcomes if not treated with immunosuppression, although outcomes were similar to C0 if these patients were treated with immunosuppressive therapy. Notably, these observational data are not sufficient to extrapolate to a recommendation that those with C1 lesions should be treated with immunosuppression. A score of C2 identifies patients at risk of a poor kidney outcome even if treated with immunosuppression.

PATHOGENESIS

Although considerable progress has been made in characterizing a number of pathogenic pathways operating in IgAN, there remains a great deal that is not understood. In particular, it remains to be established whether IgAN is a single entity or whether mesangial IgA deposition is simply the final common pathway for a number of distinct kidney diseases.

IMMUNOGLOBULIN A IN IMMUNOGLOBULIN A NEPHROPATHY

In humans, IgA is the most abundant antibody. It is predominantly present at mucosal surfaces and in secretions such as saliva and tears, where it protects against mucosal pathogens. The IgA molecule exists as two isoforms, IgA1 and IgA2, with each existing as monomers (single molecules) or polymers (most commonly dimeric IgA). It is predominantly polymeric IgA1 that is found in mesangial IgA deposits in IgAN. The major difference between IgA1 and IgA2 is that IgA1 includes a hinge region that carries a variable complement of O-linked carbohydrates (Fig. 20.4). Changes in the composition of these O-linked sugars is the most consistent finding in patients with IgAN across the world, with identical changes seen in patient cohorts from North America, Europe, and Asia.

The key change is an increase in the serum of IgA1 O-glycoforms that contain less galactose. This increase in poorly galactosylated IgA1 O-glycoforms is believed to play a central role in the pathogenesis of IgAN. Poorly galactosylated IgA1 O-glycoforms form high-molecular-weight circulating immune complexes, either through self-aggregation, aggregation with soluble CD89, or through the generation of IgG and IgA hinge region specific autoantibodies ("antiglycan" antibodies). These high-molecular-weight immune complexes are prone to mesangial deposition, resulting ultimately in mesangial cell proliferation, release of proinflammatory mediators, and glomerular injury.

ORIGINS OF MESANGIAL IMMUNOGLOBULIN A

Many of the features of mesangial IgA are those typically seen in IgA secreted at mucosal surfaces. Overabundance of this "mucosal-type" IgA in the serum in IgAN might suggest that this IgA originates from mucosal sites. However, mucosal biopsies from patients with IgAN show significantly reduced numbers of polymeric IgA-secreting plasma cells compared with healthy subjects. By comparison, increased numbers of polymeric IgA-secreting plasma cells are seen in bone marrow samples from patients with IgAN, suggesting that mesangial IgA is derived from systemically located plasma cells. This has led to the hypothesis that, in IgAN, mucosally primed IgA-committed B cells relocate to systemic sites such as the bone marrow where they secrete their poorly galactosylated polymeric IgA1 directly into the circulation rather than into the submucosa for passage across the mucosal epithelium. In addition, the systemic microenvironment is likely to be very different from the mucosal sites these plasma cells would normally inhabit, and it is possible that these plasma cells also receive cytokine signals promoting undergalactosylation of IgA1.

One of the most likely mechanisms for this displacement is incorrect homing of mucosal lymphocytes to systemic sites. Although there is emerging evidence of altered homing of B and T lymphocyte subsets in IgAN, more work needs to be undertaken to fully evaluate this hypothesis.

KEY EVENTS IN THE DEVELOPMENT OF KIDNEY SCARRING IN IMMUNOGLOBULIN A NEPHROPATHY

The Oxford Classification of IgAN publication identified four key pathologic consequences of IgA deposition that independently determine the risk of developing progressive kidney disease: mesangial cell proliferation (M), endocapillary proliferation (E), segmental glomerulosclerosis (S), and tubulointerstitial scarring (T). There is increasing evidence, predominantly from in vitro models, that circulating IgA immune complexes containing poorly galactosylated polymeric IgA1 are key drivers for all of these processes.

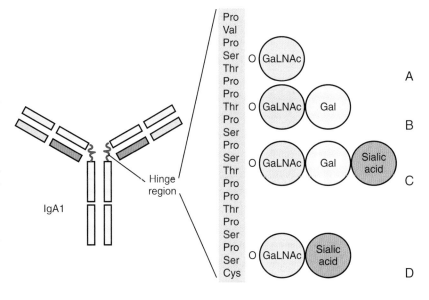

Fig. 20.4 O-glycosylation of IgA1 hinge region. IgA1 contains a 17-amino-acid hinge region that undergoes co/posttranslational modification by the addition of ≤6 O-glycan chains. (A) These chains comprise N-acetylgalactosamine (GaLNAc) in O-linkage with either serine or threonine residues. (B) Galactose can be β1,3-linked to GaLNAc by the enzyme Core 1 β-3 galactosyltransferase (C1GaLT1) and its molecular chaperone Core 1 β-3 galactosyltransferase molecular chaperone (Cosmc), which ensures its correct folding and stability. (C) Galactose may also be sialylated. (D) In addition, sialic acid (N-acetylneuraminic acid, NeuNAc) may be attached directly to GaLNAc by α-2,6 linkage to prevent further addition of galactose. *Cys*, Cysteine; *Pro*, proline; *Ser*, serine; *Thr*, threonine; *Val*, valine.

Exposure to IgA immune complexes triggers mesangial cell activation, proliferation (M), and release of proinflammatory and profibrotic mediators. These mediators, along with the direct effects of exposure to IgA immune complexes, cause podocyte injury, a process fundamental to segmental glomerular scarring (S), and proximal tubule cell activation, which drives tubulointerstitial scarring (T). Identifying the origins of these IgA immune complexes is therefore key to understanding the pathogenesis of IgAN and is paramount if effective treatments are to be developed.

GENETICS OF IMMUNOGLOBULIN A NEPHROPATHY

There is now evidence in several ethnic backgrounds to suggest that genetic factors heavily influence the composition of circulating IgA *O*-glycoforms in the serum. From these studies, it is apparent that first-degree unaffected relatives of patients with IgAN often also display high levels of poorly galactosylated IgA1, supporting the hypothesis that changes in the composition of serum IgA1 *O*-glycoforms are only one part of a "multiple-hit" pathogenic process.

Several susceptibility loci have been identified from genome-wide association studies (GWAS), and one region that has gained particular interest is the major histocompatibility complex (MHC). Polymorphisms within the MHC have been associated with several autoimmune diseases, and an association in IgAN is consistent with an autoimmune component to IgAN. This could be mediated through production of autoantibodies with specificity for the poorly galactosylated IgA1 hinge region. Other identified susceptibility risk loci implicate pathways involving mucosal immunity and complement activation, further suggesting a pathogenic role for these molecular pathways in the pathogenesis of the disease.

NATURAL HISTORY AND PROGNOSIS

Fewer than 10% of all patients with IgAN have complete resolution of urinary abnormalities. IgAN has the potential for slowly progressive CKD leading eventually to end-stage renal disease (ESRD). Approximately 25% to 30% of any cohort will require kidney replacement therapy within 20 to 25 years of presentation.

Many studies have identified clinical, laboratory, and histopathologic features at presentation that mark a poor prognosis (Table 20.2). Although the various prognostic factors listed may be informative for populations of patients, they do not as yet possess the specificity to identify an individual prognosis with complete confidence.

TREATMENT OF IMMUNOGLOBULIN A NEPHROPATHY

Management of patients with IgAN is currently limited to generic strategies applicable to all chronic glomerulonephritides: reduction of proteinuria, use of renin-angiotensin blockade, and control of hypertension (Table 20.3). As with all other causes of CKD, cardiovascular risk factors should be addressed and advice provided regarding smoking cessation, a healthy diet, and exercise.

Table 20.2 Prognostic Markers at Presentation in Immunoglobulin A Nephropathy

	Clinical	Histopathologic
Worse prognosis	Increasing age Duration of preceding symptoms Severity of proteinuria Hypertension Reduced GFR Increased body mass index Higher serum uric acid	*Light microscopy* Capsular adhesions and crescents Glomerular sclerosis Tubular atrophy Interstitial fibrosis Vascular wall thickening *Oxford Classification* M1 worse than M0 E1 worse than E0 S1 worse than S0 T2 worse than T0 C2/C1 worse than C0 *Immunofluorescence* Capillary loop IgA deposits *Ultrastructure* Capillary wall electron dense deposits Mesangiolysis GBM abnormalities
Good prognosis	Recurrent gross hematuria (possibly a result of lead time bias)	Minimal light microscopic abnormalities: M0, E0, S0, T0, C0
No effect on prognosis	Gender Ethnicity Serum IgA level	Intensity of IgA deposits Co-deposition of mesangial IgG, IgM, or C3

GBM, Glomerular basement membrane; *GFR,* glomerular filtration rate; *IgA,* immunoglobulin A; *IgG,* immunoglobulin G; *IgM,* immunoglobulin M.

Table 20.3 Treatment Recommendations for Immunoglobulin A Nephropathy According to Clinical Features

Clinical Presentation	Recommended Treatment
Recurrent visible hematuria	No specific treatment—no role for antibiotics or tonsillectomy
Proteinuria <0.5 g/24 h ± nonvisible hematuria	No specific treatment—no role for tonsillectomy
Proteinuria >0.5 g/24 h ± nonvisible hematuria	Step 1: Maximally tolerated renin-angiotensin blockade with ACE inhibitor and/or ARB Step 2: If proteinuria remains >0.5 g/24 h, then consider immunosuppression
Acute kidney injury • Acute tubular necrosis • Crescentic IgAN (with little or no chronic damage)	Supportive measures for acute tubular necrosis • Induction (~8 weeks) • Prednisolone 0.5–1 mg/kg/day • Cyclophosphamide 2 mg/kg/day • Maintenance • Prednisolone in reducing dosage • Azathioprine 2.5 mg/kg/day
Nephrotic syndrome • With minimal change on light microscopy • With structural glomerular changes	Prednisolone 0.5–1 mg/kg/day for ≤8 weeks No specific treatment
Hypertension	Target BP 125/75 if proteinuria >0.5 g/24 h ACE inhibitors/ARB first-choice agents

Note: As with all other causes of CKD, cardiovascular risk factors, including hypertension, should be addressed, and patients should be advised regarding smoking cessation, healthy diet, and exercise. Treatment of crescentic IgAN mirrors that of other systemic vasculitides with rapidly progressive GN (see Chapter 24).

ACE, Angiotensin converting enzyme; *ARB*, angiotensin receptor blocker; *BP*, blood pressure; *CKD*, chronic kidney disease; *GN*, glomerulonephritis; *IgAN*, immunoglobulin A nephropathy.

NONVISIBLE HEMATURIA AND LESS THAN 0.5 g/DAY PROTEINURIA

No specific therapy is advised for these patients, although long-term follow-up is recommended to monitor for increasing proteinuria, declining GFR, and hypertension.

RECURRENT VISIBLE HEMATURIA

No specific treatment is required for patients with recurrent visible hematuria, and there is no role for prophylactic antibiotics. Tonsillectomy reduces the frequency of acute episodes of visible hematuria when tonsillitis is the provoking factor, and tonsillectomy has its advocates, especially in Japan, as a treatment to reduce kidney disease progression. However, data from clinical trials are conflicting, and larger studies are needed before any conclusion can be drawn regarding the role of tonsillectomy in preserving long-term kidney function in IgAN.

ABOVE 0.5 g/DAY PROTEINURIA AND SLOWLY PROGRESSIVE IgAN

Several randomized controlled trials have shown that renin-angiotensin blockade, with an angiotensin-converting enzyme (ACE) inhibitor or angiotensin II receptor blocker (ARB) to control hypertension and to reduce proteinuria to less than 0.5 g/day, is beneficial in slowing progression of pro teinuric IgAN. Therefore an ACE inhibitor or ARB should be introduced and maximized to achieve this threshold. Although the combination of ACE inhibitor and ARB reduces proteinuria in IgAN, long-term beneficial effects on kidney survival have not been demonstrated, and the safety of this approach has been questioned.

There are a number of patients who will continue to experience proteinuria in excess of 0.5 g/day and declining kidney function despite maximal doses of ACE inhibitor and/or ARB. In these patients, current evidence regarding additional therapy is controversial.

CORTICOSTEROIDS

The efficacy of corticosteroids in IgAN has been tested in several studies. Overall results are equivocal, and reports showing positive outcomes have been criticized for inadequate trial design and the presence of multiple confounding factors. The risks of high-dose corticosteroid use must also be considered. The 2012 Kidney Disease Improving Global Outcomes (KDIGO) Clinical Practice Guideline suggests that a 6-month course of corticosteroids may slow progression of GFR loss in patients with persistent proteinuria greater than 1 g/day despite renin-angiotensin blockade and preserved kidney function (eGFR greater than 50 mL/min).

Since publication of the KDIGO Guidelines, two important clinical trials have questioned this approach. In the STOP-IgAN trial, patients with persistent proteinuria greater than 0.75 g/day following optimized supportive therapy for 6 months were randomized to continued supportive therapy or additional immunosuppressive therapy (corticosteroids if eGFR ≥60 mL/min, corticosteroids plus cyclophosphamide/ azathioprine if eGFR <60 mL/min). There was no difference in kidney disease progression for patients who received immunosuppression in addition to optimized intensive supportive therapy, compared with patients receiving optimized intensive supportive therapy alone. The TESTING trial (Therapeutic Evaluation of STeroids in IgA Nephropathy Global study) reported its results in 2016. While there was a suggestion of efficacy, the high-dose oral steroid therapy was associated with significantly increased rates of serious adverse outcomes in participants with IgA nephropathy at high risk of kidney disease progression.

FISH OIL

Fish oil is widely prescribed in IgAN and appears safe, although tolerability is a major issue because of a fishy odor to the breath and sweat and increased flatulence. A meta-analysis of available clinical trial data, however, failed to detect a benefit of fish oils on kidney outcomes in IgAN.

OTHER IMMUNOSUPPRESSIVE AGENTS

There is currently insufficient evidence to support the routine use of cyclophosphamide and azathioprine in IgAN. Mycophenolate mofetil (MMF) has been studied in a number of small randomized controlled trials, but results have been inconsistent, and a recent meta-analysis of these trials concluded that there is no significant benefit of MMF in reducing proteinuria in IgAN. In the most recent report providing longer follow-up data, patients with mild histologic lesions did show a benefit in reducing the composite end points of doubling of serum creatinine or ESRD. Further studies of MMF in IgAN are ongoing.

EMERGING THERAPIES

Recent studies provide new insights into key molecular pathways in IgAN including mucosal immunity, B-cell activation, and mesangial cell protein tyrosine kinase activation. This has provided the impetus for a number of phase II clinical trials of novel agents in IgAN including enteric budesonide (directed against the mucosal immune system), blisibimod (a B cell inhibitor), fostamatinib (a spleen tyrosine kinase inhibitor), and bortezomib (a proteasome inhibitor). In addition, in vitro data suggest that it may be possible to proteolytically remove mesangial and circulating immune complexes using bacterial IgA1 proteases; therefore a protease-based therapy may be a possible future treatment strategy for IgAN.

PATIENT WITH ACUTE KIDNEY INJURY

In patients with IgAN who develop AKI and fail to respond to simple supportive measures, a kidney biopsy is required to differentiate between the two most common causes of AKI in IgAN:

1. *Acute tubular necrosis with intratubular erythrocyte casts.* This requires supportive care only. Recovery to baseline GFR is usual, although some patients may be left with irreversible tubulointerstitial scarring.
2. *Crescentic IgAN.* Patients with rapidly progressive loss of kidney function, active glomerular inflammation and crescents on kidney biopsy, and no significant chronic damage may be treated similarly to other forms of crescentic GN (i.e., high-dose corticosteroids and cyclophosphamide). Evidence for treatment of crescentic IgAN is derived from small case-series and retrospective data. Response to treatment is worse in crescentic IgAN than in other forms of crescentic GN, and renal survival is estimated to be only 50% at 1 year and 20% at 5 years. This may be the consequence of significant preexisting chronic damage at the time of a crescentic transformation, thereby reducing the chances of a response to immunosuppression.

NEPHROTIC SYNDROME

Nephrotic syndrome in association with mesangial IgA deposition may be a result of advanced glomerular scarring because of longstanding IgAN, and it therefore may reflect established CKD or occasionally a second distinct coincident GN-like minimal change disease. A kidney biopsy, including electron microscopy, is key to distinguishing between these two extremes. Patients with IgAN, nephrotic syndrome, minimal glomerular scarring, and podocyte effacement typical of minimal change disease should be treated as having minimal change disease.

FOLLOW-UP

Patients with IgAN and CKD stages 1 to 3 should have kidney function, quantification of proteinuria, and blood-pressure monitoring at least annually or more frequently if higher risk features are present. Patients with more advanced CKD or high-risk features such as nephrotic range proteinuria require nephrology follow-up.

KIDNEY TRANSPLANTATION

Recurrence of IgA deposition following kidney transplantation is common, affecting up to 50% of grafts within 5 years. However, graft failure because of recurrence of IgAN is relatively rare, most often occurring in patients who had a rapidly progressive course in their native kidneys. There is little evidence that the choice of posttransplant immunosuppression protocol modifies the risk of recurrence, although a recently published analysis of the Australia and New Zealand Dialysis and Transplant Registry (ANZDATA) suggests that recurrent disease is more common in patients who undergo steroid withdrawal. There is no evidence to support any specific treatment regimen after recurrent IgAN has been diagnosed in a kidney transplant, although a single-center retrospective analysis has suggested that ACE inhibitor/ARB treatment may reduce the rate of decline in allograft function in recurrent IgAN.

IMMUNOGLOBULIN A VASCULITIS (HENOCH-SCHÖNLEIN PURPURA)

IgAV is the most common form of systemic vasculitis in children and is characterized by IgA deposition in affected blood vessels. The kidney lesion is a mesangioproliferative GN with mesangial IgA deposition that is indistinguishable from IgAN.

EPIDEMIOLOGY

Although IgAV may occur at any age, it is most common during childhood between age 3 and 15 years old. There is a slight male predominance. Most cases occur in the winter, spring, and autumn months, which may be because of its association with preceding upper respiratory tract infections.

ETIOLOGY AND PATHOGENESIS

The exact cause of IgAV remains unknown. There are, however, many factors that suggest a common pathogenic pathway operating in IgAV and IgAN. Identical twins have been reported where one presents with IgAN and the other with IgAV. IgAV developing on a background of IgAN is described in both adults and children. Both diseases share similar kidney biopsy findings, and they also share changes in the complement of serum IgA1 *O*-glycoforms. There is a similar association between mucosal infection and presentation of disease.

NATURAL HISTORY

The kidney disease that accompanies IgAV is often transient and self-limited in nature, with hematuria or proteinuria typically resolving within weeks of presentation. AKI due to crescentic IgAV is more common than crescentic IgAN (although still uncommon), and AKI tends to occur early in the course of the disease. The prognosis of patients who have transient IgAV is generally very good; however, up to 10% of patients with IgAV and nephritis will develop kidney failure.

CLINICAL FEATURES

The classic tetrad of symptoms in IgAV is a palpable purpuric rash, arthritis/arthralgia, abdominal pain, and kidney disease. Symptoms appear in any order and can evolve over days to weeks.

The rash is classically distributed on extensor surfaces, with sparing of the trunk and face (Fig. 20.5). It typically appears in crops and is symmetrically distributed. Polyarthralgia is common and is usually transient and migratory. There is often swelling and tenderness but no chronic destructive damage. Gastrointestinal symptoms often appear after the rash. Abdominal pain is usually mild and transient, but it may be severe and lead to gastrointestinal hemorrhage,

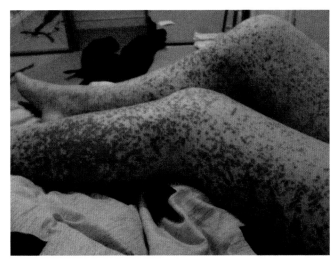

Fig. 20.5 Typical appearance of leukocytoclastic vasculitic rash of Henoch-Schönlein purpura.

bowel ischemia, intussusception, and perforation. Kidney involvement typically manifests as transient asymptomatic microscopic hematuria and/or proteinuria. More severe complications, such as nephrotic syndrome or rapidly progressive deterioration of kidney function, occur less frequently and are more common in adults than in children.

PATHOLOGY

As in IgAN, elevated serum IgA levels are found in 30% to 50% of adult patients with IgAV. Serum IgA levels do not correlate with disease activity or severity. Similarly, changes in the levels of poorly galactosylated IgA1 *O*-glycoform levels are neither sensitive nor specific enough to be used as a diagnostic test in IgAV. Confirmation of the clinical diagnosis requires histologic evidence of IgA deposition in affected tissue, often the skin or kidney.

SKIN BIOPSY

Biopsy of the skin rash typically shows a leukocytoclastic vasculitis. IgA immune complex deposition can be seen using immunofluorescence staining, but detection of IgA in the skin is unreliable. If a tissue diagnosis is required, a kidney biopsy should be performed in the presence of nephritis.

KIDNEY BIOPSY

Kidney biopsy is usually reserved for adult cases of diagnostic uncertainty or when a child presents with more severe renal involvement. Histologic features are the same as those in IgAN.

MANAGEMENT

There is little evidence to guide the treatment of IgAV with nephritis, and that which exists is derived from small retrospective case series. Patients with hematuria, proteinuria, and mildly reduced GFR do not require any specific treatment, and the nephritis usually resolves spontaneously. In patients with crescentic IgAV typified by a rapidly progressive loss of kidney function, there is limited evidence that high-dose corticosteroids are beneficial. Regimens include pulsed methylprednisolone followed by a 3-month course of oral prednisolone. There is currently no conclusive evidence that other immunosuppressive agents, including cyclophosphamide or azathioprine, or other interventions, such as plasmapheresis, have any beneficial effect on outcome.

FOLLOW-UP

Patients should be monitored in the same way as described for IgAN. Those with persistent proteinuria are at highest risk of developing progressive CKD.

TRANSPLANTATION

Kidney transplant is the treatment of choice in patients with ESRD due to IgAV. As with IgAN, recurrence of mesangial IgA deposition may occur, although loss of the graft to IgAV is less common and tends to occur in patients who had an aggressive original disease. Kidney transplant traditionally is delayed for 12 months from date of presentation.

PREGNANCY

Evidence from cohort studies of children with IgAV suggests that all women with a history of IgAV should be carefully monitored during pregnancy, even if they had no evidence of kidney disease at the time of diagnosis. These women are at increased risk of developing hypertension and proteinuria during pregnancy.

BIBLIOGRAPHY

IMMUNOGLOBULIN A NEPHROPATHY

Natural History, Epidemiology, and Diagnosis

Berger J, Hinglais N. Les depots intercapillaries d'IgA-IgG. *J Urol Nephrol (Paris)*. 1968;74:694-695.

Cattran DC, Coppo R, Cook HT, et al. The Oxford classification of IgA nephropathy: rationale, clinicopathological correlations, and classification. *Kidney Int*. 2009;76:534-545.

Lai KN, Tang SC, Schena FP, et al. IgA nephropathy. *Nat Rev Dis Primers*. 2016;2:16001. doi:10.1038/nrdp.2016.1.

Pouria S, Barratt J. Secondary IgA nephropathy. *Semin Nephrol*. 2008;28:27-37.

Wyatt RJ, Julian BA. IgA nephropathy. *N Engl J Med*. 2013;368(25):2402-2414.

Pathogenesis

Daha MR, van Kooten C. Role of complement in IgA nephropathy. *J Nephrol*. 2016;29(1):1-4. doi:10.1007/s40620-015-0245-6.

Floege J, Feehally J. The mucosa-kidney axis in IgA nephropathy. *Nat Rev Nephrol*. 2016;12(3):147-156. doi:10.1038/nrneph.2015.208.

Lechner SM, Papista C, Chemouny JM, Berthelot L, Monteiro RC. Role of IgA receptors in the pathogenesis of IgA nephropathy. *J Nephrol*. 2016;29(1):5-11. doi:10.1007/s40620-015-0246-5.

Robert T, Berthelot L, Cambier A, Rondeau E, Monteiro RC. Molecular insights into the pathogenesis of IgA nephropathy. *Trends Mol Med*. 2015;21(12):762-775. doi:10.1016/j.molmed.2015.10.003.

Genetics

Feehally J, Farrall M, Boland A, et al. HLA has strongest association with IgA nephropathy in genome-wide analysis. *J Am Soc Nephrol*. 2010;21:1791-1797.

Kiryluk K, Scolari F, Sanna-Cherchi S, et al. Discovery of new risk loci for IgA nephropathy implicates genes involved in immunity against intestinal pathogens. *Nat Genet*. 2014;46:1187-1196.

Lomax-Browne HJ, Visconti A, Pusey CD, et al. IgA1 glycosylation is heritable in healthy twins. *J Am Soc Nephrol*. 2017;28(1):64-68. doi:10.1681/ASN.2016020184.

Treatment

Eitner F, Floege J. Glomerular disease: ACEIs with or without corticosteroids in IgA nephropathy? *Nat Rev Nephrol*. 2010;6:252-254.

KDIGO. Clinical Practice Guideline for Glomerulonephritis. http://www.kdigo.org/clinical_practice_guidelines/pdf/KDIGO-GN-Guideline.pdf.

Rauen T, Eitner F, Fitzner C, et al. Intensive supportive care plus immunosuppression in IgA nephropathy. *N Engl J Med*. 2015;373:2225-2236.

Strippoli GF, Manno C, Schena FP. An "evidence-based" survey of therapeutic options for IgA nephropathy: assessment and criticism. *Am J Kidney Dis*. 2003;41:1129-1139.

Yeo SC, Liew A, Barratt J. Emerging therapies in immunoglobulin A nephropathy. *Nephrology (Carlton)*. 2015;20:788-800.

IgA VASCULITIS

Kiryluk K, Moldoveanu Z, Sanders J, et al. Aberrant glycosylation of IgA1 is inherited in pediatric IgA nephropathy and Henoch-Schönlein purpura nephritis. *Kidney Int*. 2011;80:79-87.

Ronkainen J, Nuutinen M, Koskimies O. The adult kidney 24 years after childhood Henoch-Schönlein purpura: a retrospective cohort study. *Lancet*. 2002;360:666-670.

Sanders JT, Wyatt RJ. IgA nephropathy and Henoch-Schönlein purpura nephritis. *Curr Opin Pediatr*. 2008;20:163-170.

KIDNEY IN SYSTEMIC DISEASES

21

Complement-Mediated Glomerulonephritis and Thrombotic Microangiopathy

Marina Vivarelli; Joshua M. Thurman

The complement system is a group of proteins that provide an important part of the immune defense against infection. Many components of the complement system circulate as inactive proteins in the plasma. Activation of the complement system generates peptide fragments that serve as ligands for several receptors and completes a multimeric complex (C5b-9) that forms pores in membranes resulting in cell lysis.

As with all components of the immune system, proper function of the complement system helps with the effective elimination of invasive pathogens while causing minimal inflammation or injury to host tissues. However, uncontrolled activation of the complement system can cause tissue injury, and there is clear evidence that the complement cascade is activated in many autoimmune and inflammatory diseases. The kidney is particularly susceptible to complement-mediated injury, and the complement system has been implicated in the pathogenesis of multiple kidney diseases. It is also evident that acquired and congenital defects in the complement system are important risk factors for several diseases. For the most part, these disease-associated defects impair the body's ability to regulate the complement system, thereby permitting overactivation or "dysregulation" of the complement cascade.

Uncontrolled complement alternative pathway activation appears to be central to the development of two kidney diseases: atypical hemolytic uremic syndrome (aHUS) and C3 glomerulopathy (C3G). These diseases are clinically and histologically distinct yet share similar risk factors. Our understanding of the pathogenesis of these diseases has been significantly advanced by recent discoveries. Although aHUS and C3G are both rare diseases, greater understanding of these diseases as extreme examples of complement dysregulation will likely provide greater insight into more common forms of glomerulonephritis that also involve complement activation.

BRIEF OVERVIEW OF THE COMPLEMENT SYSTEM

The complement system is composed of soluble proteins, soluble regulatory proteins, cell surface regulatory proteins, and cell surface receptors. Activation proceeds through three different pathways: the classical pathway, the mannose binding lectin (MBL) pathway, and the alternative pathway (Fig. 21.1).

Each pathway is activated by multiple different molecules. IgM and IgG containing immune complexes (ICs) activate the classical pathway, for example, but C-reactive protein, beta-amyloid fibrils, and other molecules also activate this pathway. The MBL pathway is activated when several different types of proteins, including MBLs, collectins, and ficolins, bind to targets on the surface of bacteria or damaged cells. All three pathways result in the cleavage of C3, forming C3b that can be covalently fixed to tissue surfaces.

Full activation of the complement cascade generates C3a, C3b, C5a, and C5b-9. Receptors for C3a and C5a induce several different inflammatory responses. Leukocytes also express receptors for C3b and the C3b inactivation fragments (iC3b and C3d). C5b-9 is also called the *membrane attack complex* (MAC) or the *terminal complement complex* (TCC). The insertion of C5b-9 in cell membranes can result in cell activation or lysis.

Several features of the alternative pathway are notable and may explain the link between activation of this pathway and kidney disease. Like the classical and MBL pathways, some proteins, including IgA, directly activate the alternative pathway. Tissue-bound C3b can combine with a protein called factor B to form an alternative pathway activating enzyme (C3bBb). Consequently, the deposition of C3b on tissue surfaces by the classical and MBL pathway can secondarily engage the alternative pathway, resulting in increased complement activation through an alternative pathway "amplification loop." Finally, C3 in plasma is hydrolyzed at a slow rate, forming an enzyme complex that cleaves more C3 and activates the alternative pathway unless adequately controlled. This spontaneous "tickover" process continuously generates C3b that can also bind to surfaces and be amplified through the alternative pathway.

COMPLEMENT REGULATORY PROTEINS

Because the alternative pathway of complement is continuously active in plasma and tends to self-amplify, it is crucial that the body adequately controls this process. Complement activation is controlled by a group of regulatory proteins expressed on the surface of cells or that circulate in plasma. The ability of a surface to regulate alternative pathway activation determines whether the process continues to self-amplify or is terminated (Fig. 21.2). These regulatory proteins provide a shield that protects the host from complement-mediated injury. Pathogens do not express complement regulatory

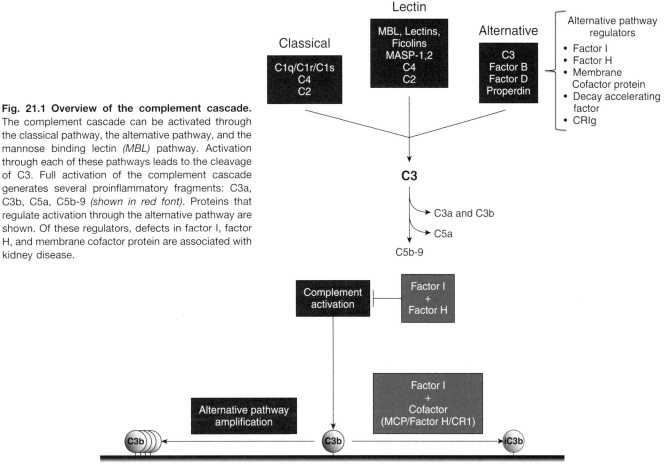

Fig. 21.1 Overview of the complement cascade. The complement cascade can be activated through the classical pathway, the alternative pathway, and the mannose binding lectin (MBL) pathway. Activation through each of these pathways leads to the cleavage of C3. Full activation of the complement cascade generates several proinflammatory fragments: C3a, C3b, C5a, C5b-9 (shown in red font). Proteins that regulate activation through the alternative pathway are shown. Of these regulators, defects in factor I, factor H, and membrane cofactor protein are associated with kidney disease.

Fig. 21.2 Activation and regulation of the alternative pathway on tissue surfaces. The cleavage of C3 by any of the activation pathways causes deposition of C3b on tissue surfaces. C3b is part of the alternative pathway C3-convertase, and this enzyme generates additional C3b unless the convertase decays or C3b is inactivated by the plasma protease factor I, generating iC3b. To inactivate C3b, factor I requires cofactor proteins. Membrane cofactor protein (MCP) and complement receptor-1 (CR1) are cell surface cofactors. Factor H is a cofactor for inactivation of C3b in the fluid phase and on cell surfaces.

proteins, and expression of these proteins is decreased on damaged host cells.

Specific activating proteins can trigger complement activation on a particular cell or surface, but the degree of activation is also determined by the local expression of complement regulatory proteins. Impaired regulation may lower the threshold for activation within a particular tissue, and local impairments of regulation may even be sufficient to permit spontaneous activation. Endothelial cells and podocytes each express several of the complement regulatory proteins, and ordinarily there is little evident complement activation within the glomerular capillary wall.

Several different proteins can regulate the complement system. Factor I is a circulating protein that cleaves (inactivates) C3b, forming iC3b (see Fig. 21.2). To function, however, factor I requires a "cofactor" protein. Several proteins with cofactor function are expressed on cell surfaces (e.g., membrane cofactor protein [MCP] and complement receptor-1 [CR1]). Factor H, a soluble alternative pathway inhibitor, also has cofactor activity. Other proteins regulate complement activation by reducing the half-life of the activating enzymes through a process termed decay acceleration. Decay accelerating

factor (DAF, or CD55) is a protein linked to the surface of cells that limits complement activation, and factor H also controls complement activation by this mechanism. Several additional proteins also control the complement system through other mechanisms. For example, carboxypeptidase N is a plasma enzyme that rapidly inactivates C3a and C5a, and CD59 is a protein that is linked to cell membranes to prevent the addition of C9 during formation of C5b-9.

Congenital or acquired defects can impair the body's ability to regulate the complement system, and these defects can increase a patient's risk of developing different autoimmune and inflammatory diseases. Mutations have been identified in the genes for the regulatory proteins factor I, factor H, and MCP. Gain-of-function mutations have also been identified in the genes for C3 and factor B. These mutations appear to reduce the ability of the regulatory proteins to inactivate the activating enzymes, so they are functionally similar to the loss-of-function mutations seen in the complement regulatory proteins. Autoantibodies to complement proteins have also been detected in patients with various diseases, and these autoantibodies tend to impair regulation of the alternative pathway.

Defects in factor H function are the most common complement abnormalities seen in aHUS, and impaired factor H function is also seen in patients with C3G. Factor H is a soluble protein that is primarily produced in the liver and circulates in plasma at a concentration of 300 to 500 µg/mL. Factor H is made of up 20 repeating structures called short consensus repeats, or SCRs. Regulation of the alternative pathway is performed at the amino terminus of the protein in the first four SCRs, whereas the last two SCRs (19 and 20) mediate binding of factor H to molecules displayed on tissue surfaces such as glycosaminoglycans (GAGs) and sialic acid. Although it is not known why impairments in factor H so frequently manifest as injury within the glomerulus, one possibility is that the glomerular basement membrane (GBM) does not contain the other regulatory proteins, so it is completely dependent on factor H to control the alternative pathway.

The complement factor H–related proteins (CFHRs) are a group of five proteins that arose through reduplication of the gene for factor H and have high structural homology with factor H. The CFHRs all contain regions that are homologous to SCRs 19 and 20 of factor H, suggesting that they can bind similar molecules and surfaces. Various deletions and mutations in the CFHR genes have been identified in patients with aHUS and C3G. Experiments have provided conflicting data regarding the function of these proteins, but some studies suggest that the CFHRs competitively inhibit factor H and cause complement dysregulation.

COMPLEMENT IN IMMUNE-COMPLEX GLOMERULONEPHRITIS

IgG and IgM containing ICs are activators of the classical pathway of complement, and there is strong evidence that the complement system is an important mediator of injury in diseases associated with glomerular IC deposition. The interaction between the complement system and ICs is complex. Some isotypes of IgG activate complement more efficiently than other isotypes. Also, the complement system helps solubilize ICs, mediating the downstream effects of ICs but also reducing their deposition in tissues. Finally, complement activation fragments affect the adaptive immune response, so the complement system may also influence disease upstream of antibody formation.

C3 GLOMERULOPATHY

C3G is a rare form of proliferative glomerulonephritis comprising two forms: C3 glomerulonephritis (C3GN) and dense-deposit disease (DDD; previously known as type II membranoproliferative glomerulonephritis [MPGN] or MPGN type II). The unifying feature of all forms of C3G is the presence of intense C3 staining, with little or no immunoglobulin staining by immunofluorescence on kidney biopsy.

EPIDEMIOLOGY

Incidence of C3G is reported as one to two per million per total population. The age of onset is highly variable. The youngest reported patient was 1 year old, and about 40% of patients presented before 16 years of age in one large cohort. There was a slight prevalence of males in this series (60%), and a family history of glomerulonephritis was reported in about 11% of cases.

ETIOLOGY AND PATHOGENESIS

A large number of molecular causes of complement alternative pathway dysregulation have been identified in patients with C3G, including autoantibodies and genetic variants that encode dysfunctional complement proteins (Table 21.1).

AUTOANTIBODIES

The most common autoantibody associated with C3G is C3 nephritic factor (C3Nef). C3Nef can be detected in approximately 70% to 80% of patients with C3G. It is more common in DDD than in C3GN and correlates with lower levels of C3. The presence of C3Nef does not correlate with clinical outcomes, however, and can be detected in healthy control subjects.

A monoclonal immunoglobulin light chain that inhibited factor H was identified in a C3G patient. This antibody blocked the regulatory function of factor H, thereby impairing regulation of the alternative pathway. Anti-factor H IgG antibodies have also been identified in additional patients with C3G. These antibodies bind to the amino terminus of the protein and block its regulatory function. Antibodies reactive to factor B and C3b have also been reported. These different autoantibodies are associated with increased alternative pathway activation, lending further support to the concept that alternative pathway activation is central to the pathogenesis of C3G. The detection of antibodies specific for the complement proteins is currently only performed in research labs and is not widely available.

GENETIC CAUSES

Disease-associated mutations and rare variants have been identified in the genes for factor H, factor I, factor B, C3, and CFHRs 1, 2, 3, and 5 (see Table 21.1). An internal reduplication of a region in CFHR5 is associated with C3G, and a deletion causing formation of a hybrid CFHR2-CFHR5 protein was found in two related patients with C3G.

The different molecular causes of C3G increase alternative pathway activation or make this system resistant to regulation. It is not known, however, whether the disease is primarily caused by systemic complement activation in the plasma or local activation directly on the mesangium and glomerular capillary wall. Complement activation in the plasma could lead to deposition of complement proteins within the glomeruli as plasma is filtered through the kidney. The GBM may be dependent upon factor H for regulating the alternative pathway. Bruch's membrane in the eye may be similarly dependent upon factor H, and patients with C3G develop retinal lesions and visual impairments.

PATHOLOGY

The identification of C3G is based on pathology and particularly on immunofluorescence (Fig. 21.3). The presence of predominant C3 staining, at least twofold greater than the intensity of staining for other immune proteins (in

Table 21.1	**Complement Abnormalities Associated With C3 Glomerulopathy**
Complement Protein	**Abnormality**
C3 convertase (C3bBb)	Autoantibody • C3Nef (70%–80% of patients). Stabilizes C3 convertase; resistance to inactivation by factor H
Factor H	Protein • Levels low in some patients Autoantibody • Mini-autoantibody to factor H (light chain dimer) blocks regulatory function. • Antibodies to factor H block regulatory function. Mutations • Heterozygous mutation • Homozygous mutations • Compound heterozygous mutation
Factor B	Protein • Levels low in some patients Autoantibody • Binds factor B and stabilizes C3 convertase (C3bBb) Mutations • Gain of function mutation in factor B reported
Factor I	Protein • Levels low in some patients Mutations • Associated with reduced levels and activity
C3	Protein • Levels low in 50%–60% of patients. C4 levels are low in only ~2% of patients. Autoantibody • Binds C3b and stabilizes C3 convertase (C3bBb) Mutations • Heterozygous C3 mutation. C3 convertases resistant to inactivation by factor H
CFHR1	Mutations • Heterozygous internal duplication in SCR • Heterozygous hybrid CFHR1-3 gene
CHFR2	Mutations • Heterozygous hybrid CFHR2-5 gene
CHFR3	Mutations • Heterozygous hybrid CFHR1-3 gene
CFHR5	Mutations • Heterozygous internal duplication in SCR1-2 • Heterozygous internal duplication of SCR1-2 with deletion of CFHR1 and 3 in one affected subject

C3Nef, C3 nephritic factor; *CFHR*, complement factor H–related protein; *CFH*, complement factor H; *SCR*, short consensus repeat.

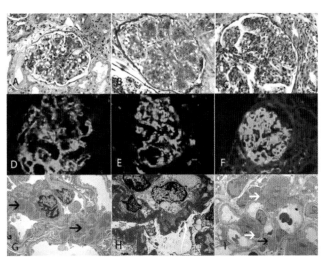

Fig. 21.3 Histologic appearance of the kidney in C3 glomerulopathy. Panel (A): Mesangial proliferation; panel (B): membranoproliferative glomerulonephritis; panel (C): diffuse endocapillary proliferation by light microscopy. Panels (D–F) show C3 immunofluorescence. Panels (G–I) show electron microscopy; (H) a typical dense-deposit disease aspect; (G and I) atypical C3GN with black arrows showing mesangial deposits and white arrows showing subepithelial deposits or "humps." (Panels [A–G] and [I] reproduced with permission from Sethi S, Fervenza FC, Zhang Y, et al. C3 glomerulonephritis: clinicopathological findings, complement abnormalities, glomerular proteomic profile, treatment, and follow-up. *Kidney Int.* 2012;82:465–473. Panel [H] courtesy Dr. Francesca Diomedi-Camassei.)

particular IgG, IgA, IgM, C1q), is necessary for diagnosis. This definition allows for discrimination between C3G and IC-mediated forms of proliferative glomerulonephritis. Positive IF staining for C4d in equal or greater magnitude than C3 suggests activation of the classical and/or lectin pathway of complement, and it has been proposed as a metric to rule out C3 glomerulopathies.

The features of C3G by light microscopy are extremely heterogeneous. It most frequently presents with a membranoproliferative pattern, although mesangial proliferation, diffuse proliferation, and, more rarely, necrotizing lesions with extracapillary proliferation may be observed. Different patterns may coexist in the same kidney biopsy, and there may be an evolution of the lesion from mesangial proliferation to MPGN. Therefore pathologists rely on the immunofluorescence pattern to distinguish forms of C3G from other glomerular diseases that may appear similar by light microscopy. The other causes of MPGN can be idiopathic or secondary to viral infections, autoimmune diseases such as systemic lupus erythematosus, malignancies, and monoclonal gammopathies. Immunofluorescence in these forms of MPGN typically shows intense immunoglobulin staining and positive staining for C4d.

Two subtypes of C3G have been identified: DDD and C3GN. The distinction of these subtypes relies on electron microscopy (see Fig. 21.3). In DDD, deposits are dense, intensely osmiophilic sausage-like ribbons located within the GBM (intramembranous). The GBM becomes altered and thickened to an extent that may be visible by light microscopy. Discrete, intensely C3-positive granular deposits are also located within the mesangium. In C3GN, the C3-positive deposits are less dense, less discrete, and more diffusely located, mostly within the mesangium and on the subendothelial side of the GBM, but also in the subepithelial and intramembranous portions of the GBM. Subepithelial deposits may closely resemble the "humps" that in the past were considered pathognomonic of acute postinfectious glomerulonephritis (PIGN).

Laser microdissection of the deposits visible by electron microscopy in C3GN and DDD and proteomic analysis of their content have shown similar profiles, with no immunoglobulin but abundant components of the alternative pathway of complement. Analysis by immunofluorescence of different components of the complement pathway in kidney biopsies from patients with C3GN and DDD has also not revealed significant differences. These results confirm that these two forms of nephropathy have a shared pathogenesis and are therefore correctly classified under the common definition of C3G.

CLINICAL AND LABORATORY FEATURES

The clinical features of C3G are extremely heterogeneous, reflecting the frequently subtle and unpredictable disease course. In one series, 41% of patients had nephrotic-range proteinuria (>3 g/day) at presentation, and 61% had microscopic hematuria. The frequency of gross hematuria was around 16% in another report. High blood pressure was present in 30.5% of patients and reduced kidney function at diagnosis in 45.5% of cases, with a mean eGFR of 69.3 mL/min/1.73 m².

The clinical presentation of disease is frequently concomitant with an infectious episode. Upper respiratory tract infection was reported in 57% children with DDD. The first manifestation of disease may be gross hematuria, with recurrent episodes of gross hematuria during intercurrent infections. These patients often have persistent proteinuria and microscopic hematuria with dysmorphic red blood cells between acute episodes. This clinical picture can resemble IgA nephropathy (IgAN) and is typical but not exclusive to C3G associated with genetic alterations of CFHR5, initially described in a cluster of families from Cyprus. C3G can also resemble classic acute PIGN in which the urinary alterations appear 2 to 3 weeks after an infectious episode, frequently accompanied by hypertension and some degree of GFR loss. The associated illness is typically an upper respiratory tract infection, and the low circulating C3 with normal C4 may lead to a clinical diagnosis of PIGN. Persistently low complement levels without resolution of hematuria and proteinuria within 3 to 6 months of infection suggest a variant of C3G (sometimes called *atypical postinfectious GN*).

Patients can also present with nephrotic syndrome and kidney failure. Hypertension is very frequent and may be severe, as is glomerular hematuria. The forms of C3G that present with nephrotic syndrome tend to have more intensely proliferative lesions at kidney biopsy, more severe kidney failure at onset, and poorer outcomes. More frequently, though, C3G has a subtle and remitting disease course, with no overt clinical symptoms. In such patients, microscopic hematuria and low-grade proteinuria are usually detected during routine urinalysis. In these cases, age at presentation is highly variable, and disease diagnosis may be very distant from actual disease onset. In about 10% of patients, the family history is positive for glomerulonephritis or for kidney failure of unknown origin.

Laboratory features mainly consist of low circulating C3 with normal C4 levels, reflecting activation of the alternative pathway of complement. This feature, however, is not always present and may be more frequent and intense in DDD compared with C3GN. In a report by Servais et al., low C3

Table 21.2 Evaluation of Patients Suspected of Having C3 Glomerulopathy

History	Family history of hematuria, glomerulonephritis, kidney failure
	Gross hematuria (if yes, concomitant or 15–20 days subsequent to infection and number of episodes)
	Infection (especially upper respiratory tract) in the preceding 2–3 weeks
	Previous urinalysis results?
Clinical examination	Signs of nephrotic syndrome (peripheral edema)
	Blood pressure
	Urine dipstick, presence of frothy urine, reduction in urinary output
	Extrarenal features: partial lipodystrophy, retinal drusen
Laboratory workup	Urinalysis, 24-hour proteinuria
	Complete blood count, urea, creatinine, protein, IgG, IgA, IgM
	Serum C3, C4
	Autoantibodies (ANA, anti-dsDNA), serology HCV, HBV, serum protein electrophoresis

plasma levels were present in 46% of all patients and 60% of those with DDD, in whom C3 levels were on average also lower. Low C4 was rare (only about 2% of cases). Therefore normal circulating C3 levels do not rule out a diagnosis of C3G. However, persistently low C3 levels with normal C4, if present, are suggestive of alternative pathway dysregulation and C3G.

A diagnosis of C3G, particularly in familial forms, warrants investigation of the alternative pathway of complement with assessment of circulating levels of different factors, measurement of C3Nef, and genetic analysis of mutations in genes coding for alternative pathway of complement proteins or regulators (Table 21.2; see also Table 21.1).

The outcome of C3G is variable but is unfavorable in a majority of patients. In both DDD and C3GN, most reports indicate that 40% to 50% of patients will reach end-stage kidney disease (ESKD) within 10 years of disease onset. Factors negatively influencing outcome are the degree of proteinuria, especially the presence of nephrotic syndrome at onset, kidney failure at onset, severe hypertension at onset, older age, and the presence of crescents on the kidney biopsy. In the CFHR5-related forms of C3G, men have a markedly poorer outcome. Forms of C3G with the clinical picture of so-called atypical PIGN generally have a favorable outcome. In general, the impression of clinicians is that DDD is more severe than C3GN, although this may change as more cases are studied.

EXTRARENAL FEATURES

Because C3G is caused by systemic defects in regulation of the alternative pathway of complement, extrarenal manifestations of disease can occur. Accumulation of C3 in the retina can give rise to drusen, an ocular abnormality visible as white or yellow dots between the retinal pigment epithelium and Bruch's membrane. Drusen are detected by electroretinogram, and patients with kidney features of C3G should be screened for their presence. Drusen may partially impair vision and are similar to the alterations seen in age-related macular degeneration, another complement-related disorder that is limited to the eye.

Another systemic feature that has been reported in patients with C3G is acquired partial lipodystrophy. This manifestation is secondary to complement-mediated destruction of adipocytes. It has a cranio-caudal distribution usually limited to the upper body, starting with the face and progressing to the neck, thorax, arms, and abdomen. Acquired partial lipodystrophy usually precedes the development of kidney symptoms.

DIFFERENTIAL DIAGNOSIS

The various clinical presentations of C3G can overlap with other glomerular diseases. The differential diagnosis, especially in young women, includes lupus nephritis, although a low C3 level in lupus nephritis is usually accompanied by low C4 due to activation of the classical pathway of complement (see Fig. 21.1). Intrainfectious recurrent gross hematuria, as seen in C3G associated with genetic mutations in CFHR5, can simulate IgAN, but IgAN is readily distinguished by IgA predominance with immunofluorescence. The kidney biopsy is less useful to distinguish PIGN from C3G, as light microscopy can be very similar, and electron microscopy can show subepithelial deposits ("humps") in both diseases. Immunofluorescence in PIGN may show more IgG than in C3G, although a recent review of 23 cases shows that this distinction may not be accurate. C4d staining is present in only about 50% of patients with PIGN, so it is of limited use in distinguishing between this disease and C3G. Clinical features suggestive of PIGN include a normalization of circulating C3 within 8 to 12 weeks from onset and the absence of disease recurrence (gross hematuria, proteinuria). Given that C3 levels may be normal in some patients with C3G, we recommend that all patients with a diagnosis of PIGN, however classic, undergo periodic urinalysis for 2 years after disease resolution.

In adults, an MPGN pattern by light microscopy warrants exclusion of an underlying monoclonal gammopathy. Furthermore, if staining for immunoglobulin is present, even if it is not predominant, it is prudent to exclude immune-mediated, infection-associated, and malignancy-related causes of MPGN.

TREATMENT

The treatment of C3G is not standardized, as there is no solid evidence of effective therapeutic options. Moreover, the extremely variable clinical picture and the often unpredictable, spontaneously remitting and relapsing natural history of the disease render the evaluation of responses to different therapeutic approaches difficult. Lastly, the fact that C3G is a recently defined disease makes analysis of long-term outcomes under different therapeutic regimens impossible.

Immunosuppression has been attempted with various approaches, but very few trials are available to guide treatment. In general, when the kidney biopsy shows abundant inflammation and proliferation with moderate or little sclerosis, immunosuppression appears reasonable even though most of these agents do not block activation of the complement alternative pathway. Prednisone is frequently used although no studies are available to confirm its effectiveness. Current guidelines based on expert opinion but not on results of clinical trials suggest that a reasonable approach may be to use alternate day 40 mg/m^2 prednisone for 6 to 12 months in patients with intense proteinuria or kidney failure, tapering and discontinuing treatment if there is no sign of improvement after 3 to 4 months.

A recent study by Rabasco et al. described a favorable response to mycophenolate mofetil in C3G. This therapeutic approach is warranted in forms with intense proliferation and inflammation. Other immunosuppressants, such as calcineurin inhibitors, appear successful in some forms of refractory MPGN, but data in DDD are conflicting and not available in C3GN. Rituximab has been proposed for forms with demonstrated C3Nef, but results have been mostly unsatisfactory. Therefore, at the present time, these therapies cannot be recommended and must be judged on a case-by-case basis.

Plasmapheresis or plasma infusions allow the removal of excess fluid-phase complement factors and the substitution of insufficient factors by fresh plasma. However, reports on the effectiveness of this approach are discordant. Its use may be recommended only for forms with rapid progression where other options seem ineffective or in the presence of CFH mutations or anti-CFH antibodies as these forms of disease seem to be most responsive to this approach.

Based on our understanding of disease pathogenesis, complement inhibition is a rational therapeutic option. However, the only complement inhibitor currently available is eculizumab, a humanized monoclonal antibody that binds C5 and blocks formation of the MAC, clearly acting downstream of the disease-initiating process. Published reports of small groups of patients or case reports have shown the clear benefit of eculizumab for reducing proteinuria in some but not all patients. A reduction in the degree of mesangial proliferation and inflammation detected by kidney biopsy has also been reported in keeping with the proinflammatory role played by C5a, while discordant results have been reported on its effect on C3 deposition. Interestingly, patients with high circulating levels of sC5b-9 appear to be more responsive to this therapeutic approach. Moreover, eculizumab appears more clearly beneficial in patients with intense proteinuria and a relatively brief disease history, and treatment seems to have little or no impact on chronic lesions, although in some cases reversal of kidney failure has been reported. However, treatment with eculizumab is expensive, requires chronic intravenous administration, and puts patients at increased risk of meningococcal infection. Thus larger and more structured clinical trials are necessary before this approach can be recommended, especially in the pediatric or young adult population.

TRANSPLANTATION

The rate of recurrence after transplantation is 60% to 85% for patients with DDD, and the risk of allograft failure is about 45% to 50% at 5 years. For C3GN, reports are scantier, but studies have shown recurrence in approximately two-thirds of recipients, with approximately one-third losing their allograft within 5 years of transplantation. Of note, patients with C3G in their native kidneys have developed thrombotic microangiopathy in their allografts after transplantation. These data are sufficient to discourage living-donor transplantation for patients with C3G-related ESKD, especially from related donors, due to the potential for genetic causes of C3G.

Published reports have shown the benefit of complement inhibition with eculizumab in treating posttransplant recurrences of disease. In general, the therapeutic approach to posttransplant recurrences should mirror the approach to native kidney disease, with a more aggressive attitude, due to the fact that these are usually rapidly progressive forms and promptly detected with routine monitoring. Plasmapheresis or complement inhibition may be considered early, particularly due to the fact that all patients are already receiving transplant-related immunosuppression.

COMPLEMENT-MEDIATED THROMBOTIC MICROANGIOPATHY

The thrombotic microangiopathies (TMAs) refer to a group of diseases that are characterized by microangiopathic hemolytic anemia, thrombocytopenia, and kidney injury. Multiple systemic diseases, infections, and drugs are associated with the development of TMA. The clinical presentation can also vary among patients, making TMAs challenging to diagnose and classify.

Over time there has been debate as to whether thrombotic thrombocytopenic purpura (TTP) and HUS are the same disease or distinct entities. The discovery that TTP is usually associated with a deficiency of ADAMTS13 lent support to the distinction of these two diseases. HUS was first identified as a distinct entity in children, and it was recognized that affected patients develop particularly severe kidney failure. The majority of cases of HUS occur in pediatric patients after infections with bacteria that produce Shiga-like toxin (Stx). Over time, HUS that is not associated with Stx-producing bacteria has been termed *diarrhea negative* and *atypical HUS*. A large body of evidence now demonstrates that the majority of these HUS patients have defects in regulation of the alternative pathway, and some experts refer to this subset of patients as having complement-mediated TMA.

There are several systemic diseases, drugs, and infections that are associated with TMAs (Table 21.3). It is not yet clear to what extent TMAs in these different settings share a common pathophysiology, but there is likely significant overlap. In patients with complement-mediated HUS, for example, disease is often triggered by systemic illness. Conversely, only a small proportion of the patients exposed to the events that can trigger TMAs go on to develop the disease, indicating that other predisposing factors must be present. For these reasons, it can be difficult to identify which patients have complement-mediated TMA. Furthermore, complement activation may be important in the pathogenesis of TMA caused by other clinical triggers. For example, underlying complement defects may be present in the majority of women who develop postpartum HUS. In this chapter, we use the term *Stx-HUS* for disease caused by Stx-producing bacteria, *secondary HUS* for patients with known causes of the disease, and *aHUS* for patients with complement-mediated disease and no identifiable cause of secondary disease. The classification of individual patients can be challenging, however, and the diagnosis and classification of the different types of TMA will undoubtedly evolve as additional studies improve our understanding of these diseases.

Table 21.3	Secondary Causes of Hemolytic Uremic Syndrome
Metabolic	Cobalamin deficiency (homozygous deficiency)
	Diacylglycerol kinase ε mutation (homozygous or compound heterozygous)
Infections	Shiga-like toxin producing bacteria (primarily *Escherichia coli* serotypes O157:H7, O111:H8, O103:H2, O123, O26 or *Shigella dysenteriae*)
	Neuraminidase producing *Streptococcus pneumoniae*
	Human immunodeficiency virus
	Hepatitis A, B, and C
	Parvovirus B19
	Cytomegalovirus
	Coxsackie B virus
	Influenza H1/N1
Autoimmune diseases	Systemic lupus erythematosus
	Scleroderma
	Antiphospholipid syndrome
	Dermatomyositis
Drugs	Calcineurin inhibitors
	Quinine
	Mitomycin
	Clopidogrel
	VEGF inhibitors
	Vincristine
	Gemcitabine
	Alemtuzumab
	Cocaine
Other systemic clinical conditions	Pregnancy
	Cancer
	Bone marrow transplantation
	Malignant hypertension
	Antibody-mediated rejection of a kidney transplant

EPIDEMIOLOGY

The incidence of aHUS is extremely low and has been estimated at approximately 3.3 cases per million children and 0.5 to 2 cases per million adults. Onset of TMA in the first 6 months of life is extremely suggestive of aHUS. Most patients present before 40 years of age, but patients have presented in their 80s. The two most critical ages for development of the disease are early childhood (before 5 years of age) and after pregnancy for women. In general, atypical complement-mediated HUS represents the majority of HUS adult cases and 5% to 10% of HUS cases in children, where Stx-HUS is predominant. Approximately 20% of patients have familial disease, and these patients are more likely to present as children. Males and females are affected equally overall, but among adults, the disease is more common in women. Approximately 40% of patients with aHUS will have a disease relapse, and the majority of relapses occur within the first year after disease onset.

ETIOLOGY AND PATHOGENESIS

An underlying complement defect can be identified in approximately 70% of patients with aHUS. The majority of

Table 21.4 Complement Defects Associated With Atypical Hemolytic Uremic Syndrome

Complement Protein	Defect
Factor H	Protein • Levels low in some patients Autoantibody • Present in ~5%–10% of patients. Usually bind carboxy terminus Mutations • Most commonly affected gene in aHUS. Majority of mutations are heterozygous. More than 150 variants described, and most affect SCR19-20 region
Membrane cofactor protein	Protein • Levels low in some patients with mutations. Can be measured by flow cytometry Mutations • Majority of mutations are heterozygous Present in 8%–10% of patients
Factor I	Mutations • Majority of mutations are heterozygous Present in 4%–8% of patients
C3	Protein • Levels low in ~50% of patients Mutations • Present in 4%–8% of patients. Can increase binding to factor B or decrease binding to regulatory proteins
Factor B	Mutations • Present in 1%–4% of patients. Mutations cause gain of function
CFHR1	Mutations • Hybrid CFH/CFHR1 gene may be present in 3%–5% of patients with aHUS
CFHR3	Mutation • Hybrid CFH/CFHR3 gene
CHFR1-3 deletion	Deletion of CFHR1 in 90% of patients with anti-factor H autoantibodies

aHUS, Atypical hemolytic uremic syndrome; *CFHR*, complement factor H–related protein; *CFH*, complement factor H; *SCR*, short consensus repeat.

complement defects are genetic mutations or rare variants in the genes of complement factors, but autoantibodies to complement proteins are seen in some patients (Table 21.4). Similar to C3G, these various molecular defects are usually associated with defective regulation or enhanced activity of the alternative pathway of complement.

GENETIC CAUSES

Mutations in the genes for many different complement proteins have been identified in patients with aHUS, including factor H, factor I, MCP, C3, the CFHRs, and factor B (see Table 21.4). Mutations in noncomplement genes have also been identified in patients with aHUS. For example, thrombomodulin mutations have been found in approximately 3% of aHUS patients. Although this protein is not usually regarded as part of the complement system, there is evidence that it has complement regulatory functions that are impaired

by these mutations. Mutations in the gene for diacylglycerol kinase ε *(DGKE)* have been identified in infants with HUS. It is not known whether *DGKE* mutations affect complement regulation or whether these patients have a distinct pathophysiology.

Functionally, most complement mutations associated with aHUS cause impaired regulation of the alternative pathway. In most patients, the mutations are heterozygous, causing only a partial defect in regulation. The mutations also tend to affect complement regulation on cell and tissue surfaces. MCP, for example, is expressed on the plasma membrane of cells. The underlying complement defects affect disease severity, and the prognosis is better for patients with *MCP* mutations than for patients with mutations in other complement genes. Even without treatment, most patients with *MCP* mutations will have self-limited disease, whereas the majority of patients with mutations in other complement genes will reach ESKD or death without treatment. Because MCP is a cell surface protein, kidney transplantation effectively corrects this molecular defect. Approximately 3% of patients have combined mutations in multiple complement genes, and the presence of multiple complement mutations increases disease penetrance.

Mutations and variants in the gene for factor H *(CFH)* are seen in more than 20% of patients with aHUS, and *CFH* is the most commonly affected complement gene. Most of the mutations in the gene for factor H that are associated with aHUS affect the carboxy terminus of the protein, a region of the protein that binds GAGs and sialic acid moieties on cell surfaces but does not directly contribute to the complement regulatory function of the protein. Consequently, mutations in this region of factor H specifically limit the ability of the protein to regulate the alternative pathway on tissue surfaces. *CFH* and the complement factor H–related *(CFHR 1-5)* genes are located next to each other on chromosome 1q32. Various hybrid genes caused by nonallelic homologous recombination of the *CFH* and *CFHR* genes have been identified. Some of the identified mutations in the CFHRs affect the tendency of these proteins to form multimers, and it is believed that some of the resultant multimers have increased affinity for surfaces and may competitively reduce the binding of factor H. Thus mutations and deletions of the *CFHRs* may affect the availability of factor H, indirectly affecting alternative pathway activation.

AUTOANTIBODIES

Approximately 10% of patients with aHUS have autoantibodies to factor H. The antibodies usually bind the carboxy terminus of factor H, the region of the protein where most of the aHUS-associated mutations are found. Interestingly, more than 90% of the patients who develop these antibodies have deletions in the *CFHR1* and *CFHR3* genes.

TRIGGERS

Disease penetrance is approximately 50% for patients carrying disease-associated complement mutations. Furthermore, many patients with congenital complement mutations present in adulthood. These observations indicate that additional factors contribute to the development of disease, even in patients with underlying impairments in their ability to regulate the alternative pathway. Approximately 30% of aHUS episodes are preceded by diarrhea, and this is the most common

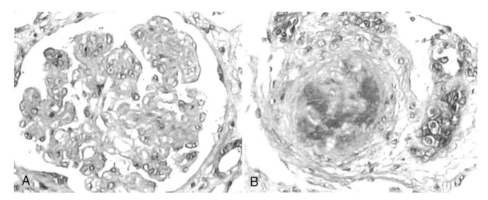

Fig. 21.4 Histologic appearance of the kidney in atypical hemolytic uremic syndrome. Panel (A) shows a typical glomerular lesion with microthrombi within the glomerular capillary lumen; panel (B) shows a small artery that is nearly entirely occluded by thrombotic material and erythrocytes and showing myointimal proliferation. (Reproduced with permission from Noris M, Remuzzi G. Glomerular diseases dependent on complement activation, including atypical hemolytic uremic syndrome, membranoproliferative glomerulonephritis, and C3 glomerulopathy: core curriculum 2015. *Am J Kidney Dis*. 2015;66:359–375.)

trigger in children. Pregnancy is the most common trigger in adults. Disease recurrence is also common in patients who receive kidney transplants, likely because the recipients have an impaired ability to control alternative pathway activation on the ischemic allograft.

PATHOLOGY

Kidney biopsy is seldom performed at disease onset, as severe hypertension and very low platelet counts make this procedure too dangerous. However, due to the importance of establishing a correct diagnosis for treatment and prognosis, a biopsy is warranted as soon as clinical conditions allow.

TMA is characterized by (1) endothelial damage with swelling and, as the lesion progresses toward chronicity, formation of double contours along the glomerular capillary walls; (2) thrombi with schistocytes in glomerular capillaries, arterioles, and small arteries; and (3) mesangiolysis (Fig. 21.4). Glomeruli can appear shrunken and ischemic, with wrinkling of the basement membrane corresponding to the injured glomerular capillaries. Obstruction of the microcirculation due to thrombi can lead to acute cortical ischemia with cortical necrosis, which is irreversible, and whose entity correlates with the degree of chronic kidney damage. Involvement of arteries is accompanied by severe hypertension. Immunofluorescence is negative for immunoglobulin and complement factors and positive for fibrinogen within blood vessels. Endothelium of arterioles and small arteries can be positive for complement activation products. Electron microscopy shows intracapillary fibrin and platelet aggregates, lucent subendothelial expansion with deposition of fluffy material and reduplication of the GBM, and no electron-dense deposits. These features are common to all forms of TMA, including TTP and Stx-HUS. Although the TMA in HUS by definition involves primarily the kidney microvasculature, other organs can be involved. The brain is the next most frequently involved organ (70%), followed by the heart, intestine, lungs, and pancreas in about 20% of patients.

CLINICAL AND LABORATORY FEATURES

Clinical onset of aHUS is usually sudden, with pallor, fatigue, general malaise, drowsiness, vomiting, and sometimes edema. Triggering events are very common. In children, these events are most frequently infections (80% of pediatric cases, 50% of cases in adults), and usually upper respiratory/pulmonary infections or diarrhea/gastroenteritis. Other triggers of HUS in adults include pregnancy (80% of these cases occur in the postpartum period), malignancies, autoimmune systemic diseases, transplants, surgical procedures, trauma, and drugs (calcineurin inhibitors, sirolimus, anti-vascular endothelial growth factor agents; see Table 21.3).

The clinical picture is characterized by the triad of (1) anemia with hemoglobin less than 10 g/dL, (2) thrombocytopenia with platelets less than 150,000/µL, and (3) reduced kidney function with oligoanuria and hypertension. If urinary output is present, proteinuria and hematuria are observed with red blood cell casts and cellular debris in the sediment.

Anemia is caused by intravascular hemolysis with platelet consumption due to formation of microthrombi, primarily in the blood vessels of the kidney and less frequently in other organs, including the brain. Therefore schistocytes are present in the peripheral blood smear, lactate dehydrogenase is markedly elevated, and haptoglobin is severely reduced or undetectable. Coombs test is negative as the hemolysis is of mechanical origin, not immune-mediated. Low circulating complement, particularly C3, may be present but is not pathognomonic.

Arterial hypertension is generally severe due to fluid overload when oligoanuria is present and to increased renin secretion due to arterial TMA. However, if the clinical condition is severe, the blood pressure can be low due to infection or to hypovolemia. Frequently, electrolyte abnormalities (hyperkalemia, hyponatremia) and metabolic acidosis are present, and about half of children and 80% of adults require dialysis at presentation.

Extrarenal symptoms are present in about 20% of patients. The patient can present with neurologic symptoms of variable intensity, ranging from mild findings in approximately 10% of cases (drowsiness, slight confusion, and irritability) to more severe signs such as seizures and profound loss of conscience with stupor and coma. Diplopia or cortical blindness, hemiparesis, and hemiplegia have also been reported. Heart failure due to cardiac involvement and fluid overload can be present and severe, leading to sudden death.

Stool must be checked for intestinal bleeding, and an abdominal ultrasound looking at the integrity of intestinal walls should be performed. Some patients (about 5%) present with fulminant multivisceral involvement, with kidney failure, seizures, intestinal bleeding, heart failure, pulmonary hemorrhage, hepatic cytolysis, and pancreatitis. Some cases present with a less acute, more subtle presentation, and fluctuating progression may be observed with mild GFR loss, proteinuria, microscopic hematuria, moderate hematologic abnormalities, and some degree of arterial hypertension. This is characteristic of HUS associated with transplantation, both of solid organ or of bone marrow. Rarely, hematologic abnormalities can be absent, with the presence of proteinuria, occasionally in the nephrotic range, microscopic hematuria, some degree of GFR loss, and arterial hypertension.

All efforts must be made to rapidly make the correct diagnosis, as aHUS is a life-threatening disease in which kidney biopsy is frequently not possible. Screening for Shiga toxin must be performed by stool or rectal swab culture and polymerase chain reaction for Shigatoxin, and serologies for antilipopolysaccharides should be sent in all children, even if diarrhea is not reported, as Stx-HUS is by far the most common form of HUS in children. Other infectious causes (*Streptococcus pneumoniae*, HIV, other viruses, etc.) must be investigated based on the presenting features and clinical history. The diagnosis of TTP is based on measurement of ADAMTS13 activity, keeping in mind that, especially in the pediatric setting, this value may be lower than the normal range, and it is considered indicative of TTP only if activity is less than 10%. In children, especially infants younger than 6 months of age, serum homocysteine levels and urinary organic acids should be measured to search for cyanocobalamin C deficiency leading to methylmalonic aciduria, a rare metabolic disorder that can cause HUS. Infants or small children, especially with concomitant nephrotic syndrome, must also be screened for DGKE mutations.

When typical HUS, TTP, and secondary forms of HUS have been excluded or appear unlikely, patients should be screened for complement abnormalities. This is particularly true in patients with reduced circulating C3 levels or a family history of kidney failure, sudden unexplained death, coagulopathies, hypertension, or glomerulopathies. Complement analysis includes measurement of circulating complement factors, anti-factor H antibodies, and screening for genetic mutations of CFH, CFI, MCP (or CD46), C3, CFB, and thrombomodulin (see Table 21.4). The age of onset, circulating C3 levels, and clinical features can be useful indicators of which complement gene or abnormality to screen first. For example, age greater than 1 year and relatively mild phenotype with a normal C3 level suggest MCP mutations, whereas a low C3 level suggests fluid phase abnormalities such as CFH, CFI, or C3 mutations. Concomitant coagulopathy or pulmonary hypertension suggests thrombomodulin mutations. Children older than 7 years with a low C3 level suggests anti-factor H antibodies.

Untreated, the natural history of the full-blown clinical syndrome is severe, with 2% to 10% of patients dying and one-third of patients progressing to ESKD. Nearly half of patients experience disease relapses. Moreover, except for patients with MCP mutations, all others have a high risk of posttransplant recurrence.

TREATMENT

Most patients with a full clinical picture of HUS are critically ill and require intensive care and hemodialysis. Every effort should be made to manage them in a setting with expertise in emergent dialysis. Infusion of platelets is contraindicated, unless there is a hemorrhagic event or a high-risk procedure is necessary. Before 2010, the use of intensive and early plasma exchange was advocated to replenish missing or malfunctioning factors and to curb the complement alternative pathway dysregulation. This approach was accompanied by significant side effects, especially in children, and it was only partially effective.

The use of the monoclonal anti-C5 antibody eculizumab, which inhibits the terminal complement pathway, has dramatically changed the natural history of this disease from a dismal prognosis to a severe but manageable condition. Eculizumab acts by binding C5 and blocking formation of C5b-9. Several clinical trials and a vast number of case reports have shown that its use is effective at all ages, both in normalizing hematologic parameters and kidney function in primary disease and in allowing successful kidney transplantation in patients who have already reached ESKD. The availability of eculizumab makes early recognition of aHUS crucial, as early initiation of therapy is essential for optimal outcome. Therefore aHUS must be considered the primary diagnosis, and eculizumab therapy, if available, must be initiated if (1) secondary HUS has been excluded (no drugs, malignancies, autoimmune diseases, etc.), especially in adults; (2) Stx-HUS has been excluded, especially in children; and (3) ADAMTS13 activity is greater than 10%, and TTP has been excluded. When these criteria are established, a complete workup of complement proteins, alternative pathway genes, and anticomplement factor H autoantibodies must be performed.

Because eculizumab blocks the terminal complement pathway, the drug makes patients more susceptible to infections by encapsulated bacteria—mainly *Neisseria meningitidis*. Therefore, when possible, all patients should receive antimenigococcal vaccination (both serotype A, C, Y, W and serotype B) 15 days before first infusion. In critically ill patients, treatment should start under antibiotic prophylaxis (with methylpenicillin or a macrolide), and vaccination should be performed when possible. Vaccination against *S. pneumoniae* and *Haemophilus influenzae* is also prudent. Moreover, in immunocompromised patients, children, and individuals at increased risk (e.g., young adults living in communities), it may be advisable to maintain antibiotic prophylaxis as long as the patient is on eculizumab therapy.

Therapy with eculizumab is not disease modifying, and treatment discontinuation entails a nonquantifiable risk of disease relapse. During therapy, a simple way to evaluate effective complement inhibition is measurement of CH50, which must be less than 10%. The issue of if and when to discontinue eculizumab is much debated and beyond the

Table 21.5 Comparison of Findings in C3 Glomerulopathy and Atypical Hemolytic Uremic Syndrome

	C3 Glomerulopathy	Atypical Hemolytic Uremic Syndrome
Membranoproliferative pattern by light microscopy/C3 deposition	+++	±
Low C3	++	±
Mutations	CFH, C3, CFI, MCP, CFHR5	CFH, MCP, CFI, CFB, C3, THBD
Type of mutations	DDD: Homozyg > Heterozyg GN-C3: Heterozyg > Homozyg	Heterozyg > Homozyg
Common polymorphisms	CFH	CFH, MCP CFHR1/CFHR3
Common haplotypes	Maybe	Yes
Autoantibodies	C3NeF Anti-FH Anti-C3b, factor B	Anti-FH
Activation of the AP	Fluid phase/?cell surfaces	Yes/cell surfaces
Activation of the terminal pathway	+	+++
Response to anti-C5	±	++++

CFHR, Complement factor H–related protein; *CFH,* complement factor H; *DDD,* dense-deposit disease; *MCP,* membrane cofactor protein.

scope of this chapter but must be assessed on a case-by-case basis, depending on age, type of mutation, risk of relapse, kidney function, and vascular access.

Of note, when anti-factor H autoantibodies are present, therapy with plasma exchange combined with immunosuppression (steroids plus azathioprine, mycophenolate mofetil, cyclophosphamide, or rituximab) is effective, though not standardized. The response to therapy can be monitored by measuring anti-factor H antibodies, which correlate closely with the risk of disease relapse.

When eculizumab is not available or ADAMTS13 activity is not readily available, plasma exchange therapy can be started at 1.5 plasma volumes (about 65 to 70 mL/kg), exchanging with fresh frozen plasma. If plasma exchange therapy is not available, plasma infusion can be considered if the patient does not present with fluid overload, heart failure, or severe hypertension. Of note, if HUS is secondary to *S. pneumoniae* infection, therapy with plasma must be avoided, as it worsens the disease. In other forms of HUS, lack of improvement of hemolysis parameters and kidney function after 3 to 5 days of daily plasma exchange or plasma infusion indicates a lack of response to this therapeutic approach.

KIDNEY TRANSPLANTATION

The risk of aHUS recurrence after transplantation varies according to the mutation type, but most experts currently agree that all patients with aHUS, with or without a known mutation, should be transplanted under eculizumab therapy. An alternative option is a combined liver-kidney transplant, as liver transplantation in aHUS due to mutations in the genes for factor H, factor I, C3, or factor B can restore the malfunctioning complement regulator. This is currently the only disease-modifying definitive cure, but plasma exchange or eculizumab should be used at the time of transplantation to protect the transplanted liver from complement-mediated injury until it can replenish these proteins.

COMPARISON OF THE UNDERLYING MECHANISMS OF C3 GLOMERULOPATHY AND ATYPICAL HEMOLYTIC UREMIC SYNDROME

C3G and aHUS are both associated with defects in regulation of the alternative pathway of complement, and it is striking that the kidney is the target of complement-mediated injury in patients with such a large number of different congenital and acquired complement defects. Yet aHUS and C3G are clinically distinct diseases—C3G typically presents as a proliferative glomerulonephritis, whereas aHUS presents as a TMA (Table 21.5). There is heterogeneity in both diseases, however. For example, the histologic patterns of injury can vary among patients with C3G. In general, the molecular complement defects in patients with aHUS tend to affect complement regulation on surfaces. Most of the mutations in CFH, for example, affect SCRs 19 and 20. Complement defects in patients with C3G, on the other hand, tend to affect complement regulation in the fluid phase. These differences are not absolute, however, and some of the mutations found in patients with C3G (e.g., mutations in *CFHR5*) are believed to reduce binding of factor H to tissue surfaces. Furthermore, some complement gene mutations have been identified in patients with both diseases, and C3G patients have developed TMA in their kidney allografts after transplantation.

It is not yet known why patients with similar defects in alternative pathway regulation manifest at different ages and with distinct clinical syndromes. It is possible that variations in other genes modify the exact location and nature of these diseases or that disease triggers or associated illnesses influence how the diseases manifest. Future work will hopefully answer these questions and improve our understanding of how best to predict, diagnose, and treat these kidney diseases.

KEY BIBLIOGRAPHY

Bresin E, Rurali E, Caprioli J, et al. Combined complement gene mutations in atypical hemolytic uremic syndrome influence clinical phenotype. *J Am Soc Nephrol.* 2013;24:475-486.

Caprioli J, Noris M, Brioschi S, et al. Genetics of HUS: the impact of MCP, CFH, and IF mutations on clinical presentation, response to treatment, and outcome. *Blood.* 2006;108:1267-1279.

Chen Q, Wiesener M, Eberhardt HU, et al. Complement factor H-related hybrid protein deregulates complement in dense deposit disease. *J Clin Invest.* 2014;124:145-155.

Dragon-Durey MA, Fremeaux-Bacchi V, Loirat C, et al. Heterozygous and homozygous factor h deficiencies associated with hemolytic uremic syndrome or membranoproliferative glomerulonephritis: report and genetic analysis of 16 cases. *J Am Soc Nephrol.* 2004;15:787-795.

Dragon-Durey MA, Sethi SK, Bagga A, et al. Clinical features of anti-factor H autoantibody-associated hemolytic uremic syndrome. *J Am Soc Nephrol.* 2010;21:2180-2187.

Fakhouri F, Roumenina L, Provot F, et al. Pregnancy-associated hemolytic uremic syndrome revisited in the era of complement gene mutations. *J Am Soc Nephrol.* 2010;21:859-867.

Fremeaux-Bacchi V, Fakhouri F, Garnier A, et al. Genetics and outcome of atypical hemolytic uremic syndrome: a nationwide French series comparing children and adults. *Clin J Am Soc Nephrol.* 2013;8:554-562.

Gale DP, de Jorge EG, Cook HT, et al. Identification of a mutation in complement factor H-related protein 5 in patients of Cypriot origin with glomerulonephritis. *Lancet.* 2010;376:794-801.

George JN, Nester CM. Syndromes of thrombotic microangiopathy. *N Engl J Med.* 2014;371:654-666.

Le Quintrec M, Zuber J, Moulin B, et al. Complement genes strongly predict recurrence and graft outcome in adult renal transplant recipients with atypical hemolytic and uremic syndrome. *Am J Transplant.* 2013;13:663-675.

Loirat C, Fakhouri F, Ariceta G, et al. An international consensus approach to the management of atypical hemolytic uremic syndrome in children. *Pediatr Nephrol.* 2015;31:15-39.

Martinez-Barricarte R, Heurich M, Valdes-Canedo F, et al. Human C3 mutation reveals a mechanism of dense deposit disease pathogenesis and provides insights into complement activation and regulation. *J Clin Invest.* 2010;120:3702-3712.

McCaughan JA, O'Rourke DM, Courtney AE. Recurrent dense deposit disease after renal transplantation: an emerging role for complementary therapies. *Am J Transplant.* 2012;12:1046-1051.

Medjeral-Thomas NR, O'Shaughnessy MM, O'Regan JA, et al. C3 glomerulopathy: clinicopathologic features and predictors of outcome. *Clin J Am Soc Nephrol.* 2014;9:46-53.

Nasr SH, Valeri AM, Appel GB, et al. Dense deposit disease: clinicopathologic study of 32 pediatric and adult patients. *Clin J Am Soc Nephrol.* 2009;4:22-32.

Noris M, Caprioli J, Bresin E, et al. Relative role of genetic complement abnormalities in sporadic and familial aHUS and their impact on clinical phenotype. *Clin J Am Soc Nephrol.* 2010;5:1844-1859.

Pickering MC, D'Agati VD, Nester CM, et al. C3 glomerulopathy: consensus report. *Kidney Int.* 2013;84:1079-1089.

Rabasco C, Cavero T, Roman E, et al. Effectiveness of mycophenolate mofetil in C3 glomerulonephritis. *Kidney Int.* 2015;88:1153-1160.

Servais A, Fremeaux-Bacchi V, Lequintrec M, et al. Primary glomerulonephritis with isolated C3 deposits: a new entity which shares common genetic risk factors with haemolytic uraemic syndrome. *J Med Genet.* 2007;44:193-199.

Servais A, Noel LH, Roumenina LT, et al. Acquired and genetic complement abnormalities play a critical role in dense deposit disease and other C3 glomerulopathies. *Kidney Int.* 2012;82:454-464.

Full bibliography can be found on www.expertconsult.com.

22 Infection-Related Glomerulonephritis

Laura Ferreira Provenzano; Leal Herlitz

In previous editions, this chapter was titled "Postinfectious Glomerulonephritis," which aptly describes classic poststreptococcal glomerulonephritis (PSGN) but is a misnomer for the increasingly recognized forms of glomerulonephritis (GN) that are manifestations of ongoing infection. Indeed, infection has a much broader role in the development of GN, sometimes serving as a trigger for a variety of common autoimmune responses including lupus, antineutrophil cytoplasmic antibody (ANCA) vasculitis, and IgA nephropathy. This chapter addresses both classic PSGN as well as forms of GN resulting from active bacterial infections. Glomerular disease due to viral hepatitis and HIV are discussed elsewhere. The change in the title from "Postinfectious" to "Infection-Related Glomerulonephritis (IRGN)" is meant to draw attention to the changing epidemiology of IRGN and to emphasize that infection may be ongoing at the time of the development of GN, which is important for guiding therapy.

CLINICAL FEATURES

The clinical presentation of IRGN is variable, ranging from a complete lack of symptoms to a rapidly progressive GN. When symptomatic, findings include hematuria, which can be either microscopic or gross; proteinuria, which is usually subnephrotic but can be in the nephrotic range; and variable degrees of hypertension, edema, and glomerular filtration rate (GFR) loss. The presentation and outcomes in children are often different from those in adults (Table 22.1).

In classic PSGN, symptomatic children usually present with acute nephritic syndrome characterized by hematuria, proteinuria, hypertension, edema, oliguria, and variable elevation of serum creatinine. The urinary sediment is usually active, with dysmorphic red cells, red blood cell casts, and leukocyturia. Hypocomplementemia is very common, with decreased C3 in up to 90% of cases and to a lesser extent depleted levels of C4. There is usually a "latent" period between the resolution of the streptococcal infection and the acute onset of the nephritic syndrome. This period is usually 7 to 10 days after oropharyngeal infections and 2 to 4 weeks after skin infections. Serologic markers of a recent streptococcal infection include elevated antistreptolysin O (ASO), antistreptokinase, antihyaluronidase, and antideoxyribonuclease B (anti-DNase B) levels. Elevation of these four markers has a yield of approximately 80% in documenting recent streptococcal infection.

In adults, most cases of IRGN no longer follow streptococcal infection, and the GN often coexists with the triggering infection. In cases of ongoing active infection, other clinical manifestations related to the specific infectious disease are common. Sites of infection can include the upper and lower respiratory tract, skin/soft tissue, bone, teeth/oral mucosa, heart, deep abscesses, shunts, and indwelling catheters. GFR loss and the nephrotic syndrome are more common in adults than in children, whereas macroscopic hematuria is less commonly seen. Hypocomplementemia is only seen in 30% to 80% of these patients. Adults more commonly present with kidney failure and with complications of hypervolemia, including decompensated heart failure. Up to 50% of adults with IRGN may require dialysis, and mortality may approach 20%.

EPIDEMIOLOGY

The incidence of PSGN has declined throughout most of the world over the past several decades, due to improvements in sanitation and infection control, but still remains a health concern in many developing countries. An effort by Carpentis and colleagues to evaluate the incidence of PSGN using 11 population-based studies suggests that approximately 472,000 cases of PSGN occur worldwide annually, resulting in approximately 5000 deaths (1% of total cases). Approximately 97% of these cases of PSGN occur in less developed countries. Other estimates of the burden of PSGN in the developing world estimate that between 9.5 and 28.5 cases of PSGN occur per 100,000 individuals per year.

In industrialized countries, much of the burden of IRGN has shifted to adults, with a lower proportion attributed to PSGN. IRGN associated with other microorganisms, including *Staphylococcus* species and gram-negative bacteria, are increasingly recognized, mainly in the adult population. In these cases, coexistence of the glomerular disease and the infection is common, and classic clinical findings such as low complement levels may be absent. The clinical course and prognosis of these newly recognized forms are also different, with more patients developing progressive chronic kidney disease (CKD), sometimes to end-stage renal disease (ESRD). Diabetes is the most commonly recognized comorbidity and is associated with poor outcomes. Other common comorbidities seen in patients with IRGN include malignancy, immunosuppression, AIDS, alcoholism, cirrhosis, malnutrition, and IV drug use. The elderly population is especially prone to IRGN, with patients over 65 years of age accounting for about 34% of

Table 22.1 Common Differences in Infection-Related Glomerulonephritis Between Children and Adults

	Onset of Nephritic Syndrome	Infection Site	Bacterial Organisms	Low C3	Prognosis
Children	After infection (typical latency 1–4 weeks)	Pharyngitis skin (impetigo)	Predominantly streptococcal	≈90% of cases	Excellent (>90% make a full recovery)
Adults	During ongoing infection	Highly variable, including respiratory tract, skin, heart, urinary tract, bone, oral/dental	Staphylococcal ≥ streptococcal, gram-negative organisms	30%–80% of cases	Guarded, with residual CKD common; elderly patients and those with diabetic nephropathy show full recovery in <25% of cases

CKD, Chronic kidney disease.

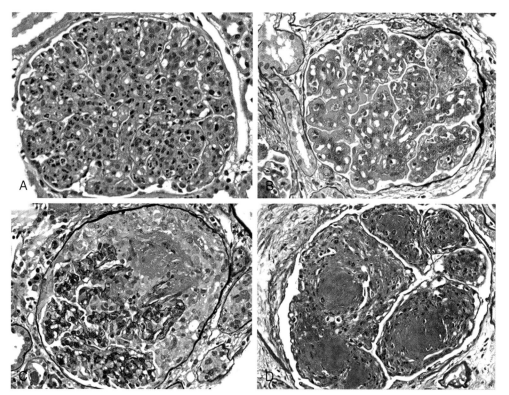

Fig. 22.1 Diverse light microscopic patterns of glomerular injury in infection-related glomerulonephritis. A diffuse endocapillary proliferative and exudative (neutrophil-rich) glomerulonephritis ([A] hematoxylin and eosin, 400× magnification) is the most common pathology encountered in infection-related glomerulonephritis. A membranoproliferative pattern ([B] Jones methenamine silver stain, 400× magnification) with large subendothelial immune deposits can be seen in cases where infection is long-standing, such as in shunt nephritis. Intravascular infections such as endocarditis may display a necrotizing crescentic glomerulonephritis with few immune deposits ([C] Jones methenamine silver stain, 400× magnification), strikingly similar to what is classically seen in ANCA vasculitis. Underlying chronic diseases, such as diabetic nephropathy, may exist and modify the appearance of glomeruli. (D) A glomerulus with large mesangial nodules due to diabetes, as well as an exudative endocapillary proliferative glomerulonephritis (periodic acid–Schiff, 400× magnification).

IRGN cases in the developed world, increased from only 4% to 6% of recognized IRGN 40 years ago.

HISTOPATHOLOGY

A spectrum of histologic findings can be seen in IRGN, and biopsy findings are influenced by the associated organism and site and duration of infection.

Light microscopy can reveal a wide range of proliferative glomerular lesions (Fig. 22.1). The most common finding in acute IRGN, including PSGN, is that of diffuse endocapillary proliferation, with significant numbers of infiltrating neutrophils. While occasional cellular crescents may be seen with these diffuse proliferative GNs, crescent formation in >50% of glomeruli is uncommon. More subacute or remote cases of IRGN may show only focal endocapillary proliferation, or simply a mesangial proliferative appearance. In longer

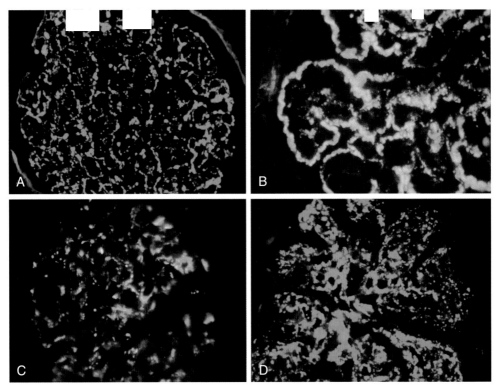

Fig. 22.2 Immunofluorescence findings in infection-related glomerulonephritis. Deposits are typically C3 dominant or co-dominant and accompanied by immunoglobulin staining of lesser intensity. (A) The classic "starry sky" appearance of C3 encountered in infection-related glomerulonephritis (IRGN), which results from the scattered combination of subepithelial, mesangial, and subendothelial deposits (400× magnification). The "garland pattern" of C3 staining is illustrated in (B) (600× magnification) and more clearly demonstrates the contour of the glomerular basement membrane, because subepithelial deposits are in abundance and nearly confluent. (C) Predominantly mesangial deposits of C3 with only rare peripheral capillary wall deposits (400× magnification). This pattern of staining is most commonly seen in the subacute and resolving stages of IRGN. The staining in (D) is for IgA (400× magnification), and a nodular, largely mesangial distribution of positive staining can be seen. This glomerulus is from a patient with a *Staphylococcus aureus*–associated IRGN superimposed on underlying diabetic nephropathy (for the corresponding light microscopic image, see Fig. 22.1D).

standing ongoing infections, such as shunt nephritis, a membranoproliferative pattern with large subendothelial deposits can be seen. Necrotizing and crescentic histology, similar to what can be seen in ANCA vasculitis, is increasingly recognized as a pattern of IRGN associated with endocarditis. In the adult population, acute GN may be superimposed on chronic conditions such as diabetic nephropathy, and this can alter the histologic appearance.

Immunofluorescence typically shows dominant or codominant staining for C3, usually accompanied by lesser degrees of immunoglobulin staining. In classic PSGN, IgG is typically seen in a similar distribution to C3. In staphylococcal infections, IgA is commonly the dominant immunoglobulin, and in up to 25% of cases, the C3 is not associated with significant amounts of immunoglobulin staining. The distribution of the deposits in glomeruli can range from the classic "starry sky" appearance, reflecting an admixture of mesangial and peripheral capillary deposits, to the "garland" appearance, in which the subepithelial deposits are confluent, to a mesangial pattern often seen in the resolving stages (Fig. 22.2). A significant portion of endocarditis-associated IRGN may have a pauci-immune appearance on immunofluorescence studies.

The classic electron microscopic finding in PSGN is the hump-shaped subepithelial electron-dense deposit (Fig. 22.3). While often present, these subepithelial deposits are not required for the diagnosis of IRGN, and their presence alone does not constitute the diagnosis of IRGN. Subendothelial deposits, though often less pronounced, are largely responsible for the prominent endocapillary proliferation that is often seen. Mesangial deposits, while sometimes sparse, are almost universally encountered in IRGN.

DIFFERENTIAL DIAGNOSIS

Given the highly variable clinical presentation, the differential diagnosis of IRGN is broad. Due to the association of IRGN with hypocomplementemia, diagnoses including lupus nephritis, C3 GN, and cryoglobulinemic GN are often considered. IgA nephropathy, because of its synpharyngitic presentation, is also frequently considered in the differential diagnosis. A combination of serologic testing and features on kidney biopsy can help distinguish these entities, but pitfalls exist. Serologic findings such as positive antinuclear antibody (ANA) and anti-DNA antibodies would typically

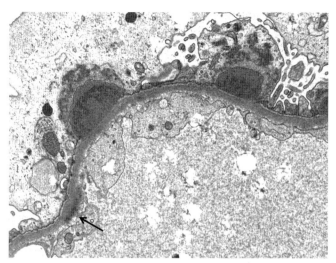

Fig. 22.3 Classic ultrastructural findings in infection-related glomerulonephritis. Subepithelial hump-shaped deposits pictured here (original magnification 9300×) are distinctive findings in many cases of infection-related glomerulonephritis (IRGN) but are neither required nor sufficient to make the diagnosis of IRGN. It is the typically smaller subendothelial deposits *(arrow)* that are likely responsible for producing much of the diffuse proliferative changes usually seen by light microscopy.

favor the diagnosis of lupus nephritis, but it is important to remember that infections such as shunt nephritis can also be accompanied by a positive ANA. Cryoglobulinemic GN is most often characterized by disproportionate lowering of C4 rather than C3, and IgA nephropathy is usually associated with normocomplementemia.

In many cases, C3 GN can be difficult or impossible to distinguish from IRGN. Both C3GN and IRGN can present with very similar clinical, pathologic, and laboratory findings, including elevated ASO levels in more than 50% of cases of C3GN. C3GN should be strongly considered in cases that have been diagnosed as IRGN if there is persistence of low C3 levels after 6 to 8 weeks. In these cases, evaluation for abnormalities of the alternative complement pathway should be considered. Histologically, C3GN is a consideration in the cases where immunoglobulin staining is sparse or absent, but sparse or absent immunoglobulin staining with prominent C3 staining is also a recognized immunofluorescence pattern in up to 25% of IRGN. One recent study proposes that C4d staining can help differentiate C3GN from IRGN, as prominent glomerular C4d positivity was detected in about half of the tested cases of IRGN but not in any of the C3GN cases, suggesting additional involvement of the classic or lectin complement pathways in IRGN. Importantly, the intensity of the C4d staining should be equal to or greater than that of C3 to be considered significant, as mild background C4d staining is routinely detected in mesangial areas of normal glomeruli.

Cases of IRGN with significant amounts of IgA deposition, as are commonly seen with IRGN due to staphylococcal organisms, can potentially be confused with IgA nephropathy or Henoch-Schönlein purpura (HSP). In one series of culture-proven staphylococcal-associated GN, 22% had an HSP-like presentation, including a purpuric skin rash over the lower extremities.

IRGN with a pauciimmune phenotype by immunofluorescence can be encountered in conjunction with a necrotizing crescentic GN histologically indistinguishable from ANCA vasculitis. This variant of IRGN is most frequently encountered in patients with endocarditis or other intravascular infections. Further complicating attempts to distinguish endocarditis-associated IRGN from a more purely ANCA-driven vasculitis is the presence of positive ANCA serologies in approximately 25% of endocarditis-associated IRGN. Ultimately, the possibility of recent or active infection should be at least considered in the differential diagnosis of almost any proliferative GN.

PATHOGENESIS

The pathogenesis of IRGN is multifactorial and far from fully understood. The development of glomerular immune complexes in IRGN is likely due to both deposition of pre-formed circulating immune complexes and the binding of antibodies directed at bacterial antigens that are planted within glomeruli, resulting in in situ formation of immune complexes. Identification of nephritogenic streptococcal antigens has been pursued for decades, and streptococcal pyrogenic exotoxin B (SPEB) appears to be the nephritogenic antigen responsible for most cases of PSGN. SPEB is cationic and therefore can more easily penetrate the anionic glomerular basement membrane, resulting in the ability of SPEB to localize subepithelially. SPEB has been demonstrated to co-localize with IgG and C3 in the subepithelial humps of many patients with PSGN, supporting the theory that in situ immune complex formation is important in the development of PSGN. In addition, SPEB can directly activate the alternative complement pathway, helping explain the disproportionate consumption of C3 in PSGN.

Outside of PSGN, the search for nephritogenic antigens is in its infancy. Staphylococcal superantigens, which have the ability to cause massive T-cell activation and high levels of proinflammatory cytokines, have been proposed to play a role in staphylococcal IRGN. Potential nephritogenic antigens associated with gram-negative bacteria and other less common organisms responsible for IRGN are yet to be identified.

The development of IRGN is also likely largely dependent on host factors that significantly influence the susceptibility of a given patient to developing IRGN. IRGN can be caused by many types and strains of bacteria, but only a small percentage of people infected with these pathogens develop clinically significant GN. The presence of hypocomplementemia and the overlapping features of C3GN and IRGN suggest that differences in the way that the alternative complement pathway is regulated likely plays a role in the development of IRGN.

TREATMENT AND PROGNOSIS

Treatment in most instances of IRGN is supportive, focusing on managing the manifestations of kidney disease (hypervolemia, hypertension, uremia) and controlling active infections when they coexist with the GN. Hypervolemia usually responds to salt restriction and loop diuretics. Volume control is often sufficient to control the new-onset hypertension, but in some cases the addition of antihypertensive medications is needed. Dialysis may be necessary, and the need for dialysis is more frequent in adults. In instances of epidemic PSGN, antibiotic prophylaxis of household or community members can help decrease the incidence of the disease. In select cases with aggressive crescentic disease and a rapidly progressive glomerulonephritis presentation, immunosuppressive therapy, typically with intravenous methylprednisolone, may be of benefit, as long as the infection is controlled; however, there are no randomized clinical trials to support this approach.

Prognosis is usually excellent in children, with more than 95% experiencing complete recovery, though it may take 4 to 8 weeks for symptoms to resolve and kidney function to return to baseline. Hematuria often lasts up to 6 months, and proteinuria might be present for years; however, only 1% will progress to ESRD. In children with an atypical presentation and limited recovery, the possibility of C3GN should be considered.

The prognosis of epidemic PSGN affecting adults is also good. In a recent 10-year follow-up study of the PSGN outbreak that occurred in Brazil after ingestion of contaminated dairy with *Streptococcus zooepidemicus*, there was no significant difference in the level of kidney function or proteinuria at 10 years compared with matched controls. However, cases had higher incidence of hypertension compared with control subjects (45% vs. 20.8%).

The prognosis for adults with sporadic IRGN cases is notably worse, with only about half experiencing complete recovery. This is not surprising, as many adult patients affected by IRGN have comorbid conditions that are also risk factors for kidney failure. Diabetes imparts a particularly poor outcome, with very high rates of progression to ESRD after IRGN (>50% in some reports). In a series focusing on elderly patients with IRGN, only 22% experienced a complete kidney recovery, 44% developed CKD, and 33% progressed to ESRD.

BIBLIOGRAPHY

Boils CL, Nasr SH, Walker PD, et al. Update on endocarditis-associated glomerulonephritis. *Kidney Int.* 2015;87:1241-1249.

Bratsford SR, Mezzano S, Mihatsch M, et al. Is the nephritogenic antigen in post-streptococcal glomerulonephritis pyrogenic exotoxin B (SPEB) or GAPDH? *Kidney Int.* 2005;68:1120-1129.

Carpentis JR, Steer AC, Mulholland EK, Weber M. The global burden of group A streptococcal diseases. *Lancet Infect Dis.* 2005;5:685-694.

Couser WG, Johnson RJ. The etiology of glomerulonephritis: roles of infection and autoimmunity. *Kidney Int.* 2014;86:905-914.

Dagan R, Cleper R, Davidovits M, et al. Post-infectious glomerulonephritis in pediatric patients over two decades: severity-associated features. *Isr Med Assoc J.* 2016;18:336-340.

Glassock RJ, Alvarado A, Prosek J, et al. *Staphylococcus*-related glomerulonephritis and poststreptococcal glomerulonephritis: why defining "post" is important in understanding and trating infection-related glomerulonephritis. *Am J Kidney Dis.* 2015;65:826-832.

Khalighi MA, Wang S, Henriksen KJ, et al. Revisiting post-infectious glomerulonephritis in the emerging era of C3 glomerulopathy. *Clin Kidney J.* 2016;9:397-402.

Kidney Disease: Improving Global Outcomes (KDIGO) Glomerulonephritis Work Group. KDIGO clinical practice guldeline for glomerulonephritis. Chapter 9: Infection-related glomerulonephritis. *Kidney Int Suppl.* 2012;2:200-208.

Nasr SH, Fidler ME, Valeri AM, et al. Post infectious glomerulonephritis in the elderly. *J Am Soc Nephrol.* 2011;22:187-195.

Nasr SH, Markowitz GS, Stokes MB, et al. Acute postinfectious glomerulonephritis in the modern era: experience with 86 adults and review of the literature. *Medicine (Baltimore).* 2008;87:21-32.

Nasr SH, Radhakrishnan J, D'Agati VD. Bacterial infection-related glomerulonephritis in adults. *Kidney Int.* 2013;83:792-803.

Nast CC. Infection-related glomerulonephritis: changing demographics and outcomes. *Adv Chronic Kidney Dis.* 2012;19:68-75.

Pinto SW, Mastroianni-Kirsztajn G, Sesso R. Ten-year follow-up of patients with epidemic post infectious glomerulonephritis. *PLoS ONE.* 2015;10:e0125313.

Rodriguez-Iturbe B, Bratsford S. Pathogenesis of poststreptococcal glomerulonephritis a century after Clemens con Pirquet. *Kidney Int.* 2007;71:1094-1104.

Rodriguez-Iturbe B, Musser JM. The current state of poststreptococcal glomerulonephritis. *J Am Soc Nephrol.* 2008;19:1855-1864.

Satoskar AA, Molenda M, Scipio P, et al. Henoch-Schonlein purpura-like presentation in IgA-dominant *Staphylococcus* infection-associated glomerulonephritis—a diagnostic pitfall. *Clin Nephrol.* 2013;79:302-312.

Satoskar AA, Nadasdy T, Silva FG. Acute postinfectious glomerulonephritis and glomerulonephritis caused by persistend bacterial infection. In: Jennette JC, Olson JL, Silva FG, D'Agati VD, eds. *Heptinstall's Pathology of the Kidney.* 7th ed. Philadelphia: Wolters Kluwer; 2015:367-436.

Sethi S, Nasr SH, De Vriese AS, Fervenza FC. C4d as a diagnostic tool in proliferative GN. *J Am Soc Nephrol.* 2015;26:2852-2859.

Stratta P, Musetti C, Marreca A, Mazzucco G. New trends of an old disease: the acute post infectious glomerulonephritis at the beginning of the new millennium. *J Nephrol.* 2014;27:229-239.

Wang SY, Bu R, Zhang Q, et al. Clinical, pathological and prognostic characteristics of glomerulonephritis related to staphylococcal infection. *Medicine (Baltimore).* 2016;95:e3386.

23

Viral Nephropathies: Human Immunodeficiency Virus, Hepatitis C Virus, and Hepatitis B Virus

Sarah Schrauben; Jeffrey S. Berns

Human immunodeficiency virus (HIV), hepatitis C virus (HCV), and hepatitis B virus (HBV) are the most important causes of viral-related kidney disease in the world. Several mechanisms are involved in the pathogenesis of virus-related kidney disease, including tropism of the virus in the kidney, direct cytopathic effects, and immune response to the virus and production of immune complexes. These lead to a spectrum of glomerular and tubulointerstitial diseases. Some of the most important features of the kidney diseases associated with these viruses are shown in Table 23.1.

HUMAN IMMUNODEFICIENCY VIRUS

Kidney disease is a frequent complication of HIV infection. The incidence of HIV-related kidney disease has decreased, and the distribution of HIV-associated kidney disease has changed with the widespread use of combined antiretroviral therapy (cART). The classic kidney disease related to HIV is a form of collapsing focal segmental glomerulosclerosis (FSGS), referred to as HIV-associated nephropathy (HIVAN). This occurs in 3.5% to 10% of HIV-infected patients. After the introduction of cART, there has been a decline in the incidence of HIVAN, with a corresponding reduction in end-stage renal disease (ESRD) attributed to HIVAN.

PATHOPHYSIOLOGY

In the setting of HIV infection, kidney disease is mediated by factors related to the virus, host genetic predisposition, host response to infection, and environmental factors.

GENETIC SUSCEPTIBILITY

Susceptibility to HIV-related kidney disease is most striking in patients of African descent. This predilection is associated with high frequencies of *APOL1* genetic polymorphisms on chromosome 22 in this population, specifically G1 (two missense mutations) and G2 (two base pair deletion). The G1 and G2 variants confer risk for HIVAN and an HIV-associated noncollapsing form of FSGS, as well as other glomerular diseases and arteriolar nephrosclerosis. The effect is largely recessive, in that homozygous (G1/G1 or G2/G2) or compound heterozygous (G1/G2) individuals have the highest

risk of HIVAN. The mechanisms by which the risk variant proteins alter kidney cell function and lead to chronic kidney disease (CKD) and ESRD remain unclear and are a matter of considerable interest and ongoing research.

DIRECT VIRAL EFFECTS

Evidence from clinical and animal studies supports a direct role of HIV infection of renal parenchymal cells in the pathogenesis of HIVAN. Exactly how HIV infection of podocytes and tubular epithelial cells occurs and the subsequent downstream process leading to cellular injury are not entirely understood. Although renal epithelial cells do not generally express viral receptors, uptake of HIV into renal epithelial cells is thought to be mediated by transfer from infected lymphocytes. The various processes that have been implicated in HIVAN, which include effects on glomerular filtration, cellular proliferation, apoptosis, de-differentiation, and immunomodulation, can be related to the presence of HIV transcripts in affected renal parenchymal cells. Expression of HIV regulatory and accessory proteins in transgenic mice produces the glomerular and tubular features of HIVAN-like pathology, even in the absence of intact virus, supporting direct effects of HIV transcript expression in glomerular (mesangial and epithelial) and tubular cells. Expression of HIV transgenes in podocytes and renal tubular epithelial cells results in de-differentiation and/or loss of expression of important proteins (e.g., nephrin) and correlates with proliferation and tubular microcyst formation. The mechanism that drives aberrant expansion of podocyte stem cells, which are located in the parietal epithelium, remains unknown.

IMMUNE REACTION

Chronic HIV infection is associated with polyclonal expansion of immunoglobulins. Immune complexes in the kidney may result from deposition from the systemic circulation or result from in situ deposition of immunoglobulins binding to HIV antigens. Subsequently, there is activation of inflammatory mediators, which results in secondary kidney damage, giving rise to HIV immune complex disease (HIV-ICD). The kidney infiltrate in HIV-ICD primarily consists of B lymphocytes, in contrast to HIVAN, in which there are mainly T lymphocytes and macrophages.

Table 23.1   Important Clinical Features of Viral Nephropathies

	HIV	HCV	HBV
Major risk groups	Infected individuals of African ancestry, HIVAN Infected individuals of European and Asian ancestry, HIV-ICD	Adults with risk factors for chronic HCV infection	Children from HBV endemic areas
Presentation	Proteinuria, nephrotic syndrome CKD with rapid progression Large, echogenic kidneys Advanced HIV (if HIVAN)	Hematuria Proteinuria Hypocomplementemia Palpable purpura Systemic vasculitis Cryoglobulinemia	Proteinuria Nephrotic syndrome
Primary kidney pathology	Collapsing FSGS Microcystic dilation of tubules Interstitial inflammation/fibrosis	MPGN	MN
Pathogenesis	Direct HIV infection Host genetic factors Immune complex deposition	Direct HCV toxicity Cryoglobulinemia	Antigen-antibody complex deposition Vasculitis
Therapy	cART ACE-I and ARBs	Antiviral therapy Rituximab Cyclophosphamide Plasmapheresis in severe cases	Antiviral therapy

ACE-I, Angiotensin converting enzyme inhibitor; *ARB,* angiotensin receptor blocker; *cART,* combined antiretroviral therapy; *CKD,* chronic kidney disease; *FSGS,* focal segmental glomerulosclerosis; *HBV,* hepatitis B virus; *HCV,* hepatitis C virus; *HIV,* human immunodeficiency virus; *HIVAN,* HIV-associated nephropathy; *HIV-ICD,* HIV immune complex disease; *MN,* membranous nephropathy; *MPGN,* membranoproliferative glomerulonephritis.

CLINICAL PRESENTATION

The classic involvement of the kidney by HIV infection is HIVAN. Other kidney diseases include HIV-ICD, HIV-related noncollapsing FSGS, thrombotic microangiopathy, and disorders associated with nephrotoxic HIV therapies. With the introduction and widespread use of cART, there has been a decline in the incidence of HIVAN and an increasing prevalence of noncollapsing FSGS. Progression to ESRD is more likely with high-grade proteinuria, severely reduced estimated glomerular filtration rate (eGFR), hepatitis B and/or C coinfection, diabetes mellitus, extensive glomerulosclerosis, and chronic interstitial fibrosis.

HUMAN IMMUNODEFICIENCY VIRUS–ASSOCIATED NEPHROPATHY

The classic presentation of HIVAN is nephrotic syndrome, GFR loss, relatively bland urinary sediment, and large, often densely echogenic, kidneys on ultrasound. Most patients are normotensive and relatively edema-free, despite advanced CKD. HIVAN occurs predominantly in those of African ancestry with advanced HIV (high viral loads, CD4 counts less than 200 cells/μL), but HIVAN is occasionally diagnosed at the time of acute HIV seroconversion. Untreated, HIVAN progresses rapidly to ESRD, often in a few months.

OTHER GLOMERULAR DISEASES

Prolonged use of cART and increased life span of HIV-infected individuals have led to increasingly common patterns of HIV-associated CKD, including noncollapsing FSGS, HIV-ICD, arteriolar nephrosclerosis, and diabetic nephropathy. Despite the suppression of HIV replication with cART, a state of chronic inflammation and dysmetabolism persists, which is linked to diabetic nephropathy, arteriolar nephrosclerosis, and possibly FSGS. HIV-ICD is the dominant glomerular disease in HIV-positive European-derived populations and is thought to be associated with HCV coinfection. One form of HIV-ICD is a glomerulonephritis with "lupus-like" features on biopsy but which lacks both serologic and clinical evidence of systemic lupus erythematosus. In general, HIV-ICD presents with less proteinuria and higher GFR and is less likely to progress to ESRD than HIVAN. HIV-related thrombotic microangiopathy presents similarly to idiopathic forms with acute kidney injury (AKI), microscopic hematuria, and nonnephrotic proteinuria, along with features of a microangiopathic hemolytic anemia.

MEDICATION TOXICITY

cART nephrotoxicity is an important clinical problem (Table 23.2). Common forms of nephrotoxicity are crystalluria and obstruction due to protease inhibitor therapy and proximal tubular damage due to tenofovir. Tenofovir-induced nephrotoxicity causes proximal tubulopathy, Fanconi syndrome, nephrogenic diabetes insipidus, AKI, and CKD. Dose adjustment of tenofovir according to eGFR is mandatory to minimize nephrotoxic effects. It is important to note that nucleoside reverse transcriptase inhibitors (NRTIs) require dose adjustment in patients with reduced GFR. Medications used to treat opportunistic infections can also cause nephrotoxicity (see Table 23.2).

DIAGNOSIS

The utility of a kidney biopsy in HIV-infected individuals has been debated, as the decision to biopsy depends on how typical or atypical the clinical presentation, which alternative diagnoses seem likely, and whether an alternative diagnosis

Table 23.2 Drug-Induced Nephrotoxicity in Patients With Human Immunodeficiency Virus-1 Infection

Class	Renal Abnormality
Nucleos(t)ide Reverse Transcriptase Inhibitors	
Abacavir	Lactic acidosis, AIN[a], Fanconi syndrome[a]
Didanosine	Lactic acidosis, AKI, proximal tubule dysfunction, Fanconi syndrome, nephrogenic diabetes insipidus
Lamivudine	Lactic acidosis, renal tubular acidosis, hypophosphatemia[a]
Stavudine	Lactic acidosis, renal tubular acidosis, hypophosphatemia[a]
Zidovudine	Lactic acidosis
Tenofovir	Proximal tubule dysfunction with Fanconi syndrome, nephrogenic diabetes insipidus, AKI, lactic acidosis, CKD, chronic tubular injury
Adefovir	Proximal tubule dysfunction with Fanconi syndrome, AKI, nephrogenic diabetes insipidus, lactic acidosis
Non-Nucleoside Reverse Transcriptase Inhibitors	
Efavirenz	Nephrolithiasis
Protease Inhibitors	
Atazanavir	Nephrolithiasis, crystal nephropathy, AIN[a]
Indinavir	Crystalluria, nephrolithiasis, interstitial nephritis (AKI, CKD), papillary necrosis, hypertension, renal atrophy
Nelfinavir	Nephrolithiasis[a]
Ritonavir	AKI, hyperuricemia
Saquinavir	AKI in association with ritonavir
Fusion or Entry Inhibitors	
Enfuvirtide	Membranoproliferative glomerulonephritis[a]
Other Antimicrobials	
Acyclovir	AKI, crystalluria, obstructive nephropathy
Aminoglycosides	AKI, renal tubular acidosis
Amphotericin	AKI, hypokalemia, hypomagnesemia, renal tubular acidosis
Cidofovir	Proximal tubular damage, bicarbonate wasting, proteinuria, AKI
Foscarnet	AKI, hypocalcemia and hypercalcemia, hypophosphatemia and hyperphosphatemia, hypomagnesemia, nephrogenic diabetes insipidus
Pentamidine	AKI, hyperkalemia, hypocalcemia
Rifampin	Interstitial nephritis
Sulfadiazine	Proximal tubule dysfunction
Valacyclovir	Thrombotic microangiopathy

[a]Case reports.
AIN, Acute interstitial nephritis; *AKI,* acute kidney injury; *CKD,* chronic kidney disease.

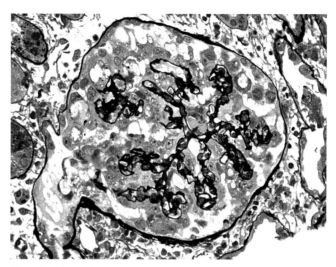

Fig. 23.1 Collapsing focal segmental glomerulonephritis in human immunodeficiency virus–associated nephropathy. (Jones methenamine silver stain, ×400 magnification.)

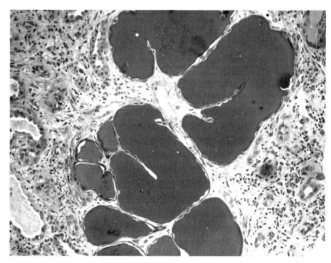

Fig. 23.2 Tubulointerstitial disease in human immunodeficiency virus–associated nephropathy, characterized by tubular atrophy, microcystic tubular dilation with proteinaceous casts, and mild interstitial inflammation. (Trichrome stain, ×200 magnification.)

HIVAN, AKI, cART-related toxicities, HIV-associated comorbidities (such as HCV infection, hypertension, and diabetes), and opportunistic infections.

GLOMERULAR DISEASES

The characteristic pathologic changes of HIVAN are observed along the full length of the nephron, including glomerular and tubulointerstitial features. Light microscopy reveals a collapse of glomerular capillaries that typically involves the entire glomerulus (Fig. 23.1), visceral glomerular epitheliosis, podocyte hypertrophy and proliferation surrounding the shrunken glomerulus, and mesangial prominence and hypercellularity. Tubular injury is marked by microcystic tubular dilation, tubular atrophy, and proteinaceous casts (Fig. 23.2). Many patients have a modest interstitial inflammation with lymphocytes, plasma cells, and monocytes. Immunofluorescence is generally nonspecific, and electron

would lead to new therapy, as well as the risks and patients' preference.

PATHOLOGY

HIV-associated kidney diseases include a broad spectrum of glomerular and tubulointerstitial pathologies secondary to

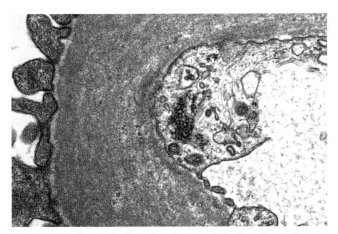

Fig. 23.3 Tubuloreticular inclusions in the endothelium classically seen on electron microscopy in human immunodeficiency virus–associated nephropathy. (Electron micrograph, ×50,000 magnification.)

microscopy shows diffuse food process effacement and possible endothelial tubuloreticular inclusions (TRIs) without immune complex deposits (Fig. 23.3). This classic HIVAN pathology is most common in the presence of advanced HIV disease, including AIDS. The clinical constellation of proteinuria, GFR loss, and low CD4 count is not sufficient for the diagnosis without a kidney biopsy.

The histology of HIV-ICD includes membranoproliferative glomerulonephritis (MPGN, types I and II), IgA nephropathy, membranous nephropathy (MN), "lupus-like" glomerulonephritis, thrombotic microangiopathy, and postinfectious glomerulonephritis; these are often seen in patients who are coinfected with hepatitis B and/or C. The predominant pattern is variable mesangial alteration with immune deposits in the mesangial and paramesangial regions. Subepithelial immune deposits are also seen and described as a "ball-in-cup" basement membrane reaction. Lupus-like features are characterized by a "full house" pattern of IgG, IgA, and IgM immunoglobulin staining and C3 and C1q complement deposits within the glomeruli, often with large subendothelial deposits. Tubulointerstitial changes are attributed to drug toxicity and superimposed viral (e.g., cytomegalovirus), fungal (e.g., candida), or mycobacterial infections (e.g., tuberculosis, histoplasmosis), resulting in interstitial nephritis.

TREATMENT

ANTIRETROVIRAL THERAPY

All patients with HIV-associated kidney disease are recommended to receive cART. Current guidelines recommend HIVAN as an indication for initiation of cART, irrespective of CD4 count. The use of cART has been associated with a lower incidence of HIVAN, improved kidney function, improvement in HIV-associated thrombotic microangiopathy, and lower risk of ESRD. There are conflicting reports on the benefit of cART in patients with HIV-ICD. Many antiretroviral medications are partially or completely eliminated by the kidney (most NRTIs) and require dose adjustment in those with reduced kidney function (eGFR <60 mL/min per 1.73 m²). Furthermore, NRTI doses may also need to be supplemented following dialysis as they are easily removed because they are not tightly protein bound and have a low-to-medium molecular weight.

Certain drug classes, such as protease inhibitors, nonnucleoside reverse transcriptase inhibitors (NNRTIs), or integrase inhibitors, do not require dose adjustment in patients with reduced kidney function. In general, fixed drug combinations are avoided in patients with moderate-to-severely reduced kidney function (i.e., eGFR <30 to 50 mL/min per 1.73 m²) because of the need for differential dose adjustments of one or more of the components.

IMMUNOSUPPRESSION

Corticosteroids are not considered standard therapy for HIVAN, as the efficacy is modest and often short-lived. A typical dose is prednisone 1 mg/kg per day, with a maximum dose of 80 mg/day for 2 months, followed by a taper over 2 to 4 months. Similar data exist for cyclosporine for inducing remission of proteinuria in children with HIVAN. If kidney function does not improve, angiotensin-converting enzyme inhibitors (ACE inhibitors) or angiotensin-receptor blockers (ARBs) may be added. However, with the availability of cART, the use of corticosteroid and other immunosuppressive therapies is rarely, if ever, indicated for the treatment of HIVAN alone.

In general, standard therapies for CKD are recommended for HIV-positive individuals, including control of blood pressure and the use of ACE inhibitors and ARBs. There is improved kidney survival associated with the use of renin-angiotensin system blockers and viral suppression.

DIALYSIS AND TRANSPLANT

Survival rates of HIV-infected patients receiving hemodialysis or peritoneal dialysis who are stable on cART are comparable to dialysis patients without HIV infection. The outcome of kidney transplantation in HIV-positive patients who receive organs from HIV-negative or HIV-positive donors is similar to the outcome of HIV-negative recipients and HIV-negative donors. Classic HIVAN does not seem to recur in allografts, but HIV-ICD recurrence has been reported. There are notable interactions between antiretroviral drugs and posttransplant immunosuppressants. Ritonavir, an inhibitor of cytochrome P450 enzyme systems, decreases metabolism of tacrolimus, resulting in an increase in blood levels up to fivefold. In contrast, the NNRTIs efavirenz and nevirapine induce P450s and increase metabolism of tacrolimus, necessitating much higher doses to maintain adequate levels.

HEPATITIS C VIRUS

EPIDEMIOLOGY

The prevalence of HCV infection is estimated to be approximately 2.4% worldwide, or 200 million individuals. In the United States, the number of new HCV infections has been relatively stable over the past decade at 17,000 per year, and the prevalence is estimated to be 2.7 to 3.5 million, reflecting a high rate of chronic infection. Worldwide, regional differences in the HCV major genotypes (1 to 6) exist because of HCV's high genetic diversity and evolution. In the United States, approximately 70% of chronic HCV infections are caused by genotype 1 (55% genotype 1a and 35% genotype 1b), 15% to 20% genotype 2, 10% to 12% genotype 3, 1%

genotype 4, and less than 1% genotype 5 or 6. Worldwide, genotype 1 is the most prevalent, and genotype 3 is the next most common, and together account for the majority of infections. The major long-term complications of chronic HCV infection are liver related (cirrhosis, liver failure, hepatocellular carcinoma), but HCV also leads to extrahepatic complications, including hematologic, dermatologic, and kidney diseases. HCV infection is the major cause of mixed cryoglobulinemia syndrome (MCS), a systemic vasculitis characterized by involvement of small-to-medium sized vessels, leading to clinical manifestations ranging from skin changes to more serious lesions with neurologic and kidney involvement. Kidney disease is considered a major cause of morbidity and mortality in MCS. The kidney disease classically associated with HCV infection is MPGN type I, usually in the context of MCS, but other glomerular diseases have been described.

PATHOPHYSIOLOGY

CRYOGLOBULIN-MEDIATED INJURY

HCV infection is implicated in 80% to 90% of the cases of MCS. HCV infection causes chronic stimulation of B lymphocytes and widespread autoantibody synthesis and production of cryoglobulins. MCS results from the production of polyclonal IgG and monoclonal (type II cryoglobulin) or polyclonal (type III cryoglobulin) IgM with rheumatoid factor (RF) activity. Cryoglobulin-associated nephrotoxicity is suggested to be due to the IgM-RF affinity for cellular fibronectin in the mesangial matrix. Cyroglobulins are deposited in the glomerular capillaries and mesangium, which can lead to complement activation, inflammatory cytokine release, vasculitis, fibrinoid necrosis, and crescent formation.

DIRECT VIRAL TOXICITY

Direct cytopathic effects of HCV play a role in HCV-related kidney disease. HCV is able to bind and penetrate into renal parenchymal cells. HCV RNA has been found in mesangial cells, tubular epithelial cells, and endothelial cells of glomerulus and peritubular capillaries. In one study, the presence of HCV-related proteins in the mesangium was associated with greater proteinuria.

CLINICAL PRESENTATION

In patients with CKD, the risks for adverse outcomes are significantly higher in HCV-infected patients than those without infection, including progression to cirrhosis, hepatocellular carcinoma, liver-related mortality, and ESRD. The association of HCV and glomerular disease has been observed in both native and transplanted kidneys. In addition, chronic HCV infection along with HIV coinfection has been associated with an accelerated course of kidney disease.

Typical kidney manifestations of HCV-infected persons include proteinuria, microscopic hematuria, and hypertension, with or without a reduction in GFR. There is an independent relationship between anti-HCV seropositive status and the presence of proteinuria. HCV infection has been associated with a large spectrum of glomerular lesions, including MCS (up to one-third), which has particular importance as cryoglobulinemic glomerulonephritis is associated with a poor prognosis.

CRYOGLOBULINEMIC GLOMERULONEPHRITIS

Cryoglobulinemia often presents with a systemic vasculitis, with palpable purpura that most commonly involves the lower limbs, arthralgias, neuropathy, and nonspecific symptoms of fever, fatigue, and malaise. However, many patients with cryoglobulinemia are asymptomatic or have mild nonspecific symptoms. Patients with HCV-associated cryoglobulinemic glomerulonephritis experience asymptomatic nonnephrotic proteinuria or nephrotic or acute nephritic syndrome with GFR loss. Most patients (80%) have severe hypertension. Laboratory evaluation demonstrates marked hypocomplementemia, with a greater reduction in C4 than C3, as well as positive anti-HCV antibodies and HCV RNA. The majority of patients are RF-positive. The natural history of this disease can be variable, with some patients having an indolent course, while others develop progressive kidney failure. ESRD requiring dialysis is relatively uncommon (10% of cases). In about 10% of patients, acute oliguric AKI is the first indicator of kidney disease. Risk factors for ESRD included older age, male sex, higher serum creatinine, and greater degrees of proteinuria at diagnosis.

POLYARTERITIS NODOSA

Polyarteritis nodosa (PAN), although classically associated with hepatitis B infection, has also been observed in patients with chronic HCV infection. Compared to cryoglobulinemic vasculitis, these patients have more severe disease at presentation but a higher rate of clinical remission.

DIAGNOSIS

Kidney disease frequently lags many years behind initial HCV infection and does not appear to correlate well with disease activity in the liver. Serologically, HCV-related MCS is characterized by circulating cryoglobulins, hypocomplementemia, and positive RF, almost invariably IgMκ. However, the presence of cryoglobulins is common in those who do not have kidney disease. Screening for urinary abnormalities and alterations in kidney function in all HCV-positive patients is strongly recommended, particularly those with cryoglobulinemia. A kidney biopsy is recommended to determine the histologic pattern of glomerular injury in those with proteinuria and/or hematuria and remains the gold standard for diagnosis of HCV-associated glomerular disease.

PATHOLOGY

The most common HCV-associated kidney disease is MPGN, usually in the context of type II MCS. Light microscopy demonstrates an expanded and hypercellular mesangium, endocapillary proliferation, monocytic infiltration, thickened capillary loops, large eosinophilic and PAS-positive intraluminal deposits, and vasculitis of small and medium-sized renal arteries. Silver staining shows double contours of the glomerular basement membranes (GBMs) resulting from immune complex deposition and mesangial cell matrix interposition between the GBM and endothelial cell, with a new basement membrane forming around these deposits (Fig. 23.4). Immunofluorescence may reveal C3, IgM, and IgG granular deposits in the capillary wall and mesangium. On electron microscopy, subendothelial deposits are usually present and may have tubular and crystalline patterns similar

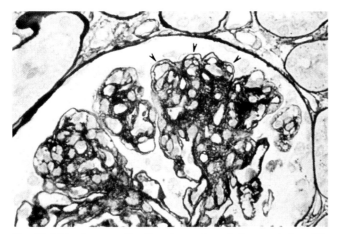

Fig. 23.4 Membranoproliferative glomerulonephritis seen in hepatitis C virus infection with typical glomerular basement membrane double contours (*arrowheads*; Jones methenamine silver stain.)

to that of cryoglobulins. Cryoglobulins are usually associated with histologic signs of vasculitis and downstream fibrinoid necrosis. One-third of these patients may have vasculitis of small renal arteries. Distinctive features of cryoglobulinemic glomerulonephritis, especially in patients with rapidly progressive deterioration of kidney function, include intraglomerular deposits, commonly observed in a subendothelial location, which might fill the capillary lumen (intraluminal thrombi).

Various other histologic types of kidney diseases are reported in association with HCV infection, including MN, FSGS, fibrillary glomerulonephritis, immunotactoid glomerulonephritis, IgA nephropathy, thrombotic microangiopathy, renal vasculitis, and interstitial nephritis. The histologic findings of HCV-associated MN are similar to that of idiopathic MN. Data are conflicting as to whether there is a real pathophysiologic link between HCV and MN. Future studies testing for antibodies to the phospholipase A2 receptor may be useful in this regard.

TREATMENT

The management of HCV-associated glomerular disease depends on the clinical presentation of the patient, with consideration of the level of kidney function and the severity of proteinuria. Three approaches can be considered for HCV-associated glomerulopathies and cryoglobulinemic kidney disease: (1) antiviral therapy to prevent further direct HCV damage to kidneys and the synthesis of immune complexes, (2) B-cell depletion therapy to prevent the formation of immune complexes and cryoglobulins, and (3) nonspecific immunosuppressive therapy targeting inflammatory cells to prevent the synthesis of immune complexes and to treat cryoglobulin-associated vasculitis. In patients with moderate proteinuria and stable kidney function, anti-HCV therapy is advised. In patients with nephrotic-range proteinuria and/or progressive kidney injury and other serious extrarenal manifestations, immunosuppressive therapy with rituximab or cyclophosphamide, corticosteroid pulses, and plasmapheresis should be considered.

ANTIVIRAL THERAPY

Antiviral therapy is recommended for patients with HCV-associated glomerulopathy whose disease severity and activity are mild to moderate, with proteinuria and gradual GFR loss. Historically, HCV drug therapy depended on interferon-α (IFN-α, in standard form or pegylated form, PEG-IFN) and ribavirin over many months and was associated with suboptimal efficacy and severe side effects. Since late 2013, several novel direct-acting antivirals (DAAs) have been approved, including NS3/4A protease inhibitors, NS5A inhibitors, and NS5B polymerase inhibitors. The first generation of DAAs included NS3/NS4A protease inhibitors (boceprevir and telaprevir) given in combination with IFN and ribavirin, but these have already been replaced by newer DAAs that provide greater efficacy and safety. The newer generation of DAAs offers shorter, IFN-free, and highly efficacious treatment options with few side effects. According to the most recent guidelines issued by the American Association of the Study of Liver Disease (AASLD) and the Infectious Diseases Society of America (IDSA) (http://www.hcvguidelines.org), sofosbuvir has replaced PEG-IFN and is currently the mainstay of IFN-free combination therapy. IFN-free regimens are now the treatment of choice for patients with chronic HCV infection. Sofosbuvir, a NS5B viral polymerase inhibitor, is effective against all six HCV genotypes in combination with other DAAs, PEG-IFN, or ribavirin. Combinations of nonnucleoside NS5B polymerase inhibitors (sofosbuvir, dasabuvir) with NS3/4A protease inhibitors (simeprevir, paritaprevir) and NS5A inhibitors (ledipasvir, daclatasvir, ombitasvir) are becoming the standard of care. The addition of ribavirin remains dependent in part on HCV genotype and subtype. Dose adjustments are recommended for several DAAs in patients with reduced kidney function (Table 23.3). In patients with creatinine clearance (CrCl) >30 mL/min, no dosage adjustment is needed when using standard dosing of daclatasvir, ledipasvir-sofosbuvir, ombiasvir-paritaprevir-ritonavir, dombiasvir-paritaprevir-ritonavir plus dasabuvir, simeprevir, and sofosbuvir. There are very limited data regarding the use of newer DAAs in patients with advanced CKD (CrCl <30 mL/min), including those on hemodialysis. In these patients, the recommended regimens vary depending on the urgency to treat, presence of cirrhosis, and likelihood of kidney transplantation. Much of the data on antiviral efficacy in this setting is with the use of PEG-IFN and ribavirin, but because of the adverse events with this combination, DAA-based, IFN-free regimens should be favored when possible. Recently, in a clinical trial of patients with HCV genotype 1 infection and stage 4 or 5 CKD, the combination of ombitasvir, paritaprevir, and ritonavir administered with dasabuvir led to a 90% viral response. In addition, a recent study of grazoprevir and elbasvir in those with CKD stage 4/5, with 75% on hemodialysis, reported responses of greater than 93%. Based on these data, fixed dose combination elbasvir and grazoprevir is recommended for the treatment of HCV-1 infection in patients with severely compromised kidney function. Clinical studies evaluating sofosbuvir dosing in patients with CrCl less than 30 mL/min are under way. The administration of sofosbuvir-containing regimens in patients with CrCl less than 30 mL/min should generally be done in consultation with an expert on HCV management.

Table 23.3   Dose-Adjustments of Hepatitis C Virus Direct-Acting Antiviral Therapy[a]

Antiviral	Excretion/Metabolism	DOSE-ADJUSTMENT			
		CrCl 50–80	CrCl 30–50	CrCl <30	ESRD on HD
Sofosobuvir[b]	Kidney	Standard	Standard	Limited data available	Limited data available
Ledipasvir	Liver and kidney (minor)	Standard	Standard	Data not available	Data not available
Daclatasvir	Liver	Standard	Standard	Standard	Standard
Ombitasvir	Liver	Standard	Standard	Limited data available	Limited data available
Dasabuvir	Liver	Standard	Standard	Limited data available	Limited data available
Paritaprevir	Liver	Standard	Standard	Limited data available	Limited data available
Simeprevir	Liver	Standard	Standard	Standard	Limited data available
Velpatasvir	Liver	Standard	Standard	Data not available	Data not available
Elbasvir	Liver	Standard	Standard	Standard	Standard
Grazoprevir	Liver	Standard	Standard	Standard	Standard

[a]For the most recent updates to guidelines, please refer to http://www.hcvguidelines.org.
[b]Renally eliminated; FDA approval is only for patients with CrCl >30 mL/min.
ESRD, End-stage renal disease; *HD,* hemodialysis.

IMMUNOSUPPRESSION

In the setting of nephrotic syndrome, rapidly progressive kidney failure, and/or acute flare of cryoglobulinemia, patients are typically treated with aggressive immunosuppressive therapy, which includes corticosteroids, cyclophosphamide or rituximab, and/or plasma exchange. Rituximab, a monoclonal antibody against CD-20 that rapidly depletes circulating and tissue B cells, interferes with the synthesis of cryoglobulins, and reduces kidney deposition of immune complexes, has been used to control severe vasculitis. Rituximab has been associated with reduction in proteinuria and cryoglobulin levels and increases in complement levels. Rituximab appears to provide effective therapy and is well tolerated, but studies do not suggest rituximab is superior to cyclophosphamide or plasmapheresis. Alternatively, pulse intravenous steroids and oral cyclophosphamide can be used. Cyclophosphamide is effective in inhibiting B-lymphocyte proliferation and thus cryoglobulin production. Corticosteroids control the acute inflammatory response (e.g., prednisone 0.5 to 1.5 mg/kg per day or IV pulses of methylprednisone 0.5 to 1.0 g/day for 3 days followed by oral prednisone). Plasma exchange is used in patients with rapidly progressive crescentic glomerulonephritis who require dialysis to remove circulating immune complexes and cryoglobulins from the plasma. When used, it should be combined with immunosuppressive therapies to prevent the reaccumulation of immune complexes and cryoglobulins. After control of the vasculitic syndrome with immunosuppression, antiviral treatment is recommended, typically, with a delay of one to four months.

DIRECT-ACTING ANTIVIRALS

Currently, antiviral therapy with new DAAs lacks data on efficacy and safety in the treatment of HCV-related glomerulonephritis. A small study comparing treatment with DAAs for MCS ($n = 12$) to that of historic controls demonstrated that patients who achieved a sustained viral response with DAAs also experienced an improvement in kidney function and a reduction in proteinuria. However, only a small number of patients ($n = 7$) in the study had evidence of glomerulonephritis. Furthermore, the limitations of antiviral therapy

remain in treating a rapidly progressive kidney disease, which includes a slow response to antiviral therapy with the development of kidney failure before clearance of the virus. The long-term outcomes of kidney disease remain unclear.

DIALYSIS AND TRANSPLANT

HCV positivity has been linked to lower graft and patient survival after kidney transplantation. HCV-associated liver disease increases the risk of graft rejection, proteinuria, infection, and diabetes. In addition, recurrence or de novo glomerulonephritis and thrombotic microangiopathy can occur after kidney transplantation in HCV-infected patients. Therefore eradication of HCV infection before transplantation can improve outcomes. Patients who are HCV infected and who are expected to undergo kidney transplantation should be evaluated for HCV treatment. Treatment of HCV before kidney transplantation is strongly preferred over treatment after transplantation. Viral eradication before transplant could reduce HCV-associated posttransplant morbidity and mortality. IFN is avoided in the postkidney transplantation setting because it can lead to acute graft rejection. Several recent reports have described successful outcomes in kidney transplant patients with sofosbuvir-based combination regimens with sustained viral responses ranging from 96% to 100%.

HEPATITIS B

EPIDEMIOLOGY

Approximately one-third of the world's population has serologic evidence of past or present infection with HBV, and more than 350 million are chronically infected. Kidney involvement is a common extrahepatic manifestation in those who have chronic HBV antigenemia, usually in the form of an immune complex–mediated glomerulopathy, such as MPGN, FSGS, minimal change disease, lupus-like nephritis, and IgA nephropathy. The most common association is with MN, especially in children with chronic HBV infection. The reported prevalence of HBV-associated nephropathy, particularly MN, closely matches the geographic patterns of HBV prevalence. The heterogeneity of presentation, pathology, and natural history makes diagnosis and therapeutic trials challenging.

PATHOPHYSIOLOGY

DIRECT TOXICITY

Indirect evidence of HBV as the causal agent for these kidney diseases comes from epidemiologic studies, including demonstration of a decrease in disease incidence following the introduction of vaccine programs. It is thought that HBV itself is not cytopathic. It carries genetic information into cells to direct synthesis of viral proteins, and studies have demonstrated viral antigens as well as viral DNA and RNA in glomerular and renal tubular epithelial cells of affected patients. This supports the hypothesis of viral transcription occurring within the kidney.

IMMUNE MEDIATED

The main pathogenic mechanism in HBV-related glomerular disease is through deposition of immune complexes in the glomerulus. The immune complexes consist of HBV antigens and host antibodies. It remains unknown if the complexes are formed in situ or are derived from circulating immune complexes. The immune complexes are predominantly deposited in the subepithelial region, where they activate complement and cause glomerular injury. The subepithelial deposits seen in this form of secondary MN are likely composed of HBe antigen (HBeAg) and anti-e antibody (anti-HBe) complex. This is supported by the clinical observation that this disease often remits if a patient undergoes clearance of the HBeAg and seroconversion to anti-HBe. In children who develop MN, there is a decreased cellular immune response to the HBV resulting in reduced clearance of the antigen compared with chronic carriers who do not develop MN. MPGN in the setting of HBV is also likely caused by deposition of immune antigen-antibody complexes within the mesangium and subepithelial space. Deposits containing both HBeAg and hepatitis B surface antigen (HBsAG) have both been reported, along with IgG and C3.

VASCULITIS

Hepatitis B virus infection is associated with PAN, and the pathogenesis has been attributed to antigen-antibody complex deposition in vessel walls, producing a clinical syndrome that is identical to idiopathic PAN. The vasculitis is characterized by arteritis in medium-sized vessels without involvement of smaller vessels (i.e., without glomerulonephritis) that can lead to glomerular ischemia with hypertension and AKI.

CLINICAL PRESENTATION

Hepatitis B virus–associated glomerular disease is more common in children than adults, and there is a male predominance, especially in children (up to 80%). Most HBV-associated glomerular disease presents with mild-to-moderate proteinuria and hematuria. Hepatitis B virus–related MN typically presents with the full nephrotic syndrome of heavy proteinuria, hyperlipidemia, hypoalbuminemia, and lower extremity edema. Adults are more likely than children to have hypertension, reduced GFR, and clinical evidence of liver disease. Patients with nephrotic syndrome and abnormal liver function tests have a greater than 50% chance of progressing to ESRD. The natural history of HBV-related MN is not well defined. In children, there is a high spontaneous remission rate (up to 60%). In adults, MN is usually progressive, with up to one-third eventually developing kidney failure. GFR loss is seen more commonly in patients with MPGN. The clinical presentation of patients with HBV-associated PAN is similar to idiopathic PAN and classically includes hypertension, reduced GFR, and systemic symptoms such as fatigue, malaise, and fever. Other organ system involvement, including the skin, the nervous system, and the gastrointestinal tract, may be present.

DIAGNOSIS

Kidney biopsy is the gold standard for diagnosing glomerular disease in the setting of HBV infection. Contrast angiography of the renal circulation showing microaneurysms is diagnostic of classic PAN.

PATHOLOGY

As stated earlier, MN and MPGN are more common. MN is characterized by thickened capillary walls and GBMs due to immune complex deposition. With silver or trichrome staining, characteristic spikes of the GBM can be seen extending around these deposits (Fig. 23.5). Immunofluorescence demonstrates granular IgG, C3, and some IgM staining in the subepithelial region (Fig. 23.6). Electron microscopy demonstrates classic intramembranous and subepithelial deposits (Fig. 23.7) and extensive effacement of the podocyte foot processes. In some cases, viral particles can be identified. MPGN is characterized by mesangial expansion and capillary wall thickening, resulting in a lobular appearance of the glomerular tuft, and the capillary walls demonstrate double contours and hypercellularity with interposition of cells. Immune deposits containing IgG, complement components, and IgM

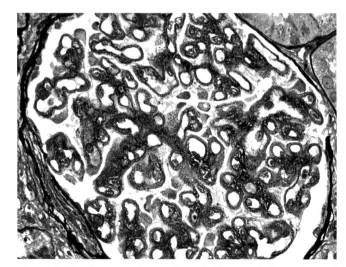

Fig. 23.5 Membranous glomerulonephritis seen in the setting of hepatitis B infection. Thickened glomerular basement membrane with spikes extending around immune deposits. (Jones methenamine silver stain, magnification ×400.)

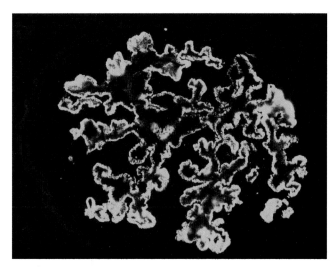

Fig. 23.6 Immunofluorescence with granular deposition of IgG in membranous glomerulonephritis resulting from hepatitis B infection. (Magnification ×400.)

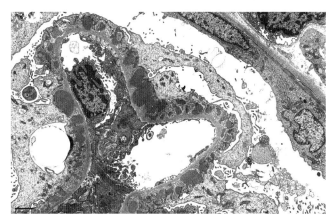

Fig. 23.7 Electron microscopy with subepithelial immune deposits in membranous glomerulonephritis resulting from hepatitis B infection. (Magnification ×6000.)

appear granular and are located in the subendothelial and mesangial areas.

LABORATORY DATA

Laboratory evaluation should include HBV DNA to confirm active replication as well as determination of antigen status, including HBeAg, HBsAg, and HBcAg. Other secondary causes of MN should be excluded, as well as common co-infections such as HCV and HIV. Unlike idiopathic MN, complement levels may be low.

TREATMENT

Antiviral treatment can promote clearance of HBV. However, little is known about the treatment of HBV-associated glomerular disease. Corticosteroids and other immunosuppressive agents (e.g., mycophenolate mofetil) have been used to treat those with nephrotic syndrome, but they can lead to active replication of HBV with worsening of liver and/or kidney disease. Given these findings, steroid monotherapy is not recommended in HBV-related kidney diseases. The

combination of glucocorticoids with antiviral therapy may be safer than steroids alone and may be reasonable for patients with vasculitis and rapidly progressive glomerulonephritis. The current options of antiviral therapies include nucleoside/nucleotide analogues (lamivudine, entacavir, telbivudine, adefovir, and tenofovir) and IFN-α (conventional or PEG-IFN), which all decrease HBV DNA levels. Entecavir has replaced lamivudine as first-line therapy in the treatment of HBV infection in naïve subjects because of the propensity of drug resistance. In the treatment of HBV-mediated glomerular disease, only lamivudine and IFN-α have demonstrated benefit thus far, with reduced proteinuria, increased HBV clearance, and stabilization of kidney function. However, there is a need for high-quality, prospective, controlled studies to address the effects of antiviral therapy in patients with HBV-associated glomerular diseases. Furthermore, there is a need to take into consideration the nephrotoxicity of the nucleoside/nucleotide analogues, such as adefovir and tenofovir, and perform dose adjustment.

DIALYSIS AND TRANSPLANTATION

HBV infection confers a significantly negative impact on the clinical outcomes of kidney transplant recipients because of increased hepatic complications. Before the availability of oral nucleoside/nucleotide analogues, chronic HBV infection was managed with IFN therapy. However, IFN should be avoided in kidney transplant recipients, as it commonly precipitates allograft dysfunction and rejection. The use of nucleoside/nucleotide analogues to effectively suppress HBV replication offers advantages of convenient administration and high tolerability, although they often require long-term use and could result in drug-resistant HBV strains. Among hepatitis B–infected transplant recipients, lamivudine therapy resulted in effective viral suppression, reduced liver complications, and improved patient survival, with patient survival rates comparable between kidney transplant recipients uninfected with HBV. A preventative approach is generally recommended to suppress reactivation of HBV. Entecavir is generally recommended because of its high resistance barrier and favorable safety profile, especially as several years of therapy may be indicated. Entecavir is effective in both treatment-naïve and lamivudine-resistant patients.

BIBLIOGRAPHY

AASLD-IDSA. Recommendations for testing, managing, and treating hepatitis C. http://www.hcvguidelines.org. Accessed 6 August 2016.
Chan T. Hepatitis B and renal disease. *Curr Hepat Rep.* 2010;9:99-105.
Elewa U, Sandri AM, Kim W, Fervenza F. Treatment of hepatitis B virus-associated nephropathy. *Nephron Clin Pract.* 2011;119:c41-c49.
Fabrizio F, Martin P, Cacoub P, et al. Treatment of hepatitis C-related kidney disease. *Expert Opin Pharmacother.* 2015;16:1815-1827.
Ferenci P. Treatment of hepatitis C in difficult-to-treat patients. *Nat Rev Gastroenterol Hepatol.* 2015;12:284-292.
Haas M, Kaul S, Eustace J. HIV-associated immune complex glomerulonephritis with "lupus-like" features: a clinicopathologic study of 14 cases. *Kidney Int.* 2005;67:1381-1390.
Lai A, Lai K. Viral nephropathy. *Nat Clin Pract Nephrol.* 2006;2:254-262.
Milburn J, Jones R, Levy J. Renal effects of novel antiretroviral drugs. *Nephrol Dial Transplant.* 2016;doi:10.1093/ndt/gfw064. [epbub ahead of print].
Muller E, Barday Z, Mendelson M, Kahn D. HIV-positive-to-HIV-positive kidney transplantation—results at 3 to 5 years. *N Engl J Med.* 2015; 372:613-620.

Naicker S, Rahmanian S, Kopp J. HIV and chronic kidney disease. *Clin Nephrol.* 2015;83(suppl 1):S32-S38.

Ozkok A, Yildiz A. Hepatitis C virus associated glomerulopathies. *World J Gastroenterol.* 2014;20:7544-7554.

Rosenberg A, Naicker S, Winkler C, Kopp J. HIV-associated nephropathies: epidemiology, pathology, mechanisms and treatment. *Nat Rev Nephrol.* 2015;11:150-160.

Ross MJ. Advances in the pathogenesis of HIV-associated kidney diseases. *Kidney Int.* 2014;86:266-274.

Sise M, Bloom A, Wisocky J, et al. Treatment of hepatitis C virus-associated mixed cryoglobulinemia with direct-acting antiviral agents. *Hepatology.* 2016;63:408-417.

Yap D, Chan T. Evolution of hepatitis B management in kidney transplantation. *World J Gastroenterol.* 2014;20:468-474.

24

Kidney Involvement in Systemic Vasculitis

Patrick H. Nachman; J. Charles Jennette; Ronald J. Falk

The kidneys are affected by many forms of system vasculitis (Fig. 24.1), which cause a wide variety of sometimes confusing clinical manifestations. Large-vessel vasculitides, such as giant cell arteritis (GCA) and Takayasu arteritis (TA), can narrow the abdominal aorta or renal arteries, resulting in renal ischemia and renovascular hypertension. Vasculitides of the medium-sized vessels, such as polyarteritis nodosa and Kawasaki disease, also can reduce flow through the renal artery and may affect intrarenal arteries, resulting in infarction and hemorrhage. Small-vessel vasculitides, such as microscopic polyangiitis (MPA), granulomatosis with polyangiitis (GPA, previously called Wegener granulomatosis), antiglomerular basement membrane (anti-GBM) disease, (also known as Goodpasture disease), immunoglobulin A (IgA) vasculitis (Henoch-Schönlein purpura), and cryoglobulinemic vasculitis, frequently involve the kidneys and especially the glomerular capillaries, resulting in glomerulonephritis. IgA vasculitis (IgAV) is discussed in Chapter 20.

PATHOLOGY

Different types of systemic vasculitis affect vessels of different caliber and type, as summarized in Fig. 24.1 and Table 24.1. Each type of vasculitis has different histologic and immuno-histologic features.

LARGE-VESSEL VASCULITIS

The large-vessel vasculitides, GCA and TA, predominantly affect the aorta and its major branches. TA preferentially involves the aorta and its primary branches and is an important cause of renovascular hypertension, especially in young patients. GCA is generally localized in more peripheral arteries and only rarely causes clinically significant kidney disease, although asymptomatic pathologic involvement is common. GCA often involves the extracranial branches of the carotid arteries, including the temporal artery. However, some patients do not have temporal artery involvement, and patients with other types of vasculitis (e.g., MPA, GPA) may have temporal artery involvement. Therefore temporal artery disease is neither a required nor a sufficient pathologic feature of GCA.

Histologically, both GCA and TA are characterized by focal chronic inflammation within the vessel wall (without perivascular lesions) that frequently has a granulomatous appearance with or without multinucleated giant cells. Aortic involvement is more likely to lead to a destructive rather than a stenotic process, leading to aneurysm formation with rupture or dissection. With chronicity, the inflammatory injury evolves into fibrosis and frequently results in vascular narrowing of the branches of the aorta, which is the basis for renovascular hypertension when a renal artery is involved.

MEDIUM-VESSEL VASCULITIS

Polyarteritis nodosa and Kawasaki disease affect medium-sized arteries (i.e., main visceral arteries), such as the mesenteric, hepatic, coronary, and main renal arteries. These diseases also may involve small arteries, such as arteries within the parenchyma of skeletal muscle, liver, heart, pancreas, spleen, and kidney (e.g., interlobar and arcuate arteries in the kidney). By the definitions in Table 24.1, polyarteritis nodosa and Kawasaki disease exclusively affect arteries and do not affect capillaries or venules. Therefore they do not cause glomerulonephritis. The presence of arteritis with glomerulonephritis indicates some form of small-vessel vasculitis rather than medium-vessel vasculitis.

Histologically, the acute arterial injury of Kawasaki disease and polyarteritis nodosa is characterized by focal artery wall necrosis and infiltration of inflammatory cells. The acute injury of polyarteritis nodosa typically includes conspicuous fibrinoid necrosis, which is absent or less apparent in Kawasaki disease. Fibrinoid necrosis results from plasma coagulation factors spilling into the necrotic areas, where they are activated to form fibrin. Early in the acute injury of polyarteritis nodosa, neutrophils predominate, but within a few days mononuclear leukocytes are most numerous. Thrombosis may occur at the site of inflammation, resulting in infarction. Focal necrotizing injury to vessels erodes into the vessel wall and adjacent tissue, producing an inflammatory aneurysm, which may rupture and cause hemorrhage. Thrombosis of the inflamed arteries causes downstream ischemia and infarction.

SMALL-VESSEL VASCULITIS

Although small-vessel vasculitides may affect medium-sized arteries, these disorders favor small vessels, such as arterioles, venules (e.g., in the dermis), and capillaries (e.g., in glomeruli and pulmonary alveoli; see Fig. 24.1). As described in Table 24.1, there are a variety of clinically and pathogenetically distinct forms of small-vessel vasculitis that have the focal necrotizing inflammation of small vessels in common. In the acute phase, this injury is characterized histologically by segmental fibrinoid necrosis and leukocyte infiltration (Fig. 24.2), sometimes with secondary thrombosis. The neutrophils often undergo karyorrhexis (leukocytoclasia). With chronicity,

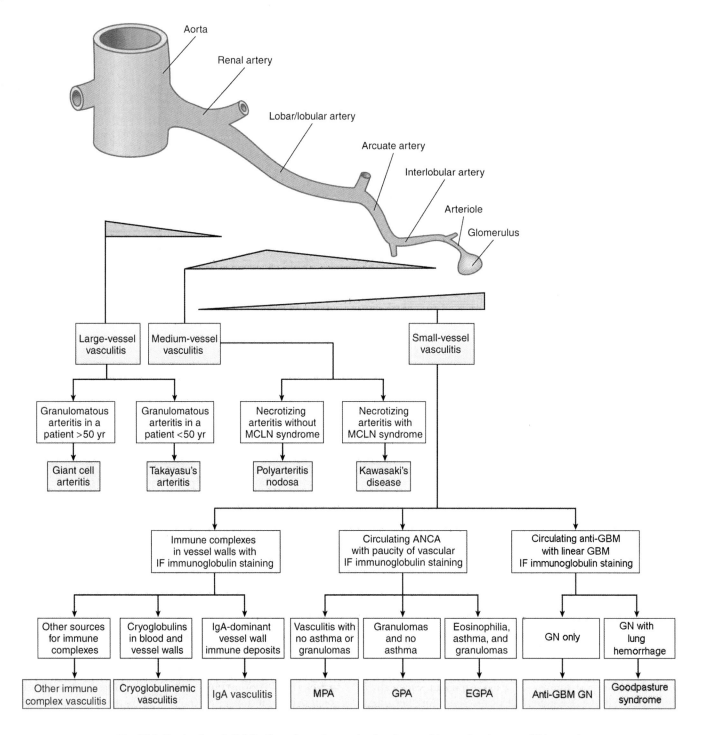

Fig. 24.1 Predominant distribution of renal vascular involvement by systemic vasculitides and the diagnostic clinical and pathologic features that distinguish among them. The width of the blue triangles indicates the predilection of small-, medium-, and large-vessel vasculitides for various portions of the renal vasculature. Note that medium-sized renal arteries can be affected by large-, medium-, or small-vessel vasculitides, but arterioles and glomeruli are affected by small-vessel vasculitides alone, based on the definitions in Table 24.1. *ANCA,* Antineutrophil cytoplasmic antibodies; *EGPA,* eosinophilic granulomatosis with polyangiitis (previously called Churg-Strauss); *GBM,* glomerular basement membrane; *GN,* glomerulonephritis; *GPA,* granulomatosis with polyangiitis (previously called Wegener granulomatosis); *IF,* immunofluorescence; *IgA,* immunoglobulin A (IgA vasculitis, previously called Henoch-Schönlein purpura); *MCLN,* mucocutaneous lymph node syndrome; *MPA,* microscopic polyangiitis; *SLE,* systemic lupus erythematosus.

Table 24.1   Partial Listing of Names and Definitions of Vasculitides Adopted by the 2012 Chapel Hill Consensus Conference on the Nomenclature of Systemic Vasculitis

Name[a]	Definition
Large-Vessel Vasculitides	
GCA	Arteritis, often granulomatous, usually affecting the aorta and/or its major branches, with a predilection for the branches of the carotid and vertebral arteries. Often involves the temporal artery. Onset usually in patients older than 50 years and often associated with polymyalgia rheumatica
TA	Arteritis, often granulomatous, predominantly affecting the aorta and/or its major branches. Onset usually in patients younger than 50 years
Medium-Vessel Vasculitides	
Polyarteritis nodosa	Necrotizing arteritis of medium or small arteries without glomerulonephritis or vasculitis in arterioles, capillaries, or venules and not associated with ANCA
Kawasaki disease	Arteritis associated with the mucocutaneous lymph node syndrome and predominantly affecting medium and small arteries. Coronary arteries are often involved. Aorta and large arteries may be involved. Usually occurs in infants and young children
Small-Vessel Vasculitides	
MPA[b,c]	Necrotizing vasculitis, with few or no immune deposits, predominantly affecting small vessels (i.e., capillaries, venules, or arterioles). Necrotizing arteritis involving small and medium arteries may be present. Necrotizing glomerulonephritis is very common. Pulmonary capillaritis often occurs. Granulomatous inflammation is absent.
GPA, formerly Wegener granulomatosis[b,c]	Necrotizing granulomatous inflammation usually involving the upper and lower respiratory tract and necrotizing vasculitis affecting predominantly small to medium vessels (e.g., capillaries, venules, arterioles, arteries, and veins). Necrotizing glomerulonephritis is common.
EGPA, formerly Churg-Strauss syndrome[b,c]	Eosinophil-rich and necrotizing granulomatous inflammation often involving the respiratory tract and necrotizing vasculitis predominantly affecting small to medium vessels and associated with asthma and eosinophilia. ANCA is more frequent when glomerulonephritis is present.
IgAV, formerly Henoch-Schönlein purpura[c]	Vasculitis, with IgA1-dominant immune deposits, affecting small vessels (predominantly capillaries, venules, or arterioles). Often involves skin and gastrointestinal tract and frequently causes arthritis. Glomerulonephritis indistinguishable from IgA nephropathy may occur.
Cryoglobulinemic vasculitis[c]	Vasculitis with cryoglobulin immune deposits affecting small vessels (predominantly capillaries, venules, or arterioles) and associated with cryoglobulins in serum. Skin, glomeruli, and peripheral nerves are often involved.
Hypocomplementemic urticarial vasculitis (Anti-C1q vasculitis)	Vasculitis accompanied by urticaria and hypocomplementemia affecting small vessels (i.e., capillaries, venules, or arterioles) and associated with anti-C1q antibodies. Glomerulonephritis, arthritis, obstructive pulmonary disease, and ocular inflammation are common.
Anti-GBM disease[c]	Vasculitis affecting glomerular capillaries, pulmonary capillaries, or both, with basement membrane deposition of antibasement membrane autoantibodies. Lung involvement causes pulmonary hemorrhage, and renal involvement causes glomerulonephritis with necrosis and crescents.

[a]The term *large vessels* refers to the aorta and the largest branches directed toward major body regions (e.g., extremities, head, and neck); *medium vessels* refers to the main visceral arteries (e.g., renal, hepatic, coronary, mesenteric); and *small vessels* refers to the distal arterial branches that connect with arterioles (e.g., renal arcuate and interlobular arteries), as well as arterioles, capillaries, and venules. Note that some small- and large-vessel vasculitides may involve medium-sized arteries, but large- and medium-vessel vasculitides do not involve vessels other than arteries.
[b]Strongly associated with antineutrophil cytoplasmic antibodies.
[c]May be accompanied by glomerulonephritis and can manifest as nephritis or pulmonary-renal vasculitic syndrome.
ANCA, Antineutrophil cytoplasmic antibody; *anti-GBM*, antiglomerular basement membrane; *EGPA*, eosinophilic granulomatosis with polyangiitis; *GCA*, giant cell arteritis; *GPA*, granulomatosis with polyangiitis; *IgAV*, immunoglobulin A vasculitis; *MPA*, microscopic polyangiitis; *TA*, Takayasu arteritis.
Modified from Jennette JC, Falk RJ, Bacon PA, et al. Revised International Chapel Hill Consensus Conference nomenclature of the vasculitides. *Arthritis Rheum.* 2013;65:1–11.

mononuclear leukocytes become predominant and fibrosis develops.

The various forms of small-vessel vasculitis differ from one another with respect to the presence or absence of distinctive features, as summarized in Table 24.1 and Fig. 24.1. For example, GPA is characterized by necrotizing granulomatous inflammation; eosinophilic granulomatosis with polyangiitis (EGPA) by eosinophil-rich granulomas, blood eosinophilia, and asthma; IgAV by IgA-dominant vascular immune deposits; and cryoglobulinemic vasculitis by circulating cryoglobulins.

The glomerular lesions of MPA, GPA, and EGPA are pathologically identical and are characterized by segmental fibrinoid necrosis, crescent formation (Fig. 24.3), and a paucity of glomerular staining for immunoglobulin (i.e., pauci-immune glomerulonephritis). Leukocytoclastic angiitis of the medullary vasa recta (Fig. 24.4) also occurs in the

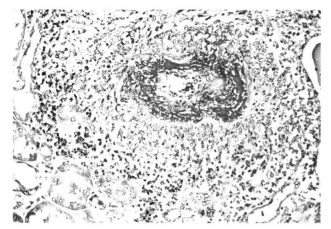

Fig. 24.2 Renal interlobular artery with fibrinoid necrosis from a patient with microscopic polyangiitis (Masson trichrome stain).

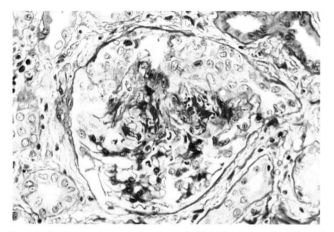

Fig. 24.3 Glomerulus with segmental fibrinoid necrosis with red (fuchsinophilic) fibrinous material and an adjacent cellular crescent, from a patient with antineutrophil cytoplasmic antibody small-vessel vasculitis (Masson trichrome stain).

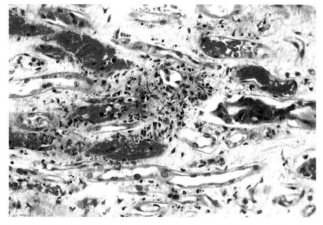

Fig. 24.4 Medullary vasa recta with leukocytoclastic angiitis, from a patient with granulomatosis with polyangiitis (hematoxylin and eosin stain).

antineutrophil cytoplasmic antibody (ANCA) vasculitides and is rarely severe enough to cause papillary necrosis. About 90% of patients with active MPA and GPA, and about 40% of patients with EGPA, have circulating ANCAs (Table 24.2).

The glomerular lesion of anti-GBM disease is also characterized by a segmental necrotizing and crescentic glomerulonephritis. It is distinguishable from the lesions of MPA, GPA, and EGPA by the presence, on immunofluorescence microscopy, of linear continuous deposits of IgG (sometimes accompanied by complement C3, IgA, or IgM) along the GBM (Fig. 24.5). No electron dense deposits are seen by electron microscopy.

The glomerulonephritis of IgAV is pathologically identical to IgA nephropathy and is characterized by the predominant mesangial deposition of IgA (mostly IgA1 subclass), and these patients have the same abnormal hinge region glycosylation of IgA1. The glomerulonephritis of cryoglobulinemic vasculitis usually manifests as type I membranoproliferative glomerulonephritis (mesangiocapillary glomerulonephritis), although other patterns of proliferative glomerulonephritis occur less often. Cryoglobulinemic vasculitis is frequently associated with hepatitis C infection.

PATHOGENESIS

Vasculitis is caused by the activation of inflammatory mediator systems in vessel walls. However, the initiating event (cause) is unknown for many forms of vasculitis. An immune response to heterologous antigens (e.g., hepatitis B or C antigens in some forms of immune complex vasculitis) or autoantigens (e.g., proteinase 3 or myeloperoxidase in ANCA vasculitis) is presumed to be the etiologic event in many patients with vasculitis. A number of types of vasculitis are categorized based on the putative or confirmed immunologic mechanisms listed in Box 24.1.

CELL-MEDIATED VASCULITIS

The pathogenesis of large-vessel vasculitis is thought to be the result of a dysregulated interaction between components of the vessel wall and the immune system. As such, stimulated vascular dendritic cells play a key role in these diseases. T cells and macrophages are recruited to the sites of vascular inflammation, leading to the formation of granulomata, whereas B cells are absent from the lesions. Infectious agents are suspected to play a role in triggering the loss of immune tolerance in the vessel wall and dendritic cell activation. Interleukin-6 (IL-6) plays an important role in mediating vascular and systemic inflammation in patients with GCA. IL-6 derives from endothelial and vascular smooth muscle cells (in addition to immune cells) and mediates the differentiation of T cells into Th17 cells. In turn, Th17 cells release a number of proinflammatory cytokines (including IL-17), which mediate the stimulation of vascular cells, the differentiation of cytotoxic cells, and the recruitment of neutrophils, macrophages, T cells, and dendritic cells. Th17 cells are present at the sites of arterial inflammation and are markedly increased in the circulation of patients with GCA. IL-6 is also implicated in downregulating antiinflammatory T regulatory (Treg) cells. Whereas the IL-6/IL-17 axis is strongly implicated in the acute phase of large-vessel vasculitis,

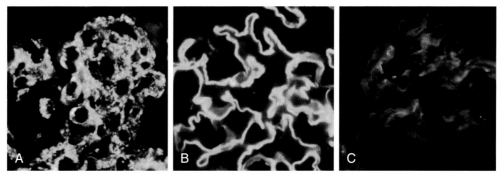

Fig. 24.5 Patterns of immunoglobulin G staining by immunofluorescence microscopy. (A) Granular staining seen in immune complex mediated disease. (B) Linear staining seen in anti-glomerular basement membrane disease. (C) No staining seen in pauci-immune glomerulonephritis typical of antineutrophil cytoplasmic antibodies-vasculitis. (Photomicrographs courtesy of Dr. J. Charles Jennette.)

Table 24.2 Approximate Frequency of Proteinase 3 Antineutrophil Cytoplasmic Antibody or Myeloperoxidase Antineutrophil Cytoplasmic Antibody in Pauci-Immune Small-Vessel Vasculitis

Antibody	MPA (%)	GPA (%)	EGPA (%)	Renal-Limited Vasculitis (Pauci-Immune Crescentic Glomerulonephritis) (%)
PR3-ANCA	40	75	5	25
MPO-ANCA	50	20	40	65
ANCA-negative	10	5	55	10

Note that more than 75% of patients with EGPA who have glomerulonephritis are ANCA-positive.
EGPA, Eosinophilic granulomatosis with polyangiitis; *GPA,* granulomatosis with polyangiitis; *MPA,* microscopic polyangiitis; *MPO-ANCA,* myeloperoxidase antineutrophil cytoplasmic antibody; *PR3-ANCA,* proteinase 3 antineutrophil cytoplasmic antibody.

Box 24.1 Putative Immunologic Causes of Vasculitis

Immune Complex–Mediated

IgA vasculitis (Henoch-Schönlein purpura)[a]
Cryoglobulinemic vasculitis
Lupus vasculitis
Serum sickness vasculitis
Hypocomplementemic urticarial vasculitis (anti-C1q vasculitis)
Anti-GBM disease

ANCA-Mediated

MPA
GPA

Cell-Mediated

Allograft cellular vascular rejection
GCA
TA

[a]May be accompanied by glomerulonephritis and can manifest as nephritis or pulmonary-renal vasculitic syndrome.
ANCA, Antineutrophil cytoplasmic antibody; *anti-GBM,* antiglomerular basement membrane; *GCA,* giant cell arteritis; *GPA,* granulomatosis with polyangiitis; *IgA,* immunoglobulin A; *MPA,* microscopic polyangiitis; *TA,* Takayasu arteritis.

and is readily suppressed by glucocorticoid treatment, the chronic phase of the disease appears to be predominantly mediated by glucocorticoid-resistant IL-12 and interferon-γ (IFN-γ). These cytokines serve as a positive amplification loop for vascular inflammation and stromal cell remodeling through a number of down-stream mediators. IFN-γ is thus implicated in the vascular wall changes leading to arterial luminal compromise.

IMMUNE COMPLEX–MEDIATED VASCULITIS

The vasculitides listed in the immune complex–mediated category in Box 24.1 all produce immunohistologic evidence for vessel wall immune complex localization—that is, granular or linear staining for immunoglobulins and complement. Antibodies bound to antigens in vessel walls activate humoral inflammatory mediator systems (complement, coagulation, plasmin, and kinin systems), which attract and activate neutrophils and monocytes. These activated leukocytes generate toxic oxygen metabolites and release enzymes that cause matrix lysis and cellular apoptosis, resulting in necrotizing inflammatory injury to the vessel walls.

This same final pathway of inflammatory injury also can be reached if antibodies bind to antigens that are integral components of vessel walls. The best-documented example is anti-GBM glomerulonephritis. In anti-GBM disease, autoantibodies develop to a specific component of the GBM referred to as the Goodpasture antigen. The GBM is formed from a network of type IV collagen molecules, of which the α3, α4, and α5 chain trimers are restricted to the GBM and certain other specialized basement membranes. The globular noncollagenous 1 (NC1) domains of the α3α4α5 trimers, in turn, form head-to-head hexamers. The Goodpasture antigen is restricted to two main epitopes colocalized in the NC1 domain of the α3 and α5 chains of type IV collagen. These epitopes are usually sequestered but become exposed to the immune system after perturbation of the quaternary structure of the α3α4α5 hexamers. It is hypothesized that such perturbation of the quaternary structure and exposure of the neo-epitopes may be the results of kidney insults from systemic inflammation (e.g., ANCA vasculitis), membranous nephropathy, or the action of reactive oxygen species on the GBM and may be associated with environmental exposures, such as industrial hydrocarbon and cigarette smoking. Although the Goodpasture antigen is also found in basement membranes of the alveoli, choroid plexus, cochlea, and eye, anti-GBM generally affects only the kidneys and lungs. The direct pathogenicity of anti-GBM antibodies has long been demonstrated by the passive transfer of sera from affected patients to squirrel monkeys reproducing the glomerulonephritis.

ANCA-MEDIATED VASCULITIS

An important group of necrotizing systemic small-vessel vasculitides, which frequently involves the kidneys, occurs without immunohistologic evidence for vascular immune complex localization or direct antibody binding. This paucity of immune deposits is the basis for the designation "pauci-immune" for this group of vasculitides, which includes MPA, GPA, and EGPA. In vitro and in vivo experimental evidence indicates that the vascular inflammation is caused by activation of neutrophils and monocytes by ANCAs. ANCAs are specific for proteins within the granules of neutrophils and the peroxidase-positive lysosomes of monocytes. When detected in patient serum by indirect immunofluorescence microscopy with alcohol-fixed normal human neutrophils as substrate, two patterns of neutrophil staining are observed that discriminate between the two major subtypes of ANCAs: cytoplasmic-staining (C-ANCA) and perinuclear-staining (P-ANCA). With the use of specific immunochemical assays, such as enzyme-linked immunosorbent assays (ELISAs), most C-ANCAs are found to be specific for a neutrophil and monocyte proteinase called proteinase 3 (PR3-ANCA), and most P-ANCAs are specific for myeloperoxidase (MPO-ANCA). Approximately 90% of patients with pauci-immune glomerulonephritis and vasculitis have circulating ANCAs. The vast majority of these patients have circulating antibodies to one or the other antigen but rarely (<5%) to both. An exception are patients with drug-associated vasculitis (e.g., levamisole-adulterated cocaine, hydralazine) who frequently present with high-titer antibodies to both antigens.

The current paradigm regarding the pathogenesis of ANCA-associated vasculitides is that ANCAs react with cytoplasmic antigens (PR3 and MPO) that are present at the surface of cytokine-stimulated leukocytes, causing the leukocytes to adhere to vessel walls, degranulate, and generate toxic oxygen metabolites. The interaction of ANCAs with neutrophils involves Fc receptor engagement, perhaps by immune complexes formed between ANCAs and ANCA antigens in the microenvironment surrounding the leukocyte. That ANCAs can directly cause vasculitis rests on the demonstration that circulating antibodies specific for MPO cause

pauci-immune crescentic glomerulonephritis and small-vessel vasculitis in mice. In vitro and animal model experiments indicate that ANCA-activated neutrophils release factors that activate the alternative complement pathway that initiates an inflammatory amplification loop, which is important for tissue injury. ANCA antigens also may become planted in vessel walls, thus providing a nidus for in situ immune complex formation. If such in situ immune complex formation is present, it occurs at a low level, as ANCA vasculitides are characteristically pauci-immune. T cells are also involved in the pathogenesis of the ANCA autoimmune response both through active B-cell help by T cells to induce a pathogenic autoantibody response with the production of IgG subclass antibodies and through ineffective suppression of the autoimmune ANCA response by regulatory T cells.

CLINICAL FEATURES

The diagnosis and management of systemic vasculitis can be challenging. The clinical features are extremely varied and are dictated by the category of vasculitis, the type of vessel involved, the organ system distribution of vascular injury, and the stage of disease. Regardless of the type of vasculitis, most patients exhibit accompanying constitutional symptoms, such as fever, arthralgias, myalgias, and weight loss.

The large-vessel vasculitides, GCA and TA, typically manifest with evidence for ischemia in tissues supplied by involved arteries. Patients with arteritis often develop claudication (especially in the upper extremities), absent pulses, and bruits. Approximately 40% of patients with TA develop renovascular hypertension, a feature that only rarely complicates GCA. GCA can affect virtually any organ in the body, but signs and symptoms of involvement of arteries in the head and neck are the most common clinical manifestations. Superficial arteries (e.g., the temporal artery) may be swollen and tender. Arterial narrowing causes ischemic manifestations in affected tissues (e.g., headache, jaw claudication, loss of vision). About half of the patients with GCA have polymyalgia rheumatica, which is characterized by aching and stiffness in the neck, shoulder girdle, or pelvic girdle.

Medium-vessel vasculitides, such as polyarteritis nodosa and Kawasaki disease, often manifest with clinical evidence for infarction in multiple organs, such as abdominal pain with occult blood in the stool and skeletal muscle and cardiac pain with elevated serum muscle enzymes. Laboratory evaluation may reveal clinically silent organ damage, such as liver injury with elevated liver function tests and pancreatic injury with elevated serum amylase.

Polyarteritis nodosa frequently causes multiple kidney infarcts and aneurysms. Unlike MPA and GPA, polyarteritis nodosa typically does not cause rapidly progressive loss of kidney function. The rupture of arterial aneurysms with massive retroperitoneal or intraperitoneal hemorrhage is a life-threatening complication of polyarteritis nodosa.

Kawasaki disease almost always occurs in children younger than 6 years of age, affects boys more often than girls, and is 20 times more common among Northeast Asians than white individuals. It has a predilection for coronary, axillary, and iliac arteries. Kawasaki disease is accompanied by the mucocutaneous lymph node syndrome that includes fever, nonpurulent lymphadenopathy, and mucosal and cutaneous inflammation.

Although the renal arteries (especially interlobar arteries) are frequently affected pathologically, clinically significant kidney involvement is rare in patients with Kawasaki disease.

Patients with small-vessel vasculitides (Table 24.1) may present with evidence of inflammation in vessels of one or multiple organs. Kidney involvement presents as hematuria, proteinuria, and impaired kidney function caused by glomerulonephritis. Other manifestations include purpura caused by leukocytoclastic angiitis in dermal venules and arterioles, abdominal pain and occult blood in the stool from mucosal and bowel wall infarcts, mononeuritis multiplex from arteritis in peripheral nerves, necrotizing sinusitis from upper respiratory tract mucosal angiitis, and pulmonary hemorrhage from alveolar capillaritis.

In addition to these features, which are shared by patients with any type of small-vessel vasculitis, patients with GPA and EGPA show distinctive clinical features that set them apart. Patients with GPA have necrotizing granulomatous inflammation, most often occurring in the upper or lower respiratory tract and rarely in other tissues (e.g., skin, orbit). In the lungs, this inflammation produces irregular nodular lesions that can be observed by radiography. These lesions may cavitate and hemorrhage; however, massive pulmonary hemorrhage in patients with GPA is usually caused by capillaritis rather than granulomatous inflammation. By definition, patients with EGPA have blood eosinophilia and a history of asthma.

Most patients with anti-GBM disease present with rapidly progressive glomerulonephritis (RPGN) and lung hemorrhage, although about one-third present with isolated glomerulonephritis. Rarely do patients present with isolated lung hemorrhage without kidney failure. Clinically, anti-GBM disease is indistinguishable from patients with ANCA vasculitis who present with a pulmonary-renal syndrome or RPGN. However, upper respiratory, musculoskeletal, neurologic, or cutaneous manifestations, which are frequent in ANCA vasculitis, are not seen in anti-GBM disease. The presence of these extrarenal and pulmonary signs points toward either ANCA vasculitis or an overlap of anti-GBM and ANCA vasculitis. Indeed, up to 30% of patients with anti-GBM also have ANCA, most commonly MPO-ANCA. These "double-positive" patients combine features of both diseases with more severe RPGN and the poorer renal prognosis typical of anti-GBM disease and a propensity of a relapsing course common in ANCA vasculitis.

DIAGNOSIS

Multisystem disease in a patient with constitutional signs and symptoms of inflammation, such as fever, arthralgias, myalgias, and weight loss, should raise suspicion of systemic vasculitis. Data to assist in resolving the differential diagnosis include the age of the patient, organ distribution of injury, concurrent syndromes (e.g., mucocutaneous lymph node syndrome in Kawasaki disease, polymyalgia rheumatica in GCA, asthma in EGPA), type of vessel involved (e.g., large artery, visceral artery, small vessel other than an artery), lesion histology (e.g., granulomatous, necrotizing), lesion immunohistology (e.g., immune deposits, pauci-immune), and serologic data (e.g., cryoglobulins, hepatitis C antibodies, hypocomplementemia, antinuclear antibodies, ANCAs, cryoglobulins, anti-C1q antibodies; Fig. 24.1).

Signs and symptoms of tissue ischemia along with imaging demonstrating irregularity, stenosis, occlusion, or, less commonly, aneurysms of large- and medium-sized arteries should suggest GCA or TA. Imaging may be based on color-duplex ultrasonography to assess superficial temporal and accessible large arteries, contrast-enhanced magnetic resonance imaging, or ^{18}F-fluorodeoxyglucose positron emission tomography (^{18}F-FDG-PET) combined with computerized tomography. ^{18}F-FDG-PET may be the most sensitive modality with early vascular inflammation but may remain "positive" in patients in clinical remission. A useful discriminator between GCA and TA is age, as the former disorder is rare in individuals younger than 50 years, whereas the latter is rare in patients older than 50 years. The presence of polymyalgia rheumatica is a clinical marker for GCA.

Polyarteritis nodosa and Kawasaki disease cause visceral ischemia, particularly in the heart, kidneys, liver, spleen, and gut. Arteritis in skeletal muscle and subcutaneous tissues causes tender erythematous nodules that can be identified on physical examination. Angiographic demonstration of aneurysms in medium-sized arteries (e.g., renal arteries) indicates that some type of vasculitis is present, but it is not disease specific, because GCA, TA, polyarteritis nodosa, Kawasaki disease, GPA, MPA, and EGPA can all produce arterial aneurysms.

A small-vessel vasculitis should be suspected if there is evidence for inflammation of vessels smaller than arteries, such as glomerular capillaries (hematuria and proteinuria), dermal venules (palpable purpura), or alveolar capillaries (hemoptysis). To discriminate among the small-vessel vasculitides, evaluation of serologic data, vessel immunohistology, or concurrent nonvasculitic disease (e.g., asthma, eosinophilia, lupus, and hepatitis) is required (see Fig. 24.1).

Evaluation of vessels in biopsy specimens, such as glomerular capillaries in kidney biopsies, alveolar capillaries in lung biopsies, or dermal venules in skin biopsies, can be helpful, especially if immunohistology is performed. The pauci-immune vasculitides lack immune deposits, anti-GBM disease produces linear immunoglobulin deposits, and immune complex vasculitides have granular immune deposits, such as the IgA-dominant deposits of IgAV.

Serology, especially ANCA analysis, is useful in differentiating among the small-vessel vasculitides. MPA, GPA, and, to a lesser extent, EGPA are associated with ANCAs (see Table 24.2). As depicted in Fig. 24.5 and listed in Table 24.2, most patients in North America and Europe with active untreated GPA have C-ANCA (PR3-ANCA), whereas a minority have P-ANCA (MPO-ANCA). Therefore PR3-ANCA is not specific for GPA, because some patients with PR3-ANCA have systemic small-vessel vasculitis without granulomatous inflammation (i.e., MPA), and others have pauci-immune necrotizing and crescentic glomerulonephritis alone. Only about 40% of patients with EGPA have circulating ANCAs and the lowest frequency of glomerulonephritis. Some patients with immunopathologic evidence for immune complex–mediated or anti-GBM–mediated vasculitis or glomerulonephritis have concurrent ANCA (see Table 24.2 and Fig. 24.6). Approximately one-third of patients with anti-GBM disease are MPO-ANCA positive, and these patients experience kidney disease that is similar in severity to anti-GBM disease (which has the worst prognosis), and they may have persistence or recurrence of ANCA disease after the anti-GBM disease remits. Rarely,

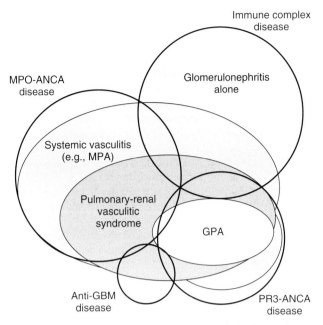

Fig. 24.6 Relationship of vasculitic clinicopathologic syndromes to immunopathologic categories of vascular injury in patients with crescentic glomerulonephritis. The circles represent the major immunopathologic categories of vascular inflammation that affect the kidneys, and the shaded ovals represent the clinicopathologic expressions of the vascular inflammation. Note that clinical syndromes can be caused by more than one immunopathologic process; for example, pulmonary-renal vasculitic syndrome can be caused by anti-GBM antibodies (i.e., Goodpasture syndrome), immune complex localization (e.g., lupus erythematosus), or ANCA-associated disease (e.g., MPA, GPA). *GBM*, Glomerular basement membrane; *GPA*, granulomatosis with polyangiitis; *MPA*, microscopic polyangiitis; *MPO-ANCA*, myeloperoxidase antineutrophil cytoplasmic antibody; *PR3-ANCA*, proteinase 3 antineutrophil cytoplasmic antibody. (Modified from Jennette JC. Anti-neutrophil cytoplasmic autoantibody-associated disease: a pathologist's perspective. *Am J Kidney Dis.* 1991;18:164–170, with permission.)

anti-GBM disease can occur in the presence of the classic linear IgG deposits along the GBM (by immunofluorescence microscopy) but in the absence of detectable circulating anti-GBM antibodies on standard ELISA tests. The vast majority of patients' anti-GBM antibodies react with the NC domain of the α3 chain of type IV collagen and, to a lesser extent, the α5 chain, with rare reports of reactivity to other collagen chains. Anti-GBM antibodies titers appear to correlate with disease activity, and their removal by plasmapheresis is associated with clinical improvement. It is important to realize that some patients with MPA, GPA, and especially EGPA are ANCA-negative. Although ANCA titers generally correlate with disease activity, they do not mirror disease activity in many patients, especially those with MPO-ANCA. Similarly, rising ANCA titers have not been demonstrated to be reliable predictors of subsequent relapse and should generally not be used as the sole indication to resume immunosuppressive medication.

The ANCA serotypes (MPO- vs. PR3-ANCA) are emerging as a better basis for categorizing patients with pauci-immune small-vessel vasculitis than the traditional phenotypes of MPA versus GPA. Not only do the serotypes correlate with clinical features and organ involvement, but also they distinguish

patients with respect to genetic predispositions based on genome-wide association studies. ANCA serotypes are also associated with different disease outcomes. Several recent studies have reported a worse renal survival in patients with MPO-ANCA, and, most notably, PR3-ANCA has consistently been associated with a significantly higher risk of relapse compared with MPO-ANCA. PR3-ANCA also may be associated with poorer patient survival.

Diagnostic serologic tests for immune complex–mediated vasculitides include assays for circulating immune complexes (e.g., cryoglobulins in cryoglobulinemic vasculitis), assays for antibodies known to participate in immune complex formation or to mark the presence of a disease that generates immune complexes (e.g., antibodies to hepatitis B or C, streptococci, DNA), and assays for the consumption or activation of humoral inflammatory mediator system components (e.g., assays for reduced complement components or for an activated membrane attack complex). Hypocomplementemia is common in patients with cryoglobulinemic vasculitis, lupus vasculitis, and hypocomplementemic urticarial vasculitis. The glomerulonephritis associated with these vasculitides is characterized by capillary wall and mesangial immune complex deposition and a proliferative or membranoproliferative pattern of injury.

THERAPY AND OUTCOME

All of the vasculitides discussed in this chapter typically respond to antiinflammatory or immunosuppressive therapy.

LARGE-VESSEL VASCULITIS

GCA and TA usually respond well to high-dose corticosteroid treatment (e.g., prednisone, 1 mg/kg body weight per day) during the acute phase of the disease, followed by tapering and low-dose maintenance for a year or more depending on disease activity. Relapses during the tapering phase, or after corticosteroids are discontinued, are reported in about 40% of patients. Patients with severe disease or steroid toxicity may benefit from other immunosuppressive agents, such as mycophenolate mofetil or azathioprine, although results have not been consistent. If present, renovascular hypertension should be controlled. After the inflammatory phase has passed and the sclerotic phase has developed, vascular surgery (stent or bypass) may be required to improve the flow to ischemic tissues, especially in patients with TA.

In patients with GCA and preserved kidney function, the use of methotrexate may be associated with a lower rate of relapse, a higher rate of corticosteroid-free remission, and a lower cumulative dose of corticosteroids. Randomized controlled trials have not demonstrated a benefit of tumor necrosis factor (TNF)-α blocking agents in the treatment of GCA. Although the majority of patients with TA respond to corticosteroid therapy, about two-thirds of patients may be dependent on this form of therapy, and a large proportion require an additional form of immunosuppression. Unlike in GCA, retrospective and uncontrolled studies suggest a possible beneficial effect of TNF-α blockers or IL-6 blockade (tocilizumab) in TA, although these results are not confirmed in controlled trials. Of note, clinically silent progression of vascular lesions has been reported while on tocilizumab therapy, and relapses appear common after its discontinuation.

MEDIUM-VESSEL VASCULITIS

Some patients with polyarteritis nodosa have a persistent viral infection, especially hepatitis B virus infection. In these cases, antiviral therapy with or without plasma exchange is recommended. In patients with no evidence for infection, management usually consists of corticosteroids with or without cytotoxic drugs.

The preferred treatment for Kawasaki disease is a combination of aspirin (80 to 100 mg/kg per day in 4 divided doses for 7 days) and a single dose of high-dose intravenous gamma globulin (IVIg) (2 g/kg). This controls the inflammatory manifestations of the disease (e.g., the mucocutaneous lymph node syndrome), prevents thrombosis of injured arteries, and markedly decreases the risk of coronary artery involvement from 20% to 25% to less than 5%. Pulse methylprednisolone (30 mg/kg per day for up to 3 days) is suggested in patients who fail to respond to two doses of IVIg. With appropriate treatment, more than 90% of patients with Kawasaki disease have complete resolution of the disease.

SMALL-VESSEL VASCULITIS

CRYOGLOBULINEMIC VASCULITIS

The treatment of symptomatic cryoglobulinemia should be adjusted according to the pathophysiologic mechanism involved (hyperviscosity vs. vasculitis) and the severity of the clinical disease. The management should include treatment of the cause of cryoglobulinemia where possible. Cryoglobulinemic vasculitis caused by hepatitis C (HCV) infection may respond to antiviral therapy. In the past, anti-HCV therapy relied on long courses of pegylated IFN plus ribavirin and were associated with sustained virologic response in 50% to 60% of patients. More recent use of triple HCV therapy with pegylated-IFN/ribavirin and a specifically targeted antiviral agent (NS3/4A protease inhibitor, e.g., boceprevir or telaprevir) led to improved response rates (65% to 70%) in HCV infection. Direct-acting antivirals, such as the NS3/4A inhibitor simeprevir and the NS5B inhibitor, sofosbuvir, are now available and have markedly improved the rates of sustained virologic response to 90% or better for certain HCV genotypes (see Chapter 23).

Rituximab is a promising therapy in mixed cryoglobulinemic vasculitis, with small controlled trials in patients with HCV-mixed cryoglobulinemic vasculitis, suggesting that the addition of rituximab to conventional therapy is associated with a shorter time to clinical remission, a better kidney response rate, and higher rates of cryoglobulin clearance. Rituximab appears to be safe in HCV-infected patients, in contrast with observations in hepatitis B virus–infected patients. Retreatment of rituximab alone at clinical relapse is effective and safe for severe manifestations of cryoglobulinemic vasculitis. Plasma exchange is reserved for severe and/or life-threatening manifestations of cryoglobulinemic vasculitis, including RPGN. For patients with severe vasculitis, control of disease with rituximab, with or without plasmapheresis, is usually required before the initiation of antiviral therapy. For non-HCV–related cryoglobulinemic vasculitis, rituximab may be used in combination with corticosteroids in patients with severe impairment of mixed cryoglobulinemia. Nevertheless, corticosteroids should be rapidly tapered to limit infectious risks, particularly in elderly patients with reduced GFR.

MICROSCOPIC POLYANGIITIS, GRANULOMATOSIS WITH POLYANGIITIS, EOSINOPHILIC GRANULOMATOSIS WITH POLYANGIITIS, AND PAUCI-IMMUNE GLOMERULONEPHRITIS

The treatments of choice for necrotizing and crescentic glomerulonephritis associated with MPA, GPA, or EGPA or for kidney-limited pauci-immune crescentic glomerulonephritis include high-dose corticosteroids and immunosuppression with cyclophosphamide or rituximab. Patients with evidence of severe pulmonary hemorrhage require emergent therapy with plasmapheresis. Plasmapheresis also improves kidney survival in patients with severe kidney disease at the time of diagnosis. Induction therapy includes pulse methylprednisolone at a dose of 7 mg/kg per day for 3 days, followed by daily oral prednisone or plasma exchange therapy for 7 to 14 days, in addition to daily oral prednisone. Prednisone dose, duration, and tapering schedules vary among centers. In our center, prednisone treatment is typically converted to alternate-day treatment during the second month of therapy, followed by a gradual taper until it is discontinued by the fourth or fifth month after diagnosis. There are a number of cyclophosphamide protocols, including intravenous or oral cyclophosphamide, which induce remission in almost 90% of patients. Once the patient has attained a clinical remission of vasculitis, treatment with cyclophosphamide can be stopped in favor of a maintenance therapy regimen. Induction therapy with rituximab has been demonstrated to be noninferior to cyclophosphamide in patients with mild or moderately severe disease; however, data on its use in patients with severe pulmonary hemorrhage or severe kidney failure are relatively scant.

About 80% of patients with ANCA vasculitis enter remission with induction immunosuppressive therapy, but subsequent relapses are common. Risk factors of relapse include PR3-ANCA serotype (vs. MPO-ANCA) and lung or upper respiratory tract disease. For this reason, a regimen of maintenance therapy is implemented with azathioprine, mycophenolate mofetil, or rituximab. The optimal duration of maintenance therapy is not well established and depends, in part, on the patient's risk factors for relapse and clinical course. Common practice is to continue maintenance therapy for about 12 months after remission is attained, followed by a gradual reduction and careful clinical follow-up. Relapses frequently occur in the same organ system as the initial disease, although relapses may involve new organ systems. Depending on the severity of the relapse, patients may be treated either with another course of corticosteroids and rituximab or cyclophosphamide. In the setting of relapsing disease, the use of rituximab may be associated with a better response than cyclophosphamide and offers the advantage of limiting exposure to cyclophosphamide.

ANTIGLOMERULAR BASEMENT MEMBRANE DISEASE

Untreated anti-GBM disease is usually rapidly fatal, and, in the absence of treatment, kidney failure is expected. However, since its introduction in the 1970s, treatment with plasmapheresis, cyclophosphamide, and corticosteroids (with dialysis when required) has resulted in most patients surviving the acute disease. The rationale behind this treatment regimen is to rapidly remove circulating anti-GBM autoantibodies (until they become undetectable) and block their synthesis. There has been only one small trial of plasma exchange compared with drug treatment alone, and it suggested a trend toward improved outcome. In addition, the widely reported improvement in mortality and kidney function after the introduction of this treatment regimen, compared with historical cases, has led to its widespread use. All patients should be considered for treatment. However, patients with extensive crescentic glomerulonephritis only (no alveolar hemorrhage) who present as dialysis dependent are least likely to respond, and the balance between risk and benefit of immunosuppressive treatment is uncertain in those cases.

When the diagnosis is suspected, treatment should be initiated as soon as possible and should not be delayed until a kidney biopsy is obtained. Daily plasmapheresis must be quickly initiated: 50 mL/kg (maximum 4L exchange) with 5% human albumin solution, or with fresh frozen plasma if within 3 days after invasive procedure (e.g., biopsy) or if there is other active bleeding, such as pulmonary hemorrhage. Plasma therapy should be continued for 14 days or until circulating anti-GBM antibody levels are undetectable. Another therapeutic option to remove circulating antibodies is immunoadsorption with a high-affinity matrix. This approach has the theoretical advantage of treating an unrestricted plasma volume.

Corticosteroids are initiated as early as possible (daily oral prednisone 1 mg/kg per day; then reduce the dose weekly to 20 mg by week 6 and then more slowly). There is no direct evidence pertaining to the use of pulse intravenous methylprednisolone; it may increase infection risk but could be of benefit if plasmapheresis is not immediately available. Corticosteroids may be tapered off after approximately 6 months. Cyclophosphamide is typically and historically administered orally at a dose of 2 to 3 mg/kg per day (decrease dose in patients >55 years and in case of leukopenia or thrombocytopenia). In general, long-term treatment is not necessary, and patients can stop cyclophosphamide after 3 months. Pulsed intravenous cyclophosphamide has not been formally tested and appears to be equivalent to daily oral dosing in ANCA-associated vasculitis with moderate kidney involvement. Also, it has been used by some practitioners in small cohorts.

Because anti-GBM disease is associated with a high risk of recurrence in the allograft when anti-GBM antibodies are still detectable in circulation, kidney transplantation should be delayed until after circulating anti-GBM antibodies become undetectable and, usually, for an additional 6 to 12 months.

KEY BIBLIOGRAPHY

Buttgereit F, Dejaco C, Matteson EL, Dasgupta B. Polymyalgia rheumatica and giant cell arteritis: a systematic review. *JAMA.* 2016;315:2442-2458.

Cacoub P, Comarmond C, Domont F, Savey L, Saadoun D. Cryoglobulinemia vasculitis. *Am J Med.* 2015;128:950-955.

Davin J-C. Henoch-Schonlein purpura nephritis: pathophysiology, treatment, and future strategy. *Clin J Am Soc Nephrol.* 2011;6:679-689.

De Vita S, Quartuccio L, Isola M, Mazzaro C, Scaini P, Lenzi M, Campanini M, Naclerio C, Tavoni A, Pietrogrande M, et al. A randomized controlled trial of rituximab for the treatment of severe cryoglobulinemic vasculitis. *Arthritis Rheum.* 2012;64:843-853.

Guillevin L, Pagnoux C, Karras A, Khouatra C, Aumaître O, Cohen P, Maurier F, Decaux O, Ninet J, Gobert P, et al. Rituximab versus azathioprine for maintenance in ANCA-associated vasculitis. *N Engl J Med.* 2014;371:1771-1780.

Hiemstra TF, Walsh M, Mahr A, Savage CO, de Groot K, Harper L, Hauser T, Neumann I, Tesar V, Wissing K-M, et al. Mycophenolate mofetil vs azathioprine for remission maintenance in antineutrophil cytoplasmic antibody–associated vasculitis: a randomized controlled trial. *JAMA.* 2010;304:2381.

Jayne D, Rasmussen N, Andrassy K, Bacon P, Tervaert JWC, Dadonienė J, Ekstrand A, Gaskin G, Gregorini G, de Groot K, et al. A randomized trial of maintenance therapy for vasculitis associated with antineutrophil cytoplasmic autoantibodies. *N Engl J Med.* 2003;349:36-44.

Jayne DRW, Gaskin G, Rasmussen N, Abramowicz D, Ferrario F, Guillevin L, Mirapeix E, Savage COS, Sinico RA, Stegeman CA, et al. Randomized trial of plasma exchange or high-dosage methylprednisolone as adjunctive therapy for severe renal vasculitis. *J Am Soc Nephrol.* 2007;18:2180-2188.

Jennette JC, Falk RJ, Bacon PA, Basu N, Cid MC, Ferrario F, Flores-Suarez LF, Gross WL, Guillevin L, Hagen EC, et al. 2012 revised International Chapel Hill Consensus Conference Nomenclature of Vasculitides. *Arthritis Rheum.* 2013;65:1-11.

Koster MJ, Matteson EL, Warrington KJ. Recent advances in the clinical management of giant cell arteritis and Takayasu arteritis. *Curr Opin Rheumatol.* 2016;28:211-217.

Kuo H-C, Yang KD, Chang W-C, Ger L-P, Hsieh K-S. Kawasaki disease: an update on diagnosis and treatment. *Pediatr Neonatol.* 2012; 53:4-11.

Newburger JW, Takahashi M, Gerber MA, Gewitz MH, Tani LY, Burns JC, Shulman ST, Bolger AF, Ferrieri P, Baltimore RS, et al. Diagnosis, treatment, and long-term management of Kawasaki disease: a statement for health professionals from the Committee on Rheumatic Fever, Endocarditis and Kawasaki Disease, Council on Cardiovascular Disease in the Young, American Heart Association. *Circulation.* 2004;110:2747-2771.

Pedchenko V, Bondar O, Fogo AB, Vanacore R, Voziyan P, Kitching AR, Wieslander J, Kashtan C, Borza DB, Neilson EG, Wilson CB, Hudson BG. Molecular architecture of the Goodpasture autoantigen in anti-GBM nephritis. *N Engl J Med.* 2010;363:343-354.

Pillebout E, Alberti C, Guillevin L, Ouslimani A, Thervet E, CESAR study group. Addition of cyclophosphamide to steroids provides no benefit compared with steroids alone in treating adult patients with severe Henoch Schönlein Purpura. *Kidney Int.* 2010;78:495-502.

Saadoun D, Resche Rigon M, Pol S, Thibault V, Blanc F, Pialoux G, Karras A, Bazin-Kara D, Cazorla C, Vittecoq D, et al. PegIFNα/ribavirin/protease inhibitor combination in severe hepatitis C virus-associated mixed cryoglobulinemia vasculitis. *J Hepatol.* 2015;62:24-30.

Srivastava A, Rao GK, Segal PE, Shah M, Geetha D. Characteristics and outcome of crescentic glomerulonephritis in patients with both antineutrophil cytoplasmic antibody and anti-glomerular basement membrane antibody. *Clin Rheumatol.* 2013;32:1317-1322.

Stone JH, Merkel PA, Spiera R, Seo P, Langford CA, Hoffman GS, Kallenberg CGM, St Clair EW, Turkiewicz A, Tchao NK, et al. Rituximab versus cyclophosphamide for ANCA-associated vasculitis. *N Engl J Med.* 2010;363:221-232.

Terrier B, Krastinova E, Marie I, Launay D, Lacraz A, Belenotti P, de Saint-Martin L, Quemeneur T, Huart A, Bonnet F, et al. Management of noninfectious mixed cryoglobulinemia vasculitis: data from 242 cases included in the CryoVas survey. *Blood.* 2012;119:5996-6004.

Walsh M, Flossmann O, Berden A, Westman K, Höglund P, Stegeman C, Jayne D, European Vasculitis Study Group. Risk factors for relapse of antineutrophil cytoplasmic antibody-associated vasculitis. *Arthritis Rheum.* 2012;64:542-548.

Xiao H, Heeringa P, Hu P, Liu Z, Zhao M, Aratani Y, Maeda N, Falk RJ, Jennette JC. Antineutrophil cytoplasmic autoantibodies specific for myeloperoxidase cause glomerulonephritis and vasculitis in mice. *J Clin Invest.* 2002;110:955-963.

Full bibliography can be found on www.expertconsult.com.

Systemic Lupus Erythematosus and the Kidney

25

Andrew S. Bomback; Vivette D. D'Agati

Systemic lupus erythematosus (SLE) is a chronic autoimmune disease that can affect multiple organs, including the skin, joints, brain, peripheral nervous system, heart, gastrointestinal tract, and kidneys. Kidney involvement in SLE, generally termed lupus nephritis (LN), is a major contributor to SLE-associated morbidity and mortality. Up to 50% of SLE patients will have clinically evident kidney disease at presentation, and, during follow-up, kidney involvement occurs in up to 75% of patients, with an even greater representation among children and young adults. LN impacts clinical outcomes in SLE both directly via target organ damage and indirectly through complications of therapy.

PRESENTATION

Most patients with SLE will have laboratory evidence of kidney involvement at some point during the course of their disease. In about one-third of SLE patients, kidney involvement first manifests with proteinuria and/or microscopic hematuria; this eventually progresses to reduction in kidney function. However, early in the course of disease, it is unusual for patients to present with decreased glomerular filtration rate (GFR), except in very aggressive cases of LN, some of which present as rapidly progressive glomerulonephritis. Instead, patients often present initially with evidence of nonkidney organ involvement, such as malar rash, arthritis, and oral ulcers. After a diagnosis of SLE is confirmed with appropriate laboratory tests, evidence of kidney disease, if present, usually emerges within the first 3 years of diagnosis.

Signs of kidney involvement tend to correlate with laboratory abnormalities. For example, patients with nephrotic range proteinuria often present with edema of the lower extremities and, if proteinuria is severe, periorbital edema in the morning. When GFR falls, as is the case with progressive forms of LN, elevated blood pressure is common. The rare development of dark or tea-colored urine is a sign of gross hematuria. A number of tools, such as the SLE Disease Activity Index (SLEDAI) and the British Isles Lupus Assessment Group (BILAG) Index, have been developed to assess the systemic severity of lupus symptoms. Although these questionnaires are primarily used to codify symptoms for clinical trial settings, they also can be very helpful to elicit a detailed history from a patient with SLE.

EVALUATION

LABORATORY FINDINGS

The American College of Rheumatology (ACR) lists 11 diagnostic criteria for SLE: antinuclear antibodies (ANA), arthritis, immunologic disorders (including anti-double-stranded DNA [dsDNA] antibody, antiphospholipid antibody, or anti-Smith antibody), malar rash, discoid rash, photosensitivity, oral ulcers, serositis, hematologic disorder, neurologic disorder, and kidney disorder (Table 25.1). Ideally, four or more of these criteria should be present to diagnose SLE, including laboratory findings of a positive ANA and/or anti-dsDNA antibody. In addition to the ANA and dsDNA antibody, serum complement (C3, C4, CH50) should be checked whenever kidney involvement is suspected, because these are often low when disease is active, as is usually the case with any severe proliferative LN. Antiphospholipid and anticardiolipin antibodies are useful in gauging the risk for clotting abnormalities that can accompany SLE.

Laboratory testing is used both to diagnose kidney involvement and to assess response to therapy in patients with SLE. Traditional parameters, such as serum creatinine and urinary protein excretion (quantified by either 24-hour collection, urine protein to creatinine ratio, or urine albumin to creatinine ratio), are supplemented by serial review of microscopic urinary sediment, changes in serum complement levels, and titers of ANA and dsDNA antibodies. Because cytopenias are often seen in active SLE, complete blood counts should be checked regularly. A number of urine and serologic tests have been studied as biomarkers for SLE and, specifically, LN disease activity. These include molecules specific to lupus (e.g., anti-C1q antibodies), mediators of chronic inflammation (e.g., TNF-like weak inducer of apoptosis [TWEAK]), and generalized markers of kidney injury (urinary neutrophil gelatinase-associated lipocalin [uNGAL]). However, the clinical utility of this approach remains unproven, and no serum or urine disease markers are able to provide as much information as a kidney biopsy. Hence, virtually all patients with SLE with suspected kidney involvement undergo one or more kidney biopsies at some point during their care.

KIDNEY BIOPSY FINDINGS

The classic pattern of LN is an immune complex–mediated glomerulonephritis; however, the pathology of LN can be

245

Table 25.1   American College of Rheumatology Criteria for the Diagnosis of Systemic Lupus Erythematosus

Criteria	Description
Malar rash	Flat or raised erythematous rash over the malar eminences
Discoid rash	Erythematous raised patches, usually circular, with adherent keratotic scaling; atrophic scarring may occur
Photosensitivity	Rash upon exposure to ultraviolet light
Oral ulcers	Oral and/or nasopharyngeal ulcerations
Arthritis	Nonerosive arthritis of at least two peripheral joints, with tenderness and/or swelling
Serositis	Pleuritis or pericarditis
Kidney disorder	Proteinuria, hematuria, and/or elevated creatinine
Neurologic disorder	Seizures or psychosis without other etiologies
Hematologic disorder	Anemia (hemolytic), leukopenia, or thrombocytopenia without other etiologies
Immunologic disorder	Anti-dsDNA, anti-Sm, and/or antiphospholipid antibodies
ANA	An abnormal ANA titer in the absence of drugs known to induce ANAs

Any combination of ≥4 criteria at any time during a patient's course suggests a diagnosis of systemic lupus erythematosus.
ANA, Antinuclear antibodies; *dsDNA,* double-stranded DNA.

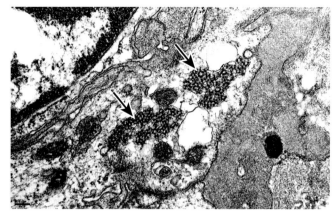

Fig. 25.1 Several large endothelial tubuloreticular inclusions *(arrows)* are located in dilated cisternae of the endoplasmic reticulum of this glomerular endothelial cell. These interanastomosing structures, which are commonly identified in systemic lupus erythemotosus, are induced in endothelial cells by exposure to ambient interferon, earning them the name "interferon footprints" (electron micrograph, ×50,000).

varied and at times can cause confusion with other immune complex–mediated glomerulonephritides. Particular biopsy findings highly characteristic of LN include (1) glomerular deposits that stain dominantly for IgG with codeposits of IgA, IgM, C3, and C1q, the so-called full house immunofluorescence (IF) pattern; (2) extraglomerular immune-type deposits within tubular basement membranes, the interstitium, and blood vessels; (3) the ultrastructural finding of coexistent mesangial, subendothelial, and subepithelial electron-dense deposits; and (4) the ultrastructural finding of tubuloreticular inclusions, which represent "interferon footprints" in the glomerular endothelial cell cytoplasm (Fig. 25.1).

Although lupus may affect all compartments of the kidney, including glomeruli, tubules, interstitium, and blood vessels, glomerular involvement is the best studied component and correlates well with presentation, course, and treatment response. Accordingly, disease classification is based largely on the glomerular alterations, as assessed by the combined modalities of light microscopy, IF, and electron microscopy (EM). Over the past 4 decades, there have been several attempts by different societies, particularly the World Health Organization (WHO), to classify the diverse glomerulopathies associated with SLE. Based on clinicopathologic correlations, a revised classification system of LN was developed by a working group of renal pathologists, nephrologists, and rheumatologists under the joint auspices of the International

Society of Nephrology (ISN) and the Renal Pathology Society (RPS) and was published in 2004 as the ISN/RPS classification. By refining and clarifying many of the deficiencies of the older WHO classification, this revised schema has eliminated ambiguities and has achieved greater reproducibility. The ISN/RPS classification recognizes six different classes of immune complex–mediated lupus glomerulonephritis based on biopsy findings (Table 25.2). These classes are not static entities but may transform from one class to another, both spontaneously and after therapy.

ISN/RPS class I represents the mildest possible glomerular lesion—immune deposits limited to the mesangium, without associated mesangial hypercellularity. In class II, the mesangial deposits detected by IF and/or EM are accompanied by mesangial hypercellularity of any degree. In class III, there is focal and predominantly segmental endocapillary proliferation and/or sclerosis, affecting less than 50% of glomeruli sampled. The active endocapillary lesions typically include infiltrating monocytes and neutrophils and may exhibit necrotizing features, including fibrinoid necrosis, rupture of glomerular basement membrane, and nuclear apoptosis, forming pyknotic or karyorrhectic debris. These segmental lesions often arise on a background of mesangial proliferation and immune deposits. In class IV, the endocapillary lesions involve ≥50% of glomeruli sampled, typically in a diffuse and global distribution (Fig. 25.2). Subendothelial immune deposits are a feature of the endocapillary lesion in class III and class IV, where they vary from focal and segmental (class III) to more diffuse and global (class IV; Fig. 25.3). Both class III and class IV may exhibit extracapillary proliferation in the form of cellular crescents, a feature that correlates best with a rapidly progressive clinical course. Subendothelial deposits that are large enough to be visible by light microscopy may form "wire loops," or intracapillary "hyaline thrombi" (Fig. 25.4). A pathognomonic, but uncommon, feature of active LN is glomerular "hematoxylin bodies," which consist of extruded nuclei from dying cells that have bound to ambient ANA to form basophilic rounded bodies ("LE bodies"; see Fig. 25.2). Class V denotes membranous LN. Subepithelial deposits are the defining feature, usually superimposed on

Table 25.2 International Society of Nephrology/Renal Pathology Society 2004 Classification of Lupus Nephritis

Designation	Description	Characteristic Clinical Features
Class I: minimal mesangial lupus nephritis	No LM abnormalities; isolated mesangial IC deposits on IF and/or EM	Normal urine or microscopic hematuria
Class II: mesangial proliferative lupus nephritis	Mesangial hypercellularity or matrix expansion with mesangial IC deposits on IF and/or EM	Microscopic hematuria and/or low-grade proteinuria
Class III: focal lupus nephritis[a]	<50% of glomeruli on LM display segmental (<50% of glomerular tuft) or global (>50% of glomerular tuft) endocapillary and/or extracapillary proliferation or sclerosis; mesangial and focal subendothelial IC deposits on IF and EM	Nephritic urine sediment and subnephrotic proteinuria
Class IV: diffuse lupus nephritis[a]	≥50% of glomeruli on LM display endocapillary and/or extracapillary proliferation or sclerosis; class IV-S denotes ≥50% of affected glomeruli have segmental lesions; class IV-G denotes ≥50% of affected glomeruli have global lesions; mesangial and diffuse subendothelial IC deposits on IF and EM	Nephritic and nephrotic syndromes, hypertension, reduced kidney function
Class V: membranous lupus nephritis[b]	Diffuse thickening of the glomerular capillary walls on LM with subepithelial IC deposits on IF and EM, with or without mesangial IC deposits	Nephrotic syndrome
Class VI: advanced sclerosing lupus nephritis	>90% of glomeruli on LM are globally sclerosed with no residual activity	Markedly reduced kidney function, hypertension

[a]Both class III and class IV may have active (proliferative), chronic, inactive (sclerosing), or combined active and chronic lesions subclassified as A, C, or A/C, respectively.
[b]Class V may coexist with class III or class IV, in which case both classes are diagnosed.
EM, Electron microscopy; *IC,* immune complex; *IF,* immunofluorescence; *LM,* light microscopy.

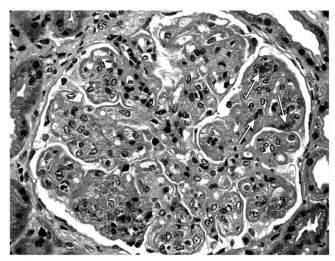

Fig. 25.2 Class IV lupus nephritis: A representative glomerulus shows global narrowing or obliteration of its capillary lumina by endocapillary proliferation, including infiltrating leukocytes. The glomerular capillary walls are thickened by eosinophilic material, forming wire loops. Rounded basophilic structures ("hematoxylin bodies," *arrows*) represent extruded nuclei altered by binding to antinuclear antibody (hematoxylin and eosin, ×400).

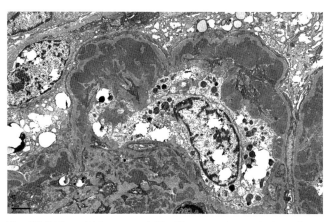

Fig. 25.3 Class IV lupus nephritis: There are large electron-dense deposits within the mesangium and in the subendothelial region. Podocyte foot processes are effaced (electron micrograph, ×6000).

a base of mesangial hypercellularity and/or mesangial immune deposits. Well-developed examples of class V typically exhibit glomerular basement membrane spikes between the subepithelial deposits (Fig. 25.5). Class V may progress to glomerulosclerosis without the development of a superimposed proliferative lesion. In those patients with combined membranous and endocapillary lesions, a diagnosis of both class V and class III or IV is made. These mixed classes carry a worse prognosis than pure class V LN. Class VI identifies

advanced chronic disease exhibiting greater than 90% sclerotic glomeruli, without residual activity.

Unusual kidney biopsy findings in SLE patients include "lupus podocytopathy," presenting as nephrotic syndrome with diffuse foot process effacement in the absence of peripheral capillary wall immune deposits. Mesangial immune deposits and variable mesangial hypercellularity may accompany the podocyte alterations. Such cases resemble minimal change disease or focal segmental glomerulosclerosis in their histopathologic findings and response to glucocorticoids. An altered systemic cytokine milieu, rather than immune complex deposition, is thought to mediate direct podocyte injury. Lupus podocytopathy with collapsing features has been associated with APOL1 risk alleles in patients of African descent and carries a poor prognosis. Rare cases of LN have predominant tubulointerstitial nephritis with abundant

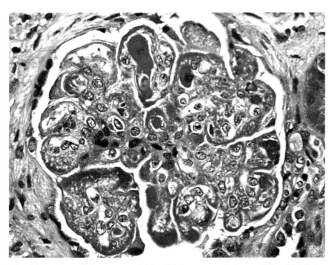

Fig. 25.4 Class IV lupus nephritis: Trichrome stain is useful to highlight fuchsinophilic *(orange)* deposits against the blue-staining glomerular basement membrane and mesangial matrix. In this glomerulus, many subendothelial "wire loops" and intracapillary "hyaline thrombi" are seen (Masson trichrome, ×600).

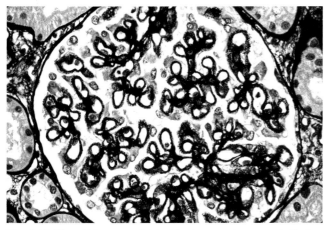

Fig. 25.5 Class V lupus nephritis: Membranous lupus nephritis has global thickening of glomerular capillary walls. Silver stain delineates the characteristic silver-positive spikes projecting from the glomerular basement membranes. These spikes form between silver-negative subepithelial deposits (Jones methenamine silver, ×600).

tubulointerstitial immune deposits in the absence of significant glomerular lesions. Some cases with necrotizing and crescentic features and a paucity of peripheral capillary wall immune deposits are associated with circulating antineutrophil cytoplasmic antibody (ANCA), in addition to ANA. This "pauci-immune" variant is particularly common in LN class IV-S, in which there are diffuse but segmental lesions of necrosis and crescent formation. In any patient with SLE who develops thrombotic microangiopathy affecting the glomeruli and/or vessels, the possibility of a circulating lupus anticoagulant or an antiphospholipid antibody should be investigated. Other unusual vascular lesions include lupus vasculopathy (a noninflammatory narrowing of arterioles by a mixture of immune deposits and fibrin) and true inflammatory arteritis.

Kidney biopsy evaluation is not complete without an assessment of both histologic activity and chronicity as a guide to therapy. Active lesions include any combination of glomerular endocapillary proliferation, leukocyte infiltration, necrotizing lesions, wire-loop deposits, cellular crescents, and interstitial inflammation, which are graded based on the proportion of glomeruli or cortical area affected. Among features of activity, necrotizing lesions and cellular crescents carry the worst prognosis. Chronic changes include global and segmental glomerular scarring (glomerulosclerosis), fibrous crescents, tubular atrophy, and interstitial fibrosis. Because lesions of activity (A) and chronicity (C) can vary widely in a given biopsy, standard approaches to therapy weigh the extent and severity of active lesions (considered potentially responsive to immunosuppressive therapy) against the extent of chronic, irreversible disease.

TREATMENT

The current approach to treating LN, as well as studying new therapeutic modalities in clinical trials, has largely been guided by histologic findings (i.e., ISN/RPS class) with appropriate consideration of presenting clinical parameters and the degree of kidney function impairment (Table 25.3). Class I and class II LN, which represent purely mesangial disease, carry a better prognosis and do not require specific therapy directed to the kidney. Rather, conservative, nonimmuno-modulatory therapy is appropriate for patients with these findings on kidney biopsy. Optimal control of blood pressure through blockade of the renin-angiotensin-aldosterone system (RAAS) is a cornerstone of conservative therapy in LN. Epidemiologic studies have suggested that ACE inhibitor use delays the development of kidney involvement in SLE and reduces overall disease activity.

CLASS III AND IV LUPUS NEPHRITIS

The treatment of active class III and class IV LN is generally divided into induction and maintenance phases of immunosuppression. Most patients with active proliferative LN are treated initially with corticosteroids, traditionally a "pulse" of intravenous steroids (500 to 1000 mg/day of methylprednisolone for 3 days), followed by a high-dose oral regimen (usually prednisone at 1 mg/kg/day, not exceeding 60 mg daily) that begins to taper at 8 weeks.

INDUCTION THERAPY

Steroids should be used in conjunction with other immunosuppressive therapy. Currently, cyclophosphamide and mycophenolate mofetil (MMF) are the two main agents used for induction phase immunosuppression. Intravenous, compared to oral, cyclophosphamide therapy involves a lower cumulative exposure to drug, less frequent cytopenias, enhanced bladder protection, and fewer problems with adherence. Several small, randomized controlled trials at the National Institutes of Health (NIH) in patients with severe proliferative LN resulted in the induction regimen widely known as the "NIH protocol," which uses six pulses of intravenous cyclophosphamide (0.5 to 1 g/m²) on consecutive months. A trial by the EuroLupus Group aimed to decrease the risk of side effects from cyclophosphamide therapy without sacrificing efficacy; their shorter treatment course (the "EuroLupus protocol") of 500 mg of intravenous cyclophosphamide every 2 weeks for 6 doses (total dose 3 g) was equally effective as the NIH protocol in various renal and extrarenal outcomes,

Table 25.3   Treatment Options for Lupus Nephritis, Stratified by International Society of Nephrology Classification and Phase of Therapy

Class	Induction Phase[a]	Maintenance Phase[a]
Class I	Conservative, nonimmunomodulatory therapy (e.g., RAAS blockade)	Not applicable
Class II	Conservative, nonimmunomodulatory therapy	Not applicable
Class III and Class IV	Pulse IV steroids followed by tapering doses of oral steroids *and* IV cyclophosphamide 0.75–1.0 g/m² IV monthly for 6 doses *or* IV cyclophosphamide 500 mg IV every 2 weeks for 6 doses *or* MMF 2000–3000 mg/day for 6 months	Lowest tolerable amount of oral steroids *and* MMF 2000 mg/day for 6 months, then 1500 mg/day for 3–6 months, then 1000 mg/day afterward assuming stable disease *or* Azathioprine 2.0 mg/kg/day for 6 months, then 1.5 mg/kg/day for 3–6 months, then 1.0 mg/kg/day afterward assuming stable disease
Class V	Pulse IV steroids followed by tapering doses of oral steroids *and* IV cyclophosphamide 0.75–1.0 g/m² IV monthly for 6 doses *or* Cyclosporine (dose adjusted to goal trough level 125–200 mcg/L) *or* Tacrolimus (dose adjusted to goal trough level 5–10 mcg/L) *or* MMF 2000–3000 mg/day for 6 months	Lowest tolerable amount of oral steroids *and* MMF 2000 mg/day for 6 months, then 1500 mg/day for 3–6 months, then 1000 mg/day afterward assuming stable disease *or* Azathioprine 2.0 mg/kg/day for 6 months, then 1.5 mg/kg/day for 3–6 months, then 1.0 mg/kg/day afterward assuming stable disease
Class VI	Conservative, nonimmunomodulatory therapy (e.g., RAAS blockade) with preparation for kidney replacement therapy	Not applicable

[a]Doses listed as mg/day are appropriate for adults. See alternate source for pediatric dosing.
IV, Intravenous; *MMF*, mycophenolate mofetil; *RAAS*, renin-angiotensin-aldosterone system.

with less toxicity and fewer total infections. Although this trial was largely performed in white subjects and may not be applicable to populations at high risk for poor kidney outcomes, reports from this trial with up to 10 years of follow-up continue to show no differences in outcome among treatment groups.

MMF has emerged as an alternative first-choice agent for inducing a remission in severe active proliferative LN. An initial report from China compared oral MMF to oral cyclophosphamide and showed similar rates of remission with lower rates of infection and overall mortality in the MMF arm at 1 and 5 years of follow-up. A larger US induction trial in a more diverse population (more than 50% black patients) of proliferative or membranous LN compared monthly intravenous cyclophosphamide pulses with oral MMF therapy, each in conjunction with a fixed tapering dose of corticosteroids, as induction therapy throughout 6 months. Although the study was powered as a noninferiority trial, complete remissions and complete plus partial remissions at 6 months were significantly more common in the MMF arm (52%) than the cyclophosphamide arm (30%). Most recently, a 370-patient, international multicenter trial of induction therapy with either MMF (goal 3 g/day) or monthly intravenous cyclophosphamide pulses showed, after 6 months of therapy, virtually identical rates of complete and partial remission (56% of patients receiving MMF vs. 53% of patients receiving IV cyclophosphamide). A subgroup analysis of those presenting with significant kidney failure (defined as GFR <30 mL/min) showed no indication that MMF was less effective than cyclophosphamide in this setting.

MAINTENANCE THERAPY

After remission has been achieved, maintenance phase therapy should focus on the long-term management of chronic disease. The goals of continued immunosuppressive therapy are to prevent relapses and flares of disease activity, to eliminate smoldering activity leading to kidney scarring, and to minimize long-term side effects of therapy. Azathioprine and MMF have replaced intravenous cyclophosphamide as the preferred immunosuppressive agents for maintenance therapy. Given the risk for long-term toxicities with all immunosuppressive agents, as well as their potential effect on fertility and risk for teratogenicity, the selection and dosage of maintenance therapy are important and modifiable choices that doctors and patients should make together. Although no clinical studies exclude the use of steroids in maintenance therapy, many clinicians will discontinue steroids within the first 1 to 6 months of maintenance therapy to minimize side effects, despite a lack of trial data for such a strategy. Until recently, most data suggested equivalence of MMF and azathioprine in sustaining remission during the maintenance phase. For example, in the MAINTAIN Nephritis trial, after standard induction therapy with steroids and cyclophosphamide, 105 subjects with class III (31%), IV (58%), or V (10%) LN underwent either azathioprine or MMF maintenance therapy. After at least 3 years of follow-up, both groups showed equal rates of remission, steroid withdrawal, and disease flares. More recently, results from the Aspreva Lupus Management Study maintenance study suggest that MMF may be more effective than azathioprine as maintenance therapy. In this study of

227 patients who had responded to induction therapy with either MMF or intravenous cyclophosphamide, 36 months of maintenance therapy with MMF appeared to be superior to azathioprine with respect to time to treatment failure, time to renal flare, and time to rescue therapy, regardless of induction therapy. Withdrawals resulting from severe adverse events were significantly more common among patients who were administered azathioprine.

CLASS V LUPUS NEPHRITIS

The treatment of class V (membranous) LN is also divided into induction and maintenance phases of immunosuppression. As with the proliferative nephritides, induction therapy options include cyclophosphamide and MMF; additionally, in class V, calcineurin inhibitors (cyclosporine or tacrolimus), which have emerged as a first-line therapy for primary membranous nephropathy, are another available treatment. Remission may occur more quickly with a calcineurin inhibitor than with cyclophosphamide or MMF, but these therapies include a higher rate of relapse after withdrawal, similar to the experience of using calcineurin inhibitors in other forms of nephrotic syndrome. One strategy, particularly when a class V lesion is superimposed on a proliferative class III or IV lesion, is to combine a calcineurin inhibitor with MMF. This multitargeted regimen, akin to those used to protect kidney transplants, was tested in a multicenter randomized trial from China that compared induction therapy with MMF, tacrolimus, and steroids versus intravenous cyclophosphamide and steroids. Intention-to-treat analysis showed a higher rate of complete remission (45.9% in the multitargeted group vs. 25.6% in the cyclophosphamide group) at 24 weeks, with no difference in adverse event rates.

ALTERNATIVE THERAPIES

Because of the unacceptably high rate of treatment failure (30% to 50%) of induction therapies as well as the high rate of relapsing disease, newer agents and treatment strategies are continuously sought for LN. Most of these therapies, when studied in a rigorous manner, are administered in addition to current standard treatment regimens of MMF or cyclophosphamide. Rituximab, an anti-CD20 monoclonal antibody that depletes B cells, was studied in a placebo-controlled trial conducted in 140 patients with severe LN, all of whom were receiving concurrent MMF (up to 3 g/day) and tapering dose of corticosteroids. Although more subjects in the rituximab group achieved complete or partial remission, there was no statistically significant difference in the primary clinical endpoint at 1 year. Other agents currently under study for treatment of LN include belimumab, a humanized monoclonal antibody that targets the B cell growth factor B lymphocyte stimulator protein; abatacept, a selective T-cell costimulation modulator; and adrenocorticotropic hormone, which has proven effective in some cases of resistant nephrotic syndrome. Plasma exchange has been added to induction therapies in several trials, without any demonstrated clear benefit in kidney or patient survival; therefore the routine use of plasma exchange is not justified in LN, although this procedure may be of value in unique individuals, such as those with a refractory antiphospholipid antibody and contraindications to anticoagulation or those with both positive lupus and ANCA serologies.

PROGNOSIS

The proliferative forms of LN—III and class IV, as well as class V superimposed on class III or IV—are progressive diseases, unless a remission is quickly achieved and sustained. In recent decades, the increasing armamentarium of immunosuppressive agents along with an improved knowledge, based on well-performed clinical trials, of how best to dose these agents has led to an improved prognosis for patients with LN. Whereas kidney survival at 5 years was as low as 20% before 1980, current treatment strategies have improved this rate to as high as 80% in the past decade. Risk factors for progressive disease include demographic variables, such as male sex, African lineage, Hispanic ethnicity, low socioeconomic status, and young age at presentation, as well as clinical and biopsy features, such as lower GFR at presentation, hypertension, anemia, higher percentage of glomeruli with necrosis or crescents, and degree of scarring or chronicity in the glomeruli and tubulointerstitium.

When LN does progress to end-stage renal disease, most patients experience a gradual complete or partial resolution of their extrarenal manifestations of lupus, including lupus serologies. Furthermore, those patients who continue to experience active disease generally have only mild to moderate symptoms. The mechanisms responsible for this apparent remission of systemic lupus in kidney failure remain unclear. Patients with end-stage renal disease due to LN should be dialyzed for at least 3 to 6 months before kidney transplantation is performed; this recommendation holds particular importance for those patients with relatively rapid progression to kidney failure. This period allows for a potential further reduction in lupus activity before transplantation and affords patients with acute kidney injury sufficient time to recover kidney function if therapy is effective. The overall graft survival in patients with lupus who receive a kidney transplant is similar to those in patients with other kidney diseases, despite a recurrence rate of LN that ranges from 5% to 30%, depending on the indications for kidney allograft biopsy. Recurrence can occur as early as the first week and as late as 10 to 15 years after transplantation. Recurrent LN does not necessarily follow the pattern of the native disease but often takes the form of a milder, nonproliferative lesion.

KEY BIBLIOGRAPHY

Appel GB, Contreras G, Dooley MA, et al. Mycophenolate mofetil versus cyclophosphamide for induction treatment of lupus nephritis. *J Am Soc Nephrol.* 2009;20:1103-1112.

Austin HA 3rd, Illei GG, Braun MJ, et al. Randomized, controlled trial of prednisone, cyclophosphamide, and cyclosporine in lupus membranous nephropathy. *J Am Soc Nephrol.* 2009;20:901-911.

Bao H, Liu ZH, Xie HL, et al. Successful treatment of class V+IV lupus nephritis with multitarget therapy. *J Am Soc Nephrol.* 2008;19:2001-2010.

Bomback AS, Appel GB. Updates on the treatment of lupus nephritis. *J Am Soc Nephrol.* 2010;21:2028-2035.

Chan TM, Li FK, Tang CS, et al. Efficacy of mycophenolate mofetil in patients with diffuse proliferative lupus nephritis. Hong Kong-Guangzhou Nephrology Study Group. *N Engl J Med.* 2000;343:1156-1162.

Dooley MA, Jayne D, Ginzler EM, et al. Mycophenolate versus azathioprine as maintenance therapy for lupus nephritis. *N Engl J Med.* 2011;365:1886-1895.

Duran-Barragan S, McGwin G Jr, Vila LM, et al. Angiotensin-converting enzyme inhibitors delay the occurrence of renal involvement and are associated with a decreased risk of disease activity in patients with systemic lupus erythematosus—results from LUMINA (LIX): a multiethnic US cohort. *Rheumatology (Oxford)*. 2008;47:1093-1096.

Ginzler EM, Dooley MA, Aranow C, et al. Mycophenolate mofetil or intravenous cyclophosphamide for lupus nephritis. *N Engl J Med*. 2005;353:2219-2228.

Gourley MF, Austin HA 3rd, Scott D, et al. Methylprednisolone and cyclophosphamide, alone or in combination, in patients with lupus nephritis. A randomized, controlled trial. *Ann Intern Med*. 1996;125:549-557.

Houssiau FA, D'Cruz D, Sangle S, et al. Azathioprine versus mycophenolate mofetil for long-term immunosuppression in lupus nephritis: results from the MAINTAIN nephritis trial. *Ann Rheum Dis*. 2010;69: 2083-2089.

Hu W, Chen Y, Wang S, et al. Clinical-morphological features and outcomes of lupus podocytopathy. *Clin J Am Soc Nephrol*. 2016;11:585-592.

Illei GG, Austin HA, Crane M, et al. Combination therapy with pulse cyclophosphamide plus pulse methylprednisolone improves long-term renal outcome without adding toxicity in patients with lupus nephritis. *Ann Intern Med*. 2001;135:248-257.

Kraft SW, Schwartz MM, Korbet SM, et al. Glomerular podocytopathy in patients with systemic lupus erythematosus. *J Am Soc Nephrol*. 2005;16:175-179.

Liu Z, Zhang H, Liu Z, et al. Multitarget therapy for induction treatment of lupus nephritis: a randomized trial. *Ann Intern Med*. 2015;162:18-26.

Miyasaka N, Kawai S, Hashimoto H. Efficacy and safety of tacrolimus for lupus nephritis: a placebo-controlled double-blind multicenter study. *Mod Rheumatol*. 2009;19:606-615.

Nasr SH, D'Agati VD, Park H-R, et al. Necrotizing and crescentic lupus nephritis with antineutrophil cytoplasmic antibody seropositivity. *Clin J Am Soc Nephrol*. 2008;3:682-690.

Ortega LM, Schultz DR, Lenz O, et al. Lupus nephritis: pathologic features, epidemiology and a guide to therapeutic decisions. *Lupus*. 2010;19:557-574.

Radhakrishnan J, Moutzouris DA, Ginzler EM, et al. Mycophenolate mofetil and intravenous cyclophosphamide are similar as induction therapy for class V lupus nephritis. *Kidney Int*. 2010;77:152-160.

Weening JJ, D'Agati VD, Schwartz MM, et al. The classification of glomerulonephritis in systemic lupus erythematosus revisited. *J Am Soc Nephrol*. 2004;15:241-250.

Wu LH, Yu F, Tan Y, et al. Inclusion of renal vascular lesions in the 2003 ISN/RPS system for classifying lupus nephritis improves renal outcome predictions. *Kidney Int*. 2013;83:715-723.

Full bibliography can be found on www.expertconsult.com.

26 Pathogenesis, Pathophysiology, and Treatment of Diabetic Nephropathy

Petter Bjornstad; Yuliya Lytvyn; Dick de Zeeuw; David Cherney

Diabetic nephropathy is the leading cause of end-stage renal disease (ESRD) in adults. In the United States, approximately half of patients initiating dialysis have diabetes mellitus, and most of these have type 2 diabetes. Patients with youth-onset type 2 diabetes, as shown in the Treatment Options for Type 2 Diabetes in Adolescents and Youth (TODAY) study, exhibit a particularly high risk of progressive diabetic nephropathy after a relatively short duration of disease. Mortality among patients with diabetic nephropathy is high, with cardiovascular diseases predominating. Once overt diabetic nephropathy is present, kidney failure can often be postponed, but in most instances not prevented, by effective antihypertensive treatment and careful glycemic control. Accordingly, there has been intensive research into the pathophysiologic mechanisms of diabetic kidney injury, predictors of risk for diabetic nephropathy, and early intervention strategies.

The classic terminology used to describe different states of urinary albumin excretion includes normoalbuminuria, microalbuminuria, and macroalbuminuria (or "overt proteinuria"). Normoalbuminuria is typically defined as urinary albumin excretion rate (UAER) less than 20 µg/min or urinary albumin to creatinine ratio (UACR) less than 30 mg/g (or 30 mg/day). Microalbuminuria is defined as UAER between 20 and 200 µg/min or UACR between 30 and 300 mg/g (30 to 300 mg/day) and macroalbuminuria as UAER greater than 200 µg/min or UACR greater than 300 mg/g (>300 mg/day). Updated guidelines now use the terms "moderately increased albuminuria" rather than microalbuminuria and "severely increased albuminuria" instead of macroalbuminuria. To promote internal validity, the authors of this chapter decided to use the classic terminology of albumin excretion (normoalbuminuria, microalbuminuria, and macroalbuminuria), unless the data of the original studies were reported differently.

PATHOPHYSIOLOGY

The pathophysiology underlying diabetic nephropathy is complex and remains incompletely understood. While other important modulating factors may contribute, the long-term deleterious impacts of hyperglycemia and insulin resistance are central to the development and progression of diabetic nephropathy. Studies in both type 1 and type 2 diabetes have shown that improved glycemic control can reduce the risk of developing diabetic nephropathy. Moreover, the development of the earliest diabetic kidney lesions can be slowed or prevented by strict glycemic control, as was demonstrated in a randomized trial in type 1 diabetic kidney transplant recipients. Similarly, intensive insulin treatment decreases the progression rates of glomerular lesions in patients with type 1 diabetes and microalbuminuria. Finally, established diabetic glomerular lesions in the native kidneys of patients with type 1 diabetes regress with prolonged normalization of glycemic levels after successful pancreas transplantation. In summary, these studies strongly suggest that hyperglycemia is necessary for the development and maintenance of diabetic nephropathy because correction of hyperglycemia allows expression of reparative mechanisms that facilitate healing of the original diabetic glomerular injury.

Hemodynamic mechanisms, including hyperfiltration, likely play a significant role in the pathogenesis of diabetic nephropathy through neurohormonal (e.g., renin-angiotensin–aldosterone system activation) and tubular (e.g., tubuloglomerular feedback) pathways. However, patients with other causes of hyperfiltration, such as unilateral nephrectomy, do not typically develop nephropathy. Furthermore, it is unlikely that all patients with diabetes and hyperfiltration develop diabetic kidney disease. Therefore glomerular hyperfiltration alone cannot fully explain the genesis of the early lesions of diabetic nephropathy. However, previous studies and clinical observations suggest that hemodynamic factors are important in modulating both the initiation of nephropathy and also the rate of progression of diabetic lesions that are already well established. Studies in adults with type 1 diabetes have also demonstrated that hyperfiltration is associated with a greater risk of experiencing rapid glomerular filtration rate (GFR) decline (>3 mL/min/1.73 m^2/year or >3.3%/year) with resultant reduced GFR (<60 mL/min/1.73 m^2). It is worth noting that the presence of reduced GFR in normo-albuminuric patients with type 1 diabetes is associated with more severe glomerular lesions, and these patients may be at increased risk of further progression.

Systemic blood pressure levels and a lack of normal nocturnal blood pressure dipping may both be implicated in the progression and genesis of diabetic nephropathy.

Supporting this hypothesis is the association between intensive blood pressure control and decreased rates of progression from normoalbuminuria to microalbuminuria, and from microalbuminuria to overt proteinuria, in both normotensive and hypertensive patients with type 2 diabetes.

Studies on human genetics offer important mechanistic insights into complex traits such as diabetic nephropathy. A genetic predisposition to diabetic nephropathy is suggested in multiple cross-sectional studies in type 1 and type 2 diabetic siblings concordant for diabetes. Importantly, diabetic sibling pairs who are concordant for diabetic nephropathy risk are also highly concordant for diabetic glomerulopathy lesions, and this risk is in part independent of glycemia. Novel loci associated with albuminuria were identified by genome-wide association study (GWAS) meta-analysis of albuminuria traits in the general population. An association between protein coding gene for cubilin (CUBN) and albuminuria was demonstrated, and gene-by-diabetes interactions were detected and confirmed for variants in HS6ST1 and near RAB38/CTSC. While there are ongoing searches for genetic loci related to diabetic nephropathy susceptibility through genomic scanning and candidate gene approaches, the search for specific variants that confer predisposition to diabetic nephropathy remains relatively unrewarding. GWAS is a promising approach to improve discovery of risk variants associated with diabetic nephropathy, as reflected by ongoing multinational efforts to compile a GWAS resource of more than 25,000 participants with diabetes, defined according to nephropathy status.

Diabetic nephropathy is characterized not only by glomerular disease but also by tubulointerstitial injury. While glomerular changes have received more attention than tubulointerstitial changes in diabetic kidney disease research, tubular injury may be more closely associated with kidney function than glomerular injury. Tubular proteinuria predates microalbuminuria in youths with type 1 diabetes, suggesting that tubular damage may occur earlier than glomerular injury in the course of diabetic nephropathy. Tubular changes associated with diabetic nephropathy include basement membrane thickening, tubular hypertrophy, epithelial–mesenchymal transition, glycogen accumulation, and interstitial inflammation. Basement membrane thickening and tubular hypertrophy are mainly related to extracellular matrix (ECM) accumulation, which reflects an imbalance between ECM synthesis and degradation, is the principal cause of mesangial expansion, and contributes to expansion of the interstitium late in the disease. Several mechanisms have been proposed to explain the link between hyperglycemia and ECM accumulation. These include increased levels of tumor growth factor (TGF)-β; activation of protein kinase C, which stimulates ECM production through the cyclic adenosine monophosphate (cAMP), pathway; increased advanced glycation end products; and increased activity of aldose reductase, leading to accumulation of sorbitol. There is also growing evidence that oxidative stress is increased in diabetes and is also related to diabetic nephropathy, mediated through altered nitric oxide production and action, and endothelial dysfunction. Importantly, many factors associated with diabetic nephropathy may act through both hemodynamic and nonhemodynamic pathways. For example, angiotensin II increases intraglomerular pressure and hyperfiltration and also increases the production of injurious

mediators such as protein kinase C. Intraglomerular hypertension, whether a consequence of angiotensin II, other neurohormones, or tubular factors, is associated with increased glomerular wall tension and shear stress, leading to the activation of proinflammatory and profibrotic pathways.

Glycocalyx dysfunction has recently attracted attention as a potential mediator of both diabetic glomerulopathy and tubulopathy. The glycocalyx is a polysaccharide gel that covers the luminal surface of the endothelium, thereby acting as a filtration barrier and regulator of endothelial vascular function. Under exposure to hyperglycemic conditions, the glycocalyx is modified, leading to exposure of heparan sulfate domains that allow chemokine binding, inflammation, and result in glycocalyx degradation. Albuminuria is likely to at least in part occur as a consequence disruption of the glycocalyx. The presence of overlapping and interrelated injurious pathways that promote diabetic nephropathy highlight the need for a multifaceted therapeutic approach, as outlined in this chapter.

PATHOLOGY

TYPE 1 DIABETES

In patients with type 1 diabetes, glomerular lesions can appear within a few years after diabetes onset. The same time frame is present when a normal kidney is transplanted into a patient with diabetes. The changes in kidney structure caused by diabetes are specific, creating a pattern not seen in any other disease, and the severity of these diabetic lesions is related to the functional disturbances of the clinical kidney disease, as well as to diabetes duration, glycemic control, and genetic factors. However, the relationship between the duration of type 1 diabetes and extent of glomerular pathology is not precise. This is consistent with the marked variability in susceptibility to this disorder, such that some patients may develop kidney failure after having diabetes for 15 years, whereas others escape kidney complications despite having type 1 diabetes for decades.

LIGHT MICROSCOPY

Kidney hypertrophy is the earliest structural change in type 1 diabetes but is not reflected in any specific light microscopic changes. In many patients, glomerular structure remains normal or near normal even after decades of diabetes, whereas others develop progressive diffuse mesangial expansion, seen mainly as increased periodic acid–Schiff (PAS)-positive ECM mesangial material. In about 40% to 50% of patients developing proteinuria, there are areas of extreme mesangial expansion called Kimmelstiel-Wilson nodules (nodular mesangial expansion). Mesangial cell nuclei in these nodules are palisaded around masses of mesangial matrix material with compression of surrounding capillary lumina. Nodules are thought to result from earlier glomerular capillary microaneurysm formation. Notably, about half of patients with severe diabetic nephropathy do not have these nodular lesions; therefore, although Kimmelstiel-Wilson nodules are diagnostic of diabetic nephropathy, they are not necessary for severe kidney disease to develop.

Early changes often include arteriolar hyalinosis lesions involving replacement of the smooth muscle cells of afferent

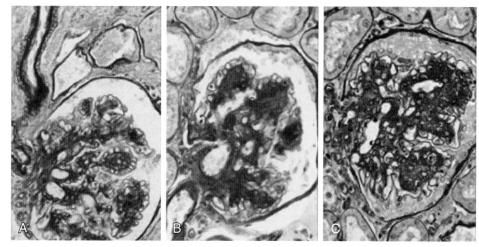

Fig. 26.1 Light microscopy photographs of glomeruli in sequential kidney biopsies performed at baseline and after 5 and 10 years of follow-up in a patient with longstanding normoalbuminuric type 1 diabetes with progressive mesangial expansion and kidney function deterioration. (A) Diffuse and nodular mesangial expansion and arteriolar hyalinosis in this glomerulus from a patient who was normotensive and normoalbuminuric at the time of this baseline biopsy, 21 years after diabetes onset (periodic acid–Schiff [PAS] stain, original magnification ×400). (B) Five-year follow-up biopsy showing worsening of the diffuse and nodular mesangial expansion and arteriolar hyalinosis in this now microalbuminuric patient with declining glomerular filtration rate (GFR) (PAS stain, ×400). (C) Ten-year follow-up biopsy showing more advanced diabetic glomerulopathy in this now proteinuric patient with further reduced GFR. Note also the multiple small glomerular (probably efferent) arterioles in the hilar region of this glomerulus (PAS stain, ×400) and in the glomerulus shown in (A).

and efferent arterioles with PAS-positive waxy, homogeneous material (Fig. 26.1). The severity of these lesions is directly related to the frequency of global glomerulosclerosis, perhaps as the result of glomerular ischemia. Glomerular basement membrane (GBM) and tubular basement membrane (TBM) thickening may be seen with light microscopy, although they are more easily seen with electron microscopy. In addition, tubular glomeruli and glomerulotubular junction abnormalities are present in proteinuric patients with type 1 diabetes and may be important in the progressive loss of GFR in diabetic nephropathy. Finally, usually quite late in the disease, tubular atrophy and interstitial fibrosis occur.

IMMUNOFLUORESCENCE

Diabetes is characterized by increased linear staining of the GBM, TBM, and Bowman capsule, especially for immunoglobulin G (mainly IgG4) and albumin. Although this staining can only be removed by strong acid conditions, consistent with strong ionic binding, the intensity of staining is not related to the severity of the underlying lesions.

ELECTRON MICROSCOPY

The first measurable change observed in diabetic nephropathy is thickening of the GBM, which can be detected as early as 1.5 to 2.5 years after onset of type 1 diabetes (Fig. 26.2). TBM thickening is also seen and parallels GBM thickening. A measurable increase in the relative area of the mesangium begins by 4 to 5 years, with the proportion of the glomerular volume that is mesangium increasing from about 20% (normal) to about 40% when proteinuria begins, and to 60% to 80% in patients with stage 3 chronic kidney disease (CKD). Immunohistochemical studies indicate that these changes in mesangium, GBM, and TBM represent

expansion of the intrinsic ECM components at these sites, most likely including types IV and VI collagen, laminin, and fibronectin.

Qualitative and quantitative changes in the renal interstitium are observed in patients with various kidney diseases. Interstitial fibrosis is characterized by an increase in ECM proteins and cellularity. Preliminary studies suggest that the pathogenesis of interstitial changes in diabetic nephropathy is different from the changes that occur in the mesangial matrix, GBM, and TBM. Whereas for all but the later stages of diabetic nephropathy, GBM, TBM, and mesangial matrix changes represent the accumulation of basement membrane ECM material, early interstitial expansion is largely a result of cellular alterations, and only later, when GFR is already compromised, is interstitial expansion associated with increased interstitial fibrillar collagen and peritubular capillary loss. Consistent with most kidney diseases affecting the glomeruli, the fraction of GBM covered by intact, nondetached foot processes is lower in proteinuric patients with diabetes, when compared with either control subjects or individuals with type 1 diabetes with low levels of albuminuria. Moreover, the fraction of the glomerular capillary luminal surface covered by fenestrated endothelium is reduced in all stages of diabetic nephropathy, with increasing severity in normoalbuminuric, microalbuminuric, and overtly proteinuric patients with type 1 diabetes, respectively, as compared with controls.

TYPE 2 DIABETES

Glomerular and tubular structures in type 2 diabetes are less well studied but overall seem more heterogeneous than those observed in type 1 diabetes. Between 30% and 50%

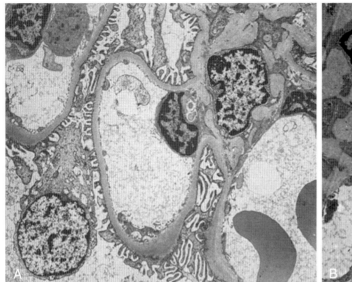
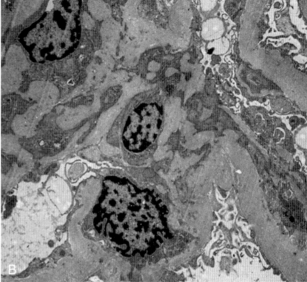

Fig. 26.2 Electron microscopy photographs of mesangial area in a normal control subject (A) and in a patient with type 1 diabetes (B) (original magnification ×3900). Note the increase in mesangial matrix and cell content, the glomerular basement membrane thickening, and the decrease in the capillary luminal space in the diabetic patient (B).

of patients with type 2 diabetes who have clinical features of diabetic nephropathy have typical changes of diabetic nephropathy, including diffuse and nodular mesangial expansion and arteriolar hyalinosis (Fig. 26.3). Notably some patients, despite the presence of albuminuria, have absent or only mild diabetic glomerulopathy, whereas others have disproportionately severe tubular and interstitial abnormalities and/or vascular lesions and/or an increased number of globally sclerosed glomeruli. Patients with type 2 diabetes with microalbuminuria more frequently have morphometric glomerular structural measures in the normal range on electron microscopy and less severe lesions compared with patients with type 1 diabetes and microalbuminuria or overt proteinuria. Interestingly, Pima Indians with type 2 diabetes, a high-risk population for ESRD, have lesions more typical of those seen in type 1 diabetes.

It is unclear why some studies show more structural heterogeneity in type 2 than in type 1 diabetes, whereas others do not. Regardless, the rate of kidney disease progression in type 2 diabetes is related, at least in part, to the severity of the classic changes of diabetic glomerulopathy. Although there are reports that patients with type 2 diabetes have an increased incidence of nondiabetic lesions, such as proliferative glomerulonephritis and membranous nephropathy, this likely reflects biopsies more often being performed in patients with atypical clinical features. When biopsies are performed for research purposes, the incidence of other definable kidney diseases is very low (<5%). It is also noteworthy that a significant proportion of patients with type 2 diabetes exhibit an accelerated GFR decline in the absence of albuminuria. Although this phenotype is not yet completely understood, it has been suggested that this may reflect a predominance of microvascular disease rather than glomerular disease, thereby attenuating albuminuria risk. GFR reduction in the absence of albuminuria highlights the need to identify alternate biomarkers that better capture early diabetic nephropathy risk.

STRUCTURAL-FUNCTIONAL RELATIONSHIPS IN DIABETIC NEPHROPATHY

Kidney disease progression rates vary greatly among individuals with diabetes. Patients with type 1 diabetes and patients with proteinuria who are biopsied for research purposes always have advanced glomerular lesions and usually have vascular, tubular, and interstitial lesions as well. There is considerable overlap in glomerular structural changes between long-standing normoalbuminuric and microalbuminuric patients, as some normoalbuminuric patients with long-standing type 1 diabetes can have quite advanced kidney lesions, whereas many patients with longstanding diabetes and normoalbuminuria have structural measurements within the normal range.

Ultimately expansion of the mesangium, mainly resulting from ECM accumulation, reduces or even obliterates the glomerular capillary luminal space, decreasing the glomerular filtration surface and therefore decreasing the GFR. Accordingly, the fraction of the glomerulus occupied by mesangium correlates with both GFR and albuminuria in patients with type 1 diabetes, reflecting in part the inverse relationship between mesangial expansion and total peripheral GBM filtration surface per glomerulus. GBM thickness is also directly related to the albumin excretion rate. Finally, the extent of global glomerulosclerosis and interstitial expansion are correlated with the clinical manifestations of diabetic nephropathy (proteinuria, hypertension, and declining GFR).

In patients with type 1 diabetes, glomerular, tubular, interstitial, and vascular lesions tend to progress more or less in parallel, whereas in patients with type 2 diabetes, this often is not the case. Current evidence suggests that, among type 2 diabetes patients with microalbuminuria, those patients with typical diabetic glomerulopathy have a higher risk of progressive GFR loss than those with lesser degrees of glomerular changes. A remarkably high frequency of glomerular tubular

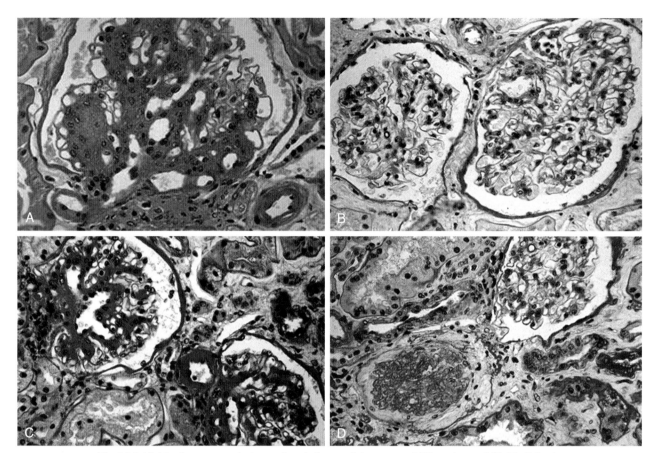

Fig. 26.3 Light microscopy photographs of glomeruli from type 1 (A) and type 2 (B–D) diabetic patients. (A) Diffuse and nodular mesangial expansion and arteriolar hyalinosis in a glomerulus from a microalbuminuric type 1 diabetic patient (periodic acid–Schiff [PAS] stain, original magnification ×400). (B) Normal or near-normal kidney structure in a glomerulus from a microalbuminuric type 2 diabetic patient (PAS stain, ×400). (C) Changes "typical" of diabetic nephropathology (glomerular, tubulointerstitial, and arteriolar changes occurring in parallel) in a kidney biopsy specimen from a microalbuminuric type 2 diabetic patient (PAS stain, ×400). (D) "Atypical" patterns of injury, with absent or only mild diabetic glomerular changes associated with disproportionately severe tubulointerstitial changes. Note also a glomerulus undergoing glomerular sclerosis (PAS stain, ×400) (B–D).

junction abnormalities can be observed in proteinuric type 1 diabetic patients. Most of these abnormalities are associated with tuft adhesions to Bowman capsule at or near the glomerular tubular junction (tip lesions). The frequency and severity of these lesions (as well as the presence of completely atubular glomeruli) predict GFR loss.

The data on structural-functional relationships in type 2 diabetes are less abundant. In several small studies, morphometric measures of diabetic glomerulopathy correlated with kidney function parameters similar to those observed in type 1 diabetes, although there seems to be a subset of patients who have normal glomerular structure despite persistent albuminuria. Overall, the relationships between kidney function and glomerular structure are less precise in patients with type 2 diabetes. It is important to note that the rate of GFR decline significantly correlates with the severity of diabetic glomerulopathy lesions. Thus kidney lesions different from those typical of diabetic glomerulopathy should be considered when investigating the nature of abnormal levels of albuminuria in type 2 diabetes. These lesions include changes in the structure of renal tubules, interstitium, arterioles, and podocytes. For example, Pima Indians with type 2 diabetes and proteinuria have fewer podocytes per glomerulus than those without nephropathy, and, in this population, a lower number of podocytes per glomerulus at baseline was the strongest predictor of greater increases in albuminuria and of progression to overt nephropathy in microalbuminuric patients. These results suggest that changes in podocyte structure and density occur early in diabetic nephropathy and might contribute to increasing albuminuria in these patients. More biopsy data are needed in people with type 1 and type 2 diabetes to better characterize DKD and rule out non-diabetes-related nephropathy.

REVERSAL OF DIABETIC NEPHROPATHY LESIONS

The lesions of diabetic nephropathy have long been considered irreversible. Theoretically, if reversal were possible, this would happen in the setting of long-term normoglycemia. Interestingly, in pancreas transplant recipients, the lesions of diabetic nephropathy were unaffected after 5 years of normoglycemia but reversed in all patients by 10 years post-transplant, with a remarkable amelioration of glomerular structure abnormalities evident by light microscopy, including total disappearance of Kimmelstiel-Wilson nodular lesions. The long time necessary for these diabetic lesions to disappear is consistent with their slow rate of development. The understanding of the molecular and cellular mechanisms involved in these repair processes could provide new directions for the treatment of diabetic nephropathy.

MEDICAL MANAGEMENT OF DIABETES

Both kidney and cardiovascular morbidity and mortality are increased in patients with type 2 diabetes, particularly in those with nephropathy. Accordingly, treatment goals in these individuals focus on slowing the rate of GFR decline and delaying the onset of kidney failure, as well as primary and secondary prevention of cardiovascular disease. This is mainly done by targeting multiple kidney and cardiovascular risk factors, such as hyperglycemia, hypertension, and dyslipidemia (Fig. 26.4). Targeting albuminuria is of specific interest for kidney protection, although not all therapies that reduce albuminuria lead to kidney or cardiovascular benefits. The remainder of this chapter reviews traditional therapeutic options to decrease the risk of kidney and cardiovascular morbidity and mortality, as well as novel risk factors for diabetic nephropathy that may provide insight into new drug targets and possibilities for new therapeutic interventions.

TRADITIONAL THERAPEUTIC STRATEGIES FOR DIABETIC NEPHROPATHY

GLYCEMIC CONTROL

Rationale

Poor glycemic control, as reflected by higher hemoglobin A1c (HbA1c) levels, is associated with markedly worse kidney

and cardiovascular outcomes in observational studies of patients with type 1 and type 2 diabetes, and targeting HbA1c values lower than 7% may delay the progression of diabetic kidney disease, including development of microalbuminuria and overt nephropathy. In patients with type 1 diabetes, the benefit of intensive glucose control in the prevention of microvascular complications (specifically retinopathy or microalbuminuria) was demonstrated in the diabetes control and complications trial (DCCT), where long-term follow-up showed a significant reduction in the risk of developing reduced GFR among individuals who were treated intensively earlier in the course of diabetes. In type 2 diabetes, the United Kingdom prospective diabetes study (UKPDS) and ADVANCE-ON documented the benefit of intensive glucose targeting on microvascular complications. Of note, although most studies of type 2 diabetes have shown a benefit in kidney outcomes, multiple trials failed to show a benefit of intensive glycemic control on mortality and cardiovascular disease, with some trials actually showing increased mortality with intensive control. In contrast with this older literature, more recent trials such as the Empagliflozin-Reduce Excess Glucose Outcome (EMPA-REG OUTCOME) trial and Liraglutide Effect and Action in Diabetes: Evaluation of Cardiovascular Outcome Results (LEADER) study demonstrate a significant reduction in cardiovascular endpoints (and kidney outcomes; EMPA-REG OUTCOME), even though HbA1c lowering effects were modest. This suggests a predominance of nonglycemic mechanisms leading to cardiorenal damage, although the underlying pathways require further study. Accordingly, a careful individualized approach is required when assigning glycemic targets in individuals with diabetes and kidney disease.

Medications of Choice

In principle, one uses the same drugs for glycemic control in patients with diabetes with and without kidney disease until late stage 3 CKD (Table 26.1). There is controversy regarding metformin use in advanced CKD, with some guidelines recommending that use be restricted to those with serum creatinine ≤1.5 mg/dL (133 μmol/L) in men and 1.4 mg/dL (124 μmol/L) in women, because of an increased risk for life-threatening lactic acidosis. However, in practice many patients with an estimated glomerular filtration rate (eGFR) of 30 to 60 mL/min/1.73 m^2 receive metformin without any problem. Although it is unlikely to occur, a randomized controlled trial assessing the efficacy and safety of metformin in patients with more advanced CKD is warranted, as metformin is an excellent glucose-lowering agent for many patients. Of note, metformin should be temporarily discontinued before surgery or administration of contrast media and during episodes of acute, significant illness.

Reduction in the doses of other oral hypoglycemic agents in later stages of CKD may also be necessary, especially for some sulfonylurea compounds that are metabolized by the kidney. Similarly, as insulin is degraded by the kidney, dose reduction may be needed to prevent hypoglycemia. Finally, thiazolidinediones, such as rosiglitazone or pioglitazone, may affect kidney water and sodium handling, thereby aggravating edema and congestive heart failure. In non-CKD populations, rosiglitazone use is associated with increased risk of heart failure and myocardial infarction compared with placebo,

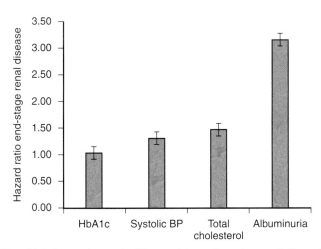

Fig. 26.4 Comparison of different risk markers for prediction of end-stage renal disease (ESRD) in patients with type 2 diabetes and nephropathy participating in the Trial to Reduce Cardiovascular Events With Aranesp Therapy (TREAT). The risk for ESRD per standard deviation increment in the risk factor is shown. Per standard deviation increment in albuminuria, the risk of ESRD markedly amplifies compared with the other kidney-disease risk factors. (Adapted from Pfeffer MA, Burdmann EA, Chen CY, et al. A trial of darbepoetin alfa in type 2 diabetes and chronic kidney disease. *N Engl J Med.* 2009;361:2019–2032.)

Table 26.1 Currently Available Oral Hypoglycemic Agents for the Management of Hyperglycemia

Class	Mechanism of Action	Examples of Drugs	Renal Clearance	HbA1c Lowering (%)	Use in Nondialysis CKD	Use in Dialysis	Advantage	Disadvantage
Biguanides (European Union 1958; United States 1995)[a]	Inhibits hepatic glucose production and increases insulin sensitivity	Metformin	Excreted unchanged in urine	1.5	Contraindicated	Contraindicated	Long-term safety; low costs; weight neutral	Risk of lactate acidosis in CKD patients; gastrointestinal side effects
Sulfonylureas (1946)[a]	Binds to SU receptor in β-cells and increases calcium influx followed by insulin release	Gliclazide Glipizide Glimepiride Glyburide	More than 90% metabolized in liver to weakly active or inactive metabolites and excreted in urine and feces	1.5	May be used	Glipizide may be used; use glimepiride and glyburide with caution	Long-term safety; low costs	Hypoglycemia; weight gain
Meglitinides (1997)[a]	Binds to SU receptor (different from SU site) and increases calcium influx followed by insulin release	Nateglinide Repaglinide	Metabolized by liver (100%) and excreted in urine (10%) and feces (90%)	1.0	May be used	No data for patients with renal clearance less than 20 mL/min	Rapid onset of action and short acting	Few long-term safety data; weight gain
Thiazolidinediones (1997)[a]	Decreases peripheral insulin resistance, thus increasing insulin sensitivity	Pioglitazone	Metabolized by liver to weakly active metabolites; excreted in urine (15%) and feces (85%)	0.6–1.5	May be used; no dose adjustments necessary; caution around edema/heart failure	May be used; no dose adjustments necessary; caution around edema/heart failure	Low-risk hypoglycemia	Pioglitazone is associated with increased risk of bladder cancer Rosiglitazone withdrawn from the market because of increased cardiovascular risk
GLP-1 receptor agonists (2005)[a]	Binds to the pancreatic GLP-1 receptor and promotes insulin secretion, decreases glucagon secretion, gastric emptying, and appetite	Exenatide Liraglutide	Metabolized by kidney, excreted in urine	0.7–1.2 on top of metformin or SU derivatives	Not recommended for patients with moderate or severe kidney failure	Not recommended for patients with moderate or severe kidney failure	Reduced rate of death from cardiovascular causes, nonfatal myocardial infarction, or nonfatal stroke (LEADER Trial)	Long-term safety data not yet known
DPP-4 inhibitors (2006)[a]	Blocks DPP-4, which inactivates endogenous incretins	Saxagliptin Sitagliptin Linagliptin	Excreted mostly unchanged in urine and feces (linagliptin metabolized and excreted in feces)	~0.8 (on top of metformin/SU derivatives)	Dose adjustments necessary for saxagliptin and sitagliptin	Dose adjustments necessary for saxagliptin and sitagliptin	Weight neutral; low risk of hypoglycemia	No proven cardiovascular benefits, possible risk of heart failure with saxagliptin
SGLT-2 inhibitors (European Union 2012)[a]	Inhibits proximal tubular glucose reabsorption	Dapagliflozin	Metabolized by liver to active metabolites, excreted in urine and feces	~0.8 (on top of metformin)	Limited clinical experience; less A1c lowering in CKD but kidney and cardiovascular benefits extended to patients with CKD	No clinical experience; not recommended	Reduced cardiac end points (death from cardiovascular causes, nonfatal myocardial infarction, or nonfatal stroke) and kidney end points (doubling of serum creatinine, ESRD and kidney death) (EMPA-REG Trial)	Increased risk of urinary or genital tract infections

[a]Year drug class became available for clinical use.

CKD, Chronic kidney disease; DPP-4, dipeptidyl peptidase-4; GLP-1, glycagon-like peptide-1; SGLT-2, sodium-glucose cotransporter-2; SU, sulfonylurea.

prompting regulatory agencies in Europe to suspend its marketing.

BLOOD PRESSURE CONTROL
Rationale

Treatment of high blood pressure is of paramount importance for preventing and delaying the progression of diabetic nephropathy. Blood pressure–lowering therapy is vital during any stage of CKD and is a mainstay of renoprotective therapy in all kidney diseases. In the UKPDS trial, where average blood pressure levels of 144/82 mm Hg were achieved, there was no threshold below which further blood pressure reduction did not reduce risk of progressive diabetic nephropathy and cardiovascular morbidity. However, recent data from the Action to Control Cardiovascular Risk in Diabetes (ACCORD) trial showed that intensive (average 119 mm Hg) versus standard blood pressure (average 134 mm Hg) control conferred no benefit on kidney outcomes in type 2 diabetes patients. Critically, patients with more than 1 g of proteinuria per day were excluded from this trial, leaving the benefits of a lower blood pressure target (<120 mm Hg systolic) for patients with type 2 diabetes and nephropathy untested. Surprisingly little evidence from randomized controlled trials demonstrates that a lower target blood pressure actually reduces kidney or cardiovascular risk in people with diabetes and CKD. Accordingly, a target of less than 140/90 mm Hg appears to be best supported by evidence, although a variety of targets are suggested by different clinical practice guidelines. For example, the Canadian Diabetes Association recommends a blood pressure target of less than 130/80 mm Hg, reflecting the lack of clear consensus in this area.

Medication of Choice

Any antihypertensive agent can be effectively used in the diabetic population, with agents that block the renin-angiotensin-aldosterone system (RAAS) being the first choice in those with diabetes and hypertension, as well as those with (normotensive) diabetes with moderately or severely increased albuminuria. Medication choice is further tailored to the need of the individual patient and the tolerability of the individual drugs. Patients with diabetic nephropathy are often volume overloaded; accordingly, diuretic therapy is often indicated. Increasing doses of loop diuretics, rather than thiazide diuretics, may become necessary to control fluid retention and accompanying hypertension at very low GFRs.

RAAS blocking agents lead to additional cardiovascular and renoprotection benefits beyond those expected with blood pressure reduction alone, leading many guidelines to advocate the use of angiotensin-converting enzyme (ACE) inhibitors or angiotensin receptor blockers (ARBs) as first-choice antihypertensive therapy to achieve renoprotection. Notably, the degree of reduction in albuminuria induced by RAAS intervention in the first months of therapy is linearly associated with the magnitude of long-term renoprotection both in early and late stages of diabetic nephropathy. The "blood pressure independent" effect of RAAS inhibitors has been attributed to a reduction in intraglomerular hypertension and consequent decrease in urine albumin excretion. Interestingly and consistent with the concept of reduced intraglomerular pressure leading to kidney protection is the observation that, in patients with type 2 diabetes, the

magnitude of the initial, acute decline in eGFR after ARB treatment is independently associated with better kidney function over time.

Angiotensin-Converting Enzyme Inhibitors

The captopril trial by the Collaborative Study Group was the first large trial to definitively show the benefit of ACE inhibitor therapy in delaying progression of kidney disease in patients with type 1 diabetes throughout a 4-year period of follow-up, with a nearly 50% reduction in the risk of doubling of serum creatinine concentration or in the combined endpoints of death, dialysis, and kidney transplantation, despite similar achieved blood pressure between the captopril and noncaptopril groups. Moreover, aggressive antihypertensive treatment with ACE inhibitors throughout a 7-year follow-up period in patients with type 1 diabetes and diabetic nephropathy was shown to induce regression or remission of nephrotic range albuminuria, slow deterioration of kidney function, and substantially improve survival. Thus ACE inhibitors should be used in patients with type 1 diabetes as soon as persistent albuminuria is documented, even if blood pressure is not elevated, to delay and/or prevent the development of overt nephropathy. In type 2 diabetes and normoalbuminuria, ACE inhibitors have consistently reduced the risk of development of microalbuminuria and reduced the rate of kidney function decline. Furthermore, patients with type 2 diabetes who received ramipril in the Heart and Outcome Protection Evaluation (HOPE) trial had significantly fewer cardiovascular events. Consequently, RAAS inhibitors can be prescribed for cardioprotective indications in all patients with type 2 diabetes, regardless of the presence or absence of kidney disease.

Angiotensin Receptor Blockers

The merits of ARBs to protect the kidney and heart beyond blood pressure control have been demonstrated in numerous randomized placebo-controlled trials, including the Irbesartan in Patients with Type 2 Diabetes and Microalbuminuria (IRMA2) and the Incipient to Overt; Angiotensin II Blocker Telmisartan Investigation on Type 2 Diabetic Nephropathy (INNOVATION) trials, where ARB-based regimens significantly reduced the number of patients with microalbuminuria who progressed to macroalbuminuria. Similarly, large-scale trials in patients with type 2 diabetes and overt nephropathy, including the Reduction in Endpoints in NIDDM with the Angiotensin-II Antagonist Losartan (RENAAL) and Irbesartan Diabetic Nephropathy Trial (IDNT) trials, have shown that ARB-based therapy reduces the risk of a composite endpoint consisting of doubling of serum creatinine, ESRD, and all-cause mortality. Irbesartan Diabetic Nephropathy Trial also established the superiority of irbesartan over the calcium channel blocker (CCB) amlodipine in this setting. Apart from kidney protection, ARBs also afford cardiovascular protection in patients with diabetes, as demonstrated in the Losartan Intervention for Endpoint Reduction in Hypertension (LIFE) trial.

Comparing Angiotensin-Converting Enzyme Inhibitors to Angiotensin Receptor Blockers

Data comparing the benefits of ACE inhibitors and ARBs for cardiovascular and/or kidney protection in patients with type 2 diabetic nephropathy are scarce. One small study directly compared the effects of telmisartan and enalapril on kidney function in type 2 diabetes and reported no difference between the two drugs. Similar results were noted in the Ongoing Telmisartan Alone and in Combination With Ramipril Trial (ONTARGET), where in people at cardiovascular risk, there was no difference in the incidence of kidney or cardiovascular outcome in subjects treated with ACE inhibitor– or ARB-based regimens in either the overall population or in the third of participants with diabetes. Accordingly, there is evidence of differential efficacy for ACE inhibitors over ARB in patients with type 2 diabetes, although the not infrequent occurrence of cough with ACE inhibitors has increased the popularity of ARB-based regimens despite higher cost.

COMBINATIONS OF BLOOD PRESSURE–LOWERING DRUGS

Rationale

More than one medication is often required to control blood pressure, and patients with overt diabetic nephropathy usually require three or four different antihypertensive drugs, including a diuretic. In addition, synergistic combinations may have the advantage that one can reduce the dose of individual components of the antihypertensive regimen, potentially retaining efficacy while reducing side effects.

Combinations of Choice

Logical combinations can be used just as in uncomplicated hypertensive patients. Because RAAS blockade will typically be the first-line agent, clinicians should use other agents, in conjunction with RAAS blockade, that have proven efficacy for preventing both surrogate and hard clinical outcomes.

The combination of a diuretic plus ACE inhibitor or ARB effectively reduces both blood pressure and proteinuria in patients with and without diabetes; however, no studies with hard outcomes have been done to compare this combination with single therapies. The ADVANCE trial showed that the combination of an ACE inhibitor (perindopril) with a diuretic (indapamide) significantly reduces blood pressure and the risk of kidney and cardiovascular complications, as compared with placebo in a broad range of patients with type 2 diabetes.

The combination of a CCB plus ACE inhibitor or ARB has been investigated in two large trials. The BENEDICT trial compared the combination of the nondihydropyridine CCB verapamil and the ACE inhibitor trandolapril versus the single use of these agents in preventing the onset of microalbuminuria in type 2 diabetes, demonstrating that the combination of verapamil and trandolapril provided no advantage over trandolapril alone, whereas trandolapril was superior to verapamil. The Avoiding Cardiovascular Events in Combination Therapy in Patients Living with Systolic Hypertension (ACCOMPLISH) trial compared benazepril plus hydrochlorothiazide versus benazepril plus amlodipine in high cardiovascular risk patients and reported that the combination of benazepril and amlodipine was superior in preventing cardiovascular and kidney outcomes. Although a prespecified analysis in the diabetic population in ACCOMPLISH (60% of the overall population) showed results similar to the main study, the small number of kidney events in ACCOMPLISH renders the interpretation of this outcome difficult.

COMBINATIONS OF RENIN-ANGIOTENSIN-ALDOSTERONE SYSTEM INTERVENTIONS

Angiotensin-Converting Enzyme Inhibitor Plus Angiotensin Receptor Blockers

The recognition of the importance of the RAAS in kidney and cardiovascular health has led to the idea that more stringent RAAS blockade by means of combination of ACE inhibitor and ARB therapy would afford additional protection. Indeed, combination therapy with ACE inhibitors and ARBs does result in additional blood pressure and albuminuria reduction. In 2013, the VA NEPHRON-D trial, which compared ARB alone to combination therapy in patients with diabetic nephropathy, was terminated early per recommendations of the Data Monitoring Committee, based on a greater number of observed acute kidney injury events and hyperkalemia in the combination therapy group. Similarly, the ONTARGET demonstrated that, despite additional blood pressure reduction and less progression of albuminuria, dual RAAS blockade did not reduce kidney or cardiovascular events in a lower kidney risk population.

Angiotensin-Converting Enzyme Inhibitor/Angiotensin Receptor Blockers and Direct Renin Inhibition

Blockade of the RAAS by renin inhibition was considered an attractive target to prevent kidney and cardiovascular outcomes. The direct renin inhibitor aliskiren is a potent inhibitor of renin, and short-term studies demonstrated its efficacy as well as its safety. However, the Aliskiren Trial in Type 2 Diabetes Using Cardiovascular and Renal Disease Endpoints (ALTITUDE) trial, which tested the combination of the direct renin-inhibitor aliskiren plus ACE inhibitor or ARB treatment, demonstrated that aliskiren was associated with adverse kidney and cardiovascular effects in patients with type 2 diabetes at cardiovascular risk, leading to premature termination of the trial and recommendations from drug regulatory agencies that aliskiren is contraindicated in patients with diabetes and moderate or severe CKD who are taking ACE inhibitors or ARBs.

Angiotensin-Converting Enzyme Inhibitor/Angiotensin Receptor Blockers and Mineralocorticoid Receptor Blockers

Adding aldosterone blockers to ACE inhibitors or ARBs is another strategy to block the deleterious effect of the RAAS in diabetic nephropathy. Because aldosterone promotes tissue fibrosis and to counteract aldosterone breakthrough, a phenomenon defined by elevations of plasma aldosterone levels during chronic ACE inhibitor or ARB treatment that occurs in approximately 40% of patients receiving these agents, mineralocorticoid receptor blocking agents may be beneficial as add-on therapy to ACE inhibitors or ARBs. A recent trial showed improvement in UACR in patients with type 2 diabetes and diabetic nephropathy treated with finerenone versus placebo for 90 days as an addition to the conventional ACE inhibitor or ARB treatment (NCT01874431). Although there were no differences observed in adverse events between the 90-day treatment with finerenone versus placebo group, long-term efficacy and safety data and the risk of hyperkalemia (in particular given the results of ONTARGET and ALTITUDE) warrant caution when combining mineralocorticoid receptor blocking agents with an ACE inhibitor or ARB. In light of the potential risk and lack of endpoint data, the combination of an ACE inhibitor or ARB or renin inhibitor with a mineralocorticoid receptor-blocking agent should not be routinely used in clinical practice until additional longer term data are available.

LIPID MANAGEMENT

Rationale

Cholesterol lowering has contributed to improved cardiovascular outcomes in a range of patient populations. However, whether lipid management delays the progression of nephropathy and decreases the risk of ESRD is subject to debate. Meta-analyses report that statin therapy may reduce proteinuria in CKD patients, but the lack of well-designed long-term trials fueled uncertainty as to whether improved lipid management reduces kidney risk. The results of the Study of Heart and Renal Protection (SHARP) trial provided much needed insight into the long-term efficacy and safety of lipid management among kidney disease patients. The SHARP results, reviewed in greater detail in Chapter 56, showed that the combination of simvastatin and ezetimibe reduced the risk of major vascular events by 16% versus placebo in individuals with advanced CKD. Of note, a recent meta-analysis of all statin trials in CKD, including SHARP, showed that the cardiovascular protective effect of statins is attenuated at lower eGFR levels, and unfortunately, the combination of simvastatin and ezetimibe in SHARP did not decrease the risk of progression to kidney failure.

Choice of Lipid-Lowering Therapy

Choosing among lipid-lowering strategies in CKD patients is challenging, given a lack of adequate data, with most studies focusing on statins. Several studies have assessed the comparative effects of statins on kidney or cardiovascular outcomes, with the results of the Prospective Evaluation of Proteinuria and Renal Function in Diabetic Patients with Progressive Renal Disease Trial (PLANET) suggesting a benefit for atorvastatin over rosuvastatin on kidney function. Further studies are needed to evaluate the long-term effects of lipid-lowering therapies, including PCSK9 inhibitors, on kidney function and the development of diabetic nephropathy.

TREATMENT OF TYPE 2 DIABETES IN PATIENTS UNDERGOING DIALYSIS

When a patient with diabetes approaches kidney failure, the various options for kidney replacement therapies should be offered: peritoneal dialysis, hemodialysis, or kidney transplantation. Survival with any kidney replacement modality is generally worse for patients with diabetes compared with nondiabetic patients, and cardiovascular complications markedly contribute to earlier deaths. In fact, more than 70% of deaths in the diabetic ESRD population are attributed to a cardiovascular cause.

Control of Hyperglycemia

While the HbA1c target associated with the best outcome among patients undergoing dialysis with type 2 diabetes has not been established, glycemic control in patients undergoing dialysis is important because (severe) hyperglycemia not only increases cardiovascular risk but also causes thirst and high fluid intake. A meta-analysis of observational studies demonstrated that a mean HbA1c ≥8.5% was associated with a

moderate increase in mortality compared with mean HbA1c values between 6.5% and 7.4% among patients on hemodialysis. Data suggest it is equally important to avoid hypoglycemia, which is also associated with increased mortality in dialysis.

The assessment of glycemic control in patients undergoing dialysis is complicated, because interpretation of the commonly used assays for HbA1c is confounded by interference with uremic toxins. In addition, altered red blood cell survival, blood transfusion, and use of erythropoietin all impact the accuracy of HbA1c measurement. The pharmacologic management of hyperglycemia in patients undergoing dialysis must take into account that dialysis reverses insulin resistance, so that the insulin requirement is generally lower than before dialysis. The glucose concentration in hemodialysate typically is 100 mg/dL (6.1 mmol/L) to avoid the risk of intradialytic hypoglycemic episodes.

Blood Pressure Control

The benefits and harm of blood pressure–lowering therapies in the dialysis population remain uncertain and likely do not differ from nondiabetic patients undergoing dialysis. Large outcome trials are needed to evaluate this further.

Lipid Control

Based on Die Deutsche Diabetes Dialysis Study (4D) and A Study to Evaluate the Use of Rosuvastatin in Subjects on Regular Hemodialysis: An Assessment of Survival and Cardiovascular Event (AURORA), patients treated with hemodialysis should not be started on a statin. Although the SHARP trial noted a benefit in a mixed CKD/ESRD population, meta-analyses of these studies have not demonstrated a substantial benefit in dialysis. Accordingly, the Kidney Disease Improving Global Outcomes guidelines recommend not initiating a statin in patients treated with dialysis but to continue statin treatment in those who are already receiving these agents at dialysis initiation.

NOVEL STRATEGIES AND AGENTS FOR DIABETIC NEPHROPATHY

Optimizing glucose, blood pressure, and lipid control in CKD patients with diabetes has undoubtedly improved their prognosis; however, a considerable proportion of patients continue to develop diabetic nephropathy and progress to kidney failure. An overview of novel agents that target well-established or novel pathophysiologic pathways is provided in the next section. Many of these novel agents not only affect the target for which they are developed (on-target risk factor) but impact multiple other risk markers as well (off-target risk factors; Table 26.2). Optimizing drug regimens to impact multiple parameters may lead to better drug use in the future.

NEWER GLYCEMIC CONTROL AGENTS

Glucagon-like Peptide-1 and Dipeptidyl Peptidase-4 Inhibitors

Glucagon-like peptide-1 (GLP-1) stimulates insulin secretion and inhibits glucagon secretion in a glucose-dependent manner. Several GLP-1 agonists, as well as dipeptidyl peptidase-4 (DPP-4) inhibitors, which block the GLP-1 degrading enzyme DPP-4, have been developed to treat

Table 26.2 On-Target and Off-Target Effects of Established and Novel Drugs Used in the Management of Diabetic Nephropathy

Drug Class	On-Target Parameter	Off-Target Parameters
Antihyperglycemic Drugs		
Metformin	Glucose ↓	VCAM ↓; ICAM ↓
DPP-4 inhibitors	Glucose ↓	Blood pressure ↓; albuminuria ↓
SGLT-2 inhibitors	Glucose ↓	Blood pressure ↓; body weight ↓; uric acid ↓; albuminuria ↓
Antihypertensive Drugs		
RAAS-intervention	Blood pressure ↓	Albuminuria ↓; K$^+$ ↑; Hb ↓; Uric acid ↓ (losartan)
Diuretics	Blood pressure ↓	K$^+$ ↓; uric acid ↑
Lipid-Lowering Drugs		
Statins	LDL cholesterol ↓	C-reactive protein ↓; albuminuria ↓
Fibrates	LDL cholesterol ↓	Uric acid ↓; albuminuria ↓
	Triglycerides ↓	

DPP-4, Dipeptidyl peptidase-4; *Hb,* hemoglobin; *HDL,* high-density lipoprotein; *ICAM,* intercellular cell adhesion molecule; *K$^+$,* potassium; *LDL,* low-density lipoprotein; *SGLT-2,* sodium-glucose cotransporter-2; *VCAM,* vascular cell adhesion molecule.

patients with type 2 diabetes (see Table 26.1). Dipeptidyl peptidase-4 inhibitors seem to exert similar effects on HbA1c as alternative agents, with decreases in the range of 0.5% to 1.0%. However, the pharmacokinetic properties vary among the different agents, which could render a specific agent particularly useful for a certain subpopulation. For example, linagliptin is mainly metabolized and eliminated by the liver, making it particularly useful for patients with lower GFR (see Table 26.1). To date, long-term cardiovascular studies of DPP4 inhibitors have generally reported neutral results. In contrast, liraglutide was recently shown to reduce composite primary outcome three-point MACE by 13% in the LEADER study. For kidney outcomes, a retrospective analysis suggested that linagliptin favorably affects a broad clinical composite outcome and also reduced albuminuria by approximately 20%. Other studies that are ongoing in this field include the MARLINA, CARMELINA, and CARO-LINA trials and include patients who are at high kidney and cardiovascular risk.

Sodium-Glucose Cotransporter-2 Inhibition

The role of the kidney in maintaining glucose homeostasis has been increasingly appreciated in the past few decades. Plasma glucose is filtered in the glomerulus and reclaimed by tubular reabsorption along with sodium ions. This process involves the sodium-glucose cotransporter-2 (SGLT-2) system, which is located in the proximal tubule. The SGLT-2 transporter accounts for the reabsorption of approximately 90% of all filtered glucose, whereas the SGLT-1 transporter, located in the more distal proximal tubule, reabsorbs the remaining 10%. SGLT-2 inhibitors reversibly inhibit the SGLT-2 transporter, leading to enhanced glucose and sodium excretion and, in turn, to reductions in plasma glucose and HbA1c of up to 0.8% (see Table 26.1). As expected based on this mechanism of action, the glycosuric effect and hence HbA1c lowering of SGLT-2 is attenuated in patients with GFR less than 60 mL/min/1.73 m^2.

Beyond effects on glucose, however, SGLT-2 inhibition has more kidney and cardiovascular protective potential than would be predicted based on glucose homeostasis effects.

The effect of SGLT-2 on kidney function may be mediated by the tubuloglomerular feedback mechanism (Fig. 26.5). In brief, overexpression of SGLT-2 in patients with diabetes leads to increased sodium reabsorption at the proximal tubule and decreased distal sodium delivery to the macula densa, which is incorrectly sensed as a reduction in effective circulating volume by the juxtaglomerular apparatus. This leads to downregulation of the tubuloglomerular feedback, vasodilation of the afferent renal arterioles, and hyperfiltration characteristic of diabetes. In the EMPA-REG OUTCOME study, a noninferiority study involving patients with type 2 diabetes and existing cardiovascular disease, the SGLT-2 inhibitor empagliflozin reduced cardiovascular disease events. Adverse kidney outcome, defined as the composite of progression to macroalbuminuria, doubling of creatinine to eGFR less than 45 mL/min/1.73 m^2, dialysis, or death, was reduced by 39%. These marked benefits were observed even though HbA1c was reduced by less than 0.4% over the course of the study, strongly implicating glucose-independent pathways, including effects on renal tubuloglomerular feedback, as well as natriuresis-related effects on plasma volume and blood pressure. Although the renal EMPA-REG OUTCOME data are interesting and could be supportive of SGLT-2 inhibition as a new kidney protective strategy (see caveats at http://www.fda.gov/downloads/AdvisoryCommittees/Committees MeetingMaterials/Drugs/EndocrinologicandMetabolicDrugs AdvisoryCommittee/UCM508422.pdf), it is important to await the results of long-term kidney outcome studies with SGLT-2 inhibitors, including CANVAS-R (NCT01989754) and CRE-DENCE (NCT02065791).

NOVEL BLOOD PRESSURE– AND LIPID-LOWERING AGENTS
Endothelin Antagonists

Endothelin receptor blockers influence hemodynamics and endothelial function and are promising drugs in development for the treatment of diabetic nephropathy. Murine diabetes models demonstrate that endothelin-1 signaling, as occurs in endothelial activation, induces heparanase expression in podocytes, with resultant damage to the glycocalyx and

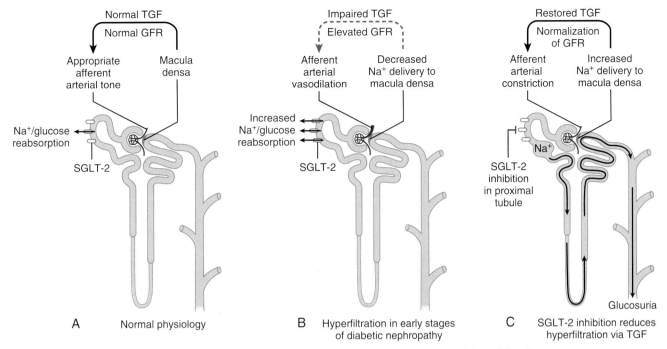

Fig. 26.5 Proposed tubuloglomerular feedback mechanisms in (A) normal physiology, (B) early stages of diabetic nephropathy, and (C) after sodium-glucose cotransporter 2 (SGLT-2) inhibition. GFR, Glomerular filtration rate; TGF, tumor growth factor. (Adapted from Cherney DZI, Perkins BA, Soleymanlou N, et al. The renal hemodynamic effect of sodium-glucose cotransporter 2 inhibition in patients with type 1 diabetes mellitus. Circulation. 2014;129:587–597.)

subsequent albuminuria, and kidney failure. The selective endothelin A receptor antagonist, atrasentan, has been shown to significantly reduce albuminuria and increase glycocalyx thickness in streptozotocin-induced diabetic mice. Furthermore, the restoration of glycocalyx with atrasentan was accompanied by increased renal nitric oxide levels and reduced expression of glomerular heparanase. Unfortunately, the first clinical trial demonstrated an increased incidence of edema and hospitalization for heart failure with avosentan, leading to the premature discontinuation of the trial. Atrasentan, a more specific inhibitor of the endothelin-1A receptor than avosentan, was recently shown to markedly lower albuminuria with fewer side effects. The renoprotective effects of this drug are currently tested in the Study of Diabetic Nephropathy with Atrasentan (SONAR; NCT01858532). This study enrolls only patients who have more than 30% albuminuria lowering in response to atrasentan and excludes patients with side effects related to sodium retention during a run-in phase.

Insulin Resistance and Lifestyle Modification

While insulin resistance is a key feature of type 2 diabetes, the role of insulin resistance in the development and progression of vascular complications in type 1 diabetes is increasingly recognized. A growing body of evidence suggests associations between insulin resistance and hemodynamic changes in the kidney, particularly elevation of glomerular hydrostatic pressure causing increased renal vascular permeability and ultimately glomerular hyperfiltration. Another possible mechanistic pathway linking insulin resistance to diabetic nephropathy is via effects on overall nonesterified fatty acid

exposure and lipotoxicity, leading to the development of vascular disease.

Despite the BARI-2D study showing no benefit of insulin sensitizing strategies compared with insulin therapy on diabetic nephropathy in older adults with type 2 diabetes and coronary artery disease, it is plausible that the long-standing vascular injury in older adults with type 2 diabetes, hypertension, and dyslipidemia may not be responsive to changes in insulin sensitivity. Early intervention before the establishment of vascular lesions may result in significant delay of clinical pathology, as suggested by the concept of "metabolic memory" in the DCCT-EDIC study. Also, clinical cardiovascular disease typically does not manifest until older ages; for example, it took 17 years of follow-up for the benefits of intensive management to manifest in DCCT. Improvements in outcomes due to adjunctive therapy in the era of intensive glycemic control may also be subtler, and long-term studies beginning in childhood or adolescence are lacking. Ongoing clinical trials investigating the effects of improving insulin sensitivity on vascular complications in type 1 diabetes include the REducing With MetfOrmin Vascular Adverse Lesions in Type 1 Diabetes (REMOVAL, NCT01483560), the Effects of Metformin on Cardiovascular Function in Adolescents With Type 1 Diabetes (EMERALD, NCT01808690), the Effect of Metformin on Vascular and Mitochondrial Function in Type 1 Diabetes (MeT1, NCT01813929), and Metformin Therapy for Overweight Adolescents with Type 1 Diabetes (NCT01881828) studies.

Dietary sodium restriction enhances the blood pressure– and albuminuria-lowering effects of ACE inhibitors and ARBs, with both RENAAL and IDNT showing that the effects of

ARBs on hard kidney and cardiovascular outcomes in patients with type 2 diabetes are greater in patients with moderately low dietary sodium intake. Dietary protein restriction has been shown in a meta-analysis of nine randomized controlled trials (seven in patients with type 1 diabetes and three in patients with type 2 diabetes) to have a small, statistically nonsignificant, long-term beneficial effect in slowing the rate of decline in GFR without demonstrable evidence of malnutrition. Currently, the ADA recommends 0.8 g/kg/day of protein restriction for patients with diabetes having increased albuminuria, which is a manageable and safe recommendation for most patients with challenging dietary prescriptions related to their diabetes and CKD. Dietary counseling by a nutritionist may be useful to assist CKD patients in safely implementing dietary changes (Chapter 54).

NOVEL TARGETS

Despite recent success with agents such as GLP-1 receptor agonists and SGLT-2 inhibitors, other therapeutic areas have been less successful. For example, raising hemoglobin targets with darbepoetin-α (via the Trial to Reduce Cardiovascular Events with Aranesp Therapy) and the use of some antiinflammatory agents such as bardoxolone methyl (Bardoxolone Methyl Evaluation in Patients with Chronic Kidney Disease and Type 2 Diabetes [BEACON]) failed to show kidney protective effects. Nevertheless, other therapeutic areas have shown promising preliminary study results and merit further consideration, including agents that target inflammation and those that influence the vitamin D receptor.

Pentoxifylline

In the past years, increasing evidence has indicated an important role for underlying, low-grade inflammatory processes in the pathogenesis of diabetic nephropathy. Consequently, research in antiinflammatory strategies may open a therapeutic window to halt the progression of disease. Pentoxifylline is a methylxanthine phosphodiesterase inhibitor with favorable antiinflammatory effects and immunoregulatory properties. Despite this theoretic benefit, most studies using this agent were until recently poorly reported, small, and methodologically flawed. The Pentoxifylline for Renoprotection in Diabetic Nephropathy study (PREDIAN), which examined the effect of pentoxifylline on eGFR decline and albuminuria over 2 years, reported a greater preservation of kidney function and a small reduction in urinary albumin excretion. The modest impact of pentoxifylline has not, to date, translated into clinical practice.

Monocyte Chemoattractant Protein-1 Inhibitors

An increasing body of evidence demonstrates that monocyte chemoattractant protein-1 (MCP-1), a potent cytokine, plays an important role in initiating and sustaining chronic inflammation in the kidney. MCP-1, secreted in response to high glucose concentrations, attracts blood monocytes and macrophages and facilitates inflammation. A prospective randomized placebo-controlled study showed that inhibition of MCP-1 synthesis further reduced albuminuria when used in addition to ACE inhibitor or ARB therapy in subjects who had macroalbuminuria, although there was no significant effect in individuals with lower levels of albuminuria. To our knowledge, there are no hard kidney outcome trials ongoing.

Uric Acid Lowering

A large body of epidemiologic and clinical evidence suggests that higher uric acid (UA) levels are associated with metabolic abnormalities, cardiovascular disease, loss of GFR, and risk of developing albuminuria. Even within the normal range, higher UA appears to exert deleterious effects on blood pressure and kidney function. Experimental work suggests that pharmacologic lowering of UA, with xanthine oxidase inhibitors like allopurinol and febuxostat, blocks the RAAS, suppresses inflammation, slows progression of kidney disease, and promotes kidney and cardiovascular protection in patients with CKD and diabetes. Although observational and prospective studies consistently suggest that UA may play a role in the pathogenesis of diabetic nephropathy, causal inferences cannot yet be made with confidence, and UA may simply represent a biomarker of kidney function. Thus adequately powered, placebo-controlled studies are needed to determine if lowering plasma UA protects the kidney from injury in patients with diabetic nephropathy. The effect of allopurinol on the reduction GFR loss among patients with type 1 diabetes over a 3-year follow-up period is being examined as part of the NIH-funded *P*rotecting *E*arly *R*enal Function *L*oss or "PERL" study (NCT02017171).

Vitamin D Receptor Activation

Emerging data suggest an important role for the vitamin D axis in kidney and cardiovascular health. The vitamin D receptor is expressed in numerous tissues, and small studies have shown that activators of this receptor may inhibit the RAAS by suppressing renin synthesis, causing a reduction in albuminuria and inflammatory markers. The Vitamin D Receptor Activator for Albuminuria Lowering (VITAL) study, designed to investigate the antialbuminuric effect of the vitamin D receptor activator paricalcitol, showed that 24 weeks of treatment with paricalcitol at 2 μg/day caused a significant fall in albuminuria over time and was well tolerated.

Novel Biomarkers

Diabetic nephropathy clinically presents as albuminuria and, once significant renal parenchymal damage has already occurred, GFR decline. Because of the presence of clinically silent disease over a long period of time, the identification of novel biomarkers of diabetic nephropathy may improve the ability of clinicians to target high-risk patients with earlier therapies prior to the development of albuminuria or kidney function decline. Recently, significant progress was achieved in developing a classifier based on 273 urinary peptides (CKD273), which likely reflects ECM turnover based on collagen peptide fragments. CKD273 is highly correlated with urine ACR and eGFR and has been validated in a number of trials for early detection of diabetic nephropathy in patients with type 1 and type 2 diabetes. Soluble tumor necrosis factor α receptors (TNFRs) are another potential biomarker at an early stage of development for diabetic nephropathy. TNFRs were shown to predict progression of CKD in patients with type 1 diabetes with normal kidney function at baseline and also to predict progression to kidney failure in proteinuric and nonproteinuric patients with type 2 diabetes. Larger multicenter trials are needed to examine promising biomarkers prior to the transition into a clinical practice.

CONCLUSION

Diabetic nephropathy is a leading cause of morbidity and mortality in people with type 1 and type 2 diabetes (T2D). The 2015 US Renal Data System reported that DKD accounted for almost half of all cases of ESRD. Despite the successful use of glycemic, lipid, and blood pressure control, including ACE inhibitor and ARB therapy, kidney risk in patients with diabetes remains very high, leaving the growing population with diabetes with a clear unmet need. Clinical trials in diabetic nephropathy have yielded disappointing results for the past 2 decades. The underlying explanation for this trend can be explained partly by the lack of valid early markers to identify and monitor high-risk individuals and the lack of interventions at an early stage of disease when benefit is most likely to be achieved. As outlined in this chapter, various promising treatment options are in development that may offer additional renoprotection and have the potential to reduce the high morbidity and mortality rates typically seen in patients with diabetes. In addition to results from trials examining the effects of novel interventions on surrogate endpoints, the nephrology community awaits the final results of the CANVAS (canagliflozin), SONAR (atrasentan), and CREDENCE (canagliflozin) studies.

KEY BIBLIOGRAPHY

Bakris GL, Agarwal R, Chan JC, et al. Effect of finerenone on albuminuria in patients with diabetic nephropathy: a randomized clinical trial. *JAMA.* 2015;314:884-894.

Barbosa J, Steffes MW, Sutherland DE, et al. Effect of glycemic control on early diabetic renal lesions: a 5-year randomized controlled clinical trial of insulin-dependent diabetic kidney transplant recipients. *JAMA.* 1994;272:600-606.

Bjornstad P, Snell-Bergeon JK, Rewers M, et al. Early diabetic nephropathy: a complication of reduced insulin sensitivity in type 1 diabetes. *Diabetes Care.* 2013;36:3678-3683.

Cherney DZ, Perkins BA, Soleymanlou N, et al. The renal hemodynamic effect of SGLT2 inhibition in patients with type 1 diabetes. *Circulation.* 2014;129:587-597.

Cho A, Noh JW, Kim JK, et al. Prevalence and prognosis of hypoglycemia in patients receiving maintenance dialysis. *Intern Med J.* 2016;46:1380-1385.

Cushman WC, Evans GW, Byington RP, et al. Effects of intensive blood-pressure control in type 2 diabetes mellitus. *N Engl J Med.* 2010;362:1575-1585.

de Boer IH, Rue TC, Cleary PA, et al. Long-term renal outcomes of patients with type 1 diabetes mellitus and microalbuminuria: an analysis of the Diabetes Control and Complications Trial/Epidemiology of diabetes interventions and complications cohort. *Arch Intern Med.* 2011;171:412-420.

de Boer IH, Sun W, Cleary PA, et al. Intensive diabetes therapy and glomerular filtration rate in type 1 diabetes. *N Engl J Med.* 2011;365:2366-2376.

de Zeeuw D, Agarwal R, Amdahl M, et al. Selective vitamin D receptor activation with paricalcitol for reduction of albuminuria in patients with type 2 diabetes (VITAL study): a randomised controlled trial. *Lancet.* 2010;376:1543-1551.

de Zeeuw D, Anzalone D, Cain V, et al. Renal effects of atorvastatin and rosuvastatin in patients with diabetes who have progressive renal disease (PLANET I): a randomized clinical trial. *Lancet Diabetes Endocrinol.* 2015;3:181-190.

Garsen M, Lenoir O, Rops AL, et al. Endothelin-1 induces proteinuria by heparanase-mediated disruption of the glomerular glycocalyx. *J Am Soc Nephrol.* 2016;27:3545-3551.

Gerstein HC, Miller ME, Byington RP, et al. Effects of intensive glucose lowering in type 2 diabetes. *N Engl J Med.* 2008;358:2545-2559.

Lewis EJ, Hunsicker LG, Clarke WR, et al. Renoprotective effect of the angiotensin-receptor antagonist irbesartan in patients with nephropathy due to type 2 diabetes. *N Engl J Med.* 2001;345:851-860.

Maahs DM, Caramori L, Cherney DZ, et al. Uric acid lowering to prevent kidney function loss in diabetes: the preventing early renal function loss (PERL) allopurinol study. *Curr Diab Rep.* 2013;13:550-559.

Nathan DM, Cleary PA, Backlund JY, et al. Intensive diabetes treatment and cardiovascular disease in patients with type 1 diabetes. *N Engl J Med.* 2005;353:2643-2653.

Parving HH, Lehnert H, Brochner-Mortensen J, et al. The effect of irbesartan on the development of diabetic nephropathy in patients with type 2 diabetes. *N Engl J Med.* 2001;345:870-878.

Patel A, MacMahon S, Chalmers J, et al. Intensive blood glucose control and vascular outcomes in patients with type 2 diabetes. *N Engl J Med.* 2008;358:2560-2572.

Saran R, Li Y, Robinson B, et al. US Renal Data System 2015 Annual Data Report: epidemiology of kidney disease in the United States. *Am J Kidney Dis.* 2016;67:Svii, S1-S305.

The Diabetes Control and Complications Trial Research Group. The effect of intensive treatment of diabetes on the development and progression of long-term complications in insulin-dependent diabetes mellitus. *N Engl J Med.* 1993;329:977-986.

TODAY Study Group. Rapid rise in hypertension and nephropathy in youth with type 2 diabetes: the TODAY clinical trial. *Diabetes Care.* 2013;36:1735-1741.

Zinman B, Wanner C, Lachin JM, et al. Empagliflozin, cardiovascular outcomes, and mortality in type 2 diabetes. *N Engl J Med.* 2015;373:2117-2128.

Full bibliography can be found on www.expertconsult.com.

27 The Kidney in Malignancy

Kevin W. Finkel; Jaya Kala

Onco-nephrology is a growing field within nephrology, with many malignancies and their treatments affecting the kidneys and kidney disease impacting the management of many malignancies. Although patients with malignancy can develop kidney diseases similar to other acutely and chronically ill patients, they are also at risk for unique kidney syndromes because of either the cancer itself or its treatment. Understanding these unique disorders is a prerequisite to providing outstanding clinical care. In addition, because patient survival has improved owing to advances in cancer treatment, chronic kidney disease (CKD) prevalence has also increased. Providing expert advice on the impact of CKD on patient survival; drug response, toxicity, and clearance; and clinical study eligibility are important considerations in onco-nephrology. Finally, patients with advanced malignancy can develop severe acute kidney injury (AKI) with multiple organ dysfunction syndrome. In these cases, the nephrologist is an essential partner in discussions about end-of-life issues and the appropriateness of initiating kidney replacement therapies.

This chapter provides an overview of kidney diseases either caused by cancer or its treatment, including AKI, CKD, electrolyte abnormalities, glomerular diseases, tumor lysis syndrome (TLS), and anticancer drug nephrotoxicity. Multiple myeloma, amyloidosis, and other dysproteinemias are discussed in Chapter 28.

ACUTE KIDNEY INJURY

In hospitalized cancer patients, AKI is associated with increased morbidity, mortality, length of stay, and costs. In a northern Denmark study with a 1.2 million population in the catchment area, incident cancer was found in 44,116 patients. The 1-year and 5-year risk of AKI in this population was 17.5% and 27.5%, respectively. The incidence of AKI was highest for kidney cancer (44%), multiple myeloma (33%), liver cancer (32%), and acute leukemia (28%).

Among critically ill patients, 20% have underlying malignancy with overall prognosis strongly dependent on the admitting diagnosis and the type of cancer. Patients with solid tumors have lower mortality (56%) than those with hematologic malignancies (67%). In the Sepsis Occurrence in Critically Ill Patients (SOAP) study, in the subset of patients with more than three failing organs, over 75% of patients with cancer died; this compares to 50% of those without cancer. In a retrospective analysis of 1009 critically ill patients with hematologic malignancies, Darmon and colleagues reported an AKI incidence of 66.5%. After adjustment, factors associated with AKI development were older age, history of

hypertension, TLS, multiple myeloma, exposure to nephrotoxins, and sequential organ failure assessment (SOFA) score.

The etiology of AKI in cancer patients is quite varied and is often multifactorial. Causes vary from those common to all hospitalized patients such as exposure to various nephrotoxins (antibiotics and radiocontrast), sepsis, and volume depletion, and factors unique to the underlying malignancy or its treatment. Table 27.1 provides a comprehensive list of causes of AKI.

CHEMOTHERAPEUTIC AGENTS

Chemotherapeutic agents can cause a variety of kidney manifestations including AKI, tubulointerstitial nephritis (TIN), acid-base and electrolyte disturbances, hypertension, proteinuria/nephrotic syndrome, and thrombotic microangiopathy (TMA). One challenge for clinicians is the vast array of new agents with unique mechanisms of action; given potentially unknown adverse kidney effects, a great degree of vigilance is needed.

The adverse kidney effects of chemotherapy can be classified by the primary site of injury. For example, these include injury to the endothelium (hypertension and TMA), visceral podocyte (proteinuria and nephrotic syndrome), renal tubules (AKI), and tubulointerstitium (renal tubular acidosis, Fanconi syndrome, and electrolyte wasting). A list of anticancer agents and their known associated kidney effects are found in Table 27.2. The nephrotoxic effects of specific anticancer drugs are reviewed in Chapter 35.

TUMOR LYSIS SYNDROME

TLS is defined by laboratory (any two of hyperuricemia, hyperphosphatemia, hypocalcemia, and hyperkalemia) and clinical (one of three among AKI, seizures, arrhythmias, and death) criteria. TLS complicated by AKI often is a dramatic presentation. It is characterized by the development of hyperphosphatemia, hypocalcemia, hyperuricemia, and hyperkalemia of varying severity. TLS can occur spontaneously during the rapid growth phase of malignancies, such as bulky lymphoblastomas and Burkitt and non-Burkitt lymphomas that have extremely rapid cell turnover rates, or when cytotoxic chemotherapy induces lysis of malignant cells in patients with large tumor burdens.

The pathophysiology of AKI associated with TLS classically is attributed to two main factors: preexisting volume depletion and the precipitation of uric acid and calcium phosphate

Table 27.1   Causes of Acute Kidney Injury in Malignancy

Prerenal	Sepsis
	Volume depletion (vomiting, diarrhea, mucositis)
	Sinusoidal occlusion syndrome
	Capillary leak (interleukin-2)
	Hypercalcemia (multifactorial including nephrogenic diabetes insipidus)
Intrinsic kidney	Acute tubular necrosis
	• ischemic
	• nephrotoxic
	Tubulointerstitial nephritis
	• tumor lysis syndrome
	• infection (BK virus)
	• pyelonephritis
	• infiltration (lymphoma and leukemia)
	• lysozymuria
	Vascular/thrombotic microangiopathy
	• underlying malignancy (gastric cancer)
	• drug induced (mitomycin C, anti-VEGF)
	• bone marrow transplantation
	• radiation
Postkidney/ obstruction	Intrarenal
	• urate
	• methotrexate
	• acyclovir
	Extrarenal
	• retroperitoneal fibrosis
	• lymphadenopathy
	• direct invasion

VEGF, Vascular endothelial growth factor.

Table 27.2   Chemotherapy and Kidney Manifestations

Chemotherapy and Miscellaneous	Kidney Effects
Cisplatin	Acute kidney injury
	Fanconi syndrome
	Nephrogenic diabetes insipidus
	Salt-wasting nephropathy
	Magnesium wasting
Ifosfamide	Acute kidney injury
	Fanconi syndrome
	Nephrogenic diabetes insipidus
Methotrexate	Acute kidney injury (crystalline nephropathy)
Pamidronate	Acute kidney injury
	Collapsing focal segmental glomerulosclerosis
Calcineurin inhibitors	Acute kidney injury
	Thrombotic microangiopathy
	Hypertension
	Hyperkalemia
Biologic Agents	
Interferon-α	Acute kidney injury
	Minimal change disease
	Focal segmental glomerulosclerosis
Interleukin-2	Acute kidney injury (prerenal)
	Capillary leak syndrome
Targeted Therapies	
Antivascular endothelial growth factor (e.g., bevacizumab, sorafenib)	Acute kidney injury
	Thrombotic microangiopathy
	Hypertension
	Proteinuria
Epidermal growth factor blockade (e.g., cetuximab, erlotinib)	Renal magnesium wasting
Check point inhibitors (e.g., nivolumab, ipilimumab)	Acute tubulointerstitial nephritis

complexes in the renal tubules and tubulointerstitium. There is also a major contribution from a "cytokine release syndrome" associated with tumor cell lysis. This leads to kidney underperfusion and AKI. Volume depletion is multifactorial and may reflect anorexia, nausea and vomiting from the malignancy or its treatment, and increased insensible losses from fever or tachypnea.

Hyperuricemia may develop despite allopurinol prophylaxis in patients with spontaneous TLS or after therapy in very chemosensitive malignancies. Excess serum uric acid is filtered into the tubular space. In general, uric acid is nearly completely ionized at physiologic pH, but it becomes progressively more insoluble in the acidic environment of the renal tubules. Precipitation of uric acid causes intratubular obstruction, while hyperuricemia may also lead to increased renal vascular resistance and decreased glomerular filtration rate (GFR). In addition, a granulomatous reaction to intraluminal uric acid crystals and necrosis of tubular epithelium may occur, resulting in inflammation and further kidney injury. Hyperphosphatemia and hypocalcemia also occur in TLS. In patients who develop AKI but do not develop hyperuricemia, kidney injury has been attributed to metastatic intrarenal calcification or acute nephrocalcinosis. Tumor lysis with release of inorganic phosphate may promote both kidney

and systemic metastatic calcification, which is complicated by acute hypocalcemia.

Optimal management of TLS can reduce the risk of AKI and of development of symptomatic electrolyte abnormalities. Key management components include ensuring a high urine output with intravenous fluids, reducing uric acid levels, and controlling serum phosphate levels. It is recommended that urine output be maintained at a rate of 200 mL/hour by infusion of isotonic crystalloid solutions. In the absence of significant hypervolemia, use of loop diuretics should be avoided because they acidify the urine and can lead to volume depletion. A consensus statement on the treatment of TLS was published by the American Society of Clinical Oncology in 2008. In patients at low risk to develop TLS, allopurinol is administered to inhibit uric acid formation. Through its metabolite oxypurinol, allopurinol inhibits xanthine oxidase and thereby blocks the conversion of hypoxanthine and xanthine to uric acid. During massive tumor lysis, excessive

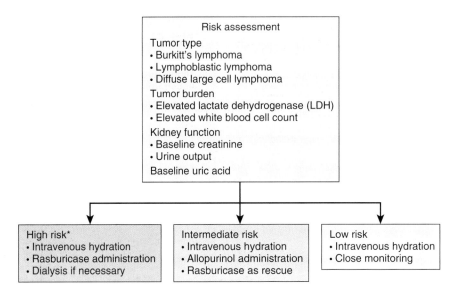

*High-risk features include: Bulky lymphadenopathy, LDH > 2x normal, White blood cell count > 25 K/mm³, Creatinine > 1.4 mg/dL, Uric acid > 7.5 mg/dL

Fig. 27.1 Management of tumor lysis syndrome.

uric acid production with increased uric acid excretion by the kidneys may occur despite allopurinol administration, making intravenous hydration necessary to prevent AKI. Because allopurinol and its metabolites are excreted by the kidneys, the starting dose should be lower in those with low GFR. Other limitations to allopurinol use include hypersensitivity reaction, drug interactions, and delayed time to lowering uric acid levels.

In the past, because uric acid is very soluble at physiologic pH, sodium bicarbonate was often added to intravenous fluids to achieve a urinary pH greater than 6.5. However, this therapy is no longer recommended for several reasons. First, systemic alkalosis from alkali administration can aggravate hypocalcemia, resulting in tetany and seizures. Second, an alkaline urine pH markedly decreases the urinary solubility of calcium phosphate, thereby promoting development of acute nephrocalcinosis from intratubular calcium-phosphate crystals.

Patients at high risk for TLS can be treated with rasburicase (recombinant urate oxidase). Risk factors for TLS include bulky lymphadenopathy, elevated lactate dehydrogenase (LDH) (>2× normal), increased white blood cell count (>25,000/mm³), baseline creatinine greater than 1.4 mg/dL, and baseline uric acid greater than 7.5 mg/dL. Rasburicase converts uric acid to water-soluble allantoin, thereby decreasing serum uric acid levels and urinary uric acid excretion. Importantly, use of rasburicase obviates the need for urinary alkalinization and its complications. However, high urine flow rates achieved with normal saline are important given the probability of preexisting volume depletion and its consequences. Rasburicase treatment should be avoided in patients with glucose-6-phosphate dehydrogenase deficiency, because hydrogen peroxide, a breakdown product of uric acid, can cause methemoglobinemia and, in severe cases, hemolytic anemia. Management of TLS is outlined in Fig. 27.1.

THROMBOTIC MICROANGIOPATHY

TMA is a disorder of multiple etiologies that manifests as nonimmune (microangiopathic) hemolytic anemia with thrombocytopenia and other organ dysfunction including AKI. In addition to anemia and thrombocytopenia, laboratory findings include elevated indirect bilirubin and LDH levels, depressed serum haptoglobin values, and schistocytes on peripheral blood smear. The characteristic kidney lesion consists of vessel wall thickening in capillaries and arterioles, with swelling and detachment of endothelial cells from the basement membranes and accumulation of subendothelial fluffy material. In the past, TMA was classified as thrombotic thrombocytopenia purpura (TTP) based on a pentad of clinical findings, diarrhea-associated (shiga-toxin) hemolytic uremic syndrome (HUS), HUS associated with an underlying condition (cancer, malignant hypertension, pregnancy), or atypical HUS. However, this classification is an oversimplification, as it is nearly impossible to differentiate these disorders based on phenotypic presentation. As such, the best approach uses classification based on pathophysiology, which ultimately will inform therapy. TTP is generally characterized by decreased enzymatic activity of the metalloprotease ADAMTS13 (a disintegrin and metalloproteinase with thrombospondin type 1 motif, member 13) and responds to therapeutic plasma exchange (TPE) whereas atypical-HUS is due to dysregulated complement activity, which responds to complement inhibition but not TPE. It is likely that there is overlap among these similar entities.

In cancer patients, malignancy itself, chemotherapy, radiation therapy, immunosuppressive agents, and stem cell transplantation all can induce endothelial injury leading to TMA and AKI. TMA has been most commonly associated with gastric carcinoma, which accounts for more than half of cases, followed by breast and lung cancer. Chemotherapeutic agents are also associated with the development of TMA. Mitomycin C is the classic drug associated with TMA with an incidence as high as 10%. Bleomycin, cisplatin, and 5-fluorouracil are less frequently reported as a cause. Gemcitabine, a nucleoside analog, and the antivascular endothelial growth factor (VEGF) agents, such as bevacizumab and sunitinib, are associated with TMA. Gemcitabine likely acts through direct, toxic endothelial injury, while the anti-VEGF agents deprive endothelial cells of VEGF, which is required to maintain endothelial health.

Treatment of AKI and TMA in cancer patients, regardless of etiology, is primarily supportive, with initiation of dialysis when indicated. Any offending agent associated with TMA should be discontinued. The role of plasma exchange is controversial for TMA unrelated to ADAMTS13 deficiency because of a lack of trial data. If stopping the culprit drug or treating the underlying cause for TMA is unsuccessful and the patient continues to deteriorate, plasma exchange should be considered; however, it is mandatory that ADAMTS13 activity be measured. If there is a delay in ascertaining the ADAMTS13 activity, plasma exchange should be started empirically. A low activity level (<5%) confirms the diagnosis of TTP, and plasma exchange should continue. If activity level is normal and TTP is excluded as a diagnosis, plasma exchange can be discontinued. If the diagnosis of atypical-HUS is likely, strong consideration should be given to administering eculizumab. This drug is a humanized monoclonal antibody that inhibits terminal complement activation by binding to complement C5 and preventing formation of the terminal membrane attack complex. The overall management of TMA is outlined in Fig. 27.2.

HEMATOPOIETIC STEM CELL TRANSPLANTATION

Hematopoietic stem cell transplantation (HSCT) can cause both AKI and CKD. The incidence of AKI is approximately 10% in autologous transplants and approximately 50% (with reduced-intensity conditioning) to 73% (with high intensity conditioning) in those who receive allogeneic transplant. Causes of AKI include acute graft-versus-host disease (GVHD), sinusoidal obstruction syndrome (SOS), TMA, use of calcineurin inhibitors, viral infections, and sepsis.

The incidence of CKD following HSCT varies from 7% to 48% and is clinically manifest anywhere from 6 months to 10 years after transplant. Risk factors for CKD are prior AKI, acute or chronic GVHD, age over 45 years at the time of transplant, hypertension, calcineurin inhibitor therapy, and exposure to total body irradiation (TBI). Kidney biopsy is generally required to diagnose the cause of CKD.

SINUSOIDAL OBSTRUCTION SYNDROME

SOS, formerly referred to as venoocclusive disease of the liver, is a unique form of AKI that occurs between 10 and 21 days after HSCT. It is characterized by tender hepatomegaly, fluid retention with ascites formation, and jaundice. It results from fibrous narrowing of small hepatic venules and sinusoids triggered by the pretransplant cytoreductive regimen and is more common after allogeneic than autologous HSCT. The development of SOS is most commonly associated with pretreatment with cyclophosphamide, busulfan, and/or TBI.

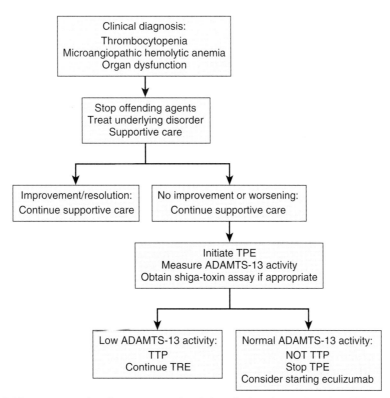

Fig. 27.2 Management of malignancy-associated thrombotic microangiopathy. *TPE*, Therapeutic plasma exchange; *TTP*, thrombotic thrombocytopenic purpura.

Table 27.3   Characteristics of Cancer-Associated Membranous Nephropathy

Age >65 year
Smoking history
Absence of antiphospholipase A2 receptor antibody
Kidney biopsy findings:
    Presence of high IgG1 and IgG2 subtype deposits
    Less than eight inflammatory cells per glomerulus observed
        in kidney biopsy specimen
Regression of glomerular lesions and proteinuria upon
    remission of cancer
No other obvious cause

IgG, Immunoglobulin G.

Table 27.4   Paraneoplastic Glomerulonephritis

Membranous Glomerulopathy
- Breast
- Colon
- Lung
- Prostate
- Graft-versus-host disease
- Others (case reports)

Minimal Change Disease
- Hodgkin lymphoma
- Non-Hodgkin lymphoma
- Graft-versus-host disease
- Others (case reports)

Case Reports
- Rapidly progressive glomerulonephritis
- Immunoglobulin A nephritis
- Focal segmental glomerulonephritis
- Membranoproliferative glomerulonephritis

AKI typically behaves similarly to hepatorenal syndrome with hyperdynamic vital signs, hyponatremia, oliguria, and low urinary sodium concentration. Urinalysis shows minimal proteinuria, and urine sediment examination reveals bile-stained renal tubular cells and granular casts possibly due to the toxicity of bile salts in the urine. Patients are usually resistant to diuretics, and spontaneous recovery is quite rare. Risk factors for the development of AKI include edema formation, hyperbilirubinemia, use of amphotericin B, vancomycin, or acyclovir, and higher pretransplant serum creatinine. AKI adversely affects survival as seen in patients who require dialysis, where the mortality rate approaches 80%. Small trials using infusions of prostaglandin E, pentoxifylline, or low-dose heparin to prevent the development of SOS have been promising. Smaller trials with defibrotide, an antithrombotic and fibrinolytic agent, have shown benefit in patients with SOS; however, use of these agents is not commonplace because of the associated risk of bleeding.

GLOMERULAR DISEASES AND PARANEOPLASTIC SYNDROMES

Several solid and hematologic malignancies are associated with glomerular diseases, thought to be the result of abnormal tumor cell products. As discussed in Chapter 19, membranous nephropathy (MN) is associated with solid malignancies, including lung and gastric tumors. Because treatment may differ, with malignancy-associated MN often responding to treatment of the malignancy, it is essential to differentiate between primary MN and MN associated with solid tumors. Table 27.3 illustrates characteristics associated with paraneoplastic MN.

Minimal change disease (MCD) is classically associated with Hodgkin lymphoma. It usually occurs at the time the malignancy is diagnosed and is associated with high rate of steroid and cyclosporine resistance. The most common glomerular disease seen with thymoma is also MCD. Focal segmental glomerulosclerosis is associated with solid malignancies, kidney cancer, and thymoma. Membranoproliferative glomerulonephritis (MPGN) is associated with lung, kidney, and stomach cancers, while immunoglobulin A nephropathy has been most frequently associated with kidney cell cancer and is also associated with T-cell lymphoma.

Glomerular lesions associated with malignancy are noted in Table 27.4.

LYMPHOMA AND LEUKEMIA

Although a variety of cancers can metastasize to the kidneys and invade the parenchyma, the most common to do so are lymphomas and leukemias. The true incidence of kidney involvement is unknown because kidney infiltration may not manifest with significantly abnormal kidney function. On autopsy, lymphomatous kidney infiltration is seen in approximately 30% of cases.

LYMPHOMA

Kidney involvement in lymphoma is often clinically silent such that patients present with slowly progressive CKD often attributed to other etiologies. Therefore a high index of suspicion is needed to make a diagnosis. Patients may present with AKI, but this is rare and is most commonly seen in highly malignant and disseminated disease. Other presentations include both nephrotic and nonnephrotic range proteinuria due to a variety of glomerular lesions including pauci-immune crescentic glomerulonephritis. Patients may also present with flank pain and hematuria, likely due to interstitial infiltration with lymphoma causing renal capsule distention and hemorrhage of small capillaries.

Kidney involvement in lymphoma may be suspected from clinical features and imaging studies. Kidney imaging, including with ultrasound or computed tomography, may reveal diffusely enlarged kidneys, multiple focal lesions, or retroperitoneal involvement with hydronephrosis. The following criteria support the diagnosis of kidney disease due to lymphomatous infiltration: (1) kidney enlargement without obstruction; (2) absence of other causes of kidney disease; and (3) rapid improvement of kidney function after radiotherapy or systemic chemotherapy. Kidney biopsy is often required to confirm the diagnosis, especially in patients with kidney-limited lymphoma.

LEUKEMIA

Leukemic cells can infiltrate any organ, and the kidneys are the most frequent extramedullary site of infiltration, with autopsy studies revealing that 60% to 90% of patients with leukemia have kidney involvement. As with lymphoma, leukemic infiltration of the kidneys is often an indolent and clinically silent aspect of leukemia. Most often, leukemic kidney infiltration is incidentally noted after autopsy or by detection of kidney enlargement on imaging often performed for other indications. Although relatively uncommon, many cases of AKI attributable to leukemic infiltration have been described. Patients may also experience hematuria or proteinuria. Occasionally, kidney enlargement is accompanied by flank pain or fullness. Patients with significantly elevated white blood cell counts, especially those with leukemic blasts, can develop AKI from intrarenal leukostasis. Treatment is directed at the type of leukemia diagnosed. Although some patients do not recover, kidney function improves in the majority of cases as the leukemia responds to systemic treatment.

RADIATION-ASSOCIATED KIDNEY INJURY

Radiation-associated kidney injury has a long latency period. With the exception of patients who undergo HSCT, there is no acute form that presents during or shortly after radiation therapy. Evidence of kidney dysfunction does not occur until at least 6 months following radiation, and it may take several years for progression to clinically apparent CKD.

Common symptoms of radiation-associated kidney injury include edema formation, fluid retention, increased weight, and malaise. In addition, symptoms can overlap with those of other kidney diseases such as malignant hypertension (headaches, vomiting, and blurry vision) and other end-organ damage (dyspnea and lethargy). It is important to recognize that these symptoms do not differentiate radiation nephropathy from many other causes of kidney failure. The complete blood count may reveal a microangiopathic hemolytic anemia with schistocytes on the peripheral smear. Thrombocytopenia may also be present. Proteinuria often is present although seldom reaches nephrotic range, while urine sediment examination reveals granular casts and red blood cells. As discussed, these clinical findings do not develop until 6 months or more after irradiation and may increase in severity as time progresses and symptoms begin to become more clinically evident.

The diagnosis of radiation nephropathy is made clinically by identifying a syndrome of progressive CKD in a cancer patient who received radiation to the total body, spine, abdomen, or pelvis. A thorough history and physical examination should be performed, and the clinician should have a strong index of suspicion in such patients. A kidney biopsy does not necessarily need to be performed. Many of the histopathologic findings in radiation nephropathy are nonspecific and common to a large host of other causes of CKD; however, kidney biopsy may demonstrate TMA. Blockade of the renin-angiotensin-aldosterone system (RAAS) is also useful once radiation-induced injury has developed, with several studies showing benefits associated with angiotensin-converting enzyme (ACE) inhibitors on the overall course of the disease.

ELECTROLYTE ABNORMALITIES

HYPONATREMIA

Hyponatremia is the most common electrolyte disorder in hospitalized patients with cancer. It is associated with higher mortality rates, longer hospital stays, and higher health care costs. In one report, the hazard ratio for 90-day mortality was 2.04 for patients with mild hyponatremia, 4.74 for moderate hyponatremia, and 3.46 for severe hyponatremia. The differential diagnosis for and evaluation and management of hyponatremia are similar to that in patients without malignancy (see Chapter 7).

The most common etiology of hyponatremia is the syndrome of inappropriate antidiuretic hormone (SIADH). SIADH is particularly common in individuals with small-cell lung cancer, with an estimated incidence of 10% to 15%. Antineoplastic drugs such as cyclophosphamide, vinblastine, and vincristine also cause SIADH. Cisplatin-associated hyponatremia is due to both a salt-wasting nephropathy and SIADH. Other factors contributing to hyponatremia in cancer patients are pain, nausea and vomiting, edema formation with third spacing (liver and heart failure), adrenal insufficiency, and hypotonic intravenous fluid administration. Therapy is determined by the cause and the severity of hyponatremia. In patients with SIADH, fluid restriction is difficult, especially during administration of chemotherapy when increased hydration is often required. Hypertonic saline acutely and salt tablets chronically may be used, with indications similar to the treatment of hyponatremia in the noncancer population. Use of vasopressin receptor antagonists such as tolvaptan has been studied in a small, randomized controlled trial treating hyponatremia in cancer patients, with 14 days of tolvaptan therapy correcting hyponatremia in 94% of patients compared with only 8% in the placebo group.

HYPERKALEMIA

Hyperkalemia in cancer patients is most commonly seen with AKI, TLS, or obstructive nephropathy (hyperkalemic or type 4 renal tubular acidosis). More rarely elevated plasma potassium levels are due to pseudohyperkalemia as a result of marked leukocytosis or thrombocytosis. Transport of blood specimens to the laboratory in an icebox to prevent cell lysis or using plasma samples for correct potassium measurements is helpful in this circumstance. Less common causes of hyperkalemia in these patients include adrenal insufficiency due to metastatic disease and exposure to ketoconazole, calcineurin inhibitors, nonsteroidal antiinflammatory agents, trimethoprim, or heparin.

HYPOKALEMIA

Hypokalemia is a common electrolyte abnormality seen in cancer patients. This disorder may result from poor oral intake, vomiting, diarrhea, ureteral diversions, diuretic use, hypercalcemia (kaliuretic effect), hypomagnesemia, various drugs, or mineralocorticoid excess. Medications such as cisplatin, ifosfamide, amphotericin B, and aminoglycosides cause hypokalemia via either proximal tubular damage or both gastrointestinal and kidney losses. Ectopic release of adrenocorticotropic hormone (ACTH) is an uncommon cause of hypokalemia. A significant association between hypokalemia and acute myelogenous leukemia has also been noted in 40% to 60% of patients. This is associated with other electrolyte abnormalities and acid-base disorders, indicating tubular injury from high concentrations of urinary lysozyme.

HYPOPHOSPHATEMIA

Dysregulation of phosphate levels is another electrolyte disorder seen with cancer, in particular hypophosphatemia. Calcium and vitamin D deficiency is often due to malnutrition in these ill patients. Phosphaturia from proximal tubular damage develops from cisplatin use, multiple myeloma (light chain proximal tubular injury), and oncogenic osteomalacia, which is associated with increased FGF23 production. Evaluation includes a thorough medical history, review of medications and nutritional status assessment, serum free light chain and urine protein electrophoresis measurement, and evaluation for tumor-associated osteomalacia.

HYPERCALCEMIA

Malignancy is the most common cause of severe hypercalcemia in hospitalized patients. In general, hypercalcemia is a late finding, occurring with very advanced cancer and carrying a poor prognosis. The major mechanisms involved in malignancy-associated hypercalcemia are (1) secretion of parathyroid hormone-related protein (PTHrP) by several solid tumors; (2) direct osteolytic metastases with release of local cytokines from multiple myeloma and breast cancer; and (3) secretion of 1,25-dihydroxy vitamin D from lymphoma.

Hypercalcemia induces a "prerenal" picture by causing volume depletion through renal sodium loss, water depletion through nephrogenic diabetes insipidus, and vasoconstriction; in addition, intratubular calcium-phosphate deposition (acute nephrocalcinosis) may result in direct tubular injury. When the serum calcium level is over 13 mg/dL, most patients will have some degree of intravascular volume depletion. In these cases, administration of isotonic saline will restore volume and increase renal calcium excretion. Furosemide or other loop diuretics sometimes are used in hypervolemic patients to further promote calcium excretion, although the benefits of this approach remain uncertain, particularly given other effective calcium-lowering therapies. At a minimum, loop diuretics should be avoided early in the course of hypercalcemia management and likely should not be part of the armamentarium for use in hypercalcemia management in the absence of symptomatic volume overload.

Bisphosphonates, which are pyrophosphate analogs with a high affinity for hydroxyapatite, may be necessary to control serum calcium, particularly in severe hypercalcemia. Pamidronate and zoledronate, two second-generation bisphosphonates, are commonly used preparations. Pamidronate can be given as a single intravenous dose of 30 to 90 mg and may maintain normal serum calcium concentrations for several weeks. However, onset of action may be delayed with a mean time to achieve normocalcemia of 4 days. Therefore other means of lowering the serum calcium level must be implemented in the immediate period. Bisphosphonates have been associated with AKI.

Calcitonin, derived from the thyroid C-cell, inhibits osteoclast activity. The onset of action of calcitonin is rapid, but this drug has a short half-life and is usually not given as a sole therapy. Tachyphylaxis to calcitonin may be seen at 48 hours because of downregulation of the calcitonin receptor. More often, calcitonin is combined with pamidronate. Concomitant administration of glucocorticoids can prolong the effective duration of action of calcitonin. Glucocorticoids are effective in the therapy of hypercalcemia in patients with hematologic malignancies or multiple myeloma. In these cases, glucocorticoids inhibit osteoclastic bone resorption by decreasing tumor production of locally active cytokines and reducing active vitamin D synthesis.

Denosumab is a more recent addition to agents used to treat hypercalcemia of malignancy. It is a humanized monoclonal antibody directed against receptor of nuclear factor κB ligand (RANKL), thereby decreasing osteoclast differentiation and proliferation. Denosumab has been effective in lowering serum calcium levels in breast and prostate cancer and in multiple myeloma. Finally, hemodialysis with a low calcium bath is the preferred method of reducing serum calcium levels in patients with severe symptomatic hypercalcemia and kidney failure.

CHRONIC KIDNEY DISEASE AND MALIGNANCY

It is well established that patients with CKD or those who have undergone kidney transplantation are at a higher risk of cancer. CKD patients are more prone to renal cell carcinoma (RCC), and cancers of the lips, thyroid, and urinary tract. Cohort studies highlight the risk of cancer in patients with estimated GFR (eGFR) of less than 55 mL/min per 1.73 m^2. For every 10 mL/min per 1.73 m^2 reduction in eGFR, there was a 29% increased risk of cancer independent of age and smoking. It is therefore essential for clinicians to be aware of the cancer risk in the CKD population and undertake prompt evaluations to detect cancers at earlier, treatable stages. Treating cancer in CKD patients is more difficult than in the general population. Mortality and morbidity due to the adverse effects of surgery and chemotherapy are higher in this group of patients. Drug dosing and toxicity are problematic in CKD patients. In addition, most cancer trials exclude advanced CKD patients, thereby denying them access to potentially beneficial therapies.

Cancer occurring after kidney transplantation is well described in the literature. There is a higher incidence of lymphoma and skin cancers. In the United States, the risk of skin cancers (excluding melanomas) was 7.4% at 3 years and that of nonskin cancers and melanomas was 7.5%. Several studies have shown that risk of death from certain cancers developing after solid organ transplant is increased as compared with the general population. Posttransplant malignancies are discussed in more detail in Chapter 61.

KIDNEY CYSTS AND KIDNEY CANCER

The rate of RCC varies globally and is more common in industrialized countries. Established risk factors for sporadic RCC are cigarette smoking, obesity, and hypertension. The overall odds ratio for cancer of ever-smokers to never-smokers is 1.38 for both sexes based on studies undertaken in North America, Europe, and Australia. Obesity as defined by the World Health Organization (WHO) as body mass index ≥30 increases risk of RCC among both sexes. In several observational trials, high blood pressure has had a dose-dependent association with RCC risk. The risk decreases with reduction in blood pressure, possibly suggesting that the risk for RCC can be modified with antihypertensive medications. Several angiogenic and other growth factors are elevated in hypertension and may be involved in renal carcinogenesis. In contrast, blood pressure control could mitigate their potential effects over time.

In patients with CKD, particularly among those receiving dialysis with acquired cystic kidney disease (ACKD), the risk of RCC is also increased. The frequency of ACKD increases with number of years on dialysis, and nearly 50% of patients on dialysis for more than 3 years will develop ACKD. As compared with the general population, there is 50-fold increased risk of developing RCC in patients with ACKD. ACKD is usually asymptomatic but can lead to complications such as bleeding, rupture, and infections. Occasionally, patients may develop erythrocytosis from cyst synthesis of erythropoietin, and, in patients undergoing dialysis, a lack of erythropoiesis stimulating agent requirement may be an important clue that triggers imaging for RCC.

BIBLIOGRAPHY

Cairo MS, Coiffier B, Reiter A, et al. Recommendations for the evaluation of risk and prophylaxis of tumour lysis syndrome (TLS) in adults and children with malignant diseases: an expert TLS panel consensus. *Br J Haematol.* 2010;149:578-586.

Christiansen CF, Johansen MB, Van Biesen W. Incidence of acute kidney injury in cancer patients: a Danish population-based cohort study. *Eur J Intern Med.* 2011;22:399-406.

Cohen EP, Krzesinski M, Launay-Vacher V, et al. Onco-nephrology: core curriculum 2015. *Am J Kidney Dis.* 2015;66:869-883.

Darmon M, Vincent F, Canet E, et al. Acute kidney injury in critically ill patients with haematological malignancies: results of a multicentre cohort study from the Groupe de Recherche en Reanimation Respiratoire en Onco-Hematologie. *Nephrol Dial Transplant.* 2015;30:2006-2013.

Dawson LA, Kavanagh B, Paulino A, et al. Radiation-associated kidney injury. *Int J Radiat Oncol Biol Phys.* 2010;76:S108-S115.

Grill V, Martin TJ. Hypercalcemia of malignancy. *Rev Endocr Metab Disord.* 2000;1:253-263.

Hingorani S. Renal complications of hematopoietic-cell transplantation. *N Engl J Med.* 2016;374:2256-2267.

Howard SC, Jones DP, Pui CH, et al. The tumor lysis syndrome. *N Engl J Med.* 2011;364:1844-1854.

Izzedine H. Anti-VEGF cancer therapy in nephrology practice. *Int J Nephrol.* 2014;2014:143426.

Izzedine H, Escudier B, Lhomme C, et al. Kidney diseases associated with anti-vascular endothelial growth factor (VEGF): an 8-year observational study at a single center. *Medicine (Baltimore).* 2014;93:333-339.

Jhaveri KD, Shah H, Patel C, et al. Glomerular diseases associated with cancer, chemotherapy, and hematopoietic stem cell transplantation. *Adv Chronic Kidney Dis.* 2014;21:48-55.

Lam AQ, Humphreys BD. Onco-nephrology: AKI in the cancer patient. *Clin J Am Soc Nephrol.* 2012;7:1692-1700.

Lameire N, Vanholder R, Van Biesen W, Benoit D. Acute kidney injury in critically ill cancer patients: an update. *Crit Care.* 2016;20:209.

McDonald GB, Hinds M, Fisher L, et al. Veno-occlusive disease of the liver and multiorgan failure after bone marrow transplantation: a cohort study of 355 patients. *Ann Intern Med.* 1993;118:255-267.

Ries F, Klastersky J. Nephrotoxicity induced by cancer chemotherapy with special emphasis on cisplatin toxicity. *Am J Kidney Dis.* 1986;8:368-379.

Rosner MH, Dalkin AC. Electrolyte disorders associated with cancer. *Adv Chronic Kidney Dis.* 2014;21:7-17.

Skinner R. Strategies to prevent nephrotoxicity of anticancer drugs. *Curr Opin Oncol.* 1995;7:310-315.

Stengel B. Chronic kidney disease and cancer: a troubling connection. *J Nephrol.* 2010;23:253-262.

Widakowich C, de Castro G, de Azambuja E, et al. Review: side effects of approved molecular targeted therapies in solid cancers. *Oncologist.* 2007;12:1443-1455.

Zager RA. Acute renal failure in the setting of bone marrow transplantation. *Kidney Int.* 1994;46:1443-1458.

28 Myeloma, Amyloid, and Other Dysproteinemias

Ala Abudayyeh; Paul W. Sanders

Paraproteinemic kidney diseases are typically the result of deposition of immunoglobulin fragments (heavy chains and light chains; Fig. 28.1) in specific parts of the nephron, and they can be divided generally into those diseases that manifest primarily as glomerular or as tubulointerstitial injury (Box 28.1). Glomerular diseases include AL-type amyloidosis (amyloid composed of light chains), AH-type amyloidosis (amyloid composed of heavy chains), monoclonal immunoglobulin deposition disease (MIDD, which includes light-chain deposition disease [LCDD], heavy-chain deposition disease, and light- and heavy-chain deposition disease), proliferative glomerulonephritis with monoclonal immunoglobulin deposition (PGMID), paraprotein-associated C3 glomerulopathy, immunotactoid glomerulopathy, and glomerulonephritis associated with type I cryoglobulinemia. In this review, AL-type amyloidosis, monoclonal LCDD, fibrillary glomerulonephritis, and immunotactoid glomerulopathy will be discussed. Patterns of tubular injury include Fanconi syndrome, proximal tubulopathy, and cast nephropathy (also known as "myeloma kidney"). In addition to these paraproteinemic kidney lesions, this chapter includes a discussion of Waldenström macroglobulinemia.

Aside from notable exceptions, such as AH-type amyloidosis and heavy-chain deposition disease, immunoglobulin light-chain deposition is directly responsible for most of the kidney pathologic alterations that occur with paraproteinemia. In one large study of multiple myeloma, kidney dysfunction was present in approximately 2% of patients who did not exhibit significant urinary free light-chain levels, while increasing urine free light-chain levels were strongly associated with kidney failure, with 48% of myeloma patients who had high urinary monoclonal free light chains having kidney failure and associated poor survival. The type of kidney lesion induced by light chains depends on the physicochemical properties of these proteins.

IMMUNOGLOBULIN LIGHT-CHAIN METABOLISM AND CLINICAL DETECTION

The original description of immunoglobulin light chains is attributed to Dr. Henry Bence Jones in 1847. He reported these unique proteins, which now bear his name, and correlated this early urinary biomarker with the disease known as multiple myeloma. More than a century later, Edelman and Gally demonstrated that Bence Jones proteins were immunoglobulin light chains.

Plasma cells synthesize light chains that become part of the immunoglobulin molecule (see Fig. 28.1). In normal states, a slight excess production of light, compared to heavy, chains appears to be required for efficient immunoglobulin synthesis, but this excess results in the release of polyclonal free light chains into the circulation. After entering the bloodstream, light chains are handled similarly to other low-molecular-weight proteins, which are usually removed from the circulation by glomerular filtration. Unlike albumin, these monomers (molecular weight ~22 kDa) and dimers (~44 kDa) are readily filtered through the glomerulus and are reabsorbed by the proximal tubule. Endocytosis of light chains into the proximal tubule occurs through a single class of heterodimeric, multiligand receptor that is composed of megalin and cubilin. After endocytosis, lysosomal enzymes hydrolyze the proteins, and the amino-acid components are returned to the circulation. The uptake and catabolism of these proteins are very efficient, with the kidney readily handling the approximately 500 mg of free light chains produced daily by the normal lymphoid system. However, in the setting of a monoclonal gammopathy, light chain production increases, and binding of light chains to the megalin-cubilin complex can become saturated, allowing light chains to be delivered to the distal nephron and to appear in the urine as Bence Jones proteins.

Light chains are modular proteins that possess two independent globular regions, termed constant (C_L) and variable (V_L) domains (see Fig. 28.1). Light chains can be isotyped as kappa (κ) or lambda (λ), based on sequence variations in the constant region of the protein. Within the globular V_L domain are four framework regions that consist of β sheets that develop a hydrophobic core. The framework regions separate three hypervariable segments that are known as complementarity determining regions (CDR1, CDR2, and CDR3; see Fig. 28.1). The CDR domains, which represent those regions of sequence variability among light chains, form loop structures that constitute part of the antigen-binding site of the immunoglobulin. Diversity among the CDR regions occurs because the V_L domain is synthesized through rearrangement of multiple gene segments. Thus, although possessing similar structures and biochemical properties, no two light chains are identical; however, there are enough sequence similarities among light chains to permit categorizing them into subgroups. There are four κ and ten λ subgroups, although, of the λ subgroups, most patients (94%) with multiple myeloma express λI, λII, λIII, or λV subgroups. Free light chains, particularly the

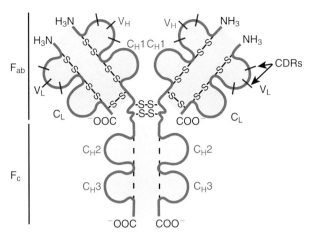

Fig. 28.1 Schematic of the immunoglobulin G molecule, which consists of two heavy chains and two light chains that are stabilized by inter- and intramolecular disulfide bonds. Light chains consist of two domains that are termed constant (C_L) and variable (V_L) regions. Within the V_L domain are the complementarity determining regions that are primarily responsible for variations in the amino-acid sequences among light chains. Heavy chains also consist of a variable domain (V_H) and three constant domains (C_H1, C_H2, C_H3). *CDRs*, Complementarity determining regions.

Box 28.1 Paraproteinemia-Associated Kidney Diseases

Glomerulopathies

AL-type and AH-type amyloidoses
Monoclonal immunoglobulin deposition disease
Proliferative glomerulonephritis with monoclonal
   immunoglobulin deposition
Paraprotein-associated C3 glomerulopathy
Paraprotein-associated fibrillary glomerulonephritis
Immunotactoid glomerulopathy
Cryoglobulinemia, type I

Tubulointerstitial Lesions

Cast nephropathy ("myeloma kidney")
Fanconi syndrome
Proximal tubulopathy
Tubulointerstitial nephritis (rare)

Vascular Lesions

Asymptomatic Bence Jones proteinuria
Hyperviscosity syndrome
Neoplastic cell infiltration (rare)

Box 28.2 Potential Causes of Monoclonal Light-Chain Proteinuria

Multiple myeloma
AL-type amyloidosis
Monoclonal light-chain deposition disease
Waldenström macroglobulinemia
MGUS
POEMS syndrome (rare)
Heavy-chain (μ) disease (rare)
Lymphoproliferative disease (rare)

MGUS, Monoclonal gammopathy of undetermined significance; *POEMS*, syndrome consisting of polyneuropathy, organomegaly, endocrinopathy, M protein, and skin changes.

λ isotype, often homodimerize before secretion into the circulation.

The multiple kidney lesions from monoclonal light chain deposition affect virtually every compartment of the kidney (see Box 28.1) and may be explained by sequence variations, particularly in the V_L domain of the offending monoclonal light chain. The light chains that are responsible for monoclonal LCDD are frequently members of the κIV subfamily and appear to possess unusual hydrophobic amino-acid residues in CDR1. In AL-type amyloidosis, sequence variations in the V_L domain of the precursor light chain confer the propensity to polymerize to form amyloid. A classic kidney presentation of multiple myeloma is Fanconi syndrome, which is produced almost exclusively by members of the κI subfamily. Unusual nonpolar residues in the CDR1 region and absence of accessible side chains in the CDR3 loop of the variable domain of κI light chains result in homotypic crystallization of the light chain in this syndrome. In cast nephropathy, the secondary structure of CDR3 is a critical determinant of cast formation. In summary, sequence variations in the V_L domain appear to determine the type of kidney lesion that occurs with monoclonal light chain deposition.

Free light chains were originally detected with turbidimetric and heat tests. Because these tests lack sensitivity, they are no longer in use. The qualitative urine dipstick test for protein also has a low sensitivity for detection of light chains. Although some Bence Jones proteins react with the chemical impregnated onto the strip, other light chains cannot be detected; the net charge of the protein may be an important determinant of this interaction. Because of the relative insensitivity of routine serum protein electrophoresis (SPEP) and urinary protein electrophoresis (UPEP) for free light chains, these tests are no longer recommended as screening tools in the diagnostic evaluation of the underlying etiology of kidney disease. SPEP is positive in 87.6% of multiple myelomas but only 73.8% of immunoglobulin light-chain (AL) amyloidosis and 55.6% of LCDD. The sensitivity of the UPEP is also low: among a population of 2799 plasma cell dyscrasia patients, only 37.7% had a positive UPEP.

Highly sensitive and reliable immunoassays now are available to detect the presence of monoclonal light chains in the urine and serum and are adequate tests for screening when both urine and serum are examined. When a clone of plasma cells exists, significant amounts of monoclonal light chains appear in the circulation and the urine. In healthy adults, the urinary concentration of polyclonal light chain proteins is about 2.5 mg/L. Causes of monoclonal light-chain proteinuria, a hallmark of plasma cell dyscrasias, are listed (Box 28.2). Urinary light chain concentration is generally between 0.02 and 0.5 g/L in patients with monoclonal gammopathy of undetermined significance (MGUS) and is often much higher (range 0.02 to 11.8 g/L) in patients with multiple myeloma or Waldenström macroglobulinemia. Immunofixation electrophoresis is sensitive and detects monoclonal light chains and immunoglobulins, even in very low concentrations, but it is a qualitative assay that may be limited by interobserver variation. A nephelometric assay that quantifies serum-free κ and λ light chains is also useful to nephrologists, because most of the kidney lesions in paraproteinemias are caused by light chain overproduction and much less commonly by heavy chains or intact immunoglobulins. Because an excess of light chains, compared with heavy chains, is synthesized and released into the circulation, this sensitive assay detects small amounts of serum polyclonal free light chains in healthy individuals. This assay can also distinguish polyclonal from monoclonal light chains and further quantifies the free light chain level in the serum. Quantifying serum light chain levels may be of use clinically, to monitor chemotherapy as well as to serve as a risk factor for development of kidney failure, because myeloma patients with baseline serum-free monoclonal light chain levels greater than 750 mg/L correlated with depressed kidney function (serum creatinine concentration ≥2 mg/dL) and more aggressive myeloma. In the evaluation of kidney disease, particularly if amyloidosis is suspected, perhaps the ideal screening tests for an associated plasma cell dyscrasia include immunofixation electrophoresis of serum and urine and quantification of serum free κ and λ light chains, which have been added as a diagnostic criterion for myeloma. The addition of serum free light chain assay to immunofixation increases detection of multiple myeloma, Waldenström macroglobulinemia, and smoldering multiple myeloma.

GLOMERULAR LESIONS OF PLASMA CELL DYSCRASIAS

AL-TYPE AMYLOIDOSIS

More than 23 different amyloid proteins have been identified. They are named according to the precursor protein that polymerizes to produce amyloid. Amyloid proteins are characterized by a misfolding event that renders them insoluble and therefore deposit in organs as fibrils, leading to dysfunction. AL-type amyloidosis, which is also known as "primary amyloidosis," represents a plasma cell dyscrasia that is characterized by organ dysfunction related to deposition of amyloid and usually only a mild increase in monoclonal plasma cells in the bone marrow. However, about 20% of patients with AL-type amyloidosis exhibit overt multiple myeloma or other lymphoproliferative disorder. In AL-type amyloidosis, the amyloid deposits are composed of immunoglobulin light chains versus AA-type amyloidosis, where the precursor protein (serum amyloid A protein) is an acute

phase reactant. The identification of the type of amyloid protein is an essential first step in the management of these patients.

AL-type amyloidosis is a systemic disease that typically involves multiple organs (Table 28.1). Cardiac infiltration frequently produces congestive heart failure and is a common presenting manifestation of primary amyloidosis. Infiltration of the lungs and gastrointestinal tract is also common but is generally asymptomatic. Dysesthesias, orthostatic hypotension, diarrhea, and bladder dysfunction from peripheral and autonomic neuropathies can occur. Amyloid deposition can also produce an arthropathy that resembles rheumatoid arthritis, a bleeding diathesis, and a variety of skin manifestations that include purpura. Kidney involvement is common in primary amyloidosis. In a retrospective review of 84 patients with biopsy-proven AL amyloid, 42% needed dialysis with median survival of less than one year following initiation of kidney replacement therapy.

PATHOLOGY

Glomerular lesions are the dominant kidney features of AL-type amyloidosis and are characterized by the presence of mesangial nodules and progressive effacement of glomerular capillaries (Fig. 28.2). In the early stage, amyloid deposits are usually found in the mesangium and are not associated with an increase in mesangial cellularity. Deposits may also be seen along the subepithelial space of capillary loops, and

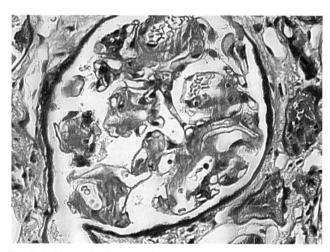

Fig. 28.2 Glomerulus from a patient with AL-type amyloidosis, showing segmentally variable accumulation of amorphous acidophilic material that is effacing portions of the glomerular architecture (PASH stain, magnification ×40).

Table 28.1   Relative Frequency of Organ Infiltration by Light Chains in AL-Type Amyloidosis and Light Chain Deposition Disease

| | | ORGAN INVOLVEMENT | | | | | |
	Isotype	Kidney	Heart	Liver	Neurologic	GI	Lung
AL-amyloid	λ > κ	+++	+++	+	+	+++	++++
LCDD	κ > λ	++++	+++	+++	+	Rare	Rare

Note: From +, uncommon but can occur during the course of the disease, through ++++, extremely common during the course of the disease. *GI*, Gastrointestinal; *LCDD*, monoclonal light-chain deposition disease.

may penetrate the glomerular basement membrane in more advanced stages. Immunohistochemistry demonstrates that the deposits consist of light chains, although the sensitivity of this test is not high. Amyloid has characteristic tinctorial properties and stains with Congo red, which produces an apple-green birefringence when the tissue section is examined under polarized light and with thioflavins T and S. On electron microscopy, the deposits are characteristic, randomly oriented, nonbranching fibrils 7 to 10 nm in diameter. In some cases of early amyloidosis, glomeruli may appear normal on light microscopy; however, careful examination can identify scattered monotypic light chains on immunofluorescence microscopy. Ultrastructural examination with immunoelectron microscopy to show the fibrils of AL-type amyloid may be required to establish the diagnosis early in the course of kidney involvement. Ultrastructural and immunohistochemical examination of biopsies of an affected organ establish the diagnosis, although tissue diagnosis of AL-type amyloidosis can also be difficult, because commercially available antibodies may not detect the presence of the light chain in the tissue. In uncertain cases, the amyloid can be extracted from tissue and examined with tandem mass spectrometry to determine the chemical composition of the amyloid. As the disease advances, mesangial deposits progressively enlarge to form nodules of amyloid protein that compress the filtering surfaces of the glomeruli and cause kidney failure. Epithelial proliferation and crescent formation are rare in AL-type amyloidosis.

CLINICAL FEATURES

Proteinuria and reduced kidney function are the major kidney manifestations of AL-type amyloidosis. Proteinuria ranges from asymptomatic nonnephrotic proteinuria to nephrotic syndrome. Isolated microscopic hematuria and nephritic syndrome are not common in AL-type amyloidosis. More than 90% of patients have monoclonal light chains either in urine or blood, but occasionally even sensitive assays will not detect a circulating monoclonal light chain in patients with documented AL-type renal amyloidosis. Reduced kidney function is present in 58% to 70% of patients at the time of diagnosis. Scintigraphy using ^{123}I-labeled serum amyloid P component, which binds to amyloid, can assess the degree of organ involvement from amyloid infiltration, but this test is not currently widely available.

PATHOGENESIS

The pathogenesis of AL-type amyloidosis is incompletely understood. Presumably, intracellular oxidation or partial proteolysis of light chains by mesangial cells allows formation of amyloid, which is then extruded into the extracellular space. With continued production of amyloid, the mesangium expands, compressing the filtering surface of the glomeruli and producing progressive kidney failure. There is evidence that amyloidogenic light chains also have intrinsic biological activity that modulates cell function independently of amyloid formation. Not all light chains are amyloidogenic. Members of the λ family are more commonly associated with AL-type amyloidosis, and sequence variations in the V_L domain appear to confer the propensity to polymerize to form amyloid.

TREATMENT AND PROGNOSIS

Patients with both multiple myeloma and AL-type amyloidosis should be managed with treatment regimens that target myeloma. For patients who experience AL-type amyloidosis and lack the criteria for multiple myeloma, the initial approach is to ensure that the patient has AL-type amyloidosis and not amyloidosis related to a nonlymphoid-derived precursor protein, because the approaches to treatment are different. Because a randomized trial suggested improved survival in patients who received chemotherapy, more aggressive anti-plasma cell therapies have been undertaken in AL-type amyloidosis, including high-dose chemotherapy with autologous peripheral stem-cell transplantation (HDT/SCT). Although reduced kidney function may not be an exclusion criteria, because of increased treatment-related mortality of HDT/SCT in higher-risk subjects, more conservative approaches should be considered for patients age ≥80 years or with decompensated heart failure, left ventricular ejection fraction below 40%, systolic blood pressure below 90 mm Hg, oxygen saturation less than 95% on room air, or significant overall functional impairment. Patients who have evidence of multiorgan system dysfunction, particularly cardiac disease, and are considered ineligible for HDT/SCT have an expected median survival of only 4 months, so delays in diagnosis and treatment can be costly. In contrast, one study reported a median survival of 4.6 years in 312 patients who underwent HDT/SCT. Almost half achieved a complete hematologic response, which portended improved long-term survival. Although carefully selected patients with AL-type amyloidosis can respond favorably to HDT/SCT, in a randomized clinical trial comparing HDT/SCT with chemotherapy, including melphalan and high-dose dexamethasone, the outcome was not superior.

Patients with AL-type amyloidosis usually die from organ decompensation due to amyloid infiltration and not from tumor burden. An important observation from these studies is that survival and organ dysfunction can improve with successful reduction in the monoclonal plasma cell population and light chain production. Other novel chemotherapeutic regimens may be of benefit in AL-type amyloidosis and are being considered, particularly given the potential toxicity of chronic treatment with alkylating agents. The recent success of thalidomide as an alternative treatment of multiple myeloma has prompted treatment of AL-type amyloidosis with this agent, although thalidomide is not well tolerated in these patients, and dosage reductions are often required. Lenalidomide, an analogue of thalidomide, is another potentially attractive therapy in AL-type amyloidosis. Bortezomib-based regimens have also provided promising results in AL-type amyloidosis. Again, randomized controlled trials are needed to determine efficacy of these pharmacologic agents in AL-type amyloidosis.

There has been increasing interest in improving amyloid-associated end-organ damage that did not recover, despite an adequate hematologic response to therapy. Novel treatment approaches are being evaluated, including methods to target precursor protein production, administration of small molecules to prevent misfolding, and introduction of agents to increase amyloid degradation. For example, NEOD001, a monoclonal antibody directed against free light chains, was shown to specifically bind soluble and insoluble aggregated light chains and mediate antibody-dependent phagocytosis. VITAL phase 3/NCT02312206 and PRONTO phase 2b are randomized, placebo-controlled, global trials that are under way to evaluate NEOD001 further.

MONOCLONAL Ig DEPOSITION DISEASE

Monoclonal Ig deposition disease (MIDD) is defined as the deposition of nonamyloid monoclonal light and/or heavy chains in a nonorganized manner in the kidney. MIDD is further categorized into three subtypes that are based on the composition of the monoclonal protein in the deposits: light chain deposition disease (LCDD), light and heavy chain deposition disease (LHCDD), and heavy chain deposition disease (HCDD). LCDD is the most common and will be further discussed; it is a systemic disease that typically presents initially with isolated kidney injury related to a glomerular lesion associated with nonamyloid electron-dense granular deposits of monoclonal light chains with or without heavy chains. It may accompany other clinical features of multiple myeloma or another lymphoproliferative disorder or may be the sole manifestation of a plasma cell dyscrasia.

PATHOLOGY

Nodular glomerulopathy with distortion of the glomerular architecture by amorphous, eosinophilic material is the most common pathologic finding observed with light microscopy (Fig. 28.3). These nodules, which are composed of light chains and extracellular matrix proteins, begin in the mesangium. The appearance is reminiscent of diabetic nephropathy. Less commonly, other glomerular morphologic changes in addition to nodular glomerulopathy can be seen in LCDD. Immunofluorescence microscopy demonstrates the presence of monotypic light chains in the glomeruli. Under electron microscopy, deposits of light chain proteins are present in a subendothelial position along the glomerular capillary wall, along the outer aspect of tubular basement membranes, and in the mesangium.

There are significant differences between amyloidosis and LCDD. For amyloid deposition to occur, amyloid P

glycoprotein must also be present. The amyloid P component is not part of the amyloid fibrils but binds them. This glycoprotein is a constituent of normal human glomerular basement membrane and elastic fibrils. In contrast to AL-type amyloid, in LCDD the light chain deposits are punctate, granular, and electron dense and are identified in the mesangium and/or subendothelial space; amyloid P component is absent. Unlike amyloid, the granular light-chain deposits of LCDD do not stain with Congo red or thioflavin T and S. Another difference between these lesions is the tendency for κ light chains to compose the granular deposits of LCDD, whereas usually λ light chains constitute AL-amyloid. Both diseases can involve organs other than the kidney (see Table 28.1).

CLINICAL FEATURES

The typical clinical presentation is reminiscent of a rapidly progressive glomerulonephritis. The major symptoms of LCDD include proteinuria, sometimes in the nephrotic range, microscopic hematuria, and kidney failure. Albumin and monoclonal free light chains are the dominant proteins in the urine. The presence of albuminuria and other findings of nephrotic syndrome are important clues to the presence of glomerular injury and not cast nephropathy. The amount of excreted light chain is usually less than that found in cast nephropathy and can be difficult to detect in some patients. Progressive kidney failure in untreated patients is common. Because kidney manifestations generally predominate and are often the sole presenting features, it is not uncommon for nephrologists to diagnose the plasma cell dyscrasia. Kidney biopsy is necessary to confirm the diagnosis. Other organ dysfunction, especially in the liver and heart, can develop and is related to deposition of light chains in those organs. Although extrarenal manifestations of overt multiple myeloma can manifest at presentation or over time, a majority (~50% to 60%) of patients with LCDD will not develop myeloma or other malignant lymphoproliferative disease.

PATHOGENESIS

LCDD represents a prototypical model of progressive kidney disease that has a pathogenesis related to glomerulosclerosis from increased production of transforming growth factor-β (TGF-β). The response to monoclonal light chain deposition includes expansion of the mesangium by extracellular matrix proteins to form nodules and eventually glomerular sclerosis. Experimental studies have shown that mesangial cells exposed to light chains obtained from patients with biopsy-proven LCDD produce TGF-β, which serves as an autacoid to stimulate these same cells to produce matrix proteins, including type IV collagen, laminin, and fibronectin. Thus TGF-β plays a central role in glomerular sclerosis from LCDD. As is true for AL-type amyloidosis, not all light chains can produce LCDD. Many offending light chains are κ, particularly the κIV subfamily, and appear to possess unusual hydrophobic amino-acid residues in the V_L domain.

Although deposition of light chain is the prominent feature of these glomerular lesions, both heavy chains and light chains can be identified in the deposits. In these specimens, the punctate electron-dense deposits appear larger and more extensive than deposits that contain only light chains, but it is unclear whether the clinical course of these patients differs from the course of isolated light chain deposition without heavy chain components, and the management is similar.

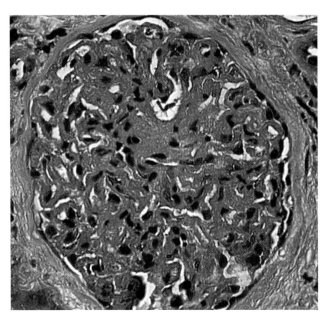

Fig. 28.3 Glomerulus from a patient with monoclonal κ light-chain deposition disease, showing expansion of the mesangium, related to matrix protein deposition, and associated compression of capillary lumens (hematoxylin-eosin stain, magnification ×40).

TREATMENT AND PROGNOSIS

For patients with both multiple myeloma and LCDD, therapy is directed toward the myeloma. The treatment of LCDD without an associated malignant lymphoproliferative disorder is difficult, because guidance from randomized controlled trials is unavailable. However, patients appear to benefit from the same therapeutic approach used for multiple myeloma. The serum creatinine concentration at presentation is an important predictor of subsequent outcome, so intervention should be early in the course of the disease.

Melphalan/prednisone therapy improves kidney prognosis, but the long-term toxicity of melphalan makes this approach less attractive. More aggressive antiplasma cell therapy in the form of HDT/SCT has been used in LCDD. In the small numbers of patients in whom HDT/SCT was performed, the procedure-related death rate was low, and when a complete hematologic response was observed, improvement in affected organ function with histologic evidence of regression of the light chain deposits occurred. This has been further confirmed in a recent study looking at overall survival and kidney outcomes in 88 patients with LCDD. Novel chemotherapeutic regimens that include thalidomide and bortezomib also appear to have efficacy in this setting.

The high incidence of progressive kidney disease in LCDD has prompted treatment with kidney transplantation, but the disease will recur in the allograft if the underlying plasma cell dyscrasia is not addressed. The study with the largest collection of patients (seven) concluded that LCDD recurred commonly in the kidney allograft, significantly impacting long-term graft survival; these findings emphasize the need to control monoclonal light chain production before kidney transplantation in LCDD.

FIBRILLARY GLOMERULONEPHRITIS AND IMMUNOTACTOID GLOMERULOPATHY

Fibrillary glomerulonephritis is a rare disorder characterized ultrastructurally by the presence of amyloid-like, randomly arranged fibrillary deposits in the capillary wall (Fig. 28.4). Unlike amyloid, these fibrils are thicker (18 to 22 nm) and Congo red, and thioflavin T stains are negative. Immunofluorescence microscopy typically shows IgG (usually IgG4) and C3. Most patients with fibrillary glomerulonephritis do not have a plasma cell dyscrasia; however, occasionally a plasma cell dyscrasia is present, so screening is advisable. Tests for cryoglobulins and hepatitis C infection should be obtained. Patients typically manifest nephrotic syndrome and varying degrees of kidney disease; progression to end-stage kidney failure is the rule. Standardized treatment for the idiopathic fibrillary glomerulonephritis is currently unavailable.

Immunotactoid, or microtubular, glomerulopathy is even less common than fibrillary glomerulonephritis and is usually associated with a plasma cell dyscrasia or another lymphoproliferative disorder. The deposits in this lesion contain thick (greater than 30 nm), organized, microtubular structures that are located in the mesangium and along capillary walls. Cryoglobulinemia, which is also discussed in Chapter 23, should be considered in the differential diagnosis and should be ruled out clinically. Treatment of the underlying plasma cell dyscrasia is indicated for this rare disorder.

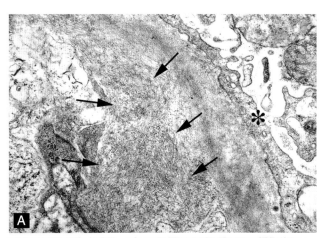

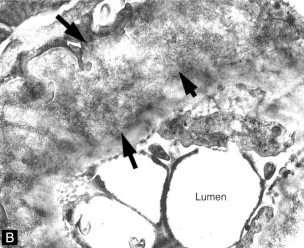

Fig. 28.4 Glomeruli. (A) Electron micrograph of a glomerulus from a patient with AL-type amyloidosis. Note the randomly arranged relatively straight fibrils with an approximate diameter of 7 to 10 nm *(arrows)*. A useful distinction from fibrillary glomerulonephritis is that amyloid fibrils will stain with Congo red or thioflavin T. Note fusion of the foot processes *(asterisk)* of the adjacent epithelial cell. (B) Electron micrograph of a glomerulus from a patient with fibrillary glomerulonephritis. The same random arrangement of nonbranching fibrils *(arrows)* is seen. Careful examination demonstrates that the fibrils are larger (approximately 20 nm in diameter). The overall ultrastructural appearance resembles amyloid, except that the fibrils are approximately twice as thick. (A, Courtesy Dr. J. Charles Jennette, Department of Pathology, University of North Carolina at Chapel Hill. B, Courtesy Dr. William Cook, Department of Pathology, University of Alabama at Birmingham.)

TUBULOINTERSTITIAL LESIONS OF PLASMA CELL DYSCRASIAS

CAST NEPHROPATHY

PATHOLOGY

Cast nephropathy is an inflammatory tubulointerstitial kidney lesion. Characteristically, multiple intraluminal proteinaceous casts are identified mainly in the distal portion of the nephrons (Fig. 28.5). The casts are usually acellular, homogeneous, and eosinophilic with multiple fracture lines. Immunofluorescence and immunoelectron microscopy confirm that the

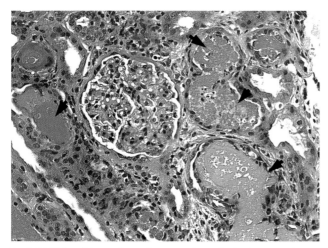

Fig. 28.5 Kidney biopsy tissue from a patient who had cast nephropathy. The findings include tubules filled with cast material *(arrows)* and presence of multinucleated giant cells. Glomeruli are typically normal in appearance (hematoxylin-eosin stain, magnification ×20).

> **Box 28.3 Standard Therapy for Cast Nephropathy**
>
> Chemotherapy to decrease light-chain production
> Increase free water intake to 2 to 3 L/day as tolerated
> Treat hypercalcemia aggressively
> Avoid exposure to diuretics, radiocontrast agents, and nonsteroidal antiinflammatory agents

casts contain light chains and Tamm-Horsfall glycoprotein. Persistence of the casts produces the giant cell inflammation and tubular atrophy that typify myeloma kidney. Glomeruli are usually normal in appearance.

CLINICAL FEATURES

Kidney failure from this lesion may present acutely or as a chronic progressive disease and may develop at any stage of myeloma. Diagnosis of multiple myeloma is usually evident when chronic bone pain, pathologic fractures, and hypercalcemia are complicated by proteinuria and kidney failure. However, many patients present to nephrologists primarily with symptoms of kidney failure or undefined proteinuria; further evaluation then confirms a malignant process. Cast nephropathy should therefore be considered when proteinuria (often more than 3 g/day), particularly without concomitant hypoalbuminemia or significant albuminuria, is found in a patient who is in the fourth decade of life or older. Hypertension is not common with cast nephropathy. Diagnosis of myeloma may be confirmed by finding monoclonal immunoglobulins or light chains in the serum and urine and by bone marrow examination, although typical intraluminal cast formation on kidney biopsy is virtually pathognomonic.

PATHOGENESIS

Intravenous infusion of nephrotoxic human light chains in rats elevates proximal tubule pressure and simultaneously decreases the single nephron glomerular filtration rate (GFR); intraluminal protein casts can be identified in these kidneys. Myeloma casts contain Tamm-Horsfall glycoprotein and occur initially in the distal nephron, which provides an optimum environment for precipitation with free light chains. Casts occur primarily because light chains coaggregate with Tamm-Horsfall glycoprotein. Tamm-Horsfall glycoprotein, which is synthesized exclusively by cells of the thick ascending limb of the loop of Henle, comprises the major fraction of total urinary protein in healthy individuals and is the predominant constituent of urinary casts. Cast-forming Bence Jones proteins bind to the same site on the peptide backbone of Tamm-Horsfall glycoprotein; binding results in coaggregation of these proteins and subsequent occlusion of the tubule lumen by the precipitated protein complexes. Intranephronal obstruction and kidney failure ensue. Light chains that bind to Tamm-Horsfall glycoprotein are potentially nephrotoxic. The CDR3 domain of the light chain determines binding affinity.

Coaggregation of Tamm-Horsfall glycoprotein with light chains also depends on the ionic environment and the physicochemical properties of the light chain, and not all patients with myeloma develop cast nephropathy, even when the urinary excretion of light chains is high. Increasing concentrations of sodium chloride or calcium, but not magnesium, facilitate coaggregation. The loop diuretic, furosemide, augments coaggregation and accelerates intraluminal obstruction in vivo in the rat. Finally, the lower tubule fluid flow rates of the distal nephron allow more time for light chains to interact with Tamm-Horsfall glycoprotein and subsequently to obstruct the tubular lumen. Conditions that further reduce flow rates, such as volume depletion, can accelerate tubule obstruction or convert nontoxic light chains into cast-forming proteins. Volume depletion and hypercalcemia are recognized factors that promote acute kidney injury (AKI) from cast nephropathy.

TREATMENT AND PROGNOSIS

The principles used to guide therapy in cast nephropathy include rapidly decreasing the concentration of circulating light chains and preventing coaggregation of light chains with Tamm-Horsfall glycoprotein (Box 28.3). Prompt and effective chemotherapy should start upon diagnosis of multiple myeloma. The traditional treatment with alkylating agents and steroids has been replaced by HDT/SCT, particularly in younger patients. An advantage with a more aggressive approach is the potential for rapid reductions in the levels of circulating monoclonal light chain. Several randomized trials showed that patients who received HDT/SCT experienced an improvement in overall survival versus patients who received conventional chemotherapy. Chemotherapy is usually initiated before HDT/SCT to reduce the plasma cell clone. Induction therapy with combinations of immunomodulatory drugs (thalidomide and lenalidomide) and proteasome inhibitors (bortezomib and carfilzomib), along with steroids, alkylators, or anthracyclines, followed by autologous hematopoietic cell transplantation (HCT), has improved the median overall survival for patients with multiple myeloma from 36 months to more than 5 years. Treatment with alkylating agents is typically avoided before HDT/SCT, because these drugs may impede peripheral stem cell harvest and are associated with myelodysplasia and acute myelogenous leukemia. Almost all patients after autologous SCT ultimately relapse and as a result need further treatment. Monoclonal antibodies, deacetylase inhibitors, kinase inhibitors, and immune checkpoint inhibitors have been tested in clinical trials with promising results; however, nephrotoxicity has been an associated complication.

Other therapeutic approaches currently lack randomized controlled trials to support their use. For example, patients with advanced kidney failure and refractory myeloma have been treated successfully with bortezomib- and thalidomide-based therapies. These agents are gaining wide acceptance and may ultimately obviate the need for HDT/SCT. Nonmyeloablative allogeneic stem-cell transplantation, so-called mini-allograft therapy, may also provide beneficial results in myeloma without the attendant complications such as severe graft-versus-host disease.

Studies suggest that interstitial fibrosis can develop rapidly in cast nephropathy, promoting persistent and ultimately irreversible kidney failure. Because clinical evidence suggests that prompt reduction in circulating free light chains accelerates kidney recovery in cast nephropathy, the delay in reduction of free light-chain levels associated with chemotherapy has provoked exploration of extracorporeal removal of circulating free light chains, with mixed results. Currently the ancillary role of plasma exchange (PLEX) in AKI in the setting of multiple myeloma is uncertain. One randomized trial suggested benefit, but two others failed to confirm a survival advantage for patients treated with PLEX along with chemotherapy. The most recent randomized trial suggested no clinical benefit from PLEX for patients with AKI, although there were limitations to this study, including potential sample size issues and the lack of kidney biopsies to document cast nephropathy as a prerequisite for study entry. In addition, serum-free light chains were not quantified either before or after PLEX. Despite these limitations, a significant theoretical issue related to PLEX is the relatively inefficient removal of light chains, which distribute throughout the extracellular fluid space. Recently, efficient removal of light chains has been achieved with high-cutoff hemodialysis treatments. Although early reports support this technique for rapid reduction in serum light-chain concentrations, ongoing randomized trials will inform medical practice. Until additional data are provided, it is probably prudent to not recommend routinely extracorporeal therapies for most patients with AKI, but rather emphasize highly effective chemotherapy, although there may be a subset of patients with AKI from cast nephropathy who will respond favorably to this additional intervention. If PLEX or high-cutoff hemodialysis is performed, demonstration of the efficacy of treatment by quantifying changes in serum free light-chain levels should be performed. Finally, hyperviscosity syndrome remains an indication for extracorporeal removal of the monoclonal proteins.

Prevention of aggregation of light chains with Tamm-Horsfall glycoprotein is a cornerstone of therapy. Volume repletion, normalization of electrolytes, and avoidance of complicating factors such as loop diuretics and nonsteroidal antiinflammatory agents are helpful in preserving and improving kidney function. Although not all patients with light-chain proteinuria develop AKI following exposure to radiocontrast agents, predicting who is at risk for this complication is difficult, suggesting caution in the use of radiocontrast agents in all patients with myeloma. Daily intake up to 3 L of electrolyte-poor fluid should be encouraged. Alkalinization of the urine with oral sodium bicarbonate (or citrate) to keep the urine pH greater than 7 may also be therapeutic but may be mitigated by the requisite sodium loading, which favors coaggregation of these proteins and also should be avoided in patients who have symptomatic extracellular fluid volume overload.

Hypercalcemia occurs during the course of the disease in more than 25% of patients with multiple myeloma. In addition to being directly nephrotoxic, hypercalcemia enhances the nephrotoxicity of light chains. Treatment of volume contraction with the infusion of saline often corrects mild hypercalcemia. Loop diuretics also increase calcium excretion, but diuretics may also facilitate nephrotoxicity from light chains and should be avoided, if possible. Glucocorticoid therapy (such as methylprednisolone) is helpful for acute management of myeloma as well as hypercalcemia. Bisphosphonates, such as pamidronate and zoledronic acid, are used to treat moderate hypercalcemia (serum calcium greater than 3.25 mmol/L, or 13 mg/dl) that is unresponsive to other measures. Bisphosphonates lower serum calcium by interfering with osteoclast-mediated bone resorption. Although hypercalcemia of myeloma responds to bisphosphonates, these agents can be nephrotoxic and should be administered only to euvolemic patients. Kidney function should be monitored closely during therapy. Treatment with pamidronate or zoledronic acid allows outpatient management of mild hypercalcemia. In addition to controlling hypercalcemia, bisphosphonates appear to inhibit growth of plasma cells and are used to treat multiple myeloma, particularly in patients with osseous lesions and bone pain.

Kidney replacement therapy as either hemodialysis or peritoneal dialysis is generally recommended in patients with kidney failure from monoclonal light-chain–related kidney diseases. Recovery of kidney function sufficient to survive without dialysis occurs in as many as 5% of patients with multiple myeloma, although in some patients, this goal requires months to achieve, probably because traditional chemotherapeutic regimens slowly reduce circulating light-chain levels. Despite the susceptibility to infection in multiple myeloma, the peritonitis rate for peritoneal dialysis, one episode every 14.4 months, is not unacceptably high. Neither peritoneal dialysis nor hemodialysis appears to provide a superior survival advantage in myeloma patients. Kidney transplant also has been performed successfully in selected myeloma patients in remission. Because the light chain is the underlying cause of cast nephropathy, tests that ensure absence of circulating free light chains are useful in the evaluation of candidacy for kidney transplantation.

OTHER TUBULOINTERSTITIAL KIDNEY LESIONS INCLUDING PROXIMAL TUBULOPATHY

Proximal tubular injury and tubulointerstitial nephritis can occur. A classic kidney presentation of multiple myeloma is Fanconi syndrome, which is characterized by type II renal tubular acidosis and defective sodium-coupled cotransport processes, producing aminoaciduria, glycosuria, and phosphaturia. Kidney biopsy typically shows crystals of light-chain protein within the epithelium of the proximal tubule. Fanconi syndrome may precede overt multiple myeloma. Plasma cell dyscrasia should therefore be considered in the differential diagnosis when this syndrome occurs in adults.

Unlike most endogenous low-molecular-weight proteins, monoclonal light chains have a propensity to produce tubular injury. Although the more common lesion is cast nephropathy, patients occasionally present with kidney failure from an isolated proximal tubulopathy that is distinct from the pathology associated with Fanconi syndrome. Kidney failure from isolated proximal tubular damage generally improves with effective chemotherapy that reduces the circulating monoclonal free light chain. A major mechanism of damage to the proximal epithelium is related to accumulation of toxic light chains in the endolysosome system. Light chains appear to catalyze sufficient amounts of hydrogen peroxide to generate intracellular oxidative stress to stimulate apoptosis and to activate NF-κB, promoting the production of inflammatory chemokines such as monocyte chemotactic factor-1. Loss of proximal tubular epithelial cells and generation of a proinflammatory milieu may also promote nephron dropout and the tubulointerstitial scarring and inflammation that are prevalent findings in cast nephropathy.

WALDENSTRÖM MACROGLOBULINEMIA

This disorder constitutes about 5% of monoclonal gammopathies and is characterized by the presence of a monoclonal B-cell malignancy consisting of lymphocytoid plasma cells. The origin of these cells is thought to be a postantigen-stimulated memory B cell that has undergone malignant transformation through somatic hypermutation. This condition clinically behaves more like lymphoma, although the malignant cell secretes IgM (macroglobulin), which usually produces most of the clinical symptoms. Lytic bone lesions are uncommon, but hepatosplenomegaly and lymphadenopathy are frequently identified. IgM is a large molecule that is not excreted and accumulates in the plasma to produce hyperviscosity syndrome, which consists of neurologic symptoms (headaches, stupor, deafness, dizziness), visual impairment (from hemorrhages and edema), bleeding diathesis (related to IgM complexing clotting factors and to platelet dysfunction), kidney failure, and symptoms of hypervolemia. Reduced GFR occurs in about 30% of patients, and hyperviscosity syndrome and precipitation of IgM in the lumen of glomerular capillaries are the most common causes. Approximately 10% to 15% of patients develop AL-type amyloidosis, but cast nephropathy is rare. Because of the typically advanced age at presentation (sixth to seventh decade) and slowly progressive course, the major therapeutic goal is relief of symptoms. All patients with IgM levels greater than 4 g/dl should have serum viscosity determined. Plasmapheresis is indicated in symptomatic patients and should be continued until symptoms resolve and serum viscosity normalizes. Kidney failure requiring kidney replacement therapy is uncommon. The course of the disease can vary but is often protracted. Factors that portend a worse outcome include age greater than 65 years and organomegaly. Patients lacking these risk factors have a median survival of 10.6 years, whereas patients with either of these risk factors have a median survival of 4.2 years. Symptomatic patients are usually treated with combination chemotherapy that includes an alkylating agent along with rituximab, because these malignant cells express CD20.

KEY BIBLIOGRAPHY

Cavo M, Rajkumar SV, Palumbo A, et al. International Myeloma Working Group consensus approach to the treatment of multiple myeloma patients who are candidates for autologous stem cell transplantation. *Blood.* 2011;117:6063-6073.

Clark WF, Stewart AK, Rock GA, et al. Plasma exchange when myeloma presents as acute renal failure: a randomized, controlled trial. *Ann Intern Med.* 2005;143:777-784.

Dember LM, Hawkins PN, Bouke PC, et al. Eprodisate for the treatment of renal disease in AA amyloidosis. *N Engl J Med.* 2007;356:2349-2360.

Deret S, Denoroy L, Lamarine M, et al. Kappa light chain-associated Fanconi's syndrome: molecular analysis of monoclonal immunoglobulin light chains from patients with and without intracellular crystals. *Protein Eng.* 1999;12:363-369.

Drayson M, Begum G, Basu S, et al. Effects of paraprotein heavy and light chain types and free light chain load on survival in myeloma: an analysis of patients receiving conventional-dose chemotherapy in Medical Research Council UK multiple myeloma trials. *Blood.* 2006;108:2013-2019.

Gertz MA. Immunoglobulin light chain amyloidosis: 2011 update on diagnosis, risk-stratification, and management. *Am J Hematol.* 2011;86:181-186.

Gertz MA, Landau H, Comenzo RL, et al. First-in-Human Phase I/II Study of NEOD001 in Patients With Light Chain Amyloidosis and Persistent Organ Dysfunction. *J Clin Oncol.* 2016;34:1097-1103.

Ghobrial IM, Fonseca R, Gertz MA, et al. Prognostic model for disease-specific and overall mortality in newly diagnosed symptomatic patients with Waldenstrom macroglobulinaemia. *Br J Haematol.* 2006;133:158-164.

Hutchison CA, Heyne N, Airia P, et al. Immunoglobulin free light chain levels and recovery from myeloma kidney on treatment with chemotherapy and high cut-off haemodialysis. *Nephrol Dial Transplant.* 2012;27:3823-3828.

Jaccard A, Moreau P, Leblond V, et al. High-dose melphalan versus melphalan plus dexamethasone for AL amyloidosis. *N Engl J Med.* 2007;357:1083-1093.

Katzmann JA, Kyle RA, Benson J, et al. Screening panels for detection of monoclonal gammopathies. *Clin Chem.* 2009;55:1517-1522.

Kourelis TV, Nasr SH, Dispenzieri A, et al. Outcomes of patients with renal monoclonal immunoglobulin deposition disease. *Am J Hematol.* 2016.

Kyle RA, Gertz MA. Primary systemic amyloidosis: clinical and laboratory features in 474 cases. *Semin Hematol.* 1995;32:45-59.

McTaggart MP, Lindsay J, Kearney EM. Replacing urine protein electrophoresis with serum free light chain analysis as a first-line test for detecting plasma cell disorders offers increased diagnostic accuracy and potential health benefit to patients. *Am J Clin Pathol.* 2013;140:890-897.

Nasr SH, Valeri AM, Cornell LD, et al. Renal monoclonal immunoglobulin deposition disease: a report of 64 patients from a single institution. *Clin J Am Soc Nephrol.* 2012;7:231-239.

Rajkumar SV, Dimopoulos MA, Palumbo A, et al. International Myeloma Working Group updated criteria for the diagnosis of multiple myeloma. *Lancet Oncol.* 2014;15:e538-e548.

Rosenstock JL, Markowitz GS, Valeri AM, et al. Fibrillary and immunotactoid glomerulonephritis: distinct entities with different clinical and pathologic features. *Kidney Int.* 2003;63:1450-1461.

van Rhee F, Bolejack V, Hollmig K, et al. High serum free-light chain levels and their rapid reduction in response to therapy define an aggressive multiple myeloma subtype with poor prognosis. *Blood.* 2007;110:827-832.

Wanchoo R, Abudayyeh A, Doshi M, et al. Renal toxicities of novel agents used for treatment of multiple myeloma. *Clin J Am Soc Nephrol.* 2017;12:176-189. doi:10.2215/CJN.06100616.

Ying WZ, Allen CE, Curtis LM, et al. Mechanism and prevention of acute kidney injury from cast nephropathy in a rodent model. *J Clin Invest.* 2012;122:1777-1785.

Full bibliography can be found on www.expertconsult.com.

Acute Cardiorenal Syndrome

Andrew A. House; Claudio Ronco

29

Cardiorenal syndromes are broadly defined as disorders of the heart and kidneys, whereby acute or chronic dysfunction in one organ induces acute or chronic dysfunction of the other. The syndromes represent the intersection and overlap of two very common conditions, heart disease and kidney disease, and an understanding of the complex bidirectional interactions of these organ systems is paramount for their management.

In this chapter, we focus on the common situation whereby patients with acute decompensated heart failure (ADHF) or acute coronary syndrome (ACS) experience abrupt worsening of kidney function known as acute kidney injury (AKI). This is termed acute cardiorenal syndrome (CRS). Other types of CRS include a more indolent form of chronic kidney disease arising in patients with longer term heart failure, termed chronic CRS. This and additional subtypes are highlighted in Box 29.1 but are not discussed in this chapter.

DEFINITION AND EPIDEMIOLOGY OF ACUTE CARDIORENAL SYNDROME

Acute CRS is defined as an acute worsening of cardiac function leading to kidney dysfunction. ADHF can represent acute presentation of de novo heart failure or, more frequently, acute decompensation of chronic heart failure and typically is characterized by rapid worsening of the typical signs and symptoms of heart failure (shortness of breath, pulmonary rales, congestion on chest radiograph, raised jugular venous pressure, and peripheral edema), as highlighted in Box 29.2 and Table 29.1. However, heart failure is a heterogeneous condition with various clinical presentations and multiple contributing factors. Although depressed left ventricular function is an important feature of heart failure, many patients presenting with ADHF have preserved left ventricular ejection fraction, and in roughly one-third of patients, ACS precipitates the decompensation. Accordingly, the hemodynamic derangements found in patients with ADHF are highly variable and to certain degrees overlapping, potentially including acute pulmonary edema with hypertension, severe peripheral fluid overload, isolated severe right heart failure with hepatic congestion, ascites and edema, cardiogenic shock, hypotension, and so on (Fig. 29.1). The European Society of Cardiology (ESC) schematic for characterizing patients based on presence or absence of congestion ("wet" or "dry") and hypoperfusion ("cold" or "warm") is depicted in Table 29.2. In addition, Table 29.3 lists the ESC diagnostic criteria and presenting clinical phenotypes of the various heart-failure syndromes as relating to reduction or preservation of ejection fraction.

Patients with acute CRS typically present with hospitalization for one of these heart-failure syndromes and meet criteria for AKI based on acute increase in serum creatinine of at least 0.3 mg/dL (26 µmol/L) and/or oliguria. The ability to detect AKI earlier (with biomarkers such as cystatin c, kidney injury molecule-1, N-acetyl-β-D-glucosaminidase, and neutrophil gelatinase-associated lipocalin) is not part of the current definition but may facilitate earlier diagnosis, perhaps affording a better opportunity to reverse or avoid acute CRS.

Heart failure itself is very common, projected to affect more than 8 million Americans by 2030 and currently implicated in one of every nine deaths in the United States. In 2012, there were more than 1 million hospitalizations for heart failure, at a total cost of nearly $30.7 billion; this cost is projected to reach nearly $70 billion by 2030. ACS as a primary admitting diagnosis is somewhat less common, although the annual incidence is much higher when secondary diagnoses are included. Of patients admitted with heart failure, acute CRS, defined as an increase in serum creatinine of ≥0.3 mg/dL (26 µmol/L), may occur in 27% to 40%. Acute CRS in this setting is associated with a nearly 50% increase in mortality, as well as increased length of hospitalization and hospital costs.

PATHOPHYSIOLOGY OF ACUTE CARDIORENAL SYNDROME

HEMODYNAMICS AND THE "TRADITIONAL" CARDIORENAL PARADIGM

One key role of a functioning cardiorenal axis is to maintain appropriate extracellular effective circulating volume, and this homeostasis is achieved through an intricate web of neurohormonal feedback loops, volume and pressure sensors, vasoactive substances, transporters, and other effector mechanisms—including the autonomic nervous system, renin-angiotensin-aldosterone system (RAAS), endothelin, arginine vasopressin, and natriuretic peptides. When these systems are functioning appropriately, they enable rapid response to changing hemodynamics and extracellular fluid volume, allowing for preserved tissue perfusion and oxygen delivery, acid-base and electrolyte homeostasis, and management of nitrogenous and other wastes.

In the past, acute CRS was believed to represent the response to falling cardiac output and renal arterial underfilling with resultant kidney hypoperfusion and diminished glomerular filtration rate (GFR). The exuberant activation of the sympathetic nervous system and RAAS then leads to significant increases in systemic angiotensin II and aldosterone, further contributing to the milieu of pressure and volume overload of the failing heart. In patients with heart failure, the kidneys release substantial amounts of renin into the circulation, and this leads in turn to production of angiotensin II. Angiotensin II has both potent systemic vasoconstrictive effects, as well as central effects on thirst and activation of the sympathetic nervous system. The vasoconstrictive effects, coupled with increased sympathetic activity, contribute to increased systemic vascular resistance, venous tone and congestion, and increased myocardial contractility, all of which may cause ventricular demand for oxygen to outstrip its supply. Angiotensin II has potent stimulatory effects on renal sodium reabsorption, and constriction of the efferent arteriole leads to an increase in the filtration fraction, causing an increase in the tubular oncotic pressure, further enhancing proximal tubular sodium and fluid reabsorption. Angiotensin II is also a potent stimulus for aldosterone release from the adrenal gland, leading to even further augmented sodium reabsorption in the distal nephron. Normally, an aldosterone escape phenomenon allows individuals with excess aldosterone to limit this salt-avid state and avoid edema formation; however, heart-failure patients lose this escape mechanism because of the neurohormonal effects that limit distal sodium delivery;

Box 29.1 Definition and Classification of the Cardiorenal Syndromes

Cardiorenal Syndromes

General Definition

Disorders of the heart and kidneys, whereby acute or chronic dysfunction in one organ may induce acute or chronic dysfunction in the other

Acute CRS (Type 1)

Acute worsening of cardiac function leading to kidney dysfunction

Chronic CRS (Type 2)

Chronic abnormalities in cardiac function leading to kidney dysfunction

Acute Renocardiac Syndrome (Type 3)

Acute worsening of kidney function causing cardiac dysfunction

Chronic Renocardiac Syndrome (Type 4)

Chronic abnormalities in kidney function leading to cardiac disease

Secondary CRS (Type 5)

Systemic conditions causing simultaneous dysfunction of the heart and kidney

CRS, Cardiorenal syndrome.

Box 29.2 Definition of Heart Failure

Heart failure is a clinical syndrome in which patients have the following features:
- **Symptoms typical of heart failure**
  - Breathlessness at rest or on exercise, fatigue, tiredness
- **Signs typical of heart failure**
  - Tachycardia, tachypnea, pulmonary rales, pleural effusion, raised jugular venous pressure, peripheral edema, hepatomegaly
- **Objective evidence of a structural or functional abnormality of the heart at rest**
  - Cardiomegaly, third heart sound, cardiac murmurs, abnormality on echocardiogram, raised concentration of natriuretic peptide

Modified from the 2008 European Society of Cardiology Guidelines for the Diagnosis and Treatment of Acute and Chronic Heart Failure.

Table 29.1 Common Clinical Manifestations of Heart Failure

Dominant Clinical Features	Symptoms	Signs
Peripheral edema/congestion	Breathlessness	Peripheral edema
	Tiredness, fatigue	Raised jugular venous pressure
	Anorexia	Pulmonary edema
		Hepatomegaly, ascites
		Fluid overload (congestion)
		Cachexia
Pulmonary edema	Severe breathlessness at rest	Pulmonary crackles, effusion
		Tachycardia, tachypnea
Cardiogenic shock (low cardiac output state)	Confusion	Poor peripheral perfusion
	Weakness	Systolic blood pressure less than 90 mm Hg
	Cold periphery	Anuria or oliguria
High blood pressure (hypertensive heart failure)	Breathlessness	Usually elevated blood pressure
		Left ventricular hypertrophy
		Preserved ejection fraction
Right heart failure	Breathlessness	Evidence of right ventricular dysfunction
	Fatigue	Raised jugular venous pulsation
		Peripheral edema, hepatomegaly

Adapted from the 2008 European Society of Cardiology Guidelines for the Diagnosis and Treatment of Acute and Chronic Heart Failure.

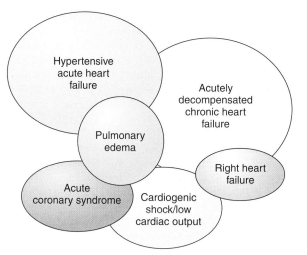

Fig. 29.1 Clinical classification of heart-failure syndromes. (Adapted from the 2008 ESC Guidelines for the Diagnosis and Treatment of Acute and Chronic Heart Failure.)

Table 29.2 Clinical Profiles of Patients With Acute Heart Failure

	Congestion Absent	Congestion Absent
Hypoperfusion absent	Warm-Dry	Warm-Wet
Hypoperfusion present	Cold-Dry	Cold-Wet

Congestion present is defined by the presence of pulmonary or peripheral edema, orthopnea or paroxysmal nocturnal dyspnea, peripheral (bilateral) edema, jugular venous dilatation, congestive hepatomegaly or hepatojugular reflux, or gut congestion or ascites. Hypoperfusion is suggested by cool and sweaty extremities, oliguria, confusion, lightheadedness, or narrow pulse pressure.
Adapted from the European Society of Cardiology; Heart Failure Association of the ESC (HFA); et al. ESC guidelines for the diagnosis and treatment of acute and chronic heart failure 2016. *Eur Heart J.* 2016;37:2129–2200.

Table 29.3 Definition of Heart Failure With Preserved, Midrange, and Reduced Ejection Fraction

Type of HF	HFrEF	HFmrEF	HFpEF
Criteria	Symptoms ± signs LV ejection fraction <40%	Symptoms ± signs LV ejection fraction 40%–49% Elevated natriuretic peptides Structural heart disease and/or diastolic dysfunction	Symptoms ± signs LV ejection fraction ≥50% Elevated natriuretic peptides Structural heart disease and/or diastolic dysfunction

HF, Heart failure; *HFmrEF,* heart failure with midrange ejection fraction; *HFpEF,* heart failure with preserved ejection fraction; *HFrEF,* heart failure with reduced ejection fraction; *LV,* Left ventricle.
Adapted from the European Society of Cardiology; Heart Failure Association of the ESC (HFA); et al. ESC guidelines for the diagnosis and treatment of acute and chronic heart failure 2016. *Eur Heart J.* 2016;37:2129–2200.

hence sodium retention continues, contributing to volume overload and edema formation.

Downstream from the activated RAAS, there is increased synthesis and activity of endothelin-1. Endothelin-1 increases renal vascular resistance, reduces renal blood flow and GFR, and may cause or amplify ischemic injury to the kidneys. Activation of the endothelin system may also enhance salt and water retention, and it causes systemic vasoconstriction, hence contributing further to volume and pressure overload. Finally, the nonosmotic release of arginine vasopressin in response to decreased effective circulating volume from heart failure leads to further enhanced vasoconstriction through the action of V1a receptors and to decreased excretion of free water because of enhanced uptake at the level of the collecting ducts mediated through V2 receptors. This in turn contributes to volume and pressure overload and development of hyponatremia (Fig. 29.2).

While this traditional "pump and filter" paradigm of cardiorenal pathophysiology is relevant to many patients with decompensated heart failure, recent observations about the types of patients developing acute CRS require us to expand our thinking. For instance, preserved ejection fraction is found in a growing proportion of patients with heart failure. In one study, almost one-half of patients developing acute

CRS exhibited preserved left ventricular ejection fraction, and a larger proportion of heart-failure patients presented with elevated blood pressure compared with patients without kidney complications. The Acute Decompensated Heart Failure Registry (ADHERE) contains information on more than 100,000 heart-failure hospitalizations in the United States, and it provides additional insights into the development of CRS. Using a more conservative definition of AKI (increase of creatinine of 0.5 mg/dL), the investigators categorized patients into four categories, with ejection fraction of less than 25%, 25% to 40%, 40% to 55%, and ≥55%, and they found small but statistically significant incremental increases in incidence of AKI with *increasing* ejection fraction at 12.1%, 14.7%, 14.9%, and 15.2%, respectively. Unsurprisingly, the groups with preserved ejection fraction had higher blood pressures on average. This disconnect between decreased cardiac performance and kidney dysfunction was recently highlighted by Hanberg et al., who examined data from the ESCAPE (Evaluation Study of Congestive Heart Failure and Pulmonary Artery Catheterization Effectiveness) trial. They found a weak but significant paradoxical *inverse* correlation between cardiac index and estimated GFR, with no association between changes in cardiac index and development of AKI.

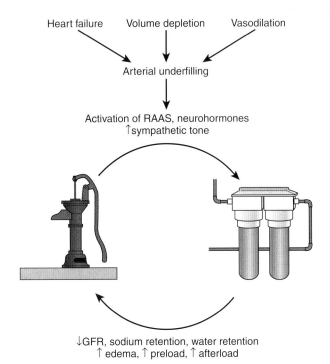

Fig. 29.2 Simplistic view of the pump and filter paradigm of the cardiorenal axis. *GFR,* Glomerular filtration rate; *RAAS,* renin-angiotensin-aldosterone system.

ADDITIONAL MECHANISMS

Beyond the traditional pump and filter paradigm, a number of additional mechanisms for acute CRS have been postulated. For instance, observations have implicated high venous pressure and raised intraabdominal pressure, leading to renal venous congestion as important contributors to impairment of kidney function. Mullens and colleagues found that raised central venous pressure, and not cardiac index, was the strongest hemodynamic predictor of AKI in the setting of ADHF. Central venous pressure is related to right heart function, blood volume, and venous capacitance, all of which are regulated by the aforementioned neurohormonal systems, and this pressure is transmitted to the draining renal veins, an observation described in heart-failure patients more than 60 years ago. As kidney perfusion and glomerular filtration are related to the arteriovenous pressure gradient, raised central venous pressure can result in decreased perfusion of the kidneys independent of arterial pressure and cardiac output, as has been shown in various animal models.

Inflammation in the setting of both chronic congestive heart failure and ADHF is increasingly recognized as playing a maladaptive role in disease progression. Inflammatory responses are designed to provide protection and to promote healing in disease states, but left unchecked, these responses may in fact promote further tissue damage or may prolong injury. Cardiac myocytes, in response to mechanical stretch or ischemia, are capable of producing a broad array of inflammatory cytokines, and elements of the innate immune response may also be upregulated. Furthermore, venous congestion may increase gut absorption of endotoxin leading to further augmentation of inflammatory responses—whereas venous congestion itself is a stimulus for peripheral synthesis and release of inflammatory mediators. Clinical evidence for this proinflammatory state is derived from observations that patients with severe heart failure experience markedly elevated levels of tumor necrosis factor-α (TNF-α); upregulation of soluble receptors for TNF; and a number of interleukins (IL), including IL-1β, IL-18, and IL-6, and upregulation of several cellular adhesion molecules. It is conceivable that these systemic responses to heart failure could contribute to distant organ damage, such as AKI. Recently, Virzi et al. demonstrated that incubating renal tubular epithelial cells with plasma from patients with acute CRS led to increased expression of proinflammatory cytokines, release of tubular damage markers, and increased apoptosis. The ischemic kidney is capable of producing a postischemic inflammatory state that can induce cardiac apoptosis and in turn contribute to ongoing apoptosis and fibrosis in the kidney. The more indolent response to this heightened proinflammatory state almost certainly contributes to chronic CRS. Furthermore, various inflammatory mediators can contribute to vascular endothelial dysfunction and capillary leak, leading to the movement of fluid into the interstitial compartment. Not only does this add to the signs and symptoms of heart failure through worsening pulmonary and peripheral edema, but movement of fluid into the interstitium further contracts the effective circulating volume, and edema within the peritubular interstitium of the kidneys contributes to tubular dysfunction and impaired GFR.

Additional considerations in the pathophysiology of acute CRS include a failure of counterregulatory systems such as natriuretic peptides; persistent renal vasoconstriction from tubuloglomerular feedback and various vasoactive substances (adenosine, endothelin); and impaired autoregulation of GFR (particularly in the setting of RAAS blockade). Natriuretic peptides are naturally occurring substances that reduce renal sodium reabsorption, promote diuresis, and work systemically to decrease sympathetic tone and RAAS activity and to cause vasodilation. Levels of natriuretic peptides are elevated in response to atrial stretch (and are certainly elevated in heart failure), yet heart-failure patients appear to lose responsiveness to these peptides, providing an additional mechanism for worsening heart and kidney failure.

Diuretics merit special mention in the pathophysiology of acute CRS. Although important for the acute management of dyspnea and pulmonary congestion, they provoke vigorous activation of both the sympathetic nervous system and RAAS, resulting in the counterproductive and maladaptive responses described earlier. Furthermore, their use is associated with diuretic resistance, requiring higher and higher doses. This resistance is multifactorial and includes decreased solute delivery to tubules because of decreased renal blood flow, decreased GFR, low albumin, and diuretic "braking" as a result of enhanced sodium reabsorption and distal tubular hypertrophy.

A pictorial overview of the complex and multifactorial pathways leading from ADHF to AKI and the acute CRS is presented in Fig. 29.3.

TREATMENT OF ACUTE CARDIORENAL SYNDROME

The management and prevention of acute CRS in the hospitalized patient with ADHF or cardiogenic shock are largely

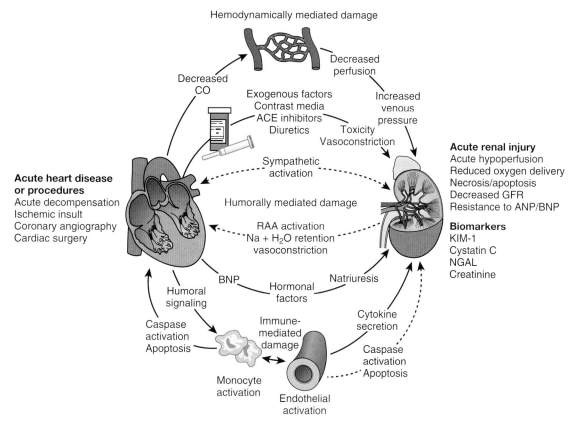

Fig. 29.3 Pathophysiologic interactions between the heart and kidney in acute cardiorenal syndrome. *ACE,* Angiotensin-converting enzyme; *ANP,* atrial natriuretic peptide; *BNP,* B-type natriuretic peptide; *CO,* cardiac output; *GFR,* glomerular filtration rate; *KIM,* kidney injury molecule; *Na,* sodium; *NGAL,* neutrophil gelatinase-associated lipocalin; *RAA,* renin angiotensin aldosterone. (Reproduced from Ronco C, Haapio M, House AA, et al. Cardiorenal syndrome. *J Am Coll Cardiol.* 2008;52:1527–1539, with permission from Elsevier. Original illustration by Rob Flewell.)

empiric, as most treatments aimed at rapid improvement of congestive symptoms or ischemia have not been studied in randomized clinical trials. Diuretics, for instance, would be difficult to withhold, but their use is often associated with worsening kidney function. High doses of diuretics have been associated with adverse outcomes, although the severity of heart failure is an obvious source of confounding. Diuretics optimally should be used in doses adequate to provide symptom relief through depletion of extracellular fluid volume at a rate that matches refilling from the interstitium to the intravascular space, balanced against the risk of further activation of neurohormonal reflexes.

Loop diuretics are preferred to thiazides as the initial choice of diuretic, because the latter produce a smaller effect in patients with more advanced kidney dysfunction. However, thiazides may need to be added to overcome diuretic resistance. Aldosterone blockade with diuretics such as spironolactone, eplerenone, and finerenone may be problematic in patients with more advanced kidney failure who are at high risk of hyperkalemia. Careful introduction and monitoring, while excluding patients with serum creatinine ≥2.5 mg/dL (220 µmol/L) or baseline hyperkalemia with potassium level ≥5.0 mEq/L, could mitigate this risk. The Diuretic Optimization Strategies Evaluation (DOSE) trial used a factorial design to compare low-dose with high-dose furosemide and administration as bolus versus infusion in 308 patients with

ADHF. The authors reported no differences in their coprimary endpoints of global assessment of symptoms and change in serum creatinine. However, bolus-group patients were twice as likely to require a dose increase compared with the infusion group, while low-dose patients were less likely to convert to oral therapy at 48 hours and more likely to require a dose increase (24% vs. 9%, *P* = .003). There was a nonsignificant trend toward greater improvement in symptoms in the high-dose group, members of which experienced greater net fluid loss, weight loss, and relief from dyspnea, although an acute rise in serum creatinine was more common in the high-dose group. Reassuringly, there were no significant differences between groups in serum creatinine and cystatin C levels at 60 days. A practical approach is to begin therapy for ADHF with bolus intravenous doses of furosemide but consider rapid conversion to infusion and/or higher doses if diuretic resistance is encountered, while closely monitoring clinical status, electrolytes, and kidney function.

As a nonpharmacologic strategy to treat patients with acute CRS more aggressively, ultrafiltration was shown in one study to be superior to diuretics, with greater fluid loss, less requirement for vasopressors, and fewer rehospitalizations and emergency room visits, although there was no difference in dyspnea, a primary study outcome, and there was no difference in secondary kidney outcomes. The subsequent Cardiorenal Rescue Study in Acute Decompensated Heart

Failure or CARRESS-HF trial did not confirm the benefits of ultrafiltration when compared with a strategy of stepped pharmacologic therapy; accordingly, ultrafiltration is generally reserved for diuretic resistance in the face of ongoing congestion.

Blockade of the RAAS is a mainstay of therapy in chronic congestive heart failure, but in acute CRS, the ability to autoregulate GFR is highly dependent on angiotensin II and its effects on the efferent arteriole. Therefore it is prudent to delay introduction of RAAS blockade (or reduce the dose in patients already receiving these drugs), particularly in low cardiac output states and/or hypotension. After kidney function stabilizes, careful introduction and titration of these agents with close monitoring of urine output and kidney function are required. Likewise, blockade of the sympathetic nervous system with beta-blockers is a reasonable goal, but if acute CRS is due to a severe low output state, beta-blockers must be used with the utmost caution if at all.

When acute CRS patients present with preserved or elevated blood pressure, vasodilators such as nitroglycerin and nitroprusside are often used to relieve symptoms and to improve hemodynamics, although their use has not been subjected to rigorous controlled study, and their effect on reversing or preventing acute CRS is unknown. Nitroglycerin is often used to relieve symptoms of congestion and ischemia, and at low doses it is a venodilator, decreasing cardiac filling pressures and reducing myocardial oxygen demand. As the dose increases, nitroglycerin can improve both preload and afterload and can increase cardiac output, although hypotension and nitrate tolerance limit its use. In a similar manner, nitroprusside has been used to dilate vascular smooth muscle in both arterial and venous systems, but because of hypotensive effects, its use is generally limited to patients with normal or elevated blood pressure. Because of the potential for accumulation of thiocyanate in patients with decreased GFR, its use in CRS is problematic, although there are reports of its safe use in ADHF patients, including those with decreased GFR and hypotension.

As mentioned previously, heart-failure patients become less responsive to endogenous natriuretic peptides. Recombinant human B-type natriuretic peptide (BNP), or nesiritide, when provided in supraphysiologic doses, can reduce levels of catecholamines, angiotensin II, and aldosterone and as a result can decrease both preload and afterload, decrease pulmonary vascular resistance, and increase cardiac output. Further, through its effects on the renal tubules, nesiritide promotes a prompt diuresis. Hence it provides rapid symptom relief in ADHF. However, studies of exogenous BNP have yielded disappointing results, with some authors suggesting increased risk of acute CRS and greater mortality. To adequately answer questions regarding safety and efficacy, the recently completed Acute Study of Clinical Effectiveness of Nesiritide in Decompensated Heart Failure (ASCEND-HF) enrolled more than 7000 patients and found no significant differences in rates of death or rehospitalization, no increased risk of acute CRS, a small improvement in dyspnea, and a near doubling of hypotension associated with nesiritide. For this reason, nesiritide cannot currently be recommended for routine treatment of patients presenting with ADHF, although studies regarding its role as a renal protective agent are ongoing.

In light of the previously described role of vasoactive substances in the pathogenesis of acute CRS, investigators have reported encouraging results related to a number of novel agents in preclinical and early clinical trials in patients with ADHF. However, as with nesiritide, subsequent larger scale trials have failed to demonstrate any substantive benefit of endothelin antagonists, vasopressin antagonists, or adenosine α1 receptor antagonists. Studies to confirm or refute the promising effects of vasodilators serelaxin and ularitide are imminently expected.

In cases of low cardiac output causing worsening heart-failure symptoms and threatening kidney function, positive inotropes such as dobutamine or phosphodiesterase inhibitors are often used, although there are serious concerns about their capacity to increase myocardial injury and to induce arrhythmias. One randomized trial of milrinone in patients with ADHF showed higher rates of hypotension and arrhythmia and no benefit related to mortality or hospitalization. Levosimendan is a phosphodiesterase inhibitor that increases myocardial sensitivity to calcium and improves hemodynamics and renal perfusion. Early studies have provided conflicting results in terms of preservation of kidney function. Levosimendan appears in the ESC guidelines for management of heart failure, adding that it may be considered to reverse effect of beta-blockade if thought to be playing a role in hypoperfusion. A recent meta-analysis suggests that it may have some beneficial effects on mortality, while another analysis suggested no short-term effect on kidney function. Levosimendan is not currently available in North America, and its precise role in the management of the prevention of acute CRS remains uncertain.

If, despite a trial of inotropic support, patients with low cardiac output and acute CRS continue to deteriorate, these patients may require more invasive treatments to serve as a bridge to recovery of kidney function, or they may require cardiac transplantation. These therapies include intraaortic balloon pulsation, ventricular assist devices, or artificial hearts; however, limited evidence supports these therapies as means to improve kidney perfusion and GFR.

SUMMARY

Acute CRS is common in patients with ADHF and/or ACS, and its appearance often heralds greater morbidity and mortality. The mechanisms behind acute CRS are complex, multifactorial, and bidirectional. Our current understanding of the pathophysiology has moved beyond the notion of the heart and kidneys operating simply as a pump and a filter, and we increasingly recognize the capacity for inflammation, apoptosis, venous congestion, and other mechanisms to contribute to the downhill spiral in the function of both organ systems. Treatment strategies are for the most part empiric, but recognition of the syndrome has led to the conduct of important, albeit largely disappointing, clinical trials as we continue to search for the optimal management of these complex cases.

KEY BIBLIOGRAPHY

Bart BA, Goldsmith SR, Lee KL, et al. Ultrafiltration in decompensated heart failure with cardiorenal syndrome. *N Engl J Med.* 2012; 367:2296-2304.

Colombo PC, Ganda A, Lin J, et al. Inflammatory activation: cardiac, renal, and cardio-renal interactions in patients with the cardiorenal syndrome. *Heart Fail Rev.* 2012;17:177-190.

Costanzo MR, Guglin ME, Saltzberg MT, et al. Ultrafiltration versus intravenous diuretics for patients hospitalized for acute decompensated heart failure. *J Am Coll Cardiol.* 2007;49:675-683.

Cuffe MS, Califf RM, Adams KF Jr, et al. Short-term intravenous milrinone for acute exacerbation of chronic heart failure: a randomized controlled trial. *JAMA.* 2002;287:1541-1547.

European Society of Cardiology; Heart Failure Association of the ESC (HFA); et al. ESC guidelines for the diagnosis and treatment of acute and chronic heart failure 2016. *Eur Heart J.* 2016;37:2129-2200.

Felker GM, Lee KL, Bull DA, et al. Diuretic strategies in patients with acute decompensated heart failure. *N Engl J Med.* 2011;364:797-805.

Forman DE, Butler J, Wang Y, et al. Incidence, predictors at admission, and impact of worsening renal function among patients hospitalized with heart failure. *J Am Coll Cardiol.* 2004;43:61-67.

Gottlieb SS, Abraham W, Butler J, et al. The prognostic importance of different definitions of worsening renal function in congestive heart failure. *J Card Fail.* 2002;8:136-141.

Hanberg JS, Sury K, Wilson FP, et al. Reduced cardiac index is not the dominant driver of renal dysfunction in heart failure. *J Am Coll Cardiol.* 2016;67:2199-2208.

House AA, Haapio M, Lassus J, et al. Therapeutic strategies for heart failure in cardiorenal syndromes. *Am J Kidney Dis.* 2010;56:759-773.

Ishihara S, Gayat E, Sato N, et al. Similar hemodynamic decongestion with vasodilators and inotropes: systematic review, meta-analysis, and meta-regression of 35 studies on acute heart failure. *Clin Res Cardiol.* 2016;105:971-980.

Kelly KJ, Burford JL, Dominguez JH. Postischemic inflammatory syndrome: a critical mechanism of progression in diabetic nephropathy. *Am J Physiol Renal Physiol.* 2009;297:F923-F931.

Landoni G, Biondi-Zoccai G, Greco M, et al. Effects of levosimendan on mortality and hospitalization: a meta-analysis of randomized controlled studies. *Crit Care Med.* 2012;40:634-646.

Mozzafarian D, Benjamin EJ, Go AS, et al. Heart disease and stroke statistics-2016 update: a report from the American Heart Association. *Circulation.* 2016;133:e38-e69.

Mullens W, Abrahams Z, Francis GS, et al. Importance of venous congestion for worsening of renal function in advanced decompensated heart failure. *J Am Coll Cardiol.* 2009;53:589-596.

Neuhofer W, Pittrow D. Role of endothelin and endothelin receptor antagonists in renal disease. *Eur J Clin Invest.* 2006;36:78-88.

O'Connor CM, Starling RC, Hernandez AF, et al. Effect of nesiritide in patients with acute decompensated heart failure. *N Engl J Med.* 2011;365:32-43.

Ronco C, Haapio M, House AA, et al. Cardiorenal syndrome. *J Am Coll Cardiol.* 2008;52:1527-1539.

Smith GL, Lichtman JH, Bracken MB, et al. Renal impairment and outcomes in heart failure: systematic review and meta-analysis. *J Am Coll Cardiol.* 2006;47:1987-1996.

Virzì GM, de Cal M, Day S, et al. Pro-apoptotic effects of plasma from patients with cardiorenal syndrome on human tubular cells. *Am J Nephrol.* 2015;41:474-484.

Full bibliography can be found on www.expertconsult.com.

30

Hepatorenal Syndrome and Other Liver-Related Kidney Diseases

Hani M. Wadei; Thomas A. Gonwa

ASSESSING KIDNEY FUNCTION IN CIRRHOTIC PATIENTS

There is no reliable method to assess kidney function in patients with cirrhosis. Serum creatinine is unreliable (especially in white women) because of their low muscle mass and because of the reduced creatine (the precursor of creatinine) generation seen in cirrhosis. Bilirubin levels also interfere with the serum creatinine measurement assessed by the Jaffé method. Because of these factors, for any given rise in serum creatinine, the glomerular filtration rate (GFR) drop is more pronounced in cirrhosis than the general population with normal muscle mass. Studies have demonstrated that almost a third of cirrhotic patients with a serum creatinine that falls in the normal range have a GFR less than 50 mL/min per 1.73 m^2. Creatinine-based equations used to estimate GFR, such as the Modification of Diet in Renal Disease (MDRD) and the Chronic Kidney Disease Epidemiology Collaboration (CKD-EPI), also overestimate GFR in the majority of patients because of the limitations of serum creatinine measurement, especially at lower levels of true GFR. Twenty-four-hour creatinine clearance is cumbersome and overestimates GFR because of increased tubular secretion of creatinine in cirrhotic patients. Cystatin C is a low-molecular-weight protein that is freely filtered by the glomerulus and subsequently metabolized in the proximal tubules. Cystatin C generation is independent of age, sex, muscle mass, or bilirubin level, which makes it an attractive biomarker to assess kidney function in cirrhosis. However, concerns regarding assay variability, interaction of cystatin C with multiple drugs, and lack of familiarity with the test have limited its use. Although the accuracy of iohexol or iothalamate clearance is lower in patients with cirrhosis than in the general population (because ascites interferes with assessment of the volume of distribution [Vd] of the radio-labeled marker), these methods are considered to be the most accurate for determining kidney function in cirrhosis.

ACUTE KIDNEY INJURY IN CIRRHOSIS: PREVALENCE AND CAUSES

Kidney dysfunction is common in patients with acute liver failure and those with cirrhosis. Studies have demonstrated that up to 50% of patients will develop one or more episodes of acute kidney injury (AKI) during the course of their illness. The risk of AKI also progressively increases with the severity of liver disease. Almost 20% of hospitalized patients with cirrhosis develop AKI during their incident hospitalization. The most common cause of AKI is volume-responsive prerenal kidney failure from diarrhea or excessive diuretic use, which accounts for almost 45% of cases. Acute tubular necrosis (ATN), from prolonged hypotension (e.g., following gastrointestinal bleeding) or exposure to nephrotoxic medications, and hepatorenal syndrome (HRS) is responsible for 32% and 23% of AKI episodes, respectively. Abdominal compartment syndrome from tense ascites (Fig. 30.1) is an increasingly recognized cause of AKI in cirrhosis. Diagnosis is based on detecting an intravesical pressure of greater than 20 mm Hg, associated with evidence of AKI. The mechanism of kidney injury is poorly understood but seems to be related to renal vein compression with subsequent decline in renal venous return, renal blood flow (RBF), and GFR. Reduction of intraabdominal pressure with paracentesis results in a brisk diuresis, increase in urine flow, and improvement in serum creatinine. Other causes of AKI, including acute interstitial nephritis and obstructive uropathy, are rare in patients with cirrhosis; obstructive uropathy accounts for less than 1% of AKI in cirrhosis.

DEFINITION OF ACUTE KIDNEY INJURY IN CIRRHOSIS

AKI in cirrhosis has been traditionally defined as a rise in serum creatinine of 50% to a level ≥1.5 mg/dL (133 µmol/L). The 1.5 mg/dL cutoff is totally arbitrary and has not been validated in any prospective study. Acute Kidney Injury Network (AKIN) criteria, which depend on percent or absolute rise in serum creatinine as well as amount of urine output, correlate with hospital and out-of-hospital mortality in patients who develop AKI in the general population. Recent studies demonstrated that AKIN criteria also predicted in-hospital as well as 6-month out-of-hospital mortality in critically ill cirrhotic patients admitted to the intensive care unit. The AKIN criteria are also better correlated with 90-day mortality than a rise of serum creatinine ≥1.5 mg/dL in patients with advanced cirrhosis. Even patients with AKIN stage 1 and a peak serum creatinine less than 1.5 mg/dL had higher mortality than those who never developed AKI. Patients presenting with higher AKIN stage (stage 2 vs. stage 1 and stage 3 vs. stage 2) and those who progressed from one AKIN stage to the next demonstrated progressively worse survival than those

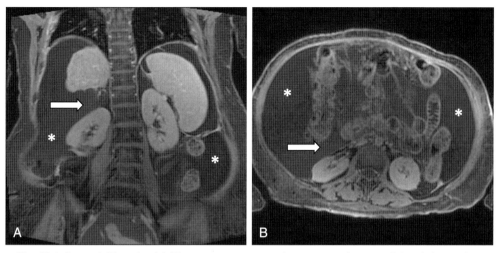

Fig. 30.1 Coronal (A) and axial (B) postcontrast magnetic resonance images of the abdomen in a cirrhotic patient. There is large volume ascites *(asterisks)* causing mass effect on the kidneys, particularly on the right *(arrows)*. Following paracentesis, serum creatinine improved, and patients reported improved urine output.

Table 30.1   International Club of Ascites Definition of Acute Kidney Injury in Patients With Cirrhosis

Subject	Definition		
Baseline sCr	A value of sCr obtained in the previous 3 months, when available, can be used as baseline sCr. In patients with more than one value within the previous 3 months, the value closest to the admission time to the hospital should be used. In patients without a previous sCr value, the sCr on admission should be used as baseline.		
Definition of AKI	• Increase in sCr ≥0.3 mg/dL (≥26.5 μmol/L) within 48 hours; or • A percentage increase sCr ≥50% from baseline that is known, or presumed, to have occurred within the previous 7 days		
Staging of AKI	• Stage 1: increase in sCr ≥0.3 mg/dL (26.5 μmol/L) or an increase in sCr ≥1.5-fold to 2-fold from baseline • Stage 2: increase in sCr >2-fold to 3-fold from baseline • Stage 3: increase of sCr >3-fold from baseline or sCr ≥4.0 mg/dL (353.6 μmol/L) with an acute increase ≥0.3 mg/dL (26.5 μmol/L) or initiation of KRT		
Progression of AKI	**Progression**		**Regression**
	Progression of AKI to higher stage and/or need for KRT		Regression of AKI to a lower stage
Response to treatment	**No Response**	**Partial Response**	**Full Response**
	No regression of AKI	Regression of AKI stage with a reduction of sCr to ≥0.3 mg/dL (26.5 μmol/L) above the baseline value	Return of sCr to a value within 0.3 mg/dL (26.5 μmol/L) of the baseline value

AKI, Acute kidney injury; *KRT,* kidney replacement therapy; *sCr,* serum creatinine.
Adapted with permission from Angeli P, et al. Diagnosis and management of acute kidney injury in patients with cirrhosis: revised consensus recommendations of the International Club of Ascites. *J Hepatol.* 2015;62:968–974.

who presented with AKIN stage 1 and whose kidney function recovered or stabilized without progression to a higher stage. In 2015, the International Club of Ascites (ICA) published a new definition for AKI in cirrhosis that aligns with the AKIN criteria for the general population. However, the urine output criterion was omitted from the ICA criteria because cirrhotic patients either are taking large doses of diuretics that affect the urine volume or are oliguric (Table 30.1).

HRS is a functional form of AKI that develops in cirrhotic patients with ascites and does not respond to volume expansion. For many years, type-1 HRS has been defined as rapid deterioration of kidney function over less than 2 weeks duration to a creatinine greater than 2.5 mg/dL, while type-2

HRS was defined as a gradual increase in serum creatinine to ≥1.5 mg/dL over weeks or months. The ICA has recently modified the definition of HRS to omit these serum creatinine cutoffs (Table 30.2). Pathophysiology and treatment of HRS are discussed later in this chapter.

IDENTIFYING THE CAUSE OF ACUTE KIDNEY INJURY IN CIRRHOSIS

Identifying the cause of AKI in cirrhotic patients can sometimes be a difficult task. Improvement of kidney function with intravascular volume expansion with albumin (1 g/kg per day) will identify patients with prerenal kidney failure from volume depletion. An intravesical pressure greater than 20 mm Hg in the setting of AKI is diagnostic of abdominal compartment syndrome and should promote measures to reduce intraabdominal pressure. Kidney ultrasound is not essential in all cases but can be used if obstructive kidney failure is suspected. The presence of granular urinary

casts, proteinuria greater than 500 mg/day, or microscopic hematuria exclude HRS. Classic teaching has advocated using fractional excretion of sodium (FENa) to differentiate between HRS and ATN, but recent studies have demonstrated that although urinary sodium excretion and FENa were lowest in patients with prerenal kidney failure, these urinary indices were also low in patients with ATN and did not differentiate between prerenal and intrinsic causes in cirrhotic patients with AKI. Because of the high risk of bleeding, kidney biopsy is rarely pursued to determine the etiology of AKI. However, there is no absolute contraindication to perform a kidney biopsy in these patients if coagulation parameters are normal, and findings from biopsy may be useful because previous studies demonstrate lack of correlation between histologic and clinical findings in cirrhosis patients. Levels of novel urinary biomarkers, including urinary neutrophil gelatinase-associated lipocalin (NGAL), are higher in patients with ATN compared with those without AKI, those with AKI from HRS, or those with prerenal kidney failure from volume depletion. However, the urinary NGAL values still show significant overlap between different causes of AKI, which limits the diagnostic accuracy of these assays. Other novel urinary biomarkers such as interleukin-18 (IL-18), kidney injury molecule-1 (KIM-1), and liver-type fatty acid-binding protein (L-FABP) are also higher in patients with ATN, but levels still overlap with those from patients with HRS. Urinary albumin excretion is also higher in patients with AKI from ATN, compared with patients with HRS, but urinary albumin excretion again shows significant overlap between these two diseases. Fig. 30.2

Table 30.2   International Club of Ascites Diagnostic Criteria of Hepatorenal Syndrome Type Acute Kidney Injury in Patients With Cirrhosis

1. Diagnosis of ascites and cirrhosis
2. Diagnosis of AKI according to the ICA-AKI criteria
3. No response after 2 consecutive days of diuretic withdrawal and plasma volume expansion with albumin 1 g/kg of body weight
4. Absence of shock
5. No current use of nephrotoxic drugs (NSAIDS, aminoglycosides, iodinated contrast media, etc.)
6. No evidence of structural kidney injury, defined as
   a. Absence of proteinuria (>500 mg/day)
   b. Absence of microhematuria (>50 RBSs per high power field)
   c. Normal findings on kidney ultrasonography

AKI, Acute kidney injury; *ICA*, International Club of Ascites; *NSAIDs*, nonsteroidal antiinflammatory drugs.

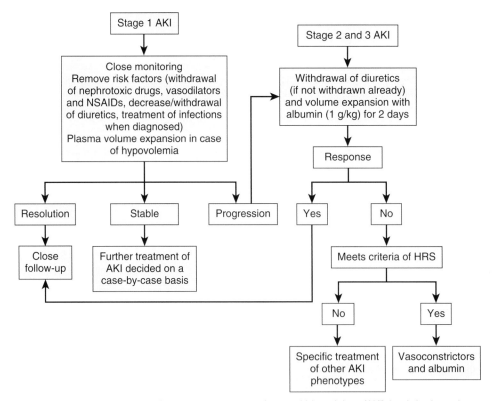

Fig. 30.2 Proposed algorithm for the management of acute kidney injury (AKI) in cirrhotic patients according to the initial Acute Kidney Injury Network stage. *NSAIDs,* Nonsteroidal antiinflammatory drugs; *HRS,* hepatorenal syndrome. (Adapted with permission from Angeli P, et al. Diagnosis and management of acute kidney injury in patients with cirrhosis: revised consensus recommendations of the International Club of Ascites. *J Hepatol.* 2015;62:968–974.)

represents a general schema for differentiating and managing cirrhotic patients with AKI according to the AKIN stage at presentation.

EFFECT OF ACUTE KIDNEY INJURY ON SURVIVAL

AKI has a strong impact on mortality in cirrhotic patients. Even after resolution of the AKI episode, patients who experienced AKI had worse survival compared with those who never developed AKI. The worst survival has been reported in patients with type-1 HRS, with some studies showing 2-week mortality as high as 80% in untreated patients. The introduction of vasoconstrictor therapy for HRS treatment and better patient care have improved survival, with one multicenter study reporting 90-day survival of 20% and 40% for patients with type-1 and type-2 HRS, respectively. Patients with volume responsive AKI and those with ATN still demonstrate lower survival compared with those without AKI episode. As alluded to earlier, progression to a higher AKI stage is associated with a progressive increase in mortality compared with those who recovered kidney function and those who did not progress to higher AKI stage.

PATHOPHYSIOLOGY OF HEPATORENAL SYNDROME

Patients with cirrhosis progress into different clinical stages. With early cirrhosis, there is increase in renal salt and water retention without any clinical evidence of ascites or peripheral edema (preascitic stage). With cirrhosis progression and further increase in renal sodium absorption, ascites starts to develop. Ascites is initially responsive to diuretics (diuretic-dependent ascites stage), but with subsequent progression of the liver disease, ascites becomes resistant to diuretics (diuretic-resistant or paracentesis-dependent ascites stage). This is the stage that precedes type-2 HRS development.

HRS is the result of a complex interplay between different pathways, including arterial vasodilatation, imbalance between vasodilator and vasoconstrictor substances, failure of renal autoregulation, systemic inflammatory response (SIRS), cardiac dysfunction, and adrenal insufficiency.

Arterial vasodilatation is the main pathophysiologic derangement that leads to HRS. Hepatic cirrhosis is associated with increased resistance of blood flow through the liver, which leads to portal hypertension, opening of portosystemic shunts, and preferential pooling of the blood volume in the splanchnic circulation. Increased production of various vasodilator mediators (e.g., nitrous oxide [NO]) that escape hepatic deactivation due to poor hepatic function and through portosystemic shunting reaches the systemic circulation, causing arterial vasodilatation, decreased systemic vascular resistance, decreased effective arterial blood volume, and hypotension. This results in off-loading of the baroreceptors in the carotid body and aortic arch and subsequent increased sympathetic nervous system (SNS) activity, increased circulating level of norepinephrine, tachycardia, and hyperdynamic circulation, with increases in cardiac output (CO). Despite the overall drop in systemic vascular resistance, vasoconstriction develops in localized vascular beds, including the brain and the kidney. In the kidney, relative arterial hypovolemia and renal vasoconstriction increase proximal sodium reabsorption and activate the renin-angiotensin-aldosterone system (RAAS), with subsequent increased aldosterone secretion, renal vasoconstriction, and salt and water retention. Nonosmotic release of vasopressin from the posterior pituitary gland helps maintain vascular tone and leads to increased free water absorption from the distal nephron and hyponatremia. In early cirrhosis (patients in the preascitic and diuretic-responsive ascites), the increase in the previously mentioned neurohumoral factors, along with the increase in CO, help maintain the effective circulating volume with no apparent change in kidney function. However, in late cirrhosis (diuretic-resistant ascites and beyond), these compensatory mechanisms fail to maintain an effective circulating volume, and renal vasoconstriction worsens, leading to HRS development. The hemodynamic and neurohumoral changes manifesting in cirrhotic patients in different stages of the liver disease are presented in Fig. 30.3.

ROLE OF SYSTEMIC INFLAMMATION

Patients with cirrhosis experience increased levels of inflammatory markers such as TNF-α, interleukin-6 (IL-6), and C-reactive protein (CRP). The levels of these inflammatory markers increase in parallel with the progression of liver disease and the increase in portal pressure. These inflammatory markers are elevated even without any clinical evidence of active infection and are probably related to the bacterial translocation to the mesenteric lymph nodes that occurs in cirrhotic patients. The level of inflammatory cytokines further increases with any infection, especially spontaneous bacterial peritonitis (SBP), leading to further deterioration of the circulatory dysfunction, decrease in CO through direct myocardial toxicity, and HRS. In one study, 41% of HRS patients showed evidence of SIRS irrespective of the presence of concomitant infection, while only 18% of patients who had AKI from hypovolemia had SIRS. Moreover, the presence of SIRS was associated with higher mortality in these patients. The role of inflammation in the pathogenesis of HRS is further supported by studies showing that gut decontamination with rifaximin leads to improvement in systemic hemodynamics and kidney function in cirrhotic patients with ascites. Norfloxacin for SBP prophylaxis has been shown to reduce the risk of HRS independent of SBP prevention. Pentoxifylline, a TNF-α inhibitor, decreases the risk of HRS in patients with alcoholic hepatitis in some but not all studies.

ROLE OF CARDIAC DYSFUNCTION

Patients with liver disease experience hyperdynamic circulation with a progressive increase in CO and decline in systemic vascular resistance, which together help maintain the effective circulatory volume. Patients with HRS have lower CO at baseline (i.e., before HRS ensues), and CO decreases further when HRS develops, implicating cardiac dysfunction as a contributor to the circulatory dysfunction that occurs in HRS. Cardiac dysfunction might explain the higher risk of

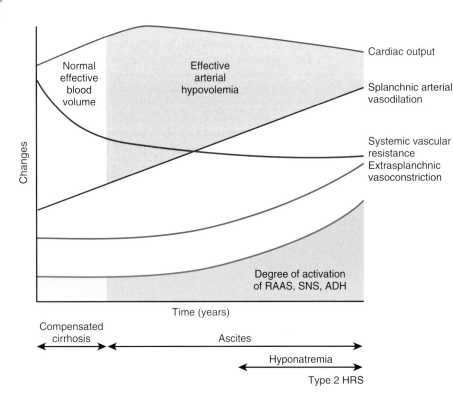

Fig. 30.3 Hemodynamic and neurohumoral changes occurring in patients with cirrhosis. *ADH,* Antidiuretic hormone; *HRS,* hepatorenal syndrome; *RAAS,* renin-angiotensin-aldosterone system; *SNS,* sympathetic nervous system. (Adapted with permission from Arroyo V, Fernández J. Management of hepatorenal syndrome in patients with cirrhosis *Nat Rev Nephrol.* 2011;7:517–526.)

HRS in patients receiving nonselective β-blockers to lower portal pressure. The etiology of HRS-related cardiac dysfunction is unclear but could be related to increased cytokine production in cirrhosis, especially in cases that are associated with sepsis and cirrhotic cardiomyopathy and in those that are due to direct sympathetic myocardial toxicity. Diastolic dysfunction is common in cirrhotic patients but is often mild and does not seem to contribute to the circulatory dysfunction or HRS.

ROLE OF RENAL PROSTAGLANDINS AND RENAL AUTOREGULATION

In response to the increase in SNS and RAAS activity, levels of intrarenal vasodilating peptides such as kallikreins and prostaglandin I2 and E2 all increase in cirrhotic patients, with higher urinary prostaglandin excretion in cirrhotic patients with ascites compared with normal controls. Urinary prostaglandin excretion is lower in HRS patients than in cirrhotic patients with preserved kidney function, and the expression of the cyclooxygenase enzyme in renal medullary tissue is lower in HRS patients compared with those with AKI from other causes. What triggers the decrease in vasodilating peptide production is unclear, but intense renal vasoconstriction and associated tissue ischemia may play a role. Another possible explanation is the increased release of local vasoconstrictors such as endothelin-1 (ET-1). Despite these known abnormalities, neither prostaglandin infusion nor ET-1 receptor blockers have proven beneficial in HRS treatment. Failure of renal autoregulation has also been observed in cirrhosis with a rightward shift of the renal perfusion pressure/RBF curve, indicating lower RBF for any given renal perfusion pressure. This rightward shift directly correlates with the circulating (endogenous) norepinephrine

level, indicating that increased SNS activity plays a role in the abnormal autoregulation seen in HRS.

ROLE OF ADRENAL INSUFFICIENCY

Relative adrenal insufficiency (as evidenced by inadequate cortisol production) has been observed in 80% of HRS patients but in only a third of cirrhotic patients with normal serum creatinine, suggesting a role for adrenal insufficiency in HRS development. Adrenal insufficiency is probably related to the arterial vasoconstriction affecting the adrenal glands. Fig. 30.4 summarizes the different pathophysiologic mechanisms involved in HRS development.

PRECIPITATING EVENTS

Almost 50% to 80% of type-1 HRS patients experience one or more precipitating events before HRS occurs. Bacterial infections, especially SBP, are the most commonly recognized factor that precede HRS. Other precipitating events include gastrointestinal bleeding, large volume paracentesis without albumin infusion, and acute alcoholic hepatitis. These precipitating events are associated with elevated levels of the aforementioned inflammatory cytokines that aggravate the circulatory dysfunction, leading to worsening renal vasoconstriction and HRS. Although most patients with gastrointestinal bleeding develop hypotension (which can precipitate ATN), there is also evidence that gastrointestinal bleeding is associated with transient increase in endotoxin levels, which can directly precipitate HRS. This could explain why antibiotic prophylaxis following gastrointestinal bleeding has been associated with a lower risk of HRS development.

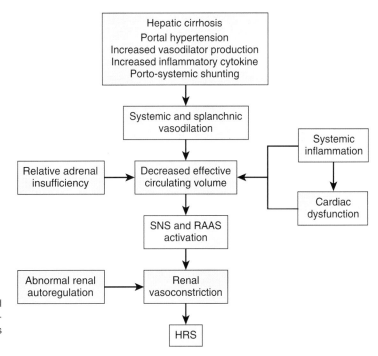

Fig. 30.4 Pathophysiologic mechanisms that lead to hepatorenal syndrome (HRS) development in cirrhotic patients. *RAAS,* Renin-angiotensin-aldosterone system; *SNS,* sympathetic nervous system.

PREVENTION OF HEPATORENAL SYNDROME

Many strategies have proven beneficial for reducing the rate of AKI and HRS in cirrhotic patients. An overall approach to the patient with kidney dysfunction in cirrhosis is outlined in Fig. 30.2 and explained in the next two sections. Patients with advanced liver disease should strictly avoid nonsteroidal antiinflammatory drugs (NSAIDs), as these medications reduce the production of vasodilator renal prostaglandins, which in turn can precipitate irreversible HRS. Other nephrotoxic medications, such as radiocontrast agents, should be used judiciously or avoided altogether, as they might precipitate AKI. Patients with ascites present a delicate treatment problem. In the early phase of cirrhosis, ascites is responsive to measures such as salt restriction and diuretic use. Loop diuretics alone or combined with aldosterone antagonists (such as spirono-lactone) may be used judiciously for comfort and treatment of compartment syndrome. However, aggressive overuse may lead to hypotension, hyper- or hypo-kalemia, AKI, and HRS. As cirrhosis progresses, the ascites becomes resistant to these measures, and treatment becomes centered on intermittent paracentesis. Diuretics should be withheld in patients with paracentesis-dependent ascites, and albumin infusion should be initiated immediately after large volume paracentesis (>5 L) at a rate of 8 g of albumin for each liter of ascitic fluid removed to avoid hypotension and postparacentesis syndrome. Concentrated 25% albumin is preferred to 5% albumin to avoid the infusion of a large volume that can precipitate acute pulmonary edema. Aggressive use can lead to the same detrimental consequences of hypotension, AKI, and irreversible HRS. Nonselective β-blockers should be used with caution in patients with paracentesis-dependent ascites, as they might precipitate postparacentesis circulatory dysfunction and aggravate myocardial dysfunction. Prophylactic antibiotics to prevent SBP are effective for reducing the risk of HRS in patients with low-protein ascites (serum albumin <1.5 g/dL). Antibiotic prophylaxis may also reduce the risk of HRS following gastrointestinal bleeding. All infections should be identified and aggressively treated with appropriate antibiotics and perhaps albumin infusion, which can improve survival and lower the HRS risk associated with certain infections compared with antibiotics alone.

TREATMENT OF HEPATORENAL SYNDROME

Vasoconstrictor agents are the cornerstone of HRS therapy and should be given together with albumin infusion, because combination treatment is more likely to be successful than vasoconstrictor therapy alone. The best-studied vasoconstrictor agent is terlipressin, which is not available in the United States or Canada. Terlipressin is metabolized by exopeptidases to lysine vasopressin, which is released slowly and allows intermittent bonus injection of the medication without the need for continuous intravenous infusion. Lysine vasopressin subsequently binds to the vasopressin (V1) receptor, which is preferentially expressed in the vascular smooth muscles of the splanchnic circulation, leading to splanchnic vasoconstriction. Studies demonstrate that terlipressin is effective in HRS reversal in almost two-thirds of cases of type-1 and type-2 HRS. Terlipressin was also associated with amelioration of the neurohumoral abnormalities and improvement in urine output, blood pressure, and hyponatremia in patients who responded to therapy. Median time to HRS reversal with terlipressin is 7 days. Importantly, all patients who responded to therapy did so in the first 14 days of treatment. High serum creatinine at the time of terlipressin initiation is associated with lower response rate, while 5 to 10 mm Hg increase in mean arterial blood pressure with terlipressin is associated with higher rates of response. Two-thirds of patients who had HRS due to infection failed to respond to traditional HRS treatment that included terlipressin and albumin. These patients had higher levels of urinary biomarkers associated with tubular damage than patients who had HRS from other causes, indicating a different pathophysiologic mechanism for kidney failure in these patients. The major side effects of terlipressin are related to ischemic events that occur at a rate between 5% and 30%. Therefore high-risk patients with a history of coronary artery disease should be treated cautiously with terlipressin. Terlipressin injections can be administered without the need for intensive care admission. However, after terlipressin discontinuation, 50% of patients will have HRS recurrence that usually responds to the reintroduction of terlipressin.

Norepinephrine is an α-1 adrenergic agonist that is as effective as terlipressin in reversing HRS. However, studies of norepinephrine and albumin infusion included a lower number of patients than those of terlipressin. The side-effect profile was also similar between the two agents. Norepinephrine is readily available for use in the United States and Canada and is less expensive than terlipressin but needs continuous monitoring in the intensive care unit. The mean effective dose of norepinephrine is 0.8 mg/hour, and in some studies dose titration to achieve a 10 mm Hg increase in mean arterial blood pressure (rather than administration of a fixed dose) was associated with response to therapy.

Midodrine is another α-adrenergic agonist that is metabolized in the liver to the active metabolite desglymidodrine. When administered as monotherapy, midodrine was associated with modest improvement in blood pressure but had no effect on improvement in kidney function in HRS patients. However, the combination of midodrine, octreotide, and albumin infusion was associated with improvement in kidney function and HRS reversal in small sample studies. However, recent studies with a large number of patients demonstrated lower efficacy of the midodrine/octreotide combination in HRS reversal compared with terlipressin. Midodrine is inexpensive, has a favorable side-effect profile, and can be given orally, which makes it an attractive option for the outpatient management of type-2 HRS patients. Midodrine can be started at a dose of 2.5 mg 3 times daily and then titrated up to 15 mg thrice daily according to response. Octreotide is injected subcutaneously at a starting dose of 50 μg thrice daily and can be increased to 200 μg thrice daily as needed.

TRANSJUGULAR INTRAHEPATIC PORTOSYSTEMIC SHUNT

Transjugular intrahepatic portosystemic shunt (TIPS) insertion reduces portal pressure and restores some of the hemodynamic and neurohumoral abnormalities observed in cirrhotic patients. In nonrandomized studies, TIPS insertion was associated with reversal of HRS in almost 50% of type-1 and type-2 HRS patients. TIPS insertion has also been successful in patients who partially responded to vasoconstrictor therapy, with further improvement in RBF, GFR, serum creatinine, and natriuresis after TIPS. The mechanism by which TIPS insertion improves kidney function is probably related to the improvement in the systemic circulatory volume and

amelioration of cardiac function. Effects of TIPS on kidney function, however, are delayed, with most studies reporting 2- to 4-week lag time from TIPS insertion to improvement in kidney function. However, TIPS is associated with worsening hepatic encephalopathy and, in some patients, cardiac decompensation. Careful patient selection for TIPS insertion is needed.

KIDNEY REPLACEMENT THERAPY

Kidney dysfunction in patients with HRS (especially type-1 HRS) may progress to the point that kidney replacement therapy (KRT) is needed. Indications for KRT include volume overload, uremia, and intractable metabolic acidosis or hyperkalemia. KRT is also indicated in patients with encephalopathy and advanced kidney dysfunction, as it is hard to differentiate if mental status changes are related to liver disease or uremia. Studies have shown that both intermittent hemodialysis (IHD) and continuous venovenous hemodiafiltration (CVVHD) or hemofiltration (CVVH) are equally effective in these patients in controlling uremia and achieving target volume balance. However, because of the tenuous hemodynamic status often seen in HRS patients, IHD can sometimes be poorly tolerated, and CVVHD or CVVH is an acceptable alternative modality. Peritoneal dialysis might be an option in stable patients, but it carries the risk of peritonitis and malnutrition from protein wasting. CVVHD and CVVH have been associated with worse survival than IHD, perhaps because of confounding by illness severity. One clear indication for continuous KRT is in patients with fulminant hepatic failure and increased intracranial pressure, as IHD can worsen intracranial pressure and cause brainstem herniation. Irrespective of the dialysis modality chosen, reasonable therapeutic goals should be set before dialysis initiation. Patients and families need to be aware of the limited chance of kidney recovery and the high mortality rates associated with HRS, especially in patients who are not candidates for liver transplantation (LT). In liver transplant candidates, the choice of dialysis modality should be individualized, depending on the patient's condition and hemodynamic status.

LIVER TRANSPLANTATION AND KIDNEY RECOVERY

Successful LT is associated with reduction in serum aldosterone and renin levels, improvement in systemic blood pressure, normalization of the renal resistive indices, and increase in renal sodium excretion. However, normalization of kidney function after LT occurs in only two-thirds of patients who required pre-LT KRT. Online calculators using clinical and demographic pre-LT information have been developed to predict who will recover kidney function after LT. However, because of the complex interplay of pre-LT and post-LT factors on kidney recovery rate, it is very difficult to accurately predict who will recover kidney function with LT alone. The most important pre-LT determinant of kidney recovery is the duration of KRT. Most studies demonstrate a precipitous drop in kidney recovery rates in patients who had KRT for 8 weeks or more before LT. In one study, 71%, 56%, 23%, and 11% of patients on KRT for less than 30 days, 31 to 60

Table 30.3 Causes of Kidney Disease in Patients With Liver Disease

Etiology of Liver Disease	Pathologic Presentation	Notes
HCV	• Membranoproliferative glomerulonephritis (MPGN) • Cryoglobulinemic glomerulonephritis (GN) • Membranous GN	—
HBV	• Membranous nephropathy • MPGN • Polyarteritis nodosa (PAN)	—
NASH	Diabetic nephropathy	—
Sarcoidosis	Granulomatous tubulointerstitial nephritis	—
Amyloidosis	Amyloidosis	—
α1-antitrypsin deficiency	MPGN	Rare association More associated with the PI*ZZ genotype
Primary sclerosing cholangitis	Drug-related nephrotoxicity	pANCA is positive in almost 80% Kidney stones Secondary hyperoxaluria
Primary biliary cirrhosis	Membranous GN Minimal change disease	Positive AMA >1:40 Other autoimmune disease such as thyroiditis, Sjögren syndrome, rheumatoid arthritis, and scleroderma may occur
Autoimmune hepatitis	Lupus-like immune-mediated glomerulonephritis Membranous GN	Only 2%–5% of autoimmune hepatitis patients; positive ASMA, ALKA
Polycystic liver disease	Autosomal dominant polycystic kidney disease	—
Congenital hepatic fibrosis	Autosomal recessive polycystic kidney disease	—
Acetaminophen toxicity	Unresolved acute tubular necrosis	— —
Schistosomiasis	Immune-mediated GN AA amyloidosis	—
Visceral leishmaniasis	Interstitial nephritis	—

AA, Amyloid A; *ALKA,* anti–liver-kidney antibodies; *AMA,* antimitochondrial antibodies; *ASMA,* antismooth muscle antibodies; *HBV,* hepatitis B virus; *HCV,* hepatitis C virus; *NASH,* nonalcoholic steatohepatitis; *pANCA,* perinuclear neutrophil antibodies.

days, 61 to 90 days, and greater than 90 days recovered kidney function, respectively. Because of the clear association between the pre-LT duration of KRT and post-LT kidney recovery, the majority of transplant centers consider that kidney recovery is unlikely in patients on KRT for 6 to 12 weeks, and will list these patients for combined liver-kidney transplantation. Pre-LT diabetes mellitus is another important factor that negatively affects post-LT kidney recovery. Other pre-LT factors that negatively affect post-LT kidney recovery include prolonged duration of kidney dysfunction and older recipient age. Intraoperative hypotension, intraoperative bleeding as measured by the number of units of packed red blood cell (PRBC) transfused, need for surgical re-exploration, older donor age, and post-LT allograft dysfunction are transplant-related factors that reduce the likelihood of kidney recovery. Delaying calcineurin inhibitor may be beneficial in enhancing kidney recovery following LT.

CAUSES OF CHRONIC KIDNEY DISEASE IN CIRRHOTIC PATIENTS

While most patients with cirrhosis and kidney dysfunction have AKI or HRS, other causes of kidney dysfunction must be evaluated and excluded. Viral infections such as hepatitis C virus (HCV) and hepatitis B virus (HBV) can cause both hepatic cirrhosis and CKD. Nonalcoholic steatohepatitis

(NASH) is now a leading cause of hepatic cirrhosis. Patients with NASH often have a prolonged history of diabetes that puts them at risk for diabetic nephropathy. With the availability of newly approved antiviral medications that appear to successfully eradicate HCV infection, the proportion of cirrhotic patients due to NASH is expected to increase. Polycystic liver and kidney disease is another important etiology of both end-stage liver and kidney diseases. Although IgA nephropathy is the most common kidney pathology in cirrhotic patients who undergo kidney biopsy, the majority of these cases do not have significantly reduced GFR. Some of the causes of CKD in patients with cirrhosis are presented in Table 30.3.

CONCLUSION

AKI is common in patients with hepatic cirrhosis and foretells a grim prognosis. HRS is a specific type of AKI that occurs only in patients with fulminant liver failure or in patients with advanced cirrhosis and ascites. HRS diagnostic criteria have recently been modified. Differentiating between HRS, other causes of AKI, and CKD in cirrhotic patients can sometimes be a difficult task. Vasoconstrictor therapy is the cornerstone of therapy for HRS and can improve outcomes in some patients, but the definitive treatment for severe HRS is liver transplantation.

KEY BIBLIOGRAPHY

Altamirano J, Fagundes C, Dominguez M, García E, Michelena J, Cárdenas A, Guevara M, Pereira G, Torres-Vigil K, Arroyo V, Caballeria J, Ginès P, Bataller R. Acute kidney injury is an early predictor of mortality for patients with alcoholic hepatitis. *Clin Gastroenterol Hepatol.* 2012;10:65-71.

Angeli P, Gines P, Wong F, Bernardi M, Boyer TD, Gerbes A, Moreau R, Jalan R, Sarin SK, Piano S, Moore K, Lee SS, Durand F, Salerno F, Caraceni P, Kim WR, Arroyo V, Garcia-Tsao G, International Club of Ascites. Diagnosis and management of acute kidney injury in patients with cirrhosis: revised consensus recommendations of the International Club of Ascites. *Gut.* 2015;64:531-537.

Angeli P, Sanyal A, Moller S, Alessandria C, Gadano A, Kim R, Sarin SK, Bernardi M, International Club of Ascites. Current limits and future challenges in the management of renal dysfunction in patients with cirrhosis: report from the International Club of Ascites. *Liver Int.* 2013; 33:16-23.

Arroyo V, Bernardi M, Epstein M, Henriksen JH, Schrier RW, Rodes J. Pathophysiology of ascites and functional renal failure in cirrhosis. *J Hepatol.* 1988;6:239-257.

Arroyo V, Fernandez J. Management of hepatorenal syndrome in patients with cirrhosis. *Nat Rev Nephrol.* 2011;7:517-526.

Belcher JM, Garcia-Tsao G, Sanyal AJ, Bhogal H, Lim JK, Ansari N, Coca SG, Parikh CR, Consortium T-A. Association of AKI with mortality and complications in hospitalized patients with cirrhosis. *Hepatology.* 2013;57:753-762.

Belcher JM, Sanyal AJ, Peixoto AJ, Perazella MA, Lim J, Thiessen-Philbrook H, Ansari N, Coca SG, Garcia-Tsao G, Parikh CR, Consortium T-A. Kidney biomarkers and differential diagnosis of patients with cirrhosis and acute kidney injury. *Hepatology.* 2014;60:622-632.

Boyer TD, Sanyal AJ, Wong F, Frederick RT, Lake JR, O'Leary JG, Ganger D, Jamil K, Pappas SC, REVERSE Study Investigators. Terlipressin plus albumin is more effective than albumin alone in improving renal function in patients with cirrhosis and hepatorenal syndrome type 1. *Gastroenterology.* 2016;150:1579-1589 e1572.

Cavallin M, Kamath PS, Merli M, Fasolato S, Toniutto P, Salerno F, Bernardi M, Romanelli R, Colletta C, Salinas F, Giacomo A, Ridola L, Fornasiere E, Caraceni P, Morando F, Piano S, Gatta A, Angeli P, Italian Association for the Study of the Liver Study Group on Hepatorenal Syndrome. Terlipressin plus albumin versus midodrine and octreotide plus albumin in the treatment of hepatorenal syndrome: a randomized trial. *Hepatology.* 2015;62:567-574.

de Carvalho JR, Villela-Nogueira CA, Luiz RR, Guzzo PL, da Silva Rosa JM, Rocha E, Moraes Coelho HS, de Mello Perez R. Acute kidney injury network criteria as a predictor of hospital mortality in cirrhotic patients with ascites. *J Clin Gastroenterol.* 2012;46:6.

Dong T, Aronsohn A, Gautham Reddy K, Te HS. Rifaximin decreases the incidence and severity of acute kidney injury and hepatorenal syndrome in cirrhosis. *Dig Dis Sci.* 2016;61:3621-3626.

Elia C, Graupera I, Barreto R, Solà E, Moreira R, Huelin P, Ariza X, Solé C, Pose E, Baiges A, Fabrellas N, Poch E, Fernández J, Arroyo V, Ginès P. Severe acute kidney injury associated with non-steroidal antiinflammatory drugs in cirrhosis: a case-control study. *J Hepatol.* 2015;63:593-600.

Fagundes C, Barreto R, Guevara M, Garcia E, Solà E, Rodríguez E, Graupera I, Ariza X, Pereira G, Alfaro I, Cárdenas A, Fernández J, Poch E, Ginès P. A modified acute kidney injury classification for diagnosis and risk stratification of impairment of kidney function in cirrhosis. *J Hepatol.* 2013;59:474-481.

Fernandez J, Navasa M, Planas R, Montoliu S, Monfort D, Soriano G, Vila C, Pardo A, Quintero E, Vargas V, Such J, Gines P, Arroyo V. Primary prophylaxis of spontaneous bacterial peritonitis delays hepatorenal syndrome and improves survival in cirrhosis. *Gastroenterology.* 2007;133:818-824.

Francoz C, Nadim MK, Durand F. Kidney biomarkers in cirrhosis. *J Hepatol.* 2016;65:809-824.

Garcia-Tsao G, Parikh CR, Viola A. Acute kidney injury in cirrhosis. *Hepatology.* 2008;48:2064-2077.

Gluud LL, Christensen K, Christensen E, Krag A. Systematic review of randomized trials on vasoconstrictor drugs for hepatorenal syndrome. *Hepatology.* 2010;51:576-584.

Gonwa TA. Combined kidney liver transplant in the MELD era: where are we going? *Liver Transpl.* 2005;11:1022-1025.

Gonwa TA, Jennings L, Mai ML, Stark PC, Levey AS, Klintmalm GB. Estimation of glomerular filtration rates before and after orthotopic liver transplantation: evaluation of current equations. *Liver Transplant.* 2004;10:301-309.

Gonwa TA, Mai ML, Melton LB, Hays SR, Goldstein RM, Levy MF, Klintmalm GB. Renal replacement therapy and orthotopic liver transplantation: the role of continuous veno-venous hemodialysis. *Transplantation.* 2001;71:1424-1428.

Full bibliography can be found on www.expertconsult.com.

ACUTE KIDNEY INJURY

31 Clinical Approach to the Diagnosis of Acute Kidney Injury

Etienne Macedo; Ravindra L. Mehta

PATHOPHYSIOLOGY

The main causes of acute kidney injury (AKI) are associated with decreased kidney perfusion resulting from conditions such as hemorrhage, vomiting, diarrhea, poor oral intake, burns, kidney losses, impaired cardiac output, decreased vascular resistance, and renal vasoconstriction. Because the kidneys receive up to 25% of the cardiac output, any decrease in mean arterial pressure may affect kidney perfusion. A decrease in oxygen delivery severe or prolonged enough to impair cellular function can cause tubular or vascular endothelium dysfunction. The mismatch between oxygen delivery and demand is more prominent in certain regions of the kidney because variations in blood flow are characteristic of renal circulation. Acute tubular necrosis (ATN) describes the pathologic result from severe or prolonged hypoperfusion or toxic injury, but it is often not present in a patient with AKI. The most common findings described in AKI—detachment of renal tubular epithelial (RTE) cells from the basement membrane, effacement and loss of brush border in proximal tubular segments, formation of tubular casts derived from sloughed cells, tubular debris, interstitial edema, and congestion of the peritubular capillaries—are not necessarily present in human biopsy sample. In addition, the degree of glomerular filtration rate (GFR) falls and these pathologic alterations in AKI are often not correlated, demonstrating the complex interplay of vascular and tubular processes that determine kidney dysfunction in AKI.

The classification of AKI into initiation, extension, maintenance, and recovery phases can be helpful for understanding the interactions of inflammation and tubular and vascular factors in determining the extent of injury. The initiation phase occurs when renal blood flow decreases to a level that results in ATP depletion, or a toxin induces acute cell injury and/or dysfunction. The severity and duration of ischemia or toxic damage define the degree of the endothelial and/or tubular cell dysfunction. During this initiation phase, upregulation of cytokines triggers the inflammatory cascade, further worsening kidney perfusion. In addition, several endothelial mechanisms may affect kidney perfusion, including the regulation of intrinsic vascular constriction and response to vasoconstrictors or vasodilators. In the extension phase, the subsequent necrosis and apoptosis defines the extent of injury and fall in GFR. Although the inflammatory cell infiltration can be detected within 24 hours following ischemia and leukocytes may appear within 2 hours, this period is the most favorable phase to allow a therapeutic

intervention to contain the amplification of the inflammatory response. In the maintenance phase, blood flow normalizes, GFR stabilizes, and the process of cell repair, migration, and proliferation initiates. In the following recovery phase, cellular differentiation continues and epithelial polarity is reestablished.

The degree of cell injury and dysfunction is heterogeneous in the kidney. While cells in the cortical region can remain viable and able to functionally and structurally recover, cells within the proximal tubule and the thick ascending limb in the outer medulla are more likely to suffer lethal injury. With sublethal injury, disruption of the actin cytoskeleton and loss of polarity lead to tubular back leak and obstruction. In more severe AKI, cell death occurs and can be confirmed by the presence of cellular debris and casts on urine microscopy. Two processes are associated with cell death; *necrosis* results in a profound inflammatory response as a trigger, while *apoptosis* initiates a regulated program leading to DNA fragmentation and cytoplasmic condensation without triggering an inflammatory response.

The remarkable efficiency of the reparative process after acute injury is attributable to the capacity of tubular epithelial cells to redifferentiate and restore the functional integrity of the kidney. New techniques of functional genomics and complementary DNA microarray have been able to demonstrate the complex pathways leading to kidney repair. Some of the genes upregulated in the reparative process are involved in cell-cycle regulation, inflammation, cell death regulation, and growth factor or cytokine production. The identification of these genes led to the discovery of early biomarkers of AKI, such as KIM-1, neutrophil gelatinase–associated lipocalin (NGAL), tissue inhibitor of metalloproteinase 2 (TIMP-2), insulin-like growth factor binding protein 7 (IGFBP7), and interleukin 18. In addition to their value for early AKI detection, these new biomarkers may also play a role in the process of injury and/or repair after AKI.

ACUTE KIDNEY INJURY DEFINITION

With the development of the classification system for AKI (RIFLE [Risk, Injury, Failure, Loss, and End-stage Kidney], AKIN [Acute Kidney Injury Network], and KDIGO [Kidney Disease International Global Outcomes]) and the introduction of the term AKI, we have seen an improved and broadly used definition of kidney injury (Fig. 31.1). The RIFLE criteria were initially proposed in 2004, with AKIN criteria released in 2007 and the KDIGO system in 2012. The criteria maintain

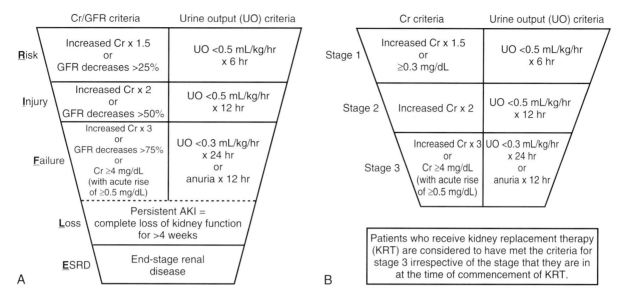

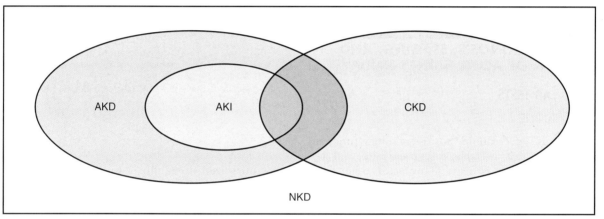

	Functional criteria	Structural criteria
AKI (acute kidney injury)	Increase in SCr by 50% within 7 days, *or* increase in SCr by 0.3 mg/dL within 2 days, *or* oliguria	No criteria
CKD (chronic kidney disease)	GFR <60 for >3 mo	Kidney damage for >3 mo
AKD (acute kidney diseases and disorders)	AKI, or GFR <60 for <3 mo, *or* decrease in GFR by ≥35% *or* increase in SCr by >50% for <3 mo	Kidney damage for <3 mo
NKD (no known kidney disease)	GFR ≥60, stable SCr	No kidney damage

C

Fig. 31.1 Risk, Injury, Failure, Loss, and End-stage Kidney (RIFLE), Acute Kidney Injury Network (AKIN), and Kidney Disease: Improving Global Outcomes (KDIGO) classification systems. (A) Risk, Injury, Failure, Loss, and End-stage Kidney. (B) AKIN, and KDIGO Classification Systems. The KDIGO definition has modified the serum creatinine criteria for Stage 1 (minimum stage for diagnosis) to include an absolute change in serum creatinine of ≥0.3 mg/dL over 48 hours or a relative change of ≥50% over 7 days. C, Definitions of kidney disease and their overlapping relationship. eGFR does not reflect measured GFR as accurately in AKI as in CKD. *AKD,* Acute kidney disease; *AKI,* acute kidney injury; *CKD,* chronic kidney disease; *Cr,* creatinine; *eGFR,* estimated glomerular filtration rate; *ESRD,* end-stage renal disease; *GFR,* glomerular filtration rate; *KRT,* kidney replacement therapy; *mGFR,* measured glomerular filtration rate; *NKD,* no known kidney disease; *SCr,* serum creatinine; *UO,* urine output.

a 48-hour time interval for absolute changes in creatinine, and a 7-day time interval for relative changes in creatinine. The KDIGO group has also proposed a new term, acute kidney disease (AKD), to address the problem that changes in creatinine may evolve over periods longer than 7 days and thus not meet the AKI definition. AKD can occur with or without other acute or chronic kidney diseases (CKDs) and disorders (see Fig. 31.1C).

Although the use of standardized definitions has greatly improved the current knowledge of AKI, there are still shortcomings with the criteria to define AKI. Serum creatinine (sCr) requires comparison to a baseline or a reference value that may not always be available. Thus to define AKI, we need two sCr values, including a "baseline" creatinine value representing the patient's underlying kidney function. In the absence of a known baseline value, a reference value after injury initiation and loss of kidney function can delay or prevent AKI detection. Conversely, a reference value days after the hospital stay affected by possible loss of muscle mass can falsely define AKI.

TOOLS FOR DIAGNOSIS, STAGING, AND EVALUATION OF ACUTE KIDNEY INJURY

STANDARD LAB TESTS

SERUM CREATININE

Although the use of creatinine to assess kidney function is not ideal, it is widely available, easy to measure, and has been used for more than 80 years. Many factors other than kidney function, such as age, sex, muscle mass, catabolic rate, and race, influence creatinine concentration. sCr has a stable concentration, which makes it inadequate to access kidney filtration, a parameter that fluctuates continually. Thus changes in GFR often correlate poorly with changes in sCr concentration. Three factors influence the sCr concentration: the actual GFR, fluctuations in creatinine production, and fluid balance affecting the volume of distribution. Furthermore, in patients with normal kidney reserve, sCr may not change, despite acute tubular injury, because of compensatory increases in function of other nephrons, creating a delay in diagnosis after injury.

In AKI, sCr generation is not equal to filtration and excretion, resulting in retention of creatinine with a rising plasma level. Until the levels of creatinine reach a plateau at a new steady state, usually 24 to 72 hours after a known injury event, assessment of sCr can overestimate kidney function. Fluid administration is another common factor delaying AKI diagnosis by sCr, as fluid accumulation increases total body water (TBW), altering the volume of distribution of creatinine and resulting in potential overestimation of kidney function (Fig. 31.2). The masking of AKI severity by volume expansion may be especially problematic in settings where the creatinine is rising relatively slowly because of either lower creatinine generation, as might be expected in the elderly or patients with less muscle mass, or to more modest overall injury. Analysis of the Fluids and Catheters Treatment Trial (FACTT) noted that sCr values corrected for fluid accumulation identified a larger number of patients with AKI who had been misclassified. These patients had outcomes similar to those with AKI.

Table 31.1 Clinical Situations Where Assessment of Glomerular Filtration Rate Is Important for Diagnosis and Management of Acute Kidney Injury

Clinical Decisions	Change in Level of GFR
Diagnosis	Extremes of age (elderly, children)
	Extremes of body size (obesity, type 2 diabetes, low body mass index <18.5 kg/m²)
	Severe malnutrition (cirrhosis, end-stage kidney disease)
	Grossly abnormal muscle mass (amputation, paralysis, myopathy)
	High or low intake of creatinine (vegetarian diet, dietary supplements)
	Pregnancy
Management	Dose and monitoring for medications cleared by the kidney
	Determine safety of diagnostic tests or procedures
	Referral to nephrologists
	Referral for kidney transplantation
	Placement of dialysis access

GFR, Glomerular filtration rate.
Adapted from Stevens LA et al. *J Am Soc Nephrol.* 2009;20: 2305-2313.

Standardized creatinine assessments with the isotope dilution mass spectrometry (IDMS) method will improve the comparison across values and will improve agreement between values across centers. However, standardizing the assays has no effect on the individual variation of sCr. A normal sCr is frequently associated with low creatinine clearance (CrCl), especially in critically ill patients.

CREATININE CLEARANCE

In critically ill patients with unstable kidney function in the nonsteady state, the loss of kidney function does not correspond to the degree of decline in estimated GFR. In those patients, the repeated measurement of CrCl may be an early indicator of AKI. For adjustment of medications, especially for toxic, antimicrobial, and chemotherapy drugs, it is fundamental to have a more reliable and accurate estimation of kidney function (Table 31.1). In those circumstances, it is necessary to consider a CrCl, which can be performed in collection periods from 1 to 24 hours. The longer the collection time, the higher the likelihood for errors caused by inaccurate time recording and incomplete urine collection. Several studies have shown that short duration (1 to 4 hours) CrCl measurements are feasible in the critically ill, and studies have validated the method compared with 24-hour clearance. The use of 4-hour CrCl in the detection of AKI is also a valuable method.

Commonly used formulas to estimate GFR are the Cockcroft-Gault and the abbreviated version of the Modification of Diet in Renal Disease (MDRD). Particularly in older, underweight, or overweight people, these equations overestimate GFR. The CKD-Epidemiology Collaboration (EPI) equation performs better in these patients. The Jelliffe

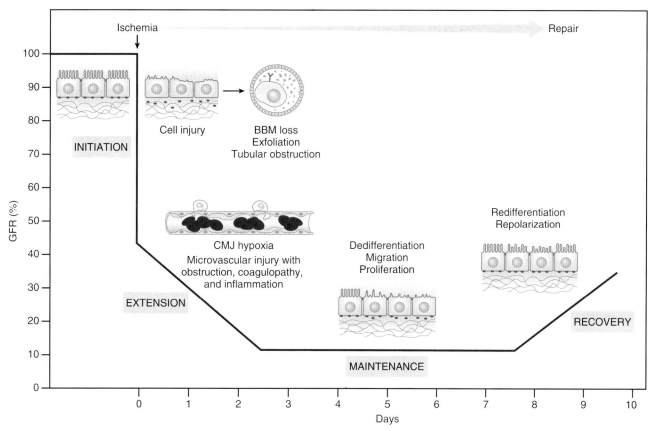

Fig. 31.2 Relationship between the clinical phases and the cellular phases of ischemic acute kidney injury (AKI), and the temporal impact on organ function as represented by glomerular filtration rate (GFR). A variety of cellular and vascular events are involved in the development of AKI. The initiation phase occurs when a reduction in renal blood flow results in cellular injury, particularly the renal tubular epithelial cells, and a decline in *GFR*. Vascular and inflammatory processes that contribute to further cell injury and further decline in *GFR* usher in the extension phase. During the maintenance phase, *GFR* reaches a stable nadir as cellular repair processes are initiated to maintain and reestablish organ integrity. The recovery phase is marked by a return of normal cell and organ function that results in an improvement in *GFR*. *BBM,* Brush border membrane; *CMJ,* corticomeduallary junction. (Data from Basile DP, Anderson MD, Sutton TA. Pathophysiology of acute kidney injury. *Compr Physiol.* 2012;2:1303-1353. Available at https://www.ncbi.nlm.nih.gov/pubmed/23798302 doi 10.1002/cphy.c110041.)

equation was developed to estimate GFR in nonsteady-state conditions; it accounts for the difference between creatinine production and excretion, using the daily changes in sCr. Creatinine production is adjusted for age and for CKD status because creatinine production generally decreases with declining kidney function. The modified Jelliffe equation accounts for the effect of positive fluid balance in variations of sCr and correlates best with measured CrCl.

BLOOD UREA NITROGEN

Blood urea nitrogen (BUN) is also used to evaluate kidney function because elevations in BUN level are often, but not always, due to a GFR decrease. Some conditions enhance urea production, such as gastrointestinal bleeding, corticosteroid therapy, and high-protein diet. In the noncatabolic patient with mildly reduced GFR, daily BUN usually increases less than 10 to 15 mg/dL/day, whereas high catabolic states and high-protein diets are associated with greater urea nitrogen production that can exceed 50 mg/dL. In the presence of a decreased intravascular effective volume, BUN increase is not proportional to the rise in sCr level and fall in GFR. Normally, the BUN:sCr ratio is about 15:1, with the BUN and sCr

increasing by 10 to 15 and 1.0 to 1.5 mg/dL/day, respectively, in the absence of glomerular filtration. In situations characterized by decreased glomerular perfusion pressure such as heart failure, BUN can increase independently from sCr.

CYSTATIN C

Cystatin C is an alternative blood marker that increases as GFR decreases. In CKD, it is an alternative to sCr for estimating GFR. Factors other than GFR affect cystatin C levels, such as glucocorticoid use, thyroid status, cancer, obesity, diabetes, and inflammation. Cystatin C has one-third of the volume of distribution of creatinine, thus reaching a new steady state three times faster than creatinine. This has the potential of predicting AKI before sCr increases. However, cystatin C and sCr have the same limitations associated with positive fluid balance.

URINE STUDIES

URINE FLOW: OLIGURIA

The normal response of the kidney to decreased effective intravascular volume and kidney perfusion is to concentrate

Table 31.2   Fractional Excretion of Sodium and Urea in Clinical Studies

Performance Measure	FE$_{Na}$ (<1% or >3%)	FE$_{Urea}$ (<35%)
Sensitivity		
For prerenal azotemia	78–96%	48–92%
For prerenal azotemia on diuretic	29–63%	79–100%
For intrinsic causes	56–75%	68–75%
Specificity		
For prerenal azotemia	67–96%	75–100%
For prerenal azotemia on diuretic	81–82%	33–91%
For intrinsic causes	78–100%	48–98%
Positive Predictive Value		
For prerenal azotemia	86–98%	79–100%
For prerenal azotemia on diuretic	86–89%	71–98%
For intrinsic causes	64–100%	43–94%
Negative Predictive Value		
For prerenal azotemia	60–86%	43–83%
For prerenal azotemia on diuretic	18–49%	44–83%
For intrinsic causes	82–86%	79–86%

Although cutoff values differ among studies, in a patient with acute kidney injury, an FE$_{Na}$ lower than 1% suggests a prerenal cause, whereas a value higher than 3% suggests an intrinsic cause. Similarly, an FE$_{Urea}$ less than 35% suggests a functional cause of altered kidney function, whereas a value higher than 50% suggests an intrinsic one. The FE$_{Na}$ can be falsely high in patients taking a diuretic; it can be falsely low in a number of intrinsic kidney conditions, such as contrast-induced nephropathy, rhabdomyolysis, and acute glomerulonephritis.

FE$_{Na}$, Fractional excretion of sodium; FE$_{Urea}$, fractional excretion of urea.

the urine and increase sodium reabsorption. As such, AKI associated with intravascular volume depletion is often accompanied by oliguria, and urinary flow can provide helpful information about the cause of AKI (Table 31.2). However, several other factors affect urine flow, including volume expansion, high-dose potent diuretic agents, and renal vasodilators. Although oliguric AKI is more frequent, nonoliguric AKI occurs in approximately 33% of cases at diagnosis. Nonoliguric states may be present in all types of AKI, including those following surgery, trauma, hypotension, nephrotoxins, and rhabdomyolysis.

Since urine output (UO) is a criterion to diagnose and stage AKI, an increasing number of studies have demonstrated that decreased UO, even without sCr elevation, is a specific marker that correlates with outcomes. However, a major barrier to the application of the UO criterion is that an accurate hourly UO measurement is difficult to obtain. Difficulties in measuring, monitoring, and accurately recording UO have resulted in a lack of identification of oliguria episodes. The nonavailability of automatic urine meters and the infectious risks associated with urinary catheters limit accurate urine volume assessment. Assessment of UO over 6- to 12-hour blocks has also been validated as an adequate parameter for AKI in epidemiologic studies; however, for prospective diagnostic and intervention studies, UO should be measured hourly.

Studies combining the UO criterion with sCr have shown an increase in AKI incidence. For example, studies adding the UO criterion to sCr reveal that up to 80% of intensive care unit (ICU) patients meet the definition of AKI. However, patients classified solely by the UO criterion are mostly stage 1 and have higher recovery rates. A systematic review, including studies using a modified UO criterion, indicated that the relative risk for death with both sCr and UO criteria tends to be lower, compared with the use of the sCr criterion alone. In a cohort of 23,866 AKI patients, those reaching both criteria for AKI, sCr and UO, had worse outcomes. Patients reaching stage 3 AKI by sCr in the absence of any UO criteria had a hospital mortality of 11.6%, but mortality increased to 38.6% when a stage 1 UO criterion was also present. Patients who met stage 3 AKI by combined criteria had the highest mortality rate, 51.1%, confirming that even small increments in sCr (stage 1) dramatically increase mortality in oliguric patients, emphasizing the importance of both UO and SCr in the assessment of AKI. Thus applying the AKI classification system without the UO criterion underestimates the incidence and grade of AKI and significantly delays the diagnosis of AKI.

URINE MICROSCOPY

In AKI, urine microscopy traditionally has been used as a tool to discriminate between functional and intrinsic kidney disorders. Cast scoring indices recently have been developed to standardize the sediment analysis and showed good performance to detect ATN. Lack of renal tubular epithelial (RTE) cells or granular casts in patients with an initial diagnosis of decreased kidney perfusion is associated with higher probability of AKI reversal, and higher scores are associated with dose-dependent increased risk of AKI worsening. In a study evaluating urine microscopy and urine NGAL levels in 363 emergency room (ER) patients of whom 76 (21%) had AKI, the presence of RTE cell, RTE cell cast, or granular cast had high specificity (93.0% to 98.6%) to discriminate AKI versus non-AKI patients. The presence of these elements as a group showed a higher sensitivity (from 6% to 22%) and good specificity (91%), determining a low negative but high positive predictive value (81.6%). In the same study, urine NGAL at ER admission had a sensitivity of 64.5% and specificity of 64.5% to predict AKI development.

When ATN is present, brownish-pigmented cellular casts and many RTE cells are observed in more than 75% of patients. Sufficient red blood cells to cause microscopic hematuria, especially if dysmorphic, are traditionally thought to result from glomerulonephritis or structural kidney disorders (stones, tumor, infection, or trauma). Red blood cell casts suggest the presence of glomerular or renal vascular inflammatory disease, and rarely, if ever, occur with ATN. Red blood cell casts, however, can rarely be seen in acute interstitial nephritis (AIN). The presence of large numbers of polymorphonuclear leukocytes, singly or in clumps, suggests acute pyelonephritis or papillary necrosis.

In AIN, white blood cell casts or eosinophilic casts on Hansel stain of urine sediment may be diagnostically helpful.

Eosinophiluria may be also present in some forms of glomerulonephritis and in atheroembolic renal disease. However, eosinophiluria is neither sensitive nor specific as a biomarker of AIN. The combination of brownish-pigmented granular casts and positive occult blood tests on urine in the absence of hematuria indicates either hemoglobinuria or myoglobinuria. The finding of large numbers of "football-shaped" uric acid crystals in fresh, warm urine may suggest a diagnosis of acute uric acid nephropathy when AKI is present, whereas the finding of large numbers of "back-of-envelope-shaped" oxalic acid crystals suggests ethylene glycol toxicity. Other agents (e.g., indinavir, atazanavir, sulfadiazine, acyclovir, and methotrexate) can also induce AKI with characteristic crystal appearance on urinalysis.

URINARY CHEMICAL INDICES

Fractional excretion of sodium (FE_{Na} = [Urine Na^+/Plasma Na^+]/[Urine creatinine/Plasma creatinine] × 100) was initially found to have a high degree of accuracy in differentiating between reversible prerenal azotemia and ATN. However, the relevance of using spot urine chemistries as a diagnostic tool has been questioned as their values are widely variable, influenced by medications (diuretics, aminoglycosides, contrast), and affected by concomitant diseases (cirrhosis, sepsis). Studies demonstrate conflicting results of these parameters for establishing the underlying pathophysiology of AKI and correlating with its duration (transient vs. persistent). In experimental studies of sepsis, decreasing urine Na and FE_{Na} have been demonstrated in the context of increasing renal blood flow. In this context, it is inappropriate to consider low urine Na and FE_{Na} as diagnostic of renal hypoperfusion, and their use to guide fluid therapy is not recommended.

Although these caveats have reduced routine use of urinary biochemistry, nearly all studies of spot chemistries were performed at a single time point, often relatively late in the course of AKI. The lack of serial data is of fundamental importance because AKI is a dynamic process. For example, in early phases of AKI, renal tubular function may be intact, while in later phases, cell injury may result in the loss of tubular cell polarity and dysfunction. The ensuing urine chemistries, therefore, are dependent on the AKI phase in which they were obtained. As shown in Table 31.2, the sensitivity, specificity, and predictive value of these tests is variable and influenced by the volume status and prior use of diuretics. The combination of sequential evaluation of these urinary indices, along with urinalysis and urine microscopy, may be more relevant in the differential diagnosis of AKI to determine if structural changes are occurring. Predicting the response to diuretic therapy may be an additional use of urinary biochemistry, as some studies suggested that oliguric patients with AKI have lower values for FE_{Na} and higher values for urine-to-plasma osmolality.

The fractional excretion of urea nitrogen (FE_{urea} = [Urine urea nitrogen/Plasma urea nitrogen]/[Urine creatinine/Plasma creatinine] × 100) has been proposed as an alternative marker to evaluate kidney dysfunction. Because intact nephrons reabsorb urea nitrogen from the urine, functional changes without nephron damage should inherently have a low FE_{urea}, with a threshold value of less than 35%. With tubular damage, FE_{urea} (>50%) is expected to parallel changes in FE_{Na}, with the possible advantage of being less affected by diuretic use. However, given the multitude of factors associated with urea production, the FE_{urea} also suffers from poor sensitivity and specificity in AKI evaluation.

CLEARANCE MEASUREMENTS

As GFR cannot be measured directly, the urinary clearance of a filtration marker is used as a surrogate. Inulin is the gold standard but is expensive and cumbersome, requiring continuous infusion and multiple blood samples. Other filtration markers, besides creatinine, are iothalamate, iohexol, and ethylenediaminetetraacetic acid (EDTA). However, inaccuracies in urine collection and analytic variations of serum and urine measurements have limited their clinical application and affected their interpretation in research studies. The development of less expensive and simpler assays may increase their utility in patients who need a more accurate estimation of kidney function.

Iothalamate is the most commonly used surrogate marker, administered as a subcutaneous injection of radioactive 125I-Iothalamate. Iothalamate urinary clearance tends to overestimate GFR because of its tubular secretion. Iohexol, a nonradioactive radiographic contrast agent delivered by bolus intravenous injection for plasma or urine clearance, is inexpensive and widely available but associated with rare adverse reactions. The main limitation is the expense of the high-performance liquid chromatography or mass spectroscopy assay. A few small studies have compared plasma clearance of iohexol to urinary clearance of inulin, showing iohexol marginally underestimates GFR, suggesting tubular reabsorption or protein binding.

51Cr-EDTA clearance underestimates GFR compared with inulin clearance by 5% to 15%, suggesting tubular reabsorption. Diethylenetriamine pentaacetic acid (DTPA), an analog of EDTA that is available for use in the United States, has a shorter half-life (5 hours) that minimizes radiation exposure. DTPA is freely filtered at the glomerulus and has minimal tubular reabsorption; however, its nonpredictable plasma protein binding and extrarenal elimination can lead to an underestimation of GFR.

NEW BIOMARKERS

Over the last decade, the concept of interventions based on "windows of opportunity" coupled with targeted therapy became more relevant with other ischemic events, such as acute chest pain syndromes and stroke. Earlier AKI diagnosis provides a wider window to perform supportive and therapeutic interventions. Several promising candidates for early biomarkers for AKI diagnosis have emerged, demonstrating reasonable performance for AKI up to 48 hours before a significant sCr change.

The first clinical studies of new biomarkers of kidney injury showed high diagnostic and prognostic ability. In heterogeneous populations in which the time of kidney injury was poorly defined, biomarker performance to detect AKI earlier declined to values similar to clinical evaluation and standard laboratory measurements. Other factors have prevented the widespread clinical use of biomarkers for AKI. The influence of inflammatory states such as sepsis, underlying kidney function, and sex imposes a challenge in determining meaningful thresholds for clinical practice. Furthermore, the pattern of elevation, in situations other than following cardiopulmonary bypass or exposure to iodinated contrast, is not completely understood.

IMAGING

Ultrasonographic evaluation of the kidney can also help in the diagnosis of AKI. Ultrasound is an excellent modality for structural imaging of renal parenchymal size, scarring, calcification, and kidney cysts. Small kidney size strongly supports a diagnosis of CKD, helping to differentiate acute from chronic kidney injury. Cortical echogenicity can be assessed, with a hyperechoic cortex (normal cortex is hypoechoic to liver) present in most causes of CKD. In ATN, ultrasound usually shows enlarged kidneys with normal cortical echogenicity and a normal or hypoechoic medulla, primarily due to interstitial edema. Obstructed kidneys are typically normal sized with a dilated pelvicalyceal system. The urine-filled structures appear as anechoic areas with posterior acoustic enhancement. Ureter and renal pelvis can be dilated without being obstructed, most commonly after previous obstruction with residual changes, normal pregnancy, or as an anatomic variant (enlarged extrarenal pelvis). False negatives can occur in the hyperacute setting if the renal collecting system has not had time to dilate, or if associated with retroperitoneal fibrosis or ureteral encasement.

Doppler ultrasonography is an emerging tool to characterize the likelihood of early AKI recovery because the renal arteries can be evaluated for the resistive index (RI). RI is defined as the systolic velocity minus diastolic velocity divided by systolic velocity ($[Vs - Vd]/Vs$). Alterations in RI (normal range ≤ 0.70) have been correlated with the severity of AKI. However, these techniques are operator dependent and have not been widely used.

Direct measurement of GFR with magnetic resonance imaging can be performed shortly after injection of gadolinium-DTPA and gadolinium-DOTA. These are widely available, and immunoassay techniques are easily performed. However, the potential risk of systemic nephrogenic fibrosis in subjects with very low GFR will limit use of these agents. Safer contrast agents may facilitate GFR measurement with MRI, but the logistics of transporting critically ill patients are difficult.

Other techniques to evaluate kidney perfusion are currently under investigation. Evaluating renal artery blood flow may identify perfusion alterations in diseases that change microcirculation. Some pathophysiologic processes may be associated with increased global renal blood flow despite loss of kidney function. Therefore correlations between kidney blood flow and GFR are not linear, and techniques evaluating the microcirculatory parameters and regional tissue oxygenation measurement may be more valuable in understanding loss of function in AKI.

KIDNEY BIOPSY

A kidney biopsy is usually considered when the cause of AKI is not obvious, heavy proteinuria and persistent hematuria are present, or with a prolonged (>2 to 3 weeks) course of AKI. In suspected glomerulonephritis or AIN, the "gold standard" diagnostic test is a kidney biopsy. In clinical practice, most nephrologists choose to perform a biopsy when they

are not confident of the cause of the AKI, or when kidney injury has an obscure etiology. Unfortunately, the lack of effective therapeutic options coupled with the risks of kidney biopsy decreases the likelihood that the clinician will perform the procedure.

Kidney biopsy should be considered when the underlying clinical AKI diagnosis is not consistent with ATN. Patients with an undefined cause of AKI may benefit from identifying a treatable form of AKI with biopsy, such as AIN. In addition, significant discordance between prebiopsy and postbiopsy diagnoses in the setting of AKI exists. In the elderly, the clinical diagnosis was incorrect in 34% of cases biopsied, many of them involving potentially treatable diseases. Among elderly patients with rapidly progressive kidney injury, 71% and 17% were noted to have crescentic glomerulonephritis and AIN, respectively. Prebiopsy and histopathologic diagnoses differed in 15% of patients, and both groups benefited from therapeutic intervention.

These data emphasize the value of the kidney biopsy in the management of AKI of uncertain origin, regardless of the age of the patient. Accurate diagnosis is important to direct appropriate treatment, especially in vasculitis and crescentic GN where delay in diagnosis may affect outcome. Given the safety of ultrasound or computed tomography (CT)-guided biopsy, unclear cases of AKI deserve consideration for kidney biopsy. The transjugular approach has also enhanced our ability to obtain tissue, particularly in patients who are at high risk for bleeding and cannot be placed in the prone position. The complication rates appear similar to ultrasound-guided biopsies. Despite this, the clinician should be aware of the major risks for kidney biopsy: bleeding, infection, creation of an intrarenal AV fistula, and injury to adjacent organs.

DIFFERENTIAL DIAGNOSIS AND EVALUATION

The definition and classification system of AKI have been standardized. Nevertheless, whether AKI refers only to ATN and other parenchymal diseases or includes reversible functional changes has not been established. Currently, reversible forms of kidney dysfunction encompassing different conditions that vary considerably in pathophysiology and course include intravascular volume depletion, relative hypotension, compromised cardiac output, and hepatorenal syndrome (Fig. 31.3). In all these situations, elevation of sCr or reduction in UO that resolves with volume resuscitation or improved renal perfusion pressure is the current accepted definition for reversible functional changes. However, there is no agreement on the amount, nature, and duration of fluid resuscitation needed to establish a prerenal state. In most cases, the response to fluid expansion or hemodynamic support on kidney function is retrospective and frequently evaluated by trial and error. The return of kidney function to the previous baseline within 24 to 72 hours is considered a prerenal or reversible condition. Diagnostic strategies are based on demonstrating a fluid-responsive change in kidney function; however, unnecessary fluid administration and fluid overload are potential complications of this approach.

Several clinical scenarios are often associated with potentially reversible AKI. The use of nonsteroidal antiinflammatory

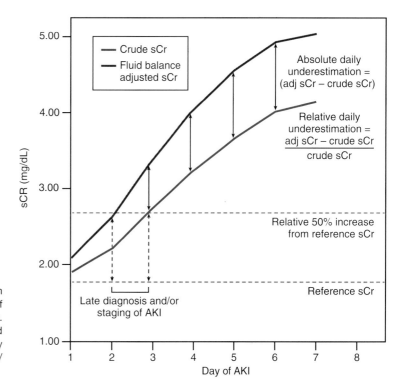

Fig. 31.3 Difference between mean crude and adjusted serum creatinine during the follow-up period (late recognition of severity group). *AKI,* Acute kidney injury; *sCr,* serum creatinine. (Data from Macedo E, Bouchard J, Soroko SH, et al. Fluid accumulation, recognition and staging of acute kidney injury in critically-ill patients. *Crit Care.* 2010;14:R82. doi 10.1186/cc9004.)

drugs (NSAIDs), volume depletion, hypoalbuminemia, an edematous disorder, advancing age, underlying CKD, or recent diuretic use are all contributing factors for prerenal AKI. A similar reversible form of AKI can complicate angiotensin-converting enzyme–inhibitor therapy in the presence of decreased renal blood flow from severe bilateral renal artery stenosis, renal artery stenosis in a solitary functioning kidney, and other high-renin/high-angiotensin II states. ACE-inhibition with a resultant decrease in both renal perfusion pressure and efferent arteriolar vasodilation can precipitously decrease GFR. About one-third of patients with severe congestive heart failure experience an abrupt rise in sCr concentration following ACE inhibitor therapy. In this setting, the increase in sCr following ACE inhibition tends to be mild and readily reversible on drug discontinuation.

With the availability of new biomarkers of kidney injury, refined paradigms for defining reversible states are emerging (Fig. 31.4). The diagnosis of reversible functional changes requires a consideration of several factors, including preexisting kidney disease, time frame for kidney function changes, and the response to interventions. There are some promising new biomarkers that may be helpful in distinguishing between reversible and established AKI. During the reversible state, persistent vasoconstriction associated with metabolic changes and inflammation promotes the release of cell functional markers that can be detected in the blood and urine. Urinary NGAL levels were evaluated in ER patients, with very little overlap in values in patients with reversible and established AKI. Alternatively, sCr values overlapped significantly. However, currently there are no specific markers identifying reversible conditions. Some studies have shown a correlation between urinary biomarker concentration and functional severity. While it is accepted that urinary biomarker concentrations increase with functional reversible injuries, the level of concentrations differs from patients with established structural damage. It is evident that as biomarkers are available for clinical use, our thresholds for these markers will be defined, and what is currently labeled as prerenal will change.

Once reversible and obstructive AKI have been excluded, a variety of kidney disorders can lead to a prolonged or sustained AKI. In hospitalized adults, many of these cases are caused by ATN. Three major categories of insults are associated with ATN: prolonged or severe renal ischemia, nephrotoxins, and pigmenturia (myoglobinuria and hemoglobinuria). ATN is often the result of multiple insults. The most common predisposing factor in the development of ATN is renal ischemia from a functional or structural reduction in renal perfusion. Sepsis, and particularly septic shock, has assumed an ever-increasing role as a major predisposing factor in the occurrence of ATN. Nephrotoxins are involved in about 20% of all cases of ATN. Contemporary nephrotoxins commonly encountered include aminoglycosides, radiographic contrast materials, NSAIDs, and antineoplasic agents. A high proportion of patients with HIV infection develop drug-induced nephrotoxicity.

DIAGNOSTIC APPROACH

Currently, clinicians classify patients with AKI as prerenal, intrinsic, or postrenal based on the clinical presentation. However, this approach may be somewhat limiting because there is usually no histopathology to confirm the diagnosis. A revised framework for approaching patients with AKI based on reversibility is noted in Table 31.3. The first step is to establish a patient's prior level of kidney function to determine whether there is de novo AKI or AKI superimposed on CKD. In several instances, information on prior kidney function is not available. Nevertheless, a detailed history including comorbidities, medication use, and prior lab tests should be obtained. Urinary abnormalities such as proteinuria can help

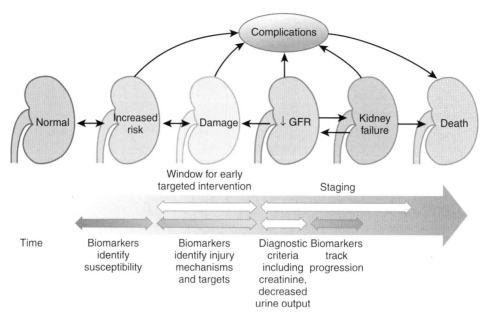

Fig. 31.4 Conceptual framework for acute kidney injury. Surveillance could be initiated for high-risk individuals on the basis of clinical and biomarker criteria. Sequential assessment of biomarkers may permit identification of a window of opportunity in which kidney injury has been initiated but has not progressed to kidney functional change. The duration of this window is inherently dependent on the type and site of injury and the nature and specificity of the biomarkers to determine the targets for intervention. Progression of kidney injury would be determined by development of functional changes staged on the basis of the severity of kidney injury. Biomarkers could further define progression, determine need for additional interventions, and predict prognosis. By combining biomarkers—for example, urine flow (functional change) and neutrophil gelatinase–associated lipocalin (structural damage)—clinicians will have better tools to characterize patients with respect to reversibility and more clearly identify phases of the disease. *GFR,* Glomerular filtration rate. (Modified from Mehta RL. Timed and targeted therapy for acute kidney injury: a glimpse of the future. *Kidney Int.* 2010;77:947-949. Available at http://www.ncbi.nlm.nih.gov/pubmed/20467432.)

Table 31.3   Clinical Approach to Acute Kidney Injury

1. *Reversible AKI*

- Decreased effective renal perfusion
- Extrarenal obstruction to urine flow

2. *Self-Limited AKI*

- Acute tubular necrosis
- Acute interstitial nephritis
- Intrarenal obstruction, drugs, uric acid
- Acute glomerulonephritis

3. *Irreversible AKI*

- Cortical necrosis
- Large vessel occlusion
- Certain nephrotoxins: methoxyflurane
- Microvascular occlusions

AKI, Acute kidney injury.

Table 31.4   Nonmodifiable and Modifiable Risk Factors for Acute Kidney Injury

Nonmodifiable	Modifiable
Chronic kidney disease	Hypertension
Diabetes mellitus	Hypoalbuminemia
Older age	Anemia
Chronic liver disease	Sepsis
Congestive heart failure	Nephrotoxic drugs
Renal artery stenosis	Mechanical ventilation
Peripheral vascular disease	Hypercholesterolemia
AIDS	Rhabdomyolysis
Prior kidney surgery	Hyponatremia

---

establish prior damage. It is preferable to consider sCr values before 3 months from the episode to determine whether a patient has CKD. However, baseline sCr is either not available or unknown in many instances. Using a surrogate such as sCr at the time of hospitalization for baseline sCr has a marked effect on the incidence and severity of AKI. Current recommendations are to assess baseline kidney function with an estimating equation. Nevertheless, this strategy will overestimate kidney function and lead to misclassification in patients with suspected CKD and long-standing diabetes or multiple risk factors for CKD. Misclassification in AKI diagnosis and severity can ultimately lead to different therapeutic approaches and influence prognosis.

Accurate identification of AKI risk factors for patients is fundamental to achieve early diagnosis and accurate assessment of AKI severity. This is essential to developing approaches for earlier intervention, correcting reversible factors, and mitigating the downstream effects of AKI (Table 31.4). Two large prospective observational studies in ICU patients have provided a better understanding of the risk factors associated with AKI: BEST and PICARD. Both BEST and PICARD found sepsis to be the most common contributing factor to ICU-related AKI, with a significant percentage of AKI patients having underlying CKD. In the BEST study, AKI was associated with septic shock in 47.5% of patients. Thirty-four percent of AKI was associated with major surgery, 27% related to cardiogenic shock, 26% related to hypovolemia, and 19% potentially drug-related. Volume depletion is another common risk factor for AKI. In addition to hypovolemia, renal hypoperfusion may be caused by decreased cardiac output, decreased plasma oncotic pressure, hypotension, and decreased renal prostaglandin production. Advanced age, which is often associated with some degree of preexisting kidney disease, is another common risk factor associated with AKI. Administration of potentially nephrotoxic drugs increases the risk of AKI, as seen with the concurrent use of furosemide and intravenous contrast agents. Congestive heart failure, nephrotic syndrome, and liver disease are common predisposing conditions associated with AKI. As shown in Table 31.4, modifiable risk factors can be targets for prevention and intervention.

Knowledge of underlying CKD status and potential risk factors should prompt a search for specific insults for AKI. While AKI associated with one specific cause is common outside the ICU, most patients have several etiologic factors contributing to AKI occurrence. The most common are failure of renal autoregulation, direct nephrotoxicity, ischemia/reperfusion, and inflammatory states. With multiple factors directly influencing kidney function, the nature and timing of the inciting event are often unknown. If a specific etiology can be identified, such as exposure to contrast agents or nephrotoxic antibiotics, the course can be somewhat predictable. However, clinicians should be vigilant in their search for additional reversible factors that may influence the course, such as volume depletion.

Diagnostic strategies using the established parameters of urinalysis, urine microscopy, urine chemistries, and imaging should be combined with newer biomarkers to better differentiate patients with functional reversible changes from those with structural kidney injury. For example, our current concepts of prerenal AKI represent conditions wherein tubular function is intact, and correction of the underlying condition reverses the kidney dysfunction. Alternatively, structural injury leads to a more protracted course, and highlights conditions where biomarkers such as NGAL and KIM1 are elevated. In the reversible conditions, markers would more likely be below thresholds associated with injury, although there will be some overlap. As we begin to use AKI biomarkers, specific combinations will provide better fingerprints to enable clinicians to more optimally assess AKI patients. Once the diagnosis and severity stage has been established, specific interventions can be further designed based on the AKI stage.

Finally, although several individual risk factors are associated with AKI occurrence, the combination of risk factors and the development of risk stratification scores could be better tools to predict AKI in specific patient populations (e.g., after cardiac surgery, contrast exposure, hospital acquired, general surgery, and high-risk surgery). Few models have examined the clinical risk factors for AKI among the ICU population, but risk profiling can be used to establish appropriate criteria for surveillance for AKI in hospitalized patients. The use of models to predict the AKI risk can help clinicians identify patients at high risk of developing AKI, perform clinical decisions based on this risk, and provide better patient counseling. A combination of risk assessment, active surveillance, early recognition, rapid response, and targeted intervention can be standardized to optimally manage these patients and improve outcomes.

Thus, as AKI is a common condition that is prevalent in outpatient and inpatient settings, a practical clinical approach to diagnosis is required. Our understanding of the pathophysiology, mechanism, and pathways has been enhanced in recent years from experimental models and epidemiologic studies. With the availability of new biomarkers, we are now better positioned to approach patients for earlier recognition, active surveillance, and targeted interventions. Strategies for management should focus on identifying reversibility and intervening early to prevent further progression. Several tools are now available to clinicians to manage patients with AKI.

KEY BIBLIOGRAPHY

Basile DP, Anderson MD, Sutton TA. Pathophysiology of acute kidney injury. *Compr Physiol.* 2012;2:1303-1353. doi:10.1002/cphy.c110041. Available at: https://www.ncbi.nlm.nih.gov/pubmed/23798302.

Bouchard J, Macedo E, Soroko S, et al. Comparison of methods for estimating glomerular filtration rate in critically ill patients with acute kidney injury. *Nephrol Dial Transplant.* 2010;25:102-107. Available at: http://www.ncbi.nlm.nih.gov/pubmed/19679558. doi: 10.1093/ndt/gfp392.

Bragadottir G, Redfors B, Ricksten SE. Assessing glomerular filtration rate (GFR) in critically ill patients with acute kidney injury—true GFR versus urinary creatinine clearance and estimating equations. *Crit Care.* 2013;17:R108.

Gotfried J, Wiesen J, Raina R, Nally JV. Finding the cause of acute kidney injury: which index of fractional excretion is better? *Cleve Clin J Med.* 2012;79:121-126. doi:10.3949/ccjm.79a.11030. Available at: https://www.ncbi.nlm.nih.gov/pubmed/22301562.

Haase M, Bellomo R, Matalanis G, Calzavacca P, Dragun D, Haase-Fielitz A. A comparison of the RIFLE and Acute Kidney Injury Network classifications for cardiac surgery-associated acute kidney injury: a prospective cohort study. *J Thorac Cardiovasc Surg.* 2009;138:1370-1376. doi:10.1016/j.jtcvs.2009.07.007. Available at: http://www.ncbi.nlm.nih.gov/entrez/query.fcgi?cmd=Retrieve&db=PubMed&dopt=Citation&list_uids=19733864. doi S0022-5223(09)00919-2.

Haase M, Devarajan P, Haase-Fielitz A, et al. The outcome of neutrophil gelatinase-associated lipocalin-positive subclinical acute kidney injury: a multicenter pooled analysis of prospective studies. *J Am Coll Cardiol.* 2011;57:1752-1761. doi:10.1016/j.jacc.2010.11.051. Available at: http://www.ncbi.nlm.nih.gov/pubmed/21511111.

Hoste EA, Damen J, Vanholder RC, et al. Assessment of renal function in recently admitted critically ill patients with normal serum creatinine. *Nephrol Dial Transplant.* 2005;20:747-753. doi:10.1093/ndt/gfh707. Available at: http://www.ncbi.nlm.nih.gov/entrez/query.fcgi?cmd=Retrieve&db=PubMed&dopt=Citation&list_uids=15701668.

Hsu RK, McCulloch CE, Dudley RA, Lo LJ, Hsu CY. Temporal changes in incidence of dialysis-requiring AKI. *J Am Soc Nephrol.* 2013;24:37-42. doi:10.1681/ASN.2012080800. Available at: http://www.ncbi.nlm.nih.gov/pubmed/23222124.

Kellum JA, Sileanu FE, Murugan R, Lucko N, Shaw AD, Clermont G. Classifying AKI by urine output versus serum creatinine level. *J Am Soc Nephrol.* 2015;26:2231-2238. doi:10.1681/ASN.2014070724. Available at: http://www.ncbi.nlm.nih.gov/pubmed/25568178.

Macedo E, Bouchard J, Soroko SH, et al. Fluid accumulation, recognition and staging of acute kidney injury in critically-ill patients. *Crit Care.* 2010;14:R82. doi:10.1186/cc9004.

Macedo E, Mehta RL. Measuring renal function in critically ill patients: tools and strategies for assessing glomerular filtration rate. *Curr Opin Crit Care.* 2013;19:560-566. doi:10.1097/MCC.0000000000000025. Available at: http://www.ncbi.nlm.nih.gov/pubmed/24240821.

Mehta RL. Timed and targeted therapy for acute kidney injury: a glimpse of the future. *Kidney Int.* 2010;77:947-949. doi:10.1038/ki.2010.79. Available at: http://www.ncbi.nlm.nih.gov/pubmed/20467432.

Perazella MA, Coca SG, Hall IE, Iyanam U, Koraishy M, Parikh CR. Urine microscopy is associated with severity and worsening of acute kidney injury in hospitalized patients. *Clin J Am Soc Nephrol.* 2010;5:402-408. doi:10.2215/CJN.06960909. Available at: http://www.ncbi.nlm.nih.gov/pubmed/20089493.

Pickering JW, Frampton CM, Walker RJ, Shaw GM, Endre ZH. Four hour creatinine clearance is better than plasma creatinine for monitoring renal function in critically ill patients. *Crit Care.* 2012;16:R107. doi:10.1186/cc11391. Available at: http://www.ncbi.nlm.nih.gov/pubmed/22713519.

Prowle JR, Kirwan CJ, Bellomo R. Fluid management for the prevention and attenuation of acute kidney injury. *Nat Rev Nephrol.* 2014;10:37-47. doi:10.1038/nrneph.2013.232. Available at: http://www.ncbi.nlm.nih.gov/pubmed/24217464.

Schneider AG, Goodwin MD, Bellomo R. Measurement of kidney perfusion in critically ill patients. *Crit Care.* 2013;17:220. doi:10.1186/cc12529. Available at: http://www.ncbi.nlm.nih.gov/pubmed/23514525.

Siew ED, Matheny ME, Ikizler TA, et al. Commonly used surrogates for baseline renal function affect the classification and prognosis of acute kidney injury. *Kidney Int.* 2010;77:536-542. doi:10.1038/ki.2009.479. Available at: http://www.ncbi.nlm.nih.gov/pubmed/20042998.

Siew ED, Ware LB, Gebretsadik T, et al. Urine neutrophil gelatinase-associated lipocalin moderately predicts acute kidney injury in critically ill adults. *J Am Soc Nephrol.* 2009;20:1823-1832. doi:10.1681/ASN.2008070673. Available at: http://www.ncbi.nlm.nih.gov/pubmed/19628673.

Stevens LA, Levey AS. Measured GFR as a confirmatory test for estimated GFR. *J Am Soc Nephrol.* 2009;20:2305-2313. doi:10.1681/ASN.2009020171. Available at: http://www.ncbi.nlm.nih.gov/pubmed/19833901.

Tangri N, Stevens LA, Schmid CH, et al. Changes in dietary protein intake has no effect on serum cystatin C levels independent of the glomerular filtration rate. *Kidney Int.* 2011;79:471-477. doi:10.1038/ki.2010.431. Available at: http://www.ncbi.nlm.nih.gov/pubmed/20980977.

Full bibliography can be found on www.expertconsult.com.

Acute Tubular Injury and Acute Tubular Necrosis

32

Jeffrey M. Turner; Steven G. Coca

While renal tubular epithelial cell (RTEC) injury can occur at any location along the nephron, damage from ischemia or nephrotoxins is usually most profound to the cells located within the proximal tubule. Once damaged, epithelial cells follow one of three pathways, depending on the extent of injury: repair, apoptosis, or necrosis. Necrosis is typically inconspicuous and restricted to highly susceptible areas, such as the outer medullary region, whereas cellular repair and cellular apoptosis typically occurs more broadly within the proximal tubule. In recent years, significant research effort has focused on understanding the mechanisms that dictate repair and apoptosis in RTECs, in hopes that this will lead to improved ways to prevent and treat acute kidney injury (AKI). As our understanding of AKI continues to evolve, so has the nomenclature we use to describe it. The term acute tubular injury (ATI) is now commonly used in place of acute tubular necrosis (ATN) to define a sudden decline in kidney function resulting from ischemic or toxin-related damage to RTECs. The main focus of this chapter is to discuss etiologies of ATI that occur secondary to ischemic insults and endogenous nephrotoxins.

ISCHEMIC ACUTE TUBULAR INJURY

AKI commonly occurs as a result of ischemic insult to RTECs. Normal function includes the ability to autoregulate blood flow and perfusion pressure within the renal microvasculature. This allows the kidney to maintain stable hemodynamics, despite fluctuations in systemic arterial pressures. In pathologic states, the ability to autoregulate is compromised, and ischemic injury can occur. The clinical manifestations of ischemia-induced insults lie on a continuum, which includes both functional changes in glomerular filtration that are traditionally labeled *prerenal* and direct tubular cell injury that is traditionally labeled *intrarenal*. However, the threshold at which prerenal insults result in tubular cell injury is not well understood. Moreover, because of normal variations in regional blood flow and differences in energy and oxygen consumption in discrete areas of the nephron, tubular injury can be patchy. Thus ATI is not an "all or none" phenomenon, and many nephrons of the kidney can endure in a prerenal functional state whereas others experience injury.

In general, the more severe the renal perfusion defect, the more severe the injury is at the cellular level. However, this association is dynamic depending on the clinical scenario. A number of comorbidities, including sepsis, chronic kidney disease (CKD), hypertension, and atherosclerosis, will lower the threshold at which cellular injury begins to occur. In addition, it has been hypothesized that reduced glomerular filtration rate (GFR) and the subsequent oliguria that occurs in the setting of AKI are protective mechanisms that attempt to limit mismatches in renal oxygen supply and demand. This creates an interesting dilemma about how we approach the importance of rapidly restoring glomerular filtration and urine output following kidney injury. In this section, we examine some of the common clinical scenarios that lead to ischemic ATI. The causes are divided into those etiologies that result from decreased systemic arterial pressures that subsequently cause end-organ hypoperfusion, and those etiologies that result in localized obstruction or constriction within the renal vasculature causing ischemia in downstream tissues.

CAUSES OF HYPOTENSION-INDUCED ISCHEMIA

In the hospital setting, ATI is the most common cause of AKI, attributable to half of all cases. The typical clinical scenario is a reduction in renal pressure and blood flow in the setting of poor effective arterial perfusion caused by a systemic disorder (Box 32.1). By various mechanisms, shock is a frequent culprit. Septic shock creates a particularly unfriendly environment for the kidney. Not only is oxygen delivery and cellular waste removal impaired because of changes in renal perfusion from systemic vasodilatation and intrarenal vasoconstriction, but the addition of direct tubular damage from endotoxins and inflammatory cytokines also contributes to the pathophysiology. Relatively modest reductions in blood pressure that occur with sepsis can still result in significant kidney impairment because of this double-hit phenomenon. Like sepsis, distributive shock results in diffuse vasodilatation of the systemic arterial system. Under normal conditions, the kidney receives 20% to 25% of the total cardiac output; however, a significant proportion of blood flow is diverted away from the kidney in this setting.

The cardinal impairment in cardiogenic shock is a reduction in cardiac output. This creates a number of unfavorable conditions for the kidney. In response to underfilling of the systemic arterial vascular bed and overfilling of the venous and splanchnic vessels, compensatory mechanisms lead to increased activity of the sympathetic nervous system and renin-angiotensin-aldosterone system, as well as increased endothelin and vasopressin. This in turn causes maladaptive vasoconstriction, particularly within the renal vasculature. The net result is a significant compromise to renal blood flow. Moreover, the venous congestion and subsequent elevations in intraabdominal pressure are also important hydraulic contributors to kidney impairment in the setting of reduced

Box 32.1   Causes of Ischemic Acute Tubular Injury/Acute Tubular Necrosis

1. **Decreased effective arterial perfusion**
   a. Shock
      i. Septic
      ii. Hypovolemic
      iii. Cardiogenic
      iv. Distributive
   b. Autonomic dysfunction
   c. Low oncotic pressure states
      i. Cirrhosis
      ii. Nephrotic syndrome
      iii. Protein-losing enteropathies
   d. Adrenal insufficiency
   e. Iatrogenic
      i. Medication induced
      ii. Perioperative
2. **Vaso-occlusion within the renal vasculature**
   a. Renal artery stenosis
   b. Thromboembolism
   c. Atheroembolic disease
3. **Vasoconstriction within the renal vasculature**
   a. Medication induced
   b. Toxin induced

systolic function. Because most patients who present with acute decompensated heart failure are overtly congested and not in frank cardiogenic shock, the venous congestion is indeed the key mechanism that manifests in most forms of "cardiorenal" syndrome.

Hypovolemic shock commonly occurs secondary to significant volume loss in the setting of diuresis, bleeding, vomiting, or diarrhea. Markedly reduced oncotic pressure from low albumin states such as cirrhosis, nephrotic syndrome, and protein-losing enteropathies can also result in severe intravascular volume depletion, despite an excess of total body water. Signs and symptoms of organ dysfunction do not typically occur until approximately 20% to 25% of effective arterial blood volume has been removed.

In addition to shock, a number of other clinical scenarios need to be considered in the etiology of ischemic ATI due to systemic hypotension. Common iatrogenic causes include medications, such as antihypertensive agents, alpha antagonists, antiarrhythmics, narcotics, and sedatives. Hypotension related to autonomic dysfunction is most commonly seen in the setting of diabetes mellitus; however, it is also associated with liver disease, Guillain-Barré syndrome, cerebral vascular accidents, dementia, and other processes. Finally, medications that interfere with the autoregulation of renal blood flow can also contribute to or exacerbate ATI from any of the previously mentioned causes. Nonsteroidal antiinflammatory drugs (NSAIDs) can reduce blood flow through the afferent arteriole and can impair medullary blood flow in patients who are prostaglandin-dependent. The role of angiotensin-converting enzyme (ACE) inhibitors and angiotensin receptor blockers (ARBs) in AKI is unclear. While these agents can reduce GFR by altering intrarenal hemodynamics, this functional change does not necessarily equate to structural changes in the kidney, and it may not be associated with the same adverse clinical consequences that occur with cell injury. There is significant research effort under way to better understand the differences in these two pathways. Thus, although it is common practice for clinicians to discontinue ACE inhibitors and ARBs in the setting of AKI, there is no clear consensus that this positively affects outcomes.

DIAGNOSIS

Ischemic ATI is usually suspected based on the clinical setting. Although one expects significant hypotension to have occurred, it is not uncommon for individuals with chronic hypertension and impaired autoregulation to experience normotensive ischemic kidney injury. In such cases, one would see a relative decrease in blood pressure as compared with baseline; however, the nadir pressure may still remain within the normal range. In contrast to prerenal AKI, in which the proximal tubules markedly increase reabsorption of sodium, urea, uric acid, and other solutes in an attempt to preserve intravascular volume, patients with ATI cannot achieve this. The laboratory data, in turn, that are consistent with ischemic ATI reflect proximal tubular dysfunction. These include a blood urea nitrogen-to-serum creatinine ratio of less than 20, a fractional excretion of sodium (FE_{Na}) greater than 2%, or a fractional excretion of urea (FE_{Urea}) greater than 50%. In states in which there is a mix of prerenal and ATI (which is patchy and not diffuse), FE_{Na} can be less than 1%. ATI also results in an inability of the distal tubules and collecting ducts to concentrate or dilute the urine effectively; thus the specific gravity will be approximately 1.010 (reflecting isosthenuria), and the urine osmolality is typically less than 350 mOsm/kg. Proteinuria can be present, but it is less than 1 g/day. In addition, it is not uncommon to have trace to 1+ heme on urine dipstick. Urine microscopy provides the most useful information to make the diagnosis. The classic finding is dense granular casts or "muddy brown casts," but additional findings include fine granular casts, RTEC casts, and RTECs. A scoring system based on the number of granular casts and RTECs seen within a low-power or high-power field, respectively, has been validated as a useful tool in differentiating ATI from pre-renal azotemia.

The application of novel biomarkers to diagnose and predict ATI continues to be an area of intense research. Such markers include neutrophil gelatinase–associated lipocalin (NGAL), interleukin-18 (IL-18), and kidney injury molecule-1 (KIM-1), among others. Their potential application includes diagnosing ATI closer to the time of the actual insult and before the rise in serum creatinine (i.e., the time ATI is typically diagnosed clinically). In addition, biomarkers can be helpful in differentiating acute GFR reductions secondary to functional changes (i.e., prerenal and hepatorenal syndrome) from those caused by true renal tubular injury. Finally, the biomarkers may be able to predict which patients with established clinical AKI will progress to more severe dysfunction, including those who may require acute kidney replacement therapy. In 2014, the FDA approved the first biomarker test to predict risk of developing moderate to severe AKI within 12 hours after the administration of the test. The NephroCheck test measures the presence of insulin-like growth-factor binding protein 7 (IGFBP7) and tissue inhibitor of metalloproteinases (TIMP-2) in the urine. These two markers were found in a high throughput screen of 300 candidate biomarkers for AKI. A recent analysis of a composite urine TIMP-2*GFBP-7 biomarker yielded an area under the curve (AUC) of 0.90 for the prediction of post-CABG AKI. However, while FDA approved, the uptake and usage of this test across the United States is still quite low, probably because there is still little that can be done to prevent or treat ATI, except for supportive care.

CHOLESTEROL ATHEROEMBOLIC KIDNEY DISEASE

Atheromatous plaques form within the walls of arterial beds throughout the body, including in the aorta and renal arteries. These structures are usually composed of smooth muscle and mononuclear cells, calcium deposits, a fibrous cap, and lipids, including cholesterol crystals. Disrupted plaques can release cholesterol crystals that flow downstream and lodge in small vessels within various organs, including the kidney. As circumstances dictate, isolated kidney involvement can occur or can be a manifestation of multiorgan involvement. Cholesterol atheroembolic kidney disease leads to ischemic kidney injury due to vessel obstruction from cholesterol crystals and the subsequently provoked immune response. Biopsy series have reported incidence rates of 1% among all patients undergoing kidney biopsy and as high as 6.5% in selected cohorts older than 65 years old. In a chart review of hospitalized nephrology consultations, 10% of all cases of AKI were attributed to atheroembolic kidney disease. It appears that widespread statin use has made cholesterol atheroembolic kidney disease a rather rare syndrome.

CLINICAL PRESENTATION

Cholesterol atheroembolic kidney disease is iatrogenic in as many as 77% of cases. The most common etiology is percutaneous coronary interventions, but other procedures include angioplasty for renal artery stenosis, vascular surgery, and cardiac surgery. These interventions involve vessel cannulation, incision, or clamping that can cause plaque disruption through mechanical trauma. A small number of case reports have also implicated thrombolytic agents or anticoagulation therapy (unfractionated heparin, low-molecular-weight [LMW] heparin, or warfarin) as the cause of spontaneous atheroemboli. These events are thought to occur when the therapeutic agent undermines an overlying stabilizing thrombus. A true cause-and-effect relationship has not been shown in clinical studies, and the absolute risk of an atheroembolic event from thrombolytics and anticoagulation appears to be small.

Patients at high risk for atheroembolic disease have extensive atherosclerosis. Typical patients are men older than 60 years with a history of smoking, diabetes, hyperlipidemia, and hypertension. When plaque disruption occurs and distal tissues are showered with cholesterol emboli, the kidney is involved in approximately 75% of all cases. Other frequently affected organs are listed in Table 32.1. After entering the bloodstream, cholesterol crystals typically settle within the arcuate and interlobular arterioles of the kidney, but they can reach the afferent arteriole and glomerular capillary as well. An inflammatory reaction ensues that is characterized

Table 32.1	Commonly Involved Organs in Cholesterol Atheroembolic Disease	
Organ	**Percentage (%)**
Kidney	75
Spleen	52
Pancreas	52
Gastrointestinal tract	31
Adrenal glands	20
Liver	17
Brain	14
Skin	6

initially by granulocyte infiltration and then is followed by mononuclear cell infiltration and giant cell formation. Endothelial proliferation occurs, which leads to intimal thickening and concentric fibrosis. Ultimately this process results in arteriole obstruction and ischemic infarction of downstream tissues, including the glomeruli, tubules, and interstitium. Kidney function may decline acutely, subacutely, or slowly over time. Approximately one-third of cases will present with fulminant AKI, typically occurring within 1 week of the triggering event. This scenario is often the result of a large burden of cholesterol emboli, and rarely is the kidney the only organ involved. The more typical presentation is a subacute decline in kidney function, with AKI appearing on average 5.3 weeks after the initial insult. Kidney dysfunction occurs in a stepwise fashion, representing ongoing crystal embolization. Finally, a chronic or delayed course, in which significant kidney impairment may not be noted until up to 6 months after the trigger, may develop. These cases are likely underrecognized and typically attributed to other causes of CKD, such as hypertensive nephrosclerosis. Large burdens of cholesterol crystals can be associated with a massive catastrophic syndrome with AKI, stroke, gastrointestinal (GI) bleeding, necrotic skin ulcerations, and rapid death. In less severe cases, GI involvement may be limited to abdominal pain, nausea, or vomiting. Skin manifestations can be helpful in making the diagnosis. These include a classic reticular rash over the lower extremities known as livedo reticularis, as well as blue or purple toes, and purpura. Acalculous cholecystitis can occur with liver involvement, and pancreatitis can also be evident. Funduscopic examination may show Hollenhorst plaques, which are refractive yellow deposits from cholesterol emboli seen within retinal arteries. Central nervous system involvement can lead to transient ischemic events, strokes, amaurosis fugax, or spinal cord infarctions.

DIAGNOSIS

The diagnosis of atheroembolic kidney disease can be elusive and requires a high index of suspicion. In addition to the clinical features described previously, laboratory data can be helpful. Initially, leukocytosis and other inflammatory markers, such as ESR or C-reactive protein, are commonly elevated in the setting of the provoked immune response. Eosinophilia is present in 25% to 50% of cases, and occasionally hypocomplementemia can be detected. The negative predictive value of these findings is low, and therefore their absence is not helpful in excluding the diagnosis. Additional lab abnormalities can implicate specific organ involvement, including elevated amylase or lipase with pancreatic involvement, increased transaminases with liver involvement, elevated lactate with bowel involvement, and increased creatine kinase (CK) concentration with muscle involvement. Urine sediment is typically bland, without cellular casts and only a minimal amount of proteinuria.

PATHOLOGY

Definitive diagnosis of atheroembolic kidney disease requires a kidney biopsy, but depending on the clinical circumstances, this may be challenging to perform. A skin or muscle biopsy can also be helpful when these tissues are involved. Often the diagnosis can be made on clinical grounds based on the presenting features, particularly when classic examination findings are present. Kidney lesions include biconvex, needle-shaped clefts within the arcuate and interlobular arterioles (Fig. 32.1). Because the cholesterol crystals dissolve during specimen processing, the clefts are empty and are referred to as "ghost cells." Within the vessels can be seen intimal thickening and concentric fibrosis; it is not uncommon for giant cells to form in the immediate vicinity of the crystal.

Vascular recanalization, endothelial proliferation, tubulointerstitial fibrosis, glomerular ischemia, and focal segmental glomerulosclerosis also characterize what can be seen on kidney biopsy.

THERAPY AND OUTCOMES

The mainstay of therapy for atheroembolic kidney disease is prevention. Paralleling conventional preventive measures for limiting atherosclerotic disease, patients should avoid smoking, hyperlipidemia, and poorly controlled hypertension or diabetes. The benefits of these modifications are extrapolated from data focusing on risk reduction for cardiovascular events, as there are no controlled trials that specifically address

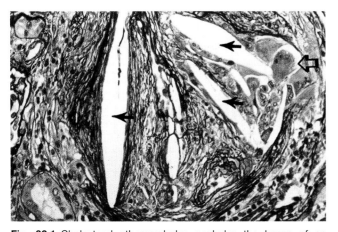

Fig. 32.1 Cholesterol atheroembolus occludes the lumen of an interlobular renal artery. Needle-like clefts *(solid arrows)* can be seen, along with a macrophage–multinucleated giant cell reaction *(open arrow)* (methenamine silver–trichrome stain, original magnification ×450). (Courtesy Dr. S.I. Bastacky. From Greenberg A, Bastacky SI, Iqbal A, et al. Focal segmental glomerulosclerosis associated with nephrotic syndrome in cholesterol atheroembolism: clinicopathologic correlations. *Am J Kidney Dis.* 1997;29:334–344, with permission.)

atheroembolic kidney disease prevention. Despite this, it is advisable to weigh the risks and benefits carefully when planning to initiate or continue anticoagulation or thrombolytic agents in subjects at high risk for cholesterol emboli. The need for elective endovascular procedures should also be critically evaluated, and when reasonable, medical management should be the preferred option. Alternatively, additional strategies that may reduce atheroembolic events include distal embolic protection devices for renovascular procedures and upper extremity approaches via the radial and brachial arteries for cardiac catheterizations. Data showing a reduction in kidney injury when these practices are implemented are sparse but suggest that the benefit may be mediated by minimizing the embolization of cholesterol plaques from the renal arteries and abdominal aorta.

After atheroembolic kidney disease has occurred, effective treatment options are limited. The use of steroids has been assessed in observational studies; however, the results have not shown consistent benefit. The largest prospective study involving 354 patients with atheroembolic kidney disease did not report a benefit in kidney outcomes in those patients treated with steroids. Another study from Spain retrospectively evaluated 45 cases and actually showed worse kidney outcomes in those who received steroids. These findings contradict results from earlier small case series and reports that showed improvement in kidney function with steroid therapy. In summary, data do not support the routine use of steroid therapy for atheroembolic kidney disease; however, they may have a role in patients with evidence of a high inflammatory burden and multiorgan involvement.

Statins have also been evaluated for their potential benefit, and it has been hypothesized that they improve kidney outcomes by way of reductions in lipid burden, plaque stabilization, and antiinflammatory effects. Again, the few observational studies involving patients treated with statins have demonstrated conflicting results regarding their effectiveness in limiting kidney injury. However, these agents should routinely be administered to patients with atheroembolic kidney disease because of their well-established ability to reduce the risk of cardiovascular events. Additionally, the routine use of ACE inhibitors or ARBs should also be implemented because of their known benefit to patients with cardiovascular risk factors. Other therapies indicating benefit in isolated reports include pentoxifylline, iloprost, low-density lipoprotein apheresis, and in some circumstances, segmental aortic replacement to remove the emboli source.

Overall, kidney prognosis is poor in atheroembolic kidney disease, with the majority of patients having progressive kidney failure. The number of subjects with severe kidney failure requiring dialysis ranges from 28% to 61% in various studies. In the largest prospective analysis, 33% of patients required dialysis at some point after diagnosis, and 25% remained on chronic dialysis at the end of 2 years. Those treated with statins had more favorable kidney outcomes, irrespective of whether therapy was initiated at the time of diagnosis or was in place before the triggering event. Important predictors of those likely to require dialysis are preexisting CKD and longstanding hypertension. However, it has been reported that as many as 39% of those who are started on dialysis recover enough kidney function to be dialysis-free at follow-up.

More recent studies have shown decreased mortality with atheroembolic disease as compared to historic case series that documented 1-year survival rates as low as 19%. Belefant et al. implemented an aggressive treatment protocol for 67 consecutive patients diagnosed with atheroembolic kidney disease in an intensive care unit, with a reported 1-year survival rate of 87%. The leading cause of death in atheroembolic kidney failure is from cardiovascular events, and improvement in survival rates in recent studies is a direct result of reducing these risks. In addition, the widespread use of dialysis has also contributed to reduced mortality rates.

KIDNEY INFARCTION

Abrupt disruption of blood supply to the kidney results in kidney infarction. Overall, this is a relatively rare event. While the literature is scant, case series estimate the annual incidence to be 0.004% to 0.007% of all hospital admissions. When kidney infarction occurs, it can involve both kidneys, one entire kidney, or a small subsection depending on the involved vessels. Because of the acute nature of the insult and the lack of collateral blood supply, these events are usually symptomatic. Patients will commonly present with flank or abdominal pain (50% to 96%), nausea and vomiting (15% to 25%), fever (10% to 20%), and microscopic hematuria (30% to 40%). When both kidneys, or a single functioning kidney, are involved, oliguric or anuric AKI may occur. Most cases (80%), however, do not present with a rise in serum creatinine or a change in urine output. Because of the renin release from infarcted tissue, an abrupt rise in blood pressure can occur. Laboratory studies show a leukocytosis and a notable rise in lactate dehydrogenase, as well as C reactive protein. Given the nonspecific nature of the clinical presentation, imaging is needed to confirm the diagnosis. Computed tomography (CT) scan with intravenous contrast is often the imaging modality used because it allows good delineation of poorly perfused areas in the renal cortex. The classic finding is a wedge-shaped lesion demarcating the area of hypoperfusion (Fig. 32.2). A renal nuclear scan with dimercaptosuccinic acid is a more sensitive study, and it is helpful when a high suspicion remains despite negative findings on CT. Finally, a renal artery angiogram is the diagnostic gold standard but is rarely needed.

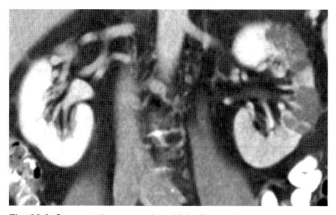

Fig. 32.2 Computed tomography with iodinated intravenous contrast demonstrating an infarction in the left kidney. Note the wedge-shaped appearance of the defect, which is typical for this finding.

A number of etiologies can lead to kidney infarction (Box 32.2). Approximately 50% of patients presenting with kidney infarction will have a cardiogenic source of thromboembolism, with the majority having atrial fibrillation. Other causes of cardiogenic emboli can occur from prosthetic mechanical valves, following myocardial infarction, paradoxical emboli from a patent foramen ovale, or thromboemboli from complex atherosclerotic plaques in the aorta. Approximately 10% of kidney infarctions occur in the setting of hypercoagulable states, and another 10% occur because of renal artery injury due to spontaneous dissection (spontaneous, traumatic, or due to fibromuscular dysplasia or Ehler-Danlos syndrome). Aortic or renal artery dissections can create false lumens that obstruct blood flow to the kidney and lead to infarction. Finally, spontaneous renal artery thrombosis can occur in the setting of atherosclerotic disease, aneurysms, or medium and large vessel vasculitides.

TREATMENT

Treatment is usually conservative. Antihypertensive therapy should be used to minimize the renin-related hypertension; typically ACE inhibitors or ARBs are the agents of choice. Volume overload states should be managed with diuretics and salt restriction. The decision to start anticoagulation is usually dictated by the underlying disorder. When cardiac thrombi or a hypercoagulable state is identified, the initiation of anticoagulation is used to prevent additional emboli. After infarction has occurred, the tissue is not salvageable. For this

---

Box 32.2   Causes of Kidney Infarction

1. **Embolism**
   a. Cardiac origin
      i. Atrial fibrillation
      ii. Valvular disease
      iii. Endocarditis
      iv. Ventricular thrombus
      v. Myxoma
   b. Noncardiac origin
      i. Paradoxical emboli
      ii. Fat emboli
      iii. Tumor emboli
2. **Thrombosis**
   a. Hypercoagulable states
      i. Nephrotic syndrome
      ii. Antiphospholipid syndrome
      iii. Antithrombin III deficiency
      iv. Homocystinuria
   b. Secondary to structural changes of the aorta or renal arteries
      i. Atherosclerotic disease
      ii. Aneurysms
      iii. Dissections
   c. Vasculitis involving the renal artery
      i. Polyarteritis nodosa
      ii. Takayasu arteritis
      iii. Kawasaki disease
      iv. Thromboangiitis obliterans
   d. Trauma
   e. As a complication of endovascular interventions

reason, revascularization with thrombolysis or angioplasty should only be considered in cases in which the diagnosis is made relatively early in the disease course, and under the assumption that restoring perfusion will prevent further tissue involvement. The largest case series published to data on kidney infarction ($n = 422$) reported that approximately 80% of patients were anticoagulated with heparin and warfarin. Only 5% of patients died, and 2% reached end-stage renal disease over a median follow-up of 20 months. However, without a comparison group, it is impossible to know what the outcomes would have been without anticoagulation. In cases of traumatic renal vascular occlusion, surgical repair of the vessel may provide kidney salvage only if the diagnosis is made within the first few hours after occurrence. In patients who develop in situ thrombi in the setting of atherosclerotic kidney disease, previous collateral blood flow has typically developed. These patients often develop ischemic kidney disease without infarction, and it is not unreasonable to use a more liberal revascularization strategy in such cases.

ACUTE TUBULAR INJURY FROM ENDOGENOUS NEPHROTOXINS

Endogenous nephrotoxins cause ATI in specific clinical circumstances. The diagnosis can sometimes be difficult, as the toxin exposure will not be readily reported by the patient or listed in his or her medical records, as is often the case with exogenous toxins. In addition, preventing further toxin exposure to the kidney is not always readily achieved at the time of diagnosis. Treatment strategies often involve manipulating the biochemical environment in which the kidney and toxin interact to limit injury.

RHABDOMYOLYSIS

The term *rhabdomyolysis* specifically refers to the clinical syndrome associated with muscle necrosis and the release of intracellular contents into the extracellular space. The clinical spectrum can range from a relatively benign course to severe systemic illness with AKI due to heme pigment nephropathy. Bywaters and Bell are credited with the initial description of kidney failure resulting from rhabdomyolysis in four cases involving crush injuries during the bombing of London in World War II. This was a landmark contribution to the understanding of heme pigment nephropathy. The incidence of AKI in rhabdomyolysis has been reported to range from 5% to 51%, and mortality rates are dramatically increased with kidney involvement.

CAUSES AND PATHOPHYSIOLOGY OF RHABDOMYOLYSIS

The etiologies of rhabdomyolysis are listed in Box 32.3. Most notable are crush injuries that accompany natural disasters such as hurricanes and earthquakes. AKI from rhabdomyolysis is one of the most common causes of mortality in these

---

Box 32.3   Causes of Rhabdomyolysis

1. Physical injury
   a. Trauma
   b. Crush injury
   c. Compartment syndrome
   d. Immobilization
2. Muscle fiber exhaustion
   a. Excessive exercise
   b. Seizures
   c. Heat stroke
   d. Neuroleptic malignant syndrome
   e. Malignant hyperthermia
3. Medications, illicit drugs, and dietary supplements
   a. Statins
   b. Fibrates
   c. Zidovudine
   d. Phenytoin
   e. Selective serotonin reuptake inhibitors
   f. Isoniazid
   g. Colchicine
   h. Antipsychotics
   i. Antimalarials
   j. Trimethoprim-sulfamethoxazole in HIV infection
   k. Cocaine
   l. Amphetamines
   m. Heroin
   n. Methadone
   o. Phencyclidine
   p. Creatine
   q. Ephedra
4. Toxins
   a. Alcohol
   b. Toluene
   c. Carbon monoxide
   d. Hydrocarbons
   e. Quail poisoning
   f. Mushroom poisoning
5. Electrolyte disturbances
   a. Hypokalemia
   b. Hypophosphatemia
   c. Excessive fluid shifts
6. Inflammatory states
   a. Dermatomyositis and polymyositis
   b. Vasculitis
   c. Systemic inflammatory response
   d. Viral infections (e.g., influenza, parainfluenza, coxsackie, HIV, EBV, CMV, herpes)
   e. Bacterial infection (e.g., Legionnaire disease, tularemia, toxic shock syndrome, streptococci, staphylococci, *Clostridium, Salmonella*)
   f. Protozoal infections (e.g., *Plasmodium falciparum* malaria)
7. Deficiencies in metabolic enzymes
   a. Muscle phosphorylase deficiency (McArdle disease)
   b. Carnitine palmitoyl transferase deficiency
   c. Phosphofructokinase deficiency in muscle (Tarui disease)

CMV, Cytomegalovirus; *EBV*, Epstein-Barr virus; *HIV*, human immunodeficiency virus.

incidents. Immediately following the 2010 earthquake in Haiti, a kidney disaster relief task force was dispatched to provide rapid treatment and dialysis support for victims. The goal of this mission was to limit the number of casualties. Compartment syndrome within a limb causes pressure necrosis that leads to tissue damage and rhabdomyolysis. This may require an emergency fasciotomy. Overexertion causes necrosis in otherwise normal muscles because of a mismatch in energy supply and demand. This is most commonly seen in poorly conditioned persons who partake in extreme exercise activities. However, even well-conditioned athletes can manifest rhabdomyolysis and develop AKI. Cases of experienced marathon runners developing kidney failure and requiring dialysis have been reported. The most frequent etiology in a series of 475 patients was from medications and toxin ingestions. Alcohol and cocaine were the two most abused substances associated with rhabdomyolysis. A number of medications also cause muscle injury; the most frequently implicated agents are antipsychotics, statins, and selective serotonin release inhibitors.

The final common pathologic pathway that leads to the disruption of the muscle-fiber integrity is the increase in the ionized calcium concentration within the cytoplasm (i.e., sarcoplasm). This results in unchecked protease activation and a fatal cascade of cellular events. The elevated intracellular calcium level is a consequence of adenosine triphosphate (ATP) depletion, and Na^+/K^+-ATPase and Ca^{2+}-ATPase failure. This inhibits the normally efficient expulsion of calcium from the cytoplasm.

After muscle cell necrosis occurs, contents in high concentration within the cell are then expelled into the extracellular fluid (ECF), specifically CK, myoglobin, organic acids, and various electrolytes. Ultimately, it is the pathophysiologic consequences of these substances that lead to morbidity and mortality in rhabdomyolysis. Significant electrolyte imbalances in rhabdomyolysis include hyperkalemia, hyperphosphatemia, and hypocalcemia. Hyperkalemia and hyperphosphatemia reflect their relatively high intracellular concentrations. Ninety-eight percent of total body stores of potassium reside intracellularly, and 70% are within skeletal muscle cells. As opposed to potassium and phosphorous, plasma calcium levels decrease during the acute phase of rhabdomyolysis. This phenomenon occurs because calcium complexes with phosphorous and precipitates within necrotic tissues in the form of calcium phosphate. As tissue recovery occurs in the following days to weeks, calcium is mobilized from necrotic tissue and can lead to significant rebound hypercalcemia late in the disease course. The release of lactate and other organic acids from muscle cells manifest as an anion gap metabolic acidosis. In addition, elevated uric acid levels may result from purine metabolism after cell injury.

DIAGNOSIS

The most striking clinical feature of patients who present with rhabdomyolysis is typically severe myalgias. However, on occasion, patients may have minimal or no symptoms, and in other situations subjects may be incapacitated. A high level of suspicion is needed in these cases. The history often shows circumstances or events that support the diagnosis. Patients should be questioned about vigorous physical activity, medication or toxin ingestion, preceding trauma, or prolonged immobilization on a hard surface.

Urine output may be decreased when AKI is significant. Because of the presence of myoglobin, the urine may appear reddish-brown in color. Under the microscope, pigmented granular casts will be seen. Urine dipstick shows significant heme protein positivity with few or no red blood cells seen on microscopy. This apparent discrepancy occurs because the dipstick test is unable to differentiate between myoglobin and hemoglobin. An additional characteristic feature of rhabdomyolysis that is unique from most other forms of ATI is an $FE_{Na} < 1\%$. This is not universal, and it is typically found early in the disease course. Approximately 50% of cases will have some level of proteinuria detected on urinalysis.

Blood tests show elevations in myoglobin and CK. Myoglobin levels are not routinely measured, because myoglobin metabolism is rapid and unpredictable and therefore unreliable. CK, on the other hand, can reach values up to 1000 times the upper limit of normal. The risk of AKI is typically not significant until the CK levels are greater than 15,000 to 20,000 U/L. Electrolyte and acid-base abnormalities, as described earlier, are also indicative of the diagnosis.

HEMOGLOBINURIA

Free circulating hemoglobin occurs in the setting of intravascular hemolysis. In small quantities, circulating hemoglobin will be completely bound by plasma haptoglobin to form a hemoglobin-haptoglobin compound that is then cleared by monocytes and macrophages. However, when significant quantities of hemoglobin are present in the plasma, the haptoglobin supply is quickly depleted. Free circulating hemoglobin exists as a tetramer (two α and two β chains; MW 68 kDa) and a dimer (one α and one β chain; MW 32 kDa). Tetrameric hemoglobin and the hemoglobin-haptoglobin complex are not readily filtered because of their large size; however, dimeric hemoglobin can undergo appreciable glomerular filtration. Filtered hemoglobin is endocytosed by proximal tubular cells or contributes to intratubular cast formation. Hemoglobinuric AKI is included in the spectrum of heme pigment nephropathies. Numerous causes of hemolysis can lead to hemoglobinuria. Common etiologies include transfusion reactions, autoimmune hemolytic anemia, mechanical shearing from prosthetic valves, glucose-6 phosphate dehydrogenase deficiency, paroxysmal nocturnal hemoglobinuria, malaria (blackwater fever), and a number of drugs or toxins.

PATHOGENESIS OF HEME PIGMENT NEPHROPATHY

In addition to the direct tubular toxicity of myoglobin and hemoglobin, additional factors including volume depletion, renal vasoconstriction, acidosis, cytokine release, and tubular cast formation all increase the nephrotoxic potential of heme pigments. Intravascular volume depletion is common with rhabdomyolysis because of fluid sequestration into tissues. In addition, the clinical settings that are associated with rhabdomyolysis often result in volume depletion (crush injury in trapped persons, overexertion, drug and alcohol abuse, immobilization). Impaired renal blood flow occurs because of a decrease in the vasodilator nitric oxide, which is avidly scavenged by heme proteins, and an increase in potent vasoconstrictors (i.e., endothelin and isoprostanes). The consequent decrease in renal perfusion results in ischemic injury to renal tubular cells. Cytokine activation also occurs. Heme-protein–mediated induction of chemokines, such as monocyte chemoattractant-1, results in leukocyte recruitment and additional epithelial cell injury. Acidosis leads to an environment that denatures heme proteins to a confirmation that promotes interaction with Tamm-Horsfall protein and urinary cast formation. Tubular obstruction subsequently occurs, which in turn prolongs the exposure of RTECs to hemoglobin and myoglobin. As a consequence, cellular uptake of heme proteins occurs, leading to renal tubular cell injury by way of lipid peroxidation and free radical formation. Ferrihemate, present in muscle injury, is a major cause of tubular injury in this setting. Finally, in the setting of marked hyperphosphatemia in rhabdomyolysis, calcium-phosphate deposition within the kidney also contributes to tubular injury.

TREATMENT

The treatment for heme pigment nephropathy is similar for both rhabdomyolysis and hemoglobinuria. Early aggressive fluid repletion is most beneficial by correcting volume depletion and subsequent kidney ischemia, but also limiting cast formation and excessive heme protein concentrations within the renal tubule. Patients may require 10 L or more of intravenous fluid daily. Although volume repletion is important for treating heme pigment nephropathy, it remains controversial whether saline is the ideal solution to use. Some experts recommend an isotonic sodium bicarbonate solution. The proposed benefits of alkalinizing the urine with sodium bicarbonate include reducing myoglobin binding with Tamm-Horsfall protein, inhibiting the reduction-oxidation (redox) cycling of myoglobin that leads to lipid peroxidation, and preventing metmyoglobin-induced vasoconstriction. These theoretical effects are mainly generated from animal studies, and there are no robust clinical data to show a clear benefit. In contrast, there is some concern regarding the potential negative effects of sodium bicarbonate administration, as the induced alkalosis may exacerbate the symptoms of hypocalcemia and increase calcium-phosphate precipitation in the kidney. The use of mannitol has also been proposed, often in combination with sodium bicarbonate. Mannitol may increase urinary flow and help flush out heme pigment by inducing an osmotic diuresis. In addition, mannitol is a free radical scavenger. Other antioxidant agents that have shown benefit in small case series include pentoxyfylline, vitamin E, and vitamin C. Kidney replacement therapy is mainly supportive when severe AKI occurs or rapid correction of electrolyte abnormalities is necessary. Despite the dense ATI that can occur in both settings and the frequent need for kidney replacement therapy, most patients recover enough kidney function to become dialysis independent, and many regain function back toward their premorbid level.

ACUTE NEPHROPATHY ASSOCIATED WITH TUMOR LYSIS SYNDROME

Tumor lysis syndrome results from the release of a large amount of intracellular contents into the ECF, following massive necrosis of tumor cells. This typically occurs after the administration of chemotherapeutic agents for the treatment of lymphomas and leukemias, but it can rarely occur spontaneously in rapidly dividing solid tumors that outgrow their blood supply.

Laboratory tests show high serum levels of potassium, phosphate, and uric acid. Acute crystalline nephropathy is a common occurrence and is a direct consequence of uric acid and calcium-phosphate precipitation within the renal tubules. Because uric acid crystal formation is enhanced in acidic urine, alkalinization of the urine with sodium bicarbonate infusion has been used to prevent or limit urate nephropathy. However, this strategy may in turn lead to more calcium-phosphate deposition and acute nephrocalcinosis. Some experts suggest management with saline alone to induce high urine flow, and only implementing sodium bicarbonate therapy when the serum uric acid level is greater than 12 mg/dL or uric acid crystals are seen on microscopy. Allopurinol and rasburicase limit the formation of uric acid by either inhibiting its production (allopurinol) or increasing its metabolism (rasburicase). These medications should be considered as prophylaxis in high-risk patients planned for chemotherapy.

OTHER ENDOGENOUS TOXINS

Given the concentrating ability of the kidney, other endogenous substances can accumulate within the renal tubules and cause ATI. Similar to the previous causes, this occurs when pathologic states lead to elevated plasma levels of substances that are relatively benign under normal conditions. In myeloma, free monoclonal light chains are filtered by the glomerulus in large quantities. After entering the tubule, they cause direct proximal tubule cellular toxicity (proximal tubulopathy) and cast injury in the distal tubule, resulting in myeloma cast nephropathy.

Plasma levels of oxalate can be elevated as a result of either endogenous production or exogenous ingestion. In primary hyperoxaluria, oxalate overproduction occurs as a result of an inborn error in the metabolism of glyoxylate. This leads to urine oxalate concentrations at supersaturated levels. Calcium oxalate precipitation occurs and results in crystal aggregation and nephrocalcinosis. The resulting tubular injury can lead to significant kidney damage. Hyperoxaluria also occurs following gastric bypass surgery and with other causes of malabsorption (pancreatitis, Crohn disease). This occurrence is a result of increased gut absorption of oxalate from dietary sources. Exogenous etiologies include ingestion of ethylene glycol (antifreeze), large doses of orlistat, and excessive amounts of vitamin C.

BIBLIOGRAPHY

Abuelo JG. Normotensive ischemic acute renal failure. *N Engl J Med.* 2007;357:797-805.

Belenfant X, Meyrier A, Jacquot C. Supportive treatment improves survival in multivisceral cholesterol crystal embolism. *Am J Kidney Dis.* 1999;33:840-850.

Bourgault M, Grimbert P, Verret C, et al. Acute renal infarction: a case series. *Clin J Am Soc Nephrol.* 2013;8:392-398.

Bywaters EG, Beall D. Crush injuries with impairment of renal function. *Br Med J.* 1941;1:427-432.

Frock J, Bierman M, Hammeke M, et al. Atheroembolic renal disease: experience with 22 patients. *Nebr Med J.* 1994;79:317-321.

Gutierrez Solis E, Morales E, Rodriguez Jornet A, et al. Atheroembolic renal disease: analysis of clinical and therapeutic factors that influence its progression. *Nefrologia.* 2010;30:317-323.

Howard SC, Jones DP, Pui CH. The tumor lysis syndrome. *N Engl J Med.* 2011;364:1844-1854.

Kashani K, Al-Khafaji A, Ardiles T, et al. Discovery and validation of cell cycle arrest biomarkers in human acute kidney injury. *Crit Care.* 2013;17:R25.

Korzets Z, Plotkin E, Bernheim J, et al. The clinical spectrum of acute renal infarction. *Isr Med Assoc J.* 2002;4:781-784.

Koyner JL, Shaw AD, Chawla LS, et al. Tissue inhibitor metalloproteinase-2 (TIMP-2)IGF binding protein-7 (IGFBP7) levels are associated with adverse long-term outcomes in patients with AKI. *J Am Soc Nephrol.* 2015;26:1747-1754.

Meersch M, Schmidt C, Van Aken H. Urinary TIMP-2 and IGFBP7 as early biomarkers of acute kidney injury and renal recovery following cardiac surgery. *PLoS ONE.* 2014;9:e93460.

Melli G, Chaudhry V, Cornblath DR. Rhabdomyolysis: an evaluation of 475 hospitalized patients. *Medicine (Baltimore).* 2005;84:377-385.

Meyrier A. Cholesterol crystal embolism: diagnosis and treatment. *Kidney Int.* 2006;69:1308-1312.

Nasr SH, D'Agati VD, Said SM, et al. Oxalate nephropathy complicating Roux-en-Y gastric bypass: an under recognized cause of irreversible renal failure. *Clin J Am Soc Nephrol.* 2008;3:1676-1683.

Oh YK, Yang CW, Kim YL, et al. Clinical characteristics and outcomes of renal infarction. *Am J Kidney Dis.* 2016;67:243-250.

Perazella MA, Coca SG, Hall IE, et al. Urine microscopy is associated with severity and worsening of acute kidney injury in hospitalized patients. *Clin J Am Soc Nephrol.* 2010;5:402-408.

Scolari F, Ravani P. Atheroembolic renal disease. *Lancet.* 2010;375: 1650-1660.

Thurau K, Boylan JW. Acute renal success: the unexpected logic of oliguria in acute renal failure. *Am J Med.* 1976;61:308-315.

Tracz MJ, Alam J, Nath KA. Physiology and pathophysiology of heme: implications for kidney disease. *J Am Soc Nephrol.* 2007;18:414-420.

33 Acute Interstitial Nephritis

Ursula C. Brewster; Randy L. Luciano

In 1898, W. T. Councilman defined acute interstitial nephritis (AIN) as "an acute inflammation of the kidney characterized by cellular and fluid exudation in the interstitial tissue, accompanied by, but not dependent on, degeneration of the epithelium; the exudation is not purulent in character, and the lesions may be both diffuse and focal." This was seen on postmortem examination of patients with scarlet fever and, less commonly, other systemic infectious diseases that had no evidence for direct bacterial invasion of the kidney parenchyma.

More than a century later, definitive diagnosis of AIN requires the pathologic findings of interstitial edema and infiltration with acute inflammatory cells, including polymorphonucleocytes (PMNs), eosinophils, and lymphocytes. In the years since Councilman's description, the causes of AIN have changed dramatically, with pharmacologic agents now being the most common etiology (more than 75%). In this chapter we will focus primarily on acute tubulointerstitial inflammation, while briefly covering direct parenchymal invasion by infectious agents.

The incidence of AIN varies greatly, depending on the clinical scenario. An incidence of 0.7% is seen in asymptomatic patients with proteinuria or hematuria, whereas hospitalized patients with acute kidney injury (AKI) of unknown etiology experience an incidence of 10% to 15%. Although AIN can occur in all age groups, it is more common in the elderly. In one report, biopsy-proven AIN was seen in 3.0% of the elderly compared with 1.9% of younger subjects. This may reflect greater exposure of elderly patients to drugs and other inciting factors.

CLINICAL PRESENTATION

The presenting symptoms of AIN include an acute or subacute decline in kidney function, often in patients exposed to multiple drugs. Although the "classic" presentation of skin rash, arthralgia, and eosinophilia is occasionally seen, this triad occurs in only 5% to 10% of unselected patients. This presentation more commonly occurs in association with certain drugs, such as penicillin derivatives, compared with nonsteroidal antiinflammatory drugs (NSAIDs). Fever, the most common clinical sign, is present in up to 50% of patients with drug-induced AIN but only in 30% of unselected patients. Skin rash is reported in one-third of patients and is usually maculopapular or morbilliform, typically involving the trunk. More often, a rash is seen when the cause of AIN is related to a drug hypersensitivity reaction. No clinical symptoms or signs are sensitive or specific enough to establish a definitive

diagnosis. Nonoliguric AKI usually accompanies AIN, but oliguric AKI with a rapid rise in creatinine also occurs. Increasingly, AIN develops in patients with underlying chronic kidney disease (CKD) and multiple comorbidities, which makes a diagnosis challenging. AIN should therefore be considered in any patient with acute or subacute decline in kidney function with no clear inciting factor.

LABORATORY FINDINGS

Common laboratory findings in AIN are summarized in Table 33.1. The most common abnormality is a slow and steady decline in the glomerular filtration rate (GFR). When dealing with drug-induced AIN, the GFR typically falls 7 to 10 days after starting the medication. Rapid and fulminant presentation of AIN occurs less often, unless there has been previous drug exposure. However, drugs such as the NSAIDs and proton pump inhibitors (PPIs) may not develop AIN for many weeks or months after initial exposure. The time course for AIN related to systemic disease, metabolic disturbances, or infection is more varied and prolonged. Other major laboratory findings include eosinophilia, eosinophiluria, and abnormal urinary sediment. Eosinophilia is common in β-lactam antibiotic–associated AIN, reported in up to 80% of cases, where only a third of other drug-induced AIN cases develop eosinophilia. Hyperkalemia, with or without hyperchloremic metabolic acidosis, is occasionally seen. Anemia is also commonly described in AIN. This finding is rather nonspecific, especially in the setting of systemic inflammation, AKI, or underlying CKD. Anemia with AIN is most likely the result of decreased erythropoietin production from the medullary interstitium and underlying erythropoietin hyporesponsiveness in the setting of inflammation or infection.

Urinalysis and the examination of the urine sediment are often the most useful laboratory tests. Low-grade proteinuria (1–2+) and positive leukocyte esterase are noted on urine dipsticks in most patients. Leukocyte esterase has been noted to be positive in approximately 80% of patients with AIN. Quantitative proteinuria measurements are usually less than 1 g/day, with the majority being nonalbumin proteinuria. (Albuminuria would be more indicative of glomerular disease.) Macroscopic hematuria is rare, whereas microscopic hematuria is present less than 50% of the time. Leukocytes are present on urine microscopy in virtually all cases of methicillin-induced AIN, but may be absent in as many as 50% of patients with AIN due to other drugs. The absence of leukocyturia, therefore, should not eliminate this diagnosis from the differential. Classically, urine microscopy will show

Table 33.1 Laboratory Findings in Acute Interstitial Nephritis

Eosinophilia	Inconsistent finding seen more commonly in drug-induced AIN
Eosinophiluria (>1% and >5%)	Sensitivity 19.8%–30.8%, specificity 68.2%–91.2%, PPV 15.6%–30%, NPV 83.7%–85.6%, positive LR 0.97–2.3, negative LR 0.9–1.01
Urinary sediment	Hematuria, leukocyteuria, leukocyte casts, RTE cells, and RTE casts
Protein excretion	Less than 1 g/24 hours
Fractional excretion of sodium (FeNa)	Greater than 1%
Proximal tubular defect	Glycosuria, phosphaturia, bicarbonaturia, aminoaciduria
Distal tubular defect	Hyperkalemia, distal RTA, sodium wasting
Medullary defect	Nephrogenic diabetes insipidus

AIN, Acute interstitial nephritis; *LR,* likelihood ratio; *NPV,* negative predictive value; *PPV,* positive predictive value; *RTA,* renal tubular acidosis; *RTE,* renal tubular epithelial.

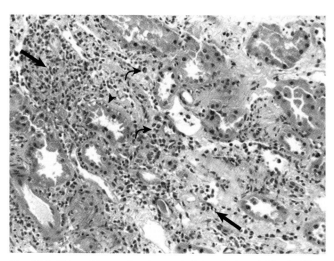

Fig. 33.2 Kidney biopsy showing acute interstitial nephritis. A diffuse interstitial infiltrate is present *(arrows)* along with severe tubular injury and tubulitis *(arrowhead),* where lymphocytes have crossed the tubular basement membrane. Also present are eosinophils *(curved arrows)* (hematoxylin and eosin ×40).

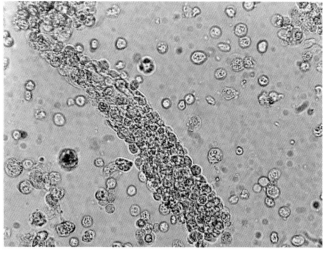

Fig. 33.1 Urine microscopy showing a white blood cell cast and surrounding white blood cells (×60).

hematuria, leukocyturia, leukocyte casts, and renal tubular epithelial (RTE) cells (Fig. 33.1). Red blood cell casts and mixed red blood cell and white blood cells casts have also been reported. Cellular casts are seen in most cases of methicillin-associated AIN and in up to 50% of patients, with AIN resulting from other etiologies. However, up to 20% of AIN cases can have a bland urinary sediment.

Eosinophiluria, once thought to be hallmark of this disease, is neither sensitive nor specific and should not be used to make a diagnosis. When using a cutoff of greater than 1% urinary eosinophils, the sensitivity and specificity are 30.8% and 68.2%, respectively. A 5% urinary eosinophil cutoff increases specificity to 91.2% but decreases sensitivity to 19.8%. Various techniques used to stain urine for eosinophils and enhance detection (Wright stain and Hansel stain) have proven unreliable and cumbersome. In addition, other disease states such as cystitis, pyelonephritis, atheroembolic kidney

disease, and rapidly progressive glomerulonephritis may present with eosinophiluria, highlighting the poor specificity of this test.

IMAGING

Kidney ultrasound in the setting of AIN typically shows normal to enlarged kidneys with normal echogenicity. However, these findings are also nonspecific and may be seen with other forms of kidney disease. Although gallium-67 scan was initially reported as highly sensitive in AIN, this has not been supported over time, and its only role may be to differentiate AIN from acute tubular necrosis (ATN) in those patients who cannot undergo a kidney biopsy. Positron emission tomography has shown diagnostic promise in several AIN cases but needs further evaluation before widespread use.

PATHOLOGY

Although suspicion of AIN is based on clinical clues, definitive diagnosis often requires a kidney biopsy. Major pathologic findings include interstitial edema, inflammation, and tubulitis without glomerular or vascular involvement (Fig. 33.2). Interstitial infiltration may be diffuse but is often patchy in nature and consists of lymphocytes, mononuclear cells, eosinophils, neutrophils, and plasma cells. T lymphocytes are primarily composed of CD4 and CD8 cells. The number of eosinophils is highly variable and is more prominent in drug-induced AIN. Granulomas are uncommon but occasionally seen, especially with sarcoidosis and drug-induced AIN. Tubulitis, characterized by the invasion of inflammatory cells though the tubular basement membrane, results in tubular injury and is often seen in association with severe inflammation. The severity of interstitial inflammation, however, does not always correlate with clinical outcome. Poor prognosis is more directly related to the degree of interstitial fibrosis and tubular atrophy. Immunofluorescence and electron microscopic studies are usually unrevealing. NSAID-associated AIN is sometimes associated with glomerular changes of minimal change disease or membranous nephropathy. In contrast to isolated AIN, full-blown nephrotic syndrome accompanies AKI in NSAID-related cases.

PATHOGENESIS

The clinical and histopathologic findings summarized earlier strongly point to an immune-mediated mechanism initiating and sustaining tubulointerstitial damage. The immunologic basis of injury is supported by the low frequency of AIN in persons exposed to a drug, lack of dose dependency, presence of systemic symptoms in some patients, and recurrence of AIN upon re-exposure. The antigens initiating the immune-mediated injury could be of endogenous origin (Tamm-Horsfall protein, megalin, and tubular base membrane components) or exogenous, such as drugs and chemicals. Exogenous antigens may be trapped directly or may circulate as immune complexes that are deposited in the kidney interstitium. They may bind to a tubular antigen acting as a hapten or mimic a normal tubular or interstitial antigen, thereby triggering an immune reaction. In animal models, both cell-mediated and humoral immunity is involved. The injury is initiated by the presentation of endogenous or exogenous antigens to antigen-presenting lymphocytes resulting in the activation of T cells. These cells induce differentiation and proliferation of other T cells responsible for delayed hypersensitivity and cytotoxicity. The resultant inflammatory infiltrates within the interstitium produce a variety of fibrinogenic cytokines and chemokines, such as transforming growth factor-β (TGF-β), platelet-derived growth factor-BB (PDGF-BB), epidermal growth factor (EGF), and fibroblast growth factor-2 (FGF-2). The fibroblasts invading the interstitium are the product of epithelial-to-mesenchymal transition. Ultimately, this inflammatory process results in the accumulation of extracellular matrix, interstitial fibrosis, and tubular loss.

NSAID-induced interstitial nephritis appears to have a different mechanism of action. NSAIDs inhibit cyclooxygenase-1 and cyclooxygenase-2, enzymes that catalyze the conversion of arachidonic acid into prostaglandin H2. When this reaction is inhibited, arachidonic acid can then be converted preferentially to leukotrienes through the action of lipoxygenase. This results in an imbalance of inflammatory mediators with an abundance of the proinflammatory leukotrienes and a paucity of prostaglandins, which serve to regulate the inflammatory cascade.

CAUSES OF ACUTE INTERSTITIAL NEPHRITIS

There are multiple causes of AIN, but pharmacologic agents are the most common (Table 33.2). Diagnosis of AIN should trigger a review of the medication list to identify culpable agents and limit further drug exposure. In addition to various drugs, certain infectious agents may induce AIN. Although less common in the antibiotic era, infectious agents must be considered when the clinical scenario is consistent. Finally, systemic diseases, primarily rheumatologic, are associated with

Table 33.2   Common Drugs Associated With Acute Interstitial Nephritis

Drug Class	Examples
Antibiotics	β-lactams, sulfonamides, fluoroquinolones, rifampin, vancomycin, erythromycin, ethambutol, chloramphenicol
Antivirals	Acyclovir, atazanavir, abacavir, indinavir
Analgesics	NSAIDs, selective COX-2 inhibitors
GI medications	PPIs, H2-receptor blockers, 5-aminosalicylates
Anticonvulsants	Phenytoin, carbamazepine, phenobarbital
Diuretics	Hydrochlorothiazide, furosemide, triamterene, chlorthalidone
Anticancer agents	Tyrosine kinase inhibitors, checkpoint inhibitors, B-RAF inhibitors
Others	Allopurinol, Chinese herbs

COX-2, Cyclooxygenase-2; *GI*, gastrointestinal; *NSAIDs*, nonsteroidal antiinflammatory drugs; *PPIs*, proton pump inhibitors.

Table 33.3   Common Diseases Associated With Acute Interstitial Nephritis

Bacterial infection	*Legionella, Staphylococcus, Streptococcus, Yersinia*
Viral infection	Hantavirus, CMV, EBV, HIV, herpes simplex, Hep C
Autoimmune	Systemic lupus erythematosis, Sjögren syndrome, sarcoidosis
Neoplastic diseases	Lymphoproliferative disorders, plasma cell dyscrasias

CMV, Cytomegalovirus; *EBV*, Epstein-Barr virus; *Hep C*, hepatitis C virus; *HIV*, human immunodeficiency virus.

the pathologic findings of AIN. These diseases are usually evident from the clinical presentation (Table 33.3).

DRUG-ASSOCIATED INTERSTITIAL NEPHRITIS

ANTIBIOTICS

β-LACTAM ANTIBIOTICS

Methicillin and other β-lactam antibiotics are common agents associated with AIN. Methicillin is immunogenic and leads to a hypersensitivity syndrome more often than other drugs, including those in the β-lactam class. The time course is variable, but AIN usually develops 10 to 14 days following drug exposure, unless previous sensitization has occurred. Patients with β-lactam–induced AIN frequently manifest systemic symptoms of fever, rash, arthralgias, and eosinophilia, along with AKI. These symptoms may be fleeting or nonexistent, making them unreliable clinical tools for diagnosing AIN. Urinalysis and urine microscopy demonstrate low-grade proteinuria, hematuria, and leukocyturia in approximately 75% of cases (see Fig. 33.1). Given its association with AIN, methicillin is rarely used because of the availability of other β-lactam agents. Cephalosporins may cause a similar clinical presentation of AIN; however, this is less common than with traditional penicillins. On withdrawal of the drug, kidney function usually recovers, although CKD may persist in some.

NON β-LACTAM ANTIBIOTICS

Rifampin-induced AIN can be severe and appears to occur more frequently with intermittent dosing as compared with continuous dosing regimens. AIN develops in a dose-dependent fashion in most but not all patients, and at times, circulating antibodies to rifampin may be detected. Systemic manifestations include fever, chills, abdominal pain, and myalgia. Laboratory abnormalities include elevated liver transaminases, hemolytic anemia, and thrombocytopenia. Kidney histopathology demonstrates interstitial inflammation with invasion of mononuclear cells and occasional eosinophils. Tubular epithelial cell injury and tubular necrosis related to vasomotor injury may also occur. Patients with a history of a severe reaction should not be re-exposed to the agent, because of the potential risk of hemodynamic collapse.

Sulfonamides are widely used antibiotics associated with kidney injury. When these drugs were introduced in the first half of the twentieth century, the most common kidney injury was tubular obstruction from crystalline deposition of insoluble drug and/or metabolite. Currently, AIN is the most common cause of kidney injury reported with these agents. Patients exposed to these drugs often present with an acute hypersensitivity syndrome characterized by fever, rash, and eosinophilia. Patients with human immunodeficiency virus (HIV) infection, kidney transplant recipients, or those with underlying CKD appear to be more susceptible to an allergic reaction, but the increased use of agents such as trimethoprim-sulfamethoxazole in these populations may account for this observation. Patients who are slow acetylators of sulfonamides may be at higher risk because of drug accumulation, even with routine dosing schedules.

Fluoroquinolones, particularly ciprofloxacin, may cause kidney injury by several mechanisms; however, AIN is the most common kidney complication. AIN often presents with a slowly progressive decline in kidney function, despite the absence of a hypersensitivity syndrome. Ciprofloxacin, based on its widespread use, is the most common agent in this class to cause AIN.

Azithromycin, erythromycin, ethambutol, gentamicin, nitrofurantoin, tetracycline, vancomycin, and multiple antiviral agents have all been associated with AIN. No drug is beyond suspicion, and every agent must be considered in the evaluation.

NONSTEROIDAL ANTIINFLAMMATORY AGENTS

Nonsteroidal antiinflammatory agents are widely used by patients, including those with chronic illness and chronic pain. Both NSAIDs and the selective cyclooxygenase-2 (COX-2) inhibitors are associated with AIN. Given the high frequency of NSAID use, AIN remains a relatively rare event, supporting an idiosyncratic drug reaction. NSAIDs cause several kidney syndromes (see Chapter 35), marked by hemodynamic AKI, electrolyte/acid-base disturbances, and nephrotic syndrome. AIN associated with NSAIDs presents more insidiously than that seen with antibiotics. It often occurs months after starting therapy, with an average onset time of 6 to 18 months. Classically patients do not develop a hypersensitivity syndrome, and fever, eosinophilia, and rash are rare. An interstitial infiltrate, which is less intense and has fewer eosinophils than that seen with other culprit agents, and tubulitis are noted on kidney histopathology. Despite multiple classes of NSAIDs with a variety of chemical structures, the pattern of kidney injury is remarkably similar across all agents, arguing against a single epitope-induced immune response.

GASTROINTESTINAL AGENTS

PPIs have emerged as the most frequent cause of AIN worldwide. In many countries, these agents are available over-the-counter, further increasing their use. Since omeprazole became available in the early 1990s, the number of prescriptions for PPIs has continued to increase. The mean time to AIN diagnosis from drug initiation is approximately 11 weeks, although it can occur after months of therapy. Only 10% of patients with PPI-induced AIN will present with the classic hypersensitivity syndrome of fever, rash, and eosinophilia, and therefore symptoms are either absent or very mild and nonspecific. Early recognition and treatment of AIN are associated with a relatively good prognosis, and AIN induced by PPIs rarely requires kidney replacement therapy. However, CKD may occur in a large percentage of these patients. CKD itself has been implicated as a complication of PPI use, with studies showing a 29% to 50% higher risk of CKD in patients exposed to PPIs.

5-Aminosalicylates are the mainstay of therapy for patients with inflammatory bowel disease. Most patients require long-term treatment and many years of drug exposure. Kidney impairment is rare with these drugs, occurring in 1 in 200 to 500 patients on therapy. A hypersensitivity reaction can occur and cause AIN. In the absence of early recognition, CKD from chronic interstitial fibrosis may develop. This reaction usually occurs within the first year of therapy, but it can develop at any time in a dose-independent fashion.

DIURETICS

Diuretic-induced AKI is almost always related to kidney hypoperfusion from decreased intravascular volume. There are, however, multiple case reports of diuretic-induced AIN from furosemide, hydrochlorothiazide, chlorthalidone, and triamterene. AIN is relatively rare, despite widespread use of these drugs. In published reports, most patients experience systemic symptoms, including fever, rash, and eosinophilia, suggesting a hypersensitivity syndrome. Drug discontinuation generally leads to kidney recovery.

INFECTIONS

INVASIVE INFECTIONS

In the preantibiotic era, streptococcal and diphtheria infections caused inflammatory reactions in the kidney in the absence of direct tissue invasion. However, infection-related AIN diminished in frequency after antibiotics became readily available. Now when AKI develops in the setting of an infection treated with antibiotics, the drug is assumed to be the culprit. If AKI persists despite antibiotic withdrawal, an acute postinfectious glomerulonephritis or AIN should be considered.

Tubulointerstitial injury can occur either from direct invasion by an organism, as in pyelonephritis, or indirectly by an immune-mediated mechanism. Unlike AIN, pyelonephritis is usually confined to one pyramid in the kidney. In the setting of urinary obstruction, it becomes more diffuse, resulting in AKI. Although clinical history and symptoms usually differentiate the two conditions readily, CT imaging showing a wedge-shaped area of inflammation supports a diagnosis of pyelonephritis rather than AIN.

A number of infectious agents have been linked with invasive AIN. These include Epstein-Barr virus (EBV), legionella, mycoplasma, cytomegalovirus, adenovirus, rickettsial Rocky Mountain spotted fever, babesiosis, and fungal infections. Leptospirosis is a classic example of invasive AIN. The spirochete enters the bloodstream through the skin or mucosa, and it transiently invades glomerular capillaries before migrating into the tubulointerstitium. Once in this compartment, the organism induces inflammation and direct tubular injury that, over time, manifests as large, edematous kidneys. In addition, ischemic ATN may coexist with AIN in patients who develop septic shock from overwhelming leptospiral infection. Eradication of infection is associated with recovery of kidney function.

Hantavirus is an RNA virus associated with interstitial edema with infiltration of polymorphonuclear leukocytes, eosinophils, and monocytes. Interstitial hemorrhage accompanies kidney inflammation and is associated with gross or microscopic hematuria. Candidemia has been associated with an interstitial inflammatory reaction initially limited to the renal cortex. With time, large fungus balls can form, obstruct the collecting system, and cause AKI as a result of obstructive uropathy.

NONINVASIVE INFECTIONS

Even without direct invasion of the kidney, infectious agents have been associated with AIN. Historically, streptococcal infections were commonly associated with AIN. The clinical syndrome associated with AIN develops early in the course of infection (9 to 12 days). Given the rapidity with which streptococcal infections are treated currently, infection-related AIN has disappeared as a clinical entity.

SYSTEMIC DISEASES

The classic lesions of acute tubulointerstitial inflammation may also complicate a variety of systemic diseases. Whereas rheumatologic diseases primarily cause immune-mediated glomerular disease, they can also induce AIN. Metabolic diseases and malignancy are also associated with interstitial inflammation and AKI.

TUBULOINTERSTITIAL NEPHRITIS AND UVEITIS

Tubulointerstitial nephritis and uveitis (TINU) is a rare condition of unclear etiology that presents most frequently in adolescent girls but may appear in adulthood. Weight loss, fever, anemia, and hyperglobulinemia occur before ocular and kidney manifestations. Fanconi syndrome with glucosuria, proteinuria, and aminoaciduria is the initial kidney manifestation, followed by a tubulointerstitial infiltrate, sometimes

with granulomas. Certain infections such as toxoplasmosis, Epstein-Barr infection, and giardiasis have been associated with TINU. However, there is no clearly elucidated immune or genetic cause. Steroids are the mainstay of therapy for both the ocular and kidney manifestations of the disease. Fortunately, the prognosis is good in treated patients.

IMMUNOLOGIC DISEASES

The vast majority of rheumatologic diseases complicated by AKI have underlying glomerular disease from antiglomerular basement membrane (GBM) antibody disease (i.e., Goodpasture disease), immune deposition diseases (lupus or IgA nephropathy among others), or antineutrophil cytoplasmic antibody (ANCA)–related pauci-immune vasculitides. However, there are some rheumatologic ailments, such as Sjögren and sarcoidosis, that may present with tubulointerstitial inflammation in the absence of glomerular involvement. In the right clinical scenario, these causes of AIN should remain high on the differential diagnosis of kidney injury.

Immune-related injury in a transplanted kidney (cellular rejection) manifests primarily as tubulointerstitial inflammation with or without vascular involvement. The workup and classification of this interstitial disease can be found in Chapter 61.

MALIGNANCY

Patients with underlying cancer are at high risk for AKI because of the malignancy itself or therapies used in its management. Primary lymphoma of the kidney is a rare cause of AKI, whereas non-Hodgkin lymphoma and acute lymphoblastic leukemias commonly invade the kidney parenchyma. Although it is seen on rare occasions in Hodgkin lymphoma, infiltrates are usually bilateral and diffuse, and kidneys may appear enlarged on imaging. Multiple myeloma and the plasma cell dyscrasias cause kidney injury when filtered light chains coalesce and obstruct tubular lumens. These obstructive "casts" are accompanied by varying degrees of tubular injury, necrosis, and an interstitial inflammatory reaction on kidney biopsy that resembles classic interstitial nephritis.

TREATMENT

Treatment of AIN depends on the underlying disease that is driving the inflammatory reaction. When the pathologic process is associated with an underlying disease such as a malignancy, therapy is directed at the identified cause. In rheumatologic disease, treatment of the inflammatory condition often improves kidney function as well. In the setting of infection-related interstitial nephritis, eradication of the infection is often associated with kidney recovery.

Treatment of drug-induced AIN is more complicated and controversial. The most important intervention is early recognition of disease and its causative agent and drug discontinuation. This can be a complicated endeavor in patients taking multiple essential medications, making it challenging to identify the culprit drug. Careful scrutiny of the medication record for exposure dates and history of previous drug treatment may point to the offending agent. When a drug is suspected, it should be immediately discontinued and replaced, if necessary, with an agent from a different class. A drug-free trial should be undertaken to determine if kidney function recovers without further intervention. If no improvement is noted after a period of observation (3 to 5 days), or if kidney function is declining rapidly, a trial of corticosteroids is reasonable. Prognosis appears to depend on the timing of diagnosis and drug withdrawal. In general, earlier is better, with data supporting a 1- to 2-week time frame. Despite this, a substantial proportion of patients (up to 35%) may develop CKD.

The data published on use of corticosteroids for AIN are incomplete. Assuming the offending drug is withdrawn, steroids improved the rate of kidney recovery in several small studies (fewer than 20 patients). A review of seven nonrandomized retrospective studies, including up to 100 patients, showed no benefit of steroids in recovery of kidney function or prevention of CKD. However, many of the retrospective studies were biased against steroids, as more severely affected patients were treated, confounding the results.

Early steroid therapy, initiated 1 to 2 weeks after diagnosis, is more likely to improve kidney function compared with those started later. In addition, it is reasonable to offer steroids to those with severe AIN, where kidney replacement therapy is or will likely be required in the absence of rapid kidney recovery. Steroid therapy is recommended for 4 to 6 weeks with a slow taper. If there is no substantial improvement in kidney function after 3 to 4 weeks, response is unlikely and steroids should be discontinued.

There are limited data available on other forms of immunosuppression. In a small case series of eight patients, mycophenolate mofetil (MMF) improved or stabilized kidney function in patients with steroid-dependent or steroid-resistant AIN. As a result, MMF may offer an alternative therapy to corticosteroids, but more data are required before this agent can be recommended.

BIBLIOGRAPHY

Baldwin DS, Levine BB, McCluskey RT, et al. Renal failure and interstitial nephritis due to penicillin and methicillin. *N Engl J Med.* 1968; 279:1245-1252.

Brewster UC, Perazella MA. Proton pump inhibitors and the kidney: critical review. *Clin Nephrol.* 2007;68:65-72.

Clarkson MR, Giblin L, O'Connell FP, et al. Acute interstitial nephritis: clinical features and response to corticosteroid therapy. *Nephrol Dial Transplant.* 2004;19:2778-2783.

Councilman WT. Acute interstitial nephritis. *J Exp Med.* 1898;3:393-420.

Fogazzi GB, Ferrari B, Garigali G, Simonini P, Consonni D. Urinary sediment findings in acute interstitial nephritis. *Am J Kidney Dis.* 2012; 60:330-332.

González E, Gutiérrez E, Galeano C, et al. Early steroid treatment improves the recovery of renal function in patients with drug-induced acute interstitial nephritis. *Kidney Int.* 2008;73:940-946.

Ivanyi B, Hamilton-Dutoit SJ, Hansen HE, et al. Acute tubulointerstitial nephritis: phenotype of infiltrating cells and prognostic impact of tubulitis. *Virchows Arch.* 1996;428:5-12.

Michel DM, Kelly CJ. Acute interstitial nephritis. *J Am Soc Nephrol.* 1998; 9:506-515.

Muriithi AK, Nasr SH, Leung N. Utility of urine eosinophils in the diagnosis of acute interstitial nephritis. *Clin J Am Soc Nephrol.* 2013;8: 1857-1862.

Nielson EG. Pathogenesis and therapy of interstitial nephritis. *Kidney Int.* 1989;35:1257-1270.

Perazella MA, Bomback AS. Urinary eosinophils in AIN: farewell to an old biomarker? *Clin J Am Soc Nephrol.* 2013;8:1841-1843.

Perazella MA, Markowitz GS. Drug-induced acute interstitial nephritis. *Nat Rev Nephrol.* 2010;6:461-470.

Praga M, González E. Acute interstitial nephritis. *Kidney Int.* 2010; 77:956-961.

Preddie DC, Markowitz GS, Radhakrishnan J, et al. Mycophenolate mofetil for the treatment of interstitial nephritis. *Clin J Am Soc Nephrol.* 2006;1:718-722.

Raghavan R, Eknoyan G. Acute interstitial nephritis—a reappraisal and update. *Clin Nephrol.* 2014;82:149-162.

Rossert J. Drug-induced acute interstitial nephritis. *Kidney Int.* 2001; 60:804-817.

Ruffing KA, Hoppes P, Blend D, et al. Eosinophils in urine revisited. *Clin Nephrol.* 1994;41:163-166.

Spanou Z, Keller M, Britschgi M, et al. Involvement of drug-specific T cells in acute drug-induced interstitial nephritis. *J Am Soc Nephrol.* 2006;17:2919-2927.

34

Management of Acute Kidney Injury

Matthew T. James; Neesh Pannu

Acute kidney injury (AKI) is defined by a decline in kidney function or reduction in urine output occurring over hours to days. It is associated with prolonged hospitalization, substantial resource utilization, high mortality, and progressive chronic kidney disease (CKD) and end-stage renal disease (ESRD) in survivors. The principles of management of AKI include timely recognition of the problem, identification and correction of the underlying cause, and steps to avoid further kidney injury. After AKI is established, current therapeutic options are limited, and mortality remains high despite recent technologic advancements. Nonetheless, regional and temporal variations in mortality among patients hospitalized for AKI suggest that several elements of management, including supportive care, management of complications, and use of renal replacement therapy (RRT), may influence outcomes. This chapter focuses on the management of early or established AKI resulting from prerenal causes or acute tubular necrosis (ATN), which contribute to the majority of cases encountered in hospitalized patients. Readers are referred elsewhere in the *Primer* for a review of specific aspects of treatment for acute interstitial nephritis, glomerulonephritis, urinary obstruction, and systemic diseases involving the kidney.

INITIAL RECOGNITION AND EARLY MANAGEMENT

Timely detection and recognition of AKI is desirable because it can allow for prompt implementation of interventions to abort kidney damage and to avoid the development of severe kidney injury and its complications (Box 34.1). AKI is usually identified based on an increase in serum creatinine; however, creatinine is an insensitive early marker of changes in kidney function, and AKI may develop before such changes become apparent. Furthermore, small changes in serum creatinine early in the course of AKI may not be readily appreciated, even though they can represent large changes in the glomerular filtration rate (GFR). Oliguria or anuria is an important sign that can identify AKI before changes in serum creatinine become apparent. Several novel biomarkers for AKI have been identified in recent years, including kidney injury molecule-1 (KIM-1), neutrophil gelatinase–associated lipocalin (NGAL), interleukin-18 (IL-18), and cystatin C, which may identify a decline in GFR or kidney damage earlier, and be more sensitive than changes in serum creatinine or urine output. However, these tests are not yet widely used in clinical practice, and their appropriate role in guiding management of patients with or at risk for AKI remains to be defined. Automated alerts for AKI based on serum creatinine or urine output changes are becoming increasingly common in electronic laboratory and medical record systems; however, whether these alerting systems improve processes of care and outcomes of AKI remains controversial.

After AKI has been identified, further clinical assessment, investigation, and intervention typically proceed simultaneously. A thorough history and examination are required to identify potential causes of AKI. Ischemia, sepsis, and exposure to nephrotoxic agents are the most common causes of AKI in hospitalized patients. A search for prerenal and postrenal causes should be performed because their correction can lead to rapid recovery of kidney function. A number of urine studies have been described to distinguish prerenal AKI from ATN, including the urine sodium concentration, fractional excretion of sodium, and fractional excretion of urea. Unfortunately, all of these tests have limitations in their diagnostic performance, and interpretation is dependent on the clinical context. Clinical examination to assess volume status remains an important aspect of early management. AKI due to hypovolemia may be rapidly reversed by the administration of intravenous fluids. Volume status should be frequently reassessed to determine the response to intravenous fluids and to avoid volume overload. Stopping medications that impair glomerular filtration, including nonsteroidal antiinflammatory drugs (NSAIDs), diuretics (when there is volume depletion), and angiotensin-converting enzyme (ACE) inhibitors/angiotensin receptor blockers (ARBs), when appropriate, can help reverse kidney dysfunction, especially in the setting of low effective arterial blood volume. Drugs that cause direct nephrotoxicity, such as aminoglycosides and intravenous radiocontrast, should be used cautiously or avoided, if possible. Selected use of kidney ultrasound is useful for identifying hydroureter and/or hydronephrosis, indicative of a postrenal cause. Lower urinary tract obstruction can be identified and treated by bladder catheterization showing a large postvoid residual urine volume, whereas nephrostomy tubes or ureteric stents can be used to treat upper urinary tract obstruction.

Urinalysis and urine microscopy provide important information about intrinsic kidney causes of AKI. Hematuria and proteinuria should prompt further investigations for causes of glomerulonephritis, whereas white bloods cell casts should prompt a careful assessment for causes of interstitial nephritis, including a review of medication exposures. The findings of granular casts and/or renal tubular epithelial cells are associated with an increased likelihood of ATN and help predict patients at highest risk for worsening kidney function, the requirement for RRT, or death.

Box 34.1   Principles of Management of Acute Kidney Injury

- Timely recognition of changes in urine output or kidney function
- Identification and reversal of underlying cause (guided by urinalysis)
- Correction of prerenal states and maintenance of hemodynamic stability
- Exclusion of postrenal causes (risk factors include history of hydronephrosis, recurrent UTIs, diagnoses consistent with obstruction, and absence of other identifiable causes such as prerenal states, heart failure, or exposure to nephrotoxic medications)
- Avoidance of nephrotoxic agents, if possible, and adjustment of medications to doses appropriate for level of kidney function
- Provision of supportive care, including nutrition and medical interventions to maintain fluid, electrolyte, and acid-base balance
- Initiation of renal replacement therapy when needed
- Assessment for recovery of kidney function, and follow-up to assess for development or progression of chronic kidney disease

UTI, Urinary tract infection.

SUPPORTIVE CARE AND MEDICAL MANAGEMENT OF COMPLICATIONS

After AKI is established, management focuses on preventing extension of kidney injury and providing supportive care while awaiting kidney recovery. Attempts are usually made to avoid further exposure to nephrotoxic agents to the greatest extent possible, without compromising management of other comorbidities. Doses of medications cleared by the kidney should be adjusted for the level of kidney function. This can be particularly important for antimicrobial agents so as to maintain appropriate therapeutic levels in patients with sepsis, while avoiding drug toxicity. The involvement of a clinical pharmacist may be helpful. Some observational reports suggest that computerized decision support tools in medication order entry systems may reduce adverse drug safety events in patients with AKI.

Supportive care in patients with AKI requires maintenance of fluid, electrolyte, and acid-base balance. Disorders of sodium and water handling, metabolic acidosis, and hyperkalemia are common complications of AKI. Hyponatremia may result from impaired free water excretion, whereas hypernatremia is common in patients with inadequate free water intake, hypotonic fluid losses, or large-volume intravenous saline infusions for resuscitation. These abnormalities may be corrected by modifying free water intake or the composition of intravenous fluids. Acid generation can be reduced by dietary protein restriction, although this may be undesirable in hypercatabolic patients. Alkaline intravenous fluids, such as sodium bicarbonate, may be provided to correct metabolic acidosis, although volume overload and pulmonary edema may limit this intervention. Hyperkalemia should be treated by discontinuing exogenous sources of potassium.

In the presence of electrocardiogram (EKG) changes, calcium gluconate may be administered. Beta-agonists, insulin, and sodium bicarbonate can shift potassium out of the plasma and into cells. Attempts to eliminate potassium through the gastrointestinal tract with ion exchange resins may be used; however, these agents are slow to take effect, have limited efficacy, have been associated with bowel necrosis or perforation, and are unlikely to be adequate in patients with severe hyperkalemia. When medical management of these abnormalities is unsuccessful, or medical interventions cannot be tolerated by the patient, RRT is usually necessary unless recovery of kidney function is imminent.

INTRAVENOUS FLUIDS AND HEMODYNAMIC SUPPORT

Hypotension is a common contributor to AKI, and after AKI is established, kidney perfusion may be further diminished through disruption of renal autoregulation. Early correction of hypovolemia and hypotension not only reverses most prerenal causes of AKI but also likely prevents extension and allows recovery from ATN. Strategies to maintain hemodynamic stability include the use of intravenous fluids, vasopressors/inotropic medications, and protocols for hemodynamic monitoring to guide the use of these therapies. Although more aggressive use of intravenous fluids in the initial phase of illness may be beneficial when AKI is volume responsive, excessive fluid repletion in oliguric patients with established ATN can have adverse effects. A positive fluid balance has been associated with increased mortality in observational studies. A restrictive fluid strategy may be more appropriate in some patients, particularly those with concomitant lung injury.

Isotonic crystalloids are the principal intravenous fluid for intravascular volume expansion of AKI patients. Normal (0.9%) saline is considered the standard crystalloid for most patients. Results from some observational studies have introduced concerns that the high chloride concentration of normal saline could itself confer a risk of AKI. However, a recent cluster randomized crossover trial comparing buffered crystalloid solution to normal saline did not detect a difference in AKI incidence in critically ill patients requiring crystalloid therapy. Colloid solutions such as albumin and starches are theoretically attractive alternatives for intravenous volume expansion, given their oncotic properties, but their appropriate use remains controversial. No differences in the incidence or duration of RRT were observed in a randomized trial of critically ill patients, comparing treatment with 4% albumin in 0.9% saline with isotonic saline alone. However, a systematic review of randomized trials suggested that the use of hyperoncotic albumin solutions may reduce the risk of AKI and be appropriate for some patients, including those with ascites, spontaneous bacterial peritonitis, or burns, or following surgery. Hydroxyethyl starch is an alternative colloid solution; however, when compared with crystalloids, hyperoncotic hydroxyethyl starch has been associated with a higher incidence of AKI, dialysis, and features of renal tubular injury (termed *osmotic nephrosis*) on kidney biopsy, suggesting these solutions may be harmful. Because colloids do not consistently reduce mortality when compared with crystalloids across all populations who are at high risk of AKI, these solutions are usually reserved for selected indications and avoided in patients with traumatic brain injury, where use has been associated with increased mortality.

Shock is a common contributor to AKI in patients with sepsis, anaphylaxis, liver failure, and burns. Appropriate fluid resuscitation remains of paramount importance in patients with AKI accompanied by these conditions, as well as those undergoing major surgical procedures. Vasopressors such as norepinephrine, dopamine, or vasopressin may be required when hypotension persists despite intravascular fluid resuscitation. Several early randomized trials using management strategies that focused on achieving specific hemodynamic and oxygenation parameters (e.g., early provision of intravenous fluids, blood transfusion, vasopressors, or inotropes based on specific goals for blood pressure, central venous pressure, serum lactate, central venous oxygen saturation, and urine output) reported improved outcomes in high-risk surgical patients or patients with septic shock. However, more recent trials of goal-directed therapeutic interventions have not replicated these findings. The need for administration of additional therapies such as blood transfusions and inotropes is typically individualized to a patient's conditions when shock is refractory to initial management with intravenous fluids and vasopressors.

DIURETICS

Oliguria has long been recognized as an important prognostic sign in AKI. The diuretic response to furosemide was recently formalized as a prognostic test for AKI, coined the "furosemide stress test," a procedure involving the administration of 1 to 1.5 mg/kg of furosemide. Failure to produce a urine output greater than 200 mL over the subsequent 2 hours outperformed several laboratory biomarkers for predicting progressive AKI. Diuretics can induce hypovolemia, leading to prerenal AKI, and their use has been associated with increased mortality and delays in kidney recovery in observational studies. However, when volume overload is present, diuretics are often prescribed to control fluid balance. Systematic review of trials that included patients with or at risk for AKI found no significant effects of furosemide on the risks of death, requirement for RRT, or number of dialysis sessions. Although furosemide facilitates diuresis, use of diuretics does not appear to improve kidney recovery among patients with AKI requiring dialysis. Nonetheless, diuretics can be used effectively to achieve fluid balance and may facilitate mechanical ventilation and improved outcomes in patients with lung injury.

VASODILATORS AND OTHER PHARMACOLOGIC AGENTS

Several pharmacologic agents with renal vasodilatory properties have been studied, with the aim of increasing renal blood flow and ameliorating ischemic damage in AKI. However, none of these agents are proven to improve the clinical outcomes of AKI. Low-dose dopamine is associated with increased renal blood flow, increased urine output, and small improvements in creatinine clearance. However, a systematic review of trials, including patients with or at risk for AKI, showed that low-dose dopamine had no significant effect on survival, need for dialysis, or adverse clinical events. Dopamine is associated with arrhythmias and intestinal ischemia and is not currently recommended to prevent or treat AKI. Fenoldopam is a dopamine type 1 receptor agonist that also increases renal blood flow, although it decreases systemic vascular resistance. A meta-analysis suggested promising results with the use of fenoldopam in critically ill patients, including reductions in AKI, need for RRT, and in-hospital mortality. However, given its risk of hypotension, along with limitations of the existing published trials, further trials are necessary to support the use of fenoldopam for this indication. Atrial natriuretic peptide (ANP) has favorable renovascular effects that increase the GFR in animals. However, large trials of ANP (0.2 μg/kg per minute) in critically ill patients with AKI showed no effects on mortality or dialysis-free survival but did show a higher incidence of hypotension. One systematic review has suggested that low-dose ANP (0.1 μg/kg per minute) is not associated with hypotension and may lead to a reduction in the requirement for RRT. Yet again, further large trials of low-dose ANP will be required before this agent can be recommended for AKI prevention or treatment.

There is inadequate efficacy and safety data to support the use of growth factors for AKI. Although insulin-like growth factor-1 showed promising results on recovery of kidney function in animals, small trials have failed to demonstrate beneficial results in humans. A small trial of erythropoietin for the prevention of AKI following cardiac surgery reported a reduction in incidence of AKI in treated patients; however, a subsequent trial in the intensive care unit (ICU) detected no effect.

NUTRITIONAL SUPPORT

Malnutrition is common in patients with AKI and has been consistently associated with mortality. Although clinical trials assessing the impact of nutrition on clinical endpoints are lacking, it is broadly accepted that appropriate nutritional support should be provided to meet the metabolic requirements of AKI patients. Total energy consumption is not increased in AKI and is only mildly increased above resting energy expenditure in patients with critical illness. A total energy intake of 20 to 30 kcal/kg per day is recommended to maintain nitrogen balance in patients with AKI and to avoid hyperglycemia, hypertriglyceridemia, and fluid accumulation observed with higher caloric provisions.

The optimal protein intake in the setting of AKI is not known. Given the association between protein-calorie malnutrition and mortality in these patients, dietary protein restriction is not considered appropriate in attempts to delay or prevent the initiation of RRT for azotemia or acidosis. Protein wasting and negative nitrogen balance may occur in AKI patients because of the inflammatory and physiologic stresses that accompany acute illnesses, particularly in critically ill patients. Nutritional protein administration is therefore usually increased to meet the greater metabolic demands of hypercatabolic patients. Furthermore, losses of amino acids and protein occur with continuous renal replacement therapy (CRRT) and peritoneal dialysis, resulting in additional nutritional requirements for patients receiving these treatments. It is reasonable to aim for a protein intake of 0.8 to 1.0 g/kg per day in noncatabolic patients not requiring RRT, increasing to a maximum of 1.7 g/kg

Table 34.1 Properties of Various Renal Replacement Therapy Modalities Used for Acute Kidney Injury

	Modality Name	Solute Removal	Blood Flow Rates	Ultrafiltration Rate	Replacement Fluid Rate	Dialysate Flow Rate	Timing
Continuous Therapies	CVVHF	Convection (ultrafiltration)	150–250 mL/min	1500–2000 mL/h	1500–2000 mL/h for neutral fluid balance. Ultrafiltration in excess of replacement fluid necessary for fluid removal	0	Continuous (24 hours per day unless interrupted)
	CVVHD	Diffusion (dialysis)	150–250 mL/min	Variable	None	1–2 L/h	
	CVVHDF	Diffusion and convection (ultrafiltration and dialysis)	150–250 mL/min	1000–1500 mL/h	1000–1500 mL/h for neutral fluid balance. Ultrafiltration in excess of replacement fluid necessary for fluid removal	1–2 L/h	
Intermittent Therapies	Conventional IHD	Diffusion (dialysis)	200–350 mL/min	Variable	None	300–800 mL/min	Typically up to 4 hours, on alternate days
	SLED or EDD	Diffusion (dialysis)	100–300 mL/min	Variable	None	100–300 mL/min	Typically daily for 6 hours or
	SLEDF or SCUF	Convection (ultrafiltration)	100–200 mL/min	Variable	None	0	longer

CVVHD, Continuous venovenous hemodialysis; *CVVHDF,* continuous venovenous hemodiafiltration; *CVVHF,* continuous venovenous hemofiltration; *EDD,* extended daily dialysis; *IHD,* intermittent hemodialysis; *SCUF,* sustained continuous ultrafiltration; *SLED,* sustained low-efficiency dialysis; *SLEDF,* sustained low-efficiency diafiltration.

per day for hypercatabolic patients receiving RRT. Consultation with a registered dietitian is valuable to estimate the appropriate energy and protein requirements for an individual patient.

Enteral nutrition is the preferred form of support for patients with AKI. If oral feeding is not possible, then enteral (tube) feeding is recommended. Electrolytes (potassium, phosphate) should be monitored following initiation of enteral feeding. Parenteral nutrition may be required in some patients to supplement the enteral route, or in patients without functional gastrointestinal tracts. Potassium, phosphate, and magnesium are usually withheld from parenteral nutrition in patients with AKI, but deficiencies can develop that may require prescription adjustment.

RENAL REPLACEMENT THERAPY

MODALITIES

Several modalities of RRT may be used in AKI, including peritoneal dialysis, CRRT, conventional intermittent hemodialysis (IHD), and prolonged IHD. Peritoneal dialysis is used for AKI in some pediatric settings and in adults in developing countries where infrastructure for hemodialysis is not available. In industrialized countries, IHD and CRRT are the mainstays of RRT for AKI. Available resources, expertise, hemodynamic stability, and patient comorbidities usually influence the decision of renal replacement modality. In institutions where both modalities are available, it is common for patients to transition between forms of CRRT and IHD, depending on various factors and the setting in which the care is being provided.

CRRT is delivered continuously and uses lower blood flow rates that result in slower fluid and solute removal than IHD. Several forms of CRRT exist, including continuous venovenous hemofiltration (CVVHF), continuous venovenous hemodialysis (CVVHD), and continuous venovenous hemodiafiltration (CVVHDF; Table 34.1). These modalities are usually only available in ICUs. Although CRRT achieves slower removal of solutes per unit time than IHD, the continuous nature of the therapy results in total clearance during a 24-hour period that may exceed that provided by IHD. Furthermore, the slower rate of solute clearance may avoid large fluid shifts between intracellular and extracellular fluid compartments. Based on these features, CRRT is often suggested for hemodynamically unstable patients and patients with brain injuries at risk of cerebral edema.

In its conventional form, IHD for AKI uses the methods, equipment, trained nursing staff, frequency, and duration of therapy in the same manner established for chronic hemodialysis in patients with ESRD. IHD achieves the fastest removal of small solutes and limits the duration a patient is exposed to the extracorporeal circuit. It is thus a good therapeutic option for many patients with severe hyperkalemia, poisoning, and tumor lysis syndrome.

In recent years, variants of IHD have been implemented that use IHD equipment but seek to achieve similar therapeutic aims as CRRT (see Table 34.1). These prolonged or "hybrid therapies" are known by a variety of names, including sustained low-efficiency dialysis (SLED) or extended daily dialysis (EDD), sustained low-efficiency diafiltration (SLEDF) or sustained continuous ultrafiltration (SCUF), and slow continuous dialysis (SCD). These modalities provide an extended duration of dialysis with a lower blood flow rate, to provide more gradual solute and fluid removal with the goal of improving hemodynamic tolerability.

Although most patients with AKI are eligible for either modality, CRRT or prolonged IHD are often viewed as preferable to conventional IHD for treatment of hemodynamically unstable patients. However, randomized comparisons of CRRT and conventional IHD have shown heterogeneous effects on hemodynamic measurements, with meta-analyses suggesting no significant differences in the risk of hypotension between modalities. Still, higher mean arterial blood pressure and fewer patients requiring escalation of vasopressor during treatment were seen with CRRT than with IHD. Experience reported from clinical trials suggests that IHD can be successfully delivered to many patients with hemodynamic instability. Strategies that may help maintain hemodynamic stability during IHD include priming of the dialysis circuit with colloid cooled dialysate, and a high dialysate sodium concentration.

Several randomized trials and meta-analyses have compared outcomes with CRRT versus conventional IHD in critically ill patients. Data from these trials have demonstrated no significant differences between these modalities in the length of hospitalization, mortality, or the requirement for chronic dialysis in survivors. Results from randomized trials comparing SLED, SLEDF, SCUF, EDD, SCD to the conventional forms of RRT for AKI are lacking, although observational reports suggest that there is a growth in dialysis programs with these modalities and that they can be applied safely and effectively.

TIMING OF RENAL REPLACEMENT THERAPY

Initiating RRT is influenced by several factors, including assessments of fluid, electrolyte, and metabolic status. It is widely accepted that hyperkalemia, metabolic acidosis, and volume overload (refractory to medical management) or overt uremic symptoms and signs constitute traditional indications for RRT. However, it is rare for uremic symptoms to develop in the setting of AKI before initiating dialysis. RRT is usually started after AKI is established and complications are deemed unavoidable. However, in the absence of imminent complications, dialysis may be deferred when there are signs of clinical improvement or kidney recovery. Many patients recover kidney function without the development of absolute indications for RRT, and in some patients, complications may be adequately managed medically. Thresholds for starting RRT appear to be lower when AKI is accompanied by multiple organ failure, the rationale being that earlier initiation will facilitate other aspects of management while maintaining fluid, solute, and metabolic control.

There is considerable practice variation for starting RRT in the absence of traditional indications (Table 34.2). In theory, earlier initiation may avoid adverse AKI consequences, including metabolic abnormalities and fluid overload, and could improve outcomes. However, earlier initiation can unnecessarily expose some patients to the risk associated with vascular access (infection, thrombosis), anticoagulation (hemorrhage), and RRT itself (hypotension, dialyzer reactions). Recent randomized trials in this area have used different Kidney Disease: Improving Global Outcomes (KDIGO) AKI stages to define early initiation of RRT and have produced conflicting findings. Although one small, single-center, unblinded randomized trial reported lower mortality in an early initiation arm (KDIGO stage 2 AKI) than a late initiation arm (KDIGO stage 3 AKI or metabolic or clinical indication), a larger, multicenter, unblinded randomized trial reported no difference in mortality between the early initiation arm (KIDGO stage 3 AKI) versus the late initiation arm (specific metabolic or clinical indication). Decisions regarding when to initiate RRT thus continue to be based on clinical judgment, with further trials needed in this area to guide practice.

Criteria	Comment
Table 34.2	**Traditional and Preemptive Criteria for Renal Replacement Therapy in Acute Kidney Injury**

Criteria	Comment
Traditional Criteria	
Volume overload	Pulmonary edema or respiratory failure that cannot be managed with medical therapy including diuretics
Electrolytes	Hyperkalemia that is refractory to medical management, severe, or associated with EKG changes
Acidemia	Usually based on severity of metabolic acidosis but no established threshold
Uremia	Pericarditis, encephalopathy, or uremic bleeding attributed to platelet dysfunction
Preemptive Criteria	
Volume management	To minimize fluid overload and to facilitate administration of nutritional support and intravenous medication that would otherwise lead to fluid accumulation
Electrolytes	Proactive use to avoid impending electrolyte disorders
Acid-base balance	To maintain arterial pH in the setting of permissive hypercapnia in patients with respiratory failure
Solute control	Severe AKI that is unlikely to recover imminently, particularly when oligoanuria is present Remove solutes that are difficult to quantify in the setting of AKI

AKI, Acute kidney injury; *EKG,* electrocardiogram; *K,* serum potassium concentration.

DOSE OF RENAL REPLACEMENT THERAPY

Several limitations exist regarding the use of urea clearance to quantify the intensity of RRT due to the high catabolic rate and changes in the volume of distribution that commonly accompany AKI. Despite these limitations, urea clearance is often used to prescribe and monitor the intensity of RRT in AKI. Urea clearance by hemodialysis is expressed as Kt/V and may be modified by increasing the surface area of the dialyzer, blood flow rate, dialysate flow rate, treatment duration, or frequency. Urea clearance by CRRT is considered equivalent to the effluent flow rate (ultrafiltrate and/or dialysate) and can be expressed as mL/kg per hour of effluent.

One small trial that evaluated the effect of daily versus alternate-day IHD in AKI reported lower mortality and shorter duration of dialysis in the daily IHD group. However, the delivered dose in the alternate-day group was lower than intended with a weekly mean Kt/V of 3.0. Two larger studies of the dose of renal replacement in AKI have provided major advances in our knowledge of this area. The Veterans Affairs ATN study was a randomized trial that evaluated the intensity of RRT while allowing patients to switch between CRRT, IHD, or SLED. In this trial, IHD treatments targeted a Kt/V of 1.4 (mean delivered dose was 1.3) and were performed 6 times weekly in the intensive arm and 3 times weekly in the less intensive arm. CRRT was performed with predilution CVVHDF targeting effluent flow rate of 35 mL/kg per hour in the intensive arm and 20 mL/kg per hour in the less intensive arm. Mortality and recovery of kidney function were similar in the intensive and less intensive groups. Similarly, the RENAL study randomized patients with AKI treated with postdilution CVVHDF to doses of 40 versus 25 mL/kg per hour and showed no difference in survival between the two groups.

Based on these results, a delivered dose equivalent to that achieved in the less intensive arm of the ATN study (weekly Kt/V 3.9) appears to be adequate for treatment of patients with IHD-requiring AKI. Moreover, a delivered effluent volume consistent with the less intensive arms of the ATN and RENAL studies (20 to 25 mL/kg per hour) has been recommended for CRRT. Hemodynamic instability, access failure, technical problems, and time off RRT to perform procedures may reduce the effective time on RRT and result in a lower delivered dose, which may require prescription adjustments. Assessment of the adequacy of RRT should also incorporate other factors in addition to small solute (urea) clearance, including fluid management, acid-base status, and electrolyte balance because these parameters may influence the prescription. Extracorporeal therapy may be required in some instances for ultrafiltration alone.

VASCULAR ACCESS FOR RENAL REPLACEMENT THERAPY

Venous access is a necessity for CRRT and IHD, and access dysfunction can limit blood flow and the delivery of dialysis. Because of their large diameter, complications of dialysis catheter insertion (arterial puncture, hematoma, pneumothorax, or hemothorax) can be serious. Indwelling catheters also predispose to bacteremia. Nontunneled catheters are the initial choice for most patients starting RRT. Cuffed, subcutaneous tunneled catheters are more complex to insert;

however, they may be less prone to dysfunction, infection, or thrombosis and thus appropriate if longer (greater than 3-week) durations of RRT are anticipated. Subclavian vein catheters are associated with the highest risk of venous stenosis. Because this may compromise future attempts at permanent vascular access, the internal jugular vein is the preferred upper body insertion site for patients at risk for progression to ESRD. Femoral catheters are another reasonable choice, but these restrict mobility and are associated with increased infection in obese patients. Ultrasound guidance is recommended to decrease the risk of insertion complications and to improve the likelihood of successful placement. Insertion should be performed according to infection control protocols, including sterile barrier precautions, skin antisepsis, and catheter use restricted to RRT to minimize the incidence of catheter-related bloodstream infection.

ANTICOAGULATION FOR RENAL REPLACEMENT THERAPY

Clotting of the dialysis filter can lead to extracorporeal blood loss, a reduction in dialysis efficiency, and procedural interruptions. Use of anticoagulation for CRRT and IHD may reduce these problems; however, the benefits of anticoagulation must be balanced against the risk of bleeding complications in acutely ill AKI patients with significant comorbidities. Patients with coagulopathy and thrombocytopenia may not benefit from additional anticoagulation, and CRRT and IHD can often be provided without anticoagulation, aided by intermittent saline flushes of the extracorporeal circuit.

Unfractionated heparin is the most widely used anticoagulant for dialysis. Low-molecular-weight heparin may also be used, although it has unpredictable clearance in patients with kidney failure. A prolonged half-life requires monitoring of factor Xa levels. Regional citrate anticoagulation has become more common in recent years, especially for anticoagulation on CRRT. Citrate is infused into the prefilter line where it chelates calcium, thereby inhibiting filter coagulation. Some citrate is removed in the extracorporeal circuit, while the citrate returning to the systemic circulation is metabolized to produce bicarbonate and calcium. Additional calcium is infused to replace extracorporeal losses and to maintain normal systemic ionized calcium concentrations. The complexity of this procedure necessitates close monitoring of acid-base status and calcium (total and ionized) levels and frequent adjustments to infusion rates. Adequately trained staff and adherence to strict protocols are required to minimize the complications of metabolic alkalosis, hypocalcemia, and citrate accumulation. Citrate anticoagulation is contraindicated in patients with severely impaired liver function or muscle hypoperfusion who are unable to metabolize citrate. Some small trials suggest that regional citrate anticoagulation reduces the requirement for transfusion and risk of hemorrhage compared with systematic heparin.

DIALYZER/HEMOFILTER MEMBRANES

Hollow fiber dialyzers used for IHD or CRRT are characterized by their surface area, composition, and flux. Synthetic dialysis membranes are associated with less activation of complement than traditional bioincompatible membranes made of unsubstituted cellulose. Meta-analyses have shown no difference in mortality with biocompatible compared with bioincompatible membranes. However, because a higher risk of death has been suggested with unsubstituted cellulose membranes, these are typically avoided in AKI. Trials to date have shown no difference in outcomes between high-flux and low-flux membranes in AKI, although the increased permeability of high-flux membranes makes them advantageous for hemofiltration.

DIALYSATE AND REPLACEMENT FLUIDS

Dialysate for IHD is produced by the dialysis machine from concentrated electrolyte solutions and treated water from a municipal source. Sterile dialysate and replacement fluid for CRRT may be purchased commercially or produced in local hospital pharmacies. Solutions containing bicarbonate, lactate, and acetate are available for use with CRRT or IHD to correct metabolic acidosis. Bicarbonate-containing solutions have become increasingly available in recent years, and they avoid lactate accumulation in patients with shock or liver failure. When citrate is used for anticoagulation, lower requirements for additional buffer in dialysate or replacement fluid are realized.

DISCONTINUING RENAL REPLACEMENT THERAPY

Many patients with AKI will experience partial or complete recovery of kidney function, although recovery is less likely in those with severe injury or preexisting CKD. Little is known about the optimal time to stop RRT; however, increasing urine output often identifies patients recovering native kidney function. Changes in interdialytic measurements of serum creatinine, urea, and urinary creatinine clearance can be used to assess native kidney function in patients receiving IHD. For patients receiving a stable prescription of CRRT for several days, urinary creatinine clearance has also been used to measure recovery of native kidney function. Because of the high mortality in patients with AKI accompanying multiorgan failure, some patients will appropriately discontinue RRT as part of withdrawal from life support measures.

LONG-TERM FOLLOW-UP

AKI is associated with an increased risk of progressive CKD and ESRD after hospital discharge. Older age, lower baseline kidney function, albuminuria, and incomplete recovery of kidney function at the time of hospital discharge are risk factors for CKD following AKI. Postdischarge follow-up of kidney function is currently recommended for survivors of AKI. Subsequent long-term management of patients with CKD after AKI usually proceeds according to the principles of CKD management.

KEY BIBLIOGRAPHY

Bouman CS, Oudemans-Van Straaten HM, Tijssen JG, et al. Effects of early high-volume continuous venovenous hemofiltration on survival and recovery of renal function in intensive care patients with acute renal failure: a prospective, randomized trial. *Crit Care Med.* 2002;30:2205-2211.

Brienza N, Giglio MT, Marucci M, et al. Does perioperative hemodynamic optimization protect renal function in surgical patients? A meta-analytic study. *Crit Care Med.* 2009;37:2079-2090.

Chawla LS, Davison DL, Brasha-Mitchell E, Koyner JL, Arthur JM, Shaw AD, Tumlin JA, Trevino SA, Kimmel PL, Seneff MG. Development and standardization of a furosemide stress test to predict the severity of acute kidney injury. *Crit Care.* 2013;17:R207.

Finfer S, Bellomo R, Boyce N, et al. A comparison of albumin and saline for fluid resuscitation in the intensive care unit. *N Engl J Med.* 2004;350:2247-2256.

Friedrich JO, Adhikari N, Herridge MS, et al. Meta-analysis: low-dose dopamine increases urine output but does not prevent renal dysfunction or death. *Ann Intern Med.* 2005;142:510-524.

Gaudry S, Hajage D, Schortgen F, Martin-Lefevre L, Pons B, Boulet E, Boyer A, Chevrel G, Lerolle N, Carpentier D, de Prost N, Lautrette A, Bretagnol A, Mayaux J, Nseir S, Megarbane B, Thirion M, Forel JM, Maizel J, Yonis H, Markowicz P, Thiery G, Tubach F, Ricard JD, Dreyfuss D, AKIKI Study Group. Initiation strategies for renal-replacement therapy in the intensive care unit. *N Engl J Med.* 2016;375:122-133.

Ho KM, Sheridan DJ. Meta-analysis of frusemide to prevent or treat acute renal failure. *BMJ.* 2006;333:420-425.

Klouche K, Amigues L, Deleuze S, et al. Complications, effects on dialysis dose, and survival of tunneled femoral dialysis catheter in acute renal failure. *Am J Kidney Dis.* 2007;49:99-108.

Landoni G, Biondi-Zoccai GG, Tumlin JA, et al. Beneficial impact of fenoldopam in critically ill patients with or at risk for acute renal failure: a meta-analysis of randomized clinical trials. *Am J Kidney Dis.* 2007;49:56-58.

Licurse A, Kim MC, Dziura J, Forman HP, et al. Renal ultrasonography in the evaluation of acute kidney injury: developing a risk stratification framework. *Arch Intern Med.* 2010;170:1900-1907.

Macias WL, Alaka KJ, Murphy MH, et al. Impact of the nutritional regimen on protein catabolism and nitrogen balance in patients with acute renal failure. *JPEN J Parenter Enteral Nutr.* 1996;20:56-62.

Marshall MR, Creamer JM, Foster M, Ma TM, Mann SL, Fiaccadori E, Maggiore U, Richards B, Wilson VL, Williams AB, Rankin AP. Mortality rate comparison after switching from continuous to prolonged intermittent renal replacement for acute kidney injury in three intensive care units from different countries. *Nephrol Dial Transplant.* 2011;26:2169-2175.

Mehta RL, Pascual MT, Soroko S, et al. Diuretics, mortality, and non-recovery of renal function in acute renal failure. *JAMA.* 2002;288:2547-2553.

Nigwekar SU, Navaneethan SD, Parikh CR, et al. Atrial natriuretic peptide for management of acute kidney injury: a systematic review and meta-analysis. *Clin J Am Soc Nephrol.* 2008;4:261-272.

Paganini EP, Sandy D, Moreno L, et al. The effect of sodium and ultra-filtration modelling on plasma volume changes and haemodynamic stability in intensive care patients receiving haemodialysis for acute renal failure: a prospective stratified, randomized, cross-over study. *Nephrol Dial Transplant.* 1996;11:32-37.

Pannu N, Klarenbach S, Wiebe N, et al. Renal replacement therapy in patients with acute renal failure: a systematic review. *JAMA.* 2008;299:793-805.

Perel P, Roberts I. Colloids versus crystalloids for fluid resuscitation in critically ill patients. *Cochrane Database Syst Rev.* 2007;(4):CD000567.

Rabindranath K, Adams J, Macleod AM, et al. Intermittent versus continuous renal replacement therapy for acute renal failure in adults. *Cochrane Database Syst Rev.* 2007;(3):CD003773.

RENAL Replacement Therapy Study Investigators, Bellomo R, Cass A, et al. Intensity of continuous renal-replacement therapy in critically ill patients. *N Engl J Med.* 2009;361:1627-1638.

Schortgen F, Lacherade JC, Bruneel F, et al. Effects of hydroxyethylstarch and gelatin on renal function in severe sepsis: a multicentre randomised study. *Lancet.* 2001;357:911-916.

Full bibliography can be found on www.expertconsult.com.

DRUGS AND THE KIDNEY

35 Kidney Disease Caused by Therapeutic Agents

Mark A. Perazella; Anushree C. Shirali

Medications are a mainstay of appropriate patient care, and new agents are being introduced into clinical practice at a rapid pace. Although most drugs are well tolerated, and therapeutic agents are often essential for medical care, kidney injury remains an unfortunate and relatively frequent adverse consequence. This bespeaks the fact that some individuals possess risk factors that predispose to drug-induced kidney toxicity. Not unexpectedly, the general population is regularly exposed to various diagnostic and therapeutic agents with nephrotoxic potential. Although most are prescribed, many other preparations are purchased over the counter. Drugs fall into the categories of diagnostic agents, therapeutic medications, alternative or complementary substances, and drugs of abuse, resulting in a variety of kidney syndromes (Table 35.1).

KIDNEY SUSCEPTIBILITY TO NEPHROTOXIC AGENTS

In addition to clearance of endogenous waste products, excretion of sodium and water, electrolyte and acid-base balance, and endocrine activity, the kidney is responsible for the metabolism and excretion of exogenously administered drugs, making it susceptible to various types of injury. There are several factors that increase the kidney's susceptibility to these potential toxins, which can be classified into three simple categories (drug-related factors, kidney-related factors, and host-related factors) and often occur in combination to promote nephrotoxicity. As we learn more about drug-induced kidney disease, it appears that these factors explain much of the variability and heterogeneity noted among patients.

Drug-related factors are the critical first step to the development of nephrotoxicity. Innate drug toxicity is important because the drug or its toxic metabolite may cause kidney injury by impairing renal hemodynamics, direct cellular injury, osmotic injury, or intratubular crystal deposition, to name a few conditions. Large doses, extended drug exposure, and nephrotoxic drug combinations further enhance nephrotoxicity.

The kidney's handling of drugs also determines why certain agents cause nephrotoxicity. As renal blood flow approximates 25% of cardiac output, the kidney is significantly exposed to nephrotoxic drugs. Kidney injury is increased in the loop of Henle where high metabolic rates coexist with a relatively hypoxic environment. Increased drug/metabolite concentrations in the kidney medulla also contribute to direct toxicity. Kidney drug metabolism from cytochrome P450 (CYP450) and other enzymes increases local toxic metabolite and reactive oxygen species (ROS) formation, which promote injury via nucleic acid oxidation/alkylation, DNA-strand breaks, lipid peroxidation, and protein damage.

The kidney pathway of excretion for many therapeutic agents involves proximal tubular cells. Extensive drug trafficking through the cell via luminal and basolateral transporters can lead to cellular injury. Some drugs are endocytosed at the luminal membrane of cells, whereas other drugs are transported into the cell via basolateral ion transporters. Such drug transport can be associated with increased cellular concentrations that injure mitochondria, phospholipid membranes, lysosomes, and other organelles.

Nonmodifiable factors such as older age and female sex increase nephrotoxic risk through reduced total body water leading to drug overdose. Unrecognized reduced glomerular filtration rate (GFR) and hypoalbuminemia, which result in increased toxic drug concentration, also enhance risk. Pharmacogenetic differences likely explain much of the variable response of patients to drugs. Liver and kidney CYP450 enzyme gene polymorphisms are associated with reduced metabolism and end-organ toxicity. Polymorphisms of genes encoding proteins involved in the metabolism and kidney elimination of drugs are correlated with nephrotoxic risk. Another important aspect of genetic makeup is a highly variable host immune response to drugs; one patient reacts with a heightened allergic response, whereas another has a limited reaction with no kidney lesion. Thus, innate host response genes tend to determine the drug reaction.

Kidney susceptibility to drug injury is also enhanced by true and effective volume depletion, including nausea/vomiting, diarrhea, and diuretic therapy, as well as heart failure, liver disease with ascites, and sepsis. This physiology enhances the nephrotoxicity of drugs that are excreted primarily by the kidney, drugs reabsorbed/secreted by the proximal tubule, and drugs that are insoluble in the urine. Nephrotoxic risk is also increased in patients with acute kidney injury (AKI) or chronic kidney disease (CKD) because of a lower number of functioning nephrons, reductions in drug clearance, and a robust kidney oxidative response to drugs and metabolites. Finally, electrolyte and acid-base disturbances present in some patients also contribute to host susceptibility to drug injury.

KIDNEY INJURY ASSOCIATED WITH MEDICATIONS

Therapeutic agents associated with kidney injury can be classified based on the category of the agent or the clinical

Table 35.1 Drug-Induced Clinical Kidney Syndromes

Kidney Syndrome	Causative Agents
Acute Kidney Injury	
Prerenal	Cyclosporine, tacrolimus, radiocontrast, Am B, ACE inhibitors, ARBs, NSAIDs, interleukin-2, exenatide
Intrarenal	
Vascular disease	Gemcitabine, anti-VEGF drugs, propylthiouracil, interferon
ATN	AGs, AmB, cisplatin, tenofovir, ifosfamide, pemetrexed, polymyxins, vancomycin, pentostat, zoledronate, warfarin
AIN	Immune checkpoint inhibitors, penicillins, cephalosporins, sulfonamides, rifampin, NSAIDs, interferon, ciprofloxacin, others
Crystal nephropathy	Methotrexate, acyclovir, sulfonamides, indinavir, atazanavir, ciprofloxacin, sodium phosphate
Osmotic nephropathy	IVIG, HES, dextran, mannitol
Postrenal	Methysergide, drug-induced stones, alpha-agonists
Proteinuria	Gold, NSAIDs, anti-VEGF drugs, penicillamine, interferon, pamidronate
Tubulopathies	AGs, tenofovir, cisplatin, ifosfamide, AmB, pemetrexed, cetuximab
Nephrolithiasis	Sulfadiazine, atazanavir, indinavir, topiramate, zonisamide
CKD	Li^+, analgesic abuse, cyclosporine, tacrolimus, cisplatin, nitrosourea

ACE, Angiotensin-converting enzyme; *AmB*, Amphotericin B; *AIN*, acute interstitial nephritis; *AGs*, aminoglycosides; *ARBs*, angiotensin receptor blockers; *ATN*, acute tubular necrosis; *CKD*, chronic kidney disease; *HES*, hydroxyethyl starch; *IVIG*, intravenous immune globulin; *Li*$^+$, lithium; *NSAIDs*, nonsteroidal antiinflammatory drugs; *VEGF*, vascular endothelial growth factor.

kidney syndrome. Recognizing that all drugs cannot be covered in this chapter, we describe drug-induced nephrotoxicity by drug category and highlight the clinical kidney syndrome and the segment of nephron injury by the drug within each category. Drug-induced acute interstitial nephritis (AIN) and CKD are discussed elsewhere in the *Primer*.

DIAGNOSTIC AGENTS

RADIOCONTRAST AGENTS

Contrast-induced nephropathy (CIN) is the third most common cause of hospital-acquired AKI and is associated with increased risk of hospital morbidity/mortality and long-term adverse outcomes. It is defined by an absolute or percentage rise in serum creatinine from the baseline within 48 to 72 hours. In general, serum creatinine begins to rise within the first 24 hours after exposure, peaks between 2 and 5 days, and returns to baseline by 7 to 14 days. The course of CIN varies depending on the overall patient risk profile.

The incidence of CIN depends on the definition used and the population studied, ranging from 5% to 40%. Two important factors drive this incidence: (1) the increased number of imaging studies and percutaneous procedures with radiocontrast throughout the past decade and (2) the ever-enlarging population of patients with underlying CKD. In the presence of reduced kidney function, the elimination ($T_{1/2}$) of radiocontrast agents is increased. Thus, the kidney undergoes prolonged contrast exposure that increases the likelihood of kidney injury. In CKD stage 3 or greater, the risk of CIN is twofold to fivefold higher compared with normal kidney function, and the risk escalates as the GFR falls.

Radiocontrast media injure the kidney via multiple mechanisms. First, vasoactive substances, such as adenosine and endothelin, mediate vasoconstriction of the afferent arterioles, thereby reducing renal blood flow and promoting kidney medullary ischemia. Second, renal epithelial cell necrosis also occurs with isoosmolar radiocontrast agents because their high viscosity causes sluggish blood flow through the peritubular capillaries and promotes hypoxic kidney injury. Lastly, radiocontrast causes direct renal tubular toxicity through hyperosmolar injury, which results in vacuolization of proximal tubular cells, and oxidative stress from free oxygen radicals with associated tubular cell apoptosis and necrosis.

The level of kidney function at the time of exposure is one of the most important determinants of the risk for CIN. In addition, patient-specific risk factors include older age, volume depletion, congestive heart failure, diabetes mellitus, both hypertension and hypotension, and anemia. The intraaortic balloon pump is associated with increased AKI risk, primarily because it is a surrogate for severe cardiac disease, tenuous cardiac output, and kidney hypoperfusion. Emergent procedures increase risk because of reduced use of contrast prophylaxis and increased severity of patient illness. The type, volume, and route of contrast administration also affects CIN risk. With regard to radiocontrast type, osmolality and viscosity are the two most important characteristics. The osmolality of a solution varies significantly from high-osmolar contrast media (HOCM) to low-osmolar media (LOCM) to isoosmolar media (IOCM). Viscosity, another contrast property, varies from one product to the next, does not correlate with osmolality, and may be associated with CIN. For example, IOCM solutions are about twice as viscous as LOCM products despite having a lower osmolality.

The incidence of CIN is higher with HOCM than with LOCM, and in CKD patients, the relative risk is doubled. As a result, LOCM and IOCM agents have replaced HOCM. A meta-analysis of 16 randomized controlled trials suggested a benefit of using IOCM instead of LOCM, with the relative risk reduction of CIN greatest in CKD patients. The maximum increase in serum creatinine was less in CKD patients given IOCM compared with LOCM. However, a randomized trial comparing IOCM with LOCM noted no significant difference in CIN incidence. Thus, the benefits of low osmolality may be counterbalanced by the detrimental properties of high viscosity, making these agents equal in their risk for CIN. A larger volume of contrast increases CIN, with a recommended upper limit of 150 mL for patients with a serum creatinine 1.5 to 3.4 mg/dL and maximum dose of 100 mL recommended for patients with a creatinine greater than 3.4 mg/dL. The smallest contrast volume required to perform the procedure should be used. Risk of CIN is highest with intraarterial injection, with the intravenous (IV) route presenting a smaller risk. Coronary angiography has an even higher CIN risk than other arterial studies. CKD outpatients have a low CIN risk with nonemergent computed tomography (CT) scans. In fact, an eGFR greater than 30 mL/min per 1.73 m^2 is not considered a substantial risk for CIN in patients receiving radiocontrast by the IV route.

As radiocontrast exposure is often predictable, measures to reduce kidney injury should be undertaken in patients at risk. In addition to limiting the contrast load and using either IOCM or nonionic LOCM, the most important intervention is IV fluid (IVF) administration. Studies have uniformly demonstrated the benefit of prophylactic isotonic IVF administered both before and after radiocontrast administration. Because urinary alkalinization is hypothesized to reduce kidney oxidative stress, IV sodium bicarbonate has been studied. In an early report, CIN developed in only 2% of CKD patients treated with bicarbonate solution as compared with 14% with IV saline. A later meta-analysis of 23 studies concluded that bicarbonate-containing solutions reduced the risk of RCIN by 38%, but the benefits were noted in small and poor-quality studies. In contrast, larger, higher-quality studies did not demonstrate a reduction in CIN. Furthermore, no benefit was demonstrated for AKI-requiring dialysis, for heart failure, or for total mortality. Thus, sodium bicarbonate is not superior to isotonic saline, and either solution is acceptable for radiocontrast prophylaxis. For outpatient studies, oral fluids with salt tablets before exposure may provide adequate volume expansion to prevent CIN in CKD, but this approach has not been extensively examined.

N-acetylcysteine (NAC) is an antioxidant that is commonly used for CIN prevention. Approximately half of the published randomized controlled trials demonstrate benefit, whereas several meta-analyses suggest either large benefit or no benefit. Beneficial studies are notable for early publication dates, small size, and low quality. Despite the enrollment of nearly 3000 patients, including CKD patients, no beneficial effect of NAC on hard clinical outcomes is noted. Given its favorable safety profile, low cost, easy administration, and wide availability, clinicians could argue for continued use of the drug as prophylaxis. However, the Acetylcysteine for Contrast-Induced Nephropathy Trial casts doubt on this conclusion. This randomized study included 2308 patients and documented no benefit with NAC therapy (the proportion developing CIN was 12.7 among both NAC and placebo recipients). Thus, NAC appears to offer no protection against CIN. Despite a lack of data, it is reasonable to avoid nonsteroidal antiinflammatory drugs (NSAIDs), calcineurin inhibitors, aminoglycosides (AGs), and osmotic agents before radiocontrast exposure. Regarding renin-angiotensin-aldosterone system (RAAS) blockers, some studies note increased CIN risk, whereas others show nephroprotection.

Based on its size, lack of protein binding, and small volume of distribution, radiocontrast is efficiently removed with hemodialysis (HD). In fact, approximately 80% is removed over 4 hours with a high-flux dialyzer. HD after radiocontrast exposure to prevent CIN, especially in patients with advanced CKD, has been examined in several studies. Although all HD studies have been negative, one small study demonstrated that prophylactic HD in stage 5 CKD patients reduced the need for an acute and chronic dialysis requirement after discharge. Hemofiltration performed 4 to 6 hours before and 18 to 24 hours after contrast reduced the incidence of CIN, in-hospital events, need for acute dialysis, and both in-hospital and 1-year mortality. In contrast, the hemofiltration post-procedure alone offered no benefit beyond standard prophylaxis. A systematic review of 11 studies with 1010 patients concluded that one or more sessions of HD, hemofiltration, or hemodiafiltration performed after contrast administration did not reduce the incidence of CIN nor the need for acute or chronic dialysis. Examination of HD and hemofiltration/hemodiafiltration separately shows that HD is associated with increased CIN risk, whereas hemofiltration/hemodiafiltration did not affect the occurrence of CIN but did reduce the receipt of acute dialysis. Therefore HD and hemodiafiltration are not recommended as a prophylactic measure for CIN.

GADOLINIUM-BASED CONTRAST AGENTS

Gadolinium-based contrast agents (GBCAs) were considered a safe and effective diagnostic agent, revolutionizing the world of imaging. However, over time, it became clear that GBCAs were not risk free. Rare reports of AKI surfaced, primarily in patients with underlying kidney disease who received large doses via direct arterial injection. Nephrotoxicity may be related to a direct effect on tubules, mediated by osmolarity or some other mechanism. In general, GBCA-induced AKI is rare and typically of minor severity, likely caused by the small volume of contrast required for imaging.

GBCAs began to be used widely for imaging patients with kidney disease in the early to mid-1990s because they offered an outstanding image without the nephrotoxicity of radiocontrast. However, nephrogenic systemic fibrosis (NSF), a severe and largely irreversible sclerosing condition of skin, joints, eyes, and internal organs, was first noted as a complication of GBCAs in 2006. Two factors were required for NSF to develop: GBCA exposure and underlying kidney disease. Other factors that likely further increased the risk for NSF included infection, inflammation, vascular disease, hypercoagulability, hypercalcemia, hyperphosphatemia, erythropoiesis-stimulating agent (ESA), and iron therapy.

The best approach to NSF is prevention because therapeutic interventions are at best suboptimal. The high-risk patient should be identified before GBCA exposure, allowing other imaging options to be explored. Such options include non-GBCA MR imaging, CT scan, ultrasonography, and other techniques that can often provide diagnostic results. When a GBCA is necessary to make the diagnosis, the following approach seems reasonable: (1) use a macrocyclic GBCA; (2) use the lowest dose required to obtain a diagnostic image; (3) optimize metabolic parameters and restrict ESA and iron use immediately before and after GBCA exposure; (4) wait for kidney recovery or stabilization in AKI; and (5) consider performing HD within hours of GBCA exposure in patients already receiving dialysis. The incidence of NSF has essentially disappeared with the implementation of prudent GBCA use in high-risk patients. However, when this disease develops, its consequences are often devastating, and therapeutic options are limited. Although a number of agents have been used, it appears that pain control and physical therapy are most important. Therapies such as extracorporeal photopheresis, sodium thiosulfate, and imatinib show promise; however, only early kidney transplant may offer stabilization or reversal of the fibrosing process.

ORAL SODIUM PHOSPHATE PREPARATION

Sodium phosphate preparations are used as purgatives for bowel cleansing before diagnostic colonoscopy and CT virtual colonoscopy. They are administered as a solution or tablets before the procedure and contain approximately 38 g of monobasic sodium phosphate and 9 g of dibasic sodium phosphate.

The adverse events associated with phosphate-containing bowel preparations occur with excessive dosing or use in patients with underlying kidney disease. Hypocalcemia and hyperphosphatemia may complicate therapy, but AKI is of greater concern. The pathogenic mechanism was described in 21 patients with AKI after a phosphate-containing bowel cleansing agent was used for colonoscopy. Patients were predominantly women, had hypertension, and were on RAAS blockade. AKI was recognized at a median of 3 months after colonoscopy. Minimal proteinuria and bland urine sediment were noted. Tubular injury and atrophy with abundant calcium phosphate deposits in distal tubules and collecting ducts were features on kidney biopsy. This entity is termed *acute phosphate nephropathy*.

Two patterns of kidney injury occur with sodium phosphate administration. First, AKI develops within days of exposure and is associated with hyperphosphatemia and hypocalcemia. A second pattern is seen when AKI is discovered incidentally in patients evaluated weeks or months after exposure. Unfortunately, acute phosphate nephropathy is frequently complicated by CKD. Thus, oral sodium phosphate-based products should not be used in patients with underlying kidney disease, volume depletion, or electrolyte abnormalities. In 2008, following an alert regarding acute phosphate nephropathy issued by the US Food and Drug Administration (FDA), over-the-counter oral phosphate-containing preparations were voluntarily withdrawn from the US market.

Recently, the possibility of CKD developing in patients receiving phosphate-containing enemas was raised. However, because there was no definitive diagnosis (i.e., kidney biopsy) to verify a relationship between the enemas and phosphate-related kidney injury, the association needs further study. Clinicians should remain vigilant for this possibility.

THERAPEUTIC AGENTS

ANALGESICS

NSAIDs, including selective cyclooxygenase-2 (COX-2) inhibitors, are widely used to treat pain, fever, and inflammation. More than 20 NSAIDs from seven major classes are approved in the United States, and many are available over the counter. Annually, more than 50 million patients ingest these drugs on an intermittent basis, whereas 15 to 25 million people in the United States use NSAIDs daily.

NSAIDs and selective COX-2 inhibitors are associated with various clinical kidney syndromes (Box 35.1). It has been

---

Box 35.1   Nonsteroidal Antiinflammatory Drug Clinical Kidney Syndromes

Acute kidney injury
    Prerenal azotemia
    Acute tubular necrosis
Glomerular disease
    Minimal change disease
    Membranous nephropathy
Acute interstitial nephritis
Hyperkalemia/metabolic acidosis (hyporeninemic hypoaldosteronism)
Hyponatremia
Hypertension/edema
Acute papillary necrosis
Analgesic nephropathy/chronic tubulointerstitial nephritis

---

estimated that 1% to 5% of patients who ingest NSAIDs develop some form of nephrotoxicity, perhaps representing as many as 500,000 persons in the United States alone. These adverse effects are caused primarily by prostaglandin (PG) inhibition; however, other effects are idiosyncratic. PGs are produced by COX enzyme metabolism and are secreted locally in the kidney to modulate the effects of various systemic and local substances. For example, PGs enhance afferent arteriolar vasodilatation in the presence of vasoconstrictors such as angiotensin-II, norepinephrine, vasopressin, and endothelin, thereby providing critical counterbalance to the vasoconstriction that predominates in hypovolemic states. Patients with decreased true or effective circulating volume are at highest risk to develop renal vasoconstriction and reduced GFR. Because CKD is a PG-dependent state, these patients are also at higher risk for NSAID-induced kidney injury. In fact, exposure to NSAIDs doubles the risk of hospitalization for AKI in patients with CKD. Similar rates of AKI with NSAID exposure are noted in the elderly, those with cardiac disease, and patients receiving angiotensin-converting enzyme (ACE) inhibitors. As noted in a nested case-control study, the adjusted relative risk of AKI was 4.1 and 3.2 in current NSAID users versus nonusers in the general population, respectively. Patients with hypertension, heart failure, and diuretic therapy had an adjusted relative risk of 11.6 with NSAIDs.

In addition to increasing arteriolar blood flow, PGs also enhance kidney sodium, potassium, and water excretion. PGs modulate kidney potassium excretion through stimulation of the RAAS. Inhibition of PGs can result in hyperkalemia when coexistent conditions such as AKI, CKD, diabetes mellitus, and therapy with certain medications (RAAS blockers, potassium-sparing diuretics) are also present. The classic syndrome of hyporeninemic hypoaldosteronism with hyperkalemic metabolic acidosis can be observed with NSAID therapy. Inhibition of PGs is associated with decreased kidney sodium excretion, and all NSAIDs cause some degree of sodium retention. This is especially common in patients with hypertension, heart disease, and other salt-retentive disease states (e.g., cirrhosis, nephrotic syndrome, AKI, and CKD), who are at highest risk for developing edema, hypertension, or heart failure. Hypertension is a particularly important complication, as small changes in blood pressure are associated with increased cardiovascular events. Hyponatremia from impaired water excretion also complicates therapy as PGs act to antagonize water reabsorption in the distal nephron, an effect that is lost with NSAIDs. Reduced GFR also contributes to water retention and hyponatremia.

Idiosyncratic effects of selective and nonselective NSAIDs include proteinuric glomerular diseases. Minimal change disease (MCD) is most common, whereas membranous nephropathy is a relatively rare complication of these drugs. Nephrotic-range proteinuria or full-blown nephrotic syndrome is the typical clinical presentation, sometimes accompanied by AKI. NSAID-induced AIN can occur alone or along with these glomerular diseases.

CHEMOTHERAPEUTIC AGENTS

Chemotherapeutic agents are critical to halting or slowing tumor growth, but adverse kidney effects often complicate treatment. They are most commonly associated with AKI, but also cause electrolyte and acid-base disturbances, proteinuria, and hypertension.

ANTIANGIOGENESIS DRUGS

Antiangiogenesis drugs target vascular endothelial growth factor (VEGF) or its tyrosine kinase receptor (VEGF-R). VEGF signaling is critical to the tumor angiogenesis, and disruption of the signaling pathways provides novel treatment options for aggressive malignancies. However, VEGF biology is also essential to renal microvasculature and glomerular integrity. Podocytes provide local VEGF to glomerular endothelial cells, preserving the integrity of the fenestrated endothelium. In animals, pharmacologic reduction in VEGF production or effect causes proteinuria, hypertension, and thrombotic microangiopathy by damaging the renal microvasculature, in particular the glomerular endothelium. A similar clinical syndrome marked by proteinuria (rarely nephrotic) and hypertension occurs in patients treated with antiangiogenesis agents such as bevacizumab and the tyrosine kinase inhibitors. Thrombotic microangiopathy is the most common pathologic lesion noted in patients who undergo kidney biopsy for AKI (Fig. 35.1).

INTERFERON

Interferon (α, β, γ) is described as causing glomerular injury and proteinuria. Early reported cases showed minimal change lesions, but more recent reports describe collapsing and noncollapsing focal segmental glomerulosclerosis (FSGS) on biopsy. Patients tend to present with nephrotic range proteinuria and/or AKI within weeks of commencing interferon therapy. The time to clinical presentation is shorter for interferon-α as compared to other subtypes. Although proteinuria declines with cessation of interferon therapy, complete reversal is uncommon. The mechanism underlying interferon-associated glomerular injury is not entirely clear, but it may include direct binding to podocyte receptors and alteration of normal cellular proliferation. Other postulated effects include macrophage activation and skewing of the cytokine profile toward IL-6 and IL-13, which are purported permeability factors in MCD and FSGS.

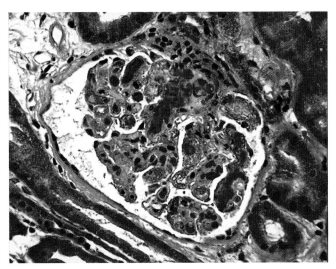

Fig. 35.1 Thrombotic microangiopathy as manifested by mesangiolysis, endothelial denudation, red blood cell congestion, and basement membrane duplication in the glomerulus on light microscopy. (Courtesy Michael Kashgarian, Yale University.)

BISPHOSPHONATES

The bisphosphonates are effectively used for malignancy-related bone disorders such as multiple myeloma, hypercalcemia of malignancy, and osteolytic metastases. They are also commonly used in Paget disease and osteoporosis. One of their major adverse effects is nephrotoxicity, seen primarily with pamidronate and zoledronate. Nephrotoxicity is more common with high-dose IV formulations than the oral or low-dose IV preparations used in osteoporosis treatment. Depending on the particular bisphosphonate, glomerular and/or tubular injury may result. Pamidronate-induced kidney injury is dose related, where high dosage and long duration increase risk. Nephrotoxic manifestations include nephrotic-range proteinuria or full-blown nephrotic syndrome associated with collapsing FSGS or MCD, consistent with a toxic podocytopathy. Acute tubular necrosis (ATN) may also accompany collapsing FSGS. Nephrotoxicity is sometimes reversible, but progressive CKD and end-stage kidney disease (ESKD) requiring chronic dialysis may develop. IV zoledronate is more commonly associated with AKI from toxic ATN, although rare cases of FSGS are described. Current evidence suggests that ibandronate has the least nephrotoxicity. As bisphosphonates undergo kidney excretion, prevention of nephrotoxicity hinges on dose reduction in patients with reduced GFR, with clinical guidelines recommending discontinuation of therapy when estimated GFR falls to less than 30 mL/min.

PLATINUM COMPOUNDS

Platinum-based agents are potent antineoplastic drugs that have a high incidence of nephrotoxicity, particularly in patients with CKD. Nonoliguric AKI from toxic ATN is the most common pattern of kidney injury. Cisplatin has the most nephrotoxic potential, although second- and third-generation drugs such as carboplatin and oxaliplatin are also nephrotoxic at high doses. Cisplatin's mechanism of nephrotoxicity is related to its drug characteristics and kidney handling. Chloride at the *cis*-position of the molecule promotes kidney injury, whereas its uptake into proximal tubular cells via OCT-2 also contributes to damage. Other mechanisms of injury are activation of intracellular injury pathways, inflammation, oxidative stress, and vascular injury. The end result is renal tubular cell apoptosis or necrosis, manifesting as clinical AKI and/or a tubulopathy. Platin drugs are also associated with Fanconi syndrome from proximal tubular injury, and sodium-wasting syndrome and hypomagnesemia from cellular injury in the loop of Henle.

In high-risk patients, carboplatin and oxaliplatin are used based on their less nephrotoxic profile. Neither of these molecules is transported by OCT-2, thereby reducing proximal tubular intracellular concentrations. In addition, the chloride at the *cis*-position in cisplatin is replaced by carboxylate and cyclobutane in carboplatin and oxaliplatin, respectively, which may further reduce toxicity. Antioxidants such as sodium thiosulfate and amifostine have been proposed as prophylactic measures against platin nephrotoxicity, but concerns of decreased anticancer activity and adverse effects limit their utility. Prevention of platin nephrotoxicity focuses on volume repletion with IV saline administration and avoidance of other nephrotoxins.

IFOSFAMIDE

Ifosfamide is an alkylating agent derived from the parent molecule cyclophosphamide. In contrast to cyclophosphamide, ifosfamide causes renal tubular injury primarily through its nephrotoxic metabolite, chloracetaldehyde. In addition, ifosfamide enters tubular cells via OCT-2, whereas cyclophosphamide does not. Nephrotoxic manifestations include tubulopathies such as isolated proximal tubular injury, Fanconi syndrome, nephrogenic diabetes insipidus (DI), and AKI from ATN, which is often reversible but can be permanent. Tubular cell injury and necrosis with swollen, dysmorphic mitochondria are noted on kidney histopathology. Risk factors for kidney injury include previous cisplatin exposure, cumulative dose greater than 90 g/m^2, and underlying CKD.

Preventive measures are limited. IV saline and dose reduction are used. Because this agent is transported into cells via OCT-2, competitive inhibition of this pathway with cimetidine is being evaluated. Treatment is supportive, addressing electrolyte deficiencies and monitoring for CKD and dialysis-requiring end-stage renal disease (ESRD). Other long-term complications include permanent proximal tubulopathy and isolated phosphaturia.

PEMETREXED

Pemetrexed is a methotrexate derivative that inhibits enzymes involved in purine and pyrimidine metabolism, impairing RNA and DNA synthesis in tumors. It is excreted unchanged by the kidneys, although pemetrexed enters proximal tubular cell via luminal and basolateral pathways. Luminal drug uptake may occur via the folate receptor-α transport pathway, whereas basolateral entry is by the reduced folate carrier. Intracellular pemetrexed is polyglutamylated, which traps the drug within the cell. The higher intracellular drug concentration more fully impairs RNA and DNA synthesis and causes cell injury. Reversible AKI occurs with high-dose therapy, with kidney lesions consisting of ATN and AIN. Tubular dysfunction

consisting of nephrogenic DI and distal renal tubular acidosis occurs. Most patients present with AKI and minimal proteinuria, which stabilizes with drug discontinuation but can lead to CKD from chronic tubulointerstitial nephritis.

EPIDERMAL GROWTH FACTOR RECEPTOR ANTAGONISTS

Monoclonal antibodies that antagonize epithelial growth factor receptor (EGFR) signaling, including cetuximab and panitumumab, offer promising biologic therapy for colorectal and head and neck tumors. Given the role of EGFR signaling in magnesium homeostasis, these antibodies induce kidney magnesium wasting. The EGFR signaling cascade is necessary for activation of transient receptor potential M6 (TRPM6), the epithelial channel in the distal nephron that facilitates magnesium reabsorption. Monoclonal antibodies against EGFR, which have a much higher affinity for EGFR than epidermal growth factor (EGF), potently inhibit placement of TRPM6 in the luminal membrane and prevent luminal magnesium reabsorption. The incidence of hypomagnesemia approaches 43% with cetuximab in clinical trials, whereas nearly all patients develop some reduction in serum magnesium level. Thus, serum magnesium monitoring should be a standard of care with anti-EGFR therapy. Panitumumab causes hypomagnesemia less commonly. The likelihood of hypomagnesemia increases with duration of therapy and may persist for several weeks after drug discontinuation before resolving. Treatment requires IV magnesium repletion, particularly in cancer patients who tend to have diarrhea, vomiting, and decreased oral intake. Because secondary hypokalemia and hypocalcemia occur with hypomagnesemia, serum potassium and calcium concentrations should be monitored and repletion undertaken when these electrolyte disorders are present.

IMMUNE CHECKPOINT INHIBITORS

Immune checkpoint inhibitors (CPIs) are a class of drugs that impair the "checkpoints" that function to suppress the adaptive immune response and prevent autoimmunity. T cells possess surface receptors such as programmed death-1 protein (PD-1) and cytotoxic T lymphocyte-associated antigen-4 (CTLA-4), which bind to their cognate ligands on antigen presenting cells leading to inhibition of T cell activation. This normally suppresses the development of autoimmunity. However, a wide variety of malignancies also employ this approach to enhance tumor survival by over-expressing ligands that bind these inhibitory T cell receptors. This leads to a decrease of infiltrating activated T cells within the tumor microenvironment and inhibits antitumor T cell responses. To combat this, monoclonal antibody drugs that block ligand binding to PD-1 and CTLA-4 receptors were designed to facilitate T cell rescue and restore antitumor immunity. Ipilimumab (anti-CTLA-4) and the anti-PD-1 drugs nivolumab and pembrolizumab are such examples. However, one potential concern of blocking immune checkpoints is that it risks the development of pathologic autoimmunity and end-organ injury, such as AIN.

In fact, this concern has been realized. In addition to other end-organ autoimmune effects, biopsy-proven AIN has been observed with these drugs (see Table 35.1). Numerous cases of AIN, some with granulomatous changes, have been described with the currently available CPIs. While some patients present clinically with rash and eosinophilia, there is no consistent clinical manifestation of drug nephrotoxicity except AKI. Urinalysis and urine microscopy findings supportive of AIN are also inconsistent, with some cases manifesting pyuria, hematuria, and low-grade proteinuria. A small number of cases have required dialysis. Most cases respond to drug discontinuation and steroid therapy. However, CKD is seen in a small number of patients.

The mechanism of CPI-induced AIN is unknown, but several are postulated. First, interference with the CTLA-4 and PD-1 pathways can lead to detrimental immune effects and autoimmunity. As has been shown in murine models, checkpoint receptor signaling blunts activation and expansion of self-reactive T cells and stimulates tolerogenic dendritic cells. When PD-1 is knocked out in mice, glomerulonephritis develops supporting the importance of checkpoint signaling in minimizing T cell–mediated kidney inflammation. Alternatively, because patients treated with CPIs are also taking other drugs capable of causing AIN, disruption of checkpoint signaling that may be critical to maintaining peripheral self-tolerance to these other drug antigens may permit reactivation of exhausted drug specific T cells previously primed by nephritogenic drugs. Suddenly, because of loss of tolerance, T cells are activated against the drug. Ultimately, CPI therapy may promote permissive environment effector T cells to migrate into the kidney and cause an inflammatory response leading to AIN.

BRAF INHIBITORS

Targeting mutations in cancer cells is an effective strategy to combat various malignancies. Melanoma frequently has a BRAF V600 mutation that can be targeted by the selective BRAF inhibitors vemurafenib and dabrafenib. Patient survival has increased with this class of anticancer drugs. However, nephrotoxicity has also been observed in treated patients. A decline in GFR at 1 and 3 months of therapy in 15/16 patients (five with proteinuria) was noted, and was complicated by persistent kidney injury after 8 months of follow-up (no kidney histology). Another series of eight patients developed AKI following vemurafenib (acute tubular injury seen on kidney biopsy in one patient). AKI in another four patients treated with vemurafenib was described. All had skin rash and two had eosinophilia, but no kidney tissue was obtained, although the clinical presentation suggested AIN. Three of four patients recovered kidney function following drug discontinuation.

A retrospective study of 74 patients exposed to vemurafenib over 3 years described AKI, primarily Kidney Disease: Improving Global Outcomes (KDIGO) stage 1 (80%), in 44 patients. AKI developed within 3 months of drug exposure and 80% recovered kidney function within 3 months of drug discontinuation. Kidney biopsy revealed tubulointerstitial injury in two patients. Examination of the FDA Adverse Events Reporting System over 3 years for BRAF inhibitor nephrotoxicity revealed evidence for nephrotoxicity. The major adverse effect noted with vemurafenib was AKI ($n = 132$) and a small number of cases of hyponatremia and hypokalemia. For dabrafenib, 13 cases of AKI, 6 cases of hyponatremia, and 2 cases of hypokalemia were noted over slightly more than a year of reporting.

Unfortunately, data on proteinuria and histology was not available from these patients.

The mechanism of kidney injury with BRAF inhibitors is unknown; they may interfere with the downstream mitogen-activated protein kinase (MAPK) pathway, increasing kidney susceptibility to ischemic tubular injury.

ANTIMICROBIAL AGENTS

Several widely prescribed antimicrobial medications can result in kidney injury, especially in hospitalized patients. Antimicrobial agents are administered to the most severely ill patients who have coexistent processes that can independently affect kidney function and potentiate nephrotoxicity.

ANTIBIOTICS

AMINOGLYCOSIDES

AGs are frequently associated with kidney injury in hospitalized patients. The reported incidence ranges between 7% and 36% of patients receiving these drugs, increases with the duration of drug administration, and may approach 50% with more than 2 weeks of therapy. AGs are freely filtered by the glomerulus and then reabsorbed by proximal tubular cells. Ultimately, kidney excretion is the major route of elimination. Their cationic and amphophilic properties enhance binding to luminal membranes of proximal tubular cells, likely via the megalin receptor, and lead to accumulation of drug within cortical tubular cells. Nephrotoxicity tracks with charge; the more cationic, the more likely the drug interacts with luminal membranes where they undergo endocytosis and accumulate within intracellular lysosomes. Myeloid bodies (Fig. 35.2) visualized on electron microscopy often develop. These structures are membrane fragments and damaged organelles that result from inhibition of lysosomal enzymes. Nephrotoxicity occurs from mechanisms such as disruption of subcellular organelle activity, induction of oxidative stress, and enhanced mitochondrial dysfunction.

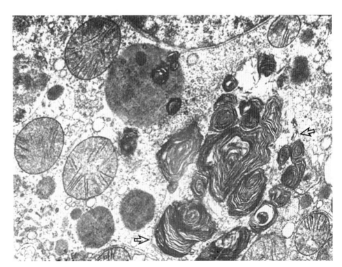

Fig. 35.2 Aminoglycoside-induced tubular cell injury manifested by myeloid bodies (arrows) as seen on electron microscopy. These bodies represent changes in tubular lysosomes caused by the accumulation of polar lipids. (Courtesy Gilbert W. Moeckel, Yale University.)

AG nephrotoxicity presents clinically as a rising serum creatinine after approximately 5 to 7 days of therapy but may occur earlier in the presence of risk factors. AKI is often preceded by a concentrating defect. Low-grade proteinuria and urine sediment containing renal tubular epithelial (RTE) cells or granular casts are seen days before clinical AKI, supporting ongoing subclinical kidney injury. Tubular dysfunction is manifested by an elevated fractional excretion of sodium (>1% to 2%), and urinary potassium, calcium, and magnesium wasting. Gentamicin has been described as causing a proximal tubulopathy or full-blown Fanconi syndrome in some patients, whereas a Bartter-like syndrome has also been noted. The latter lesion is speculated to occur from the activation of the calcium-sensing receptor by cationic gentamicin, thereby inhibiting the NaK2Cl transporter in the loop of Henle. AKI progressively worsens, but the course may be limited in severity with early drug discontinuation. Nevertheless, a time lag may occur before kidney function improves.

Several risk factors for AG nephrotoxicity have been identified (Box 35.2). This allows, when alternative antibiotics are unavailable, more intensive monitoring and modification of risk factors, such as volume depletion and electrolyte abnormalities. All members of the AG family can cause nephrotoxicity, but tobramycin exhibits less nephrotoxicity than gentamicin in animal models.

Tailoring AG doses to maintain drug levels within therapeutic range minimizes nephrotoxicity while maintaining bactericidal drug concentrations. When calculating doses, it should be recognized that changes in the serum creatinine often underestimate the true GFR reduction in elderly, cirrhotic, and malnourished patients. In addition to appropriate dose reduction, single daily-dose regimens may reduce AG nephrotoxicity because tubular absorption is saturable, although the data are mixed. Monitoring of peak and trough drug levels, along with serum creatinine concentration, every 2 to 3 days is prudent, but daily monitoring may be required in patients with serious infections and unstable kidney function. Urine microscopic findings may identify kidney injury before serum creatinine changes.

VANCOMYCIN

Vancomycin is a widely prescribed and typically well-tolerated drug. Although AKI rarely occurs as a complication, two lesions have been described. One is an idiosyncratic reaction resulting in AIN, and the other is direct tubular toxicity that occurs with excessive serum concentrations. High-dose and longer drug exposure are likely risk factors for tubular injury. Kidney biopsies in patients with AKI associated with toxic vancomycin concentrations have demonstrated toxic ATN rather than classic AIN.

POLYMYXINS

The polymyxins are a group of antibiotics generally reserved for resistant organisms, primarily because of their high nephrotoxic potential. Colistin and polymyxin B are the two agents that are employed as antimicrobials. Both have a narrow therapeutic window with nephrotoxicity related to their D-amino content and fatty acid component. This increases tubular cell membrane permeability and the influx of cations, resulting in tubular cell injury. Patients with underlying risk often develop AKI with increasing duration of therapy.

SULFONAMIDES

Sulfa-based antibiotics are effective antimicrobial agents that can cause three kidney lesions: AIN, crystal nephropathy, and vasculitis. AIN is most common, whereas crystal-induced AKI occurs primarily with high-dose sulfadiazine (and with other sulfonamides to a lesser degree). Vasculitis is probably the least common sulfonamide-related kidney lesion, typically a hypersensitivity reaction that rarely is associated with development of polyarteritis nodosa. The incidence of AKI ranges from 0.4% to 29%. Crystal-induced kidney injury occurs when insoluble sulfa-drug precipitates within the tubular lumen of the distal nephron. Because sulfa drugs are weak acids, this is more likely to happen in an acidic urine (pH <6.0), when urine flow rates are low, with hypo-albuminemia, and with excessive dose for the level of GFR.

Although patients are generally asymptomatic, vague abdominal or flank pain along with an increasing serum creatinine and oliguria occur within 7 days of starting therapy. Urine microscopy reveals strongly birefringent sulfonamide crystals (e.g., shocks of wheat and shells), sometimes admixed with white blood cells, RTE cells, and granular casts. Rarely, small radiolucent calculi may also lodge in the kidney parenchyma and/or calyces and appear as layered clusters of echogenic material on kidney ultrasonography. Treatment includes IV fluids, urinary alkalinization, and sulfonamide dose reduction or discontinuation.

CIPROFLOXACIN

The quinolone antibiotic ciprofloxacin is widely used to treat numerous bacterial infections. As noted with other antibiotics, ciprofloxacin causes AKI in patients primarily through the development of AIN. Experimental studies have demonstrated crystalluria following the administration of ciprofloxacin. Less commonly, this drug can be associated with crystal-induced AKI in humans. Ciprofloxacin is insoluble at neutral or alkaline pH (pH >7.3), and it crystallizes in alkaline urine. Intrarenal crystallization may result from excessive drug doses in elderly patients, underlying CKD, volume depletion, and/or alkaline urine. Patients are generally asymptomatic, and the first sign of kidney injury is a rise in serum creatinine after 2 to 14 days of treatment. Urine microscopy shows ciprofloxacin crystals, which appear as strongly birefringent needles, sheaves, stars, fans, butterflies, and other unusual shapes, along with other cellular elements and casts. Kidney

---

Box 35.2 Risk Factors for Aminoglycoside Nephrotoxicity

Prolonged course of treatment (>10 days)
Volume depletion
Sepsis
Preexisting kidney disease
Hypokalemia
Advanced age
Combination therapy with certain cephalosporins, particularly cephalothin
Concomitant exposure to other nephrotoxins (e.g., radiocontrast, amphotericin B, cisplatin)
Exposure to gentamicin > amikacin > tobramycin

biopsy reveals crystals within the tubules. To avoid this complication, ciprofloxacin should be dosed appropriately for the level of kidney function. To prevent AKI and crystalluria, patients receiving ciprofloxacin should be volume replete, and alkalinization of the urine should be avoided. Treatment of kidney injury is drug discontinuation or dose reduction, and volume repletion with isotonic IV fluids.

ANTIVIRAL DRUGS

ACYCLOVIR

Acyclovir is an effective antiviral agent that is widely used to treat herpes virus infections. Although generally safe, it can cause AKI from intratubular crystal deposition when administered intravenously, particularly at high doses. Acyclovir is excreted in the urine through both glomerular filtration and tubular secretion. Acyclovir is relatively insoluble in the urine, which accounts for its intratubular precipitation at high concentration or with low urine flow rates, resulting in intrarenal urinary obstruction. Isolated crystalluria and asymptomatic AKI are most common, but nausea/vomiting and flank/abdominal pain may occur. Crystal nephropathy typically develops within 24 to 48 hours of acyclovir administration, with an incidence of 12% to 48% when acyclovir is administered as a rapid IV bolus. In contrast, low-dose IV and oral acyclovir therapy rarely cause AKI unless there is severe volume depletion or underlying kidney disease. Urine microscopy usually shows both hematuria and pyuria, along with birefringent, needle-shaped crystals. Prevention hinges on avoiding rapid bolus infusion of acyclovir and by maintaining adequate intravascular volume during drug exposure. Dose reduction is critical in patients with underlying kidney disease. HD removes significant amounts of acyclovir and is sometimes indicated with severe AKI and concomitant neurotoxicity. Fortunately, most patients recover kidney function with acyclovir discontinuation and volume resuscitation.

INDINAVIR AND ATAZANAVIR

Indinavir and atazanavir are protease inhibitors used in the treatment of human immunodeficiency virus (HIV) infection. Indinavir revolutionized HIV care, but its use was complicated by a number of toxicities including crystal-induced AKI and nephrolithiasis. Atazanavir has gained widespread use, and it is also associated with crystal-related kidney injury and nephrolithiasis.

The kidney clears approximately 20% of indinavir, and intratubular crystal precipitation occurs at urine pH above 5.5 (Fig. 35.3). Intrarenal tubular obstruction and obstructing calculi can also lead to AKI. Complications include kidney colic, dysuria, back/flank pain, or gross hematuria, with an 8% incidence of urologic symptoms. Urine microscopy shows crystals of varying shapes, including plate-like rectangles, fan-shaped crystals, and starburst forms. Although most cases of indinavir-associated AKI are mild and reversible, more severe AKI from obstructing calculi and CKD occurs. Prevention of intrarenal crystal deposition requires consumption of 2 to 3 L of fluid per day. Patients with liver disease should receive a dose reduction. Discontinuation of indinavir generally reverses nephrotoxicity; however, chronic tubulointerstitial fibrosis has been noted.

Atazanavir has chemical characteristics and pharmacokinetics similar to indinavir, likely explaining its nephrotoxicity.

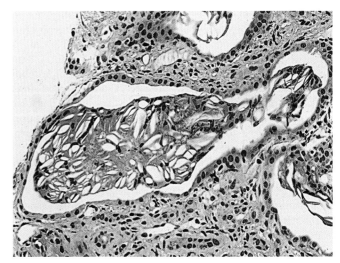

Fig. 35.3 Indinavir crystal deposition within renal tubular lumens causes acute and chronic kidney injury, an entity coined *crystal nephropathy*, as seen on light microscopy. (Courtesy Glen S. Markowitz, Columbia University.)

Crystal nephropathy, nephrolithiasis, and AIN have been described. Thirty cases of atazanavir-associated nephrolithiasis have been reported to the FDA, whereas another study estimated a 0.97% prevalence of atazanavir stones among those taking the drug. Analysis of kidney stones shows 60% atazanavir metabolite and 40% calcium apatite. Atazanavir-associated crystal nephropathy has also been described, where rod-like atazanavir crystals were noted on urine microscopy and within tubular lumens on kidney biopsy. Prevention is best achieved by avoiding intravascular volume depletion. Treatment hinges on IVF therapy and stone removal when indicated. Drug discontinuation is sometimes necessary.

TENOFOVIR

Tenofovir is an agent used to treat various viral infections, including HIV and hepatitis B virus. Animal models note that tenofovir causes proximal tubular dilatation, abnormalities in mitochondrial ultrastructure, depleted mitochondrial DNA (mtDNA), and depressed respiratory chain enzyme expression. Clinically, patients present with AKI or a proximal tubulopathy and less commonly with nephrogenic DI. AKI may require temporary dialysis, although a degree of kidney recovery often results in CKD. Kidney histology from patients with clinical nephrotoxicity demonstrates proximal tubular injury and varying degrees of chronic tubulointerstitial scarring. On light microscopy, prominent eosinophilic inclusions within proximal tubular cell cytoplasm represent giant, abnormal mitochondria. On electron microscopy, injured mitochondria vary from small and rounded to swollen with irregular contours.

Host factors that potentiate tenofovir nephrotoxicity include the HIV-infected host's mtDNA depletion, reduced GFR, and genetic defects in drug excretion pathways. Tenofovir is eliminated by a combination of glomerular filtration and proximal tubular secretion, which in part explains its compartmental toxicity. It is transported from the basolateral circulation into proximal tubular cells via organic ion transporter-1 (OAT-1), and it is subsequently translocated into the urine through luminal efflux transporters such as multidrug resistance proteins (MRP-2/-4). Reduced GFR enhances the amount of drug that is secreted, increasing traffic through proximal tubular cells. Impaired MRP-driven efflux activity can reduce drug secretion and increase intracellular concentrations. A single nucleotide polymorphism (SNP) in the MRP-2 efflux transporter gene (ABCC2) has been documented in HIV-infected patients with tenofovir-induced nephrotoxicity. Excretory pathway defects can lead to increased tenofovir concentrations within tubular cells.

Prevention of and monitoring for tenofovir-related kidney injury are important. Genetic risk factor testing (SNP in ABCC2 gene) to identify high-risk patients and targeted interventions such as probenecid to reduce OAT-1–mediated drug transport into tubular cells may reduce toxicity. Avoidance of tenofovir in patients with advanced CKD, or at least appropriate dose reduction, further reduces nephrotoxicity.

ANTIFUNGAL AGENTS

AMPHOTERICIN B

Amphotericin B is a polyene antibiotic used in treatment of many serious fungal infections, but it is also associated with nephrotoxicity. The degree of kidney injury is roughly proportional to the total cumulative dose. Because this drug is highly bound to cell membranes, it damages membrane integrity and increases permeability. Membrane injury is thought to underlie development of the characteristic clinical syndromes of potassium and magnesium wasting, inability to maximally concentrate urine, and distal tubule acidification defects. These abnormalities, along with urine microscopy findings with RTE cells/casts and granular casts, usually precede the development of clinically apparent AKI. Amphotericin B also produces acute afferent arteriolar vasoconstriction, causing a hemodynamic reduction in the GFR. Tubuloglomerular feedback triggered by increased sodium permeability has been suggested as playing a role in vasoconstriction.

Reduced kidney function is frequently nonoliguric and progressive but slowly abates after drug discontinuation. However, high doses and repetitive drug exposure can cause CKD. Volume depletion potentiates nephrotoxicity, whereas sodium loading and volume expansion can ameliorate kidney injury, perhaps by blunting tubuloglomerular feedback. Risk factors for kidney injury include a high cumulative dose, prolonged duration of therapy, intensive care unit admission when therapy is initiated, and cyclosporine therapy. Several formulations of amphotericin B in lipid vehicles, including liposomes, have been developed for clinical use and result in fewer constitutional symptoms while retaining antifungal activity. Studies have shown that these formulations are less nephrotoxic, but they can still cause AKI in high-risk patients.

MISCELLANEOUS

ANTICOAGULANT-RELATED NEPHROPATHY

A little-known complication of warfarin and other anticoagulants is AKI from severe glomerular bleeding and obstructing red blood cell (RBC) casts. This entity was initially termed *warfarin nephropathy* but can occur with any form of excessive anticoagulation in at-risk patients. It has been described in patients with and without CKD who are overanticoagulated with warfarin. The mechanism appears to be related to glomerular hemorrhage, often in patients with an underlying glomerulopathy, with subsequent obstruction of tubules by RBC casts. The cause of AKI is not known, although tubular obstruction and/or heme-related tubular injury from lysosomal overload and oxidative damage play a role. Hemoglobin may enter cells via megalin-cubilin receptor-mediated endocytosis, with free hemoglobin promoting lipid peroxidation and heme/iron-generating ROS, mitochondrial damage, and apoptosis. Treatment consists of reversal of anticoagulation initially, followed by more judicious anticoagulation in those who truly require it. Unfortunately, many patients are left with CKD, sometimes requiring chronic dialysis.

OSMOTIC AGENTS

Osmotic nephropathy refers to kidney injury seen when certain macromolecules enter proximal tubular cells through the luminal membrane. First described in animal studies, sucrose infusion was associated with tubular cell swelling and kidney dysfunction. Similar histopathology and kidney injury have been described with mannitol, dextran, and, more recently, with IV immune globulin (IVIG) and hydroxyethyl starch (HES). Tubular injury begins with drug entry into the tubular cell, followed by accumulation within lysosomes causing tubular epithelia to swell and form vacuoles. This process ultimately disrupts cellular integrity and, if tubular swelling is severe, obstructs tubular lumens and impedes urine flow causing AKI. Kidney biopsy shows characteristic histopathologic lesions such as swollen, edematous tubules filled with cytoplasmic vacuoles, which represent swollen lysosomes on electron microscopy (Fig. 35.4). With severe injury, tubules may appear degraded, similar to ischemic or toxic ATN.

Osmotic nephropathy is most commonly associated with IVIG stabilized with sucrose and HES. IVIG-related osmotic nephropathy occurs most commonly in patients

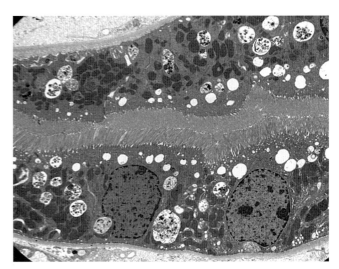

Fig. 35.4 Uptake of osmotic substances such as sucrose, hydoxyethyl starch, dextran, and radiocontrast causes acute and chronic tubular injury, an entity known as *osmotic nephropathy*. Electron microscopy demonstrates characteristic cytoplasmic vacuoles. (Courtesy Gilbert W. Moeckel, Yale University.)

with underlying kidney disease and the elderly. Nonsucrose formulations of IVIG have not been linked to AKI and thus are preferred for high-risk patients. HES is a potent volume expander with an amylopectin chain with hydroxyethyl substitutions of varying degrees. Systemic degradation of HES allows glomerular filtration of the smaller HES molecules that enter proximal tubular cells. Similar to sucrose, HES-induced kidney injury has histopathologic features typical of osmotic nephropathy including tubular cell swelling and vacuolization. Clinically, HES is associated with AKI, sometimes requiring dialysis, especially in patients with sepsis and underlying kidney disease. Prevention is based on avoiding these agents in high-risk patients, whereas therapy for osmotic nephropathy is supportive with avoidance of further exposure.

LITHIUM

Lithium (Li^+) is one of the most effective medications for the treatment of bipolar disorders, making it a cornerstone of therapy despite its various toxicities. Li^+ adversely affects several organ systems, including the kidney, which excretes this cation. Although several kidney syndromes occur, the most common complication is nephrogenic DI. This condition develops in as many as 20% to 30% of patients and is a result of kidney resistance to the actions of antidiuretic hormone (ADH). ADH resistance reduces water permeability in the distal nephron through inhibition of the generation or action of cyclic adenosine monophosphate (cyclic-AMP). This decreases expression and attenuates luminal targeting of aquaporin-2 water channels in renal epithelial cells. Although polyuria generally improves with Li^+ withdrawal, amiloride therapy can further reduce urine volume by antagonizing epithelial sodium channels, which may be useful in patients who must continue on Li^+.

Acute Li^+ intoxication can occur with intentional overdose or in patients on stable dose who suffer an acute decline in GFR. It is manifested by symptoms ranging from nausea and tremor to seizures and coma. In addition, AKI can occur. The severity of intoxication generally correlates with serum Li^+ concentrations. Along with gastric lavage and polyethylene glycol, IV saline is used to reverse volume depletion and induce diuresis, thereby facilitating Li^+ excretion. In patients with AKI or CKD, significant neurologic symptoms, and Li^+ levels greater than 4.0 mEq/L, HD should be pursued. HD efficiently clears Li^+, where a 4-hour treatment can reduce plasma levels by about 1 mEq/L.

Long-term Li^+ therapy can cause chronic tubulointerstitial nephritis, characterized by tubular atrophy and interstitial fibrosis, with cortical and medullary tubular microcysts. Rarely, patients develop high-grade proteinuria and FSGS. Although kidney function may improve after drug cessation, irreversible CKD and ESRD may be observed.

PROTON PUMP INHIBITORS

Proton pump inhibitors (PPIs) are a class of drugs that are widely used worldwide. As such, they have emerged as one of the most common causes of AIN. Recently, PPI exposure has been associated with increased risk for CKD. If this is a true PPI complication, CKD may be due to unrecognized and untreated AIN. However, this area remains unclear and needs further study. Chapter 33 describes the nephrotoxic effects of PPIs in more detail.

BIBLIOGRAPHY

Cortazar FB, Marrone KA, Troxell ML, et al. Clinicopathological features of acute kidney injury associated with immune checkpoint inhibitors. *Kidney Int.* 2016;90:638-647.

Cruz DN, Goh CY, Marenzi G, et al. Renal replacement therapies for prevention of radiocontrast-induced nephropathy: a systematic review. *Am J Med.* 2012;125:66-78.

Deray G. Amphotericin B nephrotoxicity. *J Antimicrob Chemother.* 2002;49:37-41.

Ermina V, Jefferson A, Kowalewska J, et al. VEGF inhibition and renal thrombotic microangiopathy. *N Engl J Med.* 2008;358:1129-1136.

Gurevich F, Perazella MA. Renal effects of anti-angiogenesis therapy: update for the internist. *Am J Med.* 2009;122:322-328.

Humphreys BD, Soifer RJ, Magee CC. Renal failure associated with cancer and its treatment: an update. *J Am Soc Nephrol.* 2005;16:151-161.

Izzedine H, Harris M, Perazella MA. The nephrotoxic effects of HAART. *Nat Rev Nephrol.* 2009;5:563-573.

Izzedine H, Isnard-Bagnis C, Launay-Vacher V, et al. Gemcitabine-induced thrombotic microangiopathy: a systematic review. *Nephrol Dial Transplant.* 2006;21:3038-3045.

Kintzel PE. Anticancer drug-induced kidney disorders: incidence, prevention and management. *Drug Saf.* 2001;24:19-38.

Markowitz GS, Perazella MA. Acute phosphate nephropathy. *Kidney Int.* 2009;76:1027-1034.

Markowitz GS, Perazella MA. Drug-induced renal failure: a focus on tubulointerstitial disease. *Clin Chim Acta.* 2005;351:31-47.

Perazella MA. Advanced kidney disease, gadolinium and nephrogenic systemic fibrosis: the perfect storm. *Curr Opin Nephrol Hypertens.* 2009;18:519-525.

Perazella MA. Renal vulnerability to drug toxicity. *Clin J Am Soc Nephrol.* 2009;4:1275-1283.

Perazella MA, Markowitz GS. Bisphosphonate nephrotoxicity. *Kidney Int.* 2008;74:1385-1393.

Perazella MA, Moeckel GW. Nephrotoxicity from chemotherapeutic agents: clinical manifestations, pathobiology and prevention/therapy. *Semin Nephrol.* 2010;30:570-581.

Presne C, Fakhouri F, Noel LH, et al. Lithium-induced nephropathy: rate of progression and prognostic factors. *Kidney Int.* 2003;64:585-592.

Shirali AC, Perazella MA, Gettinger S. Association of acute interstitial nephritis with programmed cell death 1 inhibitor therapy in lung cancer patients. *Am J Kidney Dis.* 2016;68:287-291.

Weisbord SD, Palevsky PM. Prevention of contrast-induced nephropathy with volume expansion. *Clin J Am Soc Nephrol.* 2008;3:273-380.

36

Principles of Drug Therapy in Patients With Reduced Kidney Function

Thomas D. Nolin; Gary R. Matzke

Reduced kidney function may be observed in many settings, including patients with chronic kidney disease (CKD), the elderly with age-related decline in glomerular filtration rate (GFR), and critically ill patients with acute kidney injury (AKI). In adults, these conditions are associated with significant medication use, making these patients particularly vulnerable to the accumulation of a drug or its active or toxic metabolites. Clinicians must have a thorough understanding of the impact of reduced kidney function (RKF) on drug disposition and the appropriate methods by which to individualize drug therapy as they strive to optimize the outcomes of their patients.

Individualization of therapy for those agents that are predominantly (>70%) eliminated unchanged by the kidney can be accomplished with a proportional dose reduction or dosing interval prolongation based on the fractional reduction in GFR or its more commonly evaluated clinical counterparts, creatinine clearance (CL_{Cr}) and estimated GFR (eGFR). However, RKF is associated with progressive alterations in the bioavailability, plasma protein binding, distribution volume, and nonrenal clearance (CL_{NR}; i.e., metabolism and transport) of many drugs. Thus a more complex adjustment scheme may be required for medications that are extensively metabolized by the liver or for which changes in protein binding and/or distribution volume have been noted. Patients with RKF may also respond to a given dose or serum concentration of a drug (e.g., phenytoin) differently from those with normal kidney function because of the physiologic and biochemical changes associated with progressive CKD.

Using a sound understanding of basic pharmacokinetic principles, the pharmacokinetic characteristics of a drug, and the pathophysiologic alterations associated with RKF, clinicians can design individualized therapeutic regimens. This chapter describes the influence of RKF resulting from CKD and, when information is available, from AKI, on drug absorption, distribution, metabolism, transport, and excretion. The chapter also provides a practical approach to drug dosage individualization for patients with RKF and those receiving continuous renal replacement therapy (CRRT), peritoneal dialysis, or hemodialysis.

DRUG ABSORPTION

There is little quantitative information about the influence of RKF in CKD patients on drug absorption. Several variables, including changes in gastrointestinal transit time and gastric pH, edema of the gastrointestinal tract, vomiting and diarrhea (frequently seen in those with stage 5 CKD), and concomitant administration of phosphate binders, have been associated with alterations in the absorption of some drugs, such as digoxin and many of the fluoroquinolone antibiotics. The fraction of a drug that reaches the systemic circulation after oral versus intravenous administration (termed *absolute bioavailability*) is rarely altered in CKD patients. However, alterations in the peak concentration (C_{max}) and in the time to which the peak concentration is attained (t_{max}) have been noted for a few drugs, suggesting that the rate, but not the extent of absorption, is altered. Although the bioavailability of some drugs, such as furosemide or pindolol, is reported as being reduced, there are no consistent findings in patients with CKD to indicate that absorption is actually impaired. However, an increase in bioavailability resulting from a decrease in metabolism during the drug's first pass through the gastrointestinal tract and liver has been noted for some β-blockers and for dextropropoxyphene and dihydrocodeine.

DRUG DISTRIBUTION

The volume of distribution of many drugs is significantly altered in patients with stages 4 or 5 CKD (Table 36.1), and changes in patients with oliguric AKI are also reported. These changes are predominantly the result of altered plasma protein or tissue binding or of volume expansion secondary to reduced kidney sodium and water excretion. The plasma protein binding of acidic drugs, such as warfarin and phenytoin, typically is decreased in patients with CKD because of decreased concentrations of albumin. Changes in the conformation of albumin binding sites and accumulation of endogenous inhibitors of binding may also contribute to decreased protein binding. In addition, the high concentrations of some drug metabolites that accumulate in CKD patients may interfere with the protein binding of the parent compound. Regardless of the mechanism, decreased protein binding increases the free or unbound fraction of the drug. On the other hand, the plasma concentration of the principal binding protein for several basic drug compounds, α_1-acid glycoprotein, is increased in kidney transplant patients and in hemodialysis patients. For this reason, the unbound fraction of some basic drugs (e.g., quinidine) may be decreased, and as a result, the volume of distribution in these patients is decreased.

Table 36.1 Volume of Distribution of Selected Drugs in Patients With Stage 5 Chronic Kidney Disease

Drug	Normal (L/kg)	Stage 5 CKD (L/kg)	Change From Normal (%)
Amikacin	0.20	0.29	45
Azlocillin	0.21	0.28	33
Cefazolin	0.13	0.17	31
Cefoxitin	0.16	0.26	63
Cefuroxime	0.20	0.26	30
Clofibrate	0.14	0.24	71
Dicloxacillin	0.08	0.18	125
Digoxin	7.3	4.0	−45
Erythromycin	0.57	1.09	91
Gentamicin	0.20	0.32	60
Isoniazid	0.6	0.8	33
Minoxidil	2.6	4.9	88
Phenytoin	0.64	1.4	119
Trimethoprim	1.36	1.83	35
Vancomycin	0.64	0.85	33

CKD, Chronic kidney disease.

The net effect of changes in protein binding is usually an alteration in the relationship between unbound and total drug concentrations, an effect frequently encountered with phenytoin. The increase in the unbound fraction, to values as high as 20% to 25% from the normal of 10%, results in increased hepatic clearance and decreased total concentrations of phenytoin. Although the unbound concentration therapeutic range is unchanged, the therapeutic range for total phenytoin concentration is reduced to 4 to 10 µg/mL (normal, 10 to 20 µg/mL) as GFR falls. Therefore the maintenance of therapeutic unbound concentrations of 1 to 2 µg/mL provides the best target for individualizing phenytoin therapy in patients with RKF.

Altered tissue binding may also affect the apparent volume of distribution of a drug. For example, the distribution volume of digoxin is reported as being reduced by 30% to 50% in patients with severe CKD. This may be the result of competitive inhibition by endogenous or exogenous digoxin-like immunoreactive substances that bind to and inhibit membrane adenosine triphosphatase (ATPase). The absolute amount of digoxin bound to the tissue digoxin receptor is reduced, and the resultant serum digoxin concentration observed after administration of any dose is greater than expected.

Therefore, in CKD patients, a normal total drug concentration may be associated with either serious adverse effects secondary to elevated unbound drug concentrations or subtherapeutic responses because of an increased plasma-to-tissue drug concentration ratio. Monitoring of unbound drug concentrations is suggested for drugs that have a narrow therapeutic range, those that are highly protein bound (>80%), and those with marked variability in the bound fraction (e.g., phenytoin, disopyramide).

DRUG METABOLISM AND TRANSPORT

CL_{NR} of drugs includes all routes of drug elimination excluding kidney excretion. Several metabolic enzymes and active transporters collectively constitute the primary pathways of CL_{NR}. Alterations in the function of and interactions between them can significantly affect the pharmacokinetic disposition and corresponding patient exposure to drugs that are substrates of nonrenal pathways. The effect of CKD on the expression or function of many of these pathways has been characterized in experimental models of kidney disease. For example, in rat models of end-stage kidney disease, hepatic expression of several cytochrome P450 (CYP) enzymes, including CYP3A1 and CYP3A2 (equivalent to human CYP3A4), is reduced by as much as 85%. CYP2C11 and CYP3A2 activity is also significantly reduced, but CYP1A1 activity is unchanged. CYP functional expression is also decreased in the intestine; CYP1A1 and CYP3A2 are reduced up to 40% and 70%, respectively.

Several hepatic reductase enzymes are also affected by kidney disease. Gene and protein expression of carbonyl reductase-1, aldo-keto reductase-3, and 11β-hydroxysteroid dehydrogenase-1 is decreased by as much as 93% and 76%, respectively, in CKD rats. Hepatic expression of the conjugative enzymes N-acetyltransferases (NAT) is also decreased, while uridine diphosphate-glucuronosyltransferases (UGT) are unchanged. Similarly, functional expression of several intestinal and hepatic transporters is altered in experimental models of kidney disease. The expression and corresponding activities of the efflux transporters P-glycoprotein (P-gp) and multidrug resistance-associated protein 2 (MRP2) are reduced by as much as 65% in the intestine, but the uptake transporter organic anion transporting polypeptide (OATP) is not affected. Conversely, in the liver, protein expression of P-gp, MRP2, and OATP is increased, unchanged, and decreased, respectively.

In humans with kidney disease, the activities of CYPs and reductases appear to be relatively unaffected. It was previously reported that CYP3A4 activity was reduced, but recent data indicate that OATP uptake activity is reduced, and thus the perceived changes in CYP3A4 activity were likely due to altered transporter activity, not an alteration in CYP activity. The reduction of CL_{NR} of several drugs that exhibit overlapping CYP and transporter substrate specificity in patients with stages 4 or 5 CKD supports this premise (Table 36.2). These studies must be interpreted with caution, however, because concurrent drug intake, age, smoking status, and alcohol intake were often not taken into consideration. Furthermore, pharmacogenetic variations in drug-metabolizing enzymes and transporters that may have been present in the individual before the onset of AKI or progression of CKD must be considered, if known. For these reasons, prediction of the effect of RKF on the metabolism and/or transport of a particular drug is difficult, and a general quantitative strategy to adjust dosage regimens for drugs that undergo extensive CL_{NR} has not yet been proposed. However, some qualitative insight may be gained if one knows which enzymes or transporters are involved in the clearance of the drug of interest and how those proteins are affected by a reduction in kidney function.

The effect of CKD on the CL_{NR} of a particular drug is difficult to predict, even for drugs within the same pharmacologic class. The reductions in CL_{NR} for CKD patients have frequently been noted to be proportional to the reductions in GFR. In the small number of studies that have evaluated CL_{NR} in critically ill patients with AKI, residual CL_{NR} was higher than

Table 36.2 Major Pathways of Nonrenal Drug Clearance and Selected Substrates

CL_{NR} Pathway	Selected Substrates
Oxidative Enzymes	
CYP	
1A2	Polycyclic aromatic hydrocarbons, caffeine, imipramine, theophylline
2A6	Coumarin
2B6	Nicotine, bupropion
2C8	Retinoids, paclitaxel, repaglinide
2C9	Celecoxib, diclofenac, flurbiprofen, indomethacin, ibuprofen, losartan, phenytoin, tolbutamide, S-warfarin
2C19	Diazepam, S-mephenytoin, omeprazole
2D6	Codeine, debrisoquine, desipramine, dextromethorphan, fluoxetine, paroxetine, duloxetine, nortriptyline, haloperidol, metoprolol, propranolol
2E1	Ethanol, acetaminophen, chlorzoxazone, nitrosamines
3A4/5	Alprazolam, midazolam, cyclosporine, tacrolimus, nifedipine, felodipine, diltiazem, verapamil, fluconazole, ketoconazole, itraconazole, erythromycin, lovastatin, simvastatin, cisapride, terfenadine
Reductase Enzymes	
11β-HSD	Bupropion, daunorubicin, prednisone, warfarin
CBR	Bupropion, daunorubicin, haloperidol, warfarin
AKR	Bupropion, daunorubicin, haloperidol, ketoprofen, nabumetone, naloxone, naltrexone, warfarin
Conjugative Enzymes	
UGT	Acetaminophen, morphine, lorazepam, oxazepam, naproxen, ketoprofen, irinotecan, bilirubin
NAT	Dapsone, hydralazine, isoniazid, procainamide
Transporters	
OATP	
1A2	Bile salts, statins, fexofenadine, methotrexate, digoxin, levofloxacin
1B1	Bile salts, statins, fexofenadine repaglinide, valsartan, olmesartan, irinotecan, bosentan
1B3	Bile salts, statins, fexofenadine, telmisartan, valsartan, olmesartan, digoxin
2B1	Statins, fexofenadine, glyburide
P-gp	Digoxin, fexofenadine, loperamide, irinotecan, doxorubicin, vinblastine, paclitaxel, erythromycin
MRP	
2	Methotrexate, etoposide, mitoxantrone, valsartan, olmesartan
3	Methotrexate, fexofenadine

AKR, Aldo keto reductase; *CYP,* cytochrome P450 isozyme; *CBR,* carbonyl reductase; *11β-HSD,* 11β-hydroxysteroid dehydrogenase; *MRP,* multidrug resistance-associated protein; *NAT,* N-acetyltransferase; *OATP,* organic anion-transporting polypeptide; *P-gp,* P-glycoprotein; *UGT,* uridine 5′-diphosphate glucuronosyltransferase.

in CKD patients with similar levels of CL_{Cr}, whether measured or estimated by the Cockcroft-Gault equation. Because an AKI patient may have a higher CL_{NR} than a CKD patient, the resultant plasma concentrations will be lower than expected and possibly subtherapeutic if classic CKD-derived dosage guidelines are followed.

KIDNEY EXCRETION OF DRUGS

Kidney clearance (CL_K) is the net result of glomerular filtration of unbound drug plus tubular secretion, minus tubular reabsorption. An acute or chronic reduction in GFR results in a decrease in CL_K. The degree of change in total body drug clearance is dependent on the fraction of the dose that is eliminated unchanged in individuals with normal kidney function, the intrarenal drug transport pathways, and the degree of functional impairment of each of these pathways. The primary kidney transport systems of clinical importance with respect to drug excretion include the organic anionic (OAT), organic cationic (OCT), P-gp, breast cancer resistance protein, and multidrug resistance-associated protein transporters. Diuretics, β-lactam antibiotics, nonsteroidal antiinflammatory drugs, and glucuronide drug metabolites are eliminated by the family of OAT transporters. The OCT transporters contribute to the secretion and excretion of cimetidine, famotidine, and quinidine. The P-gp transport system in the kidney is involved in the secretion of cationic and hydrophobic drugs (e.g., digoxin, *Vinca* alkaloids). The clearance of drugs that are secreted by the kidney (CL_K >300 mL/min) may be reduced from impairment in one or more of these kidney transporters.

Despite the different mechanisms involved in the elimination of drugs by the kidney and the availability of several methods for determining kidney function, the clinical estimation of CL_{Cr} remains the most commonly used index for guiding drug dosage regimen design. The importance of an alteration in kidney function on drug elimination usually depends primarily on two variables: (1) the fraction of drug normally eliminated by the kidney unchanged and (2) the degree of GFR loss. There are a few drugs for which a metabolite is the primary active entity; in that situation, a key variable is the degree of CL_K of the metabolite. The calculation of CL_{Cr} from a timed urine collection has been the standard clinical measure of kidney function for decades. However, urine is difficult to collect accurately in most clinical settings, and the interference of many commonly used medications with creatinine measurement limits the utility of this approach. Use of radioactive markers ([^{125}I]iothalamate, ^{51}Cr-EDTA, or ^{99m}Tc-DTPA) or nonradioactive GFR markers (iohexol, iothalamate, and inulin), although scientifically sound, is clinically impractical, because intravenous or subcutaneous marker administration and multiple timed blood and urine collections make the procedures expensive and cumbersome.

ESTIMATION OF KIDNEY FUNCTION FOR DRUG DOSING PURPOSES

The estimation of kidney function by various estimating equations for drug dosing purposes is a critically important issue. In contrast to measured approaches, estimation of CL_{Cr} or GFR requires only routinely collected laboratory and demographic data. The Cockcroft-Gault equation for CL_{Cr} and the Chronic Kidney Disease-Epidemiology Collaboration (CKD-EPI) equations for eGFR correlate well with CL_{Cr} and GFR measurements in individuals with stable kidney function and average body composition (see Chapter 3). The traditional approach of estimating CL_{Cr} and using it as a continuous variable of kidney function for drug dosing adjustment is now being supplemented and, in some institutions, replaced by eGFR. Caution is warranted since the use of eGFR as a guide for drug dosage adjustment, has not been systematically validated. Currently, there are limited prospective pharmacokinetic data and corresponding dosing recommendations based on GFR estimating equations. Because nearly all of the primary published literature to date has used CL_{Cr} to derive the relationship between kidney function and kidney and/or total body clearance of a drug, CL_{Cr} is still the standard metric for drug dosing purposes. Nevertheless, widespread availability of automatically reported eGFR affords clinicians a tool that, if validated for drug dosing, could easily be incorporated into clinical practice. Furthermore, use of eGFR for management of kidney disease and drug dosing, and harmonization of practice in this regard between physicians, pharmacists, and other clinicians, would be ideal and warrants further evaluation.

Several issues should be considered by clinicians when assessing CL_{Cr} and eGFR data for drug dosing. First, the automatically reported eGFR value provides an estimate that is normalized for body surface area (BSA) in units of mL/min per 1.73 m². When used for drug dosing, the eGFR value should be individualized (i.e., not normalized for BSA) and converted to units of mL/min, particularly in patients whose BSA is considerably larger or smaller than 1.73 m². The individualized value should be compared with CL_{Cr} estimates (mL/min). Second, when presented with various kidney function estimates that potentially translate into different drug dosing regimens, clinicians should choose the regimen that optimizes the risk-benefit ratio, given the patient-specific clinical scenario. For drugs with a narrow therapeutic range, typically more conservative kidney function estimates and corresponding doses should be used, particularly if therapeutic drug monitoring is not readily available. Because CL_{Cr} estimates are more conservative and indicate the need for dose adjustment more often than eGFR, they may be preferred when dosing narrow therapeutic window drugs, especially in high-risk subgroups such as the elderly. The use of eGFR and a more aggressive dosing strategy may be acceptable for drugs with a wide therapeutic range and a broader margin of safety. Third, when estimating equations are not expected to provide accurate measures of kidney function (i.e., because of altered creatinine generation or unstable serum creatinine concentrations) and therapeutic drug monitoring is not available, it may be reasonable to obtain an accurately timed urine collection to calculate CL_{Cr}, particularly for narrow therapeutic window drugs with high toxicity. Fourth, the limitations and the study population of the original trials from which the eGFR equations were developed, and subsequent populations in which they have been validated, must be considered before applying them to a specific patient. All of these methods are poor predictors of kidney function in individuals with liver disease, and their use is not recommended for such patients. Finally, although several methods for CL_{Cr} estimation in patients with unstable kidney function (e.g., AKI) have been proposed, the accuracy of these methods has not been rigorously assessed, and at the present time their use cannot be recommended.

STRATEGIES FOR DRUG THERAPY INDIVIDUALIZATION

Design of the optimal dosage regimen for a patient with RKF depends on the availability of an accurate characterization of the relationship between the pharmacokinetic drug parameters and kidney function. Before 1998, there was no consensus regarding the criteria for characterization of the pharmacokinetics of a drug in CKD patients. An industry guidance report issued by the US Food and Drug Administration (FDA) in May 1998 provided guidelines regarding when a study should be considered, provided recommendations for study design, data analysis, and assessment of the impact of the study results on drug dosing, and recommended use of dose adjustment categories derived from CL_{Cr}. Currently the FDA is considering including dosing tables based on eGFR and CL_{Cr} in a revised version of the 1998 FDA guideline. In the future, drug dosing recommendations based on eGFR in addition to CL_{CR} may be included in FDA-approved drug dosing labels. However, for drugs already approved by the FDA with existing dose adjustment recommendations based on CL_{CR}, it is unlikely drug manufacturers will provide additional eGFR-based dosing recommendations.

Most dosage adjustment reference sources for clinical use have proposed the use of a fixed dose or interval for patients with a broad range of kidney function. Indeed, "normal" kidney function has often been ascribed to anyone who has a CL_{Cr} greater than 50 mL/min, even though many individuals (e.g., hyperfiltering early diabetics) have values in the range of 120 to 180 mL/min. The "moderate kidney function impairment" category in many guides encompasses a fivefold range of CL_{Cr}, from 10 to 49 mL/min, whereas severe kidney function impairment or end-stage kidney disease is defined as a CL_{Cr} of less than 10 to 15 mL/min. Each of these categories encompasses a broad range of kidney function, and the calculated drug regimen may not be optimal for all patients within that range.

If specific literature recommendations or data on the relationship of the pharmacokinetic parameters of a drug to CL_{Cr} are not available, then these parameters can be estimated for a particular patient with the method of Rowland and Tozer, provided that the fraction of the drug that is eliminated unchanged by the kidney (f_e) in normal subjects is known. This approach assumes that the change in drug clearance is proportional to the change in CL_{Cr}, kidney disease does not alter the drug's CL_{NR}, any metabolites produced are inactive and nontoxic, the drug obeys first-order (linear) kinetic principles, and it is adequately described by a one-compartment model. If these assumptions are true, the kinetic parameter or dosage adjustment factor (Q) can be calculated as follows:

$$Q = 1 - [f_e(1 - KF)]$$

where KF is the ratio of the patient's CL_{Cr} to the assumed normal value of 120 mL/min. As an example, the Q factor for a patient who has a CL_{Cr} of 10 mL/min and a drug that is 85% eliminated unchanged by the kidney would be

$$Q = 1 - [0.85(1 - 10/120)]$$
$$Q = 1 - [0.85(0.92)]$$
$$Q = 1 - 0.78$$
$$Q = 0.22$$

The estimated clearance rate of the drug in this patient (CL_{PT}) would then be calculated as

$$CL_{PT} = CL_{norm} \times Q$$

where CL_{norm} is the respective value in patients with normal kidney function derived from the literature.

For antihypertensive agents, cephalosporins, and many other drugs for which there are no target values for peak or trough concentrations, attainment of an average steady-state concentration similar to that in normal subjects is appropriate. The principal means to achieve this goal is to decrease the dose or prolong the dosing interval. If the dose is reduced and the dosing interval is unchanged, the desired average steady-state concentration will be near normal; however, the peak will be lower and the trough higher. Alternatively, if the dosing interval is increased and the dose remains unchanged, the peak, trough, and average concentrations will be similar to those in the patients with normal kidney function. This interval adjustment method is often preferred because it is likely to yield significant cost savings due to less frequent drug administration. If a loading dose is not administered, it will take approximately five half-lives for the desired steady-state plasma concentrations to be achieved in any patient; this may require days rather than hours, because of the prolonged half-life of many drugs in patients with RKF. Therefore, to achieve the desired concentration rapidly, a loading dose (D_L) should be administered for most patients with RKF. D_L can be calculated as follows:

$$D_L = (C_{peak}) \times (V_D) \times (\text{Body weight in kilograms})$$

The loading dose is usually the same for patients with RKF as it is for those with normal kidney function. However, if the V_D in patients with RKF is significantly different from the V_D in patients with normal kidney function (see Table 36.1), then the modified value should be used to calculate the D_L.

The adjusted dosing interval (τ_{RKF}) or maintenance dose (D_{RKF}) for the patient can then be calculated from the normal dosing interval (τ_n) and normal dose (D_n), respectively:

$$\tau_{RKF} = \tau_n / Q$$

$$D_{RKF} = D_n \times Q$$

If these approaches yield a time interval or a dose that is impractical, a new dose can be calculated with a fixed, prespecified dose interval (τ_{FPDI}) such as 24 or 48 hours, as follows:

$$D_{RKF} = [D_n \times Q \times \tau_{FPDI}] / \tau_n$$

PATIENTS RECEIVING CONTINUOUS RENAL REPLACEMENT THERAPY

CRRT is used primarily in critically ill patients with AKI. Drug therapy individualization for the patient receiving CRRT must take into account the fact that patients with AKI may have a higher residual CL_{NR} of a drug than CKD patients with similar levels of kidney function. In addition to patient-specific differences, there are marked differences in the efficiency of drug removal among the three primary types of CRRT: continuous venovenous hemofiltration (CVVH), continuous venovenous hemodialysis (CVVHD), and continuous venovenous hemodiafiltration (CVVHDF). The primary variables that influence drug clearance during CRRT are the ultrafiltration rate (UFR), the blood flow rate (BFR), and the dialysate flow rate (DFR), as well as the type of hemofilter used. For example, clearance during CVVH is directly proportional to the UFR as a result of convective transport of drug molecules. Drug clearance in this situation is a function of the membrane permeability of the drug, which is called the sieving coefficient (SC), and the UFR. The SC can be approximated by the fraction of drug that is unbound to plasma proteins (f_u), so the clearance can be calculated as follows:

$$CL_{CVVH} = UFR \times SC$$

or

$$CL_{CVVH} = UFR \times f_u$$

Clearance during CVVHD also depends on the DFR and the SC of the drug. If UFR is negligible, CL_{CVVHD} can be estimated to be maximally equal to the product of DFR and f_u or SC. Clearance of a drug by CVVHDF is generally greater than by CVVHD, because the drug is removed by diffusion as well as by convection/ultrafiltration. CL_{CVVHDF} in many clinical settings can be mathematically approximated as

$$CL_{CVVHDF} = (UFR + DFR) \times SC$$

provided the DFR is less than 33 mL/min and BFR is at least 75 mL/min. Changes in BFR typically have only a minor effect on drug clearance by any mode of CRRT, because BFR is usually much larger than the DFR and is therefore not the limiting factor for drug removal.

Individualization of therapy for CRRT is based on the patient's residual kidney function and the drug clearance by the mode of CRRT used. The patient's residual drug clearance can be predicted as described earlier in this chapter. CRRT clearance can also be approximated from published literature reports, although many of these reports did not specify all the operating conditions, and it may thus be hard to directly apply the findings to a given patient situation. The clearances of several frequently used drugs by CVVH and CVVHDF are summarized in Tables 36.3 and 36.4, respectively. Whenever feasible, plasma drug concentration monitoring for drugs that require achievement of target concentrations to avoid toxicity or maximize efficacy (e.g., aminoglycosides, vancomycin) is highly recommended.

Table 36.3   Drug Clearance and Dosing Recommendations for Patients Receiving Continuous Venovenous Hemofiltration

Drug	Hemofilter	CL$_T$ (mL/min, Mean or Range)	CL$_{CVVH}$ (mL/min, Mean or Range)	Dosage Recommendation
Acyclovir	PS	0.39	NR	5 mg/kg q12h
Amikacin	PS	10.5	10–16	IND[a]
Amrinone	PS	40.8	2.4–14.4	None provided
Atracurium	PA	502.5	8.25	None provided
Ceftazidime	AN69, PMMA, PS	NR	7.5–15.6	500 mg q12h
Ceftriaxone	AN69, PMMA, PS	NR	NR	300 mg q12h
	PA	39.3	17	1000 mg q24h
Cefuroxime	PS	32	11	0.75–1.0 g q24h
Ciprofloxacin	AN69	84.4	12.4	400 mg q24h
Fluconazole	AN69	25.3	17.5	400–800 mg q24h
Gentamicin	PS	11.6	3.47	IND[a]
Imipenem	PS	108.3	13.3	500 mg q6–8h
Levofloxacin	AN69	42.3	11.5	250 mg q24h
Meropenem	PA	76	16–50	0.5–1.0 g q12h
Phenytoin	PS	NR	1.02	IND[a]
Piperacillin	NR	42	NR	4 g q12h
Ticarcillin	PS	29.7	12.3	2 g q8–12h
Tobramycin	PS	11.7	3.5	IND[a]
Vancomycin	PA, PMMA, PS	14–29	12–24	750–1250 mg q24h

[a]Serum concentrations may vary markedly depending on the patient's condition, therefore dose individualization is recommended.
AN69, Acrylonitrile; *CL$_{CVVH}$,* CVVH clearance; *CL$_T$,* total body clearance; *IND,* individualize; *NR,* not reported; *PA,* polyamide filter; *PMMA,* polymethylmethacrylate filter; *PS,* polysulfone filter.
Adapted from Matzke GR, Clermont G. Clinical pharmacology and therapeutics. In: Murray P, Brady HR, Hall JB, eds. *Intensive Care Nephrology.* London: Taylor and Francis; 2006.

Table 36.4   Drug Clearance and Dosing Recommendations for Patients Receiving Continuous Venovenous Hemodiafiltration

Drug	Hemofilter	CL$_T$ (mL/min, Mean or Range)	CL$_{CVVHDF}$ (mL/min, Mean or Range)	Dosage Recommendation
Acyclovir	AN69	1.2	NR	5 mg/kg q12h
Ceftazidime	AN69, PMMA, PS	25–31	13–28	0.5–1 g q24h
Ceftriaxone	AN69	—	11.7–13.2	250 mg q12h
	PMMA, PS	—	19.8–30.5	300 mg q12h
Cefuroxime	AN69	22	14–16.2	750 mg q12h
Ciprofloxacin	AN69	264	16–37	300 mg q12h
Fluconazole	AN69	21–38	25–30	400–800 mg q12h
Ganciclovir	AN69	32	13	2.5 mg/kg q24h
Gentamicin	AN69	20	5.2	IND[a]
Imipenem	AN69, PS	134	16–30	500 mg q6–8h
Levofloxacin	AN69	51	22	250 mg q24h
Meropenem	PAN	55–140	20–39	1000 mg q8–12h
Mezlocillin	AN69, PS	31–253	11–45	2–4 g q24h
Sulbactam	AN69, PS	32–54	10–23	0.5 g q24h
Piperacillin	AN69	47	22	PIP: 4 g q12h
				PIP/TAZO: 3.375 g q8–12h
Teicoplanin	AN69	9.2	3.6	LD: 800 mg
				MD: 400 mg q24h × 2, then q48–72h
Vancomycin	AN69	17–39	10–17	7.5 mg/kg q12h
	PMMA	—	15–27.0	1.0–1.5 g q24h
	PS	36	11–22	0.85–1.35 g q24h

[a]Serum concentrations may vary markedly depending on the patient's condition, therefore dose individualization is recommended.
AN69, Acrylonitrile; *CL$_{CVVHDF}$,* CVVHDF clearance; *CL$_T$,* total body clearance; *IND,* individualize; *LD,* loading dose; *MD,* maintenance dose; *NR,* not reported; *PA,* polyamide filter; *PAN,* polyacrylonitrile filter; *PMMA,* polymethylmethacrylate filter; *PS,* polysulfone filter; *TAZO,* tazobactam.
Adapted from Matzke GR, Clermont G. Clinical pharmacology and therapeutics. In: Murray P, Brady HR, Hall JB, eds. *Intensive Care Nephrology.* London: Taylor and Francis; 2006.

PATIENTS RECEIVING CHRONIC HEMODIALYSIS

Drug therapy in patients undergoing hemodialysis should be guided by careful evaluation of the patient's residual kidney function, in addition to the added clearance associated with the patient's dialysis prescription. Dosing recommendations are available for many agents, especially those with a wide therapeutic index. However, for those drugs with a narrow therapeutic index, individualization of the drug therapy regimen based on prospective serum concentration monitoring is highly recommended. Although many new hemodialyzers have been introduced in the past 20 years and the average delivered dose of hemodialysis has increased, the effect of hemodialysis on the disposition of a drug is rarely reevaluated following its initial introduction to the market. As a result, most of the published dosing guidelines underestimate the impact of hemodialysis on drug disposition, and clinicians should cautiously consider the prescription of doses that are larger than those conventionally recommended for their critically ill patients. The effect of hemodialysis on a patient's drug therapy depends on the molecular weight, protein binding, and distribution volume of the drug; the composition of the dialyzer membrane and its surface area; BFR and DFR; and whether the dialyzer is reused. Drugs that are small molecules but highly protein bound are not well dialyzed, because the two principal binding proteins (α_1-acid glycoprotein and albumin) are high-molecular-weight entities. Finally, drugs with a large volume of distribution are poorly removed by hemodialysis.

Conventional or low-flux dialyzers are relatively impermeable to drugs with a molecular weight greater than 1000 Da. High-flux hemodialyzers allow the passage of most drugs with a molecular weight of 10,000 Da or less.

The determination of drug concentrations at the start and end of dialysis, with subsequent calculation of the half-life during dialysis, has historically been used as an index of drug removal by dialysis. A more accurate means of assessing the effect of hemodialysis is to calculate the dialyzer clearance rate (CL_D) of the drug. Because drug concentrations are generally measured in plasma, the plasma clearance of the drug by hemodialysis (CL_{pD}) can be calculated as follows:

$$CL_{pD} = Q_p([A_p - V_p]/A_p)$$

where p represents plasma, A_p is arterial plasma concentration, V_p is venous plasma concentration, and Q_p is the plasma flow rate calculated as

$$Q_P = BFR \times (1 - Hematocrit)$$

This clearance calculation accurately reflects dialysis drug clearance only if the drug does not penetrate or bind to formed blood elements.

For patients receiving hemodialysis, the usual objective is to restore the amount of drug in the body at the end of dialysis to the value that would have been present if the patient had not been dialyzed. The supplementary dose (D_{postHD}) is calculated as follows:

$$D_{postHD} = [V_D \times C](e^{-k \cdot t} - e^{-k_{HD} \cdot t})$$

where ($V_D \times C$) is the amount of drug in the body at the start of dialysis, $e^{-k \cdot t}$ is the fraction of drug remaining as a result of the patient's residual total body clearance during the dialysis procedure, and $e^{-k_{HD} \cdot t}$ is the fraction of drug remaining as a result of elimination by the dialyzer:

$$k_{HD} = CL_{pD}/V_D$$

Recently, alternative dosing strategies for some drugs, such as gentamicin and vancomycin, which include drug administration before or during the dialysis procedure, were evaluated. These approaches may save time in the ambulatory dialysis setting but increase drug cost because more drugs will have to be given to compensate for the increased dialysis removal. Values for CL_{pD} of some commonly used drugs are listed in Table 36.5. This information only serves as initial dosing guidance; measurement of predialysis serum concentrations is recommended to guide subsequent drug dosing.

The impact of hemodialysis on drug therapy must not be viewed as a "generic procedure" that will result in removal of a fixed percentage of the drug from the body with each dialysis session; neither should simple "yes/no" answers on the dialyzability of drug compounds be considered sufficient information for therapeutic decisions. Compounds considered nondialyzable with low-flux dialyzers may in fact be significantly removed by high-flux hemodialyzers.

Table 36.5 Drug Disposition During Dialysis Depends on Dialyzer Characteristics

Drug	HEMODIALYSIS CLEARANCE (mL/min)		HALF-LIFE DURING DIALYSIS (h)	
	Conventional	High-Flux	Conventional	High-Flux
Ceftazidime	55–60	155 (PA)	3.3	1.2 (PA)
Cefuroxime	NR	103 (PS)	3.8	1.6 (PS)
Foscarnet	183	253 (PS)	NR	NR
Gentamicin	58.2	116 (PS)	3.0	4.3 (PS)
Tobramycin	45	119 (PS)	4.0	NR
Ranitidine	43.1	67.2 (PS)	5.1	2.9 (PS)
Vancomycin	9–21	31–60 (PAN)	35–38	12.0 (PAN)
	—	40–150 (PS)	—	4.5–11.8 (PS)
	—	72–116 (PMMA)	—	NR

NR, Not reported; *PA*, polyamide filter; *PAN*, polyacrylonitrile filter; *PMMA*, polymethylmethacrylate; *PS*, polysulfone filter.

PATIENTS RECEIVING CHRONIC PERITONEAL DIALYSIS

Peritoneal dialysis has the potential to affect drug disposition, but drug therapy individualization is often less complicated in these patients because of the relative inefficiency of the procedure per unit time. Variables that influence drug removal in peritoneal dialysis include drug-specific characteristics such as molecular weight, solubility, degree of ionization, protein binding, and volume of distribution. Patient-specific factors include peritoneal membrane characteristics such as splanchnic blood flow, surface area, and permeability. The contribution of peritoneal dialysis to total body clearance is often low and, for most drugs, markedly less than the contribution of hemodialysis per unit time. Antiinfective agents are the most commonly studied drugs because of their primary role in the treatment of peritonitis, and the dosing recommendations for peritonitis, which are regularly updated, should be consulted as necessary. Most other drugs can generally be dosed according to the patient's residual kidney function because clearance by peritoneal dialysis is small.

If there is a significant relationship between the desired peak (C_{peak}) or trough (C_{trough}) concentration of a drug for a given patient with RKF and the potential clinical response (e.g., aminoglycosides) or toxicity (e.g., quinidine, phenobarbital, phenytoin), then attainment of the target plasma concentration value is critical. In these situations, the adjusted dosage interval (τ_{RKF}) and maintenance dose (D_{RKF}) for the patient can be calculated as follows:

$$\tau_{RKF} = ([1/k_{PT}] \times \ln[C_{peak}/C_{trough}]) + t_{inf}$$

$$D_{RKF} = [k_{PT} \times V_D \times C_{peak}] \times [1 - e^{-(k_{PT})(\tau_{RKF})}/1 - e^{-(k_{PT})(t_{inf})}]$$

where t_{inf} is the infusion duration, k_{PT} is the elimination rate constant of the drug for that patient estimated as

$$k_{PT} = k_{NORM} \times Q$$

and V_D is the volume of distribution of the drug that can be obtained from literature values such as those in Table 36.1. This estimation method assumes that the drug is administered by intermittent intravenous infusion and its disposition is adequately characterized by a one-compartment linear model.

CLINICAL DECISION SUPPORT TOOLS

The availability of health information technology, namely clinical decision support tools, has increased substantially in recent years, and use of these tools may facilitate kidney drug dosing by providing consistent, accurate dosing recommendations in real time. Clinical decision support systems (CDSS) are commonplace in institutional health information computer systems and their computerized provider order entry (CPOE) systems and have been shown to improve medication use in CKD and AKI patient populations. In addition, CDSS make individual assessments and comparisons of kidney function estimates feasible. For example, CDSS can easily accommodate new equations (e.g., CKD-EPI) as they become available and facilitate conversion of eGFR values

Table 36.6   Key Recommendations for Clinicians

1. Over-the-counter and herbal products as well as prescription medications should be assessed to ensure they are indicated.
2. The least nephrotoxic agent should be used whenever possible.
3. If a drug interaction is suspected and the clinical implication is significant, alternative medications should be used.
4. Although eGFR equations such as CKD-EPI may be used for staging CKD, the Cockcroft-Gault equation remains the standard kidney function index for drug dosage adjustment.
5. The dosage of drugs that are more than 30% eliminated unchanged by the kidney should be verified to ensure that appropriate initial dosage adjustments are implemented in CKD.
6. Maintenance dosage regimens should be adjusted based on patient response and serum drug concentration determinations when indicated and available.

CKD, Chronic kidney disease; *CKD-EPI,* Chronic Kidney Disease-Epidemiology Collaboration; *eGFR,* estimated glomerular filtration rate.

to individualized values by modifying units of mL/min per 1.73 m^2 to units of mL/min.

Numerous other resources are available for kidney drug dosing information, including Internet or online resources, as well as portable handheld databases such as Epocrates, Lexicomp, and Micromedex. The American Hospital Formulary Service *Drug Information* text, the *British National Formulary,* Aronoff's *Drug Prescribing in Renal Failure,* and Martindale's *Complete Drug Reference* are excellent resources for drug dosage recommendations for patients with RKF and are all accessible electronically and/or online.

CONCLUSIONS

The adverse outcomes associated with inappropriate drug use and dosing are largely preventable if the principles illustrated in this chapter are used by the clinician in concert with reliable population pharmacokinetic estimates to design rational initial drug dosage regimens for patients with RKF and those needing dialysis. Subsequent individualization of therapy should be undertaken whenever clinical therapeutic monitoring tools, such as plasma drug concentrations, are available. These key recommendations for practice are highlighted in Table 36.6.

BIBLIOGRAPHY

Alshogran OY, Nolin TD. Implications of kidney disease on metabolic reduction. *Curr Drug Metab.* 2016;17:663-672.

Aronoff GR, Bennetl WM, Berns JS, et al. *Drug Prescribing in Renal Failure: Dosing Guidelines for Adults and Children.* 5th ed. Philadelphia: American College of Physicians-American Society of Internal Medicine; 2007.

Goldstein SL. Automated/integrated real-time clinical decision support in acute kidney injury. *Curr Opin Crit Care.* 2015;21:485-489.

Heintz BH, Matzke GR, Dager WE. Antimicrobial dosing concepts and recommendations for critically ill adult patients receiving continuous renal replacement therapy or intermittent hemodialysis. *Pharmaco-therapy.* 2009;29:562-577.

Li PK, Szeto CC, Piraino B, et al. ISPD peritonitis recommendations: 2016 update on prevention and treatment. *Perit Dial Int.* 2016;36:481-508.

Matzke GR. Status of hemodialysis of drugs in 2002. *J Pharm Pract.* 2002;15:405-418.

Matzke GR, Aronoff GR, Atkinson AJ Jr, et al. Drug dosing consideration in patients with acute and chronic kidney disease—a clinical update from Kidney Disease: Improving Global Outcomes (KDIGO). *Kidney Int.* 2011;80:1122-1137.

Matzke GR, Clermont G. Clinical pharmacology and therapeutics. In: Murray PT, Brady HR, Hall JB, eds. *Intensive Care in Nephrology.* Boca Raton, FL: Taylor and Francis; 2006:245-265.

Matzke GR, Comstock TJ. Influence of renal disease and dialysis on pharmacokinetics. In: Evans WE, Schentag JJ, Burton ME, eds. *Applied Pharmacokinetics: Principles of Therapeutic Drug Monitoring.* 4th ed. Baltimore, MD: Lippincott Williams and Wilkins; 2005.

Mueller BA, Pasko DA, Sowinski KM. Higher renal replacement therapy dose delivery influences on drug therapy. *Artif Organs.* 2003;27:808-814.

Naud J, Nolin TD, Leblond FA, Pichette V. Current understanding of drug disposition in kidney disease. *J Clin Pharmacol.* 2012;52:10S-22S.

Nigam SK, Wu W, Bush KT, et al. Handling of drugs, metabolites, and uremic toxins by kidney proximal tubule drug transporters. *Clin J Am Soc Nephrol.* 2015;10:2039-2049.

Nolin TD. A synopsis of clinical pharmacokinetic alterations in advanced CKD. *Semin Dial.* 2015;28:325-329.

Nolin TD, Aronoff GR, Fissell WH, et al. Pharmacokinetic assessment in patients receiving continuous RRT: perspectives from the kidney health initiative. *Clin J Am Soc Nephrol.* 2015;10:159-164.

Nolin TD, Frye RF, Le P, et al. ESRD impairs nonrenal clearance of fexofenadine but not midazolam. *J Am Soc Nephrol.* 2009;20:2269-2276.

Nolin TD, Naud J, Leblond FA, Pichette V. Emerging evidence of the impact of kidney disease on drug metabolism and transport. *Clin Pharmacol Ther.* 2008;83:898-903.

Nyman HA, Dowling TC, Hudson JQ, Peter WL, Joy MS, Nolin TD. Comparative evaluation of the Cockcroft-Gault equation and the modification of diet in renal disease (MDRD) study equation for drug dosing: an opinion of the nephrology practice and research network of the American College of Clinical Pharmacy. *Pharmacotherapy.* 2011;31(11):1130-1144.

Veltri MA, Neu AM, Fivush BA, et al. Drug dosing during intermittent hemodialysis and continuous renal replacement therapy: special considerations in pediatric patients. *Paediatr Drugs.* 2004;6:45-65.

Verbeeck RK, Musuamba FT. Pharmacokinetics and dosage adjustment in patients with renal dysfunction. *Eur J Clin Pharmacol.* 2009;65:757-773.

Vidal L, Shavit M, Fraser A, et al. Systematic comparison of four sources of drug information regarding adjustment of dose for renal function. *BMJ.* 2005;331:263-266.

HEREDITARY KIDNEY DISEASE

SECTION 7

37

Genetics and Kidney Disease (APOL1)

Brendan D. Crawford; Matthew G. Sampson; Rasheed A. Gbadegesin

Genetic studies of kidney diseases over the past two decades have provided novel insights into underlying pathophysiologic mechanisms and spurred progress toward the goal of precision medicine. This chapter provides a primer on genetic variation, methods for gene discovery of monogenic kidney diseases (linkage analysis and next-generation sequencing), and identification of risk loci for kidney diseases with complex inheritance (genome-wide association studies [GWAS]). The chapter also briefly discusses the challenges in interpretation of identified variants from next-generation sequencing (NGS).

GENOMIC VARIATION

Across an individual's genome, nucleotide positions can vary from the "normal" reference sequence. The simplest form of variation involves substitution of a single nucleotide base for another, known as a "single nucleotide variant" (SNV). Historically, rare SNVs that were sufficient to cause disease were called "mutations," whereas more common SNVs, occurring in greater than 1% of the population, were called "single nucleotide polymorphisms (SNPs)." The more recent SNV terminology, as it is related to disease, allows us to report SNVs as a function of their frequency in a reference population. Rare SNVs are responsible for mendelian disease, while more common SNVs increase risk for common disease. In addition to SNVs, genomic variation can include structural variation from small insertions or deletions of ten to hundreds of nucleotides (indels) to duplications or deletions of larger chromosomal segments. These larger structural variants, known as copy number variants (CNVs), are increasingly being recognized for their role in human disease.

MENDELIAN GENE DISCOVERY

Genetic discovery through the 1980s and 1990s required recruitment of families with multiple affected individuals containing a defined phenotype transmitted in a mendelian inheritance pattern (autosomal recessive, autosomal dominant, or X-linked). Family members (with and without disease) were genotyped, and linkage studies, which test for the segregation of phenotypic trait alongside genetic markers with known chromosomal location, were performed. Markers cosegregating with the phenotype "mapped" the candidate gene to a specified chromosomal region, and subsequent fine-resolution mapping narrowed the candidate region, highlighting potential genes for direct sequencing and functional analysis. Linkage studies played a pivotal role in the discovery of numerous mendelian genes, unraveling the genetic basis for kidney diseases such as polycystic kidney disease *(PKD1, PKHD1)*, congenital nephrotic syndrome *(NPHS1)*, and Alport syndrome *(COL4A5)*.

Two major advances in the 2000s revolutionized the potential for gene discovery. First, completion of the Human Genome Project increased the utility of short fragment reads because they could be aligned to the published reference genome to identify genetic variation in tested samples. Second, development of NGS technology permitted sequencing of massive quantities of short DNA fragments in parallel, increasing sequencing output by orders of magnitude. In concert, these two advances enabled whole-genome sequencing (WGS) studies, which can provide almost complete sequence data for an individual.

While sequencing costs have dropped exponentially in the first decade following development of NGS technology, the massive quantity of sequence data generated from WGS requires considerable computational resources and analysis. Thus, particularly for genetic discovery studies focusing on rare mendelian diseases, targeted sequencing strategies, such as whole-exome sequencing (WES), have been used as a method of choice for high-throughput sequencing. WES uses enrichment strategies to sequence only the exome, the 1% of the genome that encodes proteins. Linkage analysis has been coupled with WES to identify novel disease genes. For example, in two families with hereditary atypical hemolytic uremic syndrome, WES determined disease association with the gene *DGKE*, which is independent of the complement pathway, identifying a potentially novel disease mechanism. In another example, WES and genome-wide linkage analysis identified a gene *(DSTYK)* implicated in congenital urinary tract malformations that may be mechanistically important for urogenital embryologic development. In NS, application of NGS technology has accelerated gene discovery, and over 30 genes have now been implicated in mendelian monogenic disease. Such studies highlight the genetic heterogeneity within a single clinical entity and thus the potential for improved disease classification from genetic studies.

To date, over 200 monogenic genes have been identified for kidney diseases, and these monogenic genes can underlie common causes for chronic kidney disease (CKD) that often present during childhood, including steroid-resistant NS and cystic disease. The discovery of these monogenic genes has revolutionized our understanding of underlying disease pathogenesis, such as the role of cilia in cystic diseases and the role of the podocyte in NS. In addition, genetic testing can, alongside the appropriate clinical, biochemical, and/or histologic data, provide a definitive diagnosis for a patient. Results from genetic testing may enable counseling for family planning or diagnosis of affected family members. Lastly, genetic testing may facilitate personalized medical decision making, such as prognosis or therapeutic optimization.

VARIANT INTERPRETATION

Interrogation of sequencing data from high-throughput NGS has revealed the presence of significant genetic variation throughout the genome, including millions of SNVs. Initial results from the 1000 Genomes Project, a large-scale sequencing project, demonstrated that each healthy person harbors around 250 to 300 loss-of-function variants and 50 to 100 variants implicated in inherited disorders. The sheer volume of inherent genetic variation increases the false-positive discovery rate when screening for disease-associated variants. Subsequently, improper attribution of causality to a gene or variant can have significant research and clinical implications. From a research perspective, guidelines have been proposed that incorporate genetic, experimental, and bioinformatic evidence to assess confidence in attributing causality at gene level or variant level.

From a clinical perspective, multiple academic and commercial laboratories have begun genetic sequencing of isolated genes, selected gene panels, or whole exomes to aid in medical decision making. Identification of variants in sequencing results is only the first step in clinical interpretation as variants can fall along a spectrum of pathogenicity. In 2015, the American College of Medical Genetics and Genomics (ACMG) published updated Standards and Guidelines for the interpretation of identified sequence variants. A five-tier system ("pathogenic," "likely pathogenic," "uncertain significance," "likely benign," and "benign") was introduced for classification of mendelian variants. A variety of tools are used to annotate (predict the effect of) the variant, which assists the classification of pathogenicity. Population databases (i.e., Exome Aggregation Consortium [ExAC]) can provide variant allele frequencies because variants responsible for mendelian disease are predicted to be very rare in the population. Disease databases (i.e., ClinVar) can provide historical reports of the clinical significance of identified variants. For variants resulting in nonsynonymous changes to amino acid code, computational ("in silico") analyses with various software programs (e.g., SIFT, PolyPhen, CADD) can be performed to predict impact on protein function or structure.

Despite the aforementioned methods to assess pathogenicity, classification of variants remains imperfect, often necessitating other evidence to confidently define mendelian disease. For example, the presence of a variant of uncertain significance alongside a pathogenic variant in a recessive disease-causing gene raises diagnostic uncertainty, particularly because current sequencing studies cannot determine if two identified variants are located in *cis* on the same chromosome or in *trans* on different chromosomes. In such situations, genetic sequencing of the parents can provide further evidence for segregation of identified variants. Consultation with a medical geneticist can be invaluable when doubt arises regarding the interpretation of sequencing results.

MOVING BEYOND MONOGENIC DISEASE

As noted above, initial genetic studies in kidney disease focused on identifying rare causal SNVs with large effect that are responsible for disease with a mendelian inheritance pattern. However, by their nature, mendelian causes of kidney disease are rare. Thus a parallel goal in genetic nephrology research has focused on identifying low-frequency and common SNVs that may increase the risk of kidney disease. GWAS have emerged as a method to achieve this goal. In GWAS, SNPs are genotyped to determine whether the frequency of any of these markers is significantly different between unrelated cases versus unrelated controls (Fig. 37.1).

Although each individual harbors tens of millions of SNPs throughout the genome, investigators only need to test a subset of these SNPs in GWAS because of the linkage

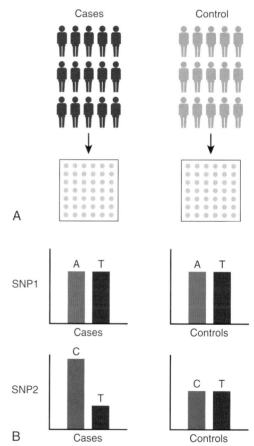

Fig. 37.1 Genome-wide association studies. (A) Rigorous phenotypic classification is used to obtain a trait- or disease-specific case cohort. A control population is carefully selected, including matching of ancestries. Subsequently, both groups undergo genotyping for hundreds of thousands to millions of single nucleotide polymorphisms (SNPs). (B) Association studies are performed comparing allele frequencies of each SNP with the phenotypic trait/disease. In the upper panel, the allele frequencies of "SNP 1" are similar between case and control cohorts, and testing does not find any association between the SNP allele and trait. In the lower panel, the allele frequencies of "SNP 2" differ, with a higher percentage of the "C" allele in the cases than controls. This implicates the C allele of SNP 2 as a risk allele for the phenotype/trait. This association should then be replicated in independent cohorts.

disequilibrium that exists in the genome. Linkage disequilibrium is the co-occurrence of specific DNA sequence variants (alleles) between nearby SNPs at a rate higher than would be expected by chance. Using these principles, a representative SNP can be selected to "tag" a haplotype—a group of variant alleles inherited together. Subsequently, the nongenotyped SNP alleles can be inferred from the analysis of reference haplotypes. Large-scale genotyping projects, such as HapMap Consortium and 1000 Genomes Project, have increased the availability of reference haplotypes, thereby facilitating GWAS.

Even with the use of tag-SNPs, case-control GWAS still consist of approximately 1 million independent tests. Thus stringent correction for multiple hypothesis testing must be used when determining whether SNPs reach a genome-wide significant association with a phenotype. In addition, the genetic variation that exists between individuals of different ethnic ancestries is greater than differences in variation attributable to disease. Thus it is very important to match cases and controls by their genetic ancestry to remove the confounding effects of population stratification.

Importantly, when SNPs are discovered to be associated with the disease trait, it does not necessarily mean that the implicated SNP is causal for the phenotype. Rather, it indicates that this "lead-SNP," or a nearby SNP in linkage disequilibrium, underlies the mechanism for the association. Unlike the highly penetrant variants responsible for mendelian disease, which almost all directly affect protein function via alteration of amino acids, GWAS SNPs are often noncoding and affect the regulation of disease-relevant genes near the GWAS allele.

Other factors affecting the success of GWAS are the underlying biology of a trait and the precision of the collected clinical phenotype. For instance, CKD can result from many different causes and can be difficult to accurately diagnose, which challenges our ability to discover a small number of SNPs that are associated with its onset. On the other hand, the discovery of GWAS alleles highly associated with membranous nephropathy (MN) in adults was facilitated because MN is a highly specific, biopsy-based diagnosis with low rates of misclassification. Despite the challenges of this method, GWAS has proven to be a powerful tool to identify susceptibility variants that may (1) promote global clinical and therapeutic advances through identification of novel biological pathways and (2) direct personalized approaches to diagnosis, prognosis, and therapeutic optimization through analysis of individualized patterns of genetic risk. However, their use in clinical care has been limited.

APOLIPOPROTEIN L-1 AS A RISK VARIANT

Successful application of GWAS in kidney disease was demonstrated by landmark studies that identified the *apolipoprotein L-1 (APOL1)* locus as a major risk allele for focal segmental glomerulosclerosis (FSGS) in individuals of African ancestry. In 2010, building upon past association studies of the high prevalence of kidney disease in individuals with African ancestry, two alleles (termed "G1" and "G2") in the *APOL1* gene were noted to be strongly associated with kidney disease. *APOL1* encodes a protein that results in lysis of trypanosomes, the parasite responsible for the lethal African sleeping sickness. In trypanosome subspecies demonstrating *APOL1* resistance, variant *APOL1* restored

trypanolytic ability. Additionally, population genomics revealed evidence of positive selection, with the risk allele providing a survival advantage similar to the advantage of sickle cell trait against malaria. The G1 allele represents two highly linked nonsynonymous variants (S342G, I384M), while the G2 allele represents a 6-bp deletion (del.N388/Y389). While the presence of one *APOL1* risk allele likely promotes a survival advantage, the presence of 2 risk alleles ("high risk" genotype) is associated with greatly increased odds of NS. In a follow-up North American study, the high-risk *APOL1* genotype led to 17-fold higher odds of FSGS and 29-fold higher odds of HIV-associated nephropathy. The high-risk genotype, which is present in 13% of individuals with African ancestry, was associated with earlier onset of FSGS and faster progression to end-stage renal disease (ESRD). The APOL1 gene product can be expressed locally in the kidney or exist as circulating form. While several lines of evidence support the role of the locally produced form in the pathogenesis of kidney disease, the exact pathophysiologic mechanism of these APOL1 variants remains under investigation. In addition, not all individuals with high-risk *APOL1* genotype develop kidney disease, suggesting that other modifier loci and/or environmental factors contribute to its penetrance for FSGS.

Nonetheless, the identification of *APOL1* risk alleles has provided a potential genetic basis for the known racial disparity in ESRD. In addition, the ability to classify disease risk by genotype leads to the possibility of precision medicine, such as the use of *APOL1* genotyping to guide decisions regarding allocation of donor allografts. Deceased donor kidney allografts from blacks with high-risk *APOL1* genotype have been associated with worse outcomes, leading some to propose routine *APOL1* genotype as part of transplant evaluation and allocation process. However, the black donor pool is limited, and the use of *APOL1* genotyping information, which may increase risk but is not deterministic, could further limit the donor pool. Consequently, there is no consensus regarding the role of *APOL1* genotyping in kidney donation.

ADDITIONAL GENOME-WIDE ASSOCIATION STUDIES IN KIDNEY DISEASE

The value of GWAS has extended beyond discovery of *APOL1* to influence our understanding of other glomerular diseases, such as MN. In 2009, Beck and colleagues reported the identification of M-type phospholipase A2 receptor 1 (PLA2R1) as the target for autoantibodies found in the serum of MN patients. From "bench-to-bedside," PLA2R1 antibody testing emerged as a potent biomarker for the diagnosis of MN with high sensitivity and specificity for trending as a correlate of remission status and for predicting recurrent disease after transplantation. In 2011, a GWAS in three separate European populations of MN patients identified two loci significantly associated with MN: *PLA2R1* and the major histocompatibility complex, *HLA-DQA1*. These genetic discoveries, combined with those from previous proteomic studies, highlight a novel potential pathophysiologic mechanism for MN and suggest that variants within HLA-DQA1 may lead to altered antigen presentation and subsequent autoantibody formation.

In another example, in immunoglobulin A nephropathy (IgAN), GWAS identified common variants significantly in several major histocompatibility complex *(HLA-DQA1)* loci and complement factor H–related-proteins *(CFHR1, CFHR3)*. A genetic risk score based on these IgAN risk alleles correlated with geospatial patterns of disease prevalence. The geospatial pattern has been hypothesized to also correlate with helminthic diversity, suggesting potential role for local pathogen exposure to disease pathophysiology.

Moving beyond glomerular disease, variants near the *UMOD* gene, which encodes uromodulin, the most abundant protein excreted into the urine, were found to be strongly associated with CKD and hypertension. Subsequently, common *UMOD* variants were shown to increase uromodulin expression, leading to salt-sensitive hypertension and histologic evidence of kidney damage in animal models, providing biologic evidence for disease susceptibility resulting from these variants.

While GWAS explores coding and noncoding regions of the genome, other types of association studies can be used, such as using genotyping chips focusing exclusively on the exome. Using this approach, variants in a major histocompatibility complex *(HLA-DQA1)* locus were associated with steroid-sensitive nephrotic syndrome (SSNS) in loci not associated with those reported in IgA and MN. Nephrotic syndrome (NS) has wide phenotypic variation, and the finding of an *HLA* locus associated with SSNS further supports an immunologic mechanism, whereby presentation of a yet-to-be identified antigen to a variant *HLA-DQA1* may lead to stimulation. Recently, the efficacy of rituximab, a B-cell depleting antibody, has highlighted a potential role for the B-cell in NS pathogenesis.

COPY NUMBER VARIANTS

Although genetic inquiry to date has primarily focused on SNVs, the contribution of CNVs, structural variations involving kilobases to megabases or more, is increasingly being studied. As with SNVs, CNVs exist in all humans, including healthy members of the population. Although CNVs can also be detected with genotyping chips, there are other technologies and analytic methods that are also used for their detection. As these approaches have matured, the role of CNVs in kidney disease has also been more understood. In a study of 522 infants with kidney hypodysplasia, a form of congenital kidney malformation, one-sixth of patients were found to have a CNV previously reported as disease causing. CNVs affecting *HNF1B* were one of the most frequently identified. Interestingly, rare exonic SNVs within *HNF1B* have been previously implicated in renal cystic dysplasia and diabetes mellitus, a syndrome encompassing a spectrum of kidney and extrarenal phenotypes. Thus we are only beginning to understand the diverse effects of structural variation and its effect on kidney development, function, and disease.

SUMMARY

In the last two decades, advances in sequencing technology and application of GWAS have enriched our understanding of the genetic architecture underlying both rare and common kidney diseases and have provided novel insights into the pathogenesis underlying these diseases. Given their potential roles as biomarkers or targets for therapeutic development, these genomic discoveries raise the promise for precision medicine. However, similar to any diagnostic test, the use of genetic sequencing results necessitates accurate interpretation of predicted pathogenicity of any identified variants and must be used within the appropriate clinical context.

KEY BIBLIOGRAPHY

1000 Genomes Project Consortium, Abecasis GR, Altshuler D, et al. A map of human genome variation from population-scale sequencing. *Nature.* 2010;467(7319):1061-1073.

Beck LH Jr, Bonegio RG, Lambeau G, et al. M-type phospholipase A2 receptor as target antigen in idiopathic membranous nephropathy. *N Engl J Med.* 2009;61(1):11-21.

Feehally J, Farrall M, Boland A, et al. HLA has strongest association with IgA nephropathy in genome-wide analysis. *J Am Soc Nephrol.* 2010; 21:1791-1797.

Freedman BI, Pastan SO, Israni AK, et al. APOL1 genotype and kidney transplantation outcomes from deceased African American donors. *Transplantation.* 2016;100:194-202.

Gbadegesin RA, Adeyemo A, Webb NJ, et al. HLA-DQA1 and PLCG2 are candidate risk loci for childhood-onset steroid-sensitive nephrotic syndrome. *J Am Soc Nephrol.* 2015;26:1701-1710.

Genovese G, Friedman DJ, Ross MD, et al. Association of trypanolytic ApoL1 variants with kidney disease in African Americans. *Science.* 2010;329:841-845.

Kiryluk K, Li Y, Sanna-Cherchi S, Rohanizadegan M, et al. Geographic differences in genetic susceptibility to IgA nephropathy: GWAS replication study and geospatial risk analysis. *PLoS Genet.* 2012;8:e1002765. doi:10.1371/journal.pgen.1002765.

Kiryluk K, Li Y, Scolari F, Sanna-Cherchi S, et al. Discovery of new risk loci for IgA nephropathy implicates genes involved in immunity against intestinal pathogens. *Nat Genet.* 2014;46:1187-1196.

Kopp JB, Nelson GW, Sampath K, et al. APOL1 genetic variants in focal segmental glomerulosclerosis and HIV-associated nephropathy. *J Am Soc Nephrol.* 2011;22:2129-2137.

Köttgen A, Glazer NL, Dehghan A, et al. Multiple loci associated with indices of renal function and chronic kidney disease. *Nat Genet.* 2009; 41:712-717.

Lemaire M, Frémeaux-Bacchi V, Schaefer F, et al. Recessive mutations in DGKE cause atypical hemolytic-uremic syndrome. *Nat Genet.* 2013; 45:531-536.

Padmanabhan S, Melander O, Johnson T, et al. Genome-wide association study of blood pressure extremes identifies variant near UMOD associated with hypertension. *PLoS Genet.* 2010;6:e1001177.

Richards S, Aziz N, Bale S, et al. Standards and guidelines for the interpretation of sequence variants: a joint consensus recommendation of the American College of Medical Genetics and Genomics and the Association for Molecular Pathology. *Genet Med.* 2015;17: 405-424.

Sampson MG, Gillies CE, Robertson CC, et al. Using population genetics to interrogate the monogenic nephrotic syndrome diagnosis in a case cohort. *J Am Soc Nephrol.* 2016;27:1970-1983.

Sampson M, Pollak M. Opportunities and challenges of genotyping patients with nephrotic syndrome in the genomic era. *Semin Nephrol.* 2015;35:212-221.

Sanna-Cherchi S, Kiryluk K, Burgess KE, et al. Copy-number disorders are a common cause of congenital kidney malformations. *Am J Hum Genet.* 2012;91:987-997.

Sanna-Cherchi S, Sampogna RV, Papeta N, et al. Mutations in DSTYK and dominant urinary tract malformations. *N Engl J Med.* 2013;369:621-629.

Stanescu HC, Arcos-Burgos M, Medlar A, et al. Risk HLA-DQA1 and PLA(2)R1 alleles in idiopathic membranous nephropathy. *N Engl J Med.* 2011;364:616-626.

Trudu M, Janas S, Lanzani C, et al. Common noncoding UMOD gene variants induce salt-sensitive hypertension and kidney damage by increasing uromodulin expression. *Nat Med.* 2013;19:1655-1660.

Zerres K, Mücher G, Bachner L, et al. Mapping of the gene for autosomal recessive polycystic kidney disease (ARPKD) to chromosome 6p21-cen. *Nat Genet.* 1994;7:429-432.

Full bibliography can be found on www.expertconsult.com.

38 Genetically Based Kidney Transport Disorders

Steven J. Scheinman

The coming of age of clinical chemistry in the latter half of the 20th century, bringing with it the routine measurement of electrolytes and minerals in patient samples, produced descriptions of distinct inherited syndromes of abnormal tubular transport in the kidney. Clinical investigation led to speculation, often ingenious and sometimes controversial, regarding the underlying causes of these syndromes. More recently, the tools of molecular biology made possible the cloning of mutated genes found in patients with monogenic disorders of renal tubular transport. These diseases represent experiments of nature, and for anyone interested in pathophysiology and specifically for renal physiologiststs, the insights they reveall are exciting. Some provide gratifying confirmation of our existing knowledge of transport mechanisms along the nephron. Examples include mutations in diuretic-sensitive transporters in the Bartter and Gitelman syndromes. In other cases, positional cloning led to the discovery of previously unknown proteins, often surprising ones that appear to play important roles in epithelial transport. For example, the chloride transporter CLC-5 (gene name *CLCN5*), the tight junction claudin 16 (paracellin 1), and the phosphaturic hormone fibroblast growth factor 23 (FGF23) were discovered through positional cloning in the study of Dent disease, inherited hypomagnesemic hypercalciuria, and autosomal-dominant hypophosphatemic rickets (ADHR), respectively.

Table 38.1 summarizes genetic diseases of renal tubular transport for which the molecular basis is known. The diseases listed are explained by abnormalities in the corresponding gene product. They are all inherited in mendelian fashion, either autosomal or X-linked, with the single exception of a syndrome of hypomagnesemia with maternal inheritance that results from mutation in a mitochondrial tRNA rather than in the nuclear genome.

DISORDERS OF PROXIMAL TUBULAR TRANSPORT FUNCTION

SELECTIVE PROXIMAL TRANSPORT DEFECTS

Sodium resorption in the proximal tubule occurs through secondary active transport processes in which the entry of sodium is coupled either to the entry of substrates (e.g., glucose, amino acids, or phosphate) or to the exit of protons. Autosomal-recessive conditions of impaired transepithelial transport of glucose and dibasic amino acids have been shown to be caused by mutations in sodium-dependent transporters that are expressed in both kidney and intestine, resulting in urinary losses and intestinal malabsorption of these solutes.

Other disorders with renal-selective transport defects result from mutations in transporters expressed specifically in kidney.

IMPAIRED PROXIMAL PHOSPHATE REABSORPTION

Hypophosphatemic rickets can be inherited in X-linked, autosomal-dominant, and autosomal-recessive patterns. All three modes are associated with renal phosphate wasting, with a reduced maximal transport capacity for phosphate. In all three, serum levels of the phosphate-regulating hormone (phosphatonin) FGF23 are elevated, and serum levels of 1,25-dihydroxyvitamin D are not elevated despite the stimulus of hypophosphatemia.

X-linked (dominant) hypophosphatemic rickets (XLHR) is the most common form of hereditary rickets. Mutations in XLHR involve a phosphate-regulating gene with homologies to a neutral endopeptidase on the X chromosome *(PHEX)* that is expressed in bone and is indirectly involved in the degradation and processing of FGF23. Elevations in FGF23 are sufficient to explain the renal phosphate wasting, but other factors independent of FGF23 appear to contribute as well to the bone demineralization and rickets.

The rare ADHR is associated with mutations in the gene encoding FGF23 that protects the phosphatonin from proteolytic cleavage. FGF23 inhibits renal phosphate reabsorption by inhibiting expression of two genes encoding sodium-dependent phosphate transporters in proximal tubule, *SLC34A1* (encoding the Na-dependent phosphate transporter Npt2a) and *SLC34A3* (encoding Npt2c). FGF23 inhibits the 1-hydroxylation of 25-hydroxyvitamin D, likely explaining why hypophosphatemia in these three conditions is not associated with either elevated levels of 1,25-dihydroxyvitamin D or hypercalciuria.

Autosomal-recessive inheritance of hypophosphatemic rickets has been reported in association with mutations in one of two genes. In ARHR type 1, the mutated gene is *DMP1*, encoding the dentin matrix protein 1 (DMP-1), a bone matrix protein that appears to play a role with PHEX in regulating bone mineralization and FGF23 production. ARHR2 is associated with mutations in *ENPP1*, encoding ectonucleotide pyrophosphatase/phosphodiesterase 1. Patients with either subtype resemble those with autosomal-dominant (i.e., FGF23 mutations) and X-linked (PHEX mutations) hypophosphatemic rickets.

Hereditary hypophosphatemic rickets with hypercalciuria (HHRH), an autosomal-recessive disorder, is different from XLHR, ADRH, and ARHR, all of which are associated with reduced urinary calcium excretion. In contrast, hypophosphatemia in HHRH is associated with appropriate elevations

Table 38.1 Molecular Bases of Genetic Disorders of Renal Transport

Inherited Disorder	Defective Gene Product
Proximal Tubule	
Glucose-galactose malabsorption syndrome	Sodium-glucose transporter 1
Dibasic aminoaciduria	Basolateral dibasic amino acid transporter (lysinuric protein intolerance)
XLHR	PHEX
ADHR	FGF23 (excess)
Autosomal recessive hypophosphatemic rickets	DMP1
	ENPP1
HHRH	Sodium-phosphate cotransporter Npt2c
Familial hyperostosis-hyperphosphatemia	FGF23 (deficiency)
	GalNac transferase 3
	Klotho (FGF23 co-receptor)
Fanconi syndrome	Aldolase B (hereditary fructose intolerance)
Fanconi-Bickel syndrome	Facilitated GLUT2
Oculocerebrorenal syndrome of Lowe	Inositol polyphosphate-5-phosphatase (OCRL1)
Dent disease (X-linked nephrolithiasis)	Chloride transporter (ClC-5)
	Inositol polyphosphate-5-phosphatase (OCRL1)
Cystinuria	Apical cystine-dibasic amino acid transporter rBAT
	Light subunit of rBAT
Autosomal recessive proximal RTA	Basolateral sodium-bicarbonate cotransporter NBC1
TAL of Loop of Henle	
Bartter syndrome	
Type I	Bumetanide-sensitive Na-K-2Cl cotransporter NKCC2
Type II	Apical potassium channel ROMK
Type III	Basolateral chloride channel ClC-Kb
Type IV, with sensorineural deafness	Barttin (ClC-Kb–associated protein)
Familial hypocalcemia with Bartter features	CaSR (activation)
Familial hypomagnesemia with hypercalciuria and nephrocalcinosis	
Without ocular abnormalities	Claudin-16 (paracellin-1)
With ocular abnormalities	Claudin-19
Familial hypocalciuric hypercalcemia[a]	CaSR (inactivation)
Neonatal severe hyperparathyroidism[b]	CaSR (inactivation)
Autosomal dominant hypercalciuric hypocalcemia	CaSR (activation) (type 1)
	$G\alpha_{11}$ G-protein (type 2)
Familial juvenile hyperuricemic nephropathy	Uromodulin (Tamm-Horsfall protein)
DCT	
Gitelman syndrome	Thiazide-sensitive NaCl cotransporter NCCT
Pseudohypoparathyroidism type Ia[c]	Guanine nucleotide-binding protein (Gs)
Familial hypomagnesemia with secondary hypocalcemia	TRPM6 cation channel[d]
Isolated recessive renal hypomagnesemia	EGF
Autosomal-dominant hypomagnesemia with hypocalciuria	γ subunit of Na/K-ATPase
	HNF1B transcription factor
	PCBD1 dimerization cofactor
SeSAME/EAST syndromes	Kir4.1 potassium channel
Dominant hypomagnesemia with ataxia	Kv1.1 potassium channel
Familial tubulopathy with hypomagnesemia	Mitochondrial tRNA[isoleucine]
Dominant or recessive hypomagnesemia	CNNM2 (cyclin M2)
Collecting Duct	
Liddle syndrome	β and γ subunits of epithelial Na channel ENaC
Pseudohypoaldosteronism	
Type 1	
Autosomal recessive	α, β, γ subunits of ENaC
Autosomal dominant	Mineralocorticoid (type I) receptor
Type 2 (Gordon syndrome)	WNK1 and WNK4 kinases
	Cullin-3 scaffold protein
	Kelch3 adaptor protein

Continued

Table 38.1   Molecular Bases of Genetic Disorders of Renal Transport—cont'd

Inherited Disorder	Defective Gene Product
Glucocorticoid-remediable aldosteronism	11β-hydroxylase and aldosterone synthase (chimeric gene)[e]
Syndrome of AME	11β-hydroxysteroid dehydrogenase type II
Distal RTA	
Autosomal dominant	Basolateral anion exchanger (AE1) (band 3 protein)
Autosomal recessive, with hemolytic anemia	Basolateral anion exchanger (AE1) (band 3 protein)
Autosomal recessive (with hearing deficit)	β1 subunit of proton ATPase
Autosomal recessive (hearing deficit variable)	α4 isoform of α subunit of proton ATPase
Carbonic anhydrase II deficiency[f]	Carbonic anhydrase type II
Nephrogenic diabetes insipidus	
X-linked	AVP 2 (V2) receptor
Autosomal	AQP-2 water channel

[a]Results from heterozygous mutation.
[b]Results from homozygous mutation.
[c]Gene also expressed in proximal tubule where functional abnormalities are clinically apparent.
[d]Gene also expressed in intestine.
[e]Gene expressed in adrenal gland.
[f]Clinical phenotype can be of proximal RTA, distal RTA, or combined.
ADHR, Autosomal-dominant hypophosphatemic rickets; *AME,* apparent mineralocorticoid excess; *AQP-2,* aquaporin 2; *AVP,* arginine vasopressin; *CaSR,* calcium-sensing receptor; *DCT,* distal convoluted tubule; *DMP1,* dentin matrix protein 1; *EAST,* epilepsy, ataxia, sensorineural deafness, and tubulopathy; *EGF,* epidermal growth factor; *ENPP1,* ectonucleotide pyrophosphatase/phosphodiesterase 1; *FGF23,* fibroblast growth factor 23; *GLUT2,* glucose transporter; *GRA,* glucocorticoid-remediable aldosteronism; *HHRH,* hereditary hypophosphatemic rickets with hypercalciuria; *NCCT,* sodium chloride cotransporter; *NKCC2,* Na⁺-K⁺-2Cl⁻ cotransporter; *PHEX,* phosphate regulating gene with homologies to endopeptidases on the X chromosome; *RTA,* renal tubular acidosis; *SeSAME,* seizures, sensorineural deafness, ataxia, mental retardation, and electrolyte imbalance; *TAL,* thick ascending limb; *XLHR,* X-linked hypophosphatemic rickets.

of 1,25-dihydroxyvitamin D levels, and FGF23 levels are normal or reduced. This profile in HHRH is consistent with a primary defect in phosphate transport, and indeed the disease is associated with mutations in *SLC34A3*, encoding the proximal tubule phosphate transporter Npt2c. Expression of this transporter, as well as that of *SLC34A1* encoding the more abundant transporter Npt2a, respond to physiologic stimuli such as parathyroid hormone (PTH) and dietary phosphate. Knockout of the mouse homologue of *SLC34A1* reproduces the features of human HHRH except for rickets; a mouse knockout of *SLC34A3* manifests hypercalcemia and hypercalciuria, but not hypophosphatemia, nephrocalcinosis, or rickets; and a double knockout of both genes produces mice with the full phenotype of hypophosphatemia, hypercalciuria, nephrocalcinosis, and rickets.

EXCESSIVE PROXIMAL PHOSPHATE REABSORPTION

Inherited hyperphosphatemia in the familial hyperostosis-hyperphosphatemia syndrome represents a mirror image of ADHR and XLHR, with excessive renal phosphate reabsorption, persistent hyperphosphatemia, inappropriately normal levels of 1,25-dihydroxyvitamin D, and low levels of FGF23. This can result from mutations in one of three genes identified to date. These genes encode FGF23 itself; a Golgi-associated biosynthetic enzyme, *N*-acetylglucosaminyl (GalNac) transferase 3, that is involved in glycosylation of FGF23 and is necessary for its secretion; and Klotho, a transmembrane protein that complexes with the FGF23 receptor and regulates its affinity for FGF23. Together, these discoveries are fleshing out our understanding of the role of bone in the complex regulation of mineral metabolism.

IMPAIRED PROXIMAL BICARBONATE TRANSPORT

Selective proximal renal tubular acidosis (RTA) is inherited in an autosomal recessive manner and is associated with mutations that inactivate the basolateral sodium bicarbonate cotransporter NBC1, encoded by the gene *SLC4A4*. These patients typically exhibit short stature and often suffer blindness from ocular abnormalities, including band keratopathy, cataracts, and glaucoma; these ocular manifestations probably are a consequence of impaired bicarbonate transport in the eye. Mutations in the *SLC4A4* gene result in impaired transporter function or aberrant trafficking of the protein to the basolateral surface. This gene belongs to the same group as the gene encoding the anion exchanger AE1 (now designated *SLC4A1*), which is mutated in distal RTA. Proximal RTA can also be inherited in an autosomal-dominant fashion, though the responsible gene(s) have not been identified.

INHERITED FANCONI SYNDROME: HEREDITARY FRUCTOSE INTOLERANCE, LOWE SYNDROME, AND DENT DISEASE

The renal Fanconi syndrome represents a generalized impairment in reabsorptive function of the proximal tubule and comprises proximal RTA with aminoaciduria, renal glycosuria, hypouricemia, and hypophosphatemia. Some or all of these abnormalities are present in individual patients with Fanconi syndrome. Inherited causes of partial or complete Fanconi syndrome include hereditary fructose intolerance, Lowe syndrome, and Dent disease.

Hereditary fructose intolerance is caused by mutations that result in deficiency of the aldolase B isoenzyme, which cleaves fructose-1-phosphate. Symptoms are precipitated by intake of sweets. Massive accumulation of fructose-1-phosphate occurs, leading to sequestration of inorganic phosphate and deficiency of adenosine triphosphate (ATP). Acute consequences can include hypoglycemic shock, severe abdominal symptoms, and impaired function of the Krebs cycle that produces metabolic acidosis; this is exacerbated by impaired renal bicarbonate reabsorption. ATP deficiency leads to impaired proximal tubular function in general, including the full expression of the Fanconi syndrome with consequent rickets and stunted growth. ATP breakdown can be so dramatic as to produce hyperuricemia, as well as hypermagnesemia from the dissolution of the magnesium-ATP complex. Avoiding dietary sources of fructose can minimize acute symptoms and chronic consequences such as liver disease.

Characteristic features of the oculocerebrorenal syndrome of Lowe include congenital cataracts, mental retardation, muscular hypotonia, and the renal Fanconi syndrome. In contrast, Dent disease is confined to the kidney. In both syndromes, low-molecular-weight (LMW) proteinuria is a prominent feature along with other evidence of proximal tubulopathy such as glycosuria, aminoaciduria, and phosphaturia. One important and puzzling difference is that proximal RTA with growth retardation can be severe in patients with Lowe syndrome, but it is not a part of Dent disease. Some patients with Lowe syndrome or Dent disease may have rickets, which is thought to be a consequence of hypophosphatemia and, in Lowe syndrome, of acidosis as well. Hypercalciuria is a characteristic feature of Dent disease and is associated with nephrocalcinosis in most and kidney stones in many patients with Dent disease; nephrocalcinosis and nephrolithiasis are less common in Lowe syndrome. Kidney failure is common in both of these conditions, typically occurring in young adulthood in Dent disease and even earlier in patients with Lowe syndrome.

Dent disease is caused in most cases by mutations that inactivate the chloride transporter CLC-5. This transport protein is expressed in the proximal tubule, the medullary thick ascending limb (MTAL) of the loop of Henle, and the alpha-intercalated cells of the collecting tubule. In the cells of the proximal tubule, CLC-5 co-localizes with the proton-ATPase in subapical endosomes. These endosomes are important in the processing of proteins that are filtered at the glomerulus and taken up by the proximal tubule through adsorptive endocytosis. The activity of the proton-ATPase acidifies the endosomal space, releasing the proteins from membrane-binding sites and making them available for proteolytic degradation. CLC-5 mediates electrogenic exchange of chloride for protons in these endosomes, facilitating endosomal acidification. Mutations that inactivate CLC-5 in patients with Dent's disease interfere with the mechanism for reabsorption of LMW proteins and explain the consistent finding of LMW proteinuria. Glycosuria, aminoaciduria, and phosphaturia occur commonly but less consistently and may reflect altered membrane protein recycling, as CLC-5 interacts directly with several trafficking proteins. Hypercalciuria appears to reflect a dysregulation of renal 1-hydroxylation of 25(OH)-vitamin D.

Lowe syndrome is associated with mutations in *OCRL1*, which encodes a phosphatidylinositol-4,5-bisphosphate-5-phosphatase. In renal epithelial cells, this phosphatase is localized to the *trans*-Golgi network, which plays an important role in directing proteins to the appropriate membrane. The CLC-5 protein and the OCRL1 phosphatase interact with the actin cytoskeleton and are involved in assembly of the endosomal apparatus. Similarities in the kidney features of these two syndromes may be the result of defective membrane trafficking. A subset of patients with mutations in *OCRL1* have no cataracts or cerebral dysfunction and no RTA ("Dent 2" disease). Such mutations occur predominantly in the 5′ end of the gene and are critical to expression of the gene in the kidney, but not to expression of transcripts in eye or brain.

DISORDERS OF TRANSPORT IN THE MEDULLARY THICK ASCENDING LIMB OF HENLE

BARTTER SYNDROME

Solute transport in the MTAL involves the coordinated functions of a set of transport proteins depicted in Fig. 38.1. These proteins are the bumetanide-sensitive Na^+-K^+-$2Cl^-$ cotransporter (NKCC2) and the renal outer medullary potassium channel (ROMK) on the apical surface of cells of the MTAL, and the chloride channel ClC-Kb on the basolateral surface. Optimal function of the ClC-Kb chloride channel requires interaction with a subunit called *barttin*. Mutations in any of the genes encoding these four proteins lead to the phenotype of Bartter syndrome. In addition, activation of the epithelial CaSR inhibits activity of the ROMK potassium channel. Mutations producing constitutive activation of the CaSR cause familial hypocalcemic hypercalciuria. Some patients with hypocalcemic hypercalciuria have the phenotype of Bartter syndrome, and mutations in the CaSR may be considered a fifth molecular cause of this syndrome. Together, these five genes still do not account for all patients with Bartter syndrome.

The ClC-Kb basolateral chloride channel provides the route for chloride exit to the interstitium. Flow of potassium through the ROMK channel ensures that potassium concentrations in the tubular lumen do not limit the activity of the NKCC2 while maintaining a positive electrical potential in the lumen of this nephron segment. This positive charge is the driving force for paracellular reabsorption of calcium and magnesium.

Bartter syndrome manifests in infancy or childhood with polyuria and failure to thrive, often occurring after a pregnancy with polyhydramnios. It is characterized by hypokalemic metabolic alkalosis, typically with hypercalciuria, and these patients resemble patients chronically taking loop diuretics that inhibit activity of NKCC2 pharmacologically. Defective function of NKCC2, ROMK, ClC-Kb, or barttin leads to impaired salt reabsorption in the MTAL, resulting in volume contraction and activation of the renin-angiotensin-aldosterone axis, which subsequently stimulates distal tubular secretion of potassium and protons, resulting in hypokalemic metabolic alkalosis. Despite impaired reabsorption of magnesium, serum magnesium levels are usually normal or only mildly reduced in patients with Bartter syndrome. Severity, age of onset of symptoms, and particular clinical features vary with the gene abnormality. For example, nephrocalcinosis as a consequence of hypercalciuria is most common in individuals with mutations in genes encoding NKCC2 and ROMK. Barttin is

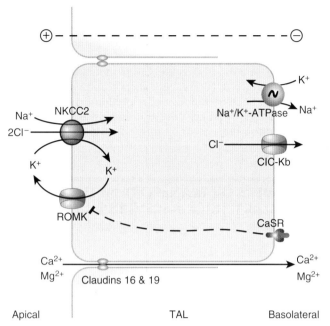

Fig. 38.1 Transport mechanisms in the thick ascending limb of loop of Henle transport proteins affected by mutations in genetic diseases. Reabsorption of sodium chloride occurs through the electroneutral activity of the bumetanide-sensitive Na^+-K^+-$2Cl^-$ cotransporter (NKCC2). Activity of the basolateral sodium-potassium adenosine triphosphatase (Na^+, K^+-ATPase) provides the driving force for this transport and also generates a high intracellular concentration of potassium, which exits through the ATP-regulated apical potassium channel, ROMK. This ensures an adequate supply of potassium for the activity of the NKCC2 and also produces a lumen-positive electrical potential, which itself is the driving force for paracellular reabsorption of calcium, magnesium, and sodium ions through the tight junctions, involving the protein paracellin 1. Chloride transported into the cell by NKCC2 exits the basolateral side of the cell through the voltage-gated chloride channel, ClC-Kb. Activation of the extracellular calcium-sensing receptor, CaSR, inhibits solute transport in the TAL by inhibiting activity of the ROMK and possibly by other mechanisms. Mutations that inactivate the CaSR are associated with enhanced calcium transport and hypocalciuria in familial benign hypercalcemia, and mutations that activate the CaSR occur in patients with familial hypercalciuria with hypocalcemia. *ROMK,* Renal outer medullary potassium channel; *TAL,* thick ascending limb.

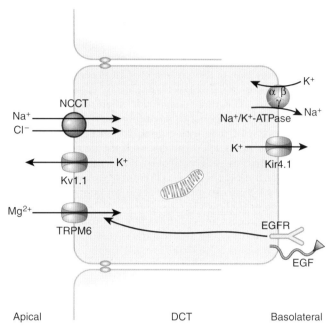

Fig. 38.2 Transport mechanisms in the distal convoluted tubule. The basolateral sodium-potassium adenosine triphosphatase (Na^+/ K^+-ATPase), composed of α, β, and γ subunits, establishes the low intracellular sodium concentration that provides the driving force for coupled sodium and chloride entry across the apical NCCT transporter. It also maintains the high intracellular potassium concentration that drives potassium exit across the apical Kv1.1 potassium channel, which establishes a positive lumen-to-cytosol electrical gradient that drives magnesium entry across the apical TRPM6 cation channel. The basolateral Kir4.1 potassium channel allows potassium exit that may serve to assure an adequate potassium supply for the Na^+/K^+-ATPase. The EGF receptor stimulates trafficking of TRPM6 to the apical membrane and stimulates activity of that transporter. Genes encoding these proteins are responsible for inherited electrolyte disturbances discussed in the text. *DCT,* Distal convoluted tubule; *EGF,* epidermal growth factor; *EGFR,* epidermal growth factor receptor; *NCCT,* sodium chloride cotransporter.

expressed in the inner ear, and patients with mutations in its gene have sensorineural deafness. Bartter syndrome is discussed further in Chapter 10.

INHERITED HYPOMAGNESEMIC HYPERCALCIURIA

Reabsorption of calcium and magnesium in the MTAL occurs through the paracellular route, driven by the positive electrical potential in the tubular lumen. The tight junctions between the epithelial cells determine the selective movement of cations (i.e., calcium, magnesium, and sodium). Disturbance of this selective paracellular barrier would be expected to produce parallel disorders in the reabsorption of calcium and magnesium.

Familial hypomagnesemia with substantial renal magnesium losses, hypercalciuria, and nephrocalcinosis (FHHNC) is inherited in an autosomal-recessive fashion. These patients develop kidney failure and kidney stones. Investigation of

families first led to identification by positional cloning of the gene encoding a tight junction protein designated claudin 16 (also called paracellin 1). This was the first instance of a disease shown to result from mutations that alter a tight junction protein. Another member of this family, claudin 19, is mutated in other pedigrees in whom FHHNC is associated with ocular abnormalities (e.g., macular colobomas, myopia, horizontal nystagmus) with severe visual impairment. Both claudin 16 and claudin 19 are expressed in the thick ascending limb (TAL; Fig. 38.2), but claudin 19 also is expressed in the retina. These two proteins interact in the tight junction to regulate cation permeability. It is unclear why a defect in tight junctions is associated with hyperuricemia, a consistent finding in this disease.

FAMILIAL HYPOCALCIURIC HYPERCALCEMIA

The extracellular CaSR is expressed in many tissues in which ambient calcium concentrations trigger cellular responses. In the parathyroid gland, activation of the CaSR suppresses synthesis and release of PTH. In the kidney, the CaSR is expressed on the basolateral surface of cells of the TAL (cortical more than medullary), on the luminal surface of the cells of the papillary collecting duct, and in other portions of the nephron. Activation of the CaSR in the TAL probably mediates the known effects of hypercalcemia to inhibit the transport of calcium, magnesium, and sodium in this nephron segment. For example, CaSR activation inhibits activity of the ROMK potassium channel (see Fig. 38.1). This can be expected to reduce the positive electrical potential in the lumen and thereby suppress the driving force for reabsorption of calcium and magnesium. The CaSR also interacts with claudins to reduce the permeability of the tight junction to Ca^{2+} and Mg^{2+}. In the papillary collecting duct, activation of the apical CaSR may explain how hypercalciuria impairs the hydroosmotic response to vasopressin, resulting in nephrogenic diabetes insipidus. Notably, the presence of a large volume of dilute urine produced in this situation is potentially protective against the development of nephrocalcinosis or nephrolithiasis in the setting of hypercalciuria due to hypercalcemia and an increased filtered load.

In familial hypocalciuric hypercalcemia (FHH), loss-of-function mutations of the *CASR* gene increase the set point for calcium sensing, resulting in hypercalcemia with relative elevation of PTH levels. Urinary calcium excretion is low because of enhanced calcium reabsorption in the TAL and PTH-stimulated calcium transport in the distal convoluted tubule (DCT). FHH occurs in patients heterozygous for such mutations. It is benign as tissues are resistant to the high serum calcium levels, although cases of pancreatitis have been reported, and chondrocalcinosis may occur in older patients. Rare cases of FHH have been reported in association with two other genes involved in signal transduction from the CaSR; these are *GNA11*, encoding $G\alpha_{11}$ (FHH type 2), and *AP2S1*, encoding $AP2\sigma$ (FHH type 3). A family history helps to differentiate FHH from primary hyperparathyroidism, which is important because parathyroidectomy should not be performed in FHH.

Infants of consanguineous parents with FHH can be homozygous for these mutations, resulting in a syndrome of severe hypercalcemia with marked hyperparathyroidism, fractures, and failure to thrive, known as *neonatal severe hyperparathyroidism.* This also occurs, albeit rarely, in infants who are compound heterozygotes for two loss-of-function CaSr alleles, without consanguinity.

In contrast, other mutations result in constitutive activation of the CaSR, producing autosomal-dominant hypocalcemia with hypercalciuria without elevated PTH concentrations. This phenotype can also occur with gain-of-function mutations in $G\alpha_{11}$. As discussed earlier, CaSR gain-of-function mutations also can produce the phenotype of Bartter syndrome. Polymorphism in the *CASR* gene producing a mild gain-of-function expression of the CaSR without frank hypocalcemia has been associated with idiopathic hypercalciuria.

DISORDERS OF TRANSPORT IN THE DISTAL CONVOLUTED TUBULE

GITELMAN SYNDROME

Reabsorption of sodium chloride in the DCT occurs through electroneutral transport mediated by the thiazide-sensitive sodium chloride cotransporter (NCCT). Mutations in the NCCT gene *(SLC12A3)* are associated with Gitelman syndrome, another condition of hypokalemic metabolic alkalosis. The phenotype of type 3 Bartter syndrome (CLC-Kb mutation) can overlap with Gitelman, particularly regarding the presence of hypomagnesemia. Gitelman syndrome once was viewed as a variant of Bartter syndrome; however, an essential distinction between these two conditions is the presence of *hypo*calciuria in Gitelman syndrome, in contrast to the *hyper*calciuria that occurs in Bartter syndrome or in patients taking loop diuretics. Hypocalciuria in Gitelman syndrome resembles the reduction in calcium excretion that occurs in patients taking thiazide diuretics. These findings are satisfying in that they connect the clinical physiology with molecular physiology. However, our understanding of kidney transport does not allow us to explain the fact that significant hypomagnesemia with renal magnesium wasting is typical of Gitelman syndrome, whereas in Bartter syndrome it is much less common and, when it does occur, milder.

IMPAIRED DISTAL MAGNESIUM REABSORPTION

Our understanding of the mechanisms involved in distal tubular magnesium transport has been substantially enriched by the identification in recent years of genes responsible for several distinct syndromes of hypomagnesemia. The TRPM6 apical magnesium channel is critical to magnesium transport in the gut as well as in the distal tubule, and mutations in the gene encoding this channel cause a hypomagnesemic syndrome sufficiently severe as to impair PTH release and function, with secondary hypocalcemia. Potassium channels expressed on the apical (Kv1.1) and basolateral (Kir4.1) membranes are also expressed in the brain, and mutations result in hypomagnesemia as well as neurologic dysfunction including ataxia. Hypomagnesemia also results from inherited defects in distal tubule basolateral membrane proteins EGF, the γ subunit of the Na^+/K^+ ATPase, and a newly discovered protein of unknown function, CNNM2.

FAMILIAL HYPOMAGNESEMIA WITH SECONDARY HYPOCALCEMIA

Patients with this syndrome experience severe hypomagnesemia, often with neonatal seizures and tetany. If not recognized and treated early, the hypomagnesemia can be fatal. Serum magnesium levels fall low enough to impair PTH release or responsiveness, and this is presumed to be the mechanism of the hypocalcemia that commonly accompanies hypomagnesemia in these patients. The primary defect appears to be in intestinal magnesium absorption, although renal magnesium conservation also is deficient. These patients have mutations in a gene *(TRPM6)* encoding the TRPM6 protein. TRPM6 is a member of the long transient receptor potential channel family and is expressed in both the intestine and the DCT. Under experimental conditions, TRPM6 forms functional heteromers with its close homologue TRPM7, which, like TRPM6, has an alpha-kinase domain. Activity of the cation channel formed by these heteromers involves a protein, RACK1, that regulates the alpha-kinase. To date, mutations have not been described in TRPM7 or RACK1.

ISOLATED RECESSIVE RENAL HYPOMAGNESEMIA

This has been described in a single consanguineous Dutch pedigree, in which two sisters presented with hypomagnesemia with renal magnesium wasting, otherwise normal serum and urinary electrolyte metabolism, and associated mental retardation. This disease is linked to the locus encompassing the gene encoding the epidermal growth factor (EGF), and both patients had homozygous mutation in this gene. This mutation leads to abnormal basolateral sorting of pro-EGF. EGF receptors are expressed on DCT cells and elsewhere in the renal epithelium and vasculature, and activation of EGF receptors stimulates activity of TRPM6 magnesium channels, whereas blockade of EGF receptors with the monoclonal antibody cetuximab prevents this stimulation. This observation is consistent with the clinical experience of hypomagnesemia seen with cetuximab use as therapy for colon cancer.

AUTOSOMAL-DOMINANT HYPOMAGNESEMIA WITH HYPOCALCIURIA

A syndrome of inherited hypomagnesemia with seizures, tetany, chondrocalcinosis, renal magnesium wasting, and hypercalciuria has been described in association with mutation in the *FXYD2* gene encoding the γ subunit of the basolateral Na^+/K^+-ATPase. The mechanism of a dominant-negative effect of heterozygous mutations in this gene is not fully understood. It has been speculated that the mutant subunit results in destabilization of the enzyme complex, leading to a reduced membrane potential in the DCT cells and a reduced drive for magnesium entry across the apical TRPM6 channel. There is also evidence that the γ subunit can mediate basolateral extrusion of magnesium.

The HNF1B transcription factor is involved in renal tubular embryonic development and tissue-specific gene expression. HNF1B interacts with FXYD2 and with a dimerization cofactor PCBD1 that is expressed in the distal collecting duct. Mutations in the genes encoding both NHF1B and PCBD1 are associated with hypomagnesemia and renal magnesium wasting.

SeSAME/EAST SYNDROMES

The *KCNJ10* gene encoding the Kir4.1 potassium channel is expressed in the brain and distal tubule, and mutations produce an autosomal-recessive syndrome that has been labeled "SeSAME syndrome" (for seizures, sensorineural deafness, ataxia, mental retardation, and electrolyte imbalance) and "EAST syndrome" (epilepsy, ataxia, sensorineural deafness, and tubulopathy). In the DCT, the Kir4.1 channel allows potassium recycling from cytosol back to the interstitium. This maintains a negative intracellular potential and also assures adequate extracellular potassium for optimal functioning of the Na^+/K^+-ATPase, which in turn provides the driving force for apical Na^+ and Cl^- influx through NCCT. Loss of function of Kir4.1 therefore results in abnormal electrolyte handling resembling that of NCCT inactivation in Gitelman syndrome, with salt-wasting, secondary activation of renin-angiotensin-aldosterone activity, hypokalemic metabolic alkalosis, and hypocalciuria, in addition to hypomagnesemia. The neurologic findings separate SeSAME/EAST syndromes from Gitelman

syndrome, and the metabolic abnormalities distinguish this from other neurodevelopmental diseases.

ISOLATED HYPOMAGNESEMIA WITH *KCNA1* MUTATION

The Kv1.1 apical potassium channel is important in establishing the negative potential across the DCT luminal membrane that provides the driving force for magnesium transport through TRPM6. Mutation is associated with autosomal-dominant inheritance of isolated hypomagnesemia, without other electrolyte disturbances. The Kv1.1 channel is also expressed in the cerebellum, and mutations in *KCNA1* are also associated with the rare episodic ataxia type 1, which, however, is not associated with hypomagnesemia. This paradox may relate to tissue-specific splice variants of the gene or differential interactions with tissue-specific Kv1 units.

HYPOMAGNESEMIA WITH MITOCHONDRIAL INHERITANCE

A single but very instructive family has been reported with maternal rather than mendelian inheritance of symptomatic hypomagnesemia with hypocalciuria and hypokalemia, associated with mutation in a mitochondrial gene encoding a tRNA for isoleucine. The DCT has the highest energy consumption of any nephron segment and is therefore presumably more susceptible to impairment in energy supply for ATP-dependent sodium transport. Electrolyte abnormalities cluster in this family with hypertension and hypercholesterolemia, suggesting a possible role for mitochondria in the metabolic syndrome.

CNNM2 MUTATIONS IN DOMINANT HYPOMAGNESEMIA

CNNM2 encodes a protein, cyclin M2, that is expressed in the brain and other organs and on the basolateral surface of TAL and DCT in the kidney. It was identified through studies of families with either dominant or recessive inheritance of symptomatic hypomagnesemia with renal magnesium wasting. Clinical manifestations include seizures and muscle weakness, but other electrolytes are normal. Its expression in cultured DCT cells is increased in magnesium deprivation, and functional studies of the mutant protein demonstrate reduction in magnesium-sensitive currents. It is speculated that cyclin M2 may represent the postulated basolateral transporter mediating magnesium efflux or a magnesium sensor.

DISORDERS OF TRANSPORT IN THE COLLECTING TUBULE

LIDDLE SYNDROME

Sodium reabsorption by the principal cells of the cortical collecting duct is physiologically regulated by aldosterone. As in other cells, low intracellular sodium concentrations are maintained by the basolateral Na^+/K^+-ATPase, and this drives sodium entry through amiloride-sensitive epithelial sodium channels (ENaC) on the apical surface. Mutations that render the ENaC persistently open produce a syndrome of excessive sodium reabsorption and low-renin hypertension (i.e., Liddle syndrome). This autosomal-dominant condition often manifests in children with severe hypertension and hypokalemic alkalosis. It resembles primary hyperaldosteronism, but serum aldosterone levels are quite low, and, for this reason, the disease also has been called *pseudohyperaldosteronism*. In their original description of the syndrome, Liddle and colleagues demonstrated that aldosterone excess was not responsible for this disease and that, although spironolactone had no effect on the hypertension, patients did respond well to triamterene or dietary sodium restriction. They proposed that the primary abnormality was excessive renal salt conservation and potassium secretion independent of mineralocorticoid. This hypothesis proved to be correct, and it is explained by excessive sodium channel activity. Renal transplantation in Liddle's original proband led to resolution of the hypertension, consistent with correction of the defect intrinsic to the kidneys.

In Liddle syndrome, gain-of-function mutations in the ENaC produce channels that are resistant to downregulation by physiologic stimuli such as volume expansion. Three homologous subunits, designated αENaC, βENaC, and γENaC, form the ENaC. Missense or truncating mutations in patients with Liddle syndrome alter the carboxyl-terminal cytoplasmic tail of the β or γ subunit in a domain that is important for interactions with the cytoskeletal protein that regulates activity of the ENaC. In addition to the severe phenotype of Liddle syndrome resulting from these mutations, it has been speculated that polymorphisms in the ENaC sequence that have less dramatic effects on sodium channel function may contribute to the much more common low-renin variant of essential hypertension.

PSEUDOHYPOALDOSTERONISM TYPES 1 AND 2

Pseudohypoaldosteronism types 1 and 2 are referred to as *pseudohypoaldosteronism,* because they feature hyperkalemia and metabolic acidosis without aldosterone deficiency. Type 1 disease is associated with salt wasting and results from mutations that inactivate either the mineralocorticoid receptor (autosomal recessive) or the ENaC (autosomal dominant). The autosomal-recessive form is milder and resolves with time, but the autosomal-dominant form is more severe and persistent. Type 2 disease differs from hypoaldosteronism in that it is a hypertensive condition. Type 2 pseudohypoaldosteronism is also known as Gordon syndrome or familial hyperkalemic hypertension. It is a mirror image of Gitelman syndrome, with hyperkalemia, metabolic acidosis, and hypercalciuria, although serum magnesium levels are normal.

The first insights into the genes responsible for Gordon syndrome emerged from the discovery that it is associated with mutations in two kinases known as WNK1 and WNK4 (with no lysine [K]). Both are expressed in the DCT and collecting duct. WNK4 downregulates the activity of both the NCCT and the ENaC. Inactivating mutations in *WNK1* result in increased activity of both pathways for sodium reabsorption. WNK4 also regulates the ROMK potassium channel, but mutations that relieve WNK4's inhibition of sodium transport enhance its inhibition of ROMK, contributing to the hyperkalemia in Gordon syndrome. WNK1 is a negative regulator of WNK4, and gain-of-function *WNK1* mutations indirectly increase NCCT activity. Coordinated regulation of distal ion transport by these WNK kinases may explain how the kidney balances the two effects of aldosterone on sodium reabsorption and potassium secretion, and polymorphisms in this pathway may be relevant to the mechanisms of essential hypertension.

More recently, it has been appreciated that the majority of families with Gordon syndrome have mutations not in these WNK proteins but in two genes encoding proteins involved in the degradation of WNK kinases: *CUL3* encoding the Cullin-3 scaffold protein in an ubiquitin-E3 ligase, and *KLHL3* encoding the adaptor protein Kelch3.

OTHER DISORDERS RESEMBLING PRIMARY HYPERALDOSTERONISM

Two other hereditary conditions produce hypertension in children with clinical features resembling primary hyperaldosteronism. The syndrome of apparent mineralocorticoid excess (AME) is an autosomal-recessive disease in which the renal isoform of the 11β-hydroxysteroid dehydrogenase enzyme is inactivated by mutation. In a sense, this is a genetic analogue of the ingestion of black licorice, which contains glycyrrhizic acid that inhibits this enzyme. Inactivation of the enzyme results in failure to convert cortisol to cortisone locally in the collecting duct, allowing cortisol to activate mineralocorticoid receptors and produce a syndrome resembling primary hyperaldosteronism but, like Liddle syndrome, with low circulating levels of aldosterone. AME presents in infancy with low birth weight, failure to thrive, severe hypertension, hypokalemia, metabolic alkalosis, hypercalciuria, and nephrocalcinosis, progressing to kidney failure. As in Liddle syndrome, kidney transplantation has resulted in resolution of hypertension in patients with AME syndrome.

The autosomal-dominant condition known as glucocorticoid-remediable aldosteronism (GRA) is caused by a chromosomal rearrangement that produces a chimeric gene in which the regulatory region of the gene encoding the steroid 11β-hydroxylase (which is part of the cortisol biosynthetic pathway and normally is regulated by adrenocorticotropic hormone [ACTH]) is fused to distal sequences of the aldosterone synthase gene. This results in production of aldosterone that responds to ACTH rather than normal regulatory stimuli. Patients with GRA may have variable elevations in plasma aldosterone levels and are often normokalemic. Aldosterone levels are suppressed by glucocorticoid therapy. Elevated urinary levels of 18-oxacortisol and 18-hydroxycortisol are characteristic of GRA.

HEREDITARY RENAL TUBULAR ACIDOSIS

Secretion of acid by the alpha-intercalated cells of the collecting duct is accomplished by the apical proton-ATPase. Cytosolic carbonic anhydrase catalyzes the formation of bicarbonate from hydroxyl ions, and the bicarbonate then exits the cell in exchange for chloride through the basolateral anion exchanger, AE1 (encoded by the gene *SLC4A1*). Mutations affecting each of these proteins have been documented in patients with hereditary forms of RTA. Autosomal-recessive distal RTA is associated with mutations in the β1 subunit of the proton-ATPase. This form of RTA is often severe, manifesting in young children, and typically is accompanied by hearing loss, consistent with the fact that this ATPase is expressed in the cochlea, endolymphatic sac of the inner ear, and kidney. Other patients with autosomal-recessive distal RTA have mutations in the gene encoding a noncatalytic α_4 isoform of the α accessory subunit of the ATPase, and these patients have less severe or no hearing deficit. Autosomal-dominant RTA, a more mild disease that often is undetected until adulthood, is associated with mutations in the AE1, which is also the band 3 erythrocyte membrane protein. In Asian patients, mutations in the AE1 occur with recessive inheritance of distal RTA and hemolytic anemia.

Other genetic loci appear to be responsible for additional familial cases of distal RTA. Familial deficiency of carbonic anhydrase II is also characterized by cerebral calcification and osteopetrosis, and the latter condition reflects the important role of carbonic anhydrase in osteoclast function. The acidification defect in carbonic anhydrase II deficiency affects bicarbonate reabsorption in the proximal tubule and the collecting duct.

NEPHROGENIC DIABETES INSIPIDUS

Reabsorption of water across the cells of the collecting duct occurs only when arginine vasopressin (AVP) is present. AVP activates V_2 receptors on the principal cells and cells of the inner medullary collecting duct, initiating a cascade that results in fusion of vesicles containing aquaporin 2 (AQP-2) water channel pores into the apical membranes of these cells (Chapter 8). A gene on the X chromosome encodes the V2 receptor, and inactivating mutations in the V2 receptor gene cause the most common form, accounting for 90% of cases of inherited nephrogenic diabetes insipidus. This results in vasopressin-resistant polyuria that typically is more severe in male patients and is associated with impaired responses to the effects of AVP that are mediated by extrarenal V_2 receptors, specifically, vasodilatation and endothelial release of factor VIIIc and von Willebrand factor. Less commonly, families have been described with autosomal-recessive inheritance of nephrogenic diabetes insipidus, and these patients have mutations in the gene encoding AQP-2 that result in either impaired trafficking of water channels to the plasma membrane or defective pore function. Rare autosomal-dominant occurrence of nephrogenic diabetes insipidus with a mutation in AQP-2 has also been reported. Patients with defective aquaporin channels can be distinguished by intact extrarenal responses to exogenous AVP.

KEY BIBLIOGRAPHY

Bockenhauer D, Bichet DG. Pathophysiology, diagnosis and management of nephrogenic diabetes insipidus. *Nat Rev Nephrol.* 2015;11:576-588.

Bockenhauer D, Feather S, Stanescu HC, et al. Epilepsy, ataxia, sensorineural deafness, tubulopathy, and KCNJ10 mutations. *N Engl J Med.* 2009;360:1960-1970.

Fry AC, Karet FE. Inherited renal acidoses. *Physiology (Bethesda).* 2007; 22:202-211.

Goldsweig BK, Carpenter TO. Hypophosphatemic rickets: lessons from disrupted FGF23 control of phosphorus homeostasis. *Curr Osteoporos Rep.* 2015;13:88-97.

Groenestege WM, Thebault S, van der Wijst J, et al. Impaired basolateral sorting of pro-EGF causes isolated recessive renal hypomagnesemia. *J Clin Invest.* 2007;117:2260-2267.

Hannan FM, Babinsky VN, Thakker RV. Disorders of the calcium-sensing receptor and partner proteins: insights into the molecular basis of calcium homeostasis. *J Mol Endocrinol.* 2016;57:127-142.

Hou J, Rajagopal M, Yu AS. Claudins and the kidney. *Annu Rev Physiol.* 2013;75:479-501.

Jonsson KB, Zahradnik R, Larsson T, et al. Fibroblast growth factor 23 in oncogenic osteomalacia and X-linked hypophosphatemia. *N Engl J Med.* 2003;348:1656-1663.

Kahle KT, Ring AM, Lifton RP. Molecular physiology of the WNK kinases. *Annu Rev Physiol.* 2007;70:329-355.

Kleta R, Bockenhauer D. Bartter syndromes and other salt-losing tubulopathies. *Nephron Physiol.* 2006;104:73-80.

Konrad M, Schlingmann KP. Inherited disorders of renal hypomagnesaemia. *Nephrol Dial Transplant.* 2014;29:iv63-iv71.

O'Shaughnessy KM. Gordon syndrome: a continuing story. *Pediatr Nephrol.* 2015;30:1903-1908.

Scheinman SJ. Dent's disease. In: Lifton R, Somlo S, Giebisch G, Seldin D, eds. *Genetic Diseases of the Kidney.* San Diego, CA: Elsevier; 2009.

Scheinman SJ, Guay-Woodford LM, Thakker RV, et al. Genetic disorders of renal electrolyte transport. *N Engl J Med.* 1999;340:1177-1187.

Simon DB, Lu Y, Choate KA, et al. Paracellin-1, a renal tight junction protein required for paracellular Mg resorption. *Science.* 1999;285:103-106.

Torres VE, Scheinman SJ. Genetic diseases of the kidney. *Nephrol Self Assess Program.* 2004; https://www.asn-online.org/education/nephsap/view.aspx?i=V3N1. Accessed July 28, 2017.

Warnock DG. Liddle syndrome: genetics and mechanisms of Na+ channel defects. *Am J Med Sci.* 2001;322:302-307.

Wilson FH, Hariri A, Farhi A, et al. A cluster of metabolic defects caused by mutation in a mitochondrial tRNA. *Science.* 2004;306:1190-1194.

Full bibliography can be found on www.expertconsult.com.

Sickle Cell Nephropathy

39

Vimal K. Derebail

Sickle cell anemia is caused by the homozygous inheritance of the sickle β-globin gene (HbSS), produced by a single point mutation in chromosome 11. The resultant β chain of the hemoglobin molecule possesses a substitution of valine for glutamic acid at position 6, leading to an unstable form of hemoglobin (hemoglobin S). Under conditions of low oxygen tension, acidity, extreme temperatures, and other stressors, the altered hemoglobin undergoes polymerization, leading to the "sickling" of red blood cells (Fig. 39.1). These red cells are rigid, leading to both microvascular obstruction and the activation of inflammation and coagulation. Sickle cell disease (SCD) is also seen in the double heterozygous inheritance of hemoglobin mutations HbS gene and another mutation, such as hemoglobin SCD and sickle β-thalassemia.

The prevalence of sickle cell trait (SCT; HbAS) in the United States is between 6% and 9% among African-Americans, with sickle cell anemia occurring in approximately 1 of 500 African-American live births. In the global population, the prevalence of the hemoglobin S mutation varies greatly and is often highest in areas where malaria is endemic because of the protection it affords against malarial infection. In 2010, an estimated 312,000 neonates were born worldwide with sickle cell anemia.

Although SCD affects multiple systems throughout the body and is characterized by acute pain crises and progressive multiorgan damage, the kidney is a particularly susceptible organ. The renal medulla, with its lower oxygen tension, high osmolarity, lower pH, and relatively sluggish blood flow, is an ideal environment for "sickling" and microvascular obstruction. As a result, kidney manifestations are common in SCD (Table 39.1).

PATHOPHYSIOLOGY

Although the classic understanding of SCD is based on microvascular obstruction, its pathophysiology is better understood in the context of recurrent vasoocclusion with ischemia-reperfusion injury and hemolytic anemia. In addition to triggering hemoglobin polymerization, inflammation and other stressors also initiate erythrocyte adhesion to endothelium and leukocytes, beginning the process of microvascular obstruction. These processes are dynamic, resulting in ischemia followed by the restoration of blood flow and the subsequent reperfusion injury, with resultant oxidative stress and inflammatory cytokine production. Intravascular hemolysis is another contributor to disease burden, with the release of free hemoglobin into the plasma generating

reactive oxygen species and depleting nitric oxide. These processes produce endothelial dysfunction and activate the coagulation system.

Disease severity in SCD appears to be modulated by the relative concentration of sickle hemoglobin (HbS). The presence of fetal hemoglobin (HbF), which can be increased with hydroxyurea therapy, reduces the relative content of hemoglobin S; accordingly, haplotypes of the mutation that correlate with lower HbF production, most notably the Central African Republic haplotype, typically have the most severe disease manifestations. Similarly, coinheritance of α-thalassemia mutations reduces intracellular HbS concentration and leads to reduced hemolysis and fewer complications.

Within the kidney, these pathologic mechanisms lead to changes in kidney hemodynamics, tubulointerstitial damage, and, in some patients, glomerular disease.

KIDNEY HEMODYNAMICS

Glomerular hyperfiltration is extraordinarily common among patients with SCD and can be detected at as early as 13 months of age. Glomerulomegaly is evident even in patients without clinical disease and may contribute to hyperfiltration. Glomerular hyperfiltration is likely driven by vasodilatation of the afferent arteriole, which may occur as a compensatory response to chronic tissue hypoxia in the renal medulla. The exact mechanisms behind this response are not fully known, but it may be mediated by up-regulation of prostaglandins and the nitric oxide systems. Indomethacin and other prostaglandin inhibitors, administered at doses that would not affect the glomerular filtration rate (GFR) in normal individuals, can reduce GFR to more normal values in patients with SCD. Hemolysis and production of free heme may also play a role in the process. Sickle cell animal models have demonstrated that hemolysis induces up-regulation of heme-oxygenase-1 (HO-1) with subsequent production of carbon monoxide (CO), a local vasodilator.

TUBULOINTERSTITIAL DISEASE

IMPAIRED URINARY CONCENTRATION

The most commonly reported kidney manifestation in patients with SCD is the loss of complete urinary concentrating ability. Typically, the generation of concentrated urine requires an intact collecting duct and a medullary concentration gradient.

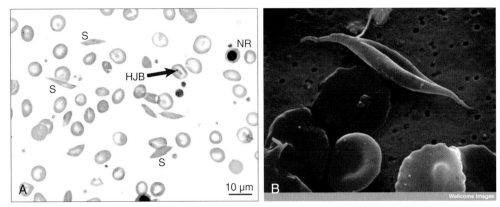

Fig. 39.1 (A) Peripheral blood smear of a patient with sickle cell anemia. This blood film shows irreversibly sickled cells (S), a nucleated red blood cell (NR), and a Howell-Jolly body (HJB); these last two features are mainly associated with hyposplenism (stained with May-Grunwald-Giemsa). (B) Scanning electron microscopic image of sickled and other red blood cells, false-colored red. Photographed with Philips 501 SEM. (A, Reprinted from Rees DC, Williams TN, Gladwin MT. Sickle cell disease. *Lancet.* 2010;376:2018–2031, with permission from Elsevier. B, With permission from EM Unit, UCL Medical School, Royal Free Campus, Wellcome Images.)

Table 39.1 Kidney Pathology in Sickle Cell Disease

Kidney Abnormality	Clinical Consequence
Glomerular	
Hyperfiltration	Increased GFR (early), albuminuria/proteinuria, sickle glomerulopathy, CKD (late)
Proximal Tubule	
Enhanced proximal tubule activity	Increased creatinine secretion, increased phosphate resorption (hyperphosphatemia)
Depressed renin	Hyporeninemic hypoaldosteronism (hyperkalemia)
Distal Tubule/Cortical Collection Duct	
Impaired hydrogen ion secretion	Metabolic acidosis (type 4 RTA)
Impaired potassium secretion	Hyperkalemia
Impaired urinary concentration	Hyposthenuria
Interstitial	
Chronic "sickling" in vasa recta	Hematuria, renal papillary necrosis (due to ischemia), renal medullary carcinoma, CKD

CKD, Chronic kidney disease; *GFR*, glomerular filtration rate; *RTA*, renal tubular acidosis.

The juxtamedullary nephrons, which extend deepest into the medulla and are most capable of producing a high concentration gradient, are also those most likely to be affected by sickling in the medullary vasa recta. Microangiographic studies demonstrate the obliteration of the vasa recta in these patients, with subsequent fibrosis and shortening of the renal papilla. The functional result of these anatomic changes ultimately manifests as an inability to achieve a urinary osmolarity above 400 mOsm/kg. Early in life, this defect is partially reversible following blood transfusions that rapidly increase normal hemoglobin A (HbA) and reduce sickling in the vasa recta. However, impaired urinary concentration becomes fixed later in life (as early as age 15) and no longer improves with transfusion. As a result, depending on water and solute intake, patients with SCD may have obligatory water losses of up to 2.0 L/day, predisposing them to higher serum osmolality and thereby potentially exacerbating sickle crises. The ability to produce a maximally dilute urine and to excrete free water remains intact.

HEMATURIA

Hematuria can be one of the most dramatic kidney presentations in patients with SCD and may range from microscopic hematuria to gross hematuria. Gross hematuria may occur in patients of any age, including young children. Although the etiology of hematuria remains unclear, vasoocclusion occurring in the acidic, hyperosmolar, low oxygen tension environment of the medulla is thought to play a central role. Studies of kidneys removed from sickle cell patients with severe hematuria demonstrate severe stasis of peritubular capillaries, particularly those in the medulla, as well as erythrocytes extravasated into the collecting tubules. In addition to the aforementioned vascular occlusion–mediated ischemia and oxidative/reperfusion injury, sickling in these vessels may also lead to vessel wall injury and necrosis, which could cause the structural changes leading to hematuria.

Typically, hematuria is unilateral and occurs nearly 4 times more often from the left kidney. The longer course and higher venous pressures of the left renal vein as it traverses between the aorta and superior mesenteric artery likely lead to this phenomenon.

Although bleeding is typically benign and self-limited, massive hemorrhage can occur and can be potentially life

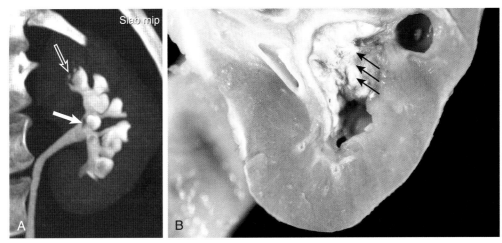

Fig. 39.2 (A) Maximum-intensity-projection (MIP) images from computed tomography urography in a 23-year-old woman with sickle cell trait presenting with intermittent gross hematuria for 5 days. Pooling of contrast material within multiple papillae bilaterally *(open arrow)* is consistent with papillary necrosis. Filling defect within left renal pelvis *(solid arrow)* was shown to represent blood clot at ureteroscopy. (B) Gross photomicrograph of a bivalved kidney demonstrating necrosis of a renal papilla *(arrows)*. Over time, this area will form a scar with cystic dilation of the calices. (A, From Chow LC, Kwan SW, Olcott EW, et al. Split-Bolus MDCT urography with synchronous nephrographic and excretory phase enhancement. *Am J Roentgenol.* 2007;189:314–322. Reprinted with permission from the American Journal of Roentgenology. B, Courtesy Vincent Moylan, Jr., MS, PA(ASCP)^{cm}, Medical Examiner–Orange County, NC, Assistant Professor, Autopsy Services, Department of Pathology and Laboratory Medicine, University of North Carolina at Chapel Hill.)

threatening. Treatment consists of conservative management, including bed-rest and the maintenance of high urine output to prevent clots. Alkalinization of the urine may help by raising medullary pH, thereby reducing sickling; however, no studies have shown a proven benefit of this intervention. Intravenous fluids may be used to ensure high urine flow but must be used with caution in patients at risk for congestive heart failure or acute chest syndrome. Diuretics can also be used to increase urine flow rates, but care must be taken to avoid volume depletion.

For those patients with massive and persistent hematuria despite conservative therapy, ε-aminocaproic acid (EACA) can be beneficial. This agent inhibits fibrinolysis and can induce clotting to halt hematuria. Reports have demonstrated improvement with EACA, although no standard dose regimen or length of therapy has been defined. However, EACA can be prothrombotic; accordingly, it must be used with caution in SCD patients who are already at risk for thrombotic events. Currently, EACA use is recommended only for a limited period and at the lowest dose necessary to achieve inhibition of urinary fibrinolytic activity. In addition to EACA, intravenous vasopressin to limit hematuria has been successful in case reports.

In patients who are refractory to medical therapy, invasive intervention may be necessary. If a source of bleeding can be localized via imaging, percutaneous embolization can be attempted. In rare cases, unilateral nephrectomy of the affected kidney may be required. In all patients presenting with hematuria, and particularly in those with persistent or massive hematuria, alternative causes should be considered, including acquired or hereditary bleeding disorders or abnormalities, such as nephrolithiasis, polycystic kidney disease, or renal medullary carcinoma (RMC; see next sections).

RENAL PAPILLARY NECROSIS

Renal papillary necrosis (RPN) is fairly common in SCD, occurring in more than 60% of patients in some series. Although often accompanied by hematuria, a similar proportion of patients may be asymptomatic. With severe sickling in the vasa recta, the renal papillae that depend on these vessels can undergo focal, repetitive infarcts leading to necrosis (Fig. 39.2). If hematuria is present, as described earlier, patients should undergo an evaluation for other potential causes, including kidney masses or nephrolithiasis. This imaging can be performed with ultrasonography, although a helical computed tomography (CT) scan may detect RPN earlier. In many patients, RPN ultimately results in calcification around the renal pelvis. Treatment, as with hematuria, is generally supportive, using similar measures. If significant sloughing occurs, necrotic and thrombotic material may lead to ureteral obstruction, which can be diagnosed by urography and relieved by stenting.

RENAL MEDULLARY CARCINOMA

RMC is extremely rare and seen almost exclusively in patients with SCT, although there are a few reports in patients with SCD (<10% of cases). The vast majority of cases have been reported in patients younger than 40 years of age, with a mean age of presentation of 24 years. Men appear to be affected more than twice as often as women. In contradistinction to hematuria and papillary necrosis, RMC has a predilection for the right kidney (>70% of cases). The typical presentation is gross hematuria, often painless but sometimes accompanied by flank or lumbar pain or abdominal masses. Malignant constitutional symptoms of weight loss, fevers, and fatigue may be present. Repetitive ischemic injuries to the tubules are postulated to drive the development of this lesion. Loss of SMARCB1, a component of chromatin remodeling and a tumor suppressor gene, has recently been identified as a feature of RMC. Regrettably, this malignancy is often metastatic at diagnosis, with survival of only 6 to 12 months and mortality of nearly 95% even with treatment. For these reasons, presentation of gross hematuria in patients with SCT or SCD should prompt consideration of imaging via ultrasonography or preferably CT scan to allow early diagnosis.

ACIDIFICATION, POTASSIUM EXCRETION, AND OTHER TUBULAR ABNORMALITIES

Acidosis is fairly uncommon in patients with SCD in the absence of kidney failure, although some patients may manifest an incomplete distal renal tubular acidosis (dRTA). Hyperkalemia may accompany this; however, this is rare without significant potassium ingestion or medications that interfere with potassium handling. The inability of the damaged distal nephron to excrete ammonium and titratable acids, as well as an inability to respond to aldosterone, lead to these findings. If necessary, treatment with potassium restriction, sodium bicarbonate, and loop diuretics can be effective.

The aforementioned abnormalities generally indicate impaired distal tubule secretory function. In contrast, the proximal tubule demonstrates enhanced activity. Sodium reabsorption is increased, leading to less urinary excretion, as well as a relative resistance to loop diuretics. Accompanying this increase in sodium reabsorption is an enhancement of proximal phosphate reabsorption that may cause hyperphosphatemia in settings of increased phosphorus loads (hemolysis, rhabdomyolysis). In addition, uric acid secretion is increased, perhaps as an adaptive mechanism to the increased uric acid load from chronic hemolysis. Finally, secretion of creatinine in the proximal tubule is also heightened, diminishing the usefulness of creatinine clearance and creatinine-based equations to estimate GFR.

SICKLE CELL GLOMERULOPATHY

The presence of glomerular involvement has long been noted in SCD, with levels of proteinuria ranging from low-level albuminuria to overt nephrotic syndrome. Initial reports of glomerular lesions were those of immune complex deposition and pathology consistent with membranoproliferative glomerulonephritis. However, more recent studies have demonstrated glomerulomegaly and development of focal segmental glomerulosclerosis (FSGS) in the majority of patients with sickle cell nephropathy. As in other forms of FSGS, immunofluorescence of biopsy samples may demonstrate minimal staining with immunoglobulin M (IgM), C1q, and C3, but electron microscopy usually fails to identify any electron-dense deposits. Collapsing lesions have also been reported, presumably due to vascular occlusion and ischemia. Hemosiderin deposition is often prominent in tubular epithelium but also may be present focally in glomerular epithelial cells (Figs. 39.3 and 39.4). Sickled erythrocytes are often noted in medullary vasculature and less commonly in glomeruli. The clinical sequelae of these composite lesions are

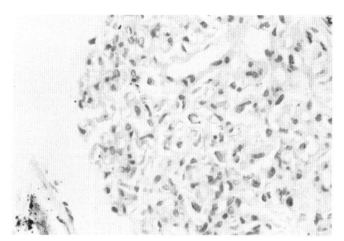

Fig. 39.3 Sickle cell nephropathy with iron deposits in glomerular visceral epithelial cells and tubular epithelial cells (*bottom left corner*; Prussian blue iron stain). (Reproduced with permission from *Am J Kidney Dis*. 2016;68[1]:e1–e3.)

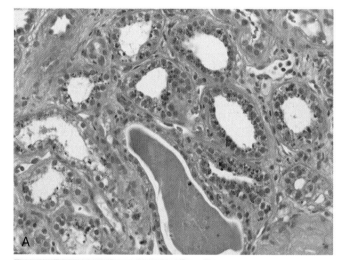

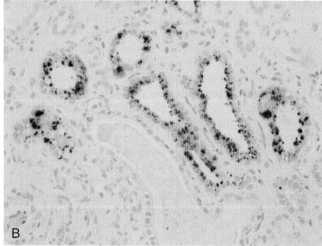

Fig. 39.4 Sickle cell nephropathy with hemosiderin in tubular epithelial cells (A, hematoxylin and eosin stain) that shows positivity by iron stain (B, Prussian blue iron stain). (Reproduced with permission from *Am J Kidney Dis*. 2016;68:e1–e3.)

thought to begin with albuminuria and evolve into overt proteinuria, loss of kidney function, and advanced chronic kidney disease (CKD).

ALBUMINURIA AND PROTEINURIA

The development of albuminuria and overt proteinuria clearly increases as patients with SCD age, with more than 60% of adults over the age of 35 exhibiting low-level albuminuria. However, children below the age of 10 rarely demonstrate this finding. Over 20% of adults with low-level albuminuria will progress to overt proteinuria and progressive GFR decline. The nephrotic syndrome itself is fairly rare, but it portends a poor kidney prognosis. An uncommon but well-recognized cause of acute onset of the nephrotic syndrome is parvovirus B19 infection, which often leads to the collapsing variant of FSGS. Abnormalities in albumin excretion are more frequent in sickle cell anemia (HbSS disease) and in sickle-β^0-thalassemia than in other sickle hemoglobinopathies (HbSC disease, HbS-β^+-thalassemia).

The severity of SCD in some series does seem to correlate with the development of albuminuria. Lower hemoglobin levels and pulmonary hypertension may be associated with the development of albuminuria. Finally, as with many other manifestations of SCD, coinheritance of α-thalassemia may attenuate the development of sickle glomerulopathy.

The underlying pathophysiology of albuminuria is multifactorial and probably related to a variety of pathologic developments in SCD. Persistence of glomerular hyperfiltration, as in other diseases with this feature, results in albuminuria and eventual GFR decline. As repetitive sickling occurs and interstitial fibrosis leads to the dropout of affected nephrons, hyperfiltration is further accentuated in the remaining glomeruli. In addition, evidence suggests that endothelial dysfunction from both direct injury related to sickling and the release of free heme during hemolysis contributes to the glomerulopathy. Subsequently, markers of hemolysis, such as reticulocyte hemoglobin and lactate dehydrogenase (LDH) may correlate with albuminuria, as do mediators of endothelial dysfunction including soluble fms-like tyrosine kinase-1 (sFLT-1). Endothelin-1 (ET-1) also appears to mediate glomerular injury via reactive oxygen species.

TREATMENT

Therapies for reducing albuminuria and proteinuria have been advocated in the hope of delaying the progression of CKD, although little prospective data exists to determine whether any therapy is truly effective. As with many diseases in which proteinuria is a feature, inhibition of the renin-angiotensin-aldosterone system forms the mainstay of therapy. Several studies have demonstrated a short-term reduction in both proteinuria and hyperfiltration with the use of angiotensin-converting enzyme (ACE) inhibitors. These effects seem to be independent of any blood pressure lowering and are likely related to the reduction of glomerular capillary hypertension. Current guidelines suggest screening for proteinuria beginning at age 10 and then annually if negative. If detected, renin-angiotensin blockade should be initiated. With the institution and dose titration of these agents, both kidney function and serum potassium must be monitored closely, because SCD patients are prone to the metabolic effects of reduced estimated glomerular filtration rate (eGFR) and impaired potassium secretion.

Hydroxyurea, or hydroxycarbamide, is indicated in SCD for those patients with acute chest syndrome, frequent pain crises, and vasoocclusive episodes. Its role in the management of albuminuria and CKD is less well defined. The mechanism of action is not completely understood but is in part due to the ability of hydroxyurea to induce HbF production and thereby reduce the overall concentration of hemoglobin S. Hydroxyurea may also affect the synthesis of nitric oxide and has other beneficial effects. Small studies have demonstrated that the addition of hydroxyurea to ACE inhibitors may provide further reduction in proteinuria. Other data have been conflicting regarding hydroxyurea use in the prevention of hyperfiltration in children with SCD. However, recent cross-sectional data and interventional studies in adults with SCD have demonstrated hydroxyurea may be associated with a reduction in albuminuria. At present, albuminuria alone in SCD is not a clear indication for hydroxyurea, but its use should be considered particularly in the setting of more traditional indications such as frequent pain crises, acute chest syndrome, or particularly severe anemia.

MANAGEMENT OF CHRONIC KIDNEY DISEASE IN SICKLE CELL DISEASE

Identification of reduced kidney function in the setting of SCD has been increasingly recognized to be somewhat difficult. Traditional methods with serum creatinine to estimate GFR are hampered in SCD because of the enhanced secretion of creatinine. Typical estimating equations when compared with radionucleotide measures of GFR demonstrated significant bias. The CKD-EPI equation seems to afford the best assessment of eGFR, although it still overestimates GFR by typically 45 mL/min per 1.73 m². Creatinine may therefore be a late indicator of CKD in patients with SCD.

The management of SCD patients who have CKD is similar to patients with CKD due to other causes, with a few exceptions. The first relates to the management of anemia. With chronic ischemic kidney insults and ongoing hemolysis, SCD patients typically have a greater stimulus for erythropoietin and exhibit higher endogenous erythropoietin levels. However, with progressive kidney disease, these patients begin to lose the ability to produce adequate endogenous erythropoietin, typically occurring when GFR falls below 60 mL/min. As with other forms of CKD, erythropoiesis-stimulating agents (ESAs) may be used to maintain hemoglobin levels and reduce the need for transfusion. SCD patients with CKD are likely to require very large doses of ESAs, and the target hemoglobin is different from what is typical in other CKD or ESKD populations. In general, a maximum achieved hemoglobin level of 10 mg/dL is recommended to avoid precipitation of vasoocclusive crises. Iron stores should be maintained to maximize erythropoiesis in those not receiving chronic transfusions, although care must be taken to avoid iron overload in this susceptible population.

Finally, even though patients with SCD are at greater risk for advanced CKD, hypertension is an uncommon feature in this population. Despite a prevalence of hypertension of 28% in the general African-American population, only about 2% to 6% of African-Americans with SCD exhibit hypertension. Various explanations for this finding have been posited, including relative volume depletion and reduced systemic vascular resistance. If hypertension is detected in patients with SCD, therapy should be initiated as in any patient with CKD or at risk for CKD. Most would consider a goal blood pressure of 130/80 mm Hg reasonable. Some suggest avoidance of diuretics given their predisposition to volume depletion, which can induce a pain crisis.

END-STAGE KIDNEY DISEASE IN SICKLE CELL DISEASE

Once patients with SCD reach ESKD, either peritoneal dialysis or hemodialysis presents viable options for kidney replacement therapy. Early referral to a nephrologist is particularly important for this population of patients. In data from the Centers for Medicare and Medicaid Services (CMS), mortality after reaching ESKD for those with SCD was 26% in the first year alone. European data suggest mortality may not be as pronounced but is still twofold higher than the non-SCD population.

Although SCD patients are less likely to be listed for kidney transplantation and less likely to receive a transplant, this option for kidney replacement therapy does appear to offer survival benefit similar to other forms of CKD. In the more recent era of kidney transplantation, the 6-year survival of SCD patients receiving kidney transplantation has approached 70% (compared with ~55% in earlier reports). Overall mortality for SCD kidney transplant recipients is now comparable to that of patients with diabetes. Further, the likelihood of graft failure does not seem to be greater in SCD recipients. After transplantation, SCD patients must be monitored for allograft thrombosis, an increase in vasoocclusive crises, and a recurrence of sickle glomerulopathy, which has been reported as early as 3 years after transplantation. Hydroxyurea and exchange transfusion have been used in the posttransplant period, and simultaneous bone marrow transplantation could be curative of the disease as a whole.

SICKLE CELL TRAIT

Patients with a single hemoglobin S mutation are deemed to have SCT, HbAS. Although generally viewed as a benign condition, SCT does have manifestations more akin to an intermediate phenotype. Kidney manifestations are by far the most commonly reported comorbidities in SCT and are similar to those seen in SCD.

Impaired urinary concentration is common, albeit not as severe as that seen in SCD. Again, the severity of the concentrating defect seems to be modulated by the coinheritance of α-thalassemia. Hematuria and RPN also occur in this population. As noted earlier, RMC, rarely described in SCD, has been nearly exclusively reported in patients with SCT.

With its numerous reported kidney abnormalities, speculation as to whether SCT contributes to the development of CKD has been longstanding. An early study demonstrated an acceleration of progression to ESKD among those with concurrent SCT and adult polycystic kidney disease (ADPKD),

and another small study has noted a high prevalence of SCT in the African-American ESKD population. Although there have been other conflicting reports, a recent population-based study of over 15,000 African-Americans has shown SCT to be associated with incident and prevalent CKD and albuminuria. This latter finding has provided more definitive evidence that SCT may be a risk factor for CKD.

KEY BIBLIOGRAPHY

Alvarez O, Miller ST, Wang WC, et al. Effect of hydroxyurea treatment on renal function parameters: results from the multi-center placebo-controlled BABY HUG clinical trial for infants with sickle cell anemia. *Pediatr Blood Cancer.* 2012;59:668-674.

Alvarez O, Rodriguez MM, Jordan L, et al. Renal medullary carcinoma and sickle cell trait: a systematic review. *Pediatr Blood Cancer.* 2015;62:1694-1699.

Asnani MR, Lynch O, Reid ME. Determining glomerular filtration rate in homozygous sickle cell disease: utility of serum creatinine based estimating equations. *PLoS ONE.* 2013;8:e69922.

Ataga KI, Derebail VK, Archer DR. The glomerulopathy of sickle cell disease. *Am J Hematol.* 2014;89:907-914.

Aygun B, Mortier NA, Smeltzer MP, et al. Hydroxyurea treatment decreases glomerular hyperfiltration in children with sickle cell anemia. *Am J Hematol.* 2013;88:116-119.

Bartolucci P, Habibi A, Stehlé T, et al. Six months of hydroxyurea reduces albuminuria in patients with sickle cell disease. *J Am Soc Nephrol.* 2016;27:1847-1853.

Boyle SM, Jacobs B, Sayani FA, et al. Management of the dialysis patient with sickle cell disease. *Semin Dial.* 2016;29:62-70.

Calderaro J, Masliah-Planchon J, Richer W, et al. Balanced translocations disrupting SMARCB1 are hallmark recurrent genetic alterations in renal medullary carcinomas. *Eur Urol.* 2016;69:1055-1061.

Day TG, Drasar ER, Fulford T, et al. Association between hemolysis and albuminuria in adults with sickle cell anemia. *Haematologica.* 2012;97:201-205.

Derebail VK, Nachman PH, Key NS, et al. High prevalence of sickle cell trait in African Americans with ESRD. *J Am Soc Nephrol.* 2010;21:413-417.

Guasch A, Navarrete J, Nass K, et al. Glomerular involvement in adults with sickle cell hemoglobinopathies: prevalence and clinical correlates of progressive renal failure. *J Am Soc Nephrol.* 2016;17:2228-2235.

Heimlich JB, Speed JS, O'Connor PM, et al. Endothelin-1 contributes to the progression of renal injury in sickle cell disease via reactive oxygen species. *Br J Pharmacol.* 2016;173(2):386-395.

Huang E, Parke C, Mehrnia A, et al. Improved survival among sickle cell kidney transplant recipients in the recent era. *Nephrol Dial Transplant.* 2013;28:1039-1046.

Key NS, Connes P. Derebail V.K. Negative health implications of sickle cell trait in high income countries: from the football field to the laboratory. *Br J Haematol.* 2015;170:5-14.

Lusco MA, Fogo AB, Najafian B, et al. AJKD atlas of renal pathology: sickle cell nephropathy. *Am J Kidney Dis.* 2016;68:e1-e3.

McClellan AC, Luthi JC, Lynch JR, et al. High one year mortality in adults with sickle cell disease and end-stage renal disease. *Br J Haematol.* 2012;159:360-367.

Nath KA, Hebbel RP. Sickle cell disease: renal manifestations and mechanisms. *Nat Rev Nephrol.* 2015;11:161-171.

Naik RP, Derebail VK, Grams ME, et al. Association of sickle cell trait with chronic kidney disease and albuminuria in African Americans. *JAMA.* 2014;312:2115-2125.

Nielsen L, Canoui-Poitrine F, Jais JP, et al. Morbidity and mortality of sickle cell disease patients starting intermittent haemodialysis: a comparative cohort study with non-sickle dialysis patients. *Br J Haematol.* 2016;174:148-152.

U.S. Department of Health and Human Services, National Institutes of Health, National Heart, Lung, and Blood Institute. 2014. *Evidence-based management of sickle cell disease: expert panel report.* Retrieved from https://www.nhlbi.nih.gov/sites/www.nhlbi.nih.gov/files/sickle-cell-disease-report.pdf.

Full bibliography can be found on www.expertconsult.com.

40

Polycystic and Other Cystic Kidney Diseases

Dana V. Rizk; Bharathi Reddy; Arlene B. Chapman

Significant advances have been made in understanding the genetic and molecular pathogenesis of inherited cystic disorders of the kidney. Many of the genes and their respective proteins have been identified (Table 40.1). Final common pathways regarding the formation and development of cysts are being elucidated. Most kidney cysts develop because of abnormal function of the primary cilium that resides in all epithelial cells. Recently developed, molecularly targeted therapies offer hope for improved outcome or cure of these disorders.

AUTOSOMAL DOMINANT POLYCYSTIC KIDNEY DISEASE

Autosomal dominant polycystic kidney disease (ADPKD) is the most common inherited kidney disorder, occurring in 1 of 400 to 1000 live births. ADPKD affects all ethnic groups equally, and it has been reported worldwide. It accounts for approximately 5% of the end-stage kidney disease (ESKD) population in the United States and 10% of those under 60 years of age. ADPKD is a systemic disorder that affects almost every organ resulting in significant extrarenal manifestations; however, its hallmark is the gradual and massive cystic enlargement of the kidneys, ultimately resulting in kidney failure.

PATHOGENESIS

At least three genes have been implicated in the pathogenesis of ADPKD. Approximately 85% of patients with ADPKD have mutations in the *PKD1* gene, close to 15% of ADPKD patients have mutations in the *PKD2* gene, and approximately 1% of patients are found to have mutations in the *GANAB* gene. Although mutations in *PKD1* and *PKD2* lead to the same phenotype, patients with *PKD2* mutations have milder disease with fewer kidney cysts, later onset of hypertension, and less ESKD than their counterparts with *PKD1* mutations (median age of onset of ESKD 74 vs. 54 years, respectively). Given the milder phenotype associated with *PKD2*, when surveillance autopsies are performed, the relative frequency of *PKD2* increases, accounting for up to 27% of all ADPKD cases. *GANAB* mutation cases are still relatively rarely reported; however, they appear to have a milder phenotype than *PKD1* with hepatic cystic disease predominating.

PKD1 is located on the short arm of chromosome 16 (16p13.3) and codes for polycystin-1 (PC1), an integral membrane protein made up of 4304 amino acids. PC1 has a large extracellular N-terminal, 11 transmembrane regions, and a short intracellular C-terminal. PC1 is located in the primary cilium, focal adhesions, tight junctions, desmosomes,

and adherens junctions. PC1 plays an important role in cell-cell interactions and cell-matrix interactions. *PKD2* is located on the long arm of chromosome 4 (4q12.2) and encodes for polycystin-2 (PC2), a 968 amino acid protein with a short cytoplasmic N-terminal, six transmembrane regions, and a short cytoplasmic C-terminal. It localizes to the endoplasmic reticulum, plasma membrane, primary cilium, centrosome, and mitotic spindles in dividing cells. PC2 belongs to the family of voltage-activated calcium channels (e.g., transient receptor potential polycystin-2 [TRPP-2]) and is involved in intracellular calcium regulation through several pathways. PC1 and PC2 are colocalized in the primary cilium of renal epithelial cells, which functions as a mechanosensor. Primary cilia create transmembrane calcium currents in the presence of stretch or luminal flow. PC1 and PC2 contribute to ciliary function, and the physical interaction between PC1 and PC2 is required for a membrane calcium channel to operate properly. Normal polycystin function increases intracellular calcium, which initiates a signaling cascade leading to vesicle fusion and a change in gene transcription. The magnitude of these changes contributing to the PKD epithelial phenotype has recently been challenged because the reservoir of calcium released from primary ciliary stimulation is relatively low.

Each polycystin affects cell proliferation, differentiation, and fluid secretion through G protein or JAK-STAT-mediated signaling pathways. The interaction of PC1 ligand on the basolateral surface with adenylate cyclase and the G protein–coupled response of adenylate cyclase to binding of vasopressin to the vasopressin V_2 receptor produce similar results. Both result in increased intracellular concentrations of cyclic adenosine monophosphate (cAMP) and ultimately in chloride secretion across the luminal membrane. This chloride-rich fluid secretion is a critical component of cystogenesis, enabling expansion of cysts even after they detach from their parent nephron. The accumulation of cyst fluid, rich in chloride and sodium, relies on the active luminal excretion of chloride primarily through the cystic fibrosis transmembrane conductor regulator (CFTR) (Fig. 40.1).

ADPKD cystic disease is focal, with less than 5% of all nephrons becoming cystic. It is thought that each kidney cyst is derived from a single, clonal hyperproliferative epithelial cell that has genetically transformed. The clonal cystic epithelia proliferate because of an additional somatic mutation in the *PKD1* or *PKD2* gene, indicating that a "second hit" is involved in cyst growth and development. Epithelial cell proliferation, fluid secretion, and alterations in extracellular matrix ultimately result in focal out-pouching from the parent nephron. Most cysts detach from the parent nephron when cyst size exceeds 2 cm and continue to secrete fluid

Table 40.1 Genes and Proteins of Inherited Cystic Disorders of the Kidney

Disease	Frequency	Chromosome	Gene Locus	Protein	Function
ADPKD	1:1000	16p13.3	PKD1	Polycystin 1, which colocalizes with polycystin 2 in the primary cilium	Regulates intracellular cAMP, mTOR, planar polarity
	1:15,000	4q21.2	PKD2	Polycystin 2, which colocalizes with polycystin 1 in the primary cilium and ER	Regulates intracellular Ca levels through ER Ca release, activates Ca channels
ARPKD	1:20,000	6q24.2	PKHD	Fibrocystin or polyductin, located throughout the primary cilium	Serves as receptor to maintain intracellular cAMP levels
VHL	1:36,000	3p25	VHL	VHL, located at the base of the primary cilium	Inhibits HIF-1α and cell turnover, maintains planar polarity, allows ciliogenesis
TSC	1:6000	9q34.3	TSC1	Hamartin	Interacts with tuberin to suppress mTOR activity
		16p13.3	TSC2	Tuberin	Interacts with hamartin to suppress mTOR activity

ADPKD, Autosomal dominant polycystic kidney disease; *ARPKD,* autosomal recessive polycystic kidney disease; *cAMP,* cyclic adenosine monophosphate; *ER,* endoplasmic reticulum; *HIF,* hypoxia inducible factor; *mTOR,* mammalian target of rapamycin; *PKHD,* polycystic kidney and hepatic disease; *TSC,* tuberous sclerosis complex; *VHL,* von Hippel-Lindau.

autonomously, resulting in cyst and kidney enlargement, and ultimately progressive loss of kidney function.

DIAGNOSIS

Kidney imaging by ultrasound remains the primary method for diagnosing ADPKD. The characteristic findings include enlarged kidneys and the presence of multiple cysts throughout the kidney parenchyma (Fig. 40.2). Unified diagnostic ultrasonographic criteria for at-risk individuals independent of genotype were developed by Pei and colleagues in 2009. In individuals aged 15 to 39, the presence of at least three (unilateral or bilateral) kidney cysts is sufficient to establish a diagnosis of ADPKD. In those individuals 40 to 59 years of age, two cysts in each kidney are required, and in those older than 60, in whom acquired cystic disease is common, four or more cysts in each kidney are required for diagnosis. For patients with no family history, the diagnostic criteria are more stringent with at least five cysts bilaterally by the age of 30 and a phenotype consistent with ADPKD required (see later).

When disease status must be determined with certainty, as when an at-risk family member is being evaluated as a potential kidney donor or for family-planning purposes, then initial computed tomography (CT) or magnetic resonance imaging (MRI) should be pursued. Genetic testing should also be considered in young individuals under the age of 40 if imaging is negative. Mutation screening with direct sequencing of the *PKD1* or *PKD2* genes is commercially available. Both the high cost of the test and its ability to detect mutations in only up to 85% of individuals restrict its use. After a genetic diagnosis is confirmed in a patient, which often requires a diagnosis in other affected members, other at-risk family members can be screened at a reduced cost by performing targeted exon-specific sequencing of the identified mutation. Current mutation detection rates are up to 86% and 95% for *PKD1* and *PKD2* genes, respectively.

KIDNEY MANIFESTATIONS AND COMPLICATIONS

Kidney enlargement is a universal feature of ADPKD, and individuals with multiple cysts in small kidneys should be screened for other cystic diseases. Kidney function among ADPKD patients remains normal for decades despite significant cyst expansion and kidney enlargement. After kidney function becomes impaired, progression is typically universal and rapid, with an average decline in glomerular filtration rate (GFR) of 4.0 to 5.0 mL/min/year. There are a number of clinical and genetic predictors for progression to ESKD in ADPKD, such as male sex, *PKD1* genotype, early age onset of hypertension, and the presence of detectable proteinuria. Total kidney volume incorporates all of the aforementioned risk factors and is the strongest predictor of future GFR loss. Significant progression of cyst growth and kidney enlargement precedes the loss of kidney function by decades in ADPKD. In the Consortium for Radiologic Imaging in the Study of Polycystic Kidney Disease (CRISP), a large multicenter study of 241 ADPKD patients with intact kidney function, patients were followed prospectively with serial MRI of their kidneys and demonstrated a 5.2%/year increase in kidney volume. Cysts accounted for the increase in total kidney volume seen, and kidney volume increased at a continuous rate resulting in an overall increase of approximately 55% over 8 years. *PKD2* patients had smaller kidney volumes at baseline (694 ± 221 vs. 986 ± 204 mL) and lower age-adjusted cyst number per kidney when compared with *PKD1* patients but demonstrated similar rates of growth (4.9 ± 2.3% vs. 5.2 ± 1.6%/year), indicating that the rate of cyst formation and cyst number rather than the rate of cyst expansion differs between the two genotypes. More recently, data from the CRISP study showed that height-adjusted total kidney volume (HtTKV) of greater than 600 mL/m accurately predicted progression to CKD stage 3 within 8 years. For each 100 mL/m change in HtTKV, there was a 48% relative risk of reaching CKD stage 3. Therefore total kidney volume is a good predictive

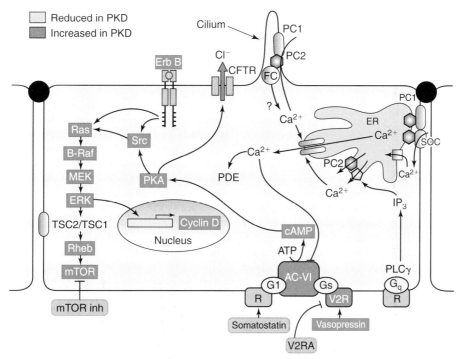

Fig. 40.1 Renal tubular epithelial cell showing location and interactions of polycystin 1 and polycystin 2. *(Top)* The luminal surface with a single cilium. *(Both sides and bottom)* The basolateral surfaces. Mutations in PC1 *(gold ovals)* or PC2 *(blue hexagons)* result in changes in the intracellular calcium level or increases in the level of cAMP. A change in the balance of these two critical intracellular components leads to alterations in the Ras pathway, the mTOR pathway, cell turnover, apoptosis, and fluid secretion through the CFTR channel. Mutations in PC1 and PC2 colocalize to the primary cilium and the basolateral membranes. PC2 resides alone in the ER. G-coupled receptor activation increases the concentration of cAMP. Interference with G-coupled receptor processes can return the increased cAMP level seen in ADPKD to normal. Blockade of the vasopressin 2 (V_2) receptor by a V_2 receptor antagonist is one example. PC1 interacts with the tuberous sclerosis complex proteins (TSC2 and TSC1) regulating the mTOR pathway. Therapies aimed at reducing G-coupled receptor, EGF receptor, CFTR channel, mTOR, and cyclin activity or increasing ER release of calcium may normalize epithelial cell function in ADPKD. *AC-VI,* Adenylate cyclase; *ADPKD,* autosomal dominant polycystic kidney disease; *B-Raf,* proto-oncogene serine/threonine-protein kinase; *cAMP,* cyclic adenosine monophosphate; *CFTR,* cystic fibrosis transmembrane conductance regulator; *EGF,* epithelial growth factor; *ER,* endoplasmic reticulum; *Erb,* epidermal growth factor (erythroblastic leukemia, viral); *ERK,* extracellular signal-regulated kinase; *Inh,* inhibitor; *IP_3,* inositol triphosphate; *MEK,* mitogen signal-regulated kinase; *mTOR,* mammalian target of rapamycin; *PC1,* polycystin 1; *PC2,* polycystin 2; *PDE,* phosphodiesterase; *PKA,* phosphokinase A; *PKD,* polycystic kidney disease; *R,* receptor; *Ras,* renin-angiotensin system; *Rheb,* Ras homolog enriched in brain; *SOC,* store-operated channels; *Src,* nonreceptor (cytoplasmic) protein tyrosine kinase; *V2R,* vasopressin V_2 receptor; *V2RA,* vasopressin V_2 receptor antagonist.

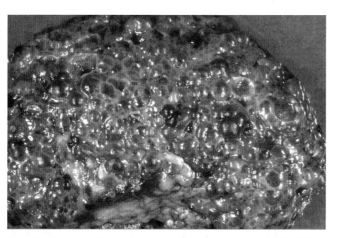

Fig. 40.2 Gross pathology of autosomal dominant polycystic kidney disease kidney.

biomarker for the development of future CKD, with potential application for risk stratification in clinical practice. Patients can now be classified into risk classes (1A to 1E) based on age, sex, serum creatinine, and measured HtTKV. Patients in class 1A and 1B are at a low risk for loss of kidney function, and patients in class 1C to 1E are at a high risk for kidney function loss and would benefit from aggressive monitoring with regard to blood pressure and diet and potentially from participating in clinical trials. TKV can be measured by ultrasound; however, ultrasound measurements are less precise, and TKV measurements are inaccurate when used over short periods of time. US measurements use the ellipsoid formula where maximum length, width, and depth are determined. This approach typically overestimates the TKV by close to 11%. Because of its lack of precision, ultrasound cannot be used to measure short-term disease progression, but single measurements can be used for risk stratification.

Similar to MRI, ultrasound measured HtTKV of greater than 650 mL/m or simply a kidney length over 16.5 cm predicts the development of CKD stage 3 within 8 years.

Hematuria, whether gross or microscopic, occurs in about 35% to 50% of patients and often precedes loss of kidney function. It is associated with increased kidney size and with worse kidney outcomes. Hematuria can be precipitated by an acute event such as trauma, heavy exertion, cyst rupture, lower urinary tract infection, pyelonephritis, cyst infection, or nephrolithiasis. Therefore ADPKD patients are typically advised to avoid heavy and high-impact exercise. Cyst hemorrhage occurs more commonly as kidneys enlarge and may be associated with hematuria and fever. However, localized pain is often the only presenting complaint. The diagnosis of a cyst hemorrhage is based on clinical evaluation and can be difficult to differentiate from kidney cyst infection. CT scan occasionally can be helpful in locating hemorrhagic cysts. The management for uncomplicated cyst hemorrhage and hematuria is supportive and includes fluid resuscitation, rest, pain control, and often withholding antihypertensive medications until the acute episode has resolved.

Lower urinary tract infections are common among ADPKD patients, as in the general population, with coliforms being the most common pathogens. The treatment is the same as in the general population. Pyelonephritis and kidney cyst infections can occur and may be challenging to differentiate. Patients with cyst infection commonly present with fever, abdominal pain, and, often, elevated C-reactive protein. Typically, blood cultures identify the offending pathogen more frequently than urine cultures. Most important, treatment of cyst infections requires a prolonged 4-week course of antibiotics that adequately penetrate into the cyst, such as quinolones, vancomycin, chloramphenicol, or trimethoprim-sulfamethoxazole. Recent reports have suggested that positron emission tomography with fluorodeoxyglucose (FDG-PET) may be a promising diagnostic tool for detecting infected cysts in challenging cases.

The incidence of nephrolithiasis is about 5 to 10 times higher among patients with ADPKD compared with the general population. About 25% of those afflicted with kidney stones are symptomatic. Increased urinary stasis and metabolic disturbances, including hypocitraturia, low urinary pH, and abnormal renal transport of ammonium, account for the high incidence of nephrolithiasis. The most common stone type in ADPKD is uric acid, responsible for approximately 50% of all stones, followed by calcium oxalate. Nephrolithiasis should be suspected in any ADPKD patient with acute flank pain. Diagnosis by imaging is difficult given the radiolucent nature of the stones and the presence of calcified cyst walls. Noncontrast CT remains the imaging modality of choice for detecting nephrolithiasis. The medical management of nephrolithiasis in ADPKD is similar to that in non-ADPKD patients. Noninvasive or minimally invasive interventions such as extracorporeal shock-wave lithotripsy and percutaneous nephrolithotomy have been performed on ADPKD patients; however, long-term studies regarding safety in this patient population are lacking.

Patients with ADPKD commonly complain of increased thirst, polyuria, nocturia, and urinary frequency. A decrease in urinary concentrating ability is one of the earliest manifestations of ADPKD. It is initially mild and worsens with increasing age and declining kidney function. The urinary concentrating defect is closely related to the severity of anatomic deformities induced by the cysts, independent of age and GFR. Approximately 60% of affected children demonstrated a decreased response to desmopressin, possibly because of disruption of tubular architecture and alterations in principal cell function.

Proteinuria is typically mild in ADPKD with an average of 260 mg of protein excretion per day, and only 18% of ADPKD adults have detectable proteinuria on dipstick or greater than 300 mg/day of protein excretion. Although the level of proteinuria is low-grade in ADPKD, the presence of proteinuria and albuminuria is associated with increased TKV and more rapid decline in kidney function.

Pain is the most common symptom in ADPKD and can be acute or chronic. Acute pain episodes are usually related to cyst rupture or hemorrhage, cyst or parenchymal infection, or nephrolithiasis. Chronic pain, on the other hand, is typically related to the massive enlargement of the kidneys and liver and their increased weight. The site of pain can be in the lower back as increased lumbar lordosis has been observed in ADPKD patients. Pain can also result from the stretching of the renal capsule or pedicle. Pain management can be challenging but should include nonpharmacologic as well as pharmacologic interventions.

Hypertension is a common and early manifestation of ADPKD affecting more than 60% of patients before any detectable decline in kidney function. Hypertension is the cause for diagnosis of ADPKD in approximately 30% of cases, with the average age of onset being 29 years. Studies show that hypertension occurs earlier and tends to be more severe among *PKD1* versus *PKD2* patients. Hypertension is also associated with a greater rate of kidney enlargement (6.2%/year vs. 4.5%/year), suggesting a relationship between cyst expansion and elevations in blood pressure. Hypertension is associated with worse kidney outcomes and increased cardiovascular morbidity and mortality. ADPKD kidneys have an attenuated vasculature with angiographic evidence of intrarenal arteriolar tapering. MRI-based measurements demonstrate a reduction of renal blood flow that correlates inversely with kidney volume and occurs before loss of kidney function. These findings suggest that renal ischemia induced by cyst expansion plays a role in the etiology of hypertension, with intrarenal activation of the renin-angiotensin-aldosterone system (RAAS). Data from the HALT-PKD trial showed that in young patients (15 to 49 years) with preserved kidney function, treatment with inhibitors of the RAAS with a goal blood pressure of <110/75 resulted in a 14.2% slower increase in TKV over 5 years, reduced urinary albumin excretion, and a greater decline in left ventricular mass index. The overall rate of decline in estimated glomerular filtration rate (eGFR) in the strict and the standard blood pressure group was similar overall but slower in the lower blood pressure group during the chronic phase of the 5-year study. The overall lack of difference in eGFR decline was due to the more rapid decline in eGFR in the strict blood pressure group during the first four months of the trial. Importantly when class 1A and 1B patients (those unlikely to progress) were excluded from the analysis, then significant benefits in change in TKV and slope of eGFR were found in the low BP control group.

Kidney transplantation remains a viable option for patients approaching ESKD. ADPKD transplant recipients tend to survive longer than those transplanted for other kidney pathologies. Native polycystic kidneys do not have to be removed before transplantation unless chronic infections are present or their large size interferes with nutritional intake or quality of life.

EXTRARENAL MANIFESTATIONS

POLYCYSTIC LIVER DISEASE

Liver cysts are the most common extrarenal manifestation in ADPKD. MRI shows presence of liver cysts in more than 80% of patients by the age of 30 (Fig. 40.3), with equal sex representation. The liver cyst burden, however, is greater in women than in men. Previous estrogen or progesterone exposure, through birth-control pills, hormone replacement therapy, or pregnancy, is associated with significant polycystic liver disease. Liver function is preserved even in the presence of massive liver cystic disease, and standard biochemical tests are normal except for mild elevation in the serum concentration of alkaline phosphatase. Isolated autosomal dominant polycystic liver disease (ADPLD) without kidney cysts exists. ADPLD is a distinct disease genetically unrelated to ADPKD and instead linked to mutations in two genes: *PRKCSH* (protein kinase C substrate 80K-H) located on chromosome 19 and *SEC 63* located on chromosome 6.

Liver enlargement is the predominant complication resulting in symptoms of shortness of breath, pain, early satiety, gastroesophageal reflux, decreased mobility, ankle swelling, and, rarely, inferior vena cava compression. Symptoms occur because of compression of surrounding organs by the enlarged liver. This severe form of polycystic liver disease is unusual, occurring in fewer than 20% of all cases. It predominantly affects women and may require surgical cyst deroofing, fenestration, partial liver resection, or, in extreme cases, liver transplantation. Recently, the use of somatostatin analogues in the treatment of polycystic liver

disease appears to be beneficial. In a small single-center, double-blind, placebo-controlled trial of long-acting somatostatin (octreotide), the investigators showed that over a 12-month period, liver volumes decreased by $4.95\% \pm 6.77\%$ in the active drug group compared with placebo. In another randomized double-blind, placebo-controlled trial, lanreotide 120 mg given monthly for 6 months demonstrated a 2.9% decrease in the liver volume as compared with 1.6% increase with placebo. Importantly, somatostatin analogues were well tolerated, and patients experienced an improved perception of pain and physical activity. The most common symptoms reported with somatostatin analogues are abdominal cramps and diarrhea. Mammalian target of rapamycin (mTOR) inhibitors have also generated a lot of interest; an observational study in ADPKD kidney transplant recipients showed that those who were treated with sirolimus had a reduction in polycystic liver volumes by 12% compared with an increase of 14% among patients not receiving sirolimus. However, in a single-center randomized controlled trial, addition of everolimus to octreotide did not provide additional benefit. In that trial, liver volume reduction during a 12-month period was 3.8% in the everolimus-octreotide group, similar to that seen in octreotide-only group.

CARDIOVASCULAR MANIFESTATIONS

Intracranial aneurysms (ICAs) are the most feared complication of ADPKD. The prevalence of ICA in patients with ADPKD is 9% to 12%, compared with 2% to 3% in the general population. The prevalence increases to 22% to 27% in patients with a family history of hemorrhagic stroke or ICA. The aneurysms occur most often in the anterior cerebral circulation, and multiple ICAs are common in ADPKD patients, similar to what is observed among non-ADPKD familial ICAs. Average age of ICA rupture in patients with ADPKD is approximately 40 years. Risk of mortality or permanent morbidity after ICA rupture is more than 50%. Ruptured aneurysms contribute to 4% to 7% of deaths among ADPKD patients. Screening is indicated in asymptomatic patients with a positive family history for ICA or with a previous history of intracranial hemorrhage, those with high-risk occupations, or before major elective surgery that would affect intracranial hemodynamics. Persons without a family history of ICAs and without these additional concerns do not warrant routine screening. Time-of-flight three-dimensional magnetic resonance angiography (MRA) without gadolinium is the imaging modality of choice. Although rupture of an ICA is associated with significant morbidity and mortality, only 50% of ADPKD individuals with ICAs have a rupture during their lifetime. Postoperative complications related to surgical clipping are common, and recovery from elective surgery can be prolonged. For larger aneurysms (greater than 10 mm), the risk of rupture is significantly increased, and the anticipated complications from rupture outweigh the benefits of no intervention; elective surgical intervention is recommended in these cases. For asymptomatic unruptured ICAs between 5 and 10 mm, the management is less straightforward and should be individualized in consultation with the treating neurosurgeon and neuroradiologist. Monitoring the rate of growth of these ICAs with periodic imaging is warranted. For those with an ICA smaller than 5 mm, longitudinal studies have not demonstrated significant growth of the ICA, and the risk of rupture is relatively small.

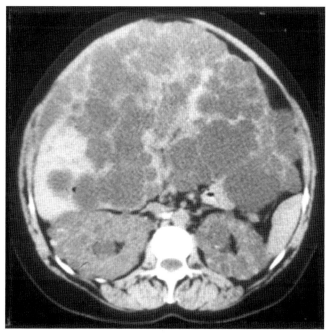

Fig. 40.3 Computed tomography scan with evidence of kidney and liver cysts in autosomal dominant polycystic kidney disease.

Stability of asymptomatic small aneurysms (<7 mm) should be assessed within 6 months to 1 year. Patients with a negative initial MRA and a positive family history of ICA or subarachnoid hemorrhage should undergo repeat evaluation every 10 years. Risk factors for aneurysmal growth include smoking and hypertension, and counseling about smoking cessation as well as blood pressure control is warranted as part of conservative management of ICA. The current indications for surgical repair of these smaller ICAs are unclear. With the development of less invasive therapies (i.e., interventional nonsurgical coiling or stenting), alternative treatment of small, asymptomatic ICAs may be used more frequently.

Left ventricular hypertrophy (LVH) with echocardiographic imaging is common in ADPKD patients, and it has been reported in as many as 48% of hypertensive individuals. More recent data derived from the HALT-PKD study using cardiac MRI in a contemporary cohort of hypertensive ADPKD patients younger than 50 years of age showed a much lower incidence of LVH (less than 4%). However, more than 50% of patients in this cohort were previously receiving long-term RAAS blockers. Other studies have shown that young normotensive ADPKD patients have increased left ventricular mass index (LVMI) and diastolic dysfunction.

Other cardiovascular manifestations of ADPKD include coronary aneurysms, valvular heart disease including mitral valve prolapse and mitral regurgitation (26% of ADPKD individuals, compared with 3% of the general population), and aortic insufficiency (11%).

EFFECTS ON FERTILITY AND PREGNANCY

Overall, fertility rates in ADPKD men and women not yet on dialysis are similar to those in the general population despite a higher incidence of ectopic pregnancies, congenital absence of the seminiferous tubules, seminal vesical cysts, and immotile spermatozoa. Affected women with a normal GFR and normal blood pressure experience pregnancy outcomes similar to those of the general population. Pregnancy-induced hypertension, worsening hypertension, and preeclampsia occur with increased frequency in women with ADPKD, and they have a higher rate of premature delivery. Patients with a decreased GFR before pregnancy are at high risk for midgestation fetal loss and progressive loss of kidney function.

AUTOSOMAL DOMINANT POLYCYSTIC KIDNEY DISEASE IN CHILDREN

Children with ADPKD are usually asymptomatic, with only about 1% to 2% of patients presenting with symptoms before the age of 15 years. TKV when regressed against age increases exponentially in children with ADPKD, and the annual growth rate in children is 7.4%. Glomerular hyperfiltration is seen early in the course of ADPKD, and children with glomerular hypertension had a faster decline in kidney function and higher rate of kidney growth.

Other kidney manifestations in children include urinary concentrating defects, present in about 60% of affected individuals. Proteinuria is usually low-grade and relatively uncommon; however, it is more common in affected children than in adults. Thirty percent of children have albuminuria, and 23% have overt proteinuria, as compared with 25% and 17% of adults, respectively. Similar to the adult population, proteinuria in children with ADPKD correlates with diastolic hypertension and more severe cystic kidney disease.

Studies in children with ADPKD show that hypertension is the earliest and most prevalent systemic feature occurring in up to 44% of cases, and children with hypertension have increased TKV and more pronounced increase in TKV compared with normotensive ADPKD children. Moreover, ADPKD children demonstrate abnormal circadian blood pressure patterns with increased nocturnal blood pressure. Other cardiovascular abnormalities found in affected children include mitral valve prolapse, increased LVMI, and hyperlipidemia, defined as a fasting cholesterol or triglyceride level above the 95th percentile for age and sex. Although rare among children, cases of ruptured cerebral aneurysms have been reported.

Extrarenal manifestations in children include liver cysts, which are typically benign. Rare cases of congenital hepatic fibrosis have been described in children with ADPKD.

At-risk offspring should have regular blood pressure measurements and urinalyses. However, there are no guidelines for systematic screening of asymptomatic ADPKD children.

THERAPY

Randomized, controlled clinical trials evaluating angiotensin-converting enzyme (ACE) inhibitors, rigorous blood pressure control, and dietary protein restriction have failed to demonstrate statistically significant kidney protection in ADPKD when studied late in the course of disease. Lifestyle and dietary changes are recommended for all patients with ADPKD. There is a positive correlation between 24-hour urine sodium excretion and rate of TKV increase in ADPKD participants of the CRISP study. Dietary salt (<2 g/day) and calorie restriction are recommended. Vasopressin stimulates the production of cAMP, which is thought to contribute to cyst development and growth, and can be inhibited by increased fluid intake. Water intake greater than 3 L/day can suppress vasopressin secretion, and patients with preserved kidney function are asked to increase fluid intake to at least this amount. Caution should be exercised in patients with more advanced stages of CKD because increasing water intake to extremely high levels can result in hyponatremia. Other dietary modifications, including limitation in caffeine intake due to its theoretical positive effects on cAMP production, have been suggested but not formally tested in prospective, randomized clinical trials.

ACE inhibitors or angiotensin receptor blockers are recommended as first-line treatment for hypertension in ADPKD. In the HALT PKD trial, strict blood pressure control of less than 110/75 mm Hg with an ACE inhibitor was associated with slower increase in TKV, reduced urinary albumin excretion, and a greater reduction of left ventricular mass index. The goal blood pressure for all patients with ADPKD is below 130/80 mm Hg, with a lower target of less than 110/75 in young adult patients with preserved kidney function.

Pravastatin showed beneficial effects on htTKV, LVMI, and urinary albumin excretion in a randomized, double-blind, placebo-controlled trial conducted in children. Statins are not currently approved for this indication.

A promising therapy aimed at reducing intracellular cAMP accumulation by blocking the vasopressin V_2 receptor has successfully slowed kidney cyst progression in four distinct genetic forms of cystic disease: the *PKD2* WS25 mouse, the Han:SPRD rat, the pcy mouse (a mouse model for familial juvenile nephronophthisis), and the polycystic kidney (pck) rat (a murine model for autosomal recessive polycystic kidney disease). Phase II studies of vasopressin V_2 receptor antagonists in ADPKD subjects demonstrated effective inhibition of the V_2 receptor, resulting in decreased water reabsorption and urinary osmolality over 24 hours. This medication was well tolerated, with patients maintaining serum sodium concentrations and tolerating mild increases in the frequency of nocturia. The Tolvaptan Efficacy and Safety Management of Autosomal Dominant Polycystic Kidney Disease and Its Outcomes (TEMPO) 3:4 trial is a phase 3, randomized, double-blind, placebo-controlled trial. Among 1445 participants over 3 years of follow-up, the tolvaptan-treated group had a slower rate of kidney volume growth (2.8% vs. 5.5%/year). The slope of kidney function decline, measured as the reciprocal of the serum creatinine, also favored tolvaptan therapy. It is worth mentioning that aside from expected side effects related to aquaresis in the tolvaptan group, a significant proportion of treated participants had liver enzyme elevations. These abnormalities were reversed when the drug was discontinued. Further studies are being planned to assess the efficacy and safety of tolvaptan in these patients. Tolvaptan is currently approved for this indication in Japan, Europe, and Canada.

Somatostatin is an inhibitor of intracellular cAMP accumulation through inhibition of the G protein and adenylate cyclase pathway. A somatostatin analogue, octreotide-long-acting repeatable depot (octreotide-LAR), was used in a randomized, single-blind, placebo-controlled trial conducted in 70 patients over a 3-year period. This trial suggested a beneficial effect with significantly less increase in TKV in the octreotide-LAR group compared with the placebo group.

Recent evidence indicates that normal PC1 interacts with the tuberous sclerosis complex (TSC1/TSC2), and this interaction plays a role in the inhibition of mTOR activity. In support of these findings, the inhibitor of mTOR, sirolimus, has been shown to decrease kidney cyst burden in the Han:SPRD rat. ADPKD patients who received sirolimus following kidney transplantation demonstrated a significant decline in the size of their native kidneys over time. However, two recent trials involving the mTOR inhibitors failed to show the anticipated benefit on kidney disease progression. In an 18-month open-label, randomized, controlled trial, 100 patients with early polycystic kidney disease were assigned to receive sirolimus versus standard of care. At the conclusion of this study, the investigators found that sirolimus therapy had no effect on kidney volume growth or GFR. However, the sirolimus dose used in this study was extremely low, raising the possibility that the drug dose chosen limited its efficacy.

In another 2-year, double-blind trial, 433 patients with ADPKD were randomly assigned to receive everolimus versus placebo. At the conclusion of this trial, everolimus significantly slowed the increase in TKV but not the progression of GFR loss. In fact, the everolimus group experienced a greater decline in the eGFR. In addition, at the end of the 2-year study, proteinuria had significantly increased in the everolimus-treated group when compared with the placebo group. Finally, everolimus use was associated with a high rate of serious adverse events (37.4% of patients who received at least one dose of the drug) and an extremely high rate

of study withdrawal (greater than 35%). Short duration of these trials and inadequate dosing may have affected the assessment of the mTOR inhibitors.

AUTOSOMAL RECESSIVE POLYCYSTIC KIDNEY DISEASE

Autosomal recessive polycystic kidney disease (ARPKD) occurs in 1 in 20,000 live births. Its etiology is linked to mutations in the polycystic kidney and hepatic disease (*PKHD1*) gene located on the short arm of chromosome 6 (6p21.1). The gene encodes for a protein product called fibrocystin (also known as polyductin), an integral membrane protein of 4074 amino acids with a large extracellular N-terminal and a short cytoplasmic tail. Fibrocystin is expressed primarily in the renal collecting ducts and ascending loop of Henle as well as biliary epithelial and pancreatic epithelial cells. The function of fibrocystin remains to be fully elucidated, but similar to other proteins involved in kidney cystic diseases, it has been localized to the basal body and primary cilia. Mutations have been identified in 42% to 87% of cases. Homozygous mutations that predict immediate stop codons or truncated proteins lead to the most severe phenotype and are associated with increased perinatal mortality. Mutations tend to be unique to each pedigree. Importantly, there is significant variability in the severity of kidney disease among patients carrying the same *PKHD1* mutation within the same family, suggesting that modifier genes and environmental factors may play contributory roles. The use of *PKHD1* sequencing data for clinical decision making or prenatal counseling is currently limited.

ARPKD is characterized by fibrocystic kidney and liver involvement of variable severity. The kidney cystic disease is a result of fusiform dilatation of renal collecting tubules. Up to 90% of collecting tubules are involved and, unlike ADPKD cysts, are diffuse and continue to retain their connection to the parent nephron. Most ARPKD patients have severely enlarged kidneys perinatally with poor corticomedullary differentiation that can be detected in utero. Affected fetuses can present with oligohydramnios secondary to poor kidney function and reduced urinary output and the Potter phenotype with pulmonary hypoplasia and deformed facies, spine, and limbs. In this setting, hypoxia due to pulmonary hypoplasia is the leading cause of death with approximately a 30% perinatal mortality. Not surprisingly, kidney survival correlates with age at diagnosis, with those diagnosed before the age of 1 having significantly higher risk of progression to ESKD. Cyst distribution also carries prognostic information. High-resolution ultrasonography is more sensitive in detecting kidney pathology limited to the medulla, and cystic anomalies limited to the medulla are associated with a milder kidney disease. Alternatively, corticomedullary anomalies that present perinatally are associated with a faster decline in kidney function. Hypertension is diagnosed in up to 80% of children with ARPKD and is usually associated with reduced GFR. Studies in animal models of ARPKD suggest intrarenal renin and ACE upregulation. The treatment of hypertension includes salt restriction and blockade of the renin-angiotensin-aldosterone system but often requires multiple agents to achieve control. Hyponatremia has been reported in about 26% of neonates diagnosed with ARPKD.

The liver disease in ARPKD consists of dilation of intrahepatic (Caroli syndrome) and extrahepatic bile ducts, which predispose them to recurrent ascending cholangitis. Patients can also have biliary dysgenesis and periportal fibrosis, known as congenital hepatic fibrosis, which leads to portal hypertension with subsequent splenomegaly and esophageal varices. Liver involvement rarely leads to hepatocellular damage with synthetic dysfunction. Although liver involvement is histologically universal, clinical manifestations of portal hypertension are variable. Therapy includes portosystemic shunts for esophageal varices. Children with advanced liver disease may be eligible for liver or combined kidney-liver transplantation.

Growth retardation is common among ARPKD children and cannot be solely attributed to chronic kidney disease or lung disease. Treatment with growth hormone can be helpful, as in other etiologies of CKD.

TUBEROUS SCLEROSIS COMPLEX

TSC is an autosomal-dominant disease estimated to occur in 1 in 6000 births. TSC results from mutations in either the *TSC1* gene, located on chromosome 9, or the *TSC2* gene, located on chromosome 16. *TSC2* is 50 base pairs away, from *PKD1*, lying in a head-to-head orientation. Deletions in both genes result in the contiguous gene syndrome characterized by severe early onset of a polycystic phenotype with cutaneous and neurologic manifestations of TSC. *TSC1* and *TSC2* are tumor suppressor genes, and, consistent with the two-hit hypothesis, a mutation in both alleles of either gene is required for disease manifestation. About 70% to 80% of patients have no family history of the disorder. Most of the spontaneous cases involve *TSC2* mutations and are associated with a more severe phenotype. In familial cases, mutations in *TSC1* are twice as likely to be the culprit. The gene products of *TSC1* and *TSC2*, hamartin and tuberin, are coexpressed in cells of many organs including the kidney, brain, lung, and pancreas. Both proteins are bound to form a heterodimer with an inhibitory effect on the mTOR complex 1. Under normal circumstances, protein kinase (Akt)-mediated inactivation of tuberin results in degradation of the tuberin-hamartin complex, allowing mTOR signaling. The mTOR pathway plays a key role in cell growth and proliferation as well as angiogenesis. In TSC cases, allelic mutations in either *TSC1* or *TSC2* followed by a second somatic mutation in the normal allele result in disruption of the tuberin-hamartin complex, resulting in unabated mTOR activation. This results in the growth of nonmalignant tumors (known as hamartomas) throughout the body. Although benign, these tumors lead to organ dysfunction characteristic of this disease.

In 1998, the National Institutes of Health sponsored a TSC consensus conference that led to the establishment of diagnostic criteria for TSC. In 2011, an international TSC consensus conference was organized with a mission to update the diagnostic criteria and provide surveillance and treatment guidelines for the disease. Currently, genetic testing alone can establish the diagnosis of TSC if a pathogenic mutation that disrupts the synthesis or function of the protein product is identified. In affected individuals, it is estimated that about 10% to 25% of genetic screening is negative, but this does not rule out the diagnosis. Clinical diagnostic criteria currently include 11 major criteria (≥3 hypomelanotic macules at least 5 mm in size, ≥3 angiofibromas or fibrous cephalic plaque, ≥2 ungual fibromas, shagreen patch, multiple retinal hamartomas, cortical dysplasias, subependymal nodules, subependymal giant cell astrocytoma, cardiac rhabdomyoma, lymphangioleiomyomatosis, and angiomyolipomas) and six minor criteria ("confetti" skin lesions, >3 dental enamel pits, ≥2 intraoral fibromas, retinal achromic patch, multiple kidney cysts, nonkidney hamartomas). The clinical diagnosis of TSC requires the presence of two major criteria, or one major and two minor.

Most features of the disease become evident after 3 years of age. Approximately 85% of TSC patients experience CNS complications that include epilepsy and cognitive impairment and are referred to as TSC-associated neuropsychiatric disorders or TAND. It is recommended that all TSC patients undergo baseline brain MRI as well as electroencephalogram. Kidney manifestations are the second most common finding. Fifty percent of patients have cystic kidney disease, and 80% have angiomyolipomas (AML) identified by noncontrast abdominal MRI. MRI is recommended for screening as well as for follow-up every 1 to 3 years. Secondary hypertension is common, and routine blood pressure checks should be performed. The abundant abnormal vascular structures in AML are prone to aneurysmal formation, and the risk of bleeding increases substantially after lesions enlarge beyond 4 cm or aneurysms enlarge beyond 5 mm in diameter. Currently the standard of care to control active bleeding is arterial embolization. Postembolectomy syndrome is common within 48 hours of the procedure and manifests as nausea, pain, fever, and hemodynamic instability and should be treated with corticosteroids. For AML larger than 3 cm, the first-line treatment is an mTOR inhibitor. Recently published results from the EXIST-2 (Everolimus for angiomyolipoma associated with tuberous sclerosis complex or sporadic lymphangioleiomyomatosis) trial showed that everolimus treatment was safe and effective in reducing the volume of AML.

Angiomyolipomas are also thought to underlie the pathogenesis of lymphangioleiomyomatosis (LAM), a devastating pulmonary complication that occurs almost exclusively among women leading to cystic and interstitial lung disease, pneumothoraces, and chylous pleural effusions. Screening high-resolution CT scans are recommended every 5 to 10 years for asymptomatic at-risk patients, but the frequency of imaging studies should increase once symptoms arise. In cases of moderate to severe lung disease, mTOR inhibitors can be used. Currently, everolimus is being investigated in clinical trials for many manifestations of TSC including dermatitis, cognitive and attention deficit disorders, seizures, and glioblastomas.

VON HIPPEL-LINDAU DISEASE

Von Hippel-Lindau (VHL) is a rare autosomal-dominant disease with an incidence of 1 in 36,000 live births characterized by benign and malignant tumors in multiple organs. The term "VHL disease" was coined in 1936 to honor Drs. Eugen von Hippel and Arvid Lindau who had respectively described retinal angiomas and spinal hemangioblastomas

(HBs) in a small group of VHL patients. Characteristic tumors in VHL include retinal and central nervous system (CNS) HB, clear cell renal carcinomas (RCCs), pheochromocytomas (PCCs), pancreatic islet tumors, and endolymphatic sac tumors (ELSTs). Other common benign findings include kidney and pancreatic cysts. The clinical diagnosis of VHL requires the presence of one of the above-mentioned tumors in the setting of a positive family history of VHL or two tumors (excluding epididymal and kidney cysts) in the absence of a family history.

Approximately 20% of VHL cases arise from de novo mutations. VHL disease is further categorized as type 1 (absence of PCC), type 2A (presence of PCC but without RCC), type 2B (presence of PCC and RCC), and type 2C (only PCC). The *VHL* gene has been mapped to chromosome 3p25 and encodes two protein isoforms: pVHL$_{30}$, a 30-kD protein of 213 amino acids, and pVHL$_{19}$, a smaller 19-kD protein lacking 53 amino acids from pVHL$_{30}$. Both isoforms are believed to have similar function. VHL is a tumor suppressor gene and, in accordance with the two hit hypothesis, a biallelic mutation is required for tumors to develop. Under normoxic conditions, the α-subunits of the hypoxia inducible factor (HIF) are hydroxylated, and pVHL binds and promotes their degradation. In conditions of hypoxia, or in the absence of functional pVHL, the HIF α-subunits are stabilized and escape degradation. They in turn form heterodimers with HIF β-subunits leading to the activation of a cascade of hypoxia-inducible genes, including vascular endothelial growth factor *(VEGF)*, erythropoietin *(EPO)*, tumor growth factor alpha *(TGFα)*, and platelet-derived growth factor *(PDGFβ)*. It is the biochemical consequence of this activation that leads to tumor formation. Another role of pVHL is its effect on microtubule orientation and stability. Cyst formation in VHL disease can be explained by pVHL effect on HIF and microtubules, both of which are essential to the integrity of the primary cilia.

Disease causing mutations can be detected in almost all patients with classic clinical features of VHL (95% to 100% detection rate). Genetic testing is recommended in at-risk relatives with a family history of VHL or those with suspected disease. Genotype-phenotype correlations have been established but so far do not affect our clinical management practice. Surprisingly, VHL mutations are also detected in a substantial number of individuals who have sporadic cases of VHL-associated tumors, including retinal HBs (30% to 50%), central nervous system hemangioblastomas (CNS HB) (4% to 40%), and ELST (20%). These observations led to the guideline recommendations by the American College of Medical Genetics and Genomics and the National Society of Genetic Counselors that patients with isolated retinal or CNS HB, PCC, or ELST, as well as clear cell RCC diagnosed before the age of 50, bilateral or multifocal tumors, or with a family history of clear cell RCC be screened for *VHL* mutations.

VHL disease is clinically characterized by the development of benign and malignant tumors in many organs. CNS HBs occur in 60% to 80% of VHL patients and most commonly occur in the cerebellum, spinal cord, and brainstem. Although benign in nature, CNS HBs enlarge over time and cause symptoms related to increased intracranial pressure and mass effect. Their biologic behavior is unpredictable with intermittent phases of growth and quiescence. These tumors tend to be multiple and recurrent, which make routine radiologic screening mandatory. MRI of the brain and cervical spine is recommended every 1 to 2 years starting at age 16. When symptomatic, CNS HBs are best treated by surgical removal. Retinal angiomas are identical histopathologically to CNS HBs and are the most common presenting feature of VHL disease. They tend to be bilateral and can lead to vision loss in 35% to 55% of cases. Annual eye examinations with indirect ophthalmoscopy are recommended from birth. Most lesions respond well to laser photocoagulation.

RCCs are the most common malignant tumors in VHL and are an important cause of death. The lifetime risk of RCC varies based on the VHL mutation but can be as high as 70%. Most RCCs are of the clear cell variety and tend to be multifocal and bilateral. The mean age at presentation is 40 years. The best management strategy remains close surveillance for RCCs with serial imaging using abdominal MRI with and without contrast every 2 years starting at age 16. When RCCs reach 3 cm in size, the risk of metastasis increases, and kidney-sparing surgery or ablation is recommended. PCC are seen in 7% to 20% of patients, with the risk varying based on the underlying mutation. They tend to be bilateral, occur at a young age (mean age 28 years), and can be extraadrenal. Screening is recommended annually starting at age 5. Asymptomatic VHL patients scheduled for elective surgery should be screened for PCC to prevent hemodynamic and cardiac complications associated with anesthesia and surgery. ELSTs arise from the membranous labyrinth of the inner ear and, when bilateral, are pathognomonic of VHL. They can lead to tinnitus, vertigo, and hearing loss. Pancreatic cysts are common but rarely lead to organ dysfunction. Pancreatic tumors occur in 5% to 10% of cases, are typically multiple, and are usually nonsecretory islet cell tumors. Surgery may be indicated when these tumors reach a size greater than 3 cm to avoid obstructive pancreatitis.

ACQUIRED CYSTIC KIDNEY DISEASE

Acquired cystic kidney disease (ACKD) refers to the sporadic, noninherited development of kidney cysts in patients with chronic kidney disease or ESKD. Its distinction from inherited cystic kidney disorder (particularly ADPKD) is important, and helpful hints include the lack of family history, the common presence of extrarenal cysts, particularly in the liver, in ADPKD, and normal parenchyma between cysts with preservation of the corticomedullary junction. Kidneys are usually small or normal in size, and the cysts tend to be of different morphology and size, although classically they are less than 3 cm.

The prevalence of ACKD increases with time on dialysis and has been reported to go from 10% to 20% after 1 to 3 years of dialysis to more than 90% after 5 to 10 years of dialysis. Men and blacks are at higher risk for developing ACKD.

Most patients with ACKD are asymptomatic, but cysts can rupture, causing hematuria or retroperitoneal hemorrhage with flank pain. This latter complication occurs mostly in patients on hemodialysis, likely related to the concomitant use of anticoagulation. RCCs remain the most feared complication affecting about 3% to 6% of patients with ACKD, which is approximately a 100-fold increase in incidence compared with the general population. The tumors tend to occur at a younger age than the general population and are more frequently multifocal and bilateral when compared with sporadic RCCs. Papillary cell carcinomas are the most common histologic variant of RCCs in ACKD, as opposed to clear cell carcinomas in sporadic cases.

More recently, two tumor types exclusive to ACKD patients have been described. Together they represent 60% of ACKD-associated RCCs. The first tumor is acquired cystic disease-associated RCC characterized by a well-circumscribed tumor that arises within cysts. A dense fibrous capsule separates the tumor from surrounding kidney tissue. The hallmark of this tumor is the presence of oxalate crystals seen under the polarizing microscope. The second type of tumor is the clear cell papillary RCC seen among ESKD patients with or without ACKD. Characteristically, tumor cells reveal signs of inverted polarity with their nuclei positioned away from the basement membrane. These two types of tumors are distinguished by morphology, cytogenetics, and immunohistochemistry. To date, there are no clear recommendations regarding the screening of ESKD patients for ACKD and RCC. A decision analysis model showed that screening provides significant benefits only for patients with a life expectancy of at least 25 years. It may, however, be beneficial to screen high-risk individuals (i.e., the young, men, blacks, patients on dialysis for more than 3 years). Ultrasound is a good screening modality; however, CT or MRI is more sensitive and recommended for patients that have signs or symptoms suggestive of carcinoma (e.g., hematuria, unexplained anemia, back pain, weight loss). When detected, tumors larger than 3 cm are treated surgically with total nephrectomy.

Screening guidelines for kidney transplant candidates or recipients are equally controversial. A study that included 516 kidney transplant recipients determined a prevalence of RCC of about 5%, and almost all cases were diagnosed in the setting of ACKD of the native kidneys. Risk factors for RCCs in that study included older age, male sex, history of heart disease, larger kidneys, and the presence of kidney calcifications. The prevalence of ACKD after transplant was lower than among ESKD patients, suggesting that better kidney function and/or immunosuppressive therapies may have a negative influence on cyst formation. A study comparing RCC diagnosed in ESKD patients on dialysis versus those transplanted suggested that tumors diagnosed after transplant have more benign features and are associated with superior clinical survival rates. It remains to be determined whether this advantage is related to more aggressive surveillance practices in transplant recipients or to an altered biology of these tumors.

KEY BIBLIOGRAPHY

Bae KT, Zhu F, Chapman AB, et al. Magnetic resonance imaging evaluation of hepatic cysts in early autosomal-dominant polycystic kidney disease: the Consortium for Radiologic Imaging Studies of Polycystic Kidney Disease cohort. *Clin J Am Soc Nephrol.* 2006;1(1):64-69.

Binderup ML, Budtz-Jørgensen E, Bisgaard ML. Risk of new tumors in von Hippel-Lindau patients depends on age and genotype. *Genet Med.* 2016;18:89-97.

Bissler J, Kingswood J, Radzikowska E, et al. Everolimus for angiomyolipoma associated with tuberous sclerosis complex or sporadic lymphangioleiomyomatosis (EXIST-2): a multicenter, randomized, double-blind, placebo-controlled trial. *Lancet.* 2013;381:817-824.

Bonsib S. Renal cystic diseases and renal neoplasms: a mini-review. *CJASN.* 2009;4:1998-2007.

Budde K, Gaedeke J. Tuberous sclerosis complex-associated angiomyolipomas: focus on mTOR inhibition. *AJKD.* 2012;59:276-283.

Cadnapaphornchai MA, George DM, McFann K, et al. Effect of pravastatin on total kidney volume, left ventricular mass index, and microalbuminuria in pediatric autosomal dominant polycystic kidney disease. *Clin J Am Soc Nephrol.* 2014;9(5):889-896.

Caroli A, Perico N, Perna A, et al. Effect of long acting somatostatin analogue on kidney and cyst growth in autosomal dominant polycystic kidney disease (ALADIN): a randomised, placebo-controlled, multicentre trial. *Lancet.* 2013;382(9903):1485-1495.

Chapman AB, Bost JE, Torres VE, et al. Kidney volume and functional outcomes in autosomal dominant polycystic kidney disease. *Clin J Am Soc Nephrol.* 2012;7(3):479-486.

Chapman AB, Devuyst O, Eckardt KU, et al. Autosomal-dominant polycystic kidney disease (ADPKD): executive summary from a kidney disease: Improving Global Outcomes (KDIGO) controversies conference. *Kidney Int.* 2015;88(1):17-27.

Chapman AB, Johnson AM, Rainguet S, Hossack K, Gabow P, Schrier RW. Left ventricular hypertrophy in autosomal dominant polycystic kidney disease. *J Am Soc Nephrol.* 1997;8(8):1292-1297.

Chapman AB, Rubinstein D, Hughes R, et al. Intracranial aneurysms in autosomal dominant polycystic kidney disease. *N Engl J Med.* 1992;327(13):916-920.

Dabora SL, Franz DN, Ashwal S, et al. Multicenter phase 2 trial of sirolimus for tuberous sclerosis: kidney angiomyolipomas and other tumors regress and VEGF-D levels decrease. *PLoS ONE.* 2011;6:e23379.

Fleming S. Renal cell carcinoma in acquired cystic kidney disease. *Histopathology.* 2010;56:395-400.

Gigante M, Neuzillet Y, Patard JJ, et al. Renal cell carcinoma (RCC) arising in native kidneys of dialyzed and transplant patients: are they different entities? *BJU Int.* 2012;110(11 Pt B):E570-E573.

Goto M, Hoxha N, Osman R, et al. The renin-angiotensin system and hypertension in autosomal recessive polycystic kidney disease. *Pediatr Nephrol.* 2010;25:2449-2457.

Grantham JJ, Torres VE, Chapman AB, et al. Volume progression in polycystic kidney disease. *N Engl J Med.* 2006;354(20):2122-2130.

Hartung EA, Guay-Woodford LM. Autosomal recessive polycystic kidney disease: a hepatorenal fibrocystic disorder with pleiotropic effects. *Pediatrics.* 2014;134(3):e833-e845.

Irazabal MV, Rangel LJ, Bergstralh EJ, et al. Imaging classification of autosomal dominant polycystic kidney disease: a simple model for selecting patients for clinical trials. *J Am Soc Nephrol.* 2015;26(1):160-172.

Krueger D, Northrup H, International Tuberous Sclerosis Complex Consensus Group. Tuberous sclerosis complex surveillance and management: recommendations of the 2012 International Tuberous Sclerosis Complex Consensus Conference. *Pediatr Neurol.* 2013;49:255-265.

Krueger DA, Care MM, Holland K, et al. Everolimus for subependymal giant-cell astrocytomas in tuberous sclerosis. *N Engl J Med.* 2010;363:1801-1811.

Full bibliography can be found on www.expertconsult.com.

Nephronophthisis and Medullary Cystic Kidney Disease

41

Daniela A. Braun; Friedhelm Hildebrandt

Nephronophthisis (NPHP) and medullary cystic kidney disease (MCKD) represent a set of rare genetic kidney diseases with a similar kidney histopathology, which includes interstitial fibrosis with tubular atrophy, changes in the tubular basement membrane (TBM), and cyst formation. These two diseases can be distinguished clinically by their inheritance pattern and often by their age of onset. NPHP has an autosomal recessive inheritance pattern and results in end-stage kidney disease (ESKD) within the first three decades of life. MCKD has an autosomal dominant inheritance pattern and usually results in ESKD between the fourth and seventh decades of life. While NPHP is frequently accompanied by defects in various other organ systems, gout is the only extrarenal manifestation described in MCKD thus far (Table 41.1).

EPIDEMIOLOGY

NPHP is recognized as a rare cause of ESKD worldwide, but it is one of the most common genetic causes of ESKD in the pediatric population. Historically, the incidence of NPHP alone has been quoted as between 1 in 50,000 and 1 in 1 million live births. The 2007 annual report of the United States Renal Data System (USRDS) indicated that the overall incidence and prevalence of ESKD related to NPHP or MCKD were both about 0.1% in the United States. For the period 2009–13, USRDS data reported a combined incidence of 1.6% for MCKD and NPHP in pediatric patients with ESKD.

The incidence and prevalence of these diseases reported in databases may be an underestimate, because patients often come to clinical attention only after reaching ESKD when the identification of the underlying diagnosis may no longer be possible. In addition, urinalysis in these disorders is typically bland without significant proteinuria or hematuria, making aggressive diagnostic procedures such as biopsy less likely to be pursued. Although a presumptive diagnosis of NPHP or MCKD can be made based on clinical features and kidney histopathology, the only way to definitively diagnose these disorders is through genetic testing. Unfortunately, despite recent advances in next-generation sequencing and drastic cost reduction, access to molecular diagnostics in clinical settings is still limited.

PATHOLOGY

The similar appearance of the kidney histology between NPHP and MCKD led to the historic association of these two disorders. The classic triad of kidney pathology, which is shared by all genetic types of NPHP except NPHP type 2 (NPHS2), includes interstitial fibrosis with tubular atrophy, TBM disruption, and corticomedullary cysts. Periglomerular fibrosis and sclerosis have also been noted. Cysts range in size from 1 to 15 mm, are typically located at the corticomedullary junction and usually arise from the distal convoluted tubule or medullary collecting duct. Kidney size is normal or reduced in these types of NPHP, and cysts may not be apparent by imaging early in the course of the disease. Although NPHP frequently presents with extrarenal involvement, cysts have not been observed in other organs in contrast to autosomal dominant polycystic kidney disease (ADPKD).

NPHP2, or infantile NPHP, is caused by mutations in the *inversin* gene *(INVS)*, and its kidney pathology and clinical course are distinct from those of other types of NPHP. NPHP2 results in ESKD in the first decade of life, often within the first 2 years, and is characterized by the cystic enlargement of the kidneys bilaterally. Kidney pathology is characterized by more remarkable cyst formation, which appears more prominently in the cortex, but it can also be present in the medulla. Cysts seem to arise from the proximal and distal tubules, and cystic enlargement of the glomerulus has occasionally been noted. Tubulointerstitial nephritis is another prominent finding in NPHP2, which it shares with the other forms of NPHP. Compared to other types of NPHP, TBM disruption is less commonly observed in the setting of NPHP2.

The gross appearance of the kidney in MCKD is normal to slightly reduced in size, similar to NPHP. Histologically, the kidney pathology of MCKD is virtually indistinguishable from NPHP, which has led to the historic nomenclature of these diseases as the *NPHP-MCKD disease complex.*

PATHOGENESIS

The molecular causes of NPHP are very heterogeneous. In addition to 20 genes that cause NPHP types 1 to 20 if mutated (Table 41.1), NPHP-like kidney involvement has been described for many of the ~90 monogenic diseases that are collectively termed ciliopathies. This term was chosen because encoded proteins localize to the primary cilium, a cellular organelle that arises from the apical surface of virtually every cell of the human body. Consequently, the genes have a broad tissue expression pattern. NPHP is inherited in an autosomal recessive manner, is fully penetrant, and typically manifests in childhood or adolescence. Disease manifestation in heterozygous carriers has never been shown. The most

385

Table 41.1   Genetic Causes of Nephronophthisis and Medullary Cystic Kidney Disease

Disease	Gene	Protein	Mode of Inheritance	Chromosomal Localization	Extrarenal Manifestations
NPHP1	*NPHP1*	Nephrocystin 1	AR	2q13	Retinitis pigmentosa, oculomotor apraxia, cerebellar vermis hypoplasia (rare)
NPHP2	*INVS*	Inversin	AR	9q31.1	Retinitis pigmentosa, *situs inversus*, liver fibrosis, pulmonary hypoplasia
NPHP3	*NPHP3*	Nephrocystin 3	AR	3q22.1	Retinitis pigmentosa, liver fibrosis, Meckel-Gruber syndrome
NPHP4	*NPHP4*	Nephroretinin	AR	1q36.22	Retinitis pigmentosa, oculomotor apraxia
NPHP5	*IQCB1*	Nephrocystin 5	AR	3q13.33	Retinitis pigmentosa (all described cases)
NPHP6	*CEP290*	Nephrocystin 6	AR	12q21.32	Retinitis pigmentosa, cerebellar vermis hypoplasia, liver fibrosis, Meckel-Gruber syndrome
NPHP7	*GLIS2*	GLIS 2	AR	16p13.3	Not reported
NPHP8	*RPGRIP1L*	Nephrocystin 8	AR	16q12.2	Retinitis pigmentosa, cerebellar vermis hypoplasia, liver fibrosis, Meckel-Gruber syndrome
NPHP9	*NEK8*	NEK8	AR	17q11.2	Liver fibrosis, congenital heart defects, Meckel-Gruber syndrome
NPHP10	*SDCCAG8*	SDCCAG8	AR	1q43–q44	Retinitis pigmentosa, Bardet-Biedl syndrome
NPHP11	*TMEM67*	Meckelin	AR	8q22.1	Retinitis pigmentosa, cerebellar vermis hypoplasia, liver fibrosis, polydactyly, Meckel-Gruber syndrome
NPHP12	*TTC21B*	TTC21B	AR	2q24.3	Cerebellar vermis hypoplasia, skeletal involvement
NPHP13	*WDR19*	WDR19/IFT144	AR	4p14	Retinitis pigmentosa, skeletal involvement, liver fibrosis
NPHP14	*ZNF423*	ZNF423	AR	16q12.1	Retinitis pigmentosa, cerebellar vermis hypoplasia
NPHP15	*CEP164*	CEP164	AR	11q23.3	Retinitis pigmentosa, cerebellar vermis hypoplasia
NPHP16	*ANKS6*	ANKS6	AR	9q22.33	Liver fibrosis, congenital heart disease
NPHP17	*IFT172*	IFT172	AR	2p23.3	Retinitis pigmentosa, skeletal involvement, liver fibrosis
NPHP18	*CEP83*	CEP83/CCDC41	AR	12q22	Retinitis pigmentosa, brain involvement
NPHP19	*DCDC2*	DCDC2	AR	6p22.3	Liver fibrosis
NPHP20	*MAPKBP1*	MAPKBP1	AR	15q15.1	None reported
MCKD1	*MUC1*	Mucin 1	AD	1q22	Hyperuricemia, gout
MCKD2	*UMOD*	Uromodulin	AD	16p12.3	Hyperuricemia, gout

AD, Autosomal dominant; *AR*, autosomal recessive; *MCKD*, medullary cystic kidney disease; *NPHP*, nephronophthisis.

common form of NPHP is type 1, which accounts for approximately 25% of all cases. Approximately 85% of mutations in *NPHP1* consist of large deletions, which typically include the whole gene. The remaining genetic causes of NPHP each account for only a small fraction of diagnosed cases.

The first monogenic causes of NPHP were identified with the help of positional cloning and linkage analysis. More recently, advances in next-generation sequencing have facilitated gene discovery and resulted in a rapid increase in the number of newly identified human disease genes. The study of NPHP genes and their related gene products, the nephrocystins, has provided important insight into pathogenic mechanisms underlying NPHP. Interestingly, all nephrocystin proteins share a common subcellular localization to the cilia-basal body-centrosome complex, suggesting that primary cilia play an essential role in the pathogenesis of cystic kidney diseases. Many nephrocystin proteins show molecular interactions with other nephrocystins, indicating that these proteins and other ciliary proteins may be part of a common functional network. Molecular research has shown that primary cilia represent signaling hubs that convert extracellular stimuli into intracellular signals. It appears that numerous different signaling pathways, including the developmental pathways Sonic Hedgehog and Wnt signaling, require primary cilia for proper function. By regulating these pathways, nephrocystin proteins seem to control kidney fibrosis and the maintenance of proper kidney architecture. More recently, it was shown

that centrosomal proteins, which give rise to NPHP and other ciliopathies if their genes are mutated, play a critical role in the regulation of cell cycle progression, mitotic spindle orientation, and DNA damage response signaling. The fact that all these signaling pathways or selective signal pathways may be defective depending on the severity of the mutation could explain the broad phenotypic spectrum and the multitude of extrarenal symptoms that can be present in patients with NPHP. Despite intense research, the exact pathogenic mechanism by which mutations in NPHP genes result in kidney disease is still unknown; however, it seems plausible that dysregulation in several pathways results in a common kidney histopathology of interstitial fibrosis, tubular atrophy, and degenerative cysts.

Two gene loci have been identified for MCKD: *MCKD1* on 1q21 and *MCKD2* on 16p12. Fifteen years after the initial description of the *MCKD1* locus and after numerous failed attempts, researchers finally identified single nucleotide insertions in very long and highly GC-rich tandem repeat areas (VNTRs) of the gene *MUC1*, encoding Mucin 1, as the molecular cause of MCKD type 1. The mutation is predicted to cause a shift of the reading frame resulting in a truncated protein that lacks several characteristic domains of the wildtype protein, including the transmembrane domain. The mutated protein was shown to be expressed in tubular epithelial and collecting duct cells, and showed subcellular mislocalization that was not observed in healthy control subjects.

Mutations in uromodulin, the Tamm-Horsfall protein, have been shown to cause MCKD2, familial juvenile hyperuricemic nephropathy (FJHN), and glomerulocystic kidney disease (GCKD). Uromodulin is expressed in the thick ascending limb of the nephron and is the most abundant protein found in the urine. The excretion of uromodulin is reduced in these patients, and pathologic intracellular accumulation of uromodulin occurs in the tubular epithelial cells of the thick ascending limb. Both types of MCKD are inherited in an autosomal-dominant manner.

CLINICAL FEATURES AND DIAGNOSIS

The age of onset of clinically apparent kidney disease and the pattern of inheritance in familial cases are different in NPHP and MCKD (see Table 41.1). Although biopsy findings in conjunction with the appropriate clinical presentation and patient history can suggest a diagnosis of NPHP or MCKD, the only definitive diagnostic modality is genetic testing. With recent technical advances and cost reduction in next-generation sequencing, molecular genetic testing has become more feasible. However, the accessibility of clinical genetic testing in certified diagnostic laboratories for patients with chronic kidney diseases is still limited, and many patients thus remain without a definitive molecular diagnosis. A list of research and clinical laboratories offering genetic testing is available at http://www.genetests.org. Considering the broad phenotypic and genetic heterogeneity of NPHP, the method of choice for genetic testing should be whole-exome sequencing rather than targeted sequencing of a limited number of candidate genes.

NEPHRONOPHTHISIS

Kidney function decline begins early in NPHP, typically progressing to ESKD within the first three decades of life. The earliest clinical manifestation of NPHP is a urinary concentrating defect that results in the clinical symptoms of polyuria, secondary enuresis, and nocturnal polydipsia. These findings may precede the onset of glomerular filtration rate (GFR) loss. A family history of affected siblings with an autosomal recessive inheritance pattern is strongly suggestive of the diagnosis, but given the rarity of the disease, sporadic cases are more common.

Historically, the age of onset has been considered an important clinical distinction amongst the various types of NPHP, leading to categorization of the disease as infantile (only NPHP2), juvenile (NPHP1 and NPHP4), or adolescent (NPHP3). However, with the exception of NPHP2, which leads to ESKD in the first decade of life, it is not clear whether there is truly a predictable difference in the age of onset for the other types of NPHP.

The extrarenal manifestations of NPHP (see Table 41.1) include retinitis pigmentosa, which has been present in all cases of NPHP5 identified thus far, but it can also be present in other types of NPHP. Many cases of NPHP6 are initially identified as Joubert syndrome, a brain developmental defect, which has the characteristic features of cerebellar vermis hypoplasia, ataxia, and other impairment of motor coordination. Beyond NPHP6, Joubert syndrome has been described in other types of NPHP. Oculomotor apraxia type Cogan is

typically associated with mutation in the genes *NPHP1* and *NPHP4*. Laterality defects, such as *situs inversus* or congenital heart defects, are frequently observed in patients with NPHP2. Liver involvement is most frequently present in patients with mutations in the genes *NPHP3*, *TMEM67* (NPHP11), *ANKS6* (NPHP16), and *DCDC2* (NPHP19). NPHP-like kidney involvement has also been described as part of several clinical syndromes, including the COACH (*C*erebellar vermis hypoplasia, *O*ligophrenia, *A*taxia, *C*oloboma, and *H*epatic fibrosis), Arima, Jeune, Sensenbrenner, and Bardet-Biedl syndromes.

Physical findings of NPHP include growth retardation and anemia. Interestingly, compared to other causes of chronic kidney disease, both symptoms have been noted as being more pronounced when adjusted to the GFR level. Conversely, elevated blood pressure is typically less prevalent than it would be expected for the given GFR.

The laboratory evaluation of NPHP patients includes a urinalysis of the first morning void, which usually is normal except for a low specific gravity reflecting a urinary concentrating defect. The absence of proteinuria or hematuria helps to distinguish NPHP from other heritable kidney diseases such as focal segmental glomerulosclerosis and Alport syndrome, respectively. Other laboratory abnormalities are commensurate with the degree of GFR loss.

The most relevant diagnostic test is ultrasound examination of the kidneys, which demonstrates normal to slightly reduced kidney size, increased echotexture, and a loss of corticomedullary differentiation. Cysts, when present, are typically located at the corticomedullary junction, but cysts that are visible on imaging are not a prerequisite for the diagnosis of NPHP. The imaging findings for patients with NPHP2 are substantially different from those of other types of NPHP: kidney size is often increased, and cysts are a prominent finding.

In summary, the diagnosis of NPHP should be entertained when an individual presents in the first three decades of life with reduced kidney function, a bland urine sediment, and normal to small kidneys on ultrasound with increased echotexture and loss of corticomedullary differentiation. The most common extrarenal manifestation associated with NPHP is retinitis pigmentosa, which often leads to blindness in the first decade of life and occurs in about 10% of patients. The occurrence of similarly affected siblings in the same family strongly suggests NPHP. The parents of affected children are not affected because NPHP is inherited as an autosomal-recessive disease. The recessive inheritance pattern differentiates NPHP from MCKD, which is transmitted as an autosomal-dominant disease (i.e., one parent of the affected individual should also be affected).

MEDULLARY CYSTIC KIDNEY DISEASE

MCKD usually presents in the fourth to seventh decade of life. Two exceptions to this pattern are FJHN and GCKD, which are allelic (i.e., caused by mutations in the same gene) to MCKD2 but manifest within the first three decades of life. MCKD, FJHN, and GCKD are all inherited in an autosomal dominant pattern. The only extrarenal manifestation associated with these diseases, aside from those attributable to reduced kidney function, is hyperuricemia with gouty arthritis.

There are no other distinctive findings on physical examination associated with MCKD. Laboratory findings are notable for a urinary concentration defect with reduced fractional excretion of uric acid, but the urinalysis is otherwise unremarkable. Ultrasound examination demonstrates normal to slightly reduced kidney size, increased echogenicity, loss of corticomedullary differentiation, and medullary cysts. However, especially in early stages of the disease, the changes may be too subtle for detection with ultrasound or computed tomography studies.

TREATMENT

Despite significant advances in understanding the molecular mechanisms of NPHP, no curative or targeted treatment is available at this point, and no systematic clinical trials have been undertaken to examine different treatment regimens for NPHP or MCKD in people. Accordingly, treatment of NPHP and MCKD centers on the sequelae of chronic kidney disease, including anemia, acidosis, electrolyte imbalance, mineral and bone disorder, and growth retardation. ESKD typically develops within the first three decades of life in patients with NPHP and between ages 40 and 70 years in patients with MCKD. Patients with NPHP and MCKD have successfully undergone kidney transplantation without evidence of recurrent disease in the transplant.

BIBLIOGRAPHY

Braun DA, Schueler M, Halbritter J, et al. Whole exome sequencing identifies causative mutations in the majority of consanguineous or familial cases with childhood-onset increased renal echogenicity. *Kidney Int.* 2016;89:468-475.

Chaki M, Airik R, Ghosh AK, et al. Exome capture reveals ZNF423 and CEP164 mutations, linking renal ciliopathies to DNA damage response signaling. *Cell.* 2012;150:533-548.

Dahan K, Devuyst O, Smaers M, et al. A cluster of mutations in *UMOD* gene causes familial hyperuricemic nephropathy with abnormal expression of uromodulin. *J Am Soc Nephrol.* 2003;14:2883-2893.

Halbritter J, Porath JD, Diaz KA, et al. Identification of 99 novel mutations in a worldwide cohort of 1,056 patients with a nephronophthisis-related ciliopathy. *Hum Genet.* 2013;132:865-884.

Hart TC, Gorry MC, Hart PS, et al. Mutations of the *UMOD* gene are responsible for medullary cystic disease 2 and familial hyperuricemic nephropathy. *J Med Genet.* 2002;39:882-892.

Hildebrandt F. Nephronophthisis-medullary cystic kidney disease. In: Avner ED, Harmon WE, Niaudet P, eds. *Pediatric Nephrology.* 5th ed. Philadelphia: Lippincott, Williams and Wilkins; 2004:665-673.

Hildebrandt F, Benzing T, Katsanis N. Ciliopathies. *N Engl J Med.* 2011; 364:1533-1543.

Hildebrandt F, Otto E. Cilia and centrosomes: a unifying pathogenetic concept for cystic kidney disease? *Nat Rev Genet.* 2005;6:928-940.

Kirby A, Gnirke A, Jaffe DB, et al. Mutations causing medullary cystic kidney disease type 1 lie in a large VNTR in MUC1 missed by massively parallel sequencing. *Nat Genet.* 2013;45:299-303.

Otto EA, Hurd TW, Airik R, et al. Candidate exome capture identifies mutation of SDCCAG8 as the cause of a retinal-renal ciliopathy. *Nat Genet.* 2012;42:840-850.

Rampoldi L, Caridi G, Santon D, et al. Allelism of MCKD, FJHN and GCKD caused by impairment of uromodulin export dynamics. *Hum Mol Genet.* 2003;12:3369-3384.

Sang L, Miller JJ, Corbit KC, et al. Mapping the NPHP-JBTS-MKS protein network reveals ciliopathy disease genes and pathways. *Cell.* 2011;145:513-528.

Simons M, Gloy J, Ganner A, et al. Inversin, the gene product mutated in nephronophthisis type II, functions as a molecular switch between Wnt signaling pathways. *Nat Genet.* 2005;37:537-543.

United States Renal Data System. *USRDS Annual Data Report: Epidemiology of Kidney Disease in the United States.* Bethesda, MD: National Institutes of Health, National Institute of Diabetes and Digestive and Kidney Diseases; 2015:2015.

Vivante A, Hildebrandt F. Exploring the genetic basis of early-onset chronic kidney disease. *Nat Rev Nephrol.* 2016;12:133-146.

Wolf MT. Nephronophthisis and related syndromes. *Curr Opin Pediatr.* 2015;27:201-211.

Alport Syndrome and Related Disorders

42

Martin C. Gregory

Alport syndrome is a disease of collagen that always affects the kidneys, usually the ears, and often the eyes. Cecil Alport described the association of hereditary hematuric nephritis with hearing loss in a family whose affected male members died in adolescence. Genetic advances have broadened the scope of the condition to include optical defects, platelet abnormalities, late-onset kidney failure, and abnormal hearing in some families. At least 85% of kindreds have X-linked disease, and most or all of those cases result from a mutation of *COL4A5*, the gene located at Xq22 that codes for the α5 chain of type IV collagen, α5(IV). Autosomal inheritance occurs in perhaps 15% of cases.

JUVENILE AND ADULT FORMS

The distinction between juvenile and adult forms is fundamental to the understanding of Alport syndrome. Kidney failure tends to occur at a broadly similar age in all male members within a family, but this age varies widely among families, with kidney failure in males occurring in childhood or adolescence in some families and in adulthood in others. Forms with early onset of kidney failure in affected males are called *juvenile*, and those with kidney failure in middle age are called *adult type*. Extrarenal manifestations tend to be more prominent in the juvenile kindreds. Because boys in juvenile kindreds do not commonly survive to reproduce, these kindreds tend to be small and frequently arise from new mutations, whereas adult-type kindreds are typically much larger, and new mutations occur infrequently (Table 42.1).

BIOCHEMISTRY

The open mesh of interlocking type IV collagen molecules that forms the framework of the glomerular basement membrane (GBM) is composed of heterotrimers of α chains. In fetal life, these heterotrimers consist of two α1(IV) chains and one α2(IV) chain, but early in postnatal development, production switches to α3(IV), α4(IV), and α5(IV) chains. The primary chemical defect in Alport syndrome involves the α5(IV) chain or, less commonly, the α3(IV) chain, but faulty assembly of the α3,4,5-heterotrimer produces similar pathology in glomerular, aural, and ocular basement membranes, regardless of which α chain is defective. As an illustration of failure of normal heterotrimer formation, most patients whose genetic defect is in the gene coding for the α5(IV) chain lack demonstrable α3(IV) chains in GBMs.

GENETICS

In most kindreds, inheritance of Alport syndrome is X-linked. This was suggested by classic pedigree analysis, strengthened by tight linkage to restriction fragment-length polymorphisms, and proved by identification of mutations.

Causative mutations of COL4A5, the gene coding for α5(IV), appear consistently in many kindreds. These mutations include deletions, point mutations, and splicing errors. There is some correlation between the mutation type and the clinical phenotype, but deletions and some splicing errors cause severe kidney disease and early hearing loss. Missense mutations may cause juvenile disease with hearing loss or adult disease with or without hearing loss. Deletions involving the 5′ end of the *COL4A5* gene and the 5′ end of the adjacent *COL4A6* gene occur consistently in families with esophageal and genital leiomyomatosis.

Homozygotes or mixed heterozygotes for mutations of the *COL4A3* or *COL4A4* genes (chromosome 2) develop autosomal-recessive Alport syndrome. Heterozygotes for these mutations account for many cases of benign familial hematuria (i.e., familial thin basement membrane disease [TBMD]).

Patients with autosomal-dominant hematuria and kidney failure with thrombocytopenia, giant platelets (Epstein syndrome), and leukocyte inclusions (Fechtner syndrome) have mutations of the *MYH9* gene on chromosome 22 (see below). These patients should no longer be considered to have Alport syndrome; they have MYH9-related disorders.

IMMUNOCHEMISTRY

Male patients with X-linked Alport syndrome and patients with autosomal-recessive Alport syndrome frequently lack the α3, α4, and α5 chains of type IV collagen in the GBM, and hemizygous males with X-linked Alport syndrome often lack α5(IV) chains in the epidermal basement membrane (EBM). Monoclonal antibodies specific to the α2 and α5 chains of type IV collagen are commercially available and can be used to assist in the diagnosis of Alport syndrome. The GBM and EBM of normal individuals, as well as those of all Alport patients, react with the α2 antibody, but most male and female patients with autosomal-recessive Alport syndrome and most male patients hemizygous for a COL4A5 mutation show no staining of the GBM with the α5 antibody. Males with X-linked disease commonly show no staining of

Table 42.1   Alport Syndrome Types With Chromosomal and Gene Locations and Relative Frequencies

Type	Chromosome	Gene	Relative Frequency[a]
X-linked	X	COL4A5	85%
Juvenile type			90% of families, 50% of patients
Adult type			8% of families, 25% of patients
Adult type with "normal" hearing			2% of families, 25% of patients
Autosomal recessive	2	COL4A3, COL4A4	15%
Autosomal dominant	2	COL4A3, COL4A4	Less than 1%

[a]Relative frequencies of the X-linked, autosomal recessive, and autosomal dominant forms are fairly well accepted. The frequencies of "juvenile" (mean age of end-stage kidney disease [ESKD] in males <30 years), "adult" (mean age of ESKD in males >30 years), and adult type with near-normal hearing are rough estimates from the numbers of patients and families known to the University of Utah Alport Study. In the United States, C1564S is a common mutation causing adult-type Alport syndrome, and L1649R is a common mutation causing adult-type Alport syndrome with near-normal hearing.

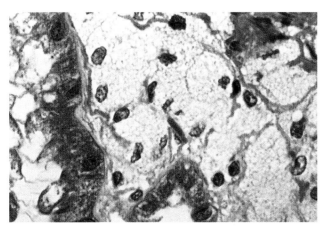

Fig. 42.1 High-power photomicrograph shows foam-filled tubular and interstitial cells in a kidney biopsy specimen from a patient with Alport syndrome. Relatively normal proximal tubular cytoplasm stains red in the tubules on the left and at the bottom. The remaining cells appear "foamy" because of the spaces left where lipids have been eluted during processing.

EBM with antibody to α5, whereas females heterozygous for a COL4A5 mutation show interrupted staining of the GBM and EBM, consistent with mosaicism.

After kidney transplantation, fewer than 5% of male patients with Alport syndrome develop anti-GBM glomerulonephritis, presumably because they are exposed for the first time to normal collagen chains including a normal 26-kDa monomer of the α3(IV) chain to which tolerance has never been acquired. Recurrences of anti-GBM glomerulonephritis are usual but not inevitable after repeat transplantation. The serum antibodies to GBM developing after transplantation are heterogeneous; all stain normal GBM, and some stain EBM.

PATHOLOGY

In young children, light microscopy of the kidneys may be normal or near normal. Glomeruli with persistent fetal morphology may be seen. As disease progresses, interstitial and tubular foam cells, which arise for reasons that are unclear, may become prominent (Fig. 42.1), although they can also be found in many other conditions. Eventually, progressive glomerulosclerosis and interstitial scarring develop; the

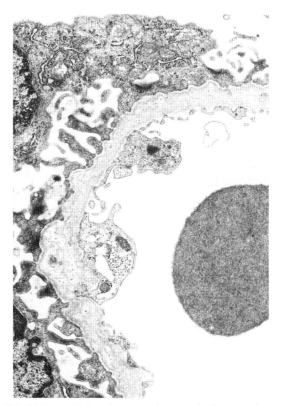

Fig. 42.2 High-resolution electron micrograph shows a glomerular basement membrane from a patient with Alport syndrome that varies in thickness. It is split into several layers, which in some areas are separated by lucencies containing small, dense granules. (Courtesy Dr. Theodore J. Pysher.)

histology may eventually be that of secondary focal segmental glomerular sclerosis (FSGS). The results of routine immunofluorescence examination for immunoglobulins and complement components are negative, but staining for the α5(IV) chain may be informative (see "Immunochemistry").

The GBM is up to 3 times its normal thickness, split into several irregular layers, and frequently interspersed with numerous electron-dense granules about 40 nm in diameter (Fig. 42.2). In florid cases of juvenile types of Alport syndrome, the basement membrane lamellae may branch and rejoin in a complex basket-weave pattern. Early in the development of the lesion, thinning of the GBM may predominate or be the only abnormality visible. The abnormalities in children or adolescents with adult-type Alport syndrome may be unimpressive or indistinguishable from those of TBMD disease (see below).

CLINICAL FEATURES

KIDNEY FEATURES

Uninterrupted microscopic hematuria occurs from birth in affected males. Hematuria may become visible after exercise or during fever; this is more common in juvenile kindreds. Microscopic hematuria has a penetrance of approximately 90% in heterozygous females in adult-type kindreds. In juvenile kindreds, the penetrance of hematuria in females has been studied less extensively but appears to be common. Urinary erythrocytes are dysmorphic, and red-cell casts usually can be found in affected males. The degree of proteinuria varies, but it occasionally reaches nephrotic levels.

Hemizygous males inevitably progress to end-stage kidney disease (ESKD). This occurs at widely different ages, but within each family, the age of ESKD is fairly constant. Heterozygous females are usually much less severely affected. About one fourth of them develop ESKD, usually after the age of 50 years, but ESKD can occur in girls in their teens or even younger.

In families with autosomal inheritance, females are affected as severely and as early as males, and kidney failure often occurs before the age of 20 in those who are homozygous for autosomal-recessive Alport syndrome.

EXTRARENAL FEATURES

HEARING LOSS

Bilateral, high-frequency cochlear hearing loss occurs in many kindreds, but X-linked disease progressing to ESKD can occur in families without overt hearing loss. It is easy to miss the diagnosis of Alport syndrome if hearing loss is expected as a constant feature (see Table 42.1). In families with juvenile-type disease, hearing loss is almost universal in male hemizygotes and common in severely affected female heterozygotes.

Patterns of hearing loss vary. Often, the most severe loss is at 2 to 6 kHz, but it may occur at a higher frequency if there has been superimposed noise damage. In adult-type Alport syndrome with hearing loss, there is typically no perceptible deficit until 20 years of age, but loss progresses to 60 to 70 dB at 6 to 8 kHz after 40 years of age. It is important to realize that about half of those with adult-type Alport syndrome will have no overt hearing loss; failure to recognize this is a common reason for overlooking the diagnosis. Hearing loss occurs earlier in juvenile kindreds. The rate at which hearing is lost is not well established in juvenile kindreds, but many adolescents require hearing aids.

OCULAR DEFECTS

Ocular defects are common in juvenile kindreds. Myopia, arcus juvenilis, and cataracts occur, but lack diagnostic specificity. Three changes that are present in a minority of kindreds but that are almost diagnostic are anterior lenticonus, posterior polymorphous corneal dystrophy, and retinal flecks. Anterior lenticonus is a forward protrusion of the anterior

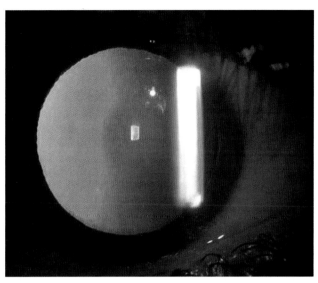

Fig. 42.3 Retroilluminated lens photography shows the "oil-drop" appearance of anterior lenticonus, a pathognomonic feature of Alport syndrome. The bulging area of the lens is the dark circular area just to the left of the vertical reflected light artifact from the slit-lamp examination. This is similar to the view obtained through a direct ophthalmoscope with a strong positive lens.

surface of the ocular lens. It results from a weakness of the type IV collagen forming the anterior lens capsule. The resulting irregularity of the surface of the lens causes an uncorrectable refractive error. The retina cannot be clearly seen by ophthalmoscopy, and with a strong positive lens in the ophthalmoscope the lenticonus often can be seen through a dilated pupil as an "oil drop," or circular smudge on the center of the lens (Fig. 42.3). Retinal flecks are small, yellow or white dots scattered around the macula or in the periphery of the retina (Fig. 42.4). If sparse, they may be difficult to distinguish from small, hard exudates. Macular holes occur rarely but can severely affect sight. Ocular manifestations are often subtle, and consultation with an ophthalmologist familiar with Alport syndrome is invaluable.

Optical coherence tomography is a simple, inexpensive test that shows retinal thinning in patients with Alport syndrome. This test appears to have high sensitivity and specificity, but more study is needed.

LEIOMYOMATOSIS

Young members of several families with X-linked Alport syndrome develop striking leiomyomas of the esophagus and female genitalia. Patients frequently have multiple large tumors, which may bleed or cause obstruction, and their resection can be difficult. All described families have had a deletion at the 5′ ends of the contiguous *COL4A5* and *COL4A6* genes.

DIAGNOSIS

No single clinical feature is pathognomonic of Alport syndrome. The diagnosis is based on finding hematuria in many family members, a history of kidney failure in related males, and a kidney biopsy showing characteristic ultrastructural changes in the proband or a relative. Immunofluorescence

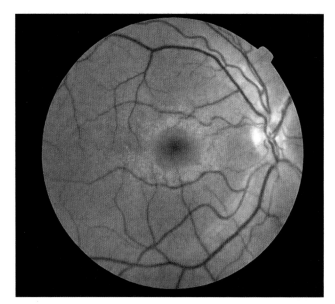

Fig. 42.4 Retinal photograph of right fundus from a 14-year-old boy with Alport syndrome shows perimacular dots and flecks that spare the foveola and are more discrete at the outer margin of the ring. Alport retinopathy varies from occasional dots and flecks in the temporal macula to this appearance. (Courtesy Dr. Judith Savige and Dr. Deb Colville.)

examination of the biopsy specimen should include staining with antibodies specific to GBM or to α5(IV); the lack of staining in most male patients with Alport syndrome helps to differentiate Alport syndrome from familial TBMD, in which staining is normal. If the skin of affected family members is known to lack immunofluorescent staining with antibodies to α5(IV), an α5(IV) immunofluorescence examination of a skin biopsy from a suspected case in the family may be diagnostic.

Molecular diagnosis is almost 100% sensitive and specific but only after a mutation has been found in the family. Sequencing the *COL4A5* gene is at least 80% sensitive for mutations, but is expensive, and sequencing of *COL4A3* and *COL4A4* may also be required if the *COL4A5* test is normal. In families with a previously defined *COL4A* mutation, molecular diagnosis of affected males and gene-carrying females is possible.

The key to diagnosis is clinical suspicion of Alport syndrome in any patient with otherwise unexplained hematuria, glomerulopathy, or kidney failure. In many cases, the familial nature of the condition is not immediately apparent. Inquiry into the family history must be detailed and complete. The patient is usually a boy or young man, and, given the X-linked transmission, he may have one or more male relatives with kidney failure in his mother's family. Urine samples from both of the patient's parents, particularly his mother, should be checked for hematuria. Although it is a helpful clue, it is crucial to remember that hearing loss is neither a sensitive nor a specific marker of Alport syndrome; it is neither necessary nor sufficient for the diagnosis. Many adults with kidney failure from Alport syndrome do not have conspicuous hearing loss, particularly those with the *COL4A5* L1649R mutation. In addition, many patients with hearing loss and kidney disease do not have Alport syndrome but instead have other kidney disorders, most often glomerulonephritis, with a more common cause for hearing loss, such as noise exposure, aminoglycoside therapy, or unrelated inherited hearing loss.

TREATMENT

There is no specific treatment for Alport syndrome, but clinical trials are currently under way. General measures to retard the progression of kidney failure, such as treatment of hypertension, specifically with angiotensin-converting enzyme (ACE) inhibitors, appear warranted. Animal studies and observational data from Europe show that ACE inhibition delays onset of kidney failure and prolongs survival, although controlled trials are still lacking. Unconfirmed reports claim benefit from cyclosporine in reducing proteinuria and retarding progression of kidney disease; however, other investigators have found little benefit with risk of cyclosporine nephrotoxicity.

Male patients should wear hearing protection in noisy surroundings. Hearing aids improve but do not completely restore hearing loss. Tinnitus is usually resistant to all forms of therapy; hearing aids may make it less disruptive by amplifying ambient sounds. Retinal lesions do not commonly affect vision and require no therapy. The serious impairment to vision caused by lenticonus or cataract cannot be corrected with spectacles or contact lenses. Lens removal with reimplantation of an intraocular lens is standard and satisfactory treatment.

RELATED DISORDERS

AUTOSOMAL-RECESSIVE ALPORT SYNDROME

A few children have homozygous or compound heterozygous mutations of the genes for the α3(IV) or α4(IV) chains of type IV collagen. Boys and girls are equally affected, and both may develop severe kidney disease before the age of 10 years. The heterozygous parents commonly have TBMD (discussed later), but not all have persistent hematuria.

AUTOSOMAL-DOMINANT ALPORT SYNDROME

Several recent studies show that families with autosomal-dominant Alport syndrome as a consequence of heterozygous mutations of the genes for the α3(IV) or α4(IV) chains of type IV collagen appear to be more common than previously reported.

ALPORT SYNDROME WITH THROMBOCYTOPATHY: EPSTEIN SYNDROME AND FECHTNER SYNDROME

The Epstein and Fechtner syndromes are uncommon autosomal-dominant syndromes of hematuria and progressive kidney failure associated with moderate thrombocytopenia and severe hearing loss in males and females. Platelets (about 7 μm in diameter) are much larger than normal (1 to 1.5 μm), and there is a mild or moderate bleeding tendency. In families with Fechtner syndrome, an additional feature is inclusion bodies (Fechtner bodies) in leukocytes. These syndromes are caused by a mutation in the nonmuscle myosin heavy chain 9 gene *(MYH9)* on chromosome 22q12.3-13.1.

FAMILIAL THIN BASEMENT MEMBRANE DISEASE

TBMD, or benign familial hematuria, is an autosomal-dominant basement membrane glomerulopathy. Many cases result from heterozygous mutations of the *COL4A3* or *COL4A4* gene at chromosome 2q35 to 2q37; those patients who carry homozygous or compound heterozygous mutations in these same genes develop autosomal-recessive Alport syndrome. Ultrastructurally, the GBM is uniformly thinned to about one half its normal thickness. There is no disruption or lamellation of the GBM, nor are any other abnormalities of the glomeruli, tubules, vessels, or interstitium visible by light, immunofluorescence, or electron microscopy. Kidney failure seldom occurs. Longevity is unaffected by this condition, with survivors into the ninth decade documented. Minor degrees of lamellation of the GBM and hearing loss have been described in some families, but these families might have had unrecognized Alport syndrome.

FAMILIAL FOCAL SEGMENTAL GLOMERULOSCLEROSIS

COL4A3, *COL4A4*, and *COL4A5* mutations are emerging as the most common cause of familial FSGS presenting in adults.

After the precise diagnosis is established, the patient and family can be spared further invasive tests, and an appropriate prognosis can be provided to them and to health insurers. However, the distinction between Alport syndrome and benign familial hematuria is not always easy to make. Being certain of the pattern of inheritance requires a large pedigree with accurate diagnoses for all family members. A single mistaken diagnosis from incidental kidney disease, inaccurate urinalysis, or incomplete penetrance may vitiate conclusions about the pattern of inheritance in the entire pedigree. Even biopsy evidence is fallible. Early cases of Alport syndrome may show ultrastructural changes indistinguishable from those of benign familial hematuria. This is particularly likely if a child from an adult-type Alport kindred is diagnosed based on a biopsy result. Stability of serum creatinine for several years in a child does not exclude adult-type Alport syndrome, and testing for mutations for the common adult types of X-linked Alport syndrome may avoid some diagnostic errors. The situation is further complicated because cases of autosomal-recessive Alport syndrome will occasionally turn up in families with TBMD. In these families, autosomal-dominant TBMD and autosomal-recessive Alport syndrome are caused by the same mutations.

APPROACH TO THE PATIENT WITH HEREDITARY NEPHRITIS

Although Alport syndrome is less common than polycystic kidney disease, it is probably more common than generally appreciated. Important conditions comprising the differential diagnoses of hematuria in young persons include IgA nephropathy or other glomerulonephritides, renal calculi, and medullary sponge kidney. The differential diagnosis of familial kidney disease with hematuria includes TBMD, familial IgA nephropathy, Fabry disease, and polycystic kidney disease. Familial kidney diseases without hematuria that may be confused with Alport syndrome include polycystic kidney disease, medullary cystic disease, and rare forms of inherited glomerular and tubulointerstitial kidney disease.

If a patient with unexplained hematuria or kidney failure has a family history of hematuria or kidney failure, the family history should be extended, concentrating particularly on the mother's male relatives. Identifying hearing loss strengthens, and finding a specific ocular lesion greatly strengthens, suspicion for Alport syndrome. Kidney biopsy is usually indicated for one family member, but after the diagnosis of a heritable basement membrane nephropathy is established in a family, it is difficult to justify biopsies in other members unless there are features that suggest another diagnosis. The extent of investigation is guided by clinical judgment and relates inversely to the strength of the family history. For example, a young man on the line of descent of a known Alport family whose urine contains dysmorphic erythrocytes needs minimal investigation. He may need no further workup other than an assessment of the glomerular filtration rate and urine protein quantification, unless there are additional clinical features suggesting a systemic disease. A patient with hematuria and an uncertain family history may merit the standard nephrologic workup for hematuria. If suspicion of Alport syndrome is moderate or strong, and the test is available, a skin biopsy with staining for the α5(IV) chain may be considered, particularly if a known affected family member is available as a positive control.

Genetic testing, if undertaken, generally will start with *COL4A5* sequencing. If this is normal, sequencing of *COL4A3* and *COL4A4* can be considered. After a mutation is defined in a family, targeted mutation analysis is an inexpensive way to determine whether other family members carry the mutant gene and may be spared the need for a kidney biopsy. In adults with late-onset kidney failure in the United States, screening with a single assay that is available for the common adult-type mutations (C1564S, L1649R, and R1677Q) can be used as an economical first step.

Patients with any hereditary nephropathy should be informed about the nature of the disease and perhaps be given a copy of the genetic analysis or kidney biopsy report to avoid unnecessary further investigation. Similar recommendations apply to family members who are potential gene carriers. Those with Alport syndrome should be followed regularly for elevation of blood pressure and changes in kidney function. The frequency of follow-up depends on the anticipated age of onset of kidney function deterioration in the family. Those with familial TBMD should be checked about every 2 years, because some may ultimately turn out to have Alport syndrome.

BIBLIOGRAPHY

Barker DF, Hostikka SL, Zhou J, et al. Identification of mutations in the *COL4A5* collagen gene in Alport's syndrome. *Science.* 1990;248:1224-1227.

Bekheirnia MR, Reed B, Gregory MC, et al. Genotype-phenotype correlation in X-linked Alport syndrome. *J Am Soc Nephrol.* 2010;21:876-883.

Gleeson MJ. Alport's syndrome: audiological manifestations and implications. *J Laryngol Otol.* 1984;98:449-465.

Govan JA. Ocular manifestations of Alport's syndrome: a hereditary disorder of basement membranes? *Br J Ophthalmol.* 1983;67:493-503.

Gregory MC. Alport's syndrome and thin basement membrane nephropathy: unraveling the tangled strands of type IV collagen. *Kidney Int.* 2004;65:1109-1110.

Gregory MC, Shamshirsam A, Kamgar M, et al. Alport's syndrome, Fabry's disease, and nail-patella syndrome. In: Schrier RW, ed. *Diseases of the Kidney.* 8th ed. Boston, MA: Little Brown; 2007;540-569.

Gross O, Licht C, Anders HJ, et al. Early angiotensin-converting enzyme inhibition in Alport syndrome delays renal failure and improves life expectancy. *Kidney Int.* 2012;81:494-501.

Heath KE, Campos-Barros A, Toren A, et al. Nonmuscle myosin heavy chain IIA mutations define a spectrum of autosomal dominant macrothrombocytopenias: May-Hegglin anomaly and Fechtner, Sebastian, Epstein, and Alport-like syndromes. *Am J Hum Genet.* 2001;69:1033-1045.

Jais JP, Knebelmann B, Giatras I, et al. X-linked Alport syndrome: natural history in 195 families and genotype-phenotype correlations in males. *J Am Soc Nephrol.* 2000;11:649-657.

Jais JP, Knebelmann B, Giatras I, et al. X-linked Alport syndrome: natural history and genotype-phenotype correlations in girls and women belonging to 195 families. A "European Community Alport Syndrome Concerted Action" study. *J Am Soc Nephrol.* 2003;14:2603-2610.

Kashtan CE, Ding J, Gregory M, et al. Clinical practice recommendations for the treatment of Alport syndrome: a statement of the Alport Syndrome Research Collaborative. *Pediatr Nephrol.* 2013;28:5-11.

Kashtan CE, Kleppel MM, Gubler M-C. Immunohistologic findings in Alport syndrome. In: Tryggvason K, ed. *Molecular Pathology and Genetics of Alport's Syndrome.* Basel: Karger; 1996;142-153.

Lemmink HH, Nielsson WN, Mochizuki T, et al. Benign familial hematuria due to mutation of the type 4 collagen gene. *J Clin Invest.* 1996;98:1114-1118.

Tiebosch TA, Frederik PM, van Breda Vriesman PJ, et al. Thin basement membrane nephropathy in adults with persistent hematuria. *N Engl J Med.* 1989;320:14-18.

Fabry Disease

43

Gere Sunder-Plassmann; Manuela Födinger; Renate Kain

Fabry disease (OMIM 301500) is an X-linked lysosomal storage disorder that results from absent or deficient activity of the enzyme α-galactosidase A (αGAL; EC 3.2.1.22). This enzyme is encoded by the *GLA* gene on Xq22 (Fig. 43.1), with more than 800 different mutations so far described. A recent newborn screening study reported the incidence of mutations in *GLA* to be 1:3859 births in Austria. The enzyme defect leads to progressive accumulation of glycosphingolipids, predominantly globotriaosylceramide (Gb3), in all organs (Fig. 43.2).

Early manifestations during childhood include pain, anhidrosis, and gastrointestinal symptoms, among others (Box 43.1). Later, chronic kidney disease (CKD; Fig. 43.3) leading to end-stage kidney disease (ESKD), hypertrophic cardiomyopathy (Fig. 43.4), and cerebral events (Fig. 43.5) are the clinically most important organ manifestations resulting in a reduced life span of hemizygous men and heterozygous women. Most male patients develop the classic phenotype with involvement of all organ systems, whereas alterations in X-inactivation lead to highly variable disease expression in women. Furthermore, kidney or heart variant phenotypes with later onset of disease, probably linked to some residual enzyme activity, have also been described. Importantly, because of the nonspecific nature of complaints, there is often a delay of more than 10 to 20 years from the earliest symptoms of disease until the correct diagnosis is established. Therefore it is prudent to include Fabry disease in the differential diagnosis if two or more of the clinical problems indicated in Box 43.2 are present in young adults.

Beyond screening individuals with a family history of Fabry disease (Fig. 43.6), many cases are identified by means of kidney biopsy on patients referred to nephrologists for proteinuria or other signs of kidney damage. Other cases are found among high-risk populations, such as patients with ESKD, left ventricular hypertrophy, or stroke. Reduced or absent activity of αGAL in leukocytes confirms the diagnosis in male patients. In women, genetic testing is mandatory because αGAL activity may be normal in a significant proportion. Urinary excretion of Gb3 is increased in many instances, and lyso-Gb3 in the plasma is a promising marker for diagnosis and treatment monitoring. Proteomics, the large-scale study of the entire complement of proteins, is another valuable research tool directed at finding biomarkers of diagnosis, disease progression, and responsiveness to therapy in the urine or serum of patients with Fabry disease.

KIDNEY MANIFESTATIONS OF FABRY DISEASE

Kidney disease is a major complication of Fabry disease related to glycosphingolipid accumulation throughout the nephron, with interstitial fibrosis and focal or segmental glomerulosclerosis observed early in the course of disease. Progression to ESKD occurs in almost all affected men around the fourth or fifth decade of life, but can also be seen in adolescents. The course of the disease is less severe in women, who may also eventually progress to ESKD.

In affected individuals, the urine sediment may show red and white blood cells, hyaline or granular casts, and lipid particles with Maltese cross appearance upon polarization. Early in the course, dysfunction of the proximal and distal tubules includes reduced net acid excretion or a urinary concentrating defect with polyuria, nocturia, and polydipsia. Albuminuria or overt proteinuria sometimes develops during childhood, but by the age of 35 years approximately 50% of men and 20% of women manifest proteinuria. Kidney imaging may show cortical or parapelvic cysts, the cause of which is unknown. Increased blood pressure above 130/80 mm Hg was present in 57% of men and 47% of women in a large analysis of 391 patients presenting with various stages of CKD. A retrospective analysis of 168 women and 279 men with Fabry disease from 27 sites in 5 countries showed a more rapid decline of estimated glomerular filtration rate (eGFR) of −6.8 mL/min per 1.73 m^2 per year in men with an eGFR less than 60 mL/min per 1.73 m^2 versus −3.0 mL/min per 1.73 m^2 in men with eGFR greater than 60 mL/min per 1.73 m^2. The corresponding progression rates for women were −2.1 and −0.9 mL/min per 1.73 m^2 per year, respectively. Similar to other nephropathies, proteinuria and hypertension are also associated with more rapid decline in kidney function. ESKD developed in 49 men and 8 women described in this report. The prevalence of Fabry disease among patients undergoing dialysis enrolled in large US and European registries was 0.017% and 0.019%, but most of the case-finding studies during the last decade have shown a prevalence of 0.2% to 0.5% among men with ESKD. In patients with an established diagnosis of Fabry disease, a routine kidney biopsy is not mandatory. Annual monitoring should include measurements of serum creatinine and urinary albumin- or protein-to-creatinine ratio.

PATHOLOGY OF KIDNEY DISEASE IN FABRY DISEASE

GROSS PATHOLOGY

There are few gross descriptions of the kidneys in Fabry disease, although enlargement caused by both storage and cysts is described.

LIGHT MICROSCOPY

Histologic changes show characteristically vacuolated "foamy" podocytes. However, other cell types, including endothelial cells, vascular myocytes, and tubular epithelial cells, may be similarly affected by accumulation of glycosphingolipid. In conventional light microscopy on formalin-fixed and paraffin-embedded material, these inclusions appear empty, as their content is removed during processing. Fixation with osmium

and embedding in epoxy resins retains the stored material that can easily be visualized by either electron microscopy or light microscopy on 1-μm thin sections with toluidine blue or methylene blue staining. The lipid content of the inclusions is sudanophilic and stains with oil red O on frozen section. It may be further characterized by immunohisto-chemistry or lectin binding. Specific histologic changes are usually accompanied by a varying degree of mesangial sclerosis, tubular atrophy, interstitial fibrosis, and sclerosis of arterial blood vessels that correlates with the stage of CKD.

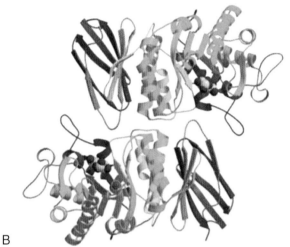

Fig. 43.1 (A) Organization of the *GLA* gene on Xq22.1. The whole gene spans 12.4 kb of genomic DNA and contains seven exons. Black boxes in the lower scheme indicate seven coding regions (exons) of the *GLA* gene. The upper scheme shows the exon position numbering according to the GenBank database entry X14448.1. (B) The structure of α-galactosidase A (αGAL). The structure of the human αGAL dimer is shown in ribbon representation. The ribbon is colored from blue to red as the polypeptide goes from *N*- to *C*-terminus. The active site is identified by the catalytic product galactose, shown in sphere Corey-Pauling-Koltun format. Each monomer in the homodimer contains two domains, a (β/α)8 barrel containing the active site *(blue to yellow)* plus a *C* terminal antiparallel β domain *(yellow to red)*. (A, From Doctoral thesis, Anita Jallitsch-Halper, Medical University of Vienna, 2012; B, From Garman SC. Structure-function relationships in alpha-galactosidase A. *Acta Paediatr Suppl*. 2007;96:6–16, Fig. 1.)

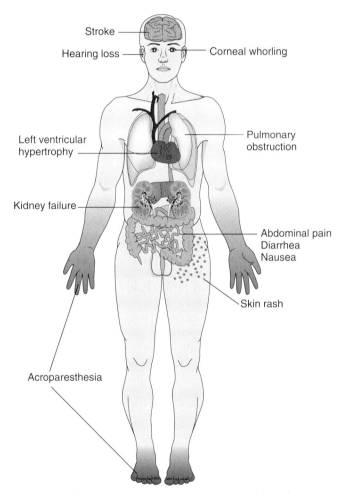

Fig. 43.2 Organ manifestations in patients with Fabry disease.

Box 43.1 Early Signs and Symptoms of Fabry Disease

Nervous System

Acroparesthesias, nerve deafness, heat intolerance, tinnitus

Gastrointestinal Tract

Nausea, vomiting, diarrhea, postprandial bloating and pain, early satiety, difficulty gaining weight

Skin

Angiokeratoma, hypohidrosis

Eyes

Corneal and lenticular opacities, vasculopathy (retina, conjunctiva)

Kidneys

Albuminuria, proteinuria, impaired concentrating ability, increased urinary Gb3 excretion

Heart

Impaired heart rate variability, arrhythmias, ECG abnormalities (shortened PR interval), mild valvular insufficiency

ECG, Electrocardiogram; *Gb3*, globotriaosylceramide.
Adapted from Germain DP. Fabry disease. *Orphanet J Rare Dis*. 2010;5:30.

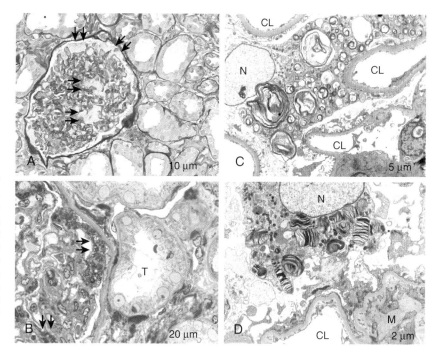

Fig. 43.3 Histopathology and electron microscopy of kidney manifestations in Fabry disease. (A) Light microscopy of formalin-fixed and paraffin-embedded material shows "foamy" podocytes *(arrows)* resulting from numerous empty cytoplasmic vacuoles (periodic acid–Schiff). Cytoplasmic inclusions are osmiophilic *(arrows)*. (B) Toluidine blue on Epon-embedded thin section. Electron microscopy showing lamellated membrane inclusion bodies with either "myelin-like" (C) or "zebroid" (D) appearance in secondary lysosomes. *CL*, Capillary lumen; *M*, mesangium; *N*, nucleus of podocytes; *T*, proximal tubule.

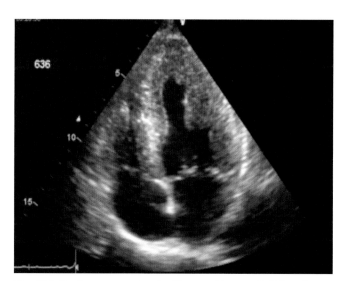

Fig. 43.4 Cardiac sonography of a 53-year-old man with Fabry disease showing cardiac hypertrophy. (Courtesy Gerald Mundigler, MD, Medical University of Vienna.)

Kidney biopsy is therefore considered a valuable instrument in the baseline assessment of Fabry nephropathy, and a validated scoring sheet has been developed to record progression on serial biopsies by light microscopy (see Fig. 43.3).

ELECTRON MICROSCOPY

Electron microscopy shows podocytes with lamellated membrane inclusion bodies in secondary lysosomes. These consist of concentric "myelin-like" rings or have a striped "zebroid" appearance (see Fig. 43.3).

DIFFERENTIAL DIAGNOSIS

Similar histologic features as seen in Fabry disease have been reported in small series of patients receiving chloroquine for autoimmune diseases. Despite the very similar appearance

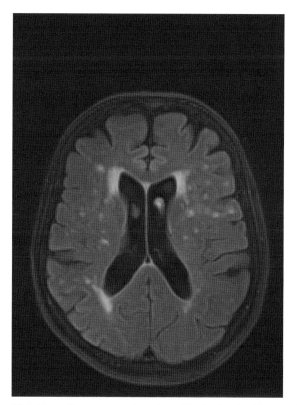

Fig. 43.5 Magnetic resonance imaging of the brain of a 63-year-old woman with Fabry disease showing typical white matter lesions on a T2-weighted image. (Courtesy Paulus Rommer, MD, Medical University of Vienna.)

of zebroid or lamellar inclusion bodies in kidney biopsies by transmission electron microscopy (TEM), curvilinear bodies (twisted microtubular structures) seem to be a unique distinguishing feature of chloroquine-induced nephropathy for which the pathogenetic mechanisms remain inconclusive. αGLA deficiency should be ruled out genetically and

Box 43.2   Signs and Symptoms Suggestive of Fabry Disease[a]

1. Acroparesthesia or neuropathic pain in hands or feet beginning in later childhood, precipitated by illness, fever, exercise, emotional stress, or exposure to heat
2. Persistent proteinuria of unknown cause
3. Hypertrophic cardiomyopathy, especially with prominent diastolic dysfunction[b]
4. Progressive CKD
5. Cryptogenic stroke or transient ischemic attack
6. Family history of ESKD, stroke, or hypertrophic cardiomyopathy showing an X-linked pattern of transmission that primarily, but not solely, affects men
7. Vague, persistent, or recurrent abdominal pain associated with nausea, diarrhea, and tenesmus

[a]Any combination of two or more of these problems is highly suggestive of Fabry disease in either sex.
[b]This may be the only clinical manifestation of Fabry disease in patients of either sex with variants of classical Fabry disease.
CKD, Chronic kidney disease; *ESKD*, end-stage kidney disease.
Adapted from Clarke JT. Narrative review: Fabry disease. *Ann Intern Med*. 2007;146:425–433.

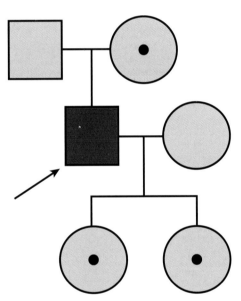

Fig. 43.6 Pedigree of a family with Fabry disease. The index case *(arrow)* was diagnosed by a nationwide case-finding study among Austrian patients undergoing dialysis. His mother and the two daughters *(dot)* carry the same mutation and were asymptomatic at the time of screening. (Case 3 from Kotanko P, et al. Results of a nationwide screening for Anderson-Fabry disease among dialysis patients. *J Am Soc Nephrol*. 2004;15:1323–1329.)

biochemically in those patients, even if systemic iatrogenic phospholipidosis is suspected.

TREATMENT ISSUES IN FABRY DISEASE

Fabry disease can affect every organ system. Therefore various symptoms may require specific therapy (Box 43.3). The most debilitating early symptom, often starting in childhood, is

Box 43.3   Concomitant Therapy in Patients With Fabry Disease

Acroparesthesia

Painful crisis: avoiding quick temperature changes, nonsteroidal antiinflammatory drugs
Chronic pain: anticonvulsants

Hypohidrosis

Appropriate temperature and environment

Angiokeratoma

Cosmetic removal with argon laser therapy

Proteinuria

ACE inhibitors or ARB

Kidney Failure

Dialysis, transplantation

Gastrointestinal Symptoms

Pain relief, H2-blockers, motility agents, pancreatic enzyme supplementation

Hypertension

Regular monitoring and rigorous surveillance following general guidelines (avoid beta-blockers because they can cause sinus bradycardia)

Hyperlipidemia

Regular routine surveillance, statin therapy

Edema

Diuretics, compression stockings, lymph drainage

Stroke Prevention

Management of hypertension, diabetes, smoking, and dyslipidemia; aspirin, clopidogrel

Depression

Selective serotonin reuptake inhibitors, serotonin norepinephrine reuptake inhibitors

ACE, Angiotensin converting enzyme; *ARB*, angiotensin receptor blockers.
Adapted from Whybra-Trümpler C. Symptomatic and ancillary therapy. In: Elstein D, Altarescu G, Beck M, eds. *Fabry Disease*. Dordrecht, Heidelberg, London, New York: Springer; 2010: 481–487.

chronic pain; this is typically triggered by vigorous exercise and temperature changes. Pain (and depression) management agents include gabapentin, carbamazepine, phenytoin, amitriptyline, and other antidepressants.

RENIN-ANGIOTENSIN-ALDOSTERONE SYSTEM BLOCKADE

The role of renin-angiotensin-aldosterone system (RAAS) blockade remains an unresolved issue in Fabry disease. One uncontrolled study of 11 patients suggested reduction of proteinuria and stabilization of kidney function with angiotensin converting enzyme (ACE) inhibitors or angiotensin receptor blockers (ARB); however, in the Fabry Outcome

Survey (FOS), 208 subjects had a nonstatistically significant reduction in eGFR with ACE inhibitor or ARB use. Furthermore, recombinant αGAL may interact with endogenous ACE and inhibit its activity, resulting in lower blood pressure during enzyme infusion.

DIALYSIS AND TRANSPLANTATION

European and US studies have shown that patients with Fabry disease receiving dialysis have a poorer 3-year survival rate as compared with nondiabetic controls. The 5-year survival after kidney transplantation is also lower than that of controls. However, Fabry nephropathy does not recur in the allograft, and transplanted Fabry patients appear to have better overall outcomes than those maintained on dialysis. Therefore kidney transplantation should be recommended as a first-choice therapy for patients with ESKD from Fabry disease.

ENZYME REPLACEMENT THERAPY

Specific enzyme replacement therapy with intravenous recombinant human αGAL has been available for treatment of Fabry disease since 2001. It can be considered for every adult male patient, for symptomatic boys, and for symptomatic women.

Two preparations are currently available, with other products in clinical development. The first, Agalsidase alfa (Replagal, Shire Human Genetic Therapies, Lexington, Massachusetts), is produced in human skin fibroblasts with gene activation technology. It is approved at a dose of 0.2 mg/kg every 2 weeks (infusion time: 40 minutes) in the European Union and many other countries, but not in the United States. The other product, agalsidase beta (Fabrazyme, Sanofi Genzyme, Cambridge, Massachusetts), is produced in Chinese hamster ovary cells and is registered for use at 1.0 mg/kg every other week (infusion time: several hours). Fabrazyme is the only currently available enzyme replacement in the United States.

Side effects of enzyme replacement therapy include fever, rigors, and chills, typically mild to moderate in nature. These occur in more than half of the patients during the first months of treatment. Infusion-related reactions may be due to IgG or IgE antibodies that have been detected in several patients. In case of reactions, the infusion rate should be decreased or stopped, and the administration of antihistamines and/ or corticosteroids should be considered. The infusion can be continued in the case of mild reactions. Some patients need premedication with antihistamines, paracetamol/ acetaminophen, or corticosteroids. In patients receiving maintenance dialysis therapy, the infusion can be administered during dialysis treatment.

The clinical effect of both products was examined in two small pivotal trials, a few controlled studies, and numerous uncontrolled studies and registry reports. In a double-blind, placebo-controlled trial, Schiffmann et al. randomized 26 men to receive Agalsidase alpha at a dosage of 0.2 mg/kg ($n = 14$) or placebo ($n = 12$) every other week for a total of 12 doses. Neuropathic pain, the primary endpoint, improved during therapy with Agalsidase alpha as assessed by a pain questionnaire. Similarly, pain-related quality-of-life improved during active treatment. Secondary endpoints included kidney function, with no significant difference in the change of measured GFR or kidney tissue Gb3 content.

In the other pivotal trial, Eng et al. examined the effect of Agalsidase beta in 58 adults (56 men, 2 women) with Fabry disease by examining the percentage of patients in whom renal microvascular endothelial Gb3 deposits were cleared. After 20 weeks of treatment (11 infusions), 20 of the 29 participants (69%) in the Agalsidase beta group had no microvascular endothelial Gb3 deposits, as compared with 0 of 29 participants in the placebo group. Among secondary endpoints, there was no difference in pain between active treatment and placebo.

A subsequent randomized controlled study by Banikazemi et al. failed to show an effect of Agalsidase beta on the primary composite endpoint (time to first clinical kidney, heart, or cerebrovascular event or death) in 82 individuals (10 women and 72 men) with advanced Fabry disease and a mean serum creatinine of 1.6 mg/dL; there were only 27 outcomes in this trial, potentially limiting power. A per-protocol analysis, adjusted for baseline proteinuria, however, suggested an effect of Agalsidase beta as compared with placebo.

Uncontrolled studies suggest stabilization or even improvement of kidney and heart disease manifestations during enzyme replacement therapy in many patients. Quality-of-life, gastrointestinal symptoms, hypohidrosis, pulmonary obstruction, and other clinical symptoms also showed improvement. Kidney function, proteinuria, and blood pressure are important predictors of the kidney response to enzyme replacement therapy. In a recent analysis of 213 patients treated with Agalsidase beta for at least 2 years enrolled in the Fabry Registry, a higher urinary protein level, worse initial kidney function, and delayed initiation of enzyme replacement therapy after the onset of symptoms were strong predictors of kidney disease progression in men. A history of cardiac or cerebral events was also associated with a steeper slope of eGFR decline. A total of 75% of the male patients had an eGFR slope of −2.8 to −15.5 mL/min per 1.73 m^2 during enzyme therapy. In a report from the FOS, kidney function was assessed in 208 patients treated with Agalsidase alpha for at least 5 years. The mean annual change in eGFR was −2.2 mL/min per 1.73 m^2 in men and −0.7 mL/min per 1.73 m^2 in women. Patients with 24-hour protein excretion greater than 1 g/24 hour had worse kidney function at baseline and follow-up compared with patients with protein excretion of 500 to 1000 mg/24 hour or less than 500 mg/24 hour. Kidney function was worse in patients with baseline hypertension, and there was a more rapid annual decline compared with normotensive patients. Taken together, these data suggest that Agalsidase alpha or Agalsidase beta cannot halt kidney disease progression in many patients. However, a comparison of treated and untreated patients suggests a somewhat attenuated slope of eGFR decline in treated patients (Fig. 43.7).

Potential reasons for disease progression during enzyme replacement therapy include low physical stability of recombinant αGAL, a short circulating half-life, and variable uptake into different tissues. Importantly, antibodies to recombinant human αGAL can be detected in about 40% of treated men and are associated with greater left ventricular mass and substantially lower GFR, among other disease manifestations, as compared with antibody-negative patients.

Thus novel therapeutic strategies are needed to improve outcomes in patients with Fabry disease. Potential strategies include higher administration frequency, other routes of

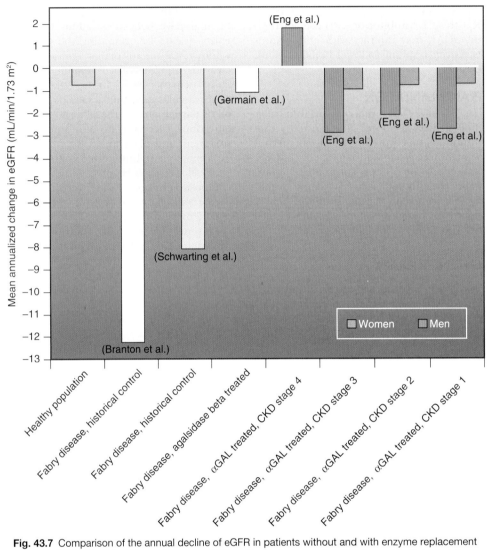

Fig. 43.7 Comparison of the annual decline of eGFR in patients without and with enzyme replacement therapy. *CKD*, Chronic kidney disease; *eGFR*, estimated glomerular filtration rate. (Adapted from Mehta A, Beck M, Elliott P, et al. Enzyme replacement therapy with agalsidase alfa in patients with Fabry's disease: an analysis of registry data. *Lancet.* 2009;374:1986–1996, Fig. 4.)

enzyme administration, and combining enzyme therapy with pharmacologic chaperones.

PHARMACOLOGIC CHAPERONES

A pharmacologic chaperone (or pharmacoperone, from "protein chaperone") is a small molecule that causes mutant proteins to fold and route correctly within the cell. Missense mutations in Fabry disease may cause misfolding of αGAL, leading to retention in the endoplasmic reticulum and subsequent degradation. A potent αGAL inhibitor, the iminosugar 1-deoxygalactonojirimycin (migalastat hydrochloride; Amicus Therapeutics, Cranbury, New Jersey) is an analogue of the terminal galactose of Gb3. It binds to the active site of αGAL, thereby improving stability and trafficking to the lysosomes (Fig. 43.8). It reduces Gb3 storage in vitro and in vivo and stabilizes wild-type and mutant forms of αGAL. Furthermore, co-administration improves the pharmacologic properties of recombinant human αGAL. It prevents denaturation and activity loss in vitro and results in substantially higher cellular αGAL and greater Gb3 reduction compared to recombinant human αGAL alone in vivo. Migalastat hydrochloride increases

enzyme activity and reduces Gb3 in the tissue of patients with specific mutations in *GLA*. An in vitro assay can be used to identify subjects with mutations that are likely to respond to chaperone treatment.

A double-blind, placebo-controlled phase III study examined the safety and efficacy of migalastat hydrochloride (150 mg orally every other day for 6 months) in 67 patients with Fabry disease. Kidney biopsy samples were available for 64 patients and showed a ≥50% reduction in the number of Gb3 inclusions per kidney interstitial capillary in 41% of patients who received migalastat hydrochloride and 28% of patients who received placebo ($P = 0.3$). Of note, among 45 patients with responsive mutations, therapy with migalastat hydrochloride was associated with a greater reduction in the mean number of Gb3 inclusions per kidney interstitial capillary compared with placebo (-0.25 ± 0.10 vs. 0.07 ± 0.13; $P = .008$). Among other secondary endpoints, therapy with migalastat hydrochloride reduced plasma levels of lyso-Gb3 and gastrointestinal symptoms but showed no effect on urinary Gb3, kidney function, or left ventricular mass. In patients who received migalastat hydrochloride for ≥18 months, kidney function remained stable and left

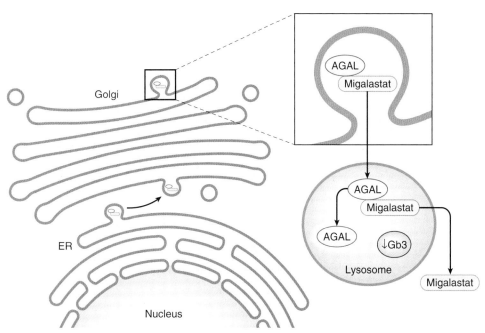

Fig. 43.8 Mechanism of action of migalastat hydrochloride. Binding of migalastat to catalytically active but unstable AGAL allows for proper folding and trafficking of the enzyme from the ER through the Golgi apparatus to the lysosome. In the lysosome, dissociation of migalastat restores enzyme activity and allows degradation of Gb3. *AGAL*, α-galactosidase A; *ER*, endoplasmic reticulum; *Gb3*, globo-triaosylceramide. (From Gaggl M, Sunder-Plassmann G. Fabry disease – a pharmacological chaperone on the horizon. *Nat Rev Nephrol.* 2016;12:653–654, Fig. 1).

ventricular mass index significantly decreased. In 2016, the European Medical Agency approved migalastat hydrochloride for the treatment of Fabry disease in patients with suitable mutations based on this trial and another phase III study that also showed stable kidney function and an improvement of left ventricular mass. Taken together, these data suggest an important clinical potential for this new therapeutic tool, alone or in combination with enzyme replacement therapy.

KEY BIBLIOGRAPHY

Banikazemi M, Bultas J, Waldek S, et al. Agalsidase-beta therapy for advanced Fabry disease: a randomized trial. *Ann Intern Med.* 2007; 146:77-86.

Benjamin ER, Khanna R, Schilling A, et al. Co-administration with the pharmacological chaperone AT1001 increases recombinant human alpha-galactosidase A tissue uptake and improves substrate reduction in Fabry mice. *Mol Ther.* 2012;20:717-726.

Branton MH, Schiffmann R, Sabnis SG, et al. Natural history of Fabry renal disease: influence of alpha-galactosidase A activity and genetic mutations on clinical course. *Medicine (Baltimore).* 2002;81:122-138.

Clarke JT. Narrative review: Fabry disease. *Ann Intern Med.* 2007;146:425-433.

Eng CM, Guffon N, Wilcox WR, et al. Safety and efficacy of recombinant human alpha-galactosidase A replacement therapy in Fabry's disease. *N Engl J Med.* 2001;345:9-16.

Fogo AB, Bostad L, Svarstad E, et al. Scoring system for renal pathology in Fabry disease: report of the International Study Group of Fabry Nephropathy (ISGFN). *Nephrol Dial Transplant.* 2010;25:2168-2177.

Gaggl M, Sunder-Plassmann G. Fabry disease—a pharmacological chaperone on the horizon. *Nat Rev Nephrol.* 2016;12:653-654.

Gal A. Molecular genetics of Fabry disease and genotype-phenotype correlation. In: Elstein D, Altarescu G, Beck M, eds. *Fabry Disease.* Dordrecht: Springer, pp. 3–19.

Germain DP, Hughes DA, Nicholls K, et al. Treatment of Fabry's Disease with the Pharmacologic Chaperone Migalastat. *N Engl J Med.* 2016;375:545-555.

Hughes DA, Nicholls K, Shankar SP, et al. Oral pharmacological chaperone migalastat compared with enzyme replacement therapy in Fabry disease: 18-month results from the randomised phase III ATTRACT study. *J Med Genet.* 2017;54:288-296.

Lenders M, Stypmann J, Duning T, et al. Serum-mediated inhibition of enzyme replacement therapy in Fabry disease. *J Am Soc Nephrol.* 2016;27:256-264.

Linhart A, Kampmann C, Zamorano JL, et al. Cardiac manifestations of Anderson-Fabry disease: results from the international Fabry outcome survey. *Eur Heart J.* 2007;28:1228-1235.

Mechtler TP, Stary S, Metz TF, et al. Neonatal screening for lysosomal storage disorders: feasibility and incidence from a nationwide study in Austria. *Lancet.* 2012;379:335-341.

Müller-Höcker J, Schmid H, Weiss M, Dendorfer U, Braun GS. Chloroquine-induced phospholipidosis of the kidney mimicking Fabry's disease: case report and review of the literature. *Hum Pathol.* 2003;34:285-289.

Schiffmann R, Kopp JB, Austin HA 3rd, et al. Enzyme replacement therapy in Fabry disease: a randomized controlled trial. *JAMA.* 2001; 285:2743-2749.

Schiffmann R, Warnock DG, Banikazemi M, et al. Fabry disease: progression of nephropathy, and prevalence of cardiac and cerebrovascular events before enzyme replacement therapy. *Nephrol Dial Transplant.* 2009;24:2102-2111.

Sunder-Plassmann G. Renal manifestations of Fabry disease. In: Mehta A, Beck M, Sunder-Plassmann G, eds. *Fabry Disease – Perspectives From 5 Years of FOS.* Oxford: Oxford PharmaGenesis, pp. 203–214.

Sunder-Plassmann G, Födinger M. Fabry disease case finding studies in high-risk populations. In: Elstein D, Altarescu G, Beck M, eds. *Fabry Disease.* Springer, pp. 153–162.

Warnock DG, Bichet DG, Holida M, et al. Oral migalastat HCl leads to greater systemic exposure and tissue levels of active alpha-galactosidase A in Fabry patients when co-administered with infused agalsidase. *PLoS ONE.* 2015;10:e0134341.

West M, Nicholls K, Mehta A, et al. Agalsidase alfa and kidney dysfunction in Fabry disease. *J Am Soc Nephrol.* 2009;20:1132-1139.

Full bibliography can be found on www.expertconsult.com.

TUBULOINTERSTITIAL DISEASES

44

Chronic Tubulointerstitial Disease

Catherine M. Meyers; Mark A. Perazella

Primary interstitial kidney disease makes up a diverse group of diseases that elicit interstitial inflammation associated with renal tubular cell damage. Traditionally, interstitial nephritis has been classified morphologically and clinically into acute and chronic forms. Acute interstitial nephritis (AIN) generally induces rapid deterioration in kidney function with a marked interstitial inflammatory response characterized by mononuclear cell infiltration, interstitial edema, and varying degrees of tubular cell damage. This process typically spares both glomerular and vascular structures, and is discussed more fully in Chapter 33. By contrast, chronic interstitial nephritis (CIN) follows a more indolent course and is characterized by interstitial mononuclear cell infiltration, tubulointerstitial fibrosis, and atrophy. Over time, glomerular and vascular structures are involved, with progressive fibrosis and sclerosis within the kidney. Overlap can occur between these two clinical conditions; AIN sometimes presents as a more insidious disease with progression to chronic kidney disease (CKD). Similarly, some forms of CIN are associated with significant cellular infiltrate.

HISTOPATHOLOGY

Histopathology of CIN is remarkably consistent despite the varied causes (Box 44.1). In addition to tubular cell damage and predominantly mononuclear cell inflammation, CIN is characterized by the development of tubulointerstitial fibrosis and scarring (Fig. 44.1). Interstitial granulomatous disease has also been observed in certain forms of CIN (e.g., sarcoidosis). Glomerular and vascular structures may be relatively preserved early in the course of disease but ultimately become involved in progressive fibrosis and sclerosis. Progressive development of tubulointerstitial fibrosis is a final common pathway to end-stage kidney disease (ESKD) observed in primary disorders of the tubulointerstitium, as well as in primary glomerular or vascular disorders. All forms of progressive kidney disease eventually result in chronic and progressive interstitial fibrosis.

Mononuclear cell infiltrates generally accompany CIN, further suggesting a pathogenic immune-mediated mechanism for disease progression. One hypothesis concerning immune recognition of the interstitium suggests that portions of infectious particles or drug molecules may cross-react with or alter endogenous kidney antigens. An immune response directed against these inciting agents would therefore also target the interstitium. Intriguing results of a study examining a series of kidney biopsy samples obtained over 8 years at a single center suggest a prominent role of Epstein-Barr virus (EBV) in cases of CIN previously deemed idiopathic. Investigators detected EBV DNA and its receptor, CD21, primarily in proximal tubular cells of all 17 patients with primary idiopathic interstitial nephritis. These findings were not apparent in 10 control kidney biopsy specimens. Such observations imply a more prominent role than previously appreciated for EBV infections in eliciting chronic deleterious immune responses that target the interstitium.

MECHANISMS OF TUBULOINTERSTITIAL FIBROSIS

Observations from the experimental literature suggest that renal tubular epithelial-mesenchymal transition (EMT) may play a role in the initiation and progression of tubulointerstitial fibrosis. As the renal epithelium develops from the metanephric mesenchyme via a process of mesenchymal-epithelial transition, observations suggest a unique paradigm of tubulointerstitial response to injury whereby dedifferentiation pathways are activated within the epithelium, resulting in a transition to cells of more mesenchymal characteristics. Dysregulation of such processes in vivo could induce more fibrogenic responses (Fig. 44.2). Renal EMT in this setting could thus facilitate accumulation of fibroblasts and myofibroblasts that are characteristic of CIN and other kidney diseases associated with tubulointerstitial fibrosis.

The ability of renal tubular epithelial cells to transform in vitro to fibroblasts and myofibroblasts is well documented. Although the processes relevant for primary CIN in humans have not been elucidated, experimental models of injury and many in vitro studies have implicated a large role for transforming growth factor-β and other fibrogenic mediators, such as fibroblast growth factor-2, advanced glycation end products, and angiotensin II. These factors regulate the renal fibrogenic responses and renal tubular EMT (Fig. 44.2). In addition, numerous human kidney biopsy studies have demonstrated the colocalization of epithelial and mesenchymal markers on tubular cells in areas of injury, supporting the notion that renal tubular EMT is associated with progressive tubulointerstitial fibrosis in a variety of kidney diseases. However, recent fate-mapping studies, which allow the tagging and tracking of renal epithelial cells in vivo in experimental models of disease, have generated apparently conflicting observations regarding the role of EMT in progressive kidney injury. Future studies will likely better characterize pathways that both initiate and propagate renal fibrogenic processes.

Box 44.1   Chronic Interstitial Nephritis

Drugs/Toxins

Analgesics
Heavy metals (lead, cadmium, mercury)
Lithium
Chinese herbs (aristolochic acid)
Calcineurin inhibitors (cyclosporine, tacrolimus)
Cisplatin
Nitrosoureas
Herbicides (glyphosate)

Hereditary Disorders

Polycystic kidney disease
Modullary cystic disease—juvenile nephronophthisis
Hereditary nephritis

Metabolic Disturbances

Hypercalcemia/nephrocalcinosis
Hypokalemia
Hyperuricemia
Hyperoxaluria
Cystinosis

Immune-Mediated Disorders

Kidney allograft rejection
Systemic lupus erythematosus
Sarcoidosis
Granulomatosis with polyangiitis (Wegener granulomatosis)
Vasculitis
Sjögren syndrome
Tubulointerstitial nephritis and uveitis (TINU) syndrome

Hematologic Disturbances

Multiple myeloma
Light chain disease
Dysproteinemias
Lymphoproliferative disease
Sickle cell disease

Infections

Kidney
Systemic

Obstruction/Mechanical Disorders

Tumors
Stones
Vesicoureteral reflux

Miscellaneous Disorders

Balkan nephropathy (aristolochic acid)
Sri Lankan agricultural nephropathy (SAN)
Mesoamerican nephropathy
Radiation nephritis
Aging
Hypertension
Kidney ischemia

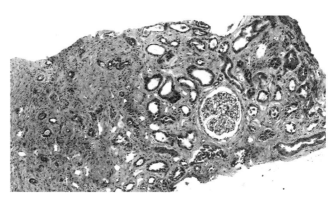

Fig. 44.1 Chronic interstitial nephritis. Light microscopy findings demonstrate focal collections of lymphocytes and pronounced loss of normal tubulointerstitial architecture. There is evidence of tubular dilation and atrophy, as well as interstitial fibrosis and relative sparing of glomerular structures. (Hematoxylin-eosin stain, courtesy Dr. James Balow, National Institutes of Health, National Institute of Diabetes, Digestive and Kidney Diseases, Bethesda, MD.)

Table 44.1   Laboratory Findings in Interstitial Nephritis

Parameter	Finding
Urinary sediment	Erythrocytes, leukocytes (eosinophils), leukocyte casts
Fractional excretion of sodium	Usually >1%
Proximal tubular defects	Glucosuria, bicarbonaturia, phosphaturia, aminoaciduria, proximal RTA
Distal tubular defects	Hyperkalemia, sodium wasting, distal RTA
Medullary defects	Sodium wasting, urine-concentrating defects

RTA, Renal tubular acidosis.

CLINICAL FEATURES

As shown in Box 44.1, CIN occurs in a variety of clinical settings, most commonly following exposure to drugs or toxins, or in settings of hereditary disorders, metabolic disorders, immune-mediated diseases, hematologic disturbances, infections, or obstruction. Because CIN tends to occur as a slowly progressive disease, most patients diagnosed with CIN present with systemic complaints of the primary underlying disease, if one exists, or with symptoms of CKD. Laboratory findings in these patients include low-grade (tubular) proteinuria, microscopic hematuria, and sterile pyuria. As listed in Table 44.1, other frequently reported urinary abnormalities, such as glucosuria, phosphaturia, and sodium wasting, reflect tubular defects. Serologic studies in CIN, such as anti-DNA antibodies, antinuclear antibodies, and complement levels, are typically normal, except when CIN occurs in the setting of a systemic autoimmune disorder.

Affected patients may also have elevated urinary excretion of low-molecular-weight (LMW) proteins that are commonly associated with tubular injury (e.g., lysozyme, β_2-microglobulin, and retinol-binding protein), and increased enzymuria with N-acetyl-β-D-glucosaminidase, alanine aminopeptidase, and intestinal alkaline phosphatase. However, routine assessment of urinary LMW proteins and enzymes is not typically conducted because they are neither diagnostic nor prognostic. Hypertension is another common clinical feature of CIN, although in many forms of CIN it is not apparent until the

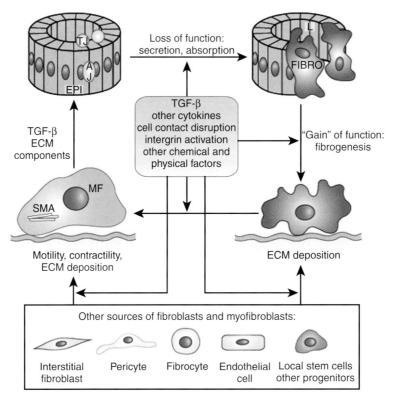

Fig. 44.2 The development and progression of kidney fibrosis. Fibroblasts and myofibroblasts (MF) originate from other cell types (as noted in the *bottom box*) and play a significant role in the process of kidney fibrosis. The paradigm of tubular epithelial-mesenchymal transition suggests an additional pathway to kidney fibrosis, in that tubular epithelium undergoes profound phenotypic changes after exposure to fibrogenic stimuli *(center box)*. This results in loss of epithelial characteristics and gain of mesenchymal characteristics. The transitioning cells might remain in the tubular wall or migrate into the interstitium. Epithelial-derived fibroblasts contribute to the deposition of extracellular matrix (ECM), and a subpopulation may begin expressing α-smooth muscle actin (SMA), a hallmark of the MF phenotype. Activated fibroblasts and MF secrete elevated amounts of transforming growth factor-β (TGF-β), whereas the enhanced contractility of MFs contributes to activation of latent TGF-β through an integrin-mediated mechanochemical pathway. Increasing TGF-β levels along with ECM accumulation might facilitate transformation of previously intact tubules, thereby creating a positive feedback loop of epithelial injury. *AJ*, Adherens junction; *EPI*, epithelium; *FIBRO*, fibroblasts; *L*, lumen; *TJ*, tight junction. (Reprinted by permission from Macmillan Publishers Ltd: Quaggin SE, Kapus A. Scar wars: mapping the fate of epithelial-mesenchymal-myofibroblast transition. *Kidney Int.* 2011;80:41-50.)

patient approaches ESKD. With progressive CIN, kidney ultrasonography in patients without significant structural abnormalities (e.g., cystic kidney disease) typically reveals shrunken, echogenic kidneys. Irregular renal contours and renal calcifications are seen in some forms of CIN.

CLINICAL COURSE AND THERAPY

Because of the slowly progressive loss of kidney function observed in most cases of CIN, general therapeutic considerations include treating an underlying systemic disorder (sarcoidosis), avoiding the drug or toxin exposure (analgesics, lead), or eliminating the condition that has induced the chronic interstitial lesion (obstruction). Interstitial fibrosis and scarring, along with the resultant impairment in kidney function, are not currently amenable to therapeutic intervention. Although definitive diagnosis of CIN requires kidney biopsy, it is probably of limited usefulness in those with

advanced CKD. Therapy is therefore largely supportive, with kidney replacement therapy initiated in ESKD patients. More specific therapies for interstitial lesions associated with lead exposure or sarcoidosis are discussed in the following section.

DISTINCT CAUSES OF CHRONIC TUBULOINTERSTITIAL NEPHRITIS

Many causes of CIN listed in Box 44.1 are more fully described in other chapters of this text. This section focuses on the common causes of primary CIN. It is also noted that progression to ESKD has been reported with all forms of AIN, which likely follow a path to CIN over time.

ANALGESIC NEPHROPATHY

Analgesic nephropathy has been considered the most common form of drug-induced CIN, particularly in the United States,

Europe, and Australia. The condition is associated with chronic excessive consumption of combined analgesic preparations over many years. Affected patients typically have regularly ingested combination analgesic products (e.g., aspirin, phenacetin, and paracetamol) that also contain codeine or caffeine. Over the last several decades, however, recognition of the association of analgesic nephropathy with chronic use of over-the-counter combination analgesic products resulted in a marked reduction in availability of these products to the public, as well as a marked reduction in the incidence of this disease. Phenacetin-containing combination products were particularly noted for their association with analgesic nephropathy, although the disorder continues to be reported even after these products were removed from the market. The subsequent removal of other combination analgesic products resulted in a further decrease in the incidence of analgesic nephropathy worldwide. Since 2002, the United States Renal Data System (USRDS) Annual Data Report indicates that approximately 180 cases of ESKD due to analgesic nephropathy are reported each year in the United States.

The nephrotoxicity of combination analgesics appears to be dose-dependent, with medullary lesions most prominent early in the disease course. Early medullary capillary and tubular changes then extend to interstitial injury and fibrosis, as well as renal papillary necrosis (RPN) with calcification. RPN is characteristic, but not diagnostic, of analgesic nephropathy, because it occurs in other kidney disorders such as diabetes mellitus, sickle cell disease, renal tuberculosis, and urinary tract obstruction. It has also been reported with use of single reagent analgesic preparations, such as nonsteroidal antiinflammatory drugs or aspirin. The mechanism of nephrotoxicity is not completely understood. Ingested compounds and their metabolites are concentrated along the medullary osmotic gradient, likely achieving chronic high levels within the medulla to facilitate the early renal medullary lesions. In addition to high local metabolite concentrations, the relatively vulnerable vascular supply in the medulla could play a major role in initiating and propagating kidney injury.

Similar to many forms of CIN, the clinical manifestations are nonspecific and insidious. Patients typically present with sterile pyuria, mild proteinuria, and slowly progressive loss of the glomerular filtration rate (GFR). As kidney disease progresses, anemia and hypertension develop. The disease has been reported more commonly in women than in men, with 50% to 80% of cases reported in women across several studies. The age range extends from 30 to 70 years of age, with a peak incidence in the early 50s. Daily use of analgesics to treat a chronic pain condition is noted, and estimates suggest that nephropathy develops after a cumulative ingestion of 2 to 3 kg of analgesic preparations. In view of the excessive regular ingestion, psychological dependence on these products has frequently been reported.

Diagnosis of analgesic nephropathy can be difficult to ascertain because patients may be reluctant to fully report the extent of chronic analgesic use, and early signs and symptoms are nonspecific. Clinicians frequently rely on clinical history, urinary findings, and kidney imaging studies to aid in diagnosis of the condition. Intravenous pyelography has not proven useful because of its low sensitivity and requirement for nephrotoxic contrast. Computerized tomography (CT) scanning without intravenous contrast is frequently used to assess kidney structures in this setting (Fig. 44.3).

Bilateral reduction in kidney volume, cortical scarring with irregular kidney contours, and evidence of papillary damage and calcification on CT scan suggests analgesic nephropathy. These typical CT features are not generally noted in other forms of CIN. Studies assessing the sensitivity and specificity of CT findings in analgesic nephropathy, however, have yielded inconsistent findings. Variability may result from different time frames of study, different geographic regions studied (European and US cohort), and distinct analgesic preparations. Noncontrast CT scan is considered a useful diagnostic test even if performed on patients who do not provide a reliable history of excessive analgesic use.

The clinical course of analgesic nephropathy is variable and depends largely on the extent of irreversible kidney scarring that has occurred at the time of diagnosis. Similar to most toxin-induced interstitial diseases, removal of the offending agent before irreversible kidney fibrosis has occurred is essential for preserving kidney function. Several reports of analgesic nephropathy have described stabilization or mild improvement in kidney function with cessation of analgesic use. Analgesic exposure is also associated with development of uroepithelial tumors later in life. Urinary tract malignancies reported are most commonly transitional cell carcinoma, although renal cell carcinoma and sarcoma have also occurred. Excessive analgesic use also appears to confer an increased risk for cardiovascular disease, specifically ischemic heart disease and renal artery stenosis.

CHRONIC LEAD NEPHROPATHY

Exposure to high levels of lead over several years to decades is associated with a progressive CIN referred to as chronic lead nephropathy. Most such exposures are occupational and seen in the manufacturing or use of lead-containing paints, ammunition, radiators, batteries, wires, ceramic glazes, solder, and metal cans. In addition, environmental lead exposure can occur in several settings, such as using lead pipes and solder joints in drinking water lines, consuming crops grown in lead-contaminated soil, or ingesting lead-based paint scraps or "moonshine" generated in lead-lined car radiators. In the developed world, it is rare to see lead exposure high enough to induce lead nephropathy because recognition of its toxicity has resulted in routine removal of lead from sources such as gasoline, paint, and industrial processing. However, this paradigm changed with the recognition of lead (and other heavy metals) intoxication from drinking water from the Flint River water in Michigan. Lead toxicity occurred when the town of Flint switched its water supply from Lake Huron to the Flint River in 2014. While acute lead toxicity has been observed, only time will tell if chronic lead nephropathy will also develop. Since the recognition of this disaster, other drinking water supplies around the United States have been noted to have excessive levels of heavy metals and other pollutants.

Because an early histologic lesion observed with chronic lead exposure consists of proximal tubular intranuclear inclusion bodies composed of a lead-protein complex, the early stage of lead-induced kidney damage probably results from proximal reabsorption with subsequent intracellular lead accumulation. Early clinical manifestations reflect proximal tubular dysfunction with hyperuricemia, aminoaciduria, and glucosuria (see Table 44.1). Because the kidney disease is

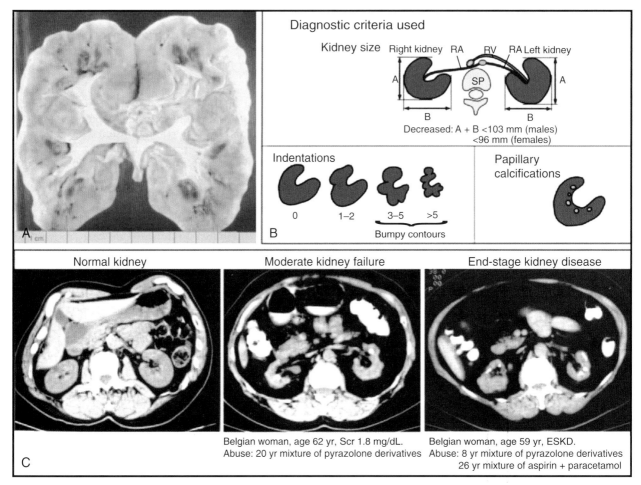

Fig. 44.3 Analgesic nephropathy. (A) Macroscopic kidney specimen from a patient who developed end-stage kidney disease as result of analgesic nephropathy. (B) Characteristic analgesic nephropathy features on computerized tomography (CT) imaging include reduced kidney size, irregular contours, and papillary calcifications. (C) Noncontrast CT findings comparing a normal subject with two cases of analgesic nephropathy, with two distinct levels of reduced kidney function. *ESKD,* End-stage kidney disease; *RA,* renal artery; *RV,* renal vein; *SP,* spine. (Reprinted by permission from the *Journal of the American Society of Nephrology*: De Broe ME, Elseviers MM. Over-the-counter analgesic use. *J Am Soc Nephrol.* 2009;20:2098-2103.)

slowly progressive, affected patients typically present with CKD, hypertension, hyperuricemia, and gout. This symptom complex might, however, suggest the diagnosis of either chronic urate nephropathy or hypertensive nephrosclerosis. Chronic urate nephropathy with tophaceous gout is currently an uncommon condition; moreover, some studies suggest that previously reported cases were associated with chronic lead exposure. By contrast, hypertensive nephrosclerosis is not typically associated with hyperuricemia and gout. Patients presenting with hypertension, hyperuricemia, and CKD should therefore be evaluated for lead exposure.

The diagnosis of chronic lead intoxication is generally established with a lead mobilization test, performed by measuring urinary lead excretion after administering ethylenediaminetetraacetic acid (EDTA). X-ray fluorescence can also be used to determine bone lead levels. The diagnosis of lead nephropathy, however, is frequently made on the basis of a history of lead exposure in the setting of hyperuricemia, hypertension, and slowly progressive kidney disease consistent with CIN. Treatment of lead intoxication consists of chelation

therapy with EDTA or oral succimer. In view of the side effects associated with EDTA administration, chelation therapy should be carefully considered, particularly if there is significant preexisting irreversible kidney fibrosis.

Recent population-based studies have observed a trend of increased blood lead levels in the general population with a related inverse trend in creatinine clearance. It is unclear, however, whether these population-based observations reflect an increase in chronic lead nephropathy or an increase in kidney disease that induces lead retention. These studies suggest that chronic low-level lead exposure in developing countries may confer additional risk for CKD progression. In addition, some studies have suggested that chelation therapy may slow progression of CKD in these patients.

ARISTOLOCHIC ACID NEPHROPATHY AND BALKAN NEPHROPATHY

Rapidly progressive fibrosing interstitial nephritis has been described in clusters of patients in weight loss programs who ingested Chinese herbal preparations tainted with a plant nephrotoxin derived from *Aristolochia fangchi* (aristolochic acid). Kidney lesions are characterized by interstitial fibrosis and tubular atrophy, with a predominance of cortical involvement. Several hundred cases have been reported in the literature thus far, although some cases were observed in patients who ingested herb preparations not containing aristolochic acid. Other reports from Asia suggest that herbal therapy–induced kidney damage is not uncommon. Kidney disease in affected individuals is typically progressive and irreversible despite withdrawal of toxin exposure, with many patients requiring dialysis therapy or transplantation within 1 year of presentation.

The putative nephrotoxin, aristolochic acid, induces tubulointerstitial fibrosis in animal models of disease following chronic daily exposure. The mechanism of aristolochic acid–induced nephrotoxicity (AAN), however, has not been delineated. The observation that some patients exposed to toxic herbs do not develop kidney disease further suggests variability in patient susceptibility to kidney injury. Women also may be at higher risk for the disorder. In addition, variability in herbal products could significantly alter toxin concentration in batched preparations. Studies in animal models indicate that both toxin exposure and concurrent renal vasoconstriction may be required to precipitate the characteristic progressive kidney disease. A frequent association of cellular atypia and urothelial cell malignancies has also been reported in experimental animals and in many affected patients. Identification of aristolactam-DNA adducts, as well as tumor suppressor *p53* gene mutations, in genitourinary tumors has implicated these factors in malignant urothelial transformation. Because many affected patients have undergone kidney transplantation with immunosuppressive therapy, routine surveillance of urinary cytology is generally recommended in view of this association with urothelial malignancy.

Balkan nephropathy (BN) is a form of CIN observed in farmers that is endemic to the areas of Bulgaria, Romania, Serbia, Croatia, Bosnia, and Herzegovina, most commonly along the confluence of the Danube River. Several recent studies suggest that BN is induced by chronic exposure to aristolochic acid in susceptible individuals. Because *Aristolochia* plants grow abundantly in agricultural areas, harvesting of crops, such as wheat, from contaminated fields could introduce aristolochic acid into the local food supply and expose the population to the nephrotoxin. BN and AAN are both linked to aristolochic acid exposure, have predominant renal cortical pathology, and are associated with urothelial tumors. A wide range of tumor incidence, from 2% to 47%, has been reported in these patients. Kidney and urothelial cancer tissue isolated from BN patients identified DNA adducts from aristolochic acid and *p53* gene mutations—two features that characterize aristolochic acid–induced tumors in experimental models and patients with AAN.

BN is a slowly progressive kidney disease that is typically observed after the fourth decade of life and rarely affects patients younger than 20 years of age. Patients generally present with normal blood pressure and either normal or slightly reduced kidney size on ultrasonography. Hematuria and tubular dysfunction may be present. Renal histologic lesions are characterized by predominant cortical fibrosis and tubular atrophy. There is not currently a specific treatment or preventive strategy for the disorder, although corticosteroids may slow progression of CKD.

SARCOIDOSIS

The most common kidney manifestation of sarcoidosis is mediated through disordered calcium metabolism resulting in hypercalcemia and hypercalciuria, occasionally presenting with nephrolithiasis and nephrocalcinosis. Although interstitial disease, at times with noncaseating granuloma formation, is relatively common in sarcoidosis (15% to 30%), autopsy series indicate that it is unusual for the interstitial abnormalities to result in clinically significant kidney dysfunction. Moreover, it is unusual to observe interstitial disease in the absence of extrarenal involvement in sarcoidosis. Although most patients with impaired kidney function respond well to corticosteroid therapy, recovery of kidney function is frequently incomplete because of chronic interstitial inflammation and fibrosis. Presentation with hypercalcemia has been associated with a more sustained response to corticosteroid therapy 1 year following therapy. Relapse of kidney functional impairment during steroid taper has been reported, but progression to ESKD is rare.

SJÖGREN SYNDROME

Sjögren syndrome, a disorder characterized by lymphocyte and plasma cell infiltration in salivary, parotid, and lacrimal glands, results in progressive organ dysfunction and the sicca syndrome. Involvement of other organs, including the kidney, is frequently reported. Circulating autoantibodies (anti-Ro and anti-La) are associated with Sjögren syndrome, and they support the diagnosis. Kidney involvement occurs in up to 67% of affected patients. The kidney lesion consists predominantly of interstitial cellular infiltrates that invade and destroy renal tubules. Cortical granuloma formation has been reported and may suggest the diagnosis of sarcoidosis or the tubulointerstitial nephritis and uveitis (TINU) syndrome. These other conditions, however, are not associated with sicca syndrome. With disease chronicity in Sjögren syndrome, tubular atrophy and interstitial fibrosis are more apparent, and patients may exhibit biochemical disorders from tubular dysfunction. As with sarcoidosis treatment, patients typically respond to a course of corticosteroids. Although rare, ESKD has been reported.

TUBULOINTERSTITIAL NEPHRITIS AND UVEITIS SYNDROME

TINU syndrome is a relatively rare autoimmune process that results in eye and kidney disease. Both acute and CIN are observed with this syndrome. It can occur at any age, but is more common in adolescents. Eye symptoms may precede, coincide, or occur up to 14 months after tubulointerstitial nephritis is noted. Fever, weight loss, fatigue, abdominal and/or flank pain, arthralgias, and polyuria may also be seen. TINU should be considered in any patient presenting with unexplained tubulointerstitial disease, which often manifests with acute or CKD, minimal proteinuria, and sterile pyuria. Typical kidney biopsy findings with chronic TINU are lymphocytic infiltrate, tubular atrophy, and interstitial fibrosis. Treatment includes prednisone 1 mg/kg per day

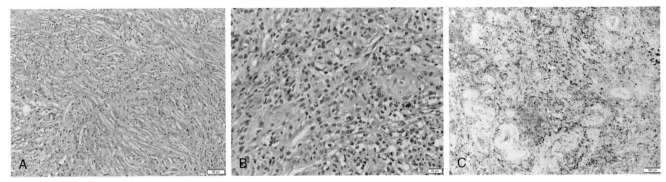

Fig. 44.4 Immunoglobulin G4 disease. (A) Hematoxylin and eosin–stained light microscopy section showing an inflammatory infiltrate on a background of fibrosis, where the fibrosis appears in bundles and sheets (20×). (B) Hematoxylin and eosin–stained light microscopy section showing an inflammatory infiltrate composed of mononuclear cells, plasma cells, and eosinophils (40×). (C) Immunohistochemistry for immunoglobulin (Ig)G4 shows that a large number of cells are positive for IgG4 (10×). (Images courtesy of Sanjeev Sethi, MD, Department of Laboratory Medicine and Pathology, Mayo Clinic, Rochester.)

for 3 to 6 months (depending on renal response) with a slow taper.

IgG4-RELATED TUBULOINTERSTITIAL NEPHRITIS

Immunoglobulin (Ig)G4-related interstitial nephritis is often part of a systemic disease process with multiorgan involvement, now known as IgG4-related disease (IgG4D). This disease is characterized by an elevated serum IgG4 level (positive in 60% of patients) and dense infiltration of IgG4-positive plasma cells within the involved organ. Predominantly affecting middle-aged to elderly men, IgG4D also involves other organs causing aortitis/periaortitis, cholangitis, sialadenitis, and hypophysitis. Other features include elevated serum IgG and IgE levels and hypocomplementemia, although these tests are not consistently positive in all patients.

Kidney involvement in IgG4D includes acute and chronic interstitial disease, membranous nephropathy, nodular masses within the kidneys, and obstructive uropathy from retroperitoneal fibrosis. CIN is characterized histopathologically by a lymphoplasmacytic infiltrate with a predominance of IgG4-positive plasma cells and T-lymphocytes and obliterative phlebitis. The interstitial fibrosis has a swirling or storiform pattern (Fig. 44.4), and IgG4 immunoperoxidase stains IgG4-positive plasma cells a brown color (see Fig. 44.4C). Interstitial nephritis is generally glucocorticoid responsive before the formation of extensive fibrosis. However, relapse occurs with steroid taper, and rituximab has been successfully used to treat steroid-dependent or steroid-resistant disease.

MESOAMERICAN NEPHROPATHY AND SRI LANKAN NEPHROPATHY

An epidemic of CKD characterized primarily by CIN (with secondary glomerulosclerosis) has been observed in young male agricultural workers in Central America. This entity, which has been called Mesoamerican nephropathy, does not have a definitive cause. Workers from the Pacific coast, especially in the sugarcane fields, have a history of manual labor under extremely hot conditions. Normal or mildly elevated blood pressure, tubular proteinuria, a progressive decline in kidney function, and often hyperuricemia and or hypokalemia are observed. The cause of the disease is unknown; however, severe heat exposure with recurrent dehydration, environmental toxin exposure, use of nonsteroidal antiinflammatory agents, and excessive hyperuricosuria are considered potential etiologies. It is likely that a combination of factors cause this chronic tubulointerstitial disease.

Another chronic interstitial disease observed in agricultural workers is Sri Lankan agricultural nephropathy (SAN). This relatively new cause of CKD was reported in Sri Lankan paddy farmers in 1994. Environmental exposure to low levels of heavy metals and the herbicide glyphosate may play a role in the pathogenesis of the disease. Patients with SAN do not have common CKD risk factors such as diabetes, hypertension, or glomerular disease. CIN associated with mononuclear cell infiltration, glomerular sclerosis, and tubular atrophy is noted on kidney histology. Slow progression of CKD, minimal proteinuria with bland sediment, and small echogenic kidneys on ultrasound are characteristic of this kidney disease.

KEY BIBLIOGRAPHY

Becker JL, Miller F, Nuovo GJ, et al. Epstein-Barr virus infection of renal proximal tubule cells: possible role in chronic interstitial nephritis. *J Clin Invest.* 1999;104:1673-1681.

Brause M, Magnusson K, Degenhardt S, et al. Renal involvement in sarcoidosis—a report of 6 cases. *Clin Nephrol.* 2002;57:142-148.

Correa-Rotter R, Wesseling C, Johnson RJ. CKD of unknown origin in Central America: the case for a Mesoamerican nephropathy. *Am J Kidney Dis.* 2014;63:506-520.

Cortazar FB, Stone JH. IgG4-related disease and the kidney. *Nat Rev Nephrol.* 2015;11(10):599-609.

De Broe ME, Elseviers MM. Over-the-counter analgesic use. *J Am Soc Nephrol.* 2009;20:2098-2103.

Ekong EB, Jaar BG, Weaver VM. Lead-related nephrotoxicity: a review of the epidemiologic evidence. *Kidney Int.* 2006;70:2074-2080.

Grollman AP, Shibutani S, Moriya M, et al. Aristolochic acid and the etiology of endemic (Balkan) nephropathy. *Proc Natl Acad Sci USA.* 2007; 104:12129-12134.

Hanna-Attisha M, LaChance J, Sadler RC, Champney Schnepp A. Elevated blood lead levels in children associated with the Flint drinking water crisis: a spatial analysis of risk and public health response. *Am J Public Health.* 2016;106(2):283-290.

Henrich WL, Clark RL, Kelly JP, et al. Non-contrast-enhanced computerized tomography and analgesic-related kidney disease: report of the national analgesic nephropathy study. *J Am Soc Nephrol.* 2006;17:1472.

Humphreys BD, Lin SL, Kobayashi A, et al. Fate tracing reveals the pericyte and not epithelial origin of myofibroblasts in kidney fibrosis. *Am J Pathol.* 2010;176:85-97.

Jayasumana C, Gunatilake S, Siribaddana S. Simultaneous exposure to multiple heavy metals and glyphosate may contribute to Sri Lankan agricultural nephropathy. *BMC Nephrol.* 2015;16:103-110.

Jelaković B, Karanović S, Vuković-Lela I, et al. Aristolacam-DNA adducts are a biomarker of environmental exposure to aristolochic acid. *Kidney Int.* 2012;81:559-567.

Kim R, Rotnitsky A, Sparrow D, et al. A longitudinal study of low-level lead exposure and impairment of renal function. The Normative Aging Study. *JAMA.* 1996;275:1177-1181.

Kritz W, Kaissling B, Le Hir M. Epithelial-mesenchymal transition (EMT) is kidney fibrosis: fact or fantasy? *J Clin Invest.* 2011;121:468-474.

Lin JL, Lin-Tan DT, Hsu KU, et al. Environmental lead exposure and progression of chronic renal diseases in patients without diabetes. *N Engl J Med.* 2003;348:277-286.

Mahévas M, Lescure FX, Boffa JJ, et al. Renal sarcoidosis: clinical, laboratory, and histologic presentation and outcome in 47 patients. *Medicine (Baltimore).* 2009;88:98-106.

Meyers CM. New insights into the pathogenesis of interstitial nephritis. *Curr Opin Nephrol Hypertens.* 1999;8:287-292.

Muntner P, He J, Vupputuri S, et al. Blood lead and chronic kidney disease in the general United States population: results from NHANES III. *Kidney Int.* 2003;63:1044-1050.

Quaggin SE, Kapus A. Scar wars: mapping the fate of epithelial-mesenchymal-myofibroblast transition. *Kidney Int.* 2011;80:41-50.

Strutz F, Okada H, Lo CS, et al. Identification and characterization of a fibroblast marker: FSP1. *J Cell Biol.* 1995;130:393-405.

Full bibliography can be found on www.expertconsult.com.

45

Obstructive Uropathy

Richard W. Sutherland

Obstruction of the urinary tract can occur anywhere between the collecting duct and the urethral meatus. Microcrystals in the collecting duct, urinary calculi, tumors, and luminal strictures may block the normal flow of urine. Regardless of the cause, the ultimate effect is the same: an increase in the hydrostatic pressure of the collecting system, which is transmitted into Bowman space. This reduces the glomerular filtration rate (GFR) and initiates a cascade of events that, if not reversed, will result in kidney scarring and loss of overall kidney function. The extent of kidney injury and the damage to the physical structures of the collecting system vary depending on the duration and completeness of the obstruction. The reduction of kidney function is determined by two components: loss of GFR and the loss of tubular function. Although both are critical, GFR is the dominant contributor. In an unobstructed kidney, tubular function collapses when glomerular filtration is disrupted. The glomerular filtrate is necessary to provide the substrate (i.e., Na^+ ions) for tubular function. In cases of prolonged obstruction to the kidney, both glomerular and tubular functions are compromised.

UNILATERAL URETERAL OBSTRUCTION

Historically, unilateral and bilateral ureteral obstructions (BUOs) are discussed separately because of distinct changes in kidney physiology. In the first hours after obstruction, differences between the two types of obstructions occur in glomerular blood flow and ureteral pressure profiles. In unilateral ureteral obstruction (UUO), a triphasic event of vascular blood flow and ureteral pressure is seen. Only two phases are seen in BUO. In UUO (Fig. 45.1), there is an initial elevation in the luminal hydrostatic pressure. GFR is maintained by a simultaneous increase in the glomerular capillary pressure induced by afferent arteriolar dilation. Prostaglandin E_2 (PGE_2) and nitrous oxide (NO) are considered the initial mediators. Studies using inhibitors of PGE_2 and NO attenuate this increase in renal blood flow and GFR. The exact triggering mechanisms for the production of PGE_2 and NO are less well understood but may be due to the decreased presentation of Na^+ and Cl^- to the macula densa. These increases in GFR and luminal pressure define the first phase.

The second phase of UUO begins with the decrease of glomerular blood flow. Between 12 and 24 hours after the initial obstruction, afferent arteriolar vasodilation transitions to vasoconstriction. Activation of the renin-angiotensin system occurs during the first phase and becomes the dominant process affecting GFR, whereupon efferent and partial afferent arteriole vasoconstriction overwhelms PGE_2- and NO-mediated vasodilation. Experimental data show that the administration of angiotensin-converting enzyme (ACE) inhibitors blunts the vasoconstriction and GFR reduction. Thromboxane A2 and endothelin reduce glomerular blood flow during UUO. This second phase of UUO is defined by a persistent elevation of hydrostatic pressure from the obstructed lumen, even with the reduction of GFR.

The third and last phase of UUO is marked by decreased luminal hydrostatic pressure and renal blood flow. Glomerular capillary blood flow and luminal pressure remain below baseline until the obstruction is relieved. It is during this last phase that the majority of permanent damage is done to the kidney. The return to baseline function is dependent on the overall duration and severity of the initial obstruction. A partial obstruction may be present for 14 days or more with complete return of function. A total obstruction will leave permanent fibrosis within a week.

BILATERAL URETERAL OBSTRUCTION

The primary difference between UUO and BUO is persistent vasoconstriction of the efferent artery, which maintains GFR in BUO. Luminal pressure remains elevated for longer than 24 hours in BUO, whereas it begins to decrease by 6 hours with UUO. To account for the persistent afferent arteriolar dilation and efferent arteriolar vasoconstriction, it is likely that additional vasoactive substances accumulate or are produced in BUO but not in UUO. One substance, atrial natriuretic peptide (ANP), is produced in the setting of volume overload and increases diuresis. Vasodilators PGE_2 and NO are likely present because blockade of their production magnifies the already blunted increase in GFR seen in BUO. This suggests that although ANP produces afferent arteriolar dilation, PGE_2 and NO enhance this process.

TUBULAR DYSFUNCTION

Loss of tubular function during obstruction occurs primarily from a decrease in GFR rather than direct hydrostatic pressure injury to the tubular cells. Sodium and potassium homeostasis, water handling, and acidification are altered. The decline in GFR initiates a series of compensatory yet maladaptive events that are mediated by vasoactive substances, cytokines, and ischemia. These maladaptive events alter the amount of filtrate, the composition of the filtrate, tubular transport proteins, and tubular blood flow (Table 45.1).

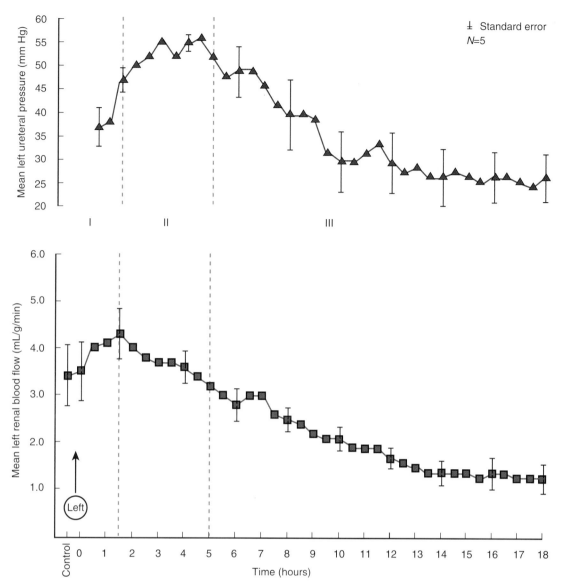

Fig. 45.1 Renal resistance in ureteral occlusion. Triphasic relationship of left ureteral luminal pressure and left renal blood flow after occlusion of the left ureter. (Moody TE, Vaughn ED Jr, Gillenwater JY. Relationship between renal blood flow and ureteral pressure during 18 hours of total unilateral urethral occlusion: implications for changing sites of increased renal resistance. *Invest Urol.* 1975;13:246–251.)

SODIUM REABSORPTION

Obstruction of the kidney impairs Na^+ reabsorption throughout the nephron. The luminal Na^+/H^+ exchanger (NHE3), the luminal $Na^+/K^+/2Cl^-$ cotransporter (NKCC2), and the basolateral Na^+/K^+-ATPase pump are downregulated in obstructed kidneys. Cell suspension studies of distinct nephron segments support this conclusion. In the proximal tubule, reduction of NHE3 activity is seen. In the loop of Henle, decreased activity of NKCC2 occurs. Diminished activity of the NKCC2 cotransporter is noted in cells studied from the thick ascending limb. Na^+ reabsorption also requires luminal movement from the lumen into the cell. This process is affected by furosemide, supporting disruption of the NKCC2 transporter. In the medullary portion of the collecting system, NHE3 has reduced energy consumption and decreased expression of NHE3. Many of these transport processes are energy dependent and require ATP. Although a reduction in the amount of available ATP has been hypothesized because of ischemia, it is the downregulation of the receptors and enzymes that appears to be the rate-limiting step in Na^+ transport.

The actual triggers for the loss of receptor and enzyme activity are still an area of research. Possible signals include decreased filtrate substrates, natriuretic substances, and direct tubular hydrostatic pressure. Decreased GFR reduces filtrate and Na^+ ion presentation to the cells. Depletion of the Na^+ ion could downregulate its receptor and transport proteins. Additionally, loss of luminal Na^+ reduces the electrochemical gradient, whereas blockade of Na^+ movement into obstructed medullary thick ascending limb cells results in a loss of ouabain-sensitive ATPase. Taken together, decreased Na^+ presentation to cells could downregulate Na^+/K^+-ATPase at the translational or posttranslational level.

PGE_2 levels change as a result of obstruction and eventually begin to affect Na^+ reabsorption. PGE_2 is released during

Table 45.1 Complications of Urinary Obstruction

1. Natriuresis
   Decreased NHE3, NKCC2, Na⁺/K⁺ ATPase activity
2. Impaired urinary concentration
   Disruption of osmotic gradient
   Damaged urea recycling
   Loss of aquaporin receptors (nephrogenic DI)
3. Metabolic acidosis
   Distal RTA
4. Renal scarring/fibrosis
   Increased extracellular matrix
   MP/TIMP imbalance
   Increased fibroblast/myofibroblast activity
   Growth factors/cytokines/enzymes/protein shifts: TGF-β, SMADs, PAI-1
5. Apoptosis
   Extrinsic pathway: TNF-α, TRADD
   Intrinsic pathway: Oxidative stress, mitochondrial breakdown

MP, Metalloproteinases; *NHE3*, Na⁺/H⁺ exchanger; *NKCC2*, Na⁺/K⁺/2Cl⁻ cotransporter; *RTA*, renal tubular acidosis; *TIMP*, tissue inhibitors of metalloproteinases; *TRADD*, tumor necrosis factor receptor type 1–associated death domain.

obstruction from increased COX-2 production. COX-2 inhibition reduces the loss of NKCC2 and Na^+/K^+-ATPase activity, implying an effect of PGE_2 to impair Na^+ reabsorption.

Na^+ reabsorption in BUO differs from UUO because of the presence of volume expansion. The addition of ANP and the loss of aldosterone reduce tubular reabsorption of Na^+. Much of the impaired Na^+ handling in UUO is amplified by the effect of ANP, which blocks release of renin and reduces the ultimate creation of angiotensin II. ANP also directly reduces Na^+ reabsorption in the collecting duct and blocks angiotensin II's effect on Na^+ reabsorption, the net effects being diuresis and natriuresis.

URINARY CONCENTRATION

Obstruction disrupts normal urinary concentration. With a reduced GFR, less Na^+ is available to create the osmolar gradient in the medullary interstitium. As with the defects in Na^+ reabsorption, there is loss of the luminal and basolateral membrane proteins, NKCC2 and Na^+/K^+-ATPase. This prevents Na^+ transport from the tubular lumen into the medullary interstitium, which is critical to the countercurrent multiplier that creates the medullary gradient. Without the ability to reabsorb Na^+ in the ascending limb and dilute the filtrate as it enters the distal convoluted tubule, the solutes required to maintain the gradient are excreted. In the collecting duct of an obstructed kidney, action of antidiuretic hormone (ADH) to increase water permeability is blunted because of decreased AQP-2 in the luminal membrane. Several studies have shown this to be a post-cAMP defect. Reduced transcription of AQP-2 mRNA and a decrease in the phosphorylation necessary to incorporate AQP-2 vesicles into the luminal membrane explain this effect. Finally, a decrease in basolateral membrane AQP-3 and AQP-4 is also noted. After obstruction is relieved, overall urinary concentration returns, paralleling the return of the AQP-2 channel to the luminal membrane.

Urea recycling is another process used by the nephron to increase the gradient for urinary concentration. Urea within the filtrate passively exits the collecting duct at its inner medullary segment and enters the interstitium. The vasa recta and the thin portion of the loop of Henle reabsorb it. A maximum medullary interstitial osmotic gradient is created with the recycling of urea. Urea permeability in the collecting duct tubules is controlled by urea transporters UT-A1 and UT-A3. ADH enhances the permeability of urea, allowing it to flow into the interstitium. Urea reabsorption by the vasa recta is stimulated by UT-B receptors under ADH control. In the obstructed kidney, expression of urea transporters UT-A1, UT-A3, and UT-B is reduced. Urea transporter defects reduce the maximal concentrating effect of the gradient by disrupting urea recycling and allowing urea to be excreted.

POTASSIUM

K^+ handling in the nephron is not affected directly by obstruction. The initial disturbance in K^+ homeostasis is explained by defects in Na^+ handling, H^+ handling, and reduced GFR. With obstruction, there is a decrease in both Na^+ reabsorption (reduced Na^+ channels) and Na^+ presentation to the distal tubule (reduced GFR). Additionally, decreased K^+ secretion occurs as a result of increased intraluminal K^+. In the low-flow state of obstruction, high urinary potassium concentrations in the collecting duct blunt the gradient between the lumen and the tubular cells, resulting in a reduction in K^+ movement into the lumen and ultimately hyperkalemia. The effect of obstruction on the renal outer medullary K^+ channel (ROMK), a K^+ secretory channel, is presently unknown.

ACIDIFICATION

Urinary obstruction produces a metabolic acidosis best understood as a form of distal (type 1) renal tubular acidosis (RTA) with hyperkalemia, or "voltage-dependent" RTA. It is characterized by a failure of distal H^+ and K^+ secretion. The Na^+ channel defects play a central role in this acidosis. Loss of Na^+ reabsorption from the distal tubule results in impaired urinary acidification in the obstructed kidney. Na^+/K^+-ATPase dysfunction on the basolateral surface of the cell ultimately disrupts Na^+ removal from the lumen of the collecting duct. This decrease in cation reabsorption reduces the passive H^+ excretion into the collecting duct lumen down the electrochemical gradient, and a "voltage-dependent acidosis" occurs. Simultaneous hyperkalemia occurs from failure of Na^+/K^+-ATPase and Na^+ reabsorption. Decreased expression of the H^+-ATPase in the collecting duct adds to the metabolic acidosis. However, a defect of the H^+-ATPase transporter cannot account completely for the acidosis seen in hyperkalemic distal RTA due to urinary obstruction. Urinary acidification occurs in the early phases of obstruction, suggesting an intact proton pump. Similarities are noted between voltage-dependent RTA and type 4 RTA. In neither of these two processes is H^+ secretion felt to be the primary defect.

FIBROSIS

Persistent obstruction produces tubulointerstitial fibrosis. The activated pathways producing fibrosis do not differ significantly from fibrosis noted with other disease processes. An imbalance in normal kidney homeostasis results in excess accumulation of extracellular matrix (ECM) with the subsequent development of tubulointerstitial fibrosis and, in later stages, glomerular and vascular sclerosis.

Maintenance of the ECM has classically been described as a balance of metalloproteinases (MMPs) and tissue inhibitors of metalloproteinases (TIMPs). The upregulation of fibroblast-produced TIMPs, which decrease the activity of the MMPs, results in a deposition of collagen I and III. Work in the last decade has shown this simple explanation is incomplete. TIMP 3 may prevent fibrosis whereas TIMP 2 may promote fibrosis through activation of MMP 2. Different classes of presenting fibroblasts produce different cytokines and growth factors.

At the cellular level, there is an increase in the number of fibroblasts and myofibroblasts. Infiltrating macrophages and fibroblasts responding to injury release cytokines, including TGF-β, BMP-7, PAI-1, interleukin (IL)-2, and IL-6. Additional fibroblasts are produced as epithelial tubular cells and endothelial cells transform into mesenchymal cells. This epithelial-mesenchymal transition (EMT) and endothelial-mesenchymal transition (EndMT) produce additional fibroblasts necessary for collagen deposition. The presence of angiotensin II, triggered by obstruction, stimulates the expression of TGF-β, a facilitator of fibrosis. TGF-β fibrosis occurs through SMAD and non-SMAD pathways. SMAD3 is the best described promoter of fibrosis. SMAD3 is counterbalanced by SMAD2, which is regulated by bone morphogenetic protein-7 (BMP-7), an ECM fibrotic protector.

Plasminogen activator inhibitor, PAI-1, appears to be an additional pathway for the creation of fibrosis. While direct inhibition of urokinase (uPA) and tissue plasminogen activator (tPA) may be one mechanism that promotes fibrosis, an independent action of PAI-1 affecting the ECM fibrosis is suspected. Additional growth factors, cytokines, and vasoactive compounds promote cell growth and fibrosis, such as TNF-α, NF-κB, platelet-derived growth factor (PDGF), vascular cell adhesion molecule-1 (VCAM-1), and basic fibroblast growth factor (bFGF).

Several therapeutic strategies to reduce fibrosis within the ECM are available not only in obstructive uropathy but also in other diseases, such as diabetes mellitus. These include manipulation of PAI-1 and TXA2 and ACE inhibition. In obstructive uropathy these continue to be hypothetical and not applicable to clinical medicine. Many of the possible treatments that would block the fibrotic pathways disrupt the very same pathways that are needed for normal wound healing, exacerbating the fibrosis. The most important therapeutic treatment is to relieve the obstruction.

APOPTOSIS

Apoptosis, programmed cell death, is a normal physiologic mechanism that occurs within the kidney and throughout other organ systems of the body. During obstruction, apoptosis is increased through external and internal cellular signals. Extrinsic activation with obstruction occurs from an increase in the tissue levels of TNF-α, which binds to its receptor, TNFR1. This complex then combines with the cell death domain (TRADD) to activate apoptotic pathways, resulting in cell death. Intrinsic activation occurs from oxidative stress, which causes intracellular release of a number of substances from damaged organelles. Mitochondrial release of cytochrome-c is a known trigger for apoptosis in many organ systems, including the kidney. Stress to the endoplasmic reticulum upregulates the apoptotic c-JUN NH2 terminal kinase, resulting in increased inflammation and subsequent fibrosis. The external and internal pathways converge on a single pathway to continue apoptosis through effector caspases, which cleave the nucleus to create apoptotic bodies. There are 12 different apoptotic caspases, with 3, 8, and 12 identified within the obstructed kidney tissue. Attempts at manipulating apoptotic pathways to ameliorate fibrosis continue to be exploratory.

POSTOBSTRUCTIVE DIURESIS

Postobstructive diuresis is a normal physiologic event in patients with prolonged BUO. The rate of diuresis is based on the severity of volume overload, urea accumulation, and electrolyte disturbances developing during obstruction. There is no rate of urine output that defines postobstructive diuresis. However, rates of 250 mL/h are common, and 750 mL/h can be seen.

Several factors facilitate the physiologic diuresis. Before release of the obstruction, there is downregulation of Na^+ transporters, and this inability to reabsorb Na^+ diminishes the osmotic gradient necessary for urinary concentration. In the distal tubule, downregulation and reduced aquaporin activity promote aquaresis. ANP is released because of activation of the cardiac atrial stretch receptors from increased preload, further increasing urine output.

Initial treatment of the postobstructive diuresis is free access to fluids. In the postsurgical patient who is unable to drink, approximately 75% of the urine volume is replaced with 0.45% (½ normal) saline. Intravenous fluids are adjusted based on volume status, subsequent urine osmolality, serum osmolality, and serum electrolyte measurements every 12 hours, depending on the rate of the diuresis and illness of the patient. The aggressive resuscitation to "chase" the volume of fluid excreted, rather than kidney pathology, results in "iatrogenic" diuresis after relief of obstruction.

Pathologic postobstructive diuresis does occur. Ongoing excretion of dilute urine can result in severe volume depletion. Initial treatment is the same as in physiologic postobstructive diuresis, with resuscitation with water and electrolytes and frequent measurement of serum and electrolytes. In severe cases, laboratory testing every 4 to 6 hours may be required until a stable balance has been created with diet, fluid, and electrolyte therapy.

SPECIFIC CAUSES OF OBSTRUCTIONS

Causes of urinary obstruction are listed in Box 45.1.

NEPHROLITHIASIS

Nephrolithiasis produces an intrinsic obstruction, anywhere from the ureteropelvic junction (UPJ) to the urethral meatus. Renal pelvic stones cause obstruction at the UPJ, with ureteral stones commonly producing an obstruction at two locations:

Box 45.1   Causes of Urinary Obstruction

Intrinsic Obstructions

Nephron

1. Uric acid crystals/stones
2. Sloughed papillae
3. Gross hematuria with clot

Renal Pelvis

1. Malignancy, primary/metastatic
2. Renal cyst
3. Ureteropelvic junction (UPJ) stenosis

Ureteral

1. Ureteral stricture
2. Ureteral stone
3. Aperistaltic ureter (i.e., megaureter or prune belly syndrome)
4. Ureterocele
5. Ectopic ureter

Bladder

1. Neurogenic (i.e., spina bifida, diabetes)
2. Malignancy, transitional cell carcinoma
3. Fibrosis (i.e., radiation, chronic inflammation)

Urethra

1. Posterior urethral valves
2. Benign prostatic hyperplasia
3. Malignancy
4. Stricture
5. Prostatic abscess
6. Phimosis

Extrinsic Compressions

Renal Pelvis

1. Peripelvic cyst
2. Cancer, primary renal or metastatic
3. Trauma

Ureter

1. UPJ crossing vessel
2. Retrocaval ureter
3. Tumor (pelvic malignancy)
4. Retroperitoneal fibrosis
5. Pregnancy
6. Endometriosis
7. Ovarian vein thrombosis

Bladder

1. Bladder neck contraction (previous surgery, malignancy)

(1) the ureter where it crosses the iliac vessels and (2) the ureterovesicular junction (UVJ). A ureteral stricture can produce a narrowing and resulting obstruction from a stone. Bladder stones can block the urethra at the bladder neck. Rarely, urethral stones, generally with prior urethral stricture disease or surgical reconstruction, occlude the urethra or urethral meatus.

Treatment of obstructing stones depends on the location and severity of illness. Stones in the calyces from infundibular stenosis produce pain and infection. The location of the infundibulum deep within the renal parenchyma makes open

surgical management difficult. Endoscopic laser incision of the stenosis may relieve the obstruction. Extended narrowing tends to re-stricture, making laser ablation of the entire calyx a consideration with partial loss of function.

Once within the renal pelvis, a small calcification can form a nidus to create a larger obstructing stone. Renal pelvis stones are excellent candidates for extracorporeal shock wave lithotripsy (ESWL). The retroperitoneal location of the kidney, away from other vital structures and bowel gas, allows for shock waves to penetrate the kidney and fragment the stone. Larger stones require prolonged and repetitive shock-wave treatment, which may damage the surrounding parenchyma. Percutaneous nephrolithotripsy (PCNL) or ureteroscopy may be a better option in these cases.

Ureteroscopy is a very effective technique (greater than 85% success) in selected cases. It treats the stone and allows for direct visualization of the ureter and renal pelvis. This ensures there is no structural pathology that may have predisposed the patient to produce the original stone. Abnormal anatomy can make ureteroscopy difficult, requiring direct access through a percutaneous nephrostomy (PCN) tube. With PCN access to the kidney, PCNL can be performed with either laser or ultrasonic probes. Treatment of larger (>2 cm) and harder stones may benefit from PCN because of the ability to use larger and more powerful instruments with better visualization.

While ESWL works well for kidney stones, it has a significantly lower success rate for mid-ureteral stones. ESWL requires focalization of a pressure wave through tissue to fragment the stone. Gas within adjacent bowel impedes shock-wave migration to the stones. Ureteroscopy becomes the treatment of choice for the majority of mid- and lower ureteral stones. Retrograde access is again the preferred choice, but antegrade access through the renal pelvis and down the ureter can be performed.

STRICTURES

Strictures found within the urinary tract suggest a previous event, such as trauma, infection, or systemic disease. They occur from the UPJ to the urethral meatus. Balloon dilation with a simultaneous full-thickness ureteral wall incision of the stricture is a good option. In short isolated strictures, a long-term success rate of 85% to 90% is expected. Postprocedure, temporary stenting facilitates drainage and minimizes extravasation of acidic urine, which can impair healing and result in restenosis. Extensive stricture disease of the ureter or urethra from tuberculosis, infection, or malignancy may require open surgical resection of the diseased portion with reanastomosis.

MALIGNANCY

There are numerous malignancies that can obstruct the urinary tract extrinsically, but few obstruct the system intrinsically. The most common internal malignancy is transitional cell carcinoma (TCC), which is derived from epithelial cells of the urinary mucosa. It is a friable, frondular tumor with a solid stalk found primarily in older patients with a history of tobacco use. Treatment of obstruction is dependent on tumor location; those that fill the renal pelvis can be treated initially with a ureteral stent. TCC can also produce obstruction at the UVJ. Initial treatment includes an attempt at local cystoscopic excision or unroofing the orifice. When unresectable by cystoscopy, a temporizing stent or nephrostomy tube can be placed until surgical reconstruction with ureteral reimplantation or a possible cystectomy can be completed.

Extrinsic compression of the ureter from malignancies occurs more frequently. The most common are primary pelvic tumors in women. Retroperitoneal adenopathy along the aorta or vena cava adjacent to the ureter can also produce obstruction. Tumors can directly invade into the ureteral wall and occlude the lumen. Initial treatment with a stent is suggested. Large pelvic masses may obliterate the normal anatomy of the bladder and ureteral orifices. This can make ureteral stent placement impossible. In this situation, an initial PCN tube can be placed with subsequent antegrade internalization of the stent.

BENIGN PROSTATIC HYPERPLASIA/PROSTATE CANCER

An enlarged prostate creates urinary obstruction through bladder decompensation and failure rather than a fixed urethral obstruction. The relatively slow and gradual prostatic enlargement can come from benign or malignant causes. Enlargement of prostate tissue produces a partial obstruction that increases the patient's voiding pressure. The chronic increase in voiding pressure produces a hydrostatic stress to the smooth muscles of the bladder, resulting in bladder muscle hypertrophy. A subsequent increase in fibroblast and smooth muscle results in bladder wall trabeculations and eventual bladder wall deterioration. The loss of muscle tone culminates in bladder dysfunction with the ultimate cause of the uropathy being urinary retention. It is this bladder deterioration that produces the functional obstruction and uropathy.

Initial treatment of symptomatic benign prostatic hyperplasia (BPH) uses α-blockers (tamsulosin, terazosin) to reduce prostatic smooth muscle tone. This increases the size of the urethral lumen and allows voiding pressures to decrease. Phosphodiesterase (PD-5) inhibitors are another class of medications that affect smooth muscle and are associated with subjective improvement in voiding symptoms. Combining the PD-5 inhibitor with an α-blocker synergistically improves symptoms better than either medication alone. If medical therapy proves inadequate, transurethral resection of the prostate, open surgical excision, and clean intermittent catheterization (CIC) may be used.

NEUROGENIC BLADDER

Patients with neurogenic bladder must be monitored closely for new-onset obstructive uropathy. This was a leading cause of morbidity and uropathy in the adult neurogenic bladder population before the acceptance of CIC in the 1970s. Spinal cord trauma and myelomeningocele are the most common causes of neurogenic bladder in the adult and pediatric population, respectively. The normal voiding reflex in the adult relaxes the urinary sphincter during bladder contraction. Loss of this coordinated reflex in patients with neurogenic bladders results in bladder contraction against a closed sphincter, known as detrusor sphincter dyssynergia (DSD). High-pressure voiding puts the patient at risk of bladder

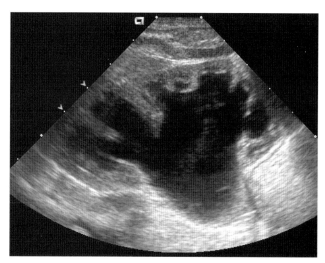

Fig. 45.2 Society of Fetal Urology grade IV hydronephrosis, which can be seen with or without vesicoureteral reflux, in a patient with a neurogenic bladder and a resting bladder pressure greater than 40 cm H_2O.

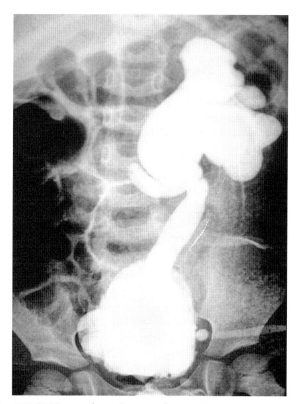

Fig. 45.3 Voiding cystourethrogram in a patient with a neurogenic bladder. High resting pressures and dysfunctional voiding result in bladder trabeculations and cellules, with the development of secondary grade 5 reflux.

deterioration and upper urinary tract damage similar to BPH (Figs. 45.2 and 45.3). Chronic elevated bladder pressure is a more significant risk factor. The bladder fills to a maximum safe volume, but the patient does not sense the continued urine production. As the volume increases further, the constant resting pressure of the bladder rises. A resting pressure above 40 cm H_2O prevents flow into the bladder by overwhelming the maximum ureteral pressure of ureteral peristalsis. This results in upper tract dilation and subsequent uropathy. Patients with a small, low-volume bladder and tight urethral sphincter are at increased risk of GFR loss.

Treatment involves lowering the resting pressure within the bladder. This can be achieved with anticholinergic medication, CIC, urethral dilation, or surgical reconstruction. Urinary diversions, such as ileal conduits or cutaneous ureterostomies, are other options. Many patients prefer a continent reconstruction with intermittent catheterization through the urethra or cutaneous stoma, such as a Mitrofanoff or Indiana pouch. Upper urinary tract deterioration with hydroureteronephrosis is generally seen before the irreversible uropathy. A screening kidney ultrasound should be considered annually in a high-risk asymptomatic patient to monitor for silent development of hydronephrosis.

CONGENITAL DEFECTS IN THE ADULT POPULATION

Congenital defects of the collecting system can present in adults. Defects of the UPJ and UVJ, ectopic ureters, uretero-celes, and even posterior urethral valves can present after childhood. Management depends on the specific signs and symptoms. Patients presenting with pain, infection, or reduced kidney function should be surgically repaired. Intervention can be endoscopic, laparoscopic, or open surgical correction. Asymptomatic abnormalities identified incidentally do not always require treatment. In the adult, there are several anatomic defects that can obstruct the urinary system. UPJ obstruction is identified when stones or infection occur as a result of urinary stasis. Chronic intermittent flank pain previously believed to be of gastrointestinal origin is another common presentation. Treatment of stones and infection will improve the symptoms, but recurrent stone formation or infection is common. Balloon dilation with simultaneous incision of the stricture with the specifically designed Acucise balloon has a success rate approaching 85% in the appropriately selected patient with a UPJ lesion. Long segments of dysplasia at the UPJ have a high failure rate with the Acucise balloon technique. Open surgery or laparoscopic/robotic pyeloplasty is an excellent option for reconstruction, approaching a 95% to 97% success rate. In asymptomatic patients with hydronephrosis from a UPJ narrowing, intervention should be reserved for those with decreased kidney function. Determination of a functional problem may require a furosemide nuclear scan to reveal if kidney dysfunction is caused by obstruction. In a cooperative adult, it is possible to recreate pain during the high urinary flow of the furosemide phase of the study. In the rare equivocal patient with intermittent pain, an indwelling double-J stent can be placed to bypass a possible obstruction to observe if the pain is relieved.

CONGENITAL DEFECTS IN THE PEDIATRIC POPULATION

Congenital obstruction in the pediatric patient occurs throughout the urinary tract. The most common locations are the UPJ, the UVJ, and the posterior urethral valves. Prenatal obstruction from a congenital defect can produce dramatic damage to the urinary tract and kidney function. Fortunately, in the majority of children with prenatal hydro-nephrosis, a continuation of normal development with growth

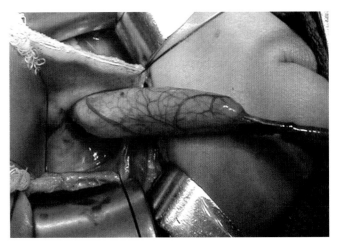

Fig. 45.4 Intraoperative megaureter reconstruction. The patient's bladder is open. Initial dissection shows the dilated ureter pulled up into the opened bladder. The distal ureteral narrowing is to the right with proximal healthy, but dilated, vascularized ureter to the left.

of the ureter occurs after birth, resulting in an unaffected urinary system. The goal of managing prenatal congenital defects is to identify the 10% to 30% that will develop progressive disease if left untreated.

Up to 80% of significant partial UPJ obstructions will resolve without loss of kidney function. Dramatic hydronephrosis with parenchymal thinning can be monitored if kidney function is comparable to the unaffected contralateral kidney. Megaureters (Fig. 45.4), associated with UVJ obstruction, correct themselves without intervention in 70% of cases. Hydronephrosis does not necessarily mean obstruction.

In the young child with symptomatic UPJ obstruction, pyeloplasty continues to be the best surgical option. A success rate of 95% to 97% should be expected. Laparoscopic pyeloplasty is an excellent technique, except in children less than 1 year old where a slightly higher failure rate is seen. Acucise balloon dilation is rarely indicated in the young child.

PREGNANCY

Hydronephrosis is commonly seen in pregnancy but is rarely pathologic. Hydronephrosis occurs in 40% to 100% of pregnant women depending on the amount of dilation considered abnormal. Postpartum dilation may be seen for up to 6 weeks and is not considered pathologic. Two mechanisms contribute to the hydroureteronephrosis of pregnancy: ureteral compression and hormonal relaxation. By the 20th week, the gravid uterus achieves adequate size to reach the pelvic rim and extrinsically compress the ureter, producing a partial mechanical obstruction. The right kidney is more likely to be dilated because of the position of the uterus. A total of 10% to 15% of women will have hydronephrosis during the first trimester. Hormones present during pregnancy, including estrogen and progesterone that relax the smooth muscle of the ureters, also contribute to hydroureteronephrosis. Identification of hydronephrosis frequently occurs during routine prenatal ultrasound. Follow-up for even moderate hydroureteronephrosis is not needed unless the individual becomes symptomatic.

Treatment of true obstruction from severe extrinsic compression or nephrolithiasis can be performed cystoscopically with ureteral stent placement. Early stent encrustation will require frequent stent exchange to prevent stent obstruction. PCN can be performed if stent placement is not possible or if the stent is not tolerated.

OBSTRUCTION WITH INFECTION

An obstructed urinary system with an active infection is a medical emergency. Active infection requires close management with early surgical intervention for any systemic progression of illness. Decompression must be accomplished to prevent significant morbidity and mortality. Regardless of the cause of the obstruction, the urgency and means of decompression are dependent on illness severity in the affected patient. Infection is a relative contraindication for many reconstructive surgeries because of the inflammatory process hindering wound healing and promoting fibrosis, scarring, and recurrent obstruction.

Treatment can be as simple as a Foley catheter in an adult man with a urethral stricture to an open pyelostomy or PCN tube in an infant with a ruptured UPJ. Ureteral obstruction from a stone or a tumor is common and is best treated early with cystoscopic stent placement. Definitive reconstruction can be done after the infection and its inflammation resolves. Voiding complaints due to stents irritating the bladder are common. Anticholinergic medications are indicated for symptomatic patients with bladder hypercontractility.

A PCN tube is particularly beneficial in the ill patient. The tube can frequently be placed with mild sedation rather than the riskier general anesthesia required for stents. An advantage of a PCN tube is the ability to monitor drainage and to ensure adequate decompression, whereas internalized stents can obstruct asymptomatically. Irrigation of the PCN tube is simple compared to a possible stent exchange. Open surgical drainage is rarely performed and is reserved for the patient with abnormal anatomy where stenting or PCN is not possible. Patients with severe contractures or ectopic kidneys are in this category. Newborn boys with small urethras will not always accept a cystoscope. If the newborn kidney is not significantly hydronephrotic, PCN placement is difficult, and an open decompression procedure may be required. Dilated distal ureters, when present, can be brought to the skin as a cutaneous ureterostomy. A pyelostomy can be performed to protect the ureter for future reconstruction.

BIBLIOGRAPHY

Batlle DC, Arrunda J, Kurtzman NA. Hyperkalemic distal renal tubular acidosis associated with obstructive uropathy. *N Engl J Med.* 1981;304:373-380.

Canbay A, Friedman S, Gores GJ. Apoptosis: the nexus of liver injury and fibrosis. *Hepatology.* 2004;39:273-278.

Edgtton KL, Gow RM, Kelly DJ, et al. Plasmin is not protective in experimental renal interstitial fibrosis. *Kidney Int.* 2004;66:68-76.

Flevaris P, Vaughan D. The role of plasminogen activator inhibitor type-1 in fibrosis. *Semin Thromb Hemost.* 2016;43(2):169-177.

Gu C, Zhang J, Noble NA, et al. An additive effect of anti-PAI-1 antibody to ACE inhibitor on the slowing the progression of diabetic kidney disease. *Am J Physiol Renal Physiol.* 2016;311:F852-F863.

Halachmi S, Pillar G. Congenital urological anomalies diagnosed in adulthood—management considerations. *J Pediatr Urol.* 2008;4:2-7.

Jensen AM, Bae EH, Fenton RA, et al. Angiotensin II regulates V2 receptor and pAQP2 during ureteral obstruction. *Am J Physiol Renal Physiol.* 2009;296:F127-F134.

Jensen AM, Li C, Praetorius HA, et al. Angiotensin II mediates downregulation of aquaporin water channels and key renal sodium transporters in response to urinary tract obstruction. *Am J Physiol Renal Physiol.* 2006;291:F1021-F1032.

Kouba E, Wallen EM, Pruthi RS. Management of ureteral obstruction due to advanced malignancy: optimizing therapeutic and palliative outcomes. *J Urol.* 2008;180:444-450.

Li C, Klein JD, Wang W, et al. Altered expression of urea transporters in response to ureteral obstruction. *Am J Physiol Renal Physiol.* 2004; 286:F1154-F1162.

McVary KT, Roehrborn CG, Avins AL, et al. Update on AUA guideline on the management of benign prostatic hyperplasia. *J Urol.* 2011; 185:1793-1803.

Meng XM, Chung AC, Lan HY. Role of the TGF-B/BMP-7/Smad pathways in renal diseases. *Clin Sci.* 2013;124:243-254.

Mirone V, Imbimbo C, Longo N, et al. The detrusor muscle: an innocent victim of bladder outlet obstruction. *Eur Urol.* 2007;51:57-66.

Misseri R, Meldrum DR, Dinarello CA, et al. TNF-alpha mediates obstruction-induced renal tubular cell apoptosis and proapoptotic signaling. *Am J Physiol Renal Physiol.* 2005;288:F406-F411.

Sands JM. Critical role of urea in the urine-concentrating mechanism. *J Am Soc Nephrol.* 2007;18:670-671.

Sands JM, Layton HE. The physiology of urinary concentration: an update. *Semin Nephrol.* 2009;29:178-195.

Stødkilde L, Nørregaard R, Fenton RA, et al. Bilateral ureteral obstruction induces early downregulation and redistribution of AQP2 and phosphorylated AQP2. *Am J Physiol Renal Physiol.* 2011;301: F226-F235.

Wang Z, Famulski K, Lee J, et al. TIMP2 and TIMP3 have divergent roles in early renal tubulointerstitial injury. *Kidney Int.* 2014;85: 82-93.

Wang G, Ring T, Li C, et al. Unilateral ureteral obstruction alters expression of acid-base transporters in rat kidney. *J Urol.* 2009;182: 2964-2973.

Wolf G. Renal injury due to renin-angiotensin-aldosterone system activation of the transforming growth factor-beta pathway. *Kidney Int.* 2006;70:1914-1919.

46 Nephrolithiasis

Megan Prochaska; Gary C. Curhan

SCOPE OF THE PROBLEM

Nephrolithiasis is a major cause of morbidity involving the urinary tract. The prevalence of nephrolithiasis in the US population increased from 3.8% in the late 1970s to 8.8% in the late 2000s. The increase in prevalence was observed in men and women and in whites and blacks. There were almost 2 million physician office visits for stone disease in 2000. It is estimated that more than $5 billion US dollars is spent on stone disease annually.

The lifetime risk of nephrolithiasis is about 19% in men and 9% in women. In men, the first episode of renal colic is most likely to occur after age 30, but it can occur earlier. The incidence for men who have never had a stone is about 0.3% per year between the ages of 30 and 60 years, and it decreases thereafter with age. For women, the rate is about 0.25% per year between the ages of 20 and 30 years and then declines to 0.15% for the next 4 decades.

The risk of the first recurrent stone after the incident stone in untreated patients remains controversial. Reported frequencies of stone recurrence in uncontrolled studies have ranged from 30% to 50% at 5 years. However, data from the control groups of randomized, controlled trials suggest much lower rates of first recurrence after an incident calcium oxalate stone, ranging from 2% to 5% per year. Sex-specific rates are not available from the randomized trials.

ACUTE RENAL COLIC

With the passage of a stone from the renal pelvis into the ureter resulting in partial or complete obstruction, there is sudden onset of unilateral flank pain of sufficient severity that the individual usually seeks medical attention. Despite the use of the misnomer "colic," the pain does not completely remit but rather waxes and wanes. Nausea and vomiting may accompany the pain. The pattern of pain depends on the location of the stone: if it is in the upper ureter, pain may radiate anteriorly to the abdomen; if it is in the lower ureter, pain may radiate to the ipsilateral testicle in men or labium in women; if it is lodged at the ureterovesical junction (UVJ), the primary symptoms may be urinary frequency and urgency. A less common acute presentation is gross hematuria without pain.

The symptoms from a ureteral stone may mimic those of several other acute conditions. A stone lodged in the right ureteropelvic junction can mimic acute cholecystitis. A stone lodged in the lower right ureter as it crosses the pelvic brim can mimic acute appendicitis. A stone lodged at the UVJ on either side can mimic acute cystitis. A stone lodged in the lower left ureter as it crosses the pelvic brim can mimic diverticulitis. An obstructing stone with proximal infection can mimic acute pyelonephritis. Note that infection in the setting of obstruction is a medical emergency ("pus under pressure") that requires emergent drainage by placement of a ureteral stent or a percutaneous nephrostomy tube. However, because nephrolithiasis is common, the simple presence of a stone in the kidney does not confirm the diagnosis of renal colic in a patient presenting with acute abdominal pain.

Other conditions to consider in the differential diagnosis of suspected renal colic include muscular or skeletal pain, herpes zoster, duodenal ulcer, abdominal aortic aneurysm, gynecologic causes, ureteral obstruction resulting from other intraluminal factors (e.g., blood clot, sloughed papilla), and ureteral stricture. Extraluminal factors causing compression tend not to result in a presentation with symptoms of renal colic.

The physical examination alone rarely allows for diagnosis, but clues guide the evaluation. The patient typically is in obvious pain and is unable to achieve a comfortable position. There may be ipsilateral costovertebral angle tenderness, or in cases of obstruction with infection, symptoms and signs of sepsis.

Although blood tests are typically normal, there may be a leukocytosis resulting from stress or infection. The GFR is typically normal, but it may be reduced in the setting of volume depletion, bilateral ureteral obstruction, or unilateral obstruction, particularly in a patient with a solitary functioning kidney. The urinalysis classically shows red blood cells and white blood cells, and occasionally crystals. If ureteral obstruction by the stone is complete, there may be no red blood cells because urine will not be flowing through that ureter into the bladder.

Because of the often nonspecific physical examination and laboratory findings, imaging studies play a crucial role in making the diagnosis. A recent study suggested that a kidney ultrasound can be used as the first imaging study in the emergency department. Ultrasonography, although avoiding radiation, can image only the kidney and proximal ureter. The imaging modality that provides the most detailed information is a noncontrast helical (spiral) computed tomography (CT), because it can detect stones as small as 1 mm. Even pure uric acid stones, traditionally considered "radiolucent," are identified. Typically the study shows a ureteral stone (Fig. 46.1) or evidence of recent passage, such as perinephric stranding or hydronephrosis. A plain abdominal radiograph of the kidney, ureter, and bladder (KUB) can miss a small stone in the ureter or kidney, even one that is radiopaque, and it provides no information on obstruction. Although KUB is often used to monitor the progress of a ureteral stone or the growth of asymptomatic kidney stones, its sensitivity is limited.

Renal colic is one of the most excruciating types of pain, and pain control is essential. Narcotics and parenteral nonsteroidal antiinflammatory drugs are effective, with the latter preferable because they cause fewer side effects. Other treatments that may be effective for promoting stone passage include α-adrenergic blockers and calcium channel blockers, which have similar reported benefits on stone passage rates. Tadalafil and silodosin have been considered, but the data on these agents are limited. In the acute setting, urinary alkalinization may be effective for dissolving a uric acid stone, but this stone type is relatively rare, and there must be adequate urine flow past the stone.

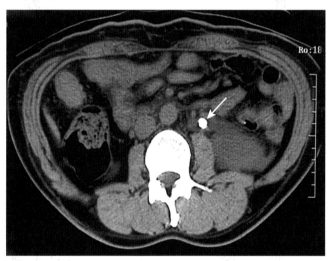

Fig. 46.1 Non–contrast-enhanced computed tomography scan shows a radioopaque obstructing stone *(arrow)* in the left ureter.

TYPES OF STONES

Almost 90% of stones in first-time stone formers contain calcium, most commonly as calcium oxalate (Fig. 46.2). Other types of stones, such as cystine, pure uric acid, and struvite, are much less common. However, these types of stones also deserve careful attention because recurrences are common.

PATHOGENESIS

The urinary concentrations of calcium, oxalate, and other solutes that influence stone formation are high enough that they should result in crystal formation in the urine of most individuals, but this is clearly not the case. This condition is termed *supersaturation*. Substances in the urine that prevent crystal formation are called *inhibitors*. The most clinically important inhibitor is citrate, which works by chelating calcium cations in the urine and decreasing the free calcium available to bind with oxalate or phosphate anions. If the supersaturation is sufficiently high or there are insufficient inhibitors, precipitation occurs with resulting crystalluria.

The causes of stone formation differ for different stone types. Cystine stones form only in individuals with the autosomal-recessive disorder of cystinuria. Uric acid stones form only in those who have persistently acidic urine, with or without hyperuricosuria. Struvite stones form only in the setting of an upper urinary tract infection with a urease-producing bacterium. These stones are seen in individuals with recurrent urinary tract infections, particularly those with abnormal urinary tract anatomy, such as patients who have urinary diversions or who require frequent catheterization. Stones may occasionally result from precipitation of medications, such as acyclovir, sulfadiazine, atazanavir, and triamterene, in the urinary tract.

Calcium-based stones have a multifactorial etiology. Traditionally, stone formation was believed to occur from (1) crystal formation in the renal tubule, followed by (2) attachment of

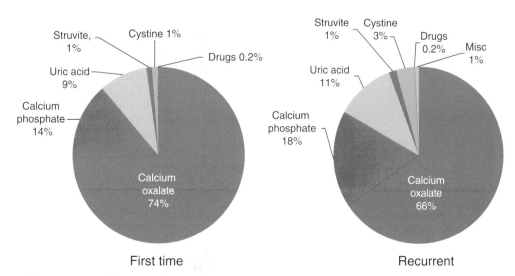

Fig. 46.2 Types of stones in first-time and recurrent stone formers. (With gratitude to Professor Michel Daudon.)

the crystal to the tubular epithelium, usually at the tip of the papilla, and (3) growth of the attached crystal by deposition of additional crystalline material. However, it now appears that the initial event occurs when calcium phosphate deposits in the medullary interstitium. The calcium phosphate material may then erode through the papillary epithelium, on which calcium oxalate is subsequently deposited.

Calcium phosphate stones are more likely to form in the presence of high urine calcium, low urine citrate, and alkaline urine (urine pH 6.5 or higher). Systemic conditions that are present more frequently in patients with calcium phosphate stones include renal tubular acidosis and primary hyperparathyroidism. The remainder of this chapter focuses on calcium oxalate stones, except where noted.

Urinary variables that increase the risk of calcium oxalate stone formation are higher levels of calcium and oxalate, whereas higher levels of citrate and higher total volume decrease the risk (Table 46.1). Risk of calcium oxalate stone formation does not vary with urine pH, unlike calcium phosphate and uric acid stones, which are pH dependent. Although higher urine uric acid concentration had been thought to increase the risk of calcium oxalate stone formation, results from a recent large study did not support this belief.

The traditional approach to urinary abnormalities is based on 24-hour urinary excretion. The reference ranges for urinary factors vary by laboratory; this is because there are no universally accepted normal ranges. Commonly used definitions of "abnormal values" are presented in Table 46.2.

Table 46.1   Risk Factors for Calcium Oxalate Stone Formation

High Levels	Low Levels
Urinary Risk Factors	
Calcium	Citrate
Oxalate	Total volume
Dietary Risk Factors	
Oxalate	Calcium, dietary
Animal protein	Potassium
Sodium	Phytate
Sucrose	Fluid
Fructose	—
Calcium, supplemental	—
Vitamin C	—
Other Risk Factors	
Obesity	—
Gout	—
Diabetes	—
Anatomic abnormalities	—

Table 46.2   Commonly Used Definitions of "Abnormal" Values

Hypercalciuria	≥200 mg/day
Hyperoxaluria	≥40 mg/day
Urine volume	<2 L/day
Hypocitraturia	≤450 mg/day

After being evaluated, patients have typically been classified into categories according to their urinary abnormalities and treatment directed at correcting the abnormalities.

Although this approach has been used for decades, it has several limitations. Stone formation is a disease of concentration. Therefore it is not just the absolute amount of substances that determines the likelihood of stone formation. The traditional definitions of "abnormal" excretion must be applied cautiously for several reasons. First, there are insufficient data supporting the cutoff points used regarding the risk of actual stone formation. For example, the traditional definition of hypercalciuria is 50 mg/day greater in men than in women, but there is no justification with respect to stone formation for having a higher upper limit of normal in men, particularly because the mean 24-hour urine volume is lower in men than in women. Similarly, another common definition of hypercalciuria is urinary calcium excretion in excess of 4 mg/kg of body weight per day. However, by this definition, an individual who is heavier or gains weight is "allowed" to excrete more calcium than someone who is thinner but still below the cutoff point. Second, an individual could have "normal" absolute excretion of calcium but still have a high urinary calcium concentration because of low urine volume. This situation has therapeutic implications, because the goal is to modify the concentration of the lithogenic factors. Finally, the risk of stone formation is a continuum, so the use of a specific cutoff point may give the false impression that a patient with "high-normal" urinary calcium excretion is not at risk for stone recurrence. Just as cardiovascular risk increases with increasing blood pressure (even in the "normal" range), the risk of stone formation increases with increasing urine calcium levels.

The underlying mechanisms for idiopathic hypercalciuria remain unknown, although hormones and their receptors involved in calcium metabolism, such as 1,25-dihydroxyvitamin D and the vitamin D receptor, likely play contributing roles. The sources of the "excess" calcium in the urine are higher intestinal absorption and higher bone resorption.

Higher urinary oxalate concentrations may result from increased gastrointestinal absorption (high dietary oxalate intake or increased fractional dietary oxalate absorption), increased endogenous production, or decreased gastrointestinal secretion. The relative contribution of exogenous and endogenous oxalate sources to urinary oxalate remains controversial. Dietary oxalate most likely contributes 30% to more than 50%, but other dietary factors (e.g., ascorbic acid) are also important.

Purines are metabolized to uric acid. Increased urinary uric acid is the result of higher purine intake and higher endogenous production from purine turnover. In the steady state, urine uric acid excretion is dependent on generation; thus the serum uric acid level does not provide any information about 24-hour urine uric acid excretion.

Low urine citrate levels are typically seen in the setting of a systemic metabolic acidosis, such as in renal tubular acidosis or excessive gastrointestinal bicarbonate losses from diarrhea. Because citrate is a potential source of bicarbonate, it is actively reclaimed in the proximal tubule after being filtered by the glomerulus.

Dietary variables associated with lower risk of incident stone formation include higher dietary intakes of calcium, potassium, and fluid; those associated with higher risk include

Table 46.3	Oxalate Content of Common Foods High in Oxalate	
Food Item	**Serving Size**	**Oxalate Content**
Spinach, raw	1 cup	656 mg
Rhubarb	½ cup	541 mg
Almonds	1 oz or 22 nuts	122 mg
Miso soup	1 cup	111 mg
Baked potato with skin	1 medium	97 mg
Corn grits	1 cup	97 mg
Beets	½ cup	76 mg
French fries	4 oz or ½ cup	51 mg
Cashews	1 oz or 18 nuts	49 mg
Raspberries	1 cup	48 mg
Mixed nuts (with peanuts)	1 oz	39 mg

Source: https://regepi.bwh.harvard.edu/health/Oxalate/files.

higher intakes of supplemental calcium, oxalate, animal protein, sodium, and sucrose (see Table 46.1). Although dietary oxalate intake has been generally believed to be important for stone formation, the magnitude of the risk is not high. Many foods contain small amounts of oxalate, but foods that are high in oxalate are less common. More recent measurements of the oxalate content of foods are much more reliable (Table 46.3).

Data from observational and randomized, controlled studies support the concept that dietary calcium intake is *inversely* associated with risk of stone formation. The mechanism by which dietary calcium may reduce the risk of stone formation is unknown, but it may involve calcium binding to oxalate in the intestine, reducing oxalate absorption.

Differences in timing of ingestion may explain the apparent contradiction between the protective effect of dietary calcium and the detrimental effect of supplemental calcium. Most people do not consume their calcium supplement with meals containing oxalate; thus the observed higher risk might rather be a result of increased urinary calcium excretion without any change in urinary oxalate excretion.

Nondietary factors that increase the risk for kidney stone formation include genitourinary anatomic abnormalities; medical conditions such as medullary sponge kidney, primary hyperparathyroidism, gout, and diabetes mellitus; and larger body size.

Several medical conditions increase the likelihood of calcium oxalate stone formation. With primary hyperparathyroidism, urinary calcium excretion is increased. Crohn disease and other malabsorptive states in which the colon is intact are associated with increased urinary oxalate excretion. With fat malabsorption, calcium is bound in the small bowel to free fatty acids, leaving a smaller amount of free calcium to bind to oxalate. An increased amount of unbound oxalate is then absorbed in the colon. These patients often lose a significant amount of fluid through the gastrointestinal tract, so the accompanying low urine volume presents an additional risk factor. Citrate reabsorption is increased by metabolic acidosis, leaving less urinary citrate to serve as a

calcium chelator. For this reason, distal renal tubular acidosis predisposes to stone formation as well.

CLINICAL EVALUATION

Evaluation after the first kidney stone appears to be cost effective, although there is some disagreement on how much should be done. The decision to proceed depends on several variables. First, what is the stone burden? Even though the episode that brought the patient to medical attention may have been the first symptomatic event, an appreciable proportion of patients has remaining stones in the kidney and could be considered "recurrent" stone formers. If such a patient had only a KUB or a kidney ultrasonogram during the acute evaluation, either of which could miss small stones, it would seem prudent to obtain a helical CT scan to determine whether there are any residual kidney stones. Second, if the initial stone was large (e.g., ≥10 mm) or required an invasive procedure to remove, an evaluation would be indicated. Finally, the patient's preferences are most important, because the recommendations often involve lifelong changes.

A detailed history provides information crucial for treatment recommendations. The following points should be covered: total number of stones, evidence of residual stones, numbers and types of procedures, types and success of previous preventive treatments, past medical history, family history of stone disease, and dietary intake and medication use before the stone event. After having experienced acute renal colic, a patient may attribute a variety of types of chronic back or flank pain to the kidney or to a residual stone. Further questioning may uncover other causes, particularly musculoskeletal. The physical examination may show findings of systemic conditions associated with stone formation, but these signs are uncommon.

LABORATORY (METABOLIC) EVALUATION

Retrieval of the stone for chemical analysis is an often overlooked but essential part of the evaluation, because treatment recommendations vary by stone type. The stone composition cannot be predicted with certainty from imaging or other laboratory studies. The decision to begin a metabolic evaluation should be guided by the patient's willingness to make lifestyle changes to prevent recurrent stone formation. Some experts advocate proceeding with an evaluation only after the second stone. However, safe and inexpensive interventions (e.g., modifying fluid intake) can be prescribed based on results of the relatively inexpensive 24-hour urine collection. If a metabolic evaluation is pursued, it is identical for first-time and recurrent stone formers. Serum chemistry values that should be measured include electrolytes, kidney function markers, and calcium and phosphorus concentrations. The decision to measure parathyroid hormone or vitamin D concentrations is based on the results of serum and urine chemistries. If the patient has high serum calcium, low serum phosphorus, or high urine calcium, then a parathyroid hormone level should be measured. The cornerstone of the evaluation is the 24-hour urine collection. Two 24-hour urine collections should be performed while the patient is consuming his or her usual diet. Because individuals often change their dietary habits soon after an episode of renal colic, a patient should wait at least 6 weeks before carrying out the collections. Two collections are needed, because there can be substantial day-to-day variability in the values.

The critical variables that should be measured in the 24-hour urine collections are total volume, calcium, oxalate, citrate, uric acid, sodium, potassium, phosphorus, pH, and creatinine. Some laboratories calculate the relative supersaturation from measurements of the urine factors, which can be used to gauge the impact of therapy.

MEDICAL TREATMENTS

Because stones can remain asymptomatic for years, the actual time of formation of the stone that brought the patient to medical attention is usually unknown. The current metabolic evaluation may, in fact, be completely normal, with no changes to lifestyle needed. Whether the patient is an active stone former influences the decision to treat. The likelihood of recurrence can be estimated but not definitely predicted from the urine chemistry results; a repeat imaging study 1 year later helps determine whether the patient is an active stone former. For patients who are at risk for stone recurrence, lifestyle modification should be attempted first, tailoring the recommendation according to stone type and urine chemistry findings. Lifelong changes are needed to prevent recurrence of this chronic condition.

DIETARY RECOMMENDATIONS

Dietary recommendations that are useful in preventing nephrolithiasis are listed in Table 46.4. There is no evidence that dietary calcium restriction is helpful in preventing stone formation, and there is substantial evidence that it is harmful. Decreasing intake of animal protein (meat, chicken, and seafood) may be helpful. Patients who have low urine citrate concentrations should increase their intake of potential alkali (fruits and vegetables) and decrease intake of acid-producing foods such as nondairy animal protein.

The role of calcium supplements deserves comment, as use of supplements is common. In someone who has never had a kidney stone, the risk attributable to supplemental calcium is low. For a patient who has had a calcium-containing stone and wishes to continue taking the supplement, 24-hour urine chemistry values should be measured while the patient is taking, and not taking, the supplement; if the urine calcium is higher while taking the supplement, then it should be discontinued. Increased fluid intake decreases the risk of stone formation and recurrence. On the basis of the urine volume, the patient should be instructed how many additional 8-ounce glasses of fluid to drink each day, with the goal of producing approximately 2 L of urine daily. Beverages associated with lower risk include coffee, orange juice, beer, and wine, while sugar sweetened beverages are associated with higher risk.

For patients with higher urine oxalate levels, a careful dietary history should be obtained. The benefit of a very low-oxalate diet is less clear because of the previously addressed issues regarding the oxalate content of food; however, spinach and rhubarb should be avoided and intake of nuts moderated. Other green leafy vegetables, such as kale, do not have a high oxalate content and therefore do not require routine avoidance. An increase in dietary calcium with meals may reduce oxalate absorption and thereby reduce urine oxalate excretion. In addition, vitamin C supplementation should be avoided, because higher vitamin C intake may increase urine oxalate excretion.

PHARMACOLOGIC OPTIONS

The use of medication is indicated if dietary recommendations are unsuccessful in adequately modifying the urine composition. The three most commonly used classes of medications for stone prevention are (1) thiazide diuretics (e.g., chlorthalidone), which reduce urinary calcium excretion; (2) alkali (e.g., potassium citrate or bicarbonate), which increase urinary citrate excretion; and (3) xanthine oxidase inhibitors (e.g., allopurinol), which reduce urinary uric acid excretion.

For patients who have higher urinary calcium levels but do not have excessive calcium intake (i.e., <1500 mg/day), a thiazide diuretic has been demonstrated to reduce the

Table 46.4 Dietary and Pharmacologic Treatments to Prevent Nephrolithiasis, According to Urinary Abnormality

Urinary Abnormality	Dietary Changes	Medication
High calcium concentration	Avoid excessive intake of calcium supplements	Thiazide diuretic
	Maintain adequate dietary calcium intake	—
	Reduce intake of animal protein	—
	Reduce sodium intake to less than 3 g/day	—
	Reduce sucrose intake	—
High oxalate concentration	Avoid high-oxalate foods	High-dose pyridoxine?
	Maintain adequate dietary calcium intake	—
	Avoid vitamin C supplements	—
High uric acid concentration	Reduce purine intake (i.e., meat, chicken, fish)	Xanthine oxidase inhibitor
Low citrate concentration	Increase intake of fruits and vegetables	Alkali (e.g., potassium citrate or potassium bicarbonate)
	Reduce intake of animal protein	
Low volume	Increase total fluid intake	Not applicable

likelihood of stone recurrence and to help maintain bone density. The dosages required to reduce urinary calcium adequately are substantially higher than those typically used for treatment of hypertension (at least 25 mg/day, and often 50 to 100 mg/day). Randomized trials of at least 3 years' duration have consistently shown a 50% reduction in the risk of recurrence. Adequate sodium restriction (to <3 g/day) is necessary to achieve maximum benefit from the thiazide diuretics; a higher sodium intake leads to greater distal sodium delivery and minimizes or negates the beneficial effect of the thiazide diuretics. For patients who are unable to increase their fluid intake, a thiazide diuretic may be helpful, even if the total urine calcium excretion is not high, because it will reduce the urinary calcium excretion and thus the calcium concentration. In addition, a thiazide diuretic may be more readily prescribed if there is evidence of low bone density.

For patients with low urine citrate levels, any form of alkali will increase the urinary citrate excretion. However, citrate is usually the first choice, because it is better tolerated than bicarbonate. Potassium salts are preferred to sodium salts because of the potential effect on urinary calcium excretion. The alkali preparations must be taken at least twice daily to maintain adequate citrate levels. Randomized trials suggest a greater than 50% reduction in risk of recurrence with alkali supplementation.

In one randomized trial, allopurinol reduced the recurrence rate by 50% among individuals with a history of recurrent calcium oxalate stones and isolated high urine uric acid. Given the epidemiologic observation that higher urine uric acid levels do not increase a person's likelihood of being a stone former, it is unclear whether the benefit was caused by the reduction in urine uric acid concentration or by some other mechanism.

NONCALCIUM STONES

For the less common types of stones (uric acid, struvite, and cystine), there is little or no information on the influence of dietary factors on actual stone formation, rather than simply changes in urine composition. The following recommendations are based on our current understanding of the pathophysiology of these stone types, but caution is warranted, because they are derived from studies of urine composition rather than actual stone formation.

URIC ACID STONES

A higher intake of nondairy animal protein may increase the risk of uric acid stone formation. Consumption of meat, chicken, and seafood increases uric acid production because of the purine content of animal flesh. Animal protein has a greater content of sulfur-containing amino acids than vegetable protein, and their metabolism leads to increased acid production with a subsequent lowering of the urinary pH. Persistently low urine pH is the major driver of uric acid crystal formation. Higher intake of fruits and vegetables, which are high in potential base, may raise the urine pH, thereby reducing the risk of uric acid crystal formation.

Alkali supplementation is the most effective treatment of existing uric acid stones. If the urine pH is maintained at 6.5 or higher (which often requires 90 to 120 mEq of supplemental alkali per day), pure uric acid stones will dissolve. Slightly lower doses may be used to prevent new uric acid stone formation. A xanthine oxidase inhibitor is the second-line choice if the patient has marked hyperuricosuria or is unable to maintain a urine pH higher than 6.5.

CYSTINE STONES

Higher sodium intake may increase urine cystine excretion. Because the solubility of cystine increases as pH rises, a higher consumption of fruits and vegetables may have a beneficial effect. Although restriction of proteins high in cystine (e.g., animal protein) seems advisable, there is little evidence to support this recommendation as a means of directly lowering urinary cystine levels; however, reducing animal protein intake may be beneficial by leading to an increase in the urine pH.

Medications such as tiopronin and penicillamine increase the solubility (not the total amount) of the filtered cystine. The effectiveness of these drugs is limited by the amount of cystine excreted daily and the high side-effect profile. If adequate amounts of the medication enter the urine, cystine stones can be dissolved. Supplemental potassium alkali salts may also provide benefit by increasing the urine pH.

STRUVITE STONES

Because struvite stones form only in the setting of an infection in the upper urinary tract with urease-producing bacteria, it is unlikely that dietary factors can directly influence struvite stone formation. Struvite stones are almost always large and may fill the renal pelvis, referred to as "staghorn calculi"; an experienced urologist should remove these stones. In addition to the complete removal of all residual fragments, prevention of urinary tract infections is the cornerstone for avoiding recurrence. Acetohydroxamic acid is the only drug available that inhibits urease; however, it should be used with extreme caution because of its common and serious side effects.

CALCIUM PHOSPHATE STONES

Information on dietary issues related to actual calcium phosphate stone formation is limited. However, on the basis of the known physicochemical aspects, nutrients that might stimulate calcium phosphate crystal formation include excessive calcium intake (resulting in higher urinary calcium excretion), higher phosphate intake (resulting in higher urinary phosphate excretion), and higher intake of fruits and vegetables (resulting in a higher urinary pH). Nonetheless, caution is advised because the "theoretical" benefits of limiting these nutrients may not be realized, and there are, of course, other reasons to maintain an adequate intake of calcium, fruits, and vegetables; higher intake of alkali-rich foods may lead to higher urine citrate.

Reduction in urine calcium can be achieved with thiazide diuretics, using an approach similar to that recommended for calcium oxalate stones. Because patients who form calcium phosphate stones may also have low urine citrate concentrations, alkali supplementation may be used with caution. Alkali supplementation often increases urine pH and therefore could increase the risk of calcium phosphate crystal formation. This risk is often outweighed by the increase in urine citrate.

SURGICAL MANAGEMENT OF STONES

In the acute setting, the urologist may assist in the management. If the stone does not pass rapidly, the patient can be sent home with appropriate oral analgesics, an α-blocker or calcium channel blocker to increase the likelihood of stone passage, and instructions to return in case of fever or uncontrollable pain. Most urologists wait several days before intervening for a ureteral stone, unless one of the following conditions exists: urinary tract infection, stone greater than 6 mm in size, presence of an anatomic abnormality that would prevent passage, or intractable pain. A cystoscopically placed ureteral stent is typically used, but anesthesia is required. The stent can be uncomfortable and not infrequently causes gross hematuria. Although it is debatable whether a stent helps with stone passage, cystoscopy or stent placement may push the stone back up into the renal pelvis, thus relieving the obstruction and permitting its management on a nonemergent basis.

The method of stone removal is determined by stone size, location, and composition; the urinary tract anatomy; availability of technology; and the experience of the urologist. Extracorporeal shock wave lithotripsy (ESWL) is the least invasive method. Cystoscopic stone removal, by either basket extraction or fragmentation, is invasive but more effective than ESWL, and newer instruments allow removal of stones even in the kidney. Percutaneous nephrostolithotomy, an approach requiring the placement of a nephrostomy tube, is more invasive but necessary for large stone burdens and for kidney stones that cannot be removed cystoscopically; this is the gold standard for making a patient "stone-free." Open procedures such as ureterolithotomy or nephrolithotomy are rarely needed.

The surgical treatment of asymptomatic stones is controversial. The availability of ESWL has lowered the threshold for treating asymptomatic stones; most urologists consider treating only asymptomatic stones that are at least 1 cm in size. While ESWL is less invasive than other approaches, potential complications include renal colic (as a result of a stone fragment entering the ureter), injury to the renal parenchyma, perirenal hematoma, and possibly a slightly higher risk of hypertension.

With the increasing prevalence of obesity in the United States, the treatment of existing stones in morbidly obese individuals deserves mention. The ability to image the urinary tract may be limited if the patient's size prohibits access to scanning by CT. ESWL may not be an option, as morbid obesity can interfere with stone localization and the ability of the shock waves to reach the calculus; therefore more invasive approaches, such as ureteroscopy, may be necessary.

LONG-TERM FOLLOW-UP

The nephrologist or primary care provider should assume responsibility for the long-term prevention program and should consult with the urologist as needed for further surgical interventions. The plan should include recommendations for prevention based on the evaluation; interventions should be followed by repeat metabolic measurements to assess their success, adjustment of recommendations, and follow-up imaging.

Adherence to recommendations frequently declines with time. In addition, the long-term sequelae of the treatments and the underlying abnormalities may have other implications for the health of the patient. For example, individuals with higher urine calcium excretion typically have lower bone density and are at increased risk for osteoporosis. With appropriate attention and evaluation, the morbidity and cost of recurrent stone disease can be dramatically reduced.

BIBLIOGRAPHY

Borghi L, Schianchi T, Meschi T, et al. Comparison of two diets for the prevention of recurrent stones in idiopathic hypercalciuria. *N Engl J Med.* 2002;346:77-84.

Coe FL, Evan A, Worcester E. Pathophysiology-based treatment of idiopathic calcium kidney stones. *Clin J Am Soc Nephrol.* 2011;6:2083-2092.

Curhan GC, Willett WC, Rimm EB, et al. A prospective study of dietary calcium and other nutrients and the risk of symptomatic kidney stones. *N Engl J Med.* 1993;328:833-838.

Evan AP, Lingeman JE, Coe FL, et al. Randall's plaque of patients with nephrolithiasis begins in basement membranes of thin loops of Henle. *J Clin Invest.* 2003;111:607-616.

Ferraro PM, Taylor EN, Eisner BH, Gambaro G, Rimm EB, Mukamal KJ, Curhan GC. History of kidney stones and the risk of coronary heart disease. *JAMA.* 2013;310(4):408-415.

Ferraro PM, Taylor EN, Gambaro G, Curhan GC, et al. Soda and other beverages and the risk of kidney stones. *Clin J Am Soc Nephrol.* 2013; 8(8):1389-1395.

Lieske JC, Rule AD, Krambeck AE, Williams JC, Bergstralh EJ, Mehta RA, Moyer TP. Stone composition as a function of age and sex. *Clin J Am Soc Nephrol.* 2014;9(12):2141-2146.

Mandeville JA, Gnessin E, Lingeman JE. Imaging evaluation in the patient with renal stone disease. *Semin Nephrol.* 2011;31:254-258.

Pearle MS, Goldfarb DS, Assimos DG, Curhan G, Denu-Ciocca CJ, Matlaga BR, Monga M, Penniston KL, Preminger GM, Turk TM, White JR. American Urological Association. Medical management of kidney stones: AUA guideline. *J Urol.* 2014;192(2):316-324.

Rule AD, Lieske JC, Li X, Melton LJ 3rd, Krambeck AE, Bergstralh EJ. The ROKS nomogram for predicting a second symptomatic stone episode. *J Am Soc Nephrol.* 2014;25(12):2878-2886.

Taylor EN, Curhan GC. Oxalate intake and the risk for nephrolithiasis. *J Am Soc Nephrol.* 2007;18:2198-2204.

Taylor EN, Stampfer MJ, Curhan GC. Obesity, weight gain, and the risk of kidney stones. *JAMA.* 2005;293:455-462.

Teichman JMH. Acute renal colic from ureteral calculus. *N Engl J Med.* 2004;350:684-693.

Urinary Tract Infection and Pyelonephritis

47

Lindsay E. Nicolle

Urinary infection is the presence of microbial pathogens within the normally sterile urinary tract. Infections are overwhelmingly bacterial, although fungi, viruses, and parasites may occasionally be pathogens (Table 47.1). Urinary infection is the most common bacterial infection in humans and can be either symptomatic or asymptomatic. Symptomatic infection is associated with a wide spectrum of morbidity, from mild irritative voiding symptoms to bacteremia, sepsis, and, occasionally, death. Asymptomatic urinary infection is defined as isolation of bacteria from urine in quantitative counts consistent with infection but without localizing genitourinary or systemic symptoms or signs attributable to the infection.

The term *bacteriuria* simply means bacteria present in the urine, although it is generally used to imply isolation of a significant quantitative count of organisms. This term is often used interchangeably with *asymptomatic urinary infection*. Recurrent urinary infection is common in individuals who experience an initial infection. It may be either relapse (i.e., recurrence after therapy with the pretherapy isolate) or reinfection (i.e., recurrence with a different organism). An important consideration in the management of urinary infection is whether the patient has a functionally and structurally normal (uncomplicated urinary infection or acute nonobstructive pyelonephritis) or abnormal (complicated urinary infection) genitourinary tract.

The microbiologic diagnosis of urinary infection requires isolation of a pathogenic organism in sufficient quantitative amounts from a urine specimen collected in a manner that minimizes contamination from vaginal or periurethral organisms. A quantitative bacterial count of $\geq 10^5$ cfu/mL is the usual standard to discriminate infection from organisms present as contaminants. The use of the quantitative urine culture is essential for the management of urinary infection, but this quantitative standard of $\geq 10^5$ cfu/mL must be interpreted in the context of the clinical presentation.

ACUTE UNCOMPLICATED URINARY INFECTION

Acute uncomplicated urinary infection, or acute cystitis, is infection occurring in individuals with a normal genitourinary tract and no recent instrumentation. It is a common syndrome that occurs virtually entirely in women; 60% of all women experience at least one infection in their lifetime. From 1% to 2% of women have frequent recurrent infection. The highest incidence is in young, sexually active women. Risk factors for infection in these women are both genetic and behavioral. Women with recurrent acute uncomplicated urinary infection are more likely to have first-degree female relatives with urinary infections and to be nonsecretors of blood group substances. Polymorphisms of genes encoding elements of the innate immune response may also contribute to the genetic propensity to recurrent infection. Sexual activity is strongly associated with infection in premenopausal women, and frequency of infection correlates with frequency of intercourse. The use of spermicides or a diaphragm for birth control also increases the risk for infection; risk is not increased by use of oral contraceptives or condoms without spermicide. Behavioral practices such as postvoid personal hygiene, type of underwear, postcoital voiding, or bathing rather than showering have no association with infection. For postmenopausal women, frequency of sexual intercourse is not a risk factor for infection. The most important predictor of infection in older women is a history of urinary infection at a younger age.

Escherichia coli is isolated from 80% to 85% of episodes. *Staphylococcus saprophyticus*, a coagulase-negative staphylococcus, occurs in 5% to 10% of episodes. This organism is rarely isolated in other clinical syndromes and has a unique seasonal variation with increased frequency in the late summer and early fall. *Klebsiella pneumoniae* and *Proteus mirabilis* are each isolated in 2% to 3% of cases. Organisms that cause infection originate from the normal gut flora, colonize the vagina and periurethral area, and ascend to the bladder. Women with urinary infection frequently have alterations in vaginal flora characterized by decreased or absent hydrogen peroxide (H_2O_2) producing lactobacilli, resulting in increased vaginal pH and facilitating colonization with *E. coli* and other potential uropathogens.

The clinical presentation, diagnosis, and recommended treatment for acute uncomplicated urinary infection are summarized in Table 47.2. New-onset frequency, dysuria, and urgency together with the absence of vaginal discharge or pain are 90% accurate to diagnose infection. From 30% to 50% of women have quantitative counts of less than 10^5 cfu/mL of a uropathogen isolated from the urine specimen. Thus, any quantitative count of a potential uropathogen with pyuria is considered sufficient for microbiologic diagnosis when accompanied by consistent clinical symptoms. Because the clinical presentation is characteristic, the bacteriology is predictable, and the quantitative microbiology is often not definitive, it is recommended that symptomatic episodes be managed with empiric antimicrobial therapy and routine pretherapy urine culture not be obtained. A urine specimen for culture should be obtained before antimicrobial treatment if there is uncertainty about the diagnosis, failure of an initial

Table 47.1 Nonbacterial Pathogens Causing Urinary Tract Infection

Fungi	Viruses	Parasites
Candida albicans	JC, BK viruses	Schistosoma
Candida parapsilosis	Adenovirus types	hematobium
Candida glabrata	11, 21	
Candida tropicalis	Mumps	
Blastomyces dermatitidis[a]	Hantavirus[b]	
Aspergillus fumigatus[a]		
Cryptococcus neoformans[a]		
Histoplasma capsulatum[a]		

[a]With disseminated infection.
[b]Hemorrhagic fever and renal syndrome.

therapeutic regimen, or early recurrence after therapy. The differential diagnosis includes urethritis due to sexually transmitted diseases such as *Neisseria gonorrhoeae* or *Chlamydia trachomatis*, yeast vulvovaginitis, or genital herpes.

Antimicrobial therapy is selected based on considerations of patient tolerance, documented efficacy for treating urinary infection, and local prevalence of resistance in community-acquired *E. coli*. Recommended therapy is nitrofurantoin for 5 days, single-dose fosfomycin trometamol, or, when available, 5 days of pivmecillinam; all of these have indications virtually limited to treatment of this syndrome. Trimethoprim-sulfamethoxazole (TMP/SMX) has been the recommended empiric therapy for many years. However, if the regional prevalence of resistance of community *E. coli* isolates to this antimicrobial is over 20%, an alternate empiric regimen should be prescribed. Fluoroquinolones and β-lactam antimicrobials are not considered first-line therapy because of the propensity to induce resistance in gut flora and, for β-lactams, a lower efficacy. The increasing global resistance of community *E. coli*, especially the widespread dissemination of extended-spectrum beta-lactamase (ESBL) or carbapenemase-producing strains, is a current concern. These organisms are also usually resistant to TMP/SMX and fluoroquinolones, but, to date, most remain susceptible to nitrofurantoin, fosfomycin, and pivmecillinam. A 3-day course of antimicrobial therapy with TMP/SMX or a fluoroquinolone is effective. A longer course of 7 days is recommended when the duration of symptoms is more than 7 days, for women with an early recurrence of symptomatic infection (<30 days) following prior antimicrobial therapy, and when treatment is with a β-lactam antimicrobial.

For women with mild to moderate symptoms, about 50% are symptom free by 7 days following initiation of antiinflammatory therapy and without antibiotics. Antibiotic therapy, however, clearly decreases symptom duration. Some women with mild symptoms may choose to delay antimicrobial therapy to see if spontaneous resolution occurs with antiinflammatory medication, but whether to delay antibiotics should be a patient decision.

Frequent recurrent acute cystitis is a disruptive and distressing problem for many women. Antimicrobial prophylaxis, given either as a long-term, low-dose regimen or after intercourse, prevents 95% or more of recurrent episodes and is usually recommended for women with two episodes in 6 months or 3 in 1 year (Table 47.3). Increasing resistance of *E. coli* strains may limit the effectiveness of TMP/SMX. Continuous low-dose prophylaxis taken at bedtime is recommended, with an initial course of 6 to 12 months. This remains effective when taken for as long as 2 to 5 years. When prophylactic therapy is discontinued, the frequency of urinary infection is similar to that observed before prophylaxis. Approximately 50% of women have recurrent infection within 3 months. Postcoital prophylaxis is, obviously, most appropriate for women who identify sexual intercourse as a precipitating factor for recurrent symptomatic episodes. An alternate approach preferred by some women, especially with less frequent recurrences or who are concerned about developing an infection while traveling, is self-treatment. This approach is effective with short-course TMP/SMX, ciprofloxacin, or ofloxacin. It is appropriate for women who are compliant with management and reliable in identifying their symptomatic episodes.

The most important nonantimicrobial intervention for prevention of recurrent urinary infection is avoidance of spermicide use. The daily intake of cranberry or lingonberry juice or cranberry tablets was previously reported to decrease the frequency of recurrent infection by 30%, but recent blinded placebo-controlled trials have not reported a benefit. Vaccines to prevent recurrent uncomplicated urinary infection and use of probiotics to reestablish normal gut or vaginal flora are being investigated, but studies to date have not shown consistent benefits with either of these approaches.

ACUTE NONOBSTRUCTIVE PYELONEPHRITIS

Acute nonobstructive pyelonephritis is a symptomatic kidney infection occurring in women with a normal genitourinary tract. Women who experience acute uncomplicated urinary infection are also at risk for nonobstructive pyelonephritis, with the frequency of episodes of cystitis relative to pyelonephritis reported to be 18–29 to 1. Risk factors for developing acute pyelonephritis are similar to those for acute cystitis for premenopausal women; frequency of sexual intercourse is the most important. *E. coli* is isolated from 85% of episodes. These strains are characterized by expression of specific virulence factors. The P fimbria, an adhesin that attaches to uroepithelial cells and induces an inflammatory response, is the most important virulence factor. Additional organism virulence factors include production of hemolysin, which may lyse host cells, and aerobactin, an iron scavenger that may promote bacterial growth.

Acute pyelonephritis presents classically with fever and costovertebral angle pain and tenderness, often associated with lower urinary tract symptoms. Fever may be low grade or, occasionally, absent. A urine specimen for culture and susceptibility testing should be obtained before the initiation of antimicrobial therapy from every woman with a suspected diagnosis of pyelonephritis. Growth of ≥10^4 cfu/mL of a uropathogen together with pyuria and consistent clinical findings is sufficient for diagnosis, although ≥10^5 cfu/mL of organisms is isolated from 95% of cases. Bacteremia occurs in about 10% of episodes and is more frequent in older

Table 47.2 Diagnosis and Management of Common Symptomatic Syndromes of Urinary Infection

Clinical Presentation	Microbiologic Diagnosis	First-Line Treatment	Second-Line Treatment	Parenteral Treatment
Acute uncomplicated urinary infection (acute cystitis) Lower tract irritative symptoms: dysuria, frequency, urgency, suprapubic discomfort, hematuria	$\geq 10^5$ cfu/mL of uropathogen with pyuria	TMP/SMX 160/180 mg bid, 3 days TMP 200 mg bid, 3 days Nitrofurantoin 50–100 mg qid, or monohydrate/macrocrystals 100 mg bid × 5 days Fosfomycin trometamol 3 g, one dose Pivmecillinam 400 mg bid,[a] 3 or 7 days	Norfloxacin 400 mg bid, 3 days Ciprofloxacin 250 mg bid, 3 days Ciprofloxacin extended-release 500 mg daily, 3 days Ofloxacin 400 mg bid, 3 days Levofloxacin 400 mg daily, 3 days Amoxicillin/clavulanic acid 500 mg bid, 7 days Cephalexin 500 mg qid, 7 days Cefixime 400 mg daily, 7 days Cefpodoxime 100 mg bid, 3 days	
Acute nonobstructive pyelonephritis Costovertebral angle pain and tenderness; ± fever, ±lower tract symptoms	$\geq 10^4$ cfu/mL (95% have $\geq 10^5$ cfu/mL)	Norfloxacin 400 mg bid Ciprofloxacin 500 mg bid Ofloxacin 400 mg bid Levofloxacin 500–750 mg daily	TMP/SMX 160/800 mg bid[b] TMP 100 mg bid[b] Amoxicillin/clavulanic acid 500 mg tid Cephalexin 500 mg qid[b] Cefixime 400 mg daily	Gentamicin 3–5 mg/kg/24 hours in one or two doses ± ampicillin 1 g q4–6h Ceftriaxone 1–2 g q24h Cefotaxime 1 g tid Ciprofloxacin 400 mg bid Levofloxacin 500–750 mg daily
Complicated urinary infection Variable symptoms, including lower tract symptoms; pyelonephritis; systemic symptoms (fever, shock)	$\geq 10^5$ cfu/mL	TMP/SMX 160/800 mg bid Norfloxacin 400 mg bid Ciprofloxacin 250–500 mg bid Ciprofloxacin extended-release, 1 g daily Ofloxacin 400 mg bid Levofloxacin 500 mg daily Amoxicillin/clavulanic acid 500 mg tid Cephalexin 500 mg qid Cefixime 400 mg PO daily		Gentamicin or tobramycin 3–5 mg/kg/24 hours in one or two doses ± Ampicillin 1 g q4–6h or piperacillin 3 g q4h Amikacin 15 mg/kg in one or two doses Piperacillin/tazobactam 3.375 g q6h Ceftazidime 1 g tid[c] Cefotaxime 1 g tid or ceftriaxone 1–2 g q24h Ertapenem 1 g q24h[c] Meropenem 500 mg q6h[c] Doripenem 500 mg q8h[c] Ceftazidime/avibactam 2.5 g q8h[c] Ceftolozane/tazobactam 1.5 g q8h[c]

bid, Twice daily; *qid*, four times daily; *tid*, three times daily; *TMP/SMX*, trimethoprim/sulfamethoxazole.
[a]Not licensed in the United States.
[b]If organism is known to be susceptible.
[c]For resistant organisms.

adult women and women with diabetes. When women with pyelonephritis present with sepsis or shock, urgent imaging should be obtained to exclude obstruction or other lesions requiring immediate intervention for source control because severe presentations are unusual with acute nonobstructive pyelonephritis.

The majority of women can be treated as outpatients with oral antimicrobial therapy (see Table 47.2). A common approach is to give a single dose of parenteral antibiotic in the emergency department, usually gentamicin 3 to 5 mg/kg or ceftriaxone 1 or 2 g, followed by a course of oral therapy. Hospitalization and initial parenteral antimicrobial therapy

Table 47.3   Prophylactic Antimicrobial Therapy for Women With Frequent Recurrence of Acute Uncomplicated Urinary Infection

| Agent | REGIMEN | |
	Long-Term	Postcoital (One Dose)
TMP/SMX[a]	80/400 mg daily or 3 × weekly	80/400 mg
TMP[a]	100 mg daily	100 mg
Nitrofurantoin[a]	50 mg daily	50–100 mg
Cephalexin	125 mg daily	250 mg
Norfloxacin	200 mg every other day	200–400 mg
Ciprofloxacin	—	250 mg

[a]Recommended first-line agents.
TMP/SMX, Trimethoprim/sulfamethoxazole.

Table 47.4   Abnormalities of the Genitourinary Tract Associated With Complicated Urinary Infection

Abnormality	Examples
Metabolic or structural	Medullary sponge kidney
	Nephrocalcinosis
	Malakoplakia
	Xanthogranulomatous pyelonephritis
Congenital	Cystic disease
	Duplicated drainage system with obstruction
	Urethral valves
Obstruction	Vesicoureteral reflux
	Pelvicalyceal obstruction
	Papillary necrosis
	Urethral fibrosis/stricture
	Bladder diverticulum
	Neurogenic bladder
	Prostatic hypertrophy
	Tumors
	Urolithiasis
Instrumentation	Indwelling catheter
	Intermittent catheterization
	Cystoscopy
	Ureteric stent
	Nephrostomy tube
Other	Immunocompromised
	Subsequent to kidney transplant
	Neutropenic

are recommended for women with hemodynamic instability, for whom oral medication may not be tolerated because of severe gastrointestinal symptoms, or when there are significant systemic signs of illness and concern regarding compliance with outpatient therapy. The parenteral antimicrobial can be replaced by oral therapy once clinical improvement has occurred, usually by 48 to 72 hours. The urine culture results are also available by this time and direct selection of a specific oral antimicrobial for continuing therapy. The total duration is usually 7 to 10 days, but ciprofloxacin or levofloxacin is effective with 5 days of therapy.

By 48 to 72 hours following initiation of effective antimicrobial therapy, there should be evidence of clinical improvement, including decreased costovertebral angle discomfort and a decrease in or resolution of fever. If there is not substantial clinical improvement by this time or if symptomatic infection recurs soon after an adequate course of therapy, a resistant bacterial strain or abnormality within the genitourinary tract causing urinary obstruction or abscess formation should be excluded. The imaging approach is individualized depending on presentation, clinical course, and access to diagnostic testing. Computed tomography (CT) scanning with contrast, however, is superior to ultrasonography or magnetic resonance imaging (MRI) for characterizing potential kidney abnormalities.

COMPLICATED URINARY INFECTION

The most important host defense preventing urinary infection is intermittent, unobstructed voiding of urine. Any abnormality of the genitourinary tract that impairs voiding increases the risk for urinary infection. Urinary infection in individuals with structural or functional abnormalities of the urinary tract, including those who have undergone instrumentation, is considered a *complicated urinary infection* (Table 47.4). The likelihood and frequency of infection are determined by the underlying abnormality and are independent of sex or age. For some abnormalities, such as an infected cyst with polycystic kidney disease, infection is infrequent but difficult to manage. In other patients, such as those with an indwelling or intermittent catheter, infection is very frequent. For patients

with chronic indwelling devices, biofilm formation on the device results in a bacterial infection rate of 5% per day, and virtually 100% of patients are bacteriuric after several weeks.

The clinical presentation of symptomatic infection varies along a spectrum from mild lower tract irritative symptoms to systemic manifestations with fever or even septic shock. Individuals with complete obstruction of urine flow or with mucosal bleeding are at greatest risk for the most severe clinical presentations.

For optimal management, a urine specimen for culture collected before initiating antimicrobial therapy is essential to identify the infecting organism and susceptibilities. A quantitative count of organisms in the urine of $\geq 10^5$ cfu/mL remains the standard for the microbiologic diagnosis of complicated urinary infection. Polymicrobial bacteriuria occurs frequently. Organisms isolated are characterized by a greater diversity of infecting species and an increased prevalence of antimicrobial resistance when compared with uncomplicated infection. They are less likely to express virulence factors because the host abnormality of impaired voiding is itself sufficient for infection. Increased antimicrobial resistance is common because of nosocomial acquisition of infecting organisms or repeated prior courses of antimicrobial therapy for recurrent infection. In cases where broad-spectrum antimicrobial therapy has been given for prolonged periods, reinfection may occur with yeast species or highly resistant bacteria, such as *Pseudomonas aeruginosa* or *Acinetobacter* species. Infections with ESBL or carbapenemase producing Enterobacteriaceae are also now frequently identified.

Similarly to acute uncomplicated urinary infection, antimicrobial treatment is selected based on clinical presentation, patient tolerance, and the known or predicted susceptibilities of the infecting organisms. When possible, antimicrobial therapy should be delayed until urine culture results are available. Patients with moderate to severe symptoms should have empiric therapy initiated pending culture results. The local antimicrobial susceptibility prevalence, recent history of antimicrobial use by the patient, and prior urine culture results in an individual patient are helpful in directing the choice of empiric therapy. Initial parenteral therapy is required for patients with severe systemic manifestations, where oral therapy is not tolerated, or when the infecting organism is suspected or known to be resistant to any available oral therapy. With a clinical presentation of lower tract symptoms, 7 days of therapy is generally adequate. In cases with fever or other systemic symptoms, 10 to 14 days of therapy are recommended, although 5 to 7 days is effective with fluoroquinolone antimicrobials such as ciprofloxacin and levofloxacin.

Complicated urinary infection can be prevented if the underlying abnormality is corrected. There may be a continuing high frequency of recurrent infections when the underlying genitourinary abnormality persists. For instance, 50% of patients with a neurogenic bladder and voiding managed by intermittent catheterization experience recurrent infection by 4 to 6 weeks after antimicrobial therapy. For hospitalized patients, the most important interventions to limit infection are avoidance of indwelling catheter use and if a catheter is indicated, to minimize the amount of time it remains in situ. Prophylactic antimicrobials are not recommended; this approach has not been shown to decrease symptomatic infections, while it does increase the risk of reinfection with organisms resistant to the administered antimicrobial. For selected patients who experience frequent, severe symptomatic recurrences and have an abnormality that cannot be corrected but do not have an indwelling device, long-term suppressive therapy may be considered. Some clinical scenarios where this may be indicated include men with recurrent symptomatic infection from chronic bacterial prostatitis or individuals with infection persisting in a nonfunctioning kidney. This approach is individualized in every case. Antimicrobial therapy is initiated at full therapeutic doses and subsequently decreased to one-half or less of the regular dose if the urine culture remains negative and the clinical course is satisfactory.

ASYMPTOMATIC URINARY INFECTION

Asymptomatic bacteriuria is isolation of one or more uropathogens in quantitative counts consistent with urinary infection ($\geq 10^5$ cfu/mL) in a patient with no localizing genitourinary signs or symptoms. Asymptomatic bacteriuria is common in many populations (Table 47.5). Pyuria is also common in these individuals, being present in 50% to 90%. Asymptomatic bacteriuria occurs with increased frequency in persons who also experience symptomatic urinary infection. This suggests that the biologic defects promoting symptomatic and asymptomatic infection are similar. Treatment is indicated only for pregnant women and patients who undergo an invasive genitourinary procedure with a high likelihood of mucosal bleeding. Identification and treatment of asymptomatic bacteriuria in early pregnancy prevent pyelonephritis and,

Table 47.5 Prevalence of Asymptomatic Bacteriuria in Selected Populations

Population	Prevalence
Healthy Girls and Women	
<10 years	1%–2%
10–50 years	3%–5%
>50 years	5%–10%
>80 years	20%
Healthy Men	
<60 years	<1%
>80 years	5%–10%
Nursing Home Residents	
Women	25%–50%
Men	15%–40%
Persons With Diabetes	
Women	5%–15%
Men	1%–10%
Catheters	
Intermittent	50%
Short Term	5%/day
Chronic	100%

possibly, adverse fetal outcomes of premature delivery and low birth weight. For patients undergoing an invasive genitourinary procedure, prophylaxis to prevent perioperative sepsis is initiated immediately before the intervention and usually requires only a single dose. For other populations, asymptomatic infection with or without pyuria does not require treatment. Long-term cohort studies do not document adverse effects attributable to bacteriuria, and prospective randomized trials have not identified any clinical benefits of antimicrobial treatment. In fact, adverse antibiotic effects and reinfection with organisms of increased resistance occur with antibiotic prophylaxis, and, in some populations, treatment of asymptomatic bacteriuria increases the short-term risk of experiencing symptomatic urinary infection.

SPECIAL POPULATIONS

URINARY INFECTION IN CHILDREN

Urinary infection occurs more frequently in boys than girls in the first year of life. Infection in boys usually occurs within 3 months of birth and is often associated with congenital anomalies of the urinary tract. The clinical presentation is of neonatal sepsis without localizing genitourinary tract signs, and these episodes are treated as neonatal sepsis. After the first year of life, urinary infection occurs more frequently in girls than boys, and the clinical presentation is with genitourinary symptoms. Most episodes in girls are acute uncomplicated urinary infection, and these girls also experience urinary infection more frequently as adults. Vesicoureteral reflux, which may lead to impaired kidney function, must be excluded. Imaging studies, including voiding cystourethrogram, ultrasonography, ^{99}Tc-dimercaptosuccinic acid (DMSA), or CT scan, are indicated for any child presenting with pyelonephritis, for a first urinary infection in a boy of any age or a girl under 3 years, for a second urinary infection in a girl older than 3 years, and for a first urinary infection at any age with a family history of urinary tract abnormalities. Other indications for imaging include urinary infection accompanied by abnormal voiding, hypertension, or poor growth.

Treatment of acute lower tract infection in young girls is for 3 to 7 days. Pyelonephritis should be treated for 10 to 14 days. Generally, the antimicrobials used are similar to those in adults with appropriate dose adjustments for weight. The fluoroquinolones are not recommended for children under the age of 16 years because of potential adverse effects on cartilage. Long-term low-dose prophylactic therapy is indicated for young girls with frequent symptomatic recurrences or with severe vesicoureteral reflux (grades IV or V) and recurrent urinary infection. Asymptomatic urinary infection is common in school-age girls. Treatment of asymptomatic urinary infection does not alter the natural history of kidney disease in young girls or prevent kidney scarring. In fact, treatment of asymptomatic bacteriuria with antimicrobials appears to increase the frequency of symptomatic infection. Thus, it is not recommended to screen for or treat asymptomatic bacteriuria in girls.

URINARY INFECTION IN PREGNANCY

Hormonal changes in pregnancy produce hypotonicity of the autonomic musculature, leading to urine stasis and ureteric reflux. In addition, obstruction at the pelvic brim—more marked on the right than the left side—occurs with the enlarging fetus. These changes are maximal at the end of the second trimester and beginning of the third trimester, correlating with the highest incidence of pyelonephritis. Acute pyelonephritis may precipitate premature labor and delivery, as may any febrile illness in later pregnancy. About 30% of women identified with asymptomatic bacteriuria in early pregnancy who are not treated with antimicrobials develop acute pyelonephritis later in the pregnancy. From 75% to 90% of these episodes are prevented by early identification and treatment of asymptomatic bacteriuria. Premature delivery and low birth weight are also decreased with treatment.

Because of these benefits of treating asymptomatic bacteriuria, pregnant women should be screened for bacteriuria by urine culture at 12 to 16 weeks' gestation. When significant bacteriuria is identified, it should be confirmed with a second urine culture and treated, if persistent. Antimicrobial therapy is selected based on the susceptibilities of the infecting organism, patient tolerance, and safety for use in pregnancy. A 3-day course of amoxicillin, nitrofurantoin, or cephalexin is usually sufficient. TMP/SMX has been widely used and is effective, but it may be associated with increased fetal abnormalities when given in the first trimester and should be avoided early in pregnancy. Fluoroquinolones are contraindicated. Women treated for an initial episode of asymptomatic bacteriuria or symptomatic urinary infection in early pregnancy should be followed with monthly urine cultures throughout the remainder of the pregnancy to identify recurrent infection. If a second episode of either symptomatic or asymptomatic infection occurs, low-dose prophylactic therapy should be initiated following treatment of the infection and continued until delivery.

URINARY INFECTION IN MEN

Men rarely present with acute uncomplicated urinary infection or acute nonobstructive pyelonephritis. Lack of circumcision, acquisition of an infecting strain from a new sexual partner, and men who have sex with men are potential risk factors in the few cases that do occur. *E. coli* is the usual infecting organism. Uncomplicated infection, however, is so uncommon in men that any man presenting with urinary infection should be investigated for the possibility of an underlying abnormality.

Older adult men have an increased frequency of urinary infection, often attributed to prostatic hypertrophy leading to obstruction and turbulent urine flow. Older men are also more likely to develop chronic bacterial prostatitis. Once bacteria are established in the prostate, poor diffusion of antibiotics into the prostate and impaired antibiotic activity in the alkaline environment of the prostate, and the frequent occurrence of prostate stones, make the infection difficult to eradicate. The prostate then serves as a nidus for recurrent symptomatic or asymptomatic bladder infection. If recurrent symptomatic infection occurs and chronic bacterial prostatitis is diagnosed, a more prolonged antimicrobial course of 4 to 6 weeks of therapy is indicated and leads to cure in 50% to 70% of cases. Fluoroquinolones are the recommended first-line agents, but TMP/SMX, tetracyclines, and azithromycin may also be used, depending on the susceptibility of the organisms isolated. When prolonged antimicrobial therapy does not cure the infection and frequent symptomatic recurrence occurs, suppressive antimicrobial therapy may be considered.

URINARY TRACT INFECTIONS IN OLDER ADULTS

Urinary infection is the most common infection occurring in both ambulatory and institutionalized older adult populations. The prevalence of bacteriuria is 5% to 10% for women and 5% in men over 65 years of age living in the community. These rates increase with advancing age. In long-term care facilities, 25% to 50% of all older adult residents have asymptomatic bacteriuria at any time. The prevalence increases with increasing functional and cognitive impairment, including dementia and bladder and bowel incontinence. Asymptomatic bacteriuria in older adult patients should not be treated with antimicrobials. Antimicrobial treatment does not decrease morbidity or mortality, but is associated with increased adverse drug effects, cost, and antimicrobial resistance. It follows that asymptomatic older adult populations should not be screened for bacteriuria.

Symptomatic infection in older adults usually has clinical presentations similar to those in younger populations. However, particularly in the functionally or cognitively impaired population, the diagnosis may not be straightforward. Difficulties in communication, comorbid illnesses with chronic symptoms, chronic genitourinary symptoms, and the high frequency of asymptomatic bacteriuria all compromise diagnostic precision. A reduced febrile response and lower frequency of leukocytosis characterize infection in older adults, and acute confusion may be a prominent presenting symptom with severe infection. Despite this, a diagnosis of symptomatic urinary infection in an older individual without an indwelling urinary catheter should not be made in the absence of localizing genitourinary symptoms. Foul-smelling or cloudy urine is not, by itself, an indication for antimicrobial treatment.

Antimicrobial regimens for therapy are similar to those in younger populations, including duration of treatment. The dosage should be adjusted for kidney function but not for age. Cure rates with any duration of therapy are lower for older women. Posttreatment urine cultures to document microbiologic cure are not recommended unless symptoms persist or recur. Some women with frequent, recurrent, symptomatic infection may have fewer infections with use of topical intravaginal estradiol, although this is less effective for prevention than prophylactic antimicrobials. Systemic estrogen therapy has been associated with an increased risk for infection.

URINARY INFECTION IN PATIENTS WITH IMPAIRED KIDNEY FUNCTION

Treatment of urinary infection requires adequate concentrations of effective antimicrobials in the kidneys or urine. There is decreased excretion of antimicrobials into the urine when kidney function is impaired, so therapeutic urinary antimicrobial levels may not be achieved. With severe kidney impairment, it is often difficult to cure urinary infection. When kidney function is impaired, antimicrobials such as nitrofurantoin and tetracyclines other than doxycycline may have increased toxicity and should be avoided. Aminoglycosides may not diffuse into nonfunctioning kidneys sufficiently to provide effective therapy. The penicillins and cephalosporins, as well as fluoroquinolones, are effective treatment for most individuals with mild or moderately impaired kidney function. Obviously, dosage adjustments appropriate for the level of kidney function are necessary. In some situations, such as infected native kidneys in transplant recipients, infection cannot be eradicated and long-term suppressive therapy may be necessary to manage frequent symptomatic recurrences.

If impaired kidney function is unilateral, the functioning kidney preferentially excretes the antimicrobial into the urine. High urinary antimicrobial levels sterilize bladder urine, but antimicrobial levels in the nonfunctioning kidney may not be therapeutic. If there is infection in the impaired kidney, relapse of infection from this source can occur once antimicrobial therapy is discontinued.

URINARY INFECTION IN PATIENTS WITH CYSTIC KIDNEY DISEASE

Patients with polycystic kidney disease may develop infection of one or more cysts. The management of these infections frequently presents diagnostic and therapeutic challenges. Symptoms usually include abdominal pain or tenderness, and bacteremia is frequent. Recurrent bacteremia is a common presentation if initial antimicrobial therapy does not cure the infection. The infected cyst should be identified and, wherever possible, cyst contents aspirated for culture. A wide variety of organisms, including yeast species, may cause infection, so optimal treatment requires knowledge of the infecting organism and susceptibilities. Magnetic resonance imaging, white cell labeled scans, or positron emission tomography (PET)/CT may be useful imaging techniques to identify

infected cysts. Treatment includes prolonged antimicrobial therapy with an agent effective against the infecting organism and with good penetration into the cyst. Potential agents that achieve therapeutic cyst levels include TMP/SMX and fluoroquinolones. At least 4 weeks of antimicrobial therapy is recommended, although clinical trials to define optimal therapy are not available. Surgery may be necessary for selected cases in which antimicrobial therapy, with or without drainage, does not lead to cure.

OTHER PRESENTATIONS OF URINARY INFECTION

FUNGAL URINARY INFECTION

Fungal urinary infection has been increasing in frequency. It is primarily a health care–acquired infection that occurs in the setting of diabetes, indwelling urethral catheters, and intense broad-spectrum antimicrobial therapy. *Candida albicans* is most frequently isolated, but other *Candida* species such as *C. glabrata, C. krusei, C. parapsilosis,* and *C. tropicalis* also occur. The clinical significance of a positive urine culture is often difficult to assess, because most of these patients have complex medical or surgical problems. When there are no genitourinary symptoms or evidence of invasive fungal infection, treatment of funguria is not beneficial and should be avoided. If an indwelling urethral catheter is present, it should be discontinued when possible. Fungus balls may develop, leading to obstruction, and should be excluded in individuals with obstruction and persistent candiduria or candidemia. If present, they must be surgically removed.

When symptoms are referable to the genitourinary tract and repeated cultures have grown yeast organisms at $\geq 10^4$ cfu/mL without other potential pathogens, treatment of funguria is indicated. Fluconazole 100 to 400 mg/day for 7 to 14 days is recommended because it is excreted in the urine and may be given as oral therapy. 5-Fluorocytosine (50 to 150 mg/kg/day for 7 days) and amphotericin B are also effective. The echinocandins (caspofungin, micafungin, anidulafungin) and other azoles (voriconazole, posaconazole) are not excreted in the urine and not recommended for therapy. *Candida* species resistant to fluconazole, such as *C. krusei* or *C. glabrata,* require treatment with amphotericin B. Amphotericin B bladder irrigation (50 mg/L continuous for 5 days) is no longer considered first-line therapy, because it requires urethral catheterization and is no more effective than other therapeutic options. In selected situations, particularly in subjects with chronic kidney disease and bladder infection, the washout method may still be useful. The cure rate with any treatment is only about 70%, but assessment of outcome is often limited by serious comorbidities.

XANTHOGRANULOMATOUS PYELONEPHRITIS

Xanthogranulomatous pyelonephritis is an uncommon subacute or chronic suppurative process of the kidney characterized by destruction of the kidney parenchyma and replacement by granulomatous tissue containing histiocytes and foamy cells. Perinephric tissues may also be involved. The etiology remains unknown, but potential contributing factors include chronic urinary tract infection, abnormal lipid metabolism, lymphatic obstruction, impaired leukocyte function, and vascular occlusion. Infection is usually present. *P. mirabilis* and *E. coli* are the most frequent organisms; *Klebsiella/Enterobacter* species, *P. aeruginosa*, and *Staphylococcus aureus* are less common. The usual clinical presentation is with subacute or chronic fever, flank or abdominal pain, weight loss, lower urinary tract symptoms, and gross hematuria. Kidney calculi are invariably present, and a history of recurrent urinary tract infections and previous urologic procedures is common. The diagnosis is usually made with a CT scan. The characteristic imaging findings are an enlarged kidney with replacement of kidney parenchyma and multiple fluid-filled cavities. Urolithiasis is also often seen. Management is nephrectomy, while antimicrobial therapy has only a secondary role. If the diagnosis is made early when only focal kidney involvement is present, partial nephrectomy may be curative.

MALAKOPLAKIA

Malakoplakia is a rare chronic granulomatous inflammatory disorder of the bladder and, occasionally, the ureter or kidneys. It occurs primarily in immunocompromised or debilitated adults but has been described in normal adults and children. Chronic infection is uniformly present, with *E. coli* isolated from 85% to 90% of cases. The pathophysiology is not fully understood, but defective macrophage lysosomal digestion of phagocytosed bacteria, particularly coliforms, is thought to play a role. The clinical presentation is variable, with chronic or subacute fever, urinary symptoms, and abdominal or pelvic pain the most frequent symptoms. Anemia and leukocytosis are common. The characteristic radiologic feature of bladder involvement is of one or more mucosal-based sessile nodular lesions less than 1 cm in diameter. Rarely, the disease presents as a kidney mass and obstruction, leading to kidney failure. Definitive diagnosis requires identification of the characteristic histopathologic findings of large histiocytes with an eosinophilic granular cytoplasm admixed with intracytoplasmic or extracellular spherical Michaelis-Gutmann bodies, which are pathognomonic for the disease. Treatment is prolonged antimicrobial therapy (8 to 12 weeks), with surgical intervention when necessary to relieve obstruction. Both TMP/SMX and fluoroquinolones have been effective. Anticholinergics and ascorbic acid are also sometimes given because they may increase cellular cyclic guanosine monophosphate (cyclic-GMP), restoring the defect in phagocytic function.

KEY BIBLIOGRAPHY

Bent S, Nallamothu BK, Simel DL. Does this woman have an acute uncomplicated urinary tract infection? *JAMA.* 2002;287:2701-2710.

Cardenas DD, Hooton TM. Urinary tract infection in persons with spinal cord injury. *Arch Phys Med Rehab.* 1995;76:272-280.

Fihn SD. Acute uncomplicated urinary tract infection in women. *N Engl J Med.* 2003;349:259-266.

Gagyor I, Bleidorn J, Kochen MM. Ibuprofen versus fosfomycin for uncomplicated urinary tract infection in women: randomized controlled trial. *BMJ.* 2015;351:h6544.

Geerlings SE, Beerepoot MAJ, Prins JM. Prevention of recurrent urinary tract infections in women: antimicrobial and nonantimicrobial strategies. *Infect Dis Clin North Am.* 2014;28:135-148.

Gould CV, Umscheid CA, Agarwal RK. Guideline for prevention of catheter-associated urinary tract infection 2009. *Infect Control Hosp Epidemiol.* 2010;31:319-326.

Gupta K, Hooton TM, Naber KG, et al. International clinical practice guidelines for acute uncomplicated cystitis and pyelonephritis in women: a 2010 update by the IDSA and ESCMID Guidelines Committee. *Clin Infect Dis.* 2011;52:e103-e120.

Hooton TM. The current management strategies for community-acquired urinary tract infection. *Infect Dis Clin North Am.* 2003;17:303-332.

Hooton TM, Bradley SF, Cardenas DD, et al. 2009 International clinical practice guideline for the diagnosis, prevention and treatment of catheter-associated urinary tract infection in adults. *Clin Infect Dis.* 2010;50:625-663.

Huttner A, Verhaegh EM, Harbath S, et al. Nitrofurantoin revisited: a systematic review and meta-analysis of controlled trials. *J Antimicrob Chemother.* 2015;70:2456-2464.

Johansen TE. The role of imaging in urinary tract infections. *World J Urol.* 2004;22:392-398.

Lipsky BA, Byren I, Hooey CT. Treatment of bacterial prostatitis. *Clin Infect Dis.* 2010;50:1641-1652.

Loffroy R, Guiu B, Watfa J, et al. Xanthogranulomatous pyelonephritis in adults: clinical and radiologic findings in diffuse and focal forms. *Clin Radiol.* 2007;62:884-890.

Mody L. Juthani-Mehta M. Urinary tract infection in older women: a clinical review. *JAMA.* 2014;311:844-854.

Montini G, Tullus K, Hewitt I. Febrile urinary tract infections in children. *N Engl J Med.* 2011;365:239-250.

Nicolle LE. Uncomplicated urinary tract infection in adults including uncomplicated pyelonephritis. *Uro Clin North Am.* 2008;35:1-12.

Nicolle LE. Urinary tract infections in special populations: diabetes, renal transplant, HIV infection, and spinal cord injury. *Infect Dis Clinics North Am.* 2014;28:91-104.

Nicolle LE, Bradley S, Colgan R, et al. IDSA guidelines for the diagnosis and treatment of asymptomatic bacteriuria in adults. *Clin Infect Dis.* 2005;40:643-654.

Rowe TA, Juthani-Mehta M. Diagnosis and management of urinary tract infection in older adults. *Infect Dis Clin N Am.* 2014;28:75-89.

Saint S, Greene MT, Krein SL, et al. A program to prevent catheter-associated urinary tract infection in acute care. *N Eng J Med.* 2016; 374:2111-2119.

Full bibliography can be found on www.expertconsult.com.

SPECIAL CIRCUMSTANCES

48

Kidney Diseases in Infants and Children

Darcy K. Weidemann; Bradley A. Warady

KIDNEY DEVELOPMENT AND MATURATION

Nephrogenesis begins in utero at approximately 5 to 6 weeks' gestation and continues until nephron formation is complete at approximately 36 weeks' gestation. Fetal urine production commences before the end of the first trimester and by the third trimester becomes the primary component of the amniotic fluid, which is essential for normal pulmonary development. Although the full-term newborn has the same number of nephrons as an adult, the glomeruli and tubules of the infant kidney are relatively immature. The neonatal tubule has a limited ability to concentrate or dilute the urine in response to different environmental or dietary conditions. Furthermore, the ability of the neonatal proximal tubule to reabsorb filtered HCO_3^- is less than that of adults. As a result, the average serum HCO_3^- concentration in preterm infants (16 to 20 mEq/L) is lower than in term infants (19 to 21 mEq/L), and older children and adults (24 to 28 mEq/L). Newborns also often have higher serum potassium concentrations (6.5 to 7.0 mEq/L) than older children as a result of a decreased glomerular filtration rate (GFR) and a relative insensitivity of the neonatal tubule to aldosterone.

The GFR of the newborn kidney is only around 20 mL/min per $1.73 m^2$ in the first few days after birth, rising to approximately 40 mL/min per $1.73 m^2$ near the end of the first week of life, and gradually reaching adult levels of 100 to 130 mL/min per $1.73 m^2$ by 2 years of age. The changes in GFR that occur after birth are the result of increased cardiac output and mean arterial blood pressure, a decrease in renal vascular resistance, and an increased surface area available for glomerular filtration. Concomitantly, blood flow is redistributed from the cortical-juxtamedullary glomeruli, which are larger but fewer in number than the more numerous glomeruli in the cortex.

In term neonates, the low GFR results in a serum creatinine (sCr) level that remains similar to the mother's for the first 24 to 48 hours of life and gradually settles to approximately 0.4 mg/dL at the fifth to seventh day of life. In preterm infants born at 28 to 30 weeks' gestation, the GFR is only approximately 12 to 13 mL/min per $1.73 m^2$ within the first few days after birth, and the sCr may take longer to normalize. The full-term newborn kidney measures 4 to 5 cm in length and continues to grow until reaching 10 to 12 cm by adolescence. Although the glomeruli do grow in size, most of this renal parenchymal expansion results from tubular growth and maturation and from an increased volume of the tubulointerstitial compartment.

ACUTE KIDNEY INJURY

Acute kidney injury (AKI) is defined as a sudden decrease in kidney function that compromises the normal regulation of fluid, electrolyte, and acid-base homeostasis. The term AKI has largely replaced the term acute renal failure (ARF). The reference to AKI emphasizes the continuum of kidney dysfunction without overt organ failure, which is clinically relevant and linked to morbidity and mortality. In practical terms, AKI is characterized by a reduction of the GFR, which results in an abrupt increase in the concentrations of sCr and blood urea nitrogen (BUN) and/or a sustained reduction in urine output. Despite its widespread use, sCr is a poor marker of kidney function in the setting of AKI, and it best correlates with GFR in steady state. In fact, patients with acute, severe AKI may still show a normal or only mildly elevated sCr concentration due to insufficient time for creatinine accumulation to occur in the serum and relatively low creatinine generation. An emerging area of research is the study of novel biomarkers useful in the prediction of AKI. Biomarkers under investigation include urinary neutrophil gelatinase-associated lipocalin (NGAL), urinary cystatin C, urinary kidney injury molecule (KIM)-1, urinary interleukin (IL)-18, and urinary liver-type fatty acid binding protein (L-FABP), although their use has not yet become part of routine clinical practice.

No current single consensus definition of pediatric AKI exists, which has resulted in substantial variability in the reported incidence, morbidity, and mortality estimates. The three most widespread definitions are the Risk Injury, Failure, Loss and End-stage (RIFLE); AKI network (AKIN); and Kidney Disease: Improving Global Outcomes (KDIGO) classifications (Table 48.1). The RIFLE criteria were developed by an international consensus panel in 2004 and were intended for use in critically ill adults. RIFLE classifies AKI into five distinct categories based upon the magnitude and direction of change in creatinine, urine output, and duration of renal replacement therapy (RRT): (R) Risk, (I) Injury, (F) Failure, (L) Loss of kidney function, and (E) End-stage renal disease. This classification system was subsequently modified for the pediatric population (pRIFLE) by the use of an estimated creatinine clearance based on the original Schwartz formula to quantify the change in GFR (rather than absolute changes in sCr used in the adult version). In addition, all children with an estimated creatinine clearance less than 35 mL/min per $1.73 m^2$ are placed in the "pRIFLE-F" category (kidney failure class) instead of waiting for the sCr

Table 48.1 **Acute Kidney Injury Definitions in Children**

pRIFLE		AKIN		KDIGO	
Stage	**Criteria**	**Stage**	**Criteria**	**Stage**	**Criteria**
Risk (R)	eCrCl ↓ 25% UOP <0.5 mL/kg/h × 8 h	1	↑ SCr ≥0.3 mg/dL or ↑ SCr ≥1.5–2×[a] UOP <0.5 mL/kg/h × 6 h	1	↑ SCr ≥0.3 mg/dL or ↑ SCr ≥1.5–2×[b] UOP <0.5 mL/kg/h × 8 h
Injury (I)	eCrCl ↓ 50% UOP <0.5 mL/kg/h × 16 h	2	↑ SCr ≥2–3× UOP <0.5 mL/kg/h × 12 h	2	↑ SCr ≥2–3× UOP <0.5 mL/kg/h × 16 h
Failure (F)	eCrCl ↓ 75% or CrCl <35 mL/min/1.73 m² UOP <0.5 mL/kg/h × 24 h or anuria for 12 h	3	↑ SCr ≥3–4× or SCr >4 (within 0.5 in 48 h) or RRT initiated UOP <0.5 mL/kg/h × 24 h or anuria × 12 h	3	↑ SCr ≥3–4× or SCr >4 (and meets criteria for AKI) or RRT initiated or eGFR <35 in patients <18 yo UOP <0.5 mL/kg/h × 24 h or anuria × 12 h
Loss (L)	Failure >4 weeks	N/A		N/A	
End-stage kidney disease (E)	Failure >3 months	N/A		N/A	

[a]Within 48 h.
[b]Within 7 days.
AKI, Acute kidney injury; *AKIN*, AKI network; *CrCl*, creatinine clearance; *KDIGO*, Kidney Disease: Improving Global Outcomes; *RRT*, renal replacement therapy; *SCr*, serum creatinine; *UOP*, urine output.
Adapted from Akcan-Arikan A, Zappitelli M, Loftis LL, et al. Modified RIFLE criteria in critically ill children with acute kidney injury. *Kidney Int.* 2007;71:1028–1035; Mehta R, Kellum J, Shah S, et al: Acute Kidney Injury Network: report of an initiative to improve outcomes in acute kidney injury. *Crit Care.* 2007;22:R31; and Kidney Disease: Improving Global Outcomes (KDIGO) Acute Kidney Injury Work Group. KDIGO clinical practice guideline for acute kidney injury. *Kidney Int Suppl.* 2012;2:1–138.

concentration to reach 4 mg/dL as proposed by the adult criteria.

The AKIN criteria are based on changes in sCr; AKIN stage 1 describes patients who experience a ≥0.3-mg/dL (26.4-µM) increase in sCr over a 48-hour period. Although AKIN was not adjusted for children, it has been used in research in pediatric AKI, as has the most recent 2012 KDIGO definition, which uses a more flexible timeline than AKIN and has a specific modification for children (see Table 48.1). The KDIGO definition and staging criteria include a 0.3-mg/dL increase in sCr over 48 hours, or a urine volume ≤0.5 mg/kg per hour for 6 hours. The diagnostic inclusion criteria for an sCr elevation ≥1.5 times baseline within the prior 7 days allows for the inclusion of patients with late-onset AKI.

Urine volume in AKI is variable: patients may be anuric, oliguric, and in some cases (particularly in neonates) polyuric. AKI develops over a period of hours to days, whereas chronic kidney disease (CKD) develops over months to years. Short stature, renal osteodystrophy, delayed puberty, normocytic anemia, and hyperparathyroidism all suggest long-standing and advanced CKD rather than AKI. However, at a single point in time of an acute clinical presentation, it may be difficult to differentiate AKI from CKD without imaging studies, extensive laboratory testing for the aforementioned complications, and possibly a kidney biopsy.

Kidney function becomes impaired when adequate blood supply and oxygenation, parenchymal integrity, and/or patency of the urinary collecting system are interrupted. Consequently, AKI can be viewed as caused by prerenal, intrinsic kidney, or postrenal factors, although substantial overlap and multifactorial etiologies can exist, particularly in hospitalized children. The likelihood of recovery from AKI depends in part on the presence or absence of urine output, the quantity of urine output, the duration of anuria, and the underlying cause and severity of kidney injury. Quantifying the urine output is essential, as this predicts the clinical course and may aid in identifying the underlying insult. Oliguria is defined as a urine output less than 1 mL/kg per hour in infants and young children and less than 0.5 mL/kg per hour in older children. Patients with nonoliguric AKI have lower complication rates and higher survival rates than those with anuric or oliguric AKI. Causes of nonoliguric AKI include acute interstitial nephritis (AIN) or nephrotoxic kidney insults, including aminoglycoside nephrotoxicity. In contrast, AKI in children with kidney hypoperfusion injury, acute glomerulonephritis, or hemolytic uremic syndrome (HUS) is usually associated with oligoanuria. In infants, oliguric AKI normally occurs as a result of either renovascular accidents (renal artery or vein thrombosis) or ischemic acute tubular necrosis (ATN) from shock.

Prerenal AKI results from kidney hypoperfusion caused by intravascular volume contraction, decreased effective circulating blood volume, or altered intrarenal hemodynamics. Intravascular volume contraction can be seen with volume depletion, acute blood loss, or extravascular accumulation of fluid (so-called third spacing of fluid), the latter most often in patients with the systemic inflammatory response syndrome (SIRS) or hypoalbuminemia. Decreased effective blood circulation occurs when the true blood volume is normal or increased, but renal perfusion is decreased, such as in left-sided heart failure, cardiac tamponade, or hepatorenal syndrome. Intrarenal afferent arteriolar vasoconstriction develops in hepatorenal syndrome, calcineurin inhibitor toxicity, and nonsteroidal antiinflammatory drug (NSAID) use; intrarenal efferent arteriolar vasodilation occurs with the use of angiotensin-converting enzyme (ACE) inhibitors and angiotensin receptor blockers. Kidney dysfunction in prerenal AKI is reversible by restoration of kidney perfusion, although severe and/or prolonged kidney hypoperfusion often leads to tubular injury and intrinsic AKI.

Intrinsic kidney injury or pathology may occur at the level of the kidney vasculature, tubules, interstitium, or glomeruli. The basic mechanisms of such injuries include hypoperfusion and ischemic cell damage, toxin-mediated cell injury, and inflammation. Vascular injury may occur in large vessels (e.g., renal artery or vein thrombosis) or in the microvasculature (e.g., HUS or thrombotic thrombocytopenic purpura, TTP). Direct tubular injury, also known as ATN, is the end result of either ischemic or toxin-mediated damage to the tubules. Ischemia-induced ATN is the result of prolonged or severe kidney hypoperfusion. Toxin-mediated intrinsic ATN may be secondary to medications (aminoglycosides, amphotericin, acyclovir, cisplatin, iodinated radiocontrast agents), endogenous toxins (e.g., heme pigments from myoglobin and hemoglobin from rhabdomyolysis or hemolysis), and exogenous toxins (e.g., mercury, crystal formation from ethylene glycol, and methanol poisoning).

Inflammatory injury in the form of AIN as a cause of intrinsic AKI most often occurs in the setting of medication exposures. Medications commonly associated with interstitial nephritis include extended-spectrum penicillins, NSAIDs, sulfonamides, and rifampin. AIN is also associated with infections, systemic diseases, tumor infiltrates, or genetic conditions. Acute glomerulonephritis is more common in school-age children but is rare before 2 years of age. Postinfectious glomerulonephritis is the most common cause of acute glomerulonephritis and AKI in childhood; however, many other conditions produce a glomerulonephritic injury as well, including antiglomerular basement membrane (anti-GBM) antibody disease, antineutrophil cytoplasmic antibody (ANCA) disease, lupus nephritis, IgA nephropathy, Henoch-Schönlein purpura (HSP) nephritis, and membranoproliferative glomerulonephritis (MPGN).

Despite the fact that congenital obstructive uropathies are among the most frequent causes of CKD in children, AKI itself is rarely the result of postrenal obstruction, except when this occurs in a solitary kidney either from aplasia, nephrectomy, or transplantation. More commonly in children with two functioning kidneys, postrenal AKI occurs in the setting of complete urethral or bladder neck obstruction, or in the unusual circumstance of bilateral ureteric obstruction. A variety of conditions can cause such unilateral or bilateral obstruction and subsequently lead to AKI, including calculi, ureteral blood clots, retroperitoneal fibrosis, neurogenic bladder, bladder or pelvic tumors, and urethral stricture.

General measures to prevent AKI include restoration of intravascular volume, avoidance of hypotension and renal ischemia by providing inotropic support in critically ill children following volume repletion, and careful readjustment of nephrotoxic medications based on close monitoring of drug levels and kidney function. Whereas several pharmacologic agents including mannitol, loop diuretics, low-dose dopamine, fenoldopam, and N-acetylcysteine have been studied in children with AKI (with no convincing evidence of benefit), none are routinely recommended to prevent AKI or its progression.

Management of AKI includes relief of obstruction if present, judicious fluid administration to maintain euvolemia, treatment of electrolyte abnormalities including hyperkalemia, metabolic acidosis, hypocalcemia, hyperphosphatemia, and blood pressure management. Loop diuretics are often used to induce diuresis in the setting of volume overload or for the treatment of hyperkalemia, but they have not been shown to prevent AKI or to substantially alter the natural history of AKI other than enhancing urine output in the nephrons that remain functional. Restriction of sodium, potassium, and phosphate intake may be indicated, as may the use of potassium-binding agents to treat for hyperkalemia and oral phosphate binders for the management of hyperphosphatemia. Metabolic acidosis should be corrected carefully; the exchange of protein-bound hydrogen ions with calcium can result in a decrease of the available ionized calcium and result in tetany. Frequent dose adjustment or elimination of potentially nephrotoxic medications is necessary when the GFR is significantly compromised, and a multidisciplinary approach among intensivists, nephrologists, and specialized pharmacists may be helpful. Polyuria and tubular dysfunction (hypokalemia, hypophosphatemia, hypomagnesemia) can be noted in the recovery phase of AKI due to a lag in the tubular reabsorptive capacity, and careful management of fluids and electrolytes during the diuretic phase is essential.

Kidney replacement therapy (KRT) is indicated when conservative measures fail. Frequent indications include fluid overload (10% to 20% excess), hyperkalemia or severe acidosis unresponsive to pharmacologic therapy, uremia (typically marked by a BUN >100 mg/dL [30 mM] or symptoms), or an inability to provide adequate nutrition. Volume overload is increasingly recognized as a predictor of unfavorable outcomes, with an overall trend in many centers toward earlier initiation of KRT. Modalities used in AKI include peritoneal dialysis (PD), hemodialysis (HD), and continuous renal replacement therapy (CRRT); the choice is dictated largely by the patient's clinical status, as well as by the availability of equipment and the center expertise. Peritoneal dialysis is advantageous in neonates and younger children and in resource-limited countries, with no requirements for systemic/regional anticoagulation, vascular access, or specialized equipment or personnel. Hemodialysis offers the advantage of being able to rapidly correct fluid or electrolyte imbalances but does require patients to tolerate a large extracorporeal volume through an adequate vascular access and mandates specially trained personnel. Finally, where equipment and trained personnel exist, CRRT may be preferred in children with multisystem organ dysfunction or hemodynamic instability; it permits gentler fluid removal rates with less dynamic fluid shifts than HD while allowing full enteral or parenteral nutrition.

CHRONIC KIDNEY DISEASE

CKD is characterized by functional or structural damage to the kidneys and/or a decrease in GFR to less than 60 mL/min per 1.73 m^2 for ≥3 months. Importantly, the GFR may be normal or near normal in the early stages of CKD (Table 48.2) when intervention is most likely to successfully prevent or slow progression and adequately treat accompanying comorbidities. Although diabetes and hypertension are the

Table 48.2 Pediatric Glomerular Filtration Rate Estimating Equations

GFR Marker	GFR Equation
SCr by alkaline picrate (Jaffe)	*Schwartz equation*[a] eGFR (mL/min/1.73 m^2) = k × Ht (cm)/Scr *Counahan-Barratt equation*[b] eGFR (mL/min/1.73 m^2) = 0.43 × Ht (cm)/Scr
SCr by IDMS traceable enzymatic methods	*CKiD bedside equation*[c] eGFR (mL/min/1.73 m^2) = 0.413 × Ht (cm)/Scr
CysC	*CKiD cystC equation*[d] eGFR (mL/min/1.73 m^2) = 70.69 (CystC)$^{-0.931}$ *Zappitelli et al. cystC equation*[e] eGFR (mL/min/1.73 m^2) = 75.94 (CystC)$^{-1.170}$ *Filler and Lepage cystC equation*[f] eGFR (mL/min/1.73 m^2) = 91.62 (CystC)$^{-1.129}$
SCr + CysC	*CKiD multivariable equation*[g] eGFR (mL/min/1.73 m^2) = 39.8 × Ht (m)/Scr)$^{0.456}$ (1.8/CystC)$^{0.418}$ (30/BUN)$^{0.079}$ (1.076)^{male} (Ht(m)/1.4)$^{0.179}$ *Zappitelli et al. equation*[h] eGFR (mL/min/1.73 m^2) = 43.82 (1/CystC)$^{0.635}$ (1/Scr)$^{0.547}$ (1.35^{height}) *Bouvet et al. equation*[i] eGFR (mL/min/1.73 m^2) = 63.2 (1.2/CystC)[(96/88.4)/(Scr)]$^{0.35}$ (weight/45)$^{0.30}$ (age/14)$^{0.40}$

Comments

[a]k is a constant, directly proportional to the muscle component of body, and varies with age. The value for k is 0.33 in premature infants through the first year of life, 0.45 for term infants through the first year of life, 0.55 in children and adolescent girls, and 0.7 in adolescent boys. Formula developed against measured inulin GFR [PMID 951142] (Schwartz et al., 1976)

[b]Jaffe reaction after adsorption onto ion exchange to remove noncreatinine chromogens. Recommendations for subtracting 0.14 mg/dL for automated Jaffe creatinine. Formula developed against measured Cr-EDTA GFR [PMID: 1008594] (Counahan et al., 1976)

[c]Formula developed against measured iohexol GFR [PMID: 19158356] (Schwartz et al., 2009)

[d]CystC by PENIA. Formula developed against single injection iohexol [PMID: 22622496] (Schwartz et al., 2012)

[e]Formula developed against cold iothalamate [PMID: 16860187] (Zappitelli et al., 2006)

[f]CystC by PENIA. Formula developed against single injection Tc-DTPA [PMID:12920638] (Filler and Lepage, 2003)

[g]Serum creatinine by IDMS traceable enzymatic method. CystC by PENIA. Formula developed against single injection iohexol [PMID: 22622496] (Schwartz et al., 2012)

[h]Serum creatinine by enzymatic creatinine. CystC by PENIA. Formula developed against nonradioactive iothalamate steady-state method [PMID: 16860187] (Zappitelli et al., 2006)

[i]Serum creatinine by noncompensated Jaffe method. CystC by PENIA. Formula developed against single injection ^{51}Cr-EDTA [PMID: 16794818] (Bouvet et al., 2006)

CKiD, Chronic kidney disease in children; *CystC*, serum cystatin C; *eGFR*, estimated glomerular filtration rate; *GFR*, glomerular filtration rate; *SCr*, serum creatinine.
Adapted from VanDeVoorde RG, Wong CS, Warady BA. Management of chronic kidney disease in children. In: Avner, ED, Harmon WE, Niadet N, Yoshikawa N, Emma F, Goldstein S. *Pediatric Nephrology*. 7th ed. Berlin: Springer; 2016:2211.

disorders that account for the vast majority of CKD cases in adult patients, approximately two thirds of childhood CKD is attributed to congenital anomalies of the kidney and urinary tract (CAKUT), including renal hypoplasia/dysplasia and obstructive uropathy (e.g., posterior urethral valves). Other common causes include focal segmental glomerulosclerosis (FSGS), chronic glomerulonephritis (lupus nephritis, IgA nephropathy, HSP, or MPGN), ciliopathies (autosomal recessive polycystic kidney disease, nephronophthisis), and HUS. Renovascular accidents, Alport syndrome, congenital nephrotic syndrome, primary hyperoxaluria, and cystinosis all remain rare but important causes of CKD in childhood.

The determination of GFR is integral to the diagnosis of CKD. The original Schwartz formula to estimate GFR in children was developed in the mid-1970s using sCr, height, and an empiric constant for age/gender. However, the sCr assay has changed from the Jaffe chromogen reaction, the assay used for the original formula, to the enzymatic method now used in most centers, requiring a refinement of pediatric GFR estimating formulas. The Schwartz estimating equation was, in turn, updated in 2009 based on results from the prospective, observational multicenter Chronic Kidney Disease in Children (CKiD) study, in which GFR was measured through the plasma disappearance of iohexol. The estimating formula is as follows:

$$eGFR = 39.1 \times [height/SCr]^{0.516} \times [1.8/cystatin\ C]^{0.294} \times [30/BUN]^{0.169} \times [1.099]^{Male} \times height/1.4]^{0.188}$$

Importantly, a simplified estimating equation was derived—the so-called bedside CKiD equation—which includes an updated constant of 0.413 (36.5 for SI units):

$$eGFR = 0.413 \times height\ (cm)/serum\ creatinine\ (in\ mg/dL)$$

Whereas this equation is used most frequently in clinical care, a variety of other equations have been published (see Table 48.2).

Accurate estimates of GFR are necessary to appropriately stage CKD. In 2002, the National Kidney Foundation's Kidney Disease Outcomes Quality Initiative (NKF-KDOQI) published a CKD classification system based on GFR that was applicable

Table 48.3 Stage of Chronic Kidney Disease

	GFR (mL/min/1.73 m²)	
Stage	KDOQI Definition	KDIGO Definition
1. Normal GFR	≥90	≥90
2. Mild CKD	60–89	60–89
3. Moderate CKD	30–59	3a: 45–59
		3b: 30–45
4. Severe CKD	15–29	15–29
5. End-stage kidney failure	<15 (or dialysis)	<15 (or dialysis)

CKD, Chronic kidney disease; *GFR,* glomerular filtration rate; *KDOQI,* Kidney Disease Outcomes Quality Initiative; *KDIGO,* Kidney Disease: Improving Global Outcomes.
Adapted from Kidney Disease Outcomes Quality Initiative (KDOQI): KDOQI clinical practice guidelines for chronic kidney disease: evaluation, classification, and stratification. Executive summaries of 2000 updates. http://www.kidney.org/professionals/KDOQI/guidelines_ckd/toc.htm and KDIGO 2012 clinical practice guideline for the evaluation and management of chronic kidney disease. *Kidney Int Suppl.* 2013;3:1.

to children and adults (Table 48.3). The KDIGO 2012 clinical practice guideline revised the 2002 KDOQI classification by defining pediatric CKD in children greater than 2 years old as GFR <60 mL/min per 1.73 m² for more than 3 months or GFR >60 mL/min per 1.73 m² that is accompanied by evidence of structural damage or other markers of functional kidney abnormalities including proteinuria, albuminuria, renal tubular disorders, or pathologic abnormalities as detected by imaging or histopathology (see Table 48.3). The 2012 KDIGO definition further subdivided stage 3 CKD into stages 3a and 3b, although current CKD staging does not stratify according to albuminuria, in contrast to criteria for adults.

Several clinical or radiologic elements in the medical history may indicate the presence of early CKD, including abnormal antenatal ultrasound, oligohydramnios or polyhydramnios, polydipsia, polyuria, nocturia, and salt craving. However, many children are often asymptomatic or have vague, nonspecific complaints, including fatigue, headaches, or gastrointestinal symptoms. Failure to thrive, short stature, delayed puberty, pallor, and difficulty concentrating with poor school performance may occur in more advanced (stages 3 to 5) CKD.

Several additional and treatable comorbidities are associated with CKD (Fig. 48.1). Hypertension may be present and can arise as a result of a number of factors including sodium

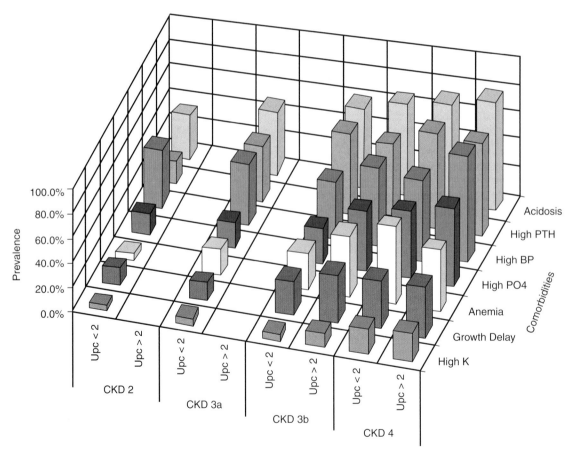

Fig. 48.1 CKD comorbidities by stage and urine protein-to-creatinine ratio. CKD3 was divided into 3a (GFR 45 to 59 mL/min per 1.73 m²) and 3b (GFR 30 to 44 mL/min per 1.73 m²) for a more detailed analysis. *BP,* Blood pressure; *CKD,* chronic kidney disease; *GFR,* glomerular filtration rate; *K,* potassium; *PTH,* parathyroid hormone; *Upc,* urine protein-to-creatinine ratio. (Adapted from Furth SL, Abraham AG, Jerry-Fluker J, et al. Metabolic abnormalities, cardiovascular risk factors and GFR decline in children with chronic kidney disease. *Clin J Am Soc Nephrol.* 2011;6:2132–2140.)

retention and extracellular volume expansion, increased activity of the renin-angiotensin system, and enhanced activity of the sympathetic nervous system. Metabolic derangements are common and include hyperkalemia, hyperphosphatemia, hypocalcemia, and metabolic acidosis. Chronic kidney disease-mineral and bone disorder (CKD-MBD, previously known as renal osteodystrophy) usually becomes evident in CKD stage 2 to 3 as a result of reduced urinary phosphate excretion; elevated serum phosphorous, parathyroid hormone (PTH), and fibroblast growth factor 23 (FGF23) levels; hypocalcemia; and reduced circulating levels of activated vitamin D (1,25-dihydroxyvitamin D). Anemia typically develops in CKD stage 3 (GFR 30 to 59 mL/min per 1.73 m^2) as a result of reduced erythropoietin production along with possible mild iron deficiency.

The overall aims of treatment for CKD are fivefold: (1) treat the underlying condition whenever possible, (2) prevent the progression of the disease, (3) treat the complications of CKD, (4) optimize conditions for normal growth and development, and (5) avoid further nephrotoxic insults. Hypertension and proteinuria are two modifiable risk factors independently associated with a more rapid progression of CKD. The ESCAPE trial, published in 2009, demonstrated that achieving the 50th percentile for mean arterial blood pressure using an intensified antihypertensive blood pressure regimen including an ACE inhibitor significantly delays CKD progression. In addition, ACE inhibitors reduced protein excretion by approximately 50% within the first 6 months of treatment initiation in children with CKD. Therefore, ACE inhibitors (or angiotensin receptor blockers [ARB]) are considered first-line therapy for hypertension or proteinuria in children with CKD, although hyperkalemia may be dose limiting in very advanced CKD.

The anemia of CKD is treated with iron supplementation and erythropoiesis-stimulating agents. CKD-MBD is primarily treated by restricting dietary phosphate intake, providing enteric phosphate binders, ensuring adequate nutritional 25-OH vitamin D stores, and administering calcitriol (synthetic 1,25-dihydroxyvitamin D). These interventions suppress PTH secretion. Recombinant growth hormone therapy may be indicated for short stature after the provider ensures the child is receiving adequate calories and the secondary hyperparathyroidism and acidosis of CKD are adequately treated. Lifestyle choices that can hasten progression of CKD, including smoking, elevated body mass index, and frequent NSAID use, should all be avoided. Children should target at least their required daily allowance of protein and calories to promote appropriate growth.

HYPERTENSION

Hypertension in children older than 1 year is defined in the 2004 *Fourth Report on the Diagnosis, Evaluation, and Treatment of High Blood Pressure in Children* as a sustained systolic or diastolic blood pressure ≥95th percentile for age, gender, and height on three or more occasions. Prehypertension is defined as a systolic or diastolic blood pressure ≥90th percentile but <95th percentile or a blood pressure exceeding 128/80 mm Hg (even if <90th percentile for age, gender, and height). Hypertension can be further staged according to severity. Stage 1 hypertension is defined as an average

blood pressure level from the 95th percentile to 5 mm Hg above the 99th percentile. Stage 2 hypertension is defined as an average blood pressure that exceeds 5 mm Hg above the 99th percentile.

Blood pressure is usually measured either through auscultation or an oscillometric device. Auscultative blood pressure assessment is considered the gold standard, and it has been used for the generation of all pediatric normative data. Oscillometric devices calculate blood pressure by proprietary unpublished formulas and are known to overestimate blood pressure in children by as much as 5 to 10 mm Hg. Although the use of oscillometric blood pressure assessment has become widespread, caution should be used when diagnosing hypertension with an automated device in children, and elevated readings should be confirmed by manual auscultation.

Ambulatory blood pressure monitoring (ABPM) is a useful diagnostic tool that has recently been introduced into the field of hypertension in children. Patients with an elevated blood pressure in the clinic but a normal ABPM study are currently designated as having isolated office hypertension, or white-coat hypertension. Those with normal conventional readings in clinic and an abnormal ABPM study are said to have masked hypertension. In turn, APBM offers the advantages of distinguishing white-coat from true hypertension, evaluating for the presence of masked hypertension, and of more precisely characterizing changes in blood pressure during daily activities, including while asleep and as a result of antihypertensive therapy.

Hypertension may also be classified by etiology. Essential hypertension is defined as hypertension without an otherwise identifiable cause. Although this condition used to be considered rare in children, it is now routinely encountered in clinical practice. Essential hypertension is usually characterized by prehypertension or stage 1 hypertension in adolescents, and is associated with obesity, a family history of hypertension, sedentary lifestyle, and black race. Secondary hypertension is, in contrast, elevated blood pressure in the context of an identifiable, underlying cause. Kidney parenchymal disorders, including glomerulonephritis, renal fibrosis, FSGS, renal dysplasia, and polycystic kidney disease, account for the vast majority of secondary causes of hypertension in children. Fibromuscular dysplasia and aortic coarctation are also relatively common causes. In neonates and premature infants, umbilical artery catheter-associated thromboembolism affecting the renal arteries is the most common cause of hypertension. In general, the likelihood of identifying a secondary cause of hypertension is directly related to the degree of hypertension (i.e., more common in stage 2) and is inversely related to the age of the child.

The evaluation of any child with hypertension largely depends on the likelihood of finding a secondary cause, and the extent of the evaluation should be individualized. Most younger children with hypertension, adolescents with stage 2 hypertension, and adolescents with stage 1 hypertension without obvious risk factors for essential hypertension will undergo an initial evaluation that consists of a basic metabolic panel, urinalysis, and a kidney ultrasound. An echocardiogram may also be recommended to assess left ventricular mass as a sign of end-organ damage and to exclude the possibility of a coarctation.

Treatment recommendations are based on the severity of the blood pressure elevation. For most patients with essential hypertension, a 6- to 12-month trial of nonpharmacologic interventions should be recommended. These recommendations include the DASH diet (Dietary Approaches to Stop Hypertension, a low-sodium plant-based diet with whole grains, low-fat dairy, and lean meats), moderate to vigorous exercise on most days of the week, achievement and maintenance of normal body mass index, and limited screen time. Pharmacologic therapy is indicated for treatment of hypertension that persists despite lifestyle changes, secondary hypertension, hypertension associated with end-organ damage such as left ventricular hypertrophy (left ventricular mass index greater than 95th percentile), and hypertension associated with chronic disorders such as diabetes or CKD. In part due to the Best Pharmaceuticals for Children Act, enacted by the FDA in 2002, the number of antihypertensive medications with pediatric-specific indications has increased considerably over the past decade and includes ACE inhibitors, ARBs, beta blockers, calcium channel blockers, and diuretics (Table 48.4). Blood pressure goals are less than the 95th percentile for age and height, although, if the patient has cardiovascular

Table 48.4 Antihypertensive Medications in Children

Drug	Initial Dose	Maximal Dose	Adverse Effects
ACE Inhibitors			
Enalapril[a]	0.08 mg/kg/day	0.6 mg/kg/day (max 40 mg/day)	Hyperkalemia, cough, angioedema, ACE fetopathy
Fosinopril[a]	0.1 mg/kg (5 or 10 mg)	0.6 mg/kg (max 40 mg/day)	
Lisinopril[a]	0.07 mg/kg/day (up to 5 mg/day)	0.6 mg/kg/day (max 40 mg/day)	
Benazepril[a]	0.2 mg/kg (up to 10 mg)	0.6 mg/kg (max 40 mg/day)	
Angiotensin-Receptor Blockers			
Losartan[a]	0.7 mg/kg/day (up to 50 mg/day)	1.4 mg/kg/day (max 100 mg/day)	Hyperkalemia; cough (less common than ACE inhibitors)
Valsartan[a]	<6 years: 5–10 mg/day; 6–17 years: 1.3 mg/kg/day (up to 40 mg/day)	<6 years: 80 mg/day; 6–17 years: 2.7 mg/kg/day (max 160 mg/day)	
Aldosterone Receptor Antagonist			
Eplerenone	25 mg/day	100 mg/day	Hyperkalemia, dizziness, gynecomastia
Spironolactone[a]	1 mg/kg/day	3.3 mg/kg/day (max 100 mg/day)	
Alpha- and Beta-Adrenergic Antagonist			
Carvedilol	0.1 mg/kg/dose (up to 6.25 mg/day)	0.5 mg/kg/dose (max 25 mg) twice daily	Caution with asthma, heart failure, diabetes; dizziness; depression; dry eyes, bradycardia, peripheral edema
Labetalol	1–3 mg/kg/day	1200 mg/day	
Beta Antagonists			
Atenolol	0.5–1 mg/kg/day	2 mg/kg/day (max 100 mg/day)	Caution with asthma, heart failure, diabetes; bradycardia; dizziness
Metoprolol[a]	1–2 mg/kg/day	6 mg/kg/day (max 600 mg/day)	
Propranolol[a]	0.5–1 mg/kg/day	8 mg/kg/day (max 640 mg/day)	
Centrally Acting Alpha Agonists			
Clonidine[a]	5–20 µg/kg/day OR 0.1-mg transdermal patch	25 µg/kg/day OR 0.3-mg transdermal patch	Sedation, bradycardia, dry eyes, dry mouth
Calcium-Channel Blockers			
Amlodipine[a]	0.06 mg/kg/day	0.3 mg/kg/day (max 10 mg/day)	Reflex tachycardia, peripheral edema
Isradipine	0.05–0.15 mg/kg/dose 3 or 4 times per day	0.8 mg/kg/day (max 20 mg/day)	
Nifedipine, extended release	0.25–0.5 mg/kg/day	3 mg/kg/day (max 120 mg/day)	
Diuretics			
Amiloride	0.4–0.625 mg/kg/day	20 mg/day	Hypokalemia, hypercholesterolemia, hyperglycemia
Chlorthalidone	0.3 mg/kg/day	2 mg/kg/day (max 50 mg/day)	
Furosemide	0.5–2 mg/kg/dose	6 mg/kg/day	
Hydrochlorothiazide[a]	0.5–1 mg/kg/day	3 mg/kg/day (max 50 mg/day)	
Vasodilators			
Hydralazine[a]	0.75 mg/kg/day divided q6–12h	7.5 mg/kg/day (max 200 mg/day)	Tachycardia, edema, hirsutism (minoxidil)
Minoxidil[a]	<12 years: 0.2 mg/kg/day; ≥12 years: 5 mg/day	<12 years: 50 mg/day; ≥12 years: 100 mg/day	

[a]Food and Drug Administration approved for use in children.
ACE, Angiotensin-converting enzyme.

disease risk factors (such as CKD or diabetes), the current recommendations are to target blood pressure to less than the 90th percentile for age and height. The long-term prognosis of pediatric hypertension depends on the underlying etiology. Overall, there is an increased risk for future cardiovascular morbidity and mortality that may be modifiable with early recognition and treatment.

KEY BIBLIOGRAPHY

Akcan-Arikan A, Zappitelli M, Loftis LL, et al. Modified RIFLE criteria in critically ill children with acute kidney injury. *Kidney Int.* 2007;71:1028-1035.

Andreoli SP. Acute renal failure: clinical evaluation and management. In: Avner ED, Harmon WE, Niaudet P, eds. *Pediatric Nephrology.* 5th ed. Baltimore: MD: Williams and Wilkins; 2009:1223-1266.

Ardissino G, Testa S, Dacco V, et al. Proteinuria as a predictor of disease progression in children with hypoplastic nephropathy. *Pediatr Nephrol.* 2004;19:172-177.

Arora P, Kher V, Rai PK, et al. Prognosis of acute renal failure in children: a multivariate analysis. *Pediatr Nephrol.* 1997;11:153-155.

Bellomo R, Ronco C, Kellum JA, et al. Acute renal failure—definition, outcome measures, animal models, fluid therapy and information technology needs: the Second International Consensus Conference of the Acute Dialysis Quality Initiative (ADQI) Group. *Crit Care.* 2004;8:R204-R212.

Brady HR, Linger GG. Acute renal failure. *Lancet.* 1995;346:1533-1540.

Brewer ED. Urinary acidification. In: Polin RA, Fox WW, Abman SH, eds. *Fetal and Neonatal Physiology.* 4th ed. Philadelphia: WB Saunders Philadelphia; 2011:1419-1422.

Copelovitch L, Meyers KEC, Kaplan BS. Acute renal failure. In: Domico SG, Canning DA, Khoury A, eds. *The Kilalis-King-Belman Textbook of Clinical Pediatric Urology.* 5th ed. London: Informa Health Care; 2007:7357-7366.

Copelovitch L, Warady BA, Furth SL. Insights from the Chronic Kidney Disease in Children (CKiD) Study. *Clin J Am Soc Nephrol.* 2007;6:2047-2053.

Fadrowski JJ, Pierce CB, Cole SR, et al. Hemoglobin decline in children with chronic kidney disease: baseline results from the chronic kidney disease in children prospective cohort study. *Clin J Am Soc Nephrol.* 2008;3:457-462.

Falkner B. Hypertension in children and adolescents: epidemiology and natural history. *Pediatr Nephrol.* 2010;25:1219-1224.

Flynn J, Daniels S, Hayman L, et al. Update: ambulatory blood pressure monitoring in children and adolescents: a scientific statement from the American Heart Association. *Hypertension.* 2014;63:1116-1135.

Furth SL, Abraham AG, Jerry-Fluker J, et al. Metabolic abnormalities, cardiovascular risk factors and GFR decline in children with chronic kidney disease. *Clin J Am Soc Nephrol.* 2011;6:2132-2140.

Garin EH, Araya CE. Treatment of systemic hypertension in children and adolescents. *Curr Opin Pediatr.* 2009;21:600-604.

Guignard JP. Postnatal development of glomerular filtration rate in neonates. In: Polin RA, Fox WW, Abman SH, eds. *Fetal and Neonatal Physiology.* 4th ed. Philadelphia: WB Saunders; 2011:1339-1348.

Hoste EA, Kellum JA. RIFLE criteria provide robust assessment of kidney dysfunction and correlate with hospital mortality. *Crit Care Med.* 2006;34:2016-2017.

Kidney Disease Outcomes Quality Initiative (K/DOQI). K/DOQI clinical practice guidelines for chronic kidney disease: evaluation, classification, and stratification. Executive summaries of 2000 updates. http://www.kidney.org/professionals/KDOQI/guidelines_ckd/toc.htm.

Lurbe E, Alvarez J, Redon J. Diagnosis and treatment of hypertension in children. *Curr Hypertens Rep.* 2010;12:480-486.

Mitsnefes M, Ho PL, McEnrey PT. Hypertension and progression of chronic renal insufficiency in children: a report of the North American Renal Transplant Cooperative Study (NAPRTCS). *J Am Soc Nephrol.* 2003;14:2618-2622.

Mogal NE, Brocklebank JT, Meadow SR. A review of acute renal failure in children: incidence, etiology, and outcome. *Clin Nephrol.* 1998;49:91-95.

Full bibliography can be found on www.expertconsult.com.

49

The Kidney in Pregnancy

Jessica Tangren; Michelle A. Hladunewich

KIDNEY ANATOMY AND PHYSIOLOGY DURING NORMAL PREGNANCY

Pregnancy produces dramatic changes in systemic hemodynamics, leading to alterations in total circulating blood volume, cardiac output, and systemic vascular resistance. The kidney itself undergoes marked changes during gestation, including alterations in kidney size, renal plasma flow (RPF), glomerular hemodynamics, and tubular function. These adaptations are critical for favorable pregnancy outcomes. Although much of our knowledge of renal anatomic and physiologic changes in human pregnancy is extrapolated from animal models and small studies in healthy pregnant women, understanding the adaptive changes that occur during pregnancy is crucial for differentiating normal from compromised pregnancies.

ANATOMIC CHANGES DURING GESTATION

Kidney size increases during pregnancy from a combination of increased kidney weight and dilatation of the urinary collecting system. In longitudinal studies of kidney size measured by ultrasound, kidney length increases by approximately 1 cm. Dilation of the collecting system is observed as early as the third month of pregnancy. The right renal pelvis is most often affected. Although traditionally believed to be the result of mechanical compression by the gravid uterus, dilatation occurs well before the uterus is large enough to cause obstruction, arguing for a hormonal contribution as well. Structural changes generally resolve by 12 weeks postpartum. Persistent hydronephrosis beyond 12 to 16 weeks postpartum suggests underlying mechanical obstruction that requires further investigation (Box 49.1).

PHYSIOLOGIC CHANGES DURING GESTATION

SYSTEMIC HEMODYNAMIC CHANGES

Systemic adaptations to normal pregnancy begin soon after conception, with the development of a low-resistance placental circulation. Changes in maternal systemic vascular resistance and cardiac output can be detected as early as 6 weeks' gestation. Pregnancy leads to systemic vasodilation, increased cardiac output, and plasma volume expansion. Despite the increase in blood volume and cardiac output, systemic blood pressure (BP) decreases over the first half of gestation and reaches a nadir between 18 and 24 weeks gestation. The mechanisms leading to systemic vasodilation in healthy human pregnancy are not fully understood but

likely reflect a balance between vasodilation and vasoconstriction mediators, such as the corpus luteum hormone, relaxin, nitric oxide (NO), and alterations of the renin-angiotensin-aldosterone system (RAAS). Systemic vasodilation results in venous pooling that triggers volume restorative responses, including increased RAAS activity and a lowered set point for antidiuretic hormone (ADH) release, leading to progressive volume expansion throughout gestation. It is interesting to note that, despite increases in RAAS activity by 2- to 10-fold, systemic BP declines.

RENAL HEMODYNAMIC CHANGES

Similar to the systemic hemodynamic changes seen in healthy pregnancies, renal vascular resistance falls, leading to increased RPF and glomerular filtration rate (GFR). Existing studies in human pregnancy physiology are challenging to interpret because of variations in GFR measurement techniques. In general, GFR and RPF increase by approximately 40%. Increased GFR is noted as early as 4 weeks' gestation, reaches peak level during the first half of pregnancy, and remains elevated until term (Fig. 49.1). The key factors that contribute to GFR are represented by the following equation:

$$GFR = K_f \times (\Delta P \cdot \pi_{GC})$$

ΔP = hydraulic pressure generated across the glomerulus
π_{GC} = glomerular intracapillary oncotic pressure
K_f = measure of surface area available for filtration and the glomerular permeability

In micropuncture studies in rats, pregnancy produces a 30% increase in single glomerular plasma flow and a 30% increase in the single nephron GFR. These single nephron measurements were proportional to whole kidney GFR and RPF measurements. Despite this increased GFR, there was *no* increase in ΔP due to proportional dilation of the afferent and efferent arterioles. Thus it appears that the glomerular hyperfiltration in normal pregnancy is accompanied by other hemodynamic adaptations that prevent interglomerular hypertension and potential glomerular damage during this period of hyperfiltration. It is not clear how applicable these physiologic changes are to a healthy human pregnancy.

VOLUME REGULATION AND ELECTROLYTE CHANGES

Total body water increases during pregnancy by 6 to 8 L, of which 4 to 6 L are extracellular. Changes in central osmostat regulation result in lower plasma osmolality (10 mOsm/L below normal), represented by a decrease in serum sodium by 4 to 5 mEq/L. Despite decreased plasma sodium concentrations, healthy pregnant women are in positive sodium balance,

Box 49.1   Normal Adaptive Changes During Pregnancy

Structural Changes in the Kidney

Increase in kidney size by approximately 1 cm
Dilation of the urinary collecting system; more prominent on the right

Hormonal Changes

10- to 20-fold increase in aldosterone
Eightfold increase in renin
Fourfold increase in angiotensin
Resistance to pressor effect of angiotensin
Decreased set point for ADH release
Increased ANP release
Increased production of prostacyclin and nitric oxide

Systemic Hemodynamic Changes

Increased cardiac output by 40%–50%
Increased plasma volume by 40%–50%
Drop in SBP by ≈9 mm and DBP by 17 mm Hg (prominent in second trimester)

Renal Hemodynamic Changes

Increase in GFR and RPF by 50% above normal
Decrease in glomerular capillary oncotic pressure

Metabolic Changes

Decrease in BUN (to <13 mg/dL) and serum creatinine (to 0.4–0.5 mg/dL)
Increase in total body water by 6–8 L
Net retention of 900 mEq of sodium
Decrease in plasma osmolality by 10 mOsm/L
Decrease in serum sodium by 4–5 mEq/L
Mild respiratory alkalosis with compensatory metabolic acidosis (bicarb of 18–22 mEq/L)
Decrease in serum uric acid levels (to 2.5–4 mg/dL)
Glucosuria irrespective of blood glucose levels

ADH, Antidiuretic hormone; *ANP,* atrial natriuretic peptide; *BUN,* blood urea nitrogen; *DBP,* diastolic blood pressure; *GFR,* glomerular filtration rate; *RPF,* renal plasma flow; *SBP,* systolic blood pressure.

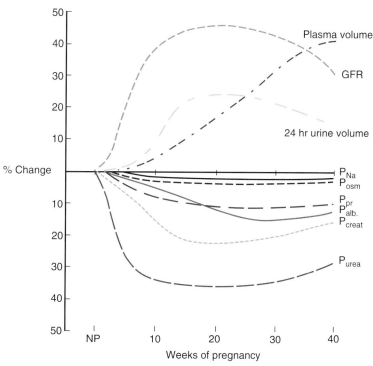

Fig. 49.1 Physiologic changes induced in pregnancy. Increments and decrements in various parameters are shown in percentage terms with reference to the nonpregnant baseline. *GFR,* Glomerular filtration rate; *NP,* nonpregnant; P_{alb}, plasma albumin; P_{creat}, plasma creatinine; P_{Na}, plasma sodium; P_{osm}, plasma osmolality; P_{pr}, plasma proteins; P_{urea}, plasma urea. (From Davison JM. The kidney in pregnancy: a review. *J Royal Soc Med.* 1983;76:485–500.)

with a net gain of 3 to 4 mEq/day. Although normal pregnancy results in increased basal metabolic rate and acid generation, plasma pH is more alkaline because of a respiratory alkalosis mediated by elevated progesterone levels. This is accompanied by an appropriate renal metabolic adaptation with reduced serum HCO_3 levels (18 to 22 mmol/L).

TUBULAR CHANGES

In the nonpregnant state, kidneys efficiently reabsorb glucose and amino acids. In a small study of euglycemic women who displayed glycosuria, the maximal tubular reabsorption capacity for glucose was significantly decreased. The precise incidence of glycosuria in pregnancy is unclear, with extensive variability noted both between women and within individual women at different times during pregnancy. There does not appear to be a relationship between glycosuria and clinical diabetes, and the majority of women with glycosuria have normal glucose screening in pregnancy. Uric acid levels drop to 2.5 to 4 mg/dL from the combined effects of increased filtration and decreased tubular reabsorption. Uric acid levels nadir in the second trimester and gradually increase as pregnancy progresses toward term. High renal clearance of uric acid is believed to be necessary to clear the increased production that occurs with fetal growth.

ASSESSMENT OF KIDNEY FUNCTION

GLOMERULAR FILTRATION RATE

Serum creatinine-based formulas are not accurate for calculating estimated GFR in pregnancy, with both the Modification of Diet in Renal Disease (MDRD) and Chronic Kidney Disease Epidemiology (CKD-EPI) underestimating GFR measured by inulin clearance by approximately 40%. Creatinine clearance (CrCl) measured in a 24-hour urine collection remains one method to estimate GFR during pregnancy, although complete collection can be difficult because of urinary retention. Cystatin C levels have been studied in a variety of clinical settings; however, their use in pregnancy is not established, as cystatin C may be released by the placenta in response to ischemia. Gestational hyperfiltration and subsequent increased GFR result in decreased blood urea nitrogen (BUN) and serum creatinine levels. A BUN greater than 13 mg/dL or serum creatinine of 0.7 to 0.8 mg/dL or higher is of concern in normal pregnancy and should be further investigated.

PROTEINURIA

Routine prenatal care includes dipstick urine protein assessment at each prenatal visit. While inexpensive, the urine dipstick has high false-positive and false-negative rates. Twenty-four-hour urine protein excretion remains the gold standard for measurement of proteinuria in pregnancy, although again it can be difficult to obtain complete collections because of incomplete bladder emptying and urinary stasis. Assessment of the urine protein-to-creatinine ratio (UPCR) or albumin-to-creatinine ratio in spot urine specimens is probably the most practical way to follow protein excretion in pregnancy.

Urinary protein excretion remains below 200 mg/24 hours in normal pregnancy despite glomerular hyperfiltration. Most obstetric guidelines define significant protein excretion as greater than 300 mg in a 24-hour period; however, this cutoff is based on small studies. In one of the largest studies, the mean 24-hour protein excretion was near 100 mg, significantly lower than the established cutoff. As such, even low levels of proteinuria should not be attributed to gestational hyperfiltration and should prompt further evaluation.

HYPERTENSIVE DISORDERS OF PREGNANCY

Hypertension in pregnancy is defined as BP ≥140/90 mm Hg, measured on at least two separate occasions. Hypertensive disorders complicate up to 10% of pregnancies and are a major cause of maternal morbidity and mortality. Hypertensive disorders in pregnancy are classified into four categories: chronic hypertension, gestational hypertension, preeclampsia, and superimposed preeclampsia. Management of hypertension in pregnancy requires the clinician to balance the effects of treatment on both the mother and developing fetus.

CHRONIC HYPERTENSION

The diagnosis of chronic hypertension is most often based on essential hypertension diagnosed before pregnancy or a BP greater than 140/90 mm Hg diagnosed before 20 weeks of gestation that does not resolve after delivery. The prevalence of chronic hypertension in pregnancy appears to be increasing because of higher pregnancy rates in women of advanced maternal age and higher rates of maternal obesity. Chronic hypertension is associated with increased risk for preeclampsia (25%), intrauterine growth restriction (IUGR; 17%), and perinatal mortality (4%), compared with the general population.

MANAGEMENT OF HYPERTENSION IN PREGNANCY

The primary management of chronic hypertension in pregnancy includes treatment of high BP and monitoring for superimposed preeclampsia. Nonpharmacologic strategies for hypertension management in nonpregnant populations, including aerobic exercise, weight loss, and dietary sodium restriction, have not been thoroughly evaluated in pregnant women. When hypertension is severe (>160/105 mm Hg), drug therapy is clearly indicated. Until recently, data on specific BP targets in mild to moderate hypertension in pregnancy were sparse. The Control of Hypertension in Pregnancy Study (CHIPS) was a recent multicenter randomized trial of women with mild to moderate nonproteinuric gestational or chronic hypertension in pregnancy. CHIPS showed no difference in adverse maternal or fetal outcomes in women with chronic hypertension treated to tight (diastolic blood pressure [DBP] target 85 mm Hg) versus less tight (DBP target 100 mm Hg) BP control during pregnancy. Women in the tight control arm did have fewer episodes of severe hypertension during pregnancy. Thus, it appears safe for the fetus to treat women with chronic or gestational hypertension to lower DBP (goal DBP 85 mm Hg), and this may prevent the acceleration of mild/moderate hypertension to severe hypertension during pregnancy. Whether tighter control of BP during pregnancy has a long-term benefit on maternal cardiovascular outcomes is unknown.

Recommended agents used to treat hypertension in pregnancy are summarized in Table 49.1. Medications used for treatment of hypertension in pregnancy include β-blockers, calcium channel blockers, methyldopa, and hydralazine. Exposure to angiotensin-converting enzyme (ACE) inhibitors and angiotensin receptor blockers (ARBs) in the second trimester is associated with fetal renal dysplasia, oligohydramnios, and pulmonary hypoplasia. ACE inhibitors and ARBs cannot be used during pregnancy. Diuretics are not first-line agents for chronic hypertension in pregnancy, but can be used if necessary to treat volume overload. They should not be used in states like preeclampsia.

GESTATIONAL HYPERTENSION

Gestational hypertension is defined as new-onset hypertension without proteinuria after 20 weeks of gestation that resolves

Table 49.1   Recommended Oral Antihypertensive Medications in Pregnancy

Medication	Initial Dose	Maximum Total Daily Dose (mg)	Side Effects
Methyldopa	250 mg twice daily	1500	Fatigue, sedation, hemolytic anemia
Labetalol	200 mg twice daily	1200	Bronchospasm, fatigue
Long-acting nifedipine	30 mg daily	120	Edema, headache
Hydralazine	50 mg three times daily	300	Tachycardia

within 3 months of delivery. Gestational hypertension and preeclampsia are likely a spectrum of disorders, with 15% to 25% of patients with gestational hypertension developing overt preeclampsia. Gestational hypertension, even in the absence of preeclampsia, is associated with adverse pregnancy outcomes. Offspring of mothers with gestational hypertension are at increased risk for preterm delivery and IUGR. Furthermore, these women are at increased risk for future development of hypertension and cardiovascular disease.

PREECLAMPSIA

Preeclampsia is a pregnancy-specific multisystem syndrome characterized by development of hypertension and proteinuria occurring after 20 weeks of gestation. It is seen in approximately 5% of pregnancies in the United States. Maternal complications of preeclampsia include liver injury (hepatitis, hepatic hepatoma, or rupture), pulmonary edema, hypertensive encephalopathy, intracerebral edema, kidney failure, and death. Fetal complications include IUGR, placental abruption, and neonatal death. Eclampsia, defined as the occurrence of seizures in a woman with preeclampsia, is now rare in the developed world because of early management of preeclampsia.

RISK FACTORS

Rates of preeclampsia vary across the globe. It is more common in nulliparous women and multiparous women with a new partner. Other risk factors include a first-degree family member with preeclampsia, multiple gestations, molar pregnancies, extremes of maternal age (<20 and >40 years), and underlying maternal medical conditions such as hypertension, diabetes, CKD, obesity, and thrombophilias, such as antiphospholipid antibody syndrome.

PATHOPHYSIOLOGY

Placental abnormalities play a central role in the development of preeclampsia (Fig. 49.2). During pregnancy, trophoblasts migrate into uterine spiral arteries, transforming thick muscular arteries into high-capacity vessels that permit greater blood flow to the uteroplacental unit. In preeclampsia, this process is impaired, and spiral arteries remain high-resistance vessels, leading to inadequate placental oxygen delivery, placental ischemia, and release of factors that induce widespread maternal vascular endothelial dysfunction. Whether placental ischemia alone is sufficient to cause preeclampsia is debatable because IUGR, also characterized by placental insufficiency, does occur without preeclampsia.

There is strong evidence for the role of placental antiangiogenic factors in pathogenesis of preeclampsia. Soluble fms-like tyrosine kinase-1 (sFlt1) is a soluble vascular endothelial growth factor (VEGF) receptor that binds to proangiogenic factors such as VEGF and placental growth factor (PlGF), neutralizing their effects. Excess production of sFlt1 from the placenta results in the widespread endothelial dysfunction characteristic of preeclampsia. Soluble endoglin (sEng) is a truncated tumor growth factor (TGF) β-coreceptor that antagonizes the action of TGF-β and augments the effects of sFlt1 on the endothelium. Both sFlt1 and sEng have been shown to increase before the onset of preeclampsia and correlate with disease severity. It is believed that preeclampsia occurs as a result of a decrease in growth factors such as VEGF and PlGF, along with overproduction of antiangiogenic factors such as sFlt1 and sEng.

Circulating levels of sFlt1 and PlGF have shown promise as predictive biomarkers of preeclampsia in several studies. Serum PlGF levels are reduced in women who go on to develop preeclampsia as early as the first trimester. In an international study of women presenting with suspected preeclampsia, low sFlt1/PlGF ratio accurately identified women at very low risk for the development of preeclampsia within the next week. A low sFlt1/PlGF had a very strong negative predictive value (99%) in this study. In the future, a negative test may allow for improved risk stratification of women who are at low risk for developing a poor outcome. In a small, open-label study, removal of sFlt1 by dextran apheresis appeared safe to both mother and fetus and prolonged pregnancy in women with early preeclampsia and elevated sflt1/PlGF ratios. Controlled studies are needed to further investigate dextran apheresis as a therapy for early onset preeclampsia, but this study highlights the potential causative role of sFlt1 in preeclampsia pathogenesis.

DEFINITIONS, DIAGNOSIS, AND CLINICAL FEATURES

The definition of preeclampsia differs by region. The American College of Obstetricians and Gynecologists (ACOG) published updated guidelines on the diagnosis of preeclampsia in 2013. Preeclampsia is characterized by a new onset of hypertension (BP of ≥140/90 mm Hg) and proteinuria after 20 weeks of gestation. However, proteinuria is no longer required for the diagnosis of preeclampsia in the most recent guidelines, and the diagnosis can be made based on new-onset hypertension with evidence of other end-organ dysfunction such as thrombocytopenia, impaired liver function tests, reduced GFR, pulmonary edema, or cerebral symptoms. HELLP syndrome is characterized by microangiopathic hemolytic anemia, elevated liver enzymes, and low platelets and occurs in 10% to 20% of patients with preeclampsia.

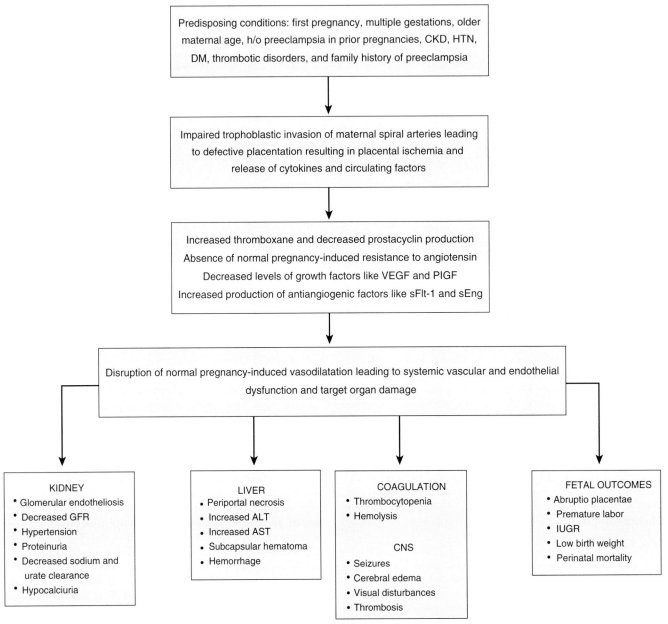

Fig. 49.2 Pathogenesis of preeclampsia. *ALT,* Alanine aminotransferase; *AST,* aspartate aminotransferase; *CKD,* chronic kidney disease; *CNS,* central nervous system; *DM,* diabetes mellitus; *GFR,* glomerular filtration rate; *HTN,* hypertension; *IUGR,* intrauterine growth restriction; *PIGF,* placental growth factor; *RPF,* renal plasma flow; *sEng,* soluble endoglin; *sFlt-1,* soluble fms-like tyrosine kinase-1; *VEGF,* vascular endothelial growth factor.

MANAGEMENT AND PREVENTION

Currently delivery of the placenta and fetus is the only definitive treatment for preeclampsia. If preeclampsia develops at or near term, immediate delivery is justified. When preeclampsia develops before fetal lung maturity, clinical decisions about delivery timing can be difficult, and a trial of expectant management is justified. Close monitoring of the fetus and mother, treatment of hypertension, and prevention of maternal seizures with intravenous magnesium are all part of expectant management of preeclampsia. In women with underlying kidney disease, magnesium infusion must be used cautiously, with frequent monitoring of serum magnesium

levels to avoid magnesium toxicity. Dose reductions are also recommended in women with advanced CKD.

Although data from early, multicenter randomized controlled trials on low-dose aspirin for the prevention of preeclampsia are conflicting, meta-analyses suggest a benefit, with a Cochrane review of 59 trials demonstrating a 17% reduction of risk for preeclampsia with low-dose aspirin. A recent meta-analysis, aimed at identifying dosage and timing of aspirin use, suggested a 43% reduction in risk for preeclampsia with low-dose aspirin when initiated before 16 weeks of gestation. As such, daily low-dose aspirin is recommended for women at high risk for preeclampsia, started ideally before 16 weeks of gestation.

Data on the role of calcium in preventing preeclampsia is similarly challenging to interpret because of inconclusive randomized controlled trials. In a Cochrane review, high-dose calcium supplementation (>1 g/day) was associated with an approximately 50% lower risk of preeclampsia, with the greatest benefit seen in women with low-calcium diets and women at high risk of preeclampsia. However, the authors stress that these data should be interpreted with caution because of the possibility of small-study effect and publication bias. Based on these results, it may be reasonable to use calcium supplements in women with low-calcium intake who are at high risk for preeclampsia.

LONG-TERM OUTCOMES AFTER PREECLAMPSIA

Hypertension and proteinuria typically improve shortly after delivery of the fetus and placenta. The majority of women have complete resolution of BP and proteinuria within 6 weeks of delivery. Despite this immediate recovery, there is strong evidence for an association between preeclampsia and future risk of cardiovascular and kidney disease, including end-stage renal disease (ESRD). Large studies, mainly from registry data, have shown increased risk of chronic hypertension (RR 3.6 to 3.7), cardiovascular disease (RR 2.2), stroke (RR 1.8 to 2.0), and ESRD (RR 4.7 to 16.0) in long-term survivors of preeclampsia. As such, appropriate counseling and postpartum follow-up are critical.

SUPERIMPOSED PREECLAMPSIA

Women with chronic hypertension who develop new-onset proteinuria after 20 weeks of gestation are diagnosed with superimposed preeclampsia. If patients have proteinuria at baseline, the diagnosis of superimposed preeclampsia is difficult, as proteinuria often increases during pregnancy in women with preexisting kidney disease. Serial fetal surveillance to assess for growth restriction and placental vascular Doppler ultrasonography can provide helpful information when distinguishing between progressive proteinuric kidney disease and superimposed preeclampsia.

SECONDARY HYPERTENSION

While secondary hypertension is a less common cause of hypertension in pregnancy than essential hypertension and gestational hypertensive disorders, secondary causes should be considered in the evaluation of new hypertension in pregnancy. Some studies have shown that up to 25% of women in whom hypertension fails to resolve 6 months after delivery may have a secondary cause of hypertension.

Undiagnosed pheochromocytoma is associated with high maternal and fetal mortality. The diagnosis can be made by 24-hour urine measurements of epinephrine, norepinephrine, and their metabolites because values are unaltered in normal pregnancy or preeclampsia. Diagnosis of primary hyperaldosteronism is difficult because of alterations in renin and aldosterone secretions during pregnancy. Renovascular hypertension from fibromuscular dysplasia can lead to severe hypertension in pregnancy, and successful control of hypertension with angioplasty has been reported. Obstructive sleep apnea is an increasingly common cause of secondary hypertension and should be considered in women with a suggestive clinical history.

> **Box 49.2 Causes of Acute Kidney Injury in Pregnancy**
>
> Volume depletion
>   Hyperemesis gravidarum
>   Postpartum bleeding
>   Placental abruption
> Sepsis
>   Septic abortion
>   Acute pyelonephritis
> Severe preeclampsia
> Bilateral cortical necrosis
> Thrombotic microangiopathies (TTP-HUS)
> Acute fatty liver of pregnancy
> Urinary tract obstruction from gravid uterus
>
> *HUS*, Hemolytic uremic syndrome; *TTP*, thrombotic thrombocytopenic purpura.

ACUTE KIDNEY INJURY IN PREGNANCY

Acute kidney injury (AKI) is a rare, but serious complication of pregnancy. The incidence of AKI in low-resource nations is decreasing, in part, because of improvement in management of sepsis (from abortions and childbirth) and postpartum hemorrhage. In high-resource nations, the rate remains very low (2 to 3/10,000 births), but has been slowly increasing because of increasing maternal age and maternal comorbidities. Although any form of AKI that affects adults in the general population can also affect pregnant women, several etiologies are more common in pregnant women (Box 49.2). The most important step in diagnosis of AKI in pregnancy is differentiating among conditions that have overlapping features, such as preeclampsia/HELLP, lupus nephritis, thrombotic thrombocytopenic purpura (TTP)/hemolytic uremic syndrome (HUS), and acute fatty liver of pregnancy (AFLP) because management strategies vary dramatically (Table 49.2).

DIFFERENTIAL DIAGNOSIS OF ACUTE KIDNEY INJURY IN PREGNANCY

The timing of AKI in gestation can often help narrow the differential diagnosis. In the first trimester, hemodynamic kidney injury (prerenal azotemia/acute tubular necrosis [ATN]) secondary to hyperemesis gravidarum or septic abortion predominate. Most cases of AKI develop in the second and third trimesters, including preeclampsia/HELLP syndromes, thrombotic microangiopathies, AFLP, or obstetric hemorrhage. Atypical HUS (aHUS) and other disorders of complement regulation typically occur near term or postpartum. Fig. 49.3 displays the main causes of AKI in pregnancy at different gestational ages. Several pregnancy-specific causes of AKI are discussed as follows.

HEMODYNAMIC KIDNEY INJURY AND BILATERAL CORTICAL NECROSIS

Hemodynamic-mediated kidney injury is a common cause of AKI in pregnancy. Injury can range from prerenal azotemia

Table 49.2   Features of Microangiopathic Syndromes Associated With Pregnancy

Features	HELLP	TTP	HUS	AFLP
Clinical onset	Third trimester	Any time	Postpartum	Third trimester
Unique to pregnancy	Yes	No	No	Yes
Underlying pathophysiology	Abnormal placentation	ADAMTS13 deficiency	Mutations in genes regulating complement function	Defective fetal mitochondrial β-oxidation of fatty acids
Hypertension	Yes	Occasional	Yes	Frequently
Kidney failure	Yes	Yes	Yes	Yes
Thrombocytopenia	Yes	Yes	Yes	Yes
Liver function tests	Abnormal	Normal	Normal	Abnormal
Antithrombin III	Low	Normal	Normal	Low
Management	Delivery	Plasma exchange	Plasma exchange, eculizumab	Delivery

AFLP, Acute fatty liver of pregnancy; *HUS,* hemolytic uremic syndrome; *TTP,* thrombotic thrombocytopenic purpura.

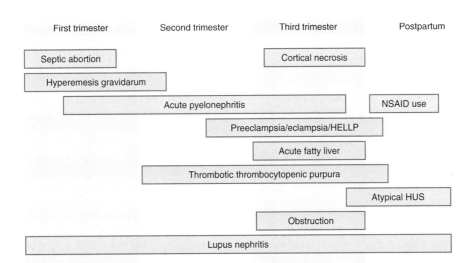

Fig. 49.3 Differential diagnosis for pregnancy-associated acute kidney injury based on timing during pregnancy. *HUS,* Hemolytic uremic syndrome; *NSAID,* nonsteroidal antiinflammatory drug.

to ischemic ATN, and rarely, to bilateral cortical necrosis hemodynamic AKI in pregnancy vary, but most commonly are seen with catastrophic pregnancy complications such as sepsis, obstetric hemorrhage, AFLP, amniotic fluid embolism, or adrenal failure.

Bilateral renal cortical necrosis, the most extreme case of hemodynamic-mediated kidney injury in pregnancy, is a pathologic diagnosis characterized by diffuse cortical necrosis on kidney biopsy, with evidence of intravascular thrombosis. The medulla is usually spared. Pregnant women with severe kidney ischemia are more likely to develop cortical necrosis than the general population. Sudden onset of oliguria/anuria in the setting of hypotension should prompt consideration of renal cortical necrosis. Computed tomography or ultrasound can help establish the diagnosis by demonstrating hypoechoic or hypodense areas in the renal cortex. Most patients require dialysis, and recovery of kidney function is unlikely.

PREECLAMPSIA/HELLP

Overt AKI is a rare complication of preeclampsia (1%) but is seen more frequently with the HELLP syndrome (7% to 15%). The pathologic kidney lesion seen in preeclampsia is glomerular endotheliosis or widespread glomerular endothelial swelling. Kidney failure in the setting of preeclampsia/HELLP has overlapping clinical features with other pregnancy-associated causes of AKI, including AFLP, lupus nephritis, TTP, and aHUS (see Table 49.2).

ACUTE FATTY LIVER OF PREGNANCY

AFLP is a rare condition that develops in the third trimester of pregnancy. Pathologically, AFLP is characterized by microvesicular fatty infiltration of maternal hepatocytes, secondary to abnormal oxidation of fatty acids by fetal mitochondria. Fetal deficiency of long-chain 3-hydroxyl CoA dehydrogenase leads to excess fetal free fatty acids that cross the placenta and are hepatotoxic to the mother. Women often present with symptoms including fatigue, vomiting, and jaundice. Laboratory findings show elevation of serum transaminases, increased bilirubin levels, and thrombocytopenia with or without disseminated intravascular coagulation (DIC). Hypoglycemia, lactic acidosis, and AKI and are common. Kidney biopsy findings in AFLP include

ATN, fatty vacuolization of tubular cells, and occlusion of capillary lumens by fibrin-like material. Definitive management is prompt delivery of the fetus. Both kidney and liver failure generally resolve postpartum, with few patients requiring liver transplant.

Distinguishing AFLP from HELLP syndrome can be challenging because both are associated with transaminitis. The most common clinical features of AFLP are malaise, nausea, vomiting, abdominal pain, and jaundice. HELLP syndrome more commonly presents with headache, abdominal or epigastric pain, and hypertension. Evidence of synthetic liver dysfunction, such as hypoglycemia and low antithrombin III, are characteristic of AFLP. DIC, AKI, ascites, and encephalopathy are also more common in AFLP.

THROMBOTIC MICROANGIOPATHIES

TTP and HUS are important causes of AKI characterized by unexplained thrombocytopenia and microangiopathic hemolytic anemia. Traditionally, TTP is considered when neurologic abnormalities are dominant and HUS when there is profound renal failure, especially in the postpartum period.

TTP results from a deficiency of von Willebrand factor cleaving protease (ADAMTS13). Most cases of pregnancy-associated TTP occur during the second or third trimester. Pregnancy appears to be a trigger for new onset or relapse of TTP, perhaps because pregnancy is associated with decreases in ADAMTS13 levels. Treatment of TTP in pregnancy is similar to the nonpregnant state with plasma exchange, which should be initiated before the diagnosis is confirmed if TTP is suspected.

Pregnancy-related aHUS, as in the nonpregnant state, is the result of complement dysregulation most often secondary to mutations in genes encoding complement regulatory proteins. Pregnancy can be a trigger for aHUS; however, unlike TTP, it most commonly presents in the peri- or postpartum period. Inhibition of C5 by eculizumab appears safe and effective in pregnant women; thus a high level of suspicion for aHUS to allow for early diagnosis and treatment is critical. Misdiagnosis is unfortunately common, and outcomes are better with shorter duration from diagnosis to treatment.

Distinguishing TTP/HUS from severe preeclampsia accompanied by HELLP syndrome can be difficult. Thrombocytopenia, microangiopathic hemolytic anemia, AKI, proteinuria, and hypertension occur in both TTP-HUS and HELLP, although elevated liver enzymes are more common in HELLP syndrome.

PYELONEPHRITIS

Although the prevalence of asymptomatic bacteriuria is similar in both pregnant and nonpregnant women, 30% to 40% of pregnant women with untreated asymptomatic bacteriuria develop symptomatic urinary tract infection, including pyelonephritis. Gestational pyelonephritis is a serious condition associated with IUGR, premature labor, and sepsis. AKI occurs in up to 25% of cases. Cephalosporins and penicillins are generally safe and effective. Treatment should be intravenous until the patient is afebrile and then continued for 14 days. Recurrent pyelonephritis occurs in 6% to 8% of women, so it is reasonable to continue suppressive therapy with low-dose antimicrobial agents for the remainder of the pregnancy.

POSTRENAL ACUTE KIDNEY INJURY

Ureteral and bladder outlet obstruction should always be considered in the differential diagnosis of AKI in pregnancy. True obstruction may be difficult to differentiate from physiologic hydronephrosis of pregnancy, which becomes more pronounced as pregnancy progresses to term. Magnetic resonance imaging can help in distinguishing physiologic hydronephrosis from obstruction in pregnancy, while ultrasound is less reliable in such a setting.

PREGNANCY IN WOMEN WITH CHRONIC KIDNEY DISEASE

Preexisting CKD increases both maternal and fetal risk. Factors associated with higher risk include CKD stage, comorbid conditions such as hypertension and diabetes, advanced maternal age, and the use of assisted reproductive technologies. Importantly, women with CKD who enter pregnancy with well-controlled BP, treated proteinuria, and stable kidney function can have excellent outcomes, making preconception kidney care critical.

The potential for pregnancy to accelerate the progression of CKD is of concern. In a recent large cohort study of women with stage 1 CKD, progression to a more advanced stage of CKD during pregnancy occurred in 8% of patients; however, the clinical significance of this change is unclear, as most progressed only to stage 2 CKD. Progression is more likely in women with advanced CKD. In a historical study of CKD pregnancies, 40% of women showed significant pregnancy-related loss of kidney function, with 20% of women progressing to kidney failure within 6 months of delivery. More recent studies suggest lower progression rates, with 16% of women with stage 3 CKD and 20% of women with stages 4 to 5 CKD progressing to a more advanced stage of CKD or ESRD. Predicting which women will experience rapid kidney function decline peri- or postpartum is challenging. Pregnancy termination does not reliably reverse the decline in kidney function.

The risk of adverse pregnancy outcomes increases with lower baseline GFR, although, even when women have preserved kidney function, normal BP, and minimal proteinuria, the risk for pregnancy complications is higher than noted in the general population. In women with advanced CKD, preterm delivery, small-for-gestational-age offspring, and need for neonatal intensive care unit care are common. Many women with advanced CKD have coexisting hypertension and proteinuria, which independently have been shown to increase the risk of adverse outcomes. Because of the detrimental effects that an unplanned pregnancy can have in women with preexisting CKD, contraception should be addressed as part of routine CKD care in reproductive-age women regardless of CKD stage.

DIABETES AND DIABETIC NEPHROPATHY

The details of pregnancy management in women with diabetes mellitus complicated by diabetic nephropathy (DN) are complex and beyond the scope of this chapter. Women with DN are at high risk of pregnancy complications because of preexisting vascular disease resulting in poor placental development and impaired autonomic functioning resulting in inadequate hemodynamic adaptation to pregnancy. There are also numerous maternal and fetal complications secondary to poor glycemic control, including increased rates of fetal malformations. Planning for pregnancy, including optimization of proteinuria with RAAS blockade before pregnancy, is essential for successful outcomes. Multiple small studies have shown that intensive hypertensive and glycemic control in women with DN before conception improves outcomes. The decision to continue RAAS blockade until women conceive is an individualized decision but appears to be a safe approach in women trying to conceive who have regular menses and can stop therapy with their first missed menstrual cycle.

LUPUS NEPHRITIS

Lupus predominantly affects women of childbearing age, with clinically significant kidney disease seen in approximately 30% of women with systemic lupus erythematosus (SLE). Pregnancy-related immunologic and hormonal changes are associated with flares. Predictors of poor pregnancy outcomes include active kidney disease, reduced GFR, hypocomplementemia, and the presence of antiphospholipid antibodies. Preeclampsia is a frequent complication, with a higher incidence in lupus nephritis compared with lupus patients with no kidney involvement and is often difficult to distinguish from a lupus nephritis flare.

A recent multicenter study showed excellent maternal and fetal outcomes in women with minimal or well-controlled kidney disease. Pregnancy may be safely planned in stable patients with quiescent kidney disease, minimal proteinuria, and controlled BP for at least 6 months on pregnancy-safe medications. Mycophenolate mofetil (MMF) is teratogenic and must be changed to azathioprine before conception. All women with SLE should be maintained on hydroxychloroquine during pregnancy because this agent reduces the frequency of lupus flares. A summary of immunosuppressive agents and whether they can be used in pregnancy is shown in Table 49.3. All women with SLE should be screened for the presence of SSA/SSB autoantibodies, which are associated with neonatal heart block and congenital lupus. Low-dose aspirin is recommended for preeclampsia prophylaxis in women with lupus. Women with antiphospholipid syndrome are at high risk for thrombosis and should be anticoagulated with low-molecular-weight heparin.

OTHER GLOMERULAR DISEASES

Immunoglobulin A (IgA) nephropathy is a common glomerular disease in reproductive-age women. In general, the risk of pregnancy is related to CKD stage alone, although the management of women with IgA complicated by kidney failure and heavy proteinuria can be challenging because of the lack of disease-specific therapies. Women with minimal proteinuria (<1 g/day) and normal GFR generally do well in pregnancy. Several studies have shown that GFR 5 years after pregnancy is similar to women who did not conceive.

Data on pregnancy in other glomerular diseases, such as membranoproliferative glomerulonephritis (MPGN), primary focal segmental glomerulosclerosis (FSGS), membranous nephropathy (MN) and anti–glomerular basement membrane (anti-GBM) disease, are even more limited. Antineutrophil cytoplasmic antibody (ANCA)-associated vasculitis is uncommon in reproductive-age women compared with older adults, and data on outcomes in pregnancy are limited to case reports. In one of the largest case series, 8 out of 21 women with disease in remission relapsed during pregnancy. Induction therapy during pregnancy is challenging because of teratogenicity of many first-line agents. In a study of long-term follow-up in women with primary glomerular disease on kidney biopsy with preserved GFR, women who became pregnant after clinical onset of disease were no more likely to progress to ESRD than women who did not conceive.

NEPHROTIC SYNDROME

The most common cause of new-onset nephrotic range proteinuria in late pregnancy is preeclampsia. However, new-onset primary nephrotic syndrome can present during pregnancy. Evaluation for secondary causes of nephrotic syndrome including serologic testing should be done in all women with de novo nephrotic syndrome that is not clearly related to preeclampsia. Severe proteinuria, hypoalbuminemia, edema, and hypercoagulability can be especially detrimental during pregnancy. Peripheral volume overload may require the use of diuretics. As pregnancy itself produces a hypercoagulable state, additional urinary losses of antithrombotic proteins in the nephrotic syndrome amplify this risk. Thromboprophylaxis

Table 49.3 Immunosuppressive Medications in Pregnancy

Medication	Side Effects	Dosing Adjustments
Cyclosporine/tacrolimus	Increased incidence of maternal diabetes, hypertension, and preeclampsia	Higher doses required because of increased metabolism
Sirolimus	Contraindicated in pregnancy	Stopped 6 weeks before conception
Mycophenolic acid	Contraindicated in pregnancy	Stopped 12 weeks before conception
Azathioprine	Widely used despite being category D; low birth weights and leukopenia reported in newborns	No dosing adjustments required
Cyclophosphamide	Increased risk for congenital anomalies and childhood cancer	Should be avoided; used with extreme caution only late in pregnancy
Rituximab	Limited human data; crosses placenta; B-cell lymphocytopenia reported in neonates	Limited data

with low-molecular-weight heparin should be considered in women with heavy proteinuria, especially in those with a serum albumin less than 2.0 mg/dL or less than 2.5 mg/dL in the context of other risk factors for thrombosis (e.g., immobility, obesity, membranous nephropathy, etc.). Although anticoagulation may be temporarily suspended to reduce peripartum bleeding, it should be continued for at least 6 weeks postpartum.

AUTOSOMAL-DOMINANT POLYCYSTIC KIDNEY DISEASE

Advanced kidney disease in women with autosomal-dominant polycystic kidney disease (ADPKD) generally develops after childbearing age. Fertility is normal in women with preserved kidney function. When compared with pregnancies in unaffected family members, women with ADPKD have higher rates of preeclampsia. The presence of preexisting hypertension was the most important risk factor for adverse outcomes. Women with ADPKD and hypertension who had multiple pregnancies (≥4) were at higher risk for CKD progression. Normotensive women with ADPKD in general have uncomplicated pregnancies, although pregnant women with ADPKD may experience an increased incidence of asymptomatic bacteriuria, more severe urinary tract infections, and an increase in the size and number of cysts due to estrogen stimulation. Preimplantation genetic testing is available in some centers for at-risk couples.

DIALYSIS

Historically, women dependent on dialysis were unlikely to conceive and often counseled against pregnancy because of the association with poor outcomes. Emerging data suggest that intensive dialysis results in improved outcomes and may be a viable option for women receiving dialysis who are unlikely to receive a kidney transplant during their reproductive years. Early menopause is common in women treated with standard thrice-weekly dialysis regimens. Ovulatory cycles may be restored in women who begin intensified hemodialysis regimens such as home or nocturnal hemodialysis.

Pregnancy outcomes have significantly improved since the report of the first successful pregnancy in a patient undergoing dialysis in 1971. In 1998, only 50% of pregnancies in women conceiving after starting dialysis resulted in surviving infants; however, more recent series note live birth rates in excess of 85%. This improvement likely reflects near universal adaptation of intensified dialysis practices in pregnant women.

Because amenorrhea is common during dialysis, diagnosing pregnancy can be difficult. A pregnancy diagnosis should be confirmed with ultrasound. Medications should be carefully reviewed and teratogenic medications promptly discontinued. Hemodialysis should be intensified to a minimum of 36 hours per week, targeting predialysis BUN less than 50 mg/dL (Box 49.3). Because weight should increase by 0.5 kg/week in the third trimester, weight gain should be expected. Determination of dry weight can be difficult and should be made by clinical examination and assessment of fetal growth. Pregnancy should be managed by a multidisciplinary team that includes high-risk obstetricians and nephrologists.

KIDNEY TRANSPLANTATION

Sexual dysfunction and infertility often reverse post transplantation. Ovulation can occur within the first month after transplant. Optimal contraception should be initiated during the peritransplant period. Oral contraceptive pills are a reasonable choice if BP is adequately controlled. Intrauterine devices (IUDs), previously believed to require an intact immune system, appear to be a safe and effective option.

The consensus opinion of the American Transplant Society is that pregnancy can be planned when the patient reaches 1 year posttransplantation, as long as the following criteria

---

Box 49.3 Management of Pregnant Patients Undergoing Hemodialysis

Dialysis Dose

At least 36 hours of dialysis per week; goal BUN of <50 mg/dL

Dialysate Composition

Sodium: 130–135 mEq/L based on serum Na
Potassium: 3.0–4.0 mmol/L
Bicarbonate: 25 mEq/L

Diet/Vitamin Supplementation

Double dose of MVI
Folic acid 5 mg/daily
Unrestricted diet
Protein intake: 1.5–1.8 g/kg/day

Dry Weight

Assess weekly
Increases by 0.5 kg/week in second and third trimesters

Anemia

Increase in ESA and iron doses
Target hemoglobin of 10 g/dL

Hypertension

Target postdialysis BP of 140/90 mm Hg

Diagnosis of Preeclampsia

Difficult to diagnose; must rely on worsening BP control and fetal assessments
Low-dose aspirin (75–81 mg) daily for prophylaxis of preeclampsia

Metabolic Bone Disease

Vitamin D analogs to maintain PTH levels, as in general patients undergoing dialysis
Dialysate calcium: 2.5–3.0 mmol/L
Oral phosphorus binders generally not required

BP, Blood pressure; *BUN,* blood urea nitrogen; *ESA,* erythropoiesis-stimulating agent; *MVI,* multiple vitamin for infusion; *PTH;* parathyroid hormone.

are met: adequate kidney function on stable, pregnancy-safe immunosuppressive medication, and no evidence of fetotoxic infections, including cytomegalovirus (CMV). The major concerns are the effect of pregnancy on maternal allograft function and potential side effects of medications on fetal growth. Preeclampsia, premature delivery, and low birth weight are more common in transplant recipients than in the general population.

Many studies comparing kidney transplant recipients with and without pregnancies report no difference in long-term allograft survival. In studies from the United States and United Kingdom, women with allograft loss had higher mean pre-pregnancy creatinine. Recent data from the US Renal Data System (USRDS) showed a 10% incidence of allograft loss at 1 year and a 37% incidence of allograft loss at 5 years in women who conceived after transplant. Conceiving within the first and second year after transplant was a risk factor for accelerated allograft loss, while conceiving during the third posttransplant year was not associated with accelerated allograft loss. These estimates were higher than previously reported in US transplant recipients. Kidney allograft biopsy can be safely performed to evaluate for graft dysfunction during pregnancy.

All immunosuppressive medications cross the placenta; however, steroids, calcineurin inhibitors, and azathioprine have an acceptable safety profile. Much remains to be learned about the pharmacokinetics and pharmacodynamics of immunosuppressive medications during pregnancy, and, as expected, most of the available information is from retrospective review and clinical experience (see Box 49.3). Maintenance immunosuppression in pregnant transplant patients generally includes cyclosporine or tacrolimus, azathioprine, and prednisone. Mycophenolate should be discontinued in transplant patients planning to become pregnant. Antibodies used to treat rejection, such as thymoglobulin and alemtuzumab, cross the placenta, and there is insufficient experience with these agents in pregnancy.

KIDNEY BIOPSY IN PREGNANCY

Kidney biopsy in pregnancy is recommended only when there is suspicion of significant disease in which diagnosis will alter therapy. The most common indications are to diagnose unexplained rapid decline in GFR or new-onset nephrotic syndrome in the absence of preeclampsia or other systemic conditions. If necessary, the biopsy should be performed before 32 weeks' gestational age. Kidney biopsies become technically challenging as gestation progresses, because the gravid uterus prevents prone positioning. Biopsy is never indicated when preeclampsia is part of the differential diagnosis, as hypertension and abnormal coagulation indices can significantly hamper the safety of the procedure.

KEY BIBLIOGRAPHY

American College of Obstetricians and Gynecologists. Task Force on Hypertension in Pregnancy. Report of the American College of Obstetricians and Gynecologists' task force on hypertension in pregnancy. *Obstet Gynecol.* 2013;122:1122-1131.

Bartsch E, Medcalf KE, Park AL, Ray JG. Clinical risk factors for preeclampsia determined in early pregnancy: systematic review and meta-analysis of large cohort studies. *BMJ.* 2016;353:i1753.

Bramham K, Nelson-Piercy C, Gao H, et al. Pregnancy in renal transplant recipients: a UK national cohort study. *Clin J Am Soc Nephrol.* 2013;8:290-298.

Buyon JP, Kim MY, Guerra MM, et al. Predictors of pregnancy outcomes in patients with lupus: a cohort study. *Ann Intern Med.* 2015;163: 153-163.

Chapman AB, Johnson AM, Gabow PA. Pregnancy outcome and its relationship to progression of renal failure in autosomal dominant polycystic kidney disease. *J Am Soc Nephrol.* 1994;5:1178-1185.

Fakhouri F, Roumenina L, Provot F, et al. Pregnancy-associated hemolytic uremic syndrome revisited in the era of complement gene mutations. *J Am Soc Nephrol.* 2010;21:859-867.

Hildebrand AM, Liu K, Shariff SZ, et al. Characteristics and outcomes of AKI treated with dialysis during pregnancy and the postpartum period. *J Am Soc Nephrol.* 2015;26:3085-3091.

Hladunewich MA, Hou S, Odutayo A, et al. Intensive hemodialysis associates with improved pregnancy outcomes: a Canadian and United States cohort comparison. *J Am Soc Nephrol.* 2014;25:1103-1109.

Hofmeyr GJ, Lawrie TA, Atallah AN, Duley L, Torloni MR. Calcium supplementation during pregnancy for preventing hypertensive disorders and related problems. *Cochrane Database Syst Rev.* 2014; Cd001059.

Jungers P, Houillier P, Forget D, et al. Influence of pregnancy on the course of primary chronic glomerulonephritis. *Lancet.* 1995;346: 1122-1124.

Levine RJ, Maynard SE, Qian C, et al. Circulating angiogenic factors and the risk of preeclampsia. *N Engl J Med.* 2004;350:672-683.

Lindheimer MD, Davison JM. Renal biopsy during pregnancy: "to b ... or not to b ... ?" *Br J Obstet Gynaecol.* 1987;94:932-934.

Magee LA, von Dadelszen P, Rey E, et al. Less-tight versus tight control of hypertension in pregnancy. *N Engl J Med.* 2015;372:407-417.

Odutayo A, Hladunewich M. Obstetric nephrology: renal hemodynamic and metabolic physiology in normal pregnancy. *Clin J Am Soc Nephrol.* 2012;7:2073-2080.

Piccoli GB, Cabiddu G, Attini R, et al. Risk of adverse pregnancy outcomes in women with CKD. *J Am Soc Nephrol.* 2015;26:2011-2022.

Rana S, Powe CE, Salahuddin S, et al. Angiogenic factors and the risk of adverse outcomes in women with suspected preeclampsia. *Circulation.* 2012;125:911-919.

Roberge S, Nicolaides K, Demers S, Hyett J, Chaillet N, Bujold E. The role of aspirin dose on the prevention of preeclampsia and fetal growth restriction: systematic review and meta-analysis. *Am J Obstet Gynecol.* 2017;216:110-120, e6.

Rose C, Gill J, Zalunardo N, Johnston O, Mehrotra A, Gill JS. Timing of pregnancy after kidney transplantation and risk of allograft failure. *Am J Transplant.* 2016;16:2360-2367.

Thadhani R, Hagmann H, Schaarschmidt W, et al. Removal of soluble Fms-like tyrosine kinase-1 by dextran sulfate apheresis in preeclampsia. *J Am Soc Nephrol.* 2016;27:903-913.

Vikse BE, Irgens LM, Leivestad T, Skjaerven R, Iversen BM. Preeclampsia and the risk of end-stage renal disease. *N Engl J Med.* 2008;359: 800-809.

Full bibliography can be found on www.expertconsult.com.

Kidney Disease in the Elderly

50

Ann M. O'Hare; C. Barrett Bowling; Manjula Kurella Tamura

AGE AND THE PREVALENCE OF CHRONIC KIDNEY DISEASE

The prevalence of chronic kidney disease (CKD) increases markedly with age, and available data suggest that the number of older adults with advanced kidney disease will continue to increase over time. Among adults in the general population, CKD prevalence increases from less than 5% for those under the age of 40% to 47% among those age 70 and older. While the high prevalence of CKD in older adults may in part reflect a high prevalence of comorbidities associated with CKD at older ages (e.g., diabetes and hypertension), a strong age-associated increase in the prevalence of CKD is present even among those without these conditions.

The marked increase in prevalence of CKD at older ages largely reflects the estimated glomerular filtration rate (eGFR) threshold of 60 mL/min per 1.73 m^2 used to define CKD and the distribution of eGFR within the population. Estimates of GFR in the general population follow a normal distribution with a median value around 80 to 90 mL/min per 1.73 m^2. The midpoint of this distribution decreases with age and moves close to 60 mL/min per 1.73 m^2 in some groups. For example, in women without comorbidity participating in a community-based cohort study in the Netherlands, median eGFR ranged from 90 mL/min per 1.73 m^2 for those aged 18 to 24 years to 60 mL/min per 1.73 m^2 for those aged 85 and older. Less than 5% of women aged 85+ without comorbidity had eGFR close to 90 mL/min per 1.73 m^2, the median value for the youngest age group. In summary, median eGFR decreases with age, but there is substantial heterogeneity in eGFR values among patients of the same age.

The amount of urinary protein excretion also increases with age. However, the distribution of albumin-to-creatinine ratio (ACR) and its relationship to the threshold value of 30 mg/g selected for defining CKD are both quite different than for eGFR. Almost half of adults in the general population have ACR below the level of detection, whereas values of 30 mg/g or higher occur in a small minority. Because the percentage of patients who meet ACR criteria for CKD varies less as a function of age than the percentage who meet eGFR criteria for CKD, the majority of older adults with CKD have a low eGFR without significant albuminuria, whereas the majority of younger adults have albuminuria but normal eGFR (Fig. 50.1).

Prevalence estimates for CKD in older adults vary widely depending on the methods used to estimate GFR (see

Chapter 3). The Cockcroft-Gault and Modification of Diet in Renal Disease (MDRD) equations were not developed in populations that included a representative sample of older adults and also rely on serum creatinine, which is a marker of muscle mass. Small improvements in the accuracy of GFR estimation can substantially affect the estimated prevalence of CKD, because a disproportionately large number of patients with a low eGFR have levels that are only slightly less than 60 mL/min per 1.73 m^2. In recent years, the Chronic Kidney Disease Epidemiology Collaboration (CKD-EPI) equation has supplanted the MDRD equation in clinical practice, resulting in slightly lower prevalence estimates of CKD in the general population, particularly for younger populations.

PROGRESSION TO END-STAGE RENAL DISEASE

Patients with CKD are at risk for progressive loss of kidney function and of end-stage renal disease (ESRD), traditionally defined as initiation of chronic dialysis or receipt of a kidney transplant. The burden of kidney failure is particularly high in older adults: in the United States the mean age of new patients undergoing dialysis is 65 years, and the crude incidence of ESRD is highest among adults aged 75 and older. The high incidence of ESRD at older ages parallels the high prevalence of CKD in the elderly. However, among patients with similar levels of eGFR, those who are older are actually less likely to go on to initiate kidney replacement therapy. This phenomenon likely reflects a number of different factors, including a greater competing risk of death, lower uptake of kidney replacement therapy, differences in the accuracy of eGFR estimates, and perhaps slower loss of kidney function among older compared with younger adults.

HIGH COMPETING RISK OF DEATH AT OLDER AGES

The incidence of ESRD increases exponentially as eGFR decreases. Mortality rates also increase with falling eGFR, but this increase is more linear and far less dramatic. Most patients with CKD have eGFR between 45 and 59 mL/min per 1.73 m^2, and because death is more common than ESRD at this level of kidney function, most patients with CKD will die before they reach ESRD. At lower levels of eGFR, the risk of ESRD eventually exceeds the risk of death for most patient groups; however, the threshold level of eGFR at which this transition occurs varies depending on age. For example, among a cohort of US veterans, the threshold level of eGFR

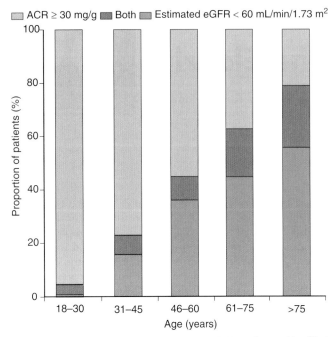

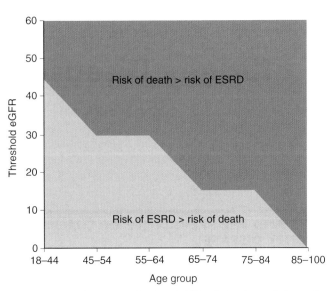

Fig. 50.1 Proportions of patients with chronic kidney disease identified by albumin-to-creatinine ratio (ACR), estimated glomerular filtration rate (eGFR), or both in the US population. (From James MT, Hemmelgarn BR, Tonelli M. Early recognition and prevention of chronic kidney disease. *Lancet*. 2010;375:1296–1309. Adapted from McCullough PA, Li S, Jurkovitz CT, et al. CKD and cardiovascular disease in screened high-risk volunteer and general populations: the Kidney Early Evaluation Program [KEEP] and National Health and Nutrition Examination Survey [NHANES] 1999–2004. *Am J Kidney Dis*. 2008;51:S38–S45.)

Fig. 50.2 Age differences in the threshold level of estimated glomerular filtration rate (eGFR) at which risk of end-stage renal disease (ESRD) exceeds risk of death among a US cohort of veterans. (From O'Hare AM, Choi AI, Bertenthal D, et al. Age affects outcomes in chronic kidney disease. *J Am Soc Nephrol*. 2007;18:2758–2765.)

at which the incidence of ESRD exceeded that of death was as high as 30 to 44 mL/min per 1.73 m^2 for some younger age groups but as low as 15 mL/min per 1.73 m^2 for some older age groups (Fig. 50.2). Similar patterns are present when ESRD is defined more broadly to include patients with sustained eGFR less than 15 mL/min per 1.73 m^2 who do not receive kidney replacement therapy. The relationships among eGFR, ESRD, and the competing risk of death are probably also modified by other factors, such as level of proteinuria, sex, race, and other comorbidity.

AGE DIFFERENCES IN LOSS OF KIDNEY FUNCTION

The relationship between age and rate of loss of eGFR is less straightforward than the relationship between age and treated ESRD described previously, and it may vary depending on the method used to estimate progression, the method for ascertaining repeated measures of kidney function (e.g., systematic collection at regular intervals vs. as part of clinical care), and the population studied. Some studies, mostly in patients with early stages of CKD, report more rapid loss of kidney function among older populations, while other studies, mostly among patients with lower levels of eGFR, reported slower loss of kidney function among older populations. A recent study from Alberta, Canada, found a similar incidence of kidney failure, defined as initiation of dialysis or sustained eGFR less than 15 mL/min per 1.73 m^2, for older and younger adults.

AGE DIFFERENCES IN END-STAGE RENAL DISEASE TREATMENT DECISIONS

Because most ESRD registries include only patients treated with kidney replacement therapy, little is known about those patients with advanced CKD who either prefer not to undergo dialysis or are not offered dialysis. A growing number of single-center studies outside the United States have described relatively high rates of conservative management among older adults with advanced kidney disease. Joly and colleagues reported that, among 146 consecutive patients aged 80 years or older referred to a renal unit in Paris between 1989 and 2000 with an estimated creatinine clearance less than 10 mL/min, conservative nondialytic management was recommended in 37 (25%). Similarly, among 321 patients referred to a renal unit in Britain, palliative nondialytic care was recommended in 20%. Those receiving nondialysis care were older, had lower functional status, and were more likely to have diabetes. An Australian study reported that older patients were more likely to receive information on conservative care and also were more likely to choose not to receive dialysis.

Because many elderly patients with advanced kidney disease are not referred to nephrologists, single-center studies in referred populations likely underestimate the number and percentage of elderly patients with advanced kidney disease who either prefer not to receive or are not offered dialysis. Using laboratory and administrative data from Alberta, Canada, Hemmelgarn et al. found that, while the incidence of ESRD treated with dialysis was lower in older compared with younger patients with similar levels of eGFR, the incidence of sustained eGFR less than 15 mL/min per 1.73 m^2 not treated with dialysis was higher in older adults. These results suggest that there are age differences in treatment practices for advanced kidney disease.

Little is currently known about treatment practices for advanced kidney disease in the United States; however, several

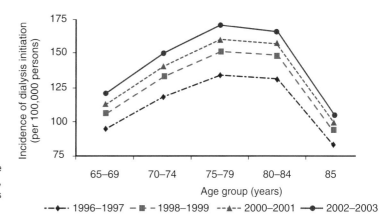

Fig. 50.3 Incidence of treated end-stage renal disease by age group over time. (From Kurella M, Covinsky KE, Collins AJ, Chertow GM. Octogenarians and nonagenarians starting dialysis in the United States. *Ann Intern Med.* 2007;146:177–183.)

lines of indirect evidence support the possibility that a substantial number of elderly US patients with advanced CKD do not receive dialysis. First, across hospital referral regions in the United States, there are large differences in the incidence of treated ESRD among older adults that are not accounted for by differences in age, race, and sex. Hospital referral regions with the highest levels of health care spending in general have the highest incidence of treated ESRD. Furthermore, regional differences in the incidence of treated ESRD are most pronounced in the very elderly. Second, despite an increasing prevalence of CKD at older ages, the incidence of ESRD per million of population among US adults peaks in the 75 to 79 age group and decreases thereafter (Fig. 50.3). Similar trends across age groups appear to exist for treatment of acute kidney injury (AKI) among hospitalized patients. Hsu and colleagues described age differences in the management of AKI among members of a large health maintenance organization in northern California from 1996 to 2003. While the incidence of AKI not treated with dialysis increased linearly with age, the incidence of AKI treated with dialysis peaked among those aged 70 to 79 and declined at older ages. More recently, Wong and colleagues described dialysis initiation practices in US veterans with advanced kidney disease and found that, although an implicit decision not to pursue dialysis was relatively rare among members of this cohort (<15% of patients), it was far more common in older than in younger patients. Nevertheless, even among the oldest patients with the highest level of comorbidity, most were either treated with dialysis or were preparing to be treated with dialysis at the most recent follow-up. The percentage of older patients in this study treated with dialysis was much higher than for other developed countries, suggesting that there are marked international variations in kidney failure treatment practices for older patients.

CLINICAL SIGNIFICANCE OF MODERATELY REDUCED ESTIMATED GLOMERULAR FILTRATION RATE

Adults older than 70 years account for approximately half of all US adults with CKD; however, more than half of these older adults with CKD have only moderate reductions in eGFR in the 45 to 59 mL/min per 1.73 m² range. For many of these older patients, eGFR in this range falls close to the median value for their peers. Because eGFR is thought to

decline as part of "normal" aging, some have questioned the clinical significance of such moderate reductions in eGFR in older adults.

Because death is far more common than progression to ESRD among patients with moderately reduced eGFR, the debate about the clinical significance of eGFR in older adults largely revolves around mortality risk. On a population level, the same increase in relative risk of death will be associated with a greater number of deaths in patients with higher background mortality rates (e.g., older patients). However, among individual patients, the same increase in the relative risk of death will translate into a smaller difference in life expectancy among those with more limited life expectancy. For example, a 10% increase in mortality risk translates into 1-year reduction in survival for a patient with a life expectancy of 10 years, as compared with 1-month reduction in survival for a patient with a life expectancy of 10 months. This distinction becomes clinically relevant when considering mortality risk among older patients with very moderate reductions in eGFR, in whom the relative risk of death is only modestly increased compared with the referent of patients with normal kidney function. Such modest increases in relative mortality risk may not translate into a meaningful difference in life expectancy in populations with very high baseline mortality rates.

Consistent with this possibility, several studies have demonstrated that the time to death (or relative hazard of death) associated with a given level of eGFR is attenuated at older ages. In a large national cohort of veterans, O'Hare and colleagues found that at each level of eGFR, the relative hazard of death was attenuated with increasing age. Members of this cohort aged 65 and older with GFR in the 50 to 59 mL/min per 1.73 m² range (comprising nearly half of the cohort designated as CKD) did not have an increased relative risk of death compared with their age peers with GFR ≥60 mL/min per 1.73 m². On the other hand, younger members of this cohort with moderate reductions in eGFR did have a higher risk of death compared with the referent group. Similar results were reported by Raymond et al. for a large UK cohort. More recently, attenuation of the relative hazard of death associated with a given level of eGFR was reported in a large pooled analysis. This study provides the added insight that the threshold level of eGFR, above which mortality risk increases, seems to vary depending on the population studied, the referent category used, the equation used to estimate GFR, and whether analyses include information on level of proteinuria.

Table 50.1   Relevance and Significance of Select Geriatric Syndromes in Older Adults With Chronic Kidney Disease

Geriatric Syndromes	Relevance and Significance in Older Adults With CKD
Cognitive impairment	The prevalence and incidence of cognitive impairment increases at lower levels of eGFR and is common in older adults receiving chronic dialysis. In both the general population and in ESRD patients, cognitive impairment is associated with increased mortality.
Depressive symptoms	Depression is more common in patients with CKD and is associated with worsening kidney function and incident kidney failure. Among patients with ESRD, depression is associated with an increased risk of mortality.
Falls	CKD complications such as neuropathy, muscle weakness, and anemia are associated with falls. CKD patients have higher risk of fractures.
Polypharmacy	CKD patients take an average of eight medications and have decreased renal clearance of many drugs. Among older adults, polypharmacy is associated with increased mortality. Drug dosing is based on creatinine clearance, which may be a poor marker for kidney function in older adults with decreased muscle mass.
Poor physical performance	CKD is associated with poor physical performance. In the general population, poor physical performance predicts mortality and functional decline.
Frailty	Frailty is more prevalent in older adults with CKD than among those without CKD. Among patients undergoing dialysis, frailty is common even among younger patients and is associated with an increased risk of mortality.

CKD, Chronic kidney disease; *eGFR*, estimated glomerular filtration rate; *ESRD*, end-stage renal disease.

Given the very large numbers of older adults with moderate reductions in eGFR and uncertainty about the clinical implications of such modest reductions in eGFR, there is growing interest in efforts to distinguish high- from low-risk members of this group. Several studies suggest that information on other disease markers, such as level of albuminuria, eGFR trajectory, and cystatin C, might be useful in identifying a higher risk subgroup within the large population of older adults with moderate reductions in eGFR. While these measures may be helpful on a population level, it is important to keep in mind that there can be substantial heterogeneity in life expectancy among patients of the same age with similar levels of eGFR and proteinuria. Among a national cohort of older VA patients, the interquartile range in survival time among patients with similar levels of eGFR and proteinuria rivaled differences in median survival across strata. For example, in those aged 80 to 84 years with eGFR of 30 to 44 mL/min per 1.73 m^2 and negative to trace proteinuria, median survival time was 5.3 years, but with an interquartile range of more than 6 years (2.6 to 8.7 years).

COMORBIDITY AND GERIATRIC SYNDROMES

CKD is associated with metabolic abnormalities among older adults. Two large studies found that, similar to younger adults, lower eGFR was associated with a higher prevalence of anemia, hyperkalemia, acidosis, hyperphosphatemia, and hyperparathyroidism among older adults. Patients with CKD are also at higher risk for geriatric syndromes such as cognitive impairment, functional limitation, and falls. These syndromes are conceptualized as heterogeneous conditions that aggregate in older adults and result from a shared risk factor or factors. Geriatric syndromes contribute to frailty, a phenotype characterized as rendering patients vulnerable to situational challenges, which in turn leads to disability, dependence,

and death (Table 50.1). The burden of geriatric syndromes and frailty among older adults with CKD is quite high. For example, in several studies, more than 20% of adults with stage 4 CKD have evidence of cognitive impairment and frailty, while, among patients undergoing dialysis over the age of 65, more than 30% have cognitive impairment and more than 75% are frail. In contrast to the general population, geriatric syndromes and frailty are relatively common, even among younger patients with CKD. These observations have led some investigators to describe CKD as a process of accelerated aging.

OUTCOMES AMONG OLDER ADULTS WITH ADVANCED CHRONIC KIDNEY DISEASE

Treatment options for advanced CKD are similar for older as compared with younger adults. However, advanced age and the associated high burden of comorbidity and disability have important implications for determining the relative benefits and burdens of available treatment options. For some older adults, quality of life may be equally important or even more important than length of life in making ESRD treatment choices.

DIALYSIS VERSUS CONSERVATIVE THERAPY

Median survival after dialysis initiation for adults ages 75 to 79, 80 to 84, 85 to 89, and ≥90 years is 1.7 years, 1.3 years, 0.9 years, and 0.6 years, respectively; however, considerable heterogeneity in survival exists among patients of similar ages, highlighting the limitations of age alone to predict outcomes. For example, among adults ages 75 to 79 starting dialysis, 25% survive more than 3 years, while 25% survive less than 6 months, most of whom die in the first 3 months following initiation. In addition to advanced age, a number of negative prognostic factors have been identified in epidemiologic studies, including frailty or reduced functional status, low body weight or serum albumin concentration, number and severity of comorbidities, and late referral or unplanned dialysis initiation. Validated prognostic models incorporating several of these factors have been developed and may help refine estimates of life expectancy.

Given these estimates and the slow rate of progression of CKD among many older adults, many providers question whether dialysis can be expected to extend life or improve quality of life for older adults with high levels of comorbidity and/or disability. Unfortunately, relatively little information is available about outcomes of conservative management among older adults with advanced CKD. Earlier studies should be interpreted cautiously in light of the selection biases present (i.e., healthier patients are more likely to receive dialysis and sicker patients are more likely to receive conservative management). Most studies show that overall survival for patients selected for dialysis exceeds survival of patients selected for conservative management; however, the magnitude of this effect varies across studies. Among a French cohort of octogenarians, patients who initiated dialysis survived on average 20 months longer than those who received conservative therapy, while, among a British cohort of septuagenarians, those for whom dialysis was recommended survived 24 months longer than those for whom conservative therapy was recommended. However, those who chose dialysis also spent more days in the hospital and were more likely to die in the hospital. Notably, several studies suggest that a subgroup of older adults do not experience a survival benefit from dialysis.

Older adults continue to experience a high burden of comorbidity and symptoms after starting dialysis. For example, older adults with ESRD are hospitalized approximately 2 times per year and an average of 25 days per year. Functional decline is common and especially prominent around the time of dialysis initiation or hospitalization. In one study of US nursing home residents, there was a marked decline in functional status at the time of dialysis initiation. As a result, fewer than 13% of nursing home patients starting dialysis survived for 1 year and maintained their predialysis functional abilities. Similar patterns have been noted among ambulatory older adults starting chronic dialysis and among prevalent ESRD patients after hospitalization. Adverse physical symptoms may also be prominent and interfere with daily functioning or quality of life.

Just as decisions to start dialysis vary nationally and internationally, so too do rates of dialysis withdrawal. Annually, 8% of US patients undergoing dialysis withdraw from dialysis, a figure that rises to 13% among those over the age of 75. Comorbidity and recent hospitalizations are linked to dialysis withdrawal. Hospice utilization is low among patients with ESRD compared with other life-limiting conditions such as advanced dementia, heart failure, and cancer. In addition, fewer than half of all patients who withdraw from dialysis use hospice services before death. Low utilization may reflect restrictions on Medicare coverage for concurrent hospice and dialysis if kidney failure is the indication for hospice and poor knowledge about hospice as a treatment option.

Despite substantial morbidity, available data suggest that quality of life is acceptable for many older adults receiving chronic dialysis. In the North Thames Study, older adults with ESRD had lower physical quality of life but similar mental quality of life to the age-matched general population. Similar results were noted in the Dialysis Outcomes and Practice Patterns Study. In the HEMO trial, older adults with ESRD had similar changes in quality of life over 3 years to their younger counterparts. These studies included only prevalent patients undergoing dialysis, so it is possible that quality of life was overestimated due to exclusion of sicker patients who withdrew from dialysis or died of other causes soon after initiating dialysis.

How should clinicians reconcile this information? One suggestion has been to rethink the process of obtaining informed consent for dialysis. This is especially true among patients with substantial comorbidity, disability, or cognitive impairment. Important elements of obtaining informed consent include discussions of anticipated prognosis and clearly delineating treatment alternatives. While quality of life on dialysis is necessarily subjective, estimates of survival, functional status, and expected lifestyle changes can inform the decision-making process for many patients. A second suggestion has been to increase integration of palliative care services into routine dialysis care. Such an approach may help patients address the symptoms of ESRD and dialysis therapy and prepare for end-of-life decisions.

TRANSPLANTATION

At the other end of the spectrum of treatment options for kidney failure, the demand for kidney transplantation continues to increase among older adults. Over the last two decades, the number of patients over the age of 60 on the US kidney transplant waiting list has increased 20-fold, such that adults over the age of 60 now comprise approximately 30% of all wait-listed patients and 25% of all kidney transplant recipients. In these individuals, transplantation extends life by 1 to 4 years on average compared with remaining on dialysis. More recent studies suggest these benefits extend to selected patients over the age of 75. One study showed that kidney transplantation was cost-effective for patients over the age of 65, but that the attractiveness of transplantation declined as waiting time increased. Short-term allograft survival is slightly lower among older adults, but generally excellent.

The expanded criteria donor (ECD) list shortens waiting times at the cost of a higher risk of allograft loss. For older patients and those in regions with long waiting times, the benefits of an ECD kidney appear to outweigh the risks. As a result, this option is common among older transplant recipients. As the demand for transplantation among older adults rises, the selection of candidates and allocation of limited organs have become increasingly challenging. Perhaps as a result, the criteria for accepting an older patient to the transplant wait list vary greatly from center to center. Allocation of organs by more closely matching donor and recipient age has been implemented in Europe and is being considered in the United States.

MANAGEMENT OF OLDER ADULTS WITH CHRONIC KIDNEY DISEASE

The last decade has seen the evolution of a disease-based approach to CKD, along with the development of clinical practice guidelines that both define CKD and provide an evidence-based approach to patient care. Clinical practice guidelines for CKD present a standardized approach to management, prioritizing interventions to reduce mortality and cardiovascular events and to prevent and slow disease progression at earlier stages of disease. At later stages of CKD, a greater focus is placed on management of disease complications and preparation for kidney failure. The goal of clinical practice guidelines is to provide a simplified model to guide management rather than to address the many complex questions that may arise in individual patients. Contemporary guidelines for the management of patients with CKD do not distinguish among patients of different ages; however, in older patients with multiple comorbid conditions, there is often a tension between what might be recommended by clinical practice guidelines and what might be most beneficial for an individual patient.

HIGH BURDEN OF COMPLEX COMORBIDITY COMPLICATING MANAGEMENT

At older ages, patients often have more than one disease process. This is particularly true for older adults with CKD. The presence of multiple comorbid conditions may generate competing health priorities and conflicting treatment recommendations (Fig. 50.4). Clinical practice guidelines rarely acknowledge the possibility that patients may have more than one condition, and most do not provide guidance on how to manage the multiple competing health priorities that often arise in older adults with complex comorbidity. Boyd et al. provided a hypothetical case to illustrate how disease-based guidelines may be harmful in older adults with complex comorbidity. In an older patient with a fairly standard set of

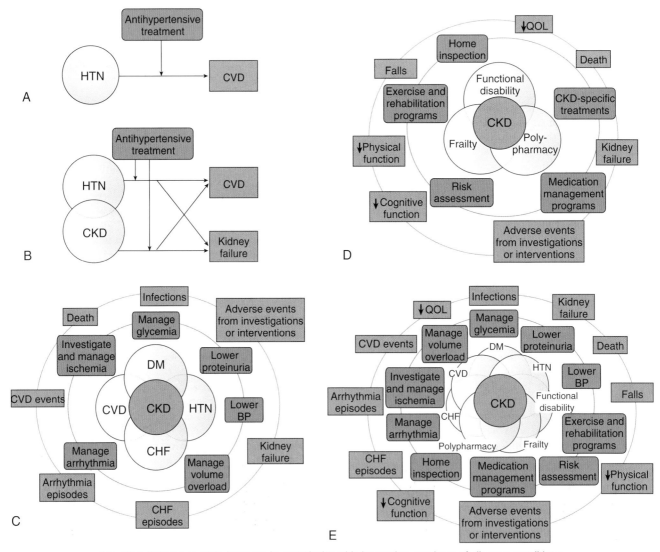

Fig. 50.4 Disease models increase in complexity with increasing numbers of disease conditions, treatments, and outcomes considered, such as in patients with chronic kidney disease (CKD) or of older age. *Circles* indicate diseases, *rectangles* outcomes, and *rounded rectangles* treatments. Disease models show treatment of (A) hypertension (HTN) without CKD; (B) HTN in patients with CKD; (C) CKD and a cluster of additional common comorbid conditions; (D) CKD along with a cluster of geriatric syndromes; and (E) CKD in older patients, incorporating clusters of common comorbid conditions, as well as geriatric syndromes (the overlap of C and D). *BP*, Blood pressure; *CHF*, congestive heart failure; *CVD*, cardiovascular disease; *DM*, diabetes mellitus; *QOL*, quality of life. (From Uhlig K, Boyd C. Guidelines for the older adult with CKD. *Am J Kidney Dis*. 2011;58:162–165.)

comorbidities, these authors modeled the onerous pharmacologic and nonpharmacologic treatment regimen with multiple potential drug interactions and competing treatment priorities that would result if all relevant practice guidelines were followed.

DIFFERENCES IN OUTCOMES BY AGE AND IMPACT ON TREATMENT EFFECTS

Guidelines for patients with CKD assume a uniform relationship between level of kidney function and clinical outcomes among patients of all ages; however, the relative and absolute frequency of different clinical outcomes varies among older and younger patients with the same level of eGFR. Such differences in outcomes are likely to affect the benefit of many recommended interventions for individual patients. For example, while interventions intended to lower cardiovascular risk have the potential to prevent the greatest number of events among high-risk groups (e.g., older patients with CKD), in patients with more limited life expectancy, such interventions will provide more modest gains in life expectancy or event-free survival. Similarly, interventions to slow progression to ESRD may prevent the greatest number of cases of ESRD in older adults, due to the higher crude incidence of ESRD at older ages; however, the benefit of interventions to prevent nondeath outcomes such as ESRD may be more limited in patients with a shorter life expectancy who are less likely to survive long enough to experience the relevant outcome. Similar principles may apply to treatment decisions undertaken to prepare for dialysis, including, for example, vascular access placement in a patient unlikely to survive long enough to require maintenance dialysis. Thus clinical practice guidelines and the evidence on which these are based must be interpreted within the context of each patient's life expectancy, baseline risk for the outcome of interest, and individual goals and preferences.

LIMITED EVIDENCE TO SUPPORT RECOMMENDED INTERVENTIONS

Evidence for interventions recommended in clinical practice guidelines are often based on the results of clinical trials that did not enroll a representative sample of older adults, and it can be difficult to extrapolate available evidence from younger trial populations to real-world populations of older adults. Thus the benefits and harms of many recommended interventions are unknown in older adults.

Similar to the general population, evidence supporting the efficacy for many recommended interventions is often lacking in older adults with CKD. For example, most trials of angiotensin-converting enzyme (ACE) inhibitors and angiotensin-receptor blockers (ARBs) cited in support of contemporary practice guidelines for the use of these agents in CKD did not enroll any adults older than 70. The relevance of these trials to older adults with CKD is especially uncertain, because most selected for patients with proteinuria, whereas the majority of older adults with CKD have a low eGFR without substantial proteinuria. A subgroup analysis among older participants in the Reduction of Endpoints in NIDDM with the Angiotensin II Antagonist Losartan (RENAAL) Trial, which enrolled 1513 adults with diabetes and proteinuria,

suggests that renin-angiotensin system blockade slows progression to ESRD in older adults with diabetes and proteinuria; however, the results of another trial, the Antihypertensive and Lipid Lowering Therapy to Prevent Heart Attack Trial (ALLHAT), may be of much greater relevance to the majority of older adults with CKD. ALLHAT differed from most other trials examining the effect of ACE inhibitors and ARBs on progression of kidney disease, as approximately half of the participants in this trial with CKD were 70 years or older and participants were not selected for proteinuria (in fact, the trial did not even ascertain level of proteinuria). Among ALLHAT participants with eGFR below 60 mL/min per 1.73 m^2, lisinopril was no more effective than either chlorthalidone or amlodipine in slowing progression to ESRD. Thus, in evaluating the relative benefits and harms of different interventions recommended for older adults with CKD, clinicians should consider not only the strength of available evidence but also its relevance to individual older patients.

HETEROGENEITY IN HEALTH STATUS, LIFE EXPECTANCY, AND PREFERENCES

The marked heterogeneity in health status, life expectancy, and preferences among older adults may be difficult to accommodate within the disease-based framework embodied in clinical practice guidelines. The disease-based approach assumes a direct causal relationship for clinical signs and symptoms with underlying disease pathophysiology. Thus treatment plans often target pathophysiologic mechanisms relevant to the disease process with the goal of improving disease-related outcomes. Outcomes prioritized by a disease-based approach to CKD include survival, cardiovascular events, and kidney function decline; however, these outcomes might not always be meaningful to individual patients. For patients with limited life expectancy, interventions intended to lengthen life might not be as important as those that allow them to maintain independence, improve quality of life, or optimize pain control—outcomes that may not always be tied to a specific underlying disease process. When faced with competing health priorities, patients may be willing to make tradeoffs to achieve those outcomes that matter most to them. Because those outcomes prioritized by clinical practice guidelines for CKD may not align with those outcomes that matter most to an individual older patient with CKD, eliciting individual patient goals and priorities is a crucial step in determining the relevance and potential benefits of guideline-recommended treatment strategies for individual patients.

INDIVIDUALIZED APPROACH TO MANAGEMENT

The individualized approach avoids some of the inherent tensions that arise when applying a strict disease-based approach to complex older patients (Fig. 50.5). The individualized approach prioritizes outcomes that matter to the patient and that can be modified by available interventions. While the disease-oriented approach assumes that signs and symptoms can be explained by one or more underlying disease processes and are best addressed by interventions targeting those processes, the individualized approach embraces the notion that signs and symptoms might not be directly explained by an underlying disease process and might reflect a variety of different intrinsic and extrinsic

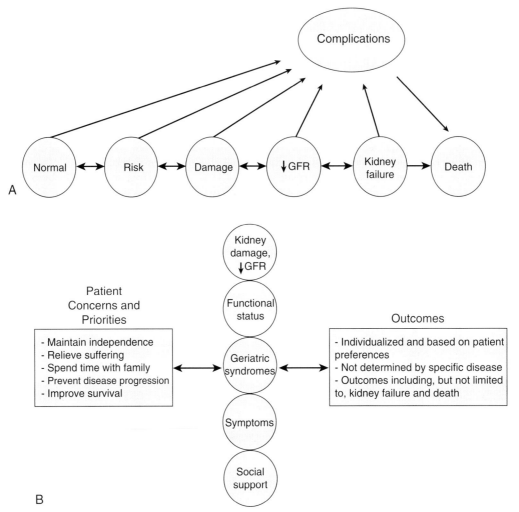

Fig. 50.5 Conceptualization of (A) disease-based and (B) individualized approaches to chronic kidney disease. *GFR*, Glomerular filtration rate. (From Bowling CB, O'Hare AM. Managing older adults with CKD: individualized versus disease-based approaches. *Am J Kidney Dis*. 2012;59:293–302.)

processes. Under the individualized approach, signs and symptoms are often considered legitimate targets for intervention, in many instances requiring complex multifaceted interventions that do not target a specific underlying disease process.

OPTIMIZING INDIVIDUALIZED TREATMENT DECISIONS

Many older adults with CKD will benefit from some interventions recommended under a disease-oriented approach. Information on prognosis and the comparative effectiveness of different therapies is often very helpful in structuring individualized treatment plans and helping patients evaluate the benefits and harms of interventions recommended under a disease-based approach. Walter and Covinsky developed a framework to support individualized decisions about cancer screening in older adults. This framework uses information on life expectancy and baseline risk of dying from a screen-detectable cancer to generate quantitative estimates of each patient's likelihood of developing the outcome of interest during their remaining lifetime, thus determining how much

they will benefit from interventions to prevent this outcome. Because patients may weigh the same information on risks and benefits differently, patient preferences are critical in determining how quantitative information on life expectancy, baseline risk of disease outcomes, and the efficacy of clinical interventions will ultimately inform treatment decisions.

A similar approach can be used to evaluate the benefit of recommended treatments in older adults with CKD. In applying this approach, it is important to recognize that although the presence and severity of CKD carries prognostic significance in older adults, many other factors can affect prognosis, leading to substantial heterogeneity in life expectancy, despite similar levels of kidney function. In addition, while life expectancy and disease-related outcomes such as slowing progression of kidney disease are often important, other outcomes such as independence and quality of life may matter more to patients. By accounting for differences in prognosis, baseline risk, and patient goals and preferences, the individualized approach is expected to yield diverse treatment plans in older adults with very similar levels of kidney function.

ACKNOWLEDGMENTS

Support was through a Beeson Career Development Award from the NIA to Dr. Kurella Tamura and the Birmingham/Atlanta GRECC Special Fellowship in Advanced Geriatrics and John A. Hartford Foundation/Southeast Center of Excellence in Geriatric Medicine to Dr. Bowling.

KEY BIBLIOGRAPHY

Bowling CB, O'Hare AM. Managing older adults with CKD: individualized versus disease-based approaches. *Am J Kidney Dis.* 2012;59:293-302.

Bowling CB, Sharma P, Fox CS, O'Hare AM, Muntner P. Prevalence of reduced estimated glomerular filtration rate among the oldest old from 1988–1994 through 2005–2010. *JAMA.* 2013;310:1284-1286.

Boyd CM, Darer J, Boult C, Fried LP, Boult L, Wu AW. Clinical practice guidelines and quality of care for older patients with multiple comorbid diseases: implications for pay for performance. *JAMA.* 2005;294:716-724.

Hemmelgarn BR, James MT, Manns BJ, et al. Rates of treated and untreated kidney failure in older vs younger adults. *JAMA.* 2012;307:2507-2515.

Jassal SV, Chiu E, Hladunewich M. Loss of independence in patients starting dialysis at 80 years of age or older. *N Engl J Med.* 2009;361:1612-1613.

Johansen KL, Chertow GM, Jin C, Kutner NG. Significance of frailty among dialysis patients. *J Am Soc Nephrol.* 2007;18:2960-2967.

Kurella M, Chertow GM, Fried LF, et al. Chronic kidney disease and cognitive impairment in the elderly: the health, aging, and body composition study. *J Am Soc Nephrol.* 2005;16:2127-2133.

Kurella M, Covinsky KE, Collins AJ, Chertow GM. Octogenarians and nonagenarians starting dialysis in the United States. *Ann Intern Med.* 2007;146:177-183.

Kurella Tamura M, Covinsky KE, Chertow GM, Yaffe K, Landefeld CS, McCulloch CE. Functional status of elderly adults before and after initiation of dialysis. *N Engl J Med.* 2009;361:1539-1547.

Kurella Tamura M, Tan JC, O'Hare AM. Optimizing renal replacement therapy in older adults: a framework for making individualized decisions. *Kidney Int.* 2012;82:261-269.

Murray AM, Arko C, Chen SC, Gilbertson DT, Moss AH. Use of hospice in the United States dialysis population. *Clin J Am Soc Nephrol.* 2006; 1:1248-1255.

Murtagh FE, Marsh JE, Donohoe P, Ekbal NJ, Sheerin NS, Harris FE. Dialysis or not? A comparative survival study of patients over 75 years with chronic kidney disease stage 5. *Nephrol Dial Transplant.* 2007;22:1955-1962.

O'Hare AM, Bertenthal D, Covinsky KE, et al. Mortality risk stratification in chronic kidney disease: one size for all ages? *J Am Soc Nephrol.* 2006;17:846-853.

O'Hare AM, Choi AI, Bertenthal D, et al. Age affects outcomes in chronic kidney disease. *J Am Soc Nephrol.* 2007;18:2758-2765.

O'Hare AM, Rodriguez RA, Bowling CB. Caring for patients with kidney disease: shifting the paradigm from evidence-based medicine to patient-centered care. *Nephrol Dial Transplant.* 2016;31:368-375.

O'Hare AM, Rodriguez RA, Hailpern SM, Larson EB, Kurella Tamura M. Regional variation in health care intensity and treatment practices for end-stage renal disease in older adults. *JAMA.* 2010;304: 180-186.

Rao PS, Merion RM, Ashby VB, Port FK, Wolfe RA, Kayler LK. Renal transplantation in elderly patients older than 70 years of age: results from the Scientific Registry of Transplant Recipients. *Transplantation.* 2007;83:1069-1074.

Uhlig K, Boyd C. Guidelines for the older adult with CKD. *Am J Kidney Dis.* 2011;58:162-165.

Walter LC, Covinsky KE. Cancer screening in elderly patients: a framework for individualized decision making. *JAMA.* 2001;285:2750-2756.

Wong SP, Hebert PL, Laundry RJ, et al. Decisions about renal replacement therapy in patients with advanced kidney disease in the US Department of Veterans Affairs, 2000–2011. *Clin J Am Soc Nephrol.* 2016; 11:1825-1833.

Full bibliography can be found on www.expertconsult.com.

CHRONIC KIDNEY DISEASE

51

Development and Progression of Chronic Kidney Disease

William L. Whittier; Ed Lewis

Chronic kidney disease (CKD) is defined as abnormal measurements of the actual or estimated glomerular filtration rate (GFR) for a minimum of 3 months (Box 51.1), or situations where the GFR is normal but pathology in the kidney is still present, such as radiographically imaged cysts in polycystic kidney disease or isolated proteinuria in early glomerular disease (see Chapter 52). The most commonly reported causes of CKD and end-stage renal disease (ESRD) (Table 51.1) are diabetic nephropathy (Fig. 51.1) and hypertensive nephrosclerosis, although the diagnosis of "hypertensive nephrosclerosis" has recently been questioned in reference to APOL1 genetic abnormalities (Chapter 37). However, many other conditions can cause CKD, including primary glomerular diseases (e.g., IgA nephropathy, membranous glomerulopathy), secondary glomerular diseases (e.g., lupus nephritis, amyloidosis), and tubulointerstitial, vascular, cystic, and hereditary kidney diseases. Each of these has specific pathophysiologic mechanisms for kidney damage; therefore the treatments developed for these diseases are unique and aimed at controlling or reversing the primary disease process.

The idea, then, that CKD could be generalized into one disease process is an oversimplification, because the primary processes causing kidney damage are protean. However, the pathophysiology of progression of many of these disorders involves similar pathways, and generic treatments aimed at slowing this progression have been applied across a wide variety of kidney diseases effectively and safely. Over the last 20 years, treatments have been developed and proven to delay progression to ESRD, and other therapies continue to be studied. Therefore early recognition of CKD becomes important to help implement therapy that may delay or reverse this progression and reduce the associated morbidity and mortality.

PATHOPHYSIOLOGIC MECHANISMS OF CHRONIC KIDNEY DISEASE

The pathophysiology of CKD is complex and in large part dependent on the primary cause. After a primary acute or chronic insult occurs, such as in diabetic nephropathy or lupus nephritis, many common pathways are activated to perpetuate and exacerbate glomerular and tubulointerstitial injury (Fig. 51.2). These harmful adaptations, occurring because of an initial injury, can be broadly categorized into those that are hemodynamically mediated or those that are nonhemodynamic.

HEMODYNAMIC INJURY

Much of the work in hemodynamic-mediated injury stems from the 5/6 nephrectomy animal model. Following unilateral nephrectomy and 2/3 removal of the contralateral kidney in rats, hypertension, proteinuria, and progressive decline in GFR ensue. Pathologic examination of the remaining tissue exhibits hyperfiltration injury, as evidenced by glomerular hypertrophy and focal segmental glomerular sclerosis (FSGS). The process occurs at a linear rate in proportion to the greater reduction in kidney mass. Micropuncture techniques reveal an increase in renal plasma flow and hyperfiltration of the remaining nephrons. Systemic and glomerular hypertension, from activation of the renin-angiotensin-aldosterone system (RAAS), causes progressive glomerular damage and proteinuria. As a result of these changes, efferent arteriolar tone increases more than afferent tone. This net efferent vasoconstriction increases intraglomerular and filtration pressure further, perpetuating hyperfiltration injury. Animal models of other primary kidney diseases, such as that of diabetic nephropathy in the rat, reveal similar pathophysiologic changes of glomerular hypertension, hypertrophy, and hyperfiltration.

These maladaptive hemodynamic effects are mediated by the RAAS (Figs. 51.2 and 51.3). With nephron loss, adaptation leads to release of renin from the juxtaglomerular apparatus because of decreased perfusion pressure and low solute delivery to the macula densa. Renin converts angiotensinogen to angiotensin I, which is converted to angiotensin II (AII) under the influence of angiotensin converting enzyme (ACE). AII, in addition to increasing aldosterone production from the adrenal gland, is the main perpetrator of glomerular hemodynamic maladaptation. Through an increase in sympathetic activity, AII is a potent vasoconstrictor, especially predominant in the efferent arterioles. It also exhibits a role in salt and water retention, both directly through proximal tubular sodium reabsorption and indirectly through aldosterone-dependent distal sodium reabsorption. Finally, it stimulates the posterior pituitary to release antidiuretic hormone (ADH).

The net effect of all these mechanisms is an integral component of autoregulation, helping to maintain GFR when perfusion is decreased. However, in the setting of nephron loss through a primary kidney insult or CKD, the effect of continuous AII overactivity is perpetual maladaptation by creating systemic and, notably, glomerular hypertension. This glomerular hypertension increases the filtration fraction, increases the radius of the pores in the glomerular basement membrane (GBM) through an increase in hydrostatic pressure, and eventually results in clinical proteinuria and glomerular destruction.

Box 51.1   Important Characteristics of Chronic Kidney Disease

1. Chronic kidney disease (CKD) is currently defined by a reduction in glomerular filtration rate over a period of time or evidence of kidney damage.
2. The most commonly reported causes of CKD are diabetes mellitus and hypertension, and less frequent causes are primary glomerular, tubulointerstitial, and cystic diseases.
3. The pathophysiology of chronic kidney damage is related to the underlying disease, but it is accelerated by glomerular hypertension, systemic hypertension, inflammation, and fibrosis.
4. Risk factors for progression are hypertension, proteinuria, and recurrent acute kidney injury.
5. Treatment for CKD is disease specific, but several generalized methods can be applied to almost all kidney diseases. The goal is slowing or reversing progression with therapies aimed at correcting the pathophysiologic patterns. These involve blocking the renin-angiotensin-aldosterone system (RAAS) with medications, controlling blood pressure, and reducing albuminuria when present. This goal is attempted while also targeting cardiovascular risk reduction. Novel methods, which require further study, involve attacking the inflammatory and fibrotic effects of the pathophysiology.

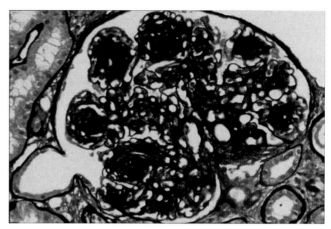

Fig. 51.1 Glomerulus from a patient with overt diabetic nephropathy, termed "The Face of the Enemy" by Dr. Edmund J. Lewis. There is marked expansion with nodular glomerular sclerosis, consistent with Kimmelstiel-Wilson nodules. Note the hypertrophied glomerulus, prominent mesangium, and aneurysmal features of the capillary walls, giving the appearance of a daisy flower (methenamine silver stain; magnification ×230).

Table 51.1   Frequency of Reported Primary Disease Causing End-Stage Renal Disease

Disease	Percentage (%)
Diabetes mellitus type 1	3.9
Diabetes mellitus type 2	41.0
Hypertension	27.2
Primary glomerulonephritis	8.2
Tubulointerstitial	3.6
Hereditary or cystic	3.1
Secondary glomerulonephritis or vasculitis	2.1
Neoplasm or plasma cell dyscrasias	2.1
Miscellaneous	4.6
Unknown	5.2

The best example of a human model of decreased nephron mass or number is unilateral renal agenesis. Ashley and Mostofi originally reported 232 patients with unilateral renal agenesis in the 1960s, and, although the pathology was not described, 16% of the patients died from kidney failure. Later, in the 1980s, autopsy series and case series confirmed the association of unilateral renal agenesis with hypertension, proteinuria, progressive kidney disease, glomerulomegaly, and FSGS (Fig. 51.4). Besides renal agenesis, another human example is the condition known as oligomeganephronia. This is a form of congenital renal hypoplasia in which the number of nephrons is reduced. The glomeruli hypertrophy in compensation for the reduced nephron number. The sequelae of this include hypertension, proteinuria, and FSGS related to hyperfiltration and progressive kidney failure. Other

clinical human examples of disease that support this mechanism of kidney injury include obesity-related glomerulomegaly and nephropathy, dysplastic solitary kidney, or partial nephrectomy in the setting of a solitary kidney.

Because animal models and human congenital diseases of reduced nephron mass lead to hemodynamic maladaptation and morphologic evidence of FSGS, it is natural to speculate that a transplant donor would be at risk for this same pathophysiology. Fortunately, the development of hypertension or kidney damage in the remaining kidney in transplant donors is infrequent. This may reflect extensive screening of potential donors, resulting in a sufficiently healthy population with minimal vascular disease, such that the donor can readily compensate for a 50% reduction in kidney mass. Similar results are seen in experimental models where adult rats with unilateral nephrectomy rarely develop hypertension or kidney disease; however, when a single kidney is removed from immature rats, the glomerular lesion FSGS manifests in the remaining kidney. Therefore hemodynamic injury may be present or clinically apparent only when the kidney is undergoing normal growth. Another explanation of this benign clinical course in patients donating a kidney is that the development of clinical pathology is directly linked to the length of time and degree of reduction of nephron mass. Indeed, there are studies demonstrating an increased risk for hypertension, proteinuria, and progressive kidney disease in patients who have more than a 50% reduction in kidney mass, such as those with bilateral partial nephrectomy for carcinoma, and a greater likelihood of progressive kidney disease with a longer duration of nephron mass reduction.

NONHEMODYNAMIC INJURY

Besides the hemodynamic effects of systemic vasoconstriction, sodium retention, and efferent arteriolar vasoconstriction, activation of the RAAS leads to several nonhemodynamic maladaptive pathways (see Fig. 51.2), which in turn result

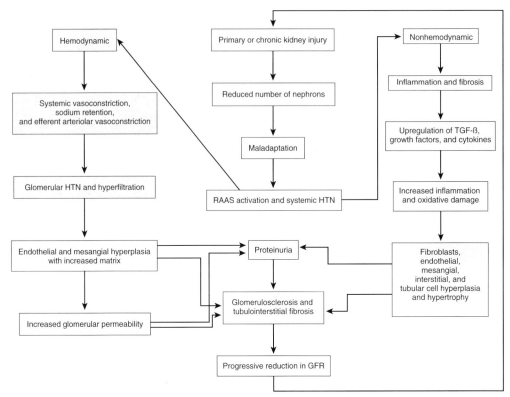

Fig. 51.2 Schematic diagram of the pathogenesis of progressive chronic kidney disease. After a primary or chronic injury occurs, activation of the renin-angiotensin-aldosterone system leads to hemodynamic and nonhemodynamic injury. *GFR,* Glomerular filtration rate; *HTN,* hypertension; *RAAS,* renin-angiotensin-aldosterone system; *TGF-β,* transforming growth factor-β.

in inflammation and fibrosis. AII has been demonstrated in high concentrations in virtually every compartment of the kidney in CKD, including the mesangial cells, endothelial cells, podocytes, the urinary space (Bowman capsule), and the tubulointerstitium.

Activation of the RAAS eventually results in fibrosis and a progressive decline in GFR. This fibrosis manifests with up regulation of several growth factors and their receptors, such as connective tissue growth factor (CTGF), epidermal growth factor (EGF), insulin-like growth factor-1 (IGF-1), platelet-derived growth factor (PDGF), vascular endothelial growth factor (VEGF), transforming growth factor-β (TGF-β), and monocyte chemotactic protein-1 (MCP-1). The activation of these factors by AII and aldosterone leads to cellular proliferation and hypertrophy of glomerular endothelial cells, mesangial cells, podocytes, tubulointerstitial cells, and fibroblasts. AII and TGF-β also upregulate other factors that lead to the overproduction of extracellular matrix, such as type 1 procollagen, plasminogen activator inhibitor 1, and fibronectin. In addition, excess adhesion molecules, such as integrins or vascular cellular adhesion molecule 1, allow the increased extracellular matrix and hypercellularity to accumulate and persist. This leads to cell proliferation, extracellular matrix accumulation, adhesion of these cells, and functional changes with eventual fibrosis (Fig. 51.5).

Inflammation is also a key component in the progression of kidney disease (see Fig. 51.2). This may seem obvious in diseases in which inflammation is the primary insult, such as postinfectious glomerulonephritis or severe lupus nephritis,

because it is apparent by light microscopy of kidney biopsy specimens. However, inflammation is an important factor in the progression of almost all types of kidney diseases and is mediated in part by the RAAS. AII recruits T cells and macrophages by stimulating endothelin-1 (ET-1) and increases production of nuclear factor κ–light-chain enhancer of activated B cells (NF-κB); these molecules release cytokines, creating more inflammation. Increased expression of TGF-β also induces cellular recruitment. Finally, free radical oxygen species lead to additional injury, which enables further inflammation and fibrosis.

Experimental evidence also supports the idea that proteinuria itself contributes to progressive nephrosclerosis. Through hyperfiltration, the increased glomerular permeability to albumin allows reabsorption of more albuminuria by the proximal tubular cells. Experimental models show that when this protein becomes prevalent in the interstitium, macrophages and inflammatory mediators, such as ET-1, MCP-1, and other chemokines, are upregulated, which eventually leads to inflammation and subsequent tubulointerstitial and glomerular fibrosis.

Through primary stimulation of the RAAS, predominantly through TGF-β, a cascade of events occurs that begins with inflammation, is perpetuated by accumulation of cells and matrix, is exacerbated by adhesion and persistence of these cells and matrix, and ends with injury, glomerulosclerosis, and tubulointerstitial fibrosis (see Fig. 51.2). This creates a progressive course of CKD, proteinuria, GFR loss, and a vicious cycle of continuous RAAS activation.

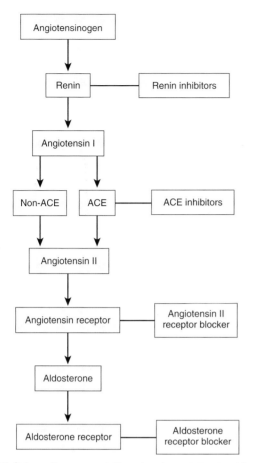

Fig. 51.3 Schematic representation of renin-angiotensin-aldosterone activation and targeted therapies that interrupt the pathway. *ACE,* Angiotensin-converting enzyme.

RISK FACTORS FOR PROGRESSION

Risk factors for progression include nonmodifiable characteristics such as older age, male sex, and black race. One study of younger patients with CKD estimated the lifetime risk for ESRD for a 20-year-old person to be 7.8% for black women, 7.3% for black men, 1.8% for white women, and 2.5% for white men. Conversely, other risk factors such as hypertension, proteinuria, and recurrent acute kidney injury (AKI) are all potentially modifiable and deserve attention (Box 51.2).

By means of increased activity of the RAAS with vasoconstriction and sodium retention, hypertension continues the cycle of progressive CKD. In patients who have diabetic nephropathy from type 2 diabetes mellitus (DM), the most common cause of CKD, elevated blood pressure, is a clear risk factor for a progressive decline in GFR and, notably, treating this hypertension reduces this progression. The effect of therapy is even more pronounced in this patient population when treatment is with angiotensin receptor blockade (Fig. 51.6). Early in the 1980s, Mogensen established that in patients with diabetic nephropathy, treating elevated blood pressure (mean 162/103 mm Hg) to an achieved level of 144/95 mm Hg reduced the rate of GFR loss from 1.23 mL/min per month to 0.49 mL/min per month. Since that time, other observational studies and well-designed clinical trials have demonstrated that hypertension is clearly a risk factor for ESRD in diabetic nephropathy, and that blood pressure reduction, especially with RAAS blockade, attenuates this risk.

Hypertension is also an established risk factor for progression of nondiabetic kidney disease. The Multiple Risk Factor Intervention Trial (MRFIT), which used various interventions to treat patients with multiple cardiovascular risk factors, such

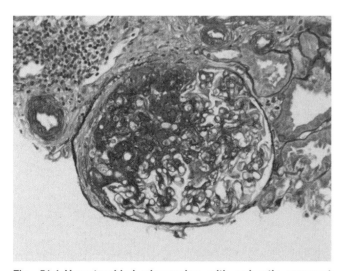

Fig. 51.4 Hypertrophied glomerulus with sclerotic segment encompassing almost 50% of the glomerular surface area from a patient with unilateral dysplastic kidney, hypertension, and proteinuria. The uninvolved segment of the glomerulus has patent capillaries and normal architecture. The glomerular diameter was measured to be 270 μm (periodic acid–Schiff stain; magnification ×230). Normal glomerular diameter is 144 ± 11 μm.

Box 51.2   Risk Factors for the Development or Progression of Kidney Disease

Albuminuria
Hypertension
Episodes of acute kidney injury
Underlying cause of kidney disease (e.g., diabetic nephropathy)
Obesity
Hyperlipidemia
Smoking
High-protein diet
Metabolic acidosis
Hyperphosphatemia
Hyperuricemia
Hyperglycemia
Elevated plasma soluble urokinase receptor (suPAR)
APOL1 alleles
Black or Native American race
Male sex
Older age
Family history of DM, CKD, or ESRD
Low birth weight

CKD, Chronic kidney disease; *DM,* diabetes mellitus.

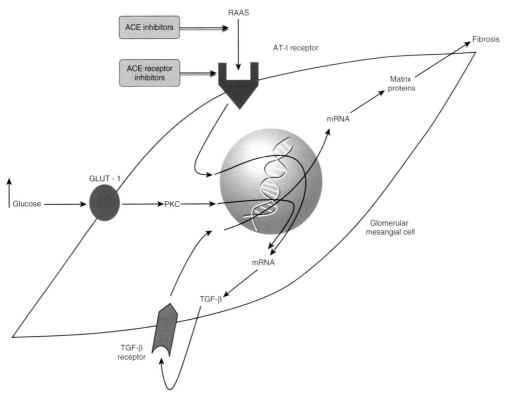

Fig. 51.5 Schematic representation of a glomerular mesangial cell in chronic kidney disease due to diabetic nephropathy. Activation of renin-angiotensin-aldosterone system upregulates TGF-β, which leads to matrix accumulation, inflammation, and fibrosis. Hyperglycemia also perpetuates this fibrosis via increased activity of protein kinase C. Through interruption of this cascade, angiotensin-converting enzyme inhibitors and angiotensin receptor blockers are effective treatments, delaying progression of chronic kidney disease in diabetic nephropathy. *ACE*, Angiotensin-converting enzyme; *AT-I*, angiotensin I; *GLUT-1*, glucose transporter; *mRNA*, messenger ribonucleic acid; *PKC*, protein kinase C; *RAAS*, renin-angiotensin-aldosterone system; *TGF-β*, transforming growth factor-β.

as smoking, hypertension, obesity, and hyperlipidemia, demonstrated that elevated blood pressure was an independent risk factor for the development of kidney failure. Other studies of nondiabetic kidney disease, such as the African American Study of Kidney Disease (AASK), reveal a similar pattern, indicating that patients with nondiabetic CKD benefited from a lower achieved blood pressure, especially if proteinuria was present. Similarly, observational studies suggest slower progression in patients with other causes of CKD, such as polycystic kidney disease, when blood pressure is controlled.

Albuminuria is another well-established risk factor for progression of CKD. In patients with overt diabetic nephropathy, the degree of baseline albuminuria is directly correlated with a more rapid decline in GFR (Fig. 51.7). This is also true in nondiabetic kidney diseases, such as IgA nephropathy or lupus nephritis. In the Modification of Diet in Renal Disease (MDRD) study, which is a population that is predominantly nondiabetic, those with albuminuria had the highest risk for progressive kidney disease. The Ramipril Efficacy in Nephropathy (REIN) study similarly noted that, in nondiabetic CKD, the baseline level of albuminuria was the strongest predictor of kidney failure, independent of the baseline GFR. Even in patients with earlier stages of CKD, with an estimated GFR of greater than 60 mL/min per 1.73 m², those that demonstrate albuminuria by ≥2+ on dipstick or greater than 300 mg albumin/g of creatinine are over 3 times more likely to double the serum creatinine over

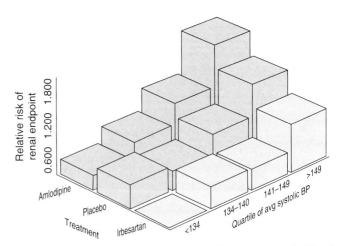

Fig. 51.6 Simultaneous impact to quartile of achieved systolic blood pressure and treatment modality on the relative risk for reaching a kidney endpoint (doubling of baseline serum creatinine or ESRD, defined as serum creatinine ≥6.0 mg/dL or renal replacement therapy). avg, Average; BP, blood pressure. (Reproduced with permission from Pohl MA, Blumenthal S, Cordonnier DJ, et al. Independent and additive impact of blood pressure control and angiotensin II receptor blockade on renal outcomes in the irbesartan diabetic nephropathy trial: clinical implications and limitations. *J Am Soc Nephrol.* 2005;16:3031.)

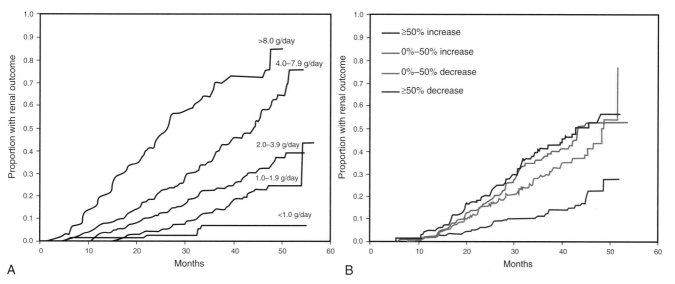

Fig. 51.7 (A) Kaplan-Meier analysis of doubling of a baseline serum creatinine level, serum creatinine level of ≥6.0 mg/dL, or the development of ESRD by baseline proteinuria values. (B) Kaplan-Meier analysis of doubling of a baseline serum creatinine level, serum creatinine level of ≥6.0 mg/dL, or the development of ESRD by level of proteinuria change in the first 12 months. (Reproduced from Atkins RC, Briganti EM, Lewis JB, et al. Proteinuria reduction and progression to renal failure in patients with type 2 diabetes mellitus and overt nephropathy. *Am J Kidney Dis.* 2005;45:283.)

time compared with those with lower levels (30 to 300 mg albumin/g creatinine). This trend is also true when comparing patients who have 30 to 300 mg albumin/g with those who have less than 30 mg/g.

Despite these robust data, controversy exists as to whether albuminuria is truly a pathogenic risk factor or just a marker of kidney disease severity. If albuminuria were a simple manifestation of advanced disease, such as a cough in the setting of pneumonia, then treating the symptom would have minimal to no effect on improving the disease outcome. However, targeting and reducing albuminuria is highly effective at improving kidney outcomes, both in diabetic (see Fig. 51.7) and nondiabetic kidney diseases.

The idea that recurrent or episodic AKI leads to progressive chronic kidney dysfunction is sound based on the pathophysiology of the disease (see Fig. 51.2). Multiple studies have now shown that in patients with preexisting CKD, AKI is a risk factor for the development of chronic kidney failure. The degree of preexisting CKD, severity of AKI, advanced age, presence of DM, and low serum albumin amplify this risk. In a retrospective study by Ishani et al., the hazard ratio of developing ESRD for older adult patients (>67 years) who had CKD without AKI was 8.4, whereas for those patients who had CKD and AKI, the hazard ratio for progressing to ESRD was 41.2.

Knowledge that AKI affects CKD is important so that future therapies can be developed and evaluated in an attempt to retard this progression. It is also relevant at present, as minimizing episodes of iatrogenic AKI in CKD patients can often be achieved. It is sensible to avoid, if possible, situations that may cause AKI, such as iatrogenic hypotension or nephrotoxic injury from polypharmacy, iodinated contrast exposure, atheroemboli, and nonsteroidal antiinflammatory agents in vulnerable patients.

Many other factors have been associated with a progressive decline in GFR (see Box 51.2). The primary kidney disease affects the rate of progression, as glomerular diseases and polycystic kidney diseases tend to progress faster than most tubulointerstitial diseases. Evidence exists for the APOL1 genetic mutations as not only a cause of CKD, but also a factor for progression. Elevated levels of the soluble urokinase-type plasminogen activator receptor (suPAR) have also been linked to the development and progression of CKD. Although evidence establishing hyperlipidemia, tobacco dependence, or obesity as risk factors is not as robust as that pointing to hypertension or proteinuria, these associations do exist, and targeting these risk factors when present is prudent.

TREATMENT AND PREVENTION OF CHRONIC KIDNEY DISEASE PROGRESSION

Based on the underlying pathophysiology, therapies have been developed and studied in an attempt to safely slow or reverse the vicious cycle of RAAS activation, glomerular hypertension, systemic hypertension, proteinuria, inflammation, and progressive fibrosis (Table 51.2). In addition, therapies have targeted other clinically modifiable risk factors, all with the goal of safely reducing or reversing the progression of CKD.

ANTAGONISM OF THE RENIN-ANGIOTENSIN-ALDOSTERONE SYSTEM

Based on the animal models of 5/6 nephrectomy and diabetic glomerulosclerosis, it is plausible that interruption of the RAAS cascade (see Fig. 51.3) could lead to renoprotection. In animal models, AII selectively causes hemodynamic-mediated injury through efferent arteriolar vasoconstriction, whereas the use of ACE inhibitors and angiotensin receptor blockers (ARBs) effectively dilates the efferent arteriole, leading to glomerular relaxation and subsequent reduction in glomerular hypertrophy and injury (Fig. 51.8). RAAS blockade also mediates improvements in systemic hypertension, which further reduces glomerular hypertension. In addition to the hemodynamic

Table 51.2 Therapies for Slowing Progression of Chronic Kidney Disease

Proven Benefit	Preliminary Evidence
Angiotensin-converting enzyme inhibitors	Aldosterone receptor antagonists
Angiotensin receptor antagonists	Renin inhibitors
	Dietary measures
	Exercise
Blood pressure goal between 120 and 140 mm Hg systolic and 80 and 90 mm Hg diastolic	Weight loss in obesity
	Smoking cessation
	Glycemic control in diabetes mellitus
	Empagliflozin
	Reduction of hyperuricemia, hyperlipidemia, hyperphosphatemia, albuminuria
	Folate
	Vitamin D
	Acid-base balance
	Endothelin-1 antagonists
	Pirfenidone
	Inhibitors of advanced glycation end products

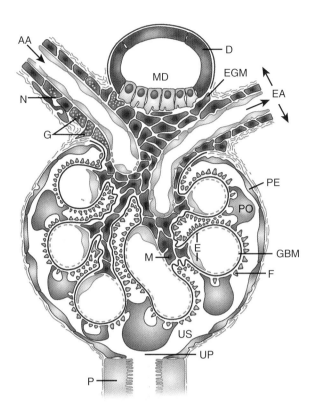

Fig. 51.8 Schematic representation of glomerular hemodynamic changes with blockade of the renin-angiotensin-aldosterone system. Angiotensin-converting enzyme inhibitors and angiotensin receptor blockers blunt the intrarenal arteriolar effects of angiotensin II, which leads to net dilation of the efferent arteriole (EA) *(black arrows)* and reduction in glomerular hypertension. This reduction in glomerular capillary pressure reduces glomerular hyperpermeability, leading to reduced urinary protein excretion and renoprotection. *AA,* Afferent arteriole; *D,* distal tubule; *E,* endothelial cell; *EGM,* extraglomerular mesangial cell; *F,* foot process; *G,* juxtaglomerular granular cell; *GBM,* glomerular basement membrane; *M,* mesangial cell; *MD,* macula densa; *N,* sympathetic nerve endings; *P,* proximal tubule; *PE,* parietal epithelial cell; *PO,* epithelial podocyte; *UP,* urinary pole; *US,* urinary space.

reduction in glomerular damage, blockade of the RAAS in animals has been shown to impair the inflammatory and fibrosing effects of the various cytokines, including TGF-β. The net effect of RAAS antagonism is therefore renoprotective on multiple levels: hemodynamic, antifibrotic, and antiproteinuric.

Lewis and colleagues tested the hypothesis that this could lead to renoprotection in humans in 1993. In a randomized controlled clinical trial, 409 patients with overt type 1 diabetic nephropathy received either the ACE inhibitor captopril or placebo with achievement of equivalent systemic blood pressures between the two groups. This study found a dramatic 43% reduction in the doubling of the serum creatinine and a significant reduction in the time to death, dialysis, or transplantation with captopril compared with placebo. Thus for the first time in human patients, ACE inhibitors established renoprotection by slowing progressive CKD independent of lowering blood pressure and clinical remission in advanced diabetic nephropathy.

RAAS blockade has also been evaluated in type 2 diabetic nephropathy. In the Irbesartan for Microalbuminuria in Type 2 Diabetes (IRMA-2) trial of patients with type 2 DM, preserved GFR, and low-level albuminuria, irbesartan was more effective at reducing the progression to overt proteinuria from low-level albuminuria than placebo at identical blood pressure levels. Two large randomized studies subsequently validated the use of ARBs in overt type 2 diabetic nephropathy. In the Irbesartan Diabetic Nephropathy Trial (IDNT), 1715 hypertensive patients with overt diabetic nephropathy (median baseline serum creatinine 1.67 mg/dL; median baseline urine protein excretion 2.9 g/24 hours) were randomized to receive one of three different treatment regimens: irbesartan 300 mg daily, the calcium channel blocker amlodipine 10 mg daily, or placebo. The achieved blood pressure was not different among the three groups. With irbesartan, the risk for reaching the composite endpoint of doubling of the serum creatinine, ESRD, or death was 20% lower when compared with placebo and 23% lower compared with amlodipine. In addition to use of the ARB, lower systolic blood pressure was also associated with a decreased relative risk in doubling of the serum creatinine or ESRD (see Fig. 51.6). Analogous results were demonstrated with the ARB losartan in the Reduction in Endpoints in non–insulin-dependent diabetes mellitus (NIDDM) with the Angiotensin-II Antagonist Losartan (RENAAL) trial. In this randomized controlled trial, 1513 patients with overt type 2 diabetic nephropathy were randomized to receive either losartan or placebo. Once again, both groups achieved equivalent blood pressure levels, with losartan reducing the incidence of doubling of the serum creatinine by 25% and the risk for ESRD by 28%. In both trials, there was a significant reduction in albuminuria with use of the ARB. Given the nearly identical results, these trials provide remarkable support for the use of ARBs for renoprotection in overt diabetic nephropathy.

In addition to systemic and glomerular hypertension, albuminuria is also reduced in patients with diabetic nephropathy treated with RAAS blockade. In both IDNT and RENAAL, baseline albuminuria was directly correlated with the risk of doubling of the serum creatinine or ESRD. More important, those patients who had a decrease in albuminuria experienced improved kidney outcomes (see Fig. 51.7), emphasizing that albuminuria may be an independent risk factor to the development of progressive kidney disease and suggesting that reducing albuminuria might be an appropriate surrogate target for an overall benefit in kidney outcomes.

Similar results are seen in nondiabetic kidney disease, where a meta-analysis by Jafar and colleagues demonstrated that RAAS inhibition slows progression, particularly in individuals with proteinuria exceeding 1000 mg/day. To confirm this finding, investigators for the REIN trial randomized 352 patients with hypertension and albuminuria but without diabetic nephropathy to receive either the ACE inhibitor ramipril or conventional antihypertensive therapy, achieving identical blood pressure control in both groups. Notably, patients randomized to receive ramipril had a 50% lower risk for progression to ESRD during the 3 years of follow-up. Similar to prior findings, patients who had greater degrees of albuminuria and received ramipril had a slower decline in GFR compared with patients receiving conventional antihypertensive therapy.

In nonproteinuric and nondiabetic nephropathy, the data for use of RAAS blockade are not as strong. Primarily in black patients with kidney disease previously attributed to "hypertensive nephrosclerosis," those without albuminuria have failed to show independent renoprotection with RAAS blockade. The mechanism of progression is linked to APOL1 genetic mutations and the development of focal and global glomerulosclerosis. Treatments targeting this specific mechanism are an area of future research.

In summary, clinical trial data reveal that inhibition of the RAAS with ACE inhibitors or ARBs provides the strongest renoprotection available to date, especially in patients with diabetic nephropathy or proteinuric CKD not due to DM, and these agents should be first-line therapy in these clinical settings. Critically, advanced CKD does not preclude their use.

The question that naturally follows is whether additive or dual blockade would provide synergistic renoprotection. Most of the trials performed with dual blockade with use of ACE inhibitors, ARBs, renin inhibitors, or aldosterone antagonists have broadly demonstrated reduction in albuminuria. However, despite the improvement in albuminuria, these trials have not demonstrated a benefit of dual therapy on "hard" outcomes, such as a decrease in the rate of decline of GFR or a decrease in the incidence of kidney failure, and have been associated with adverse events such as hyperkalemia, hypotension, and AKI. Currently, dual blockade of the RAAS is not recommended, and it may incur harm, particularly in individuals with diabetic nephropathy or in those without substantial albuminuria. In addition, care must be taken to monitor and treat the potential development of hyperkalemia when using any agent to block the RAAS. Because many of these patients have a decreased GFR and a reduced capacity to excrete potassium, blocking the RAAS at multiple sites may contribute to hyperkalemia; accordingly, it is prudent to check the serum potassium 7 to 14 days after initiating or modifying therapy with these agents. Gastrointestinal cation exchangers, such as patiromer, sodium polystyrene sulfonate, or zirconium cyclosilicate, are of particular importance to

help control hyperkalemia, because they can allow for uninterrupted RAAS blockade in advancing CKD.

BLOOD PRESSURE CONTROL

Blockade of the RAAS exerts its beneficial effect by reducing glomerular hypertension while simultaneously reducing systemic blood pressure. This clearly makes them first-line agents in most patients with hypertension, albuminuria, and CKD. Observational studies and randomized controlled trials have shown that lowering blood pressure in patients with hypertension and CKD slows the rate of disease progression. However, the ideal goal blood pressure in patients with CKD remains controversial. Guidelines suggest the target of less than 140/90 mm Hg for patients with CKD or DM. Notably, blood pressure control often requires at least two to four antihypertensive medications, including an agent to block the RAAS and usually a diuretic.

Previous guidelines had recommended a lower goal (<130/80) based on several studies revealing that "intensive" blood pressure control has substantial benefits in CKD for the treatment of nephropathy and/or cardiovascular disease. But how far should blood pressure be lowered, and is there a detrimental effect in lowering blood pressure too much in patients with CKD? This concern was raised in 1988, when the concept of the "J-curve" was introduced. The J-curve implies that lowering blood pressure reduces cardiovascular disease and death to a point, below which a plateau is achieved where lower blood pressure no longer confers a benefit and may result in increased risk for adverse events. A post hoc analysis of the IDNT trial described the J-curve in diabetic nephropathy: worse outcomes were seen in patients with overt diabetic nephropathy at both high and very low systolic blood pressures. The lowest risk for kidney outcomes was seen at achieved systolic blood pressures between 120 and 130 mm Hg, and the risk for death was increased below an achieved systolic blood pressure of 120 mm Hg. In 2010, investigators for the Action to Control Cardiovascular Risks in Diabetes (ACCORD) trial reported the results of a trial consisting of 4733 patients with type 2 DM, relatively preserved kidney function (serum creatinine ≤1.5 mg/dL), and either increased cardiovascular disease risk or a history of cardiovascular disease. These patients were randomized to an intensive systolic blood pressure goal of less than 120 mm Hg compared with a systolic blood pressure goal of less than 140 mm Hg. The achieved blood pressure in the intensive group was 119/64 mm Hg, while in the standard control group, it was 134/71 mm Hg. Over an average follow-up of nearly 5 years, there was no difference in cardiovascular disease or stroke between the two groups; however, the intensive therapy group demonstrated more hypotension, higher serum creatinine, and lower estimated GFR, as well as a tenfold higher rate of hyperkalemia, suggesting that the beneficial effects of hypertension treatment reach a plateau somewhere between a systolic blood pressure of 120 and 140 mm Hg.

Evidence for a plateau also exists in patients without diabetic nephropathy based on data from the AASK trial, where there was no difference in outcomes, including doubling of serum creatinine, ESRD, or death in patients with the lower achieved mean arterial blood pressure (94.7 mm Hg), unless proteinuria (defined as a urine protein/creatinine ratio of >0.22 g of protein per g of creatinine) was present at baseline. More data on blood pressure goals in nondiabetic patients comes from the Systolic Blood Pressure Intervention Trial (SPRINT). Similar to the ACCORD trial, investigators randomized 9361 patients with high cardiovascular risk but without diabetes mellitus to a systolic blood pressure goal of less than 120 (intensive) versus less than 140 (standard) mm Hg. Although not designed to study hypertension in CKD specifically (mean eGFR 72 mL/min per 1.73 m^2; patients with eGFR <20 mL/min per 1.73 m^2 and/or proteinuria >1 g/d were excluded), 28% of the patients had CKD (eGFR 20 to 60 mL/min per 1.73 m^2). The trial was stopped early (mean duration 3.3 years) because of a benefit of 25% relative risk reduction in the primary outcomes of cardiovascular events, heart failure, and stroke, and a 27% relative risk reduction in mortality in the intensive blood pressure group. Although this benefit extended to patients with CKD (eGFR 20 to 60 mL/min per 1.73 m^2), there were more episodes of AKI and electrolyte abnormalities in the intensive group. In addition, the absolute risk reduction of intensive blood pressure lowering was only 0.6% (2.17% to 1.56%), leading to a large number needed to treat (NNT) of 90. Therefore in patients without diabetic nephropathy who have nonproteinuric mild to moderate CKD, evidence to target a lower systolic blood pressure goal exists, taking care to monitor for AKI and electrolyte abnormalities.

However, at the present time, lowering blood pressure to less than 120/80 mm Hg in patients with proteinuric CKD or diabetic nephropathy with pharmacologic therapy is not warranted. Consistent blood pressures above 140/90 mm Hg should be treated, and the first-line agent in people with diabetes or with proteinuria should be an ACE inhibitor or ARB. The exact blood pressure goal in patients with CKD remains controversial, but the present guideline of less than 140/90 mm Hg for patients with diabetic nephropathy and/or proteinuria is reasonable.

LIFESTYLE MODIFICATION

Based on the pathophysiology for acute and CKD, glomerular hyperfiltration due to altered hemodynamics plays a role. Theoretically, decreasing elevated intraglomerular pressure by any means may have a benefit. Dietary protein restriction is a proposed method, and in the animal model of 5/6 nephrectomy, dietary protein restriction demonstrated reduced kidney injury by decreasing afferent arteriolar vasodilation, glomerular hypertension, and oncotic pressure. Unfortunately, contrary to RAAS blockade, human studies on dietary protein restriction have not shown substantial benefits of renoprotection.

The current recommended diet for people with diabetes, consisting of low sodium, low fat, and moderately low protein with high fiber, has been shown to decrease blood pressure in patients with hypertension and type 2 DM in the absence of CKD or albuminuria. Based on available evidence, a prudent diet for a patient with CKD is to limit protein intake to approximately 0.8 to 1.0 g/kg of body weight per day and to limit dietary sodium to less than 2.4 g a day. This is discussed in further detail in Chapter 53. In addition, as discussed in Chapter 26, control of blood glucose levels in patients who have DM is important to reduce microvascular and cardiovascular complications, although few data support intensive glycemic control for reducing the rate of GFR

decline in patients with diabetic nephropathy. The method of glucose control may also be important for progressive diabetic nephropathy. Empagliflozin, which exerts its glucose-lowering effects by inducing glycosuria, has been shown to lower blood pressure and weight and delay progression of CKD compared to placebo.

Obesity and obesity-related glomerulopathy are increasing in prevalence. Obesity is a risk factor for developing CKD, and in patients with CKD, obesity is a risk factor for progression. Preexisting albuminuria is exacerbated by weight gain and decreases with weight loss; in addition, patients achieving sustained weight loss with bariatric surgery have a slower decline in eGFR over time compared to those who have not lost weight. These findings fit well into the model of hyperfiltration and glomerular hypertension with subsequent albuminuria and provide evidence that intervention can be renoprotective.

Hyperlipidemia, similar to obesity, may be a modifiable risk factor to slow progressive CKD. Hyperlipidemia may contribute to CKD progression through proinflammatory and profibrotic mechanisms because low-density lipoproteins (LDL) have these properties. Animal models reveal that rats fed high-cholesterol diets exhibit a greater degree of glomerulosclerosis and interstitial disease compared with those fed a low-cholesterol diet. In the same animal models, 3-hydroxy-3-methyl-glutaryl-CoA reductase inhibitors (statins) have been shown to limit inflammatory cytokines and adhesion molecules and slow the rate of GFR loss. Observational studies in humans also support this hypothesis; however, unlike blockade of the RAAS, human clinical trials investigating the use of statin therapy to decrease the progression of CKD have been discouraging. In the Study of Heart and Renal Protection (SHARP) trial, 6247 patients with moderate to severe CKD were randomized to receive a statin and ezetimibe or placebo, and although there was a cardiovascular benefit, no difference was seen in the development of kidney failure in the active therapy arm.

ALBUMINURIA REDUCTION

As noted earlier, in patients with or without reduced GFR, albuminuria is an independent risk factor for progressive kidney injury, and there is some evidence that reductions in albuminuria lead to better kidney and cardiovascular outcomes. Therefore reducing proteinuria to the lowest possible amount would seem beneficial. However, in one study in which patients with vascular disease or high-risk DM were randomized to receive either the ARB telmisartan or the ACE inhibitor ramipril, or both, combination therapy reduced albuminuria to a greater degree than solitary therapy, but it was associated with a greater decline in estimated GFR. In another study of overt diabetic nephropathy, the renin inhibitor aliskiren was found to lower albuminuria to a greater degree when used in combination with losartan compared with losartan alone; however, a follow-up study of dual therapy with aliskiren and valsartan was halted early because of increased risk for stroke, kidney complications, hyperkalemia, and hypotension in the dual therapy group. Therefore although patients who achieve lower levels of albuminuria have better clinical outcomes than those who do not, it is unknown whether therapies that specifically target lower albuminuria per se (such as blocking the RAAS system at multiple different sites; see Fig. 51.3) is beneficial. Thus, dual therapy, especially in diabetic nephropathy, is not recommended.

Notably, the severity of albuminuria may be helpful in defining optimal blood pressure goals. Nondiabetic patients in the MDRD trial, the AASK trial, and the REIN trial with higher levels of proteinuria had a greater benefit from a lower blood pressure goal. In the REIN study, the beneficial effect in the intensive blood pressure arm was more pronounced with use of ACE inhibitors.

NOVEL METHODS

Novel therapies attempting to reduce the progression of CKD exist; these target the inflammatory and/or fibrotic effects that occur in the pathophysiology of CKD progression. Pirfenidone is an agent that acts on the fibrosing pathway of CKD, and has beneficial effects in animal models of CKD and diabetic nephropathy. However, positive, large, long-term human clinical trials showing a reduction in the progression of CKD have not yet been completed. Endothelin antagonists are another promising area for the future as ET-1 contributes to kidney damage via both vasoconstrictive properties and promotion of interstitial fibrosis. Animal models have demonstrated a benefit of endothelin antagonists with a reduction in proteinuria and improvement in creatinine clearance. At present, positive safety and efficacy data from clinical trials evaluating these agents is lacking.

Another novel medication, pyridoxamine, exerts its effect through antioxidant properties and impairment in advanced glycation end products (AGEs). Pyridoxamine has been evaluated in a multicenter randomized controlled trial of patients with overt diabetic nephropathy. In that trial, the drug failed to reduce GFR loss at 1 year, but there was a stabilization noted in the group of patients with the most preserved baseline kidney function. Sulodexide, a glycosaminoglycan, was rigorously tested in clinical trials of patients with diabetic nephropathy and failed to show a benefit. Bardoxolone methyl, an activator of nuclear 1 factor (erythroid derived 2)–related factor 2 (Nrf2), showed a reduction in serum creatinine over a 1-year period in humans, but unfortunately it was associated with more cardiovascular events in a randomized controlled trial.

Treatment of hyperuricemia, hyperphosphatemia, hyperhomocysteinemia, and folate and vitamin D deficiency, and maintaining appropriate acid-base balance with sodium bicarbonate therapy have been shown in observational studies and/or small clinical trials to be associated with a reduction in albuminuria and/or the progression of CKD. In a large population in China, in an area without folic acid fortification, administration of folate with the ACE-I enalapril was found to slow the rate of eGFR decline compared to enalapril alone. These therapies may hold promise for the future, but validated long-term controlled trials are currently lacking.

CARDIOVASCULAR RISK REDUCTION

The leading cause of death in patients with CKD is cardiovascular disease. Hypertension, sodium and volume retention, anemia, hyperphosphatemia, high prevalence of DM and vascular disease, and electrolyte disturbances including hyperkalemia are all reported risk factors to this effect. Consequently, it is prudent to reduce this risk with lifestyle modifications, smoking cessation, use of aspirin, and pharmacologic therapy for hypertension, dyslipidemia, albuminuria, and hyperglycemia (when present), because there appears to be synergy between the development and progression of cardiovascular disease and the development and progression of CKD.

CONCLUSION

The pathophysiology of CKD is largely dependent on the primary insult, but common pathways exist across almost all subsets of kidney disorders. These include hemodynamic-mediated hyperfiltration and eventual nephron loss and inflammatory and cellular-mediated fibrosis. Much of the pathophysiology arises from maladaptation to autoregulation with hyperactivation of the RAAS. Theoretically, blocking these pathways will interrupt this progression; in fact, the most robust clinical evidence for slowing or reversing the progression is with disruption of the RAAS system. Controlling blood pressure, interrupting the RAAS, avoiding AKI, and attempting cardiovascular risk reduction are important goals for the physicians treating patients with CKD. Exciting novel therapies are eagerly anticipated, but these must be tested through rigorous clinical study for safety, tolerability, and efficacy.

KEY BIBLIOGRAPHY

Brenner BM, Cooper ME, de Zeeuw D, et al. Effects of losartan on renal and cardiovascular outcomes in patients with type 2 diabetes and nephropathy. *N Engl J Med.* 2001;345:861-869.

Cushman WC, Evans GW, Byington RP, et al. Effects of intensive blood-pressure control in type 2 diabetes mellitus. *N Engl J Med.* 2010;362:1575-1585.

GISEN Group (Gruppo Italiano di Studi Epidemiologici in Nefrologia). Randomised placebo-controlled trial of effect of ramipril on decline in glomerular filtration rate and risk of terminal renal failure in proteinuric, non-diabetic nephropathy. *Lancet.* 1997;349:1857-1863.

Jafar TH, Stark PC, Schmid CH, et al. Progression of chronic kidney disease: the role of blood pressure control, proteinuria, and angiotensin-converting enzyme inhibition: a patient-level meta-analysis. *Ann Intern Med.* 2003;139:244-252.

Klahr S, Levey AS, Beck GJ, et al. The effects of dietary protein restriction and blood-pressure control on the progression of chronic renal disease. Modification of Diet in Renal Disease Study Group. *N Engl J Med.* 1994;330:877-884.

Lewis EJ, Hunsicker LG, Bain RP, Rohde RD. The effect of angiotensin-converting-enzyme inhibition on diabetic nephropathy. The Collaborative Study Group. *N Engl J Med.* 1993;329:1456-1462.

Lewis EJ, Hunsicker LG, Clarke WR, et al. Renoprotective effect of the angiotensin-receptor antagonist irbesartan in patients with nephropathy due to type 2 diabetes. *N Engl J Med.* 2001;345:851-860.

Mogensen CE. The effect of blood pressure intervention on renal function in insulin-dependent diabetes. *Diabete Metab.* 1989;15:343-351.

Parving HH, Brenner BM, McMurray JJ, et al. Cardiorenal end points in a trial of aliskiren for type 2 diabetes. *N Engl J Med.* 2012;367:2204-2213.

Parving HH, Lehnert H, Brochner-Mortensen J, Gomis R, Andersen S, Arner P. The effect of irbesartan on the development of diabetic nephropathy in patients with type 2 diabetes. *N Engl J Med.* 2001;345:870-878.

Tonelli M, Muntner P, Lloyd A, et al. Using proteinuria and estimated glomerular filtration rate to classify risk in patients with chronic kidney disease: a cohort study. *Ann Intern Med.* 2011;154:12-21.

Full bibliography can be found on www.expertconsult.com.

52

Staging and Management of Chronic Kidney Disease

Lesley A. Inker; Andrew S. Levey

Chronic kidney disease (CKD) is a growing worldwide public health problem, characterized by increasing prevalence, high cost, and poor outcomes. The poor outcomes include progression of kidney disease leading to chronic kidney failure, increased risk for acute kidney injury (AKI), cardiovascular disease (CVD), and mortality, as well as a wide variety of other complications.

In 2002 the Kidney Disease Outcomes Quality Initiative (KDOQI) of the National Kidney Foundation (NKF) sponsored guidelines for the definition, classification, evaluation, and risk stratification of CKD. The purpose of these guidelines was to create uniform terminology to improve communications among all involved in the care and management of CKD, including patients, physicians, researchers, and policy makers. The guidelines were adopted with minor modification by Kidney Disease: Improving Global Outcomes (KDIGO) in 2005. In response to controversy and accumulation of new data, KDIGO sponsored a Controversies Conference in 2009, followed by an update of the guidelines in 2012, which maintained the definition of CKD but modified the classification. Subsequent reviews by national and international guideline workgroups have endorsed maintaining the CKD definition but expressed reservations about some aspects of the classification. The goals of this chapter are to describe the conceptual model for CKD, the revised 2012 KDIGO guideline recommendations for the definition and stages of CKD, and the associated prevalence and clinical action plan, along with commentary by other national and international guideline workgroups. We also provide an overview of detection, evaluation, predicting prognosis, and management, with comments on the role of nephrologists in the care of these patients.

COURSE, DEFINITION, CLASSIFICATION, AND PREVALENCE OF CHRONIC KIDNEY DISEASE

COURSE OF CHRONIC KIDNEY DISEASE

Fig. 52.1 shows a conceptual model for CKD, and Table 52.1 outlines the outcomes. This model describes the natural history of CKD, beginning with antecedent conditions associated with increased risk for developing kidney disease, followed by the stages of CKD (kidney damage, decreased glomerular filtration rate [GFR], and kidney failure), and associated complications.

Risk factors for the development of CKD include exposure to factors that cause kidney disease, such as hypertension,

diabetes, autoimmune diseases, and kidney stones, and characteristics that increase susceptibility to kidney disease, such as older age, minority racial and ethnic status, and reduced nephron mass. The mechanisms underlying increased susceptibility have not been completely described or proven. For example, minority race or ethnicity may imply an underlying genetic tendency, or it may be a marker for lack of access to health care. Susceptibility factors may explain why a family history of kidney disease, regardless of the cause, places an individual at increased risk for development of kidney disease.

The horizontal arrows in Fig. 52.1 indicate transitions among kidney outcomes. The arrows pointing from left to right emphasize the progressive nature of CKD. However, the rate of progression is variable, and not all CKD progresses; thus not all patients with CKD develop kidney failure. Early stages of kidney disease may be reversible, and individuals with kidney failure can revert to earlier stages through kidney transplantation, shown as dashed arrowheads pointing from right to left. Studies suggest that CKD is a risk factor for development of AKI and that episodes of AKI may increase the risk for progression of CKD. The earlier stages and the risk factors for progression to later stages can be identified, permitting improvements in outcome by prevention, earlier detection, and initiation of therapies that can slow progression and prevent the development of kidney failure.

The diagonal arrows emphasize complications of CKD other than kidney outcomes. It is well accepted that both decreased GFR and albuminuria are associated with an independent risk of CVD and all-cause mortality. Metabolic and endocrine complications of decreased GFR, including anemia, bone and mineral disorders, malnutrition, and neuropathy, have long been recognized as consequences of kidney failure, but these abnormalities may appear with lesser reduction in GFR. Similarly, nephrotic syndrome occurs in patients with marked albuminuria, but hyperlipidemia and hypercoagulability may be observed with lesser increases in albuminuria. Other complications include threats to patient safety from systemic toxicity from drugs and procedures, as well as an increased risk of infections and impaired cognitive and physical function. Strategies for prevention, early detection, and treatment of CKD complications may prolong survival and improve quality of life, even if there is no effect on kidney disease progression.

DEFINITION OF CHRONIC KIDNEY DISEASE

The 2012 KDIGO guideline update defines CKD as abnormalities of kidney structure or function, present for longer than 3 months, with implications for health. Criteria for CKD

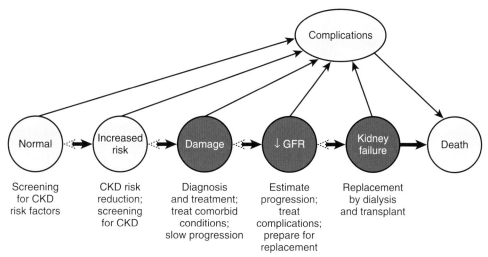

Fig. 52.1 Conceptual model for chronic kidney disease. The continuum of development, progression, and complications of chronic kidney disease (CKD) and strategies to improve outcomes. *Dark green circles,* Stages of CKD; *light green circles,* potential antecedents of CKD; *lavender circles,* consequences of CKD; *thick arrows between circles,* development, progression, and remission of CKD. *Complications* refers to all complications of CKD, including decreased glomerular filtration rate (GFR) and cardiovascular disease. Complications may also arise from adverse effects of interventions to prevent or treat the disease. Horizontal arrows pointing from left to right emphasize the progressive nature of CKD. Dashed arrowheads pointing from right to left signify that remission is less frequent than progression. (Reproduced with modifications from the National Kidney Foundation. K/DOQI clinical practice guidelines for chronic kidney disease: evaluation, classification, and stratification. *Am J Kidney Dis.* 2002;39:S1–S266; Levey AS, Stevens LA, Coresh J. Conceptual model of CKD: applications and implications, *Am J Kidney Dis.* 2009;53:S4–S16.)

Table 52.1 Outcomes of Chronic Kidney Disease and Relationship to Kidney Disease Characteristics

Outcomes of Chronic Kidney Disease	KIDNEY DISEASE CHARACTERISTICS		
	Glomerular Filtration Rate	Albuminuria	Cause
Kidney Outcomes			
CKD progression (GFR decline and worsening albuminuria)	+	+++	+++
AKI	+++	+	+
Chronic kidney failure	+++	+	+++
Complications (Current and Future)			
CVD and mortality	+++	+++	++
Systemic drug toxicity	+++	+	+
Metabolic/endocrine (anemia, bone and mineral disorders, malnutrition, and neuropathy)	+++	+	+
Infections, cognitive impairment, frailty	++	++	++

Number of + indicates the strength of the risk relationship between the kidney disease characteristic and the outcome.
AKI, Acute kidney injury; *CKD,* chronic kidney disease; *CVD,* cardiovascular disease; *GFR,* glomerular filtration rate.

include either kidney damage or GFR of less than 60 mL/min per 1.73 m² of body surface area lasting for longer than 3 months (90 days; Table 52.2). Of note, CKD can be diagnosed without knowledge of its cause.

Kidney damage can be within the parenchyma, large blood vessels, or collecting systems, and it is usually inferred from markers rather than direct examination of kidney tissue. The markers of kidney damage often provide a clue to the likely site of damage within the kidney and, in association with other clinical findings, the cause of kidney disease. Because most kidney diseases in North America are caused by diabetes or hypertension, persistent albuminuria is the principal marker. Other markers of damage include abnormalities in urine sediment (e.g., blood cells, tubular cells, or casts), abnormal findings on imaging studies (e.g., hydronephrosis, asymmetry in kidney size, polycystic kidney disease, stones, small echogenic kidneys), and abnormalities in blood and urine chemistry measurements (related to altered tubular function, such as renal tubular acidosis). A history of kidney transplantation is also defined as a marker of kidney damage, and patients with a functioning transplant are considered to have CKD, irrespective of the presence of other markers of kidney damage or the level of GFR.

Decreased GFR for more than 3 months, specifically GFR less than 60 mL/min per 1.73 m², represents CKD, irrespective of age. The level of GFR is usually accepted as the best overall index of kidney function in health and disease. GFR less than 60 mL/min per 1.73 m² represents the loss of half or more of the adult level of normal kidney function, and it is associated with an increased prevalence of systemic complications. The normal level of GFR varies according to age, gender, and body size. Normal GFR is approximately 120 to 130 mL/min per 1.73 m^2 in a young adult and declines with age by approximately 1 mL/min per 1.73 m^2 per year after the third decade. More than 25% of individuals aged 70 years and older have GFR of less than 60 mL/min per 1.73 m^2; whether this results from normal aging or the high prevalence of systemic vascular diseases that cause kidney disease remains controversial. Whatever its cause, GFR less than 60 mL/min per 1.73 m^2 in the elderly is an independent predictor of adverse outcomes such as death and CVD.

Kidney failure is defined either as a GFR less than 15 mL/min per 1.73 m^2 or initiation of kidney replacement therapy (dialysis or transplantation). A number of terms refer to severe decrease in kidney function, which is not synonymous with kidney failure. *Uremia* is defined as elevated concentrations within the blood of urea, creatinine, and other nitrogenous end products of amino acid and protein metabolism that are normally excreted in the urine. The *uremic syndrome*, the terminal clinical manifestation of kidney failure, is the constellation of symptoms, physical signs, and abnormal findings on diagnostic studies that result from the failure of the kidneys to maintain adequate function. *End-stage kidney disease* (ESKD) generally refers to kidney failure treated by dialysis or transplantation, regardless of the level of kidney function, and is used administratively in the United States and elsewhere. The availability of dialysis and transplantation for the treatment of kidney failure varies around the world, and not all patients with kidney failure choose to receive kidney replacement therapy. Therefore populations defined as having ESKD might not include patients with kidney failure who are not treated with dialysis or transplantation.

CLASSIFICATION OF CHRONIC KIDNEY DISEASE

The NKF-KDOQI classification system for stages of CKD was based on the severity of the disease defined only by the level of GFR. The KDIGO classification adds cause of the disease and level of albuminuria to the level of GFR (CGA classification). Because recent epidemiologic data demonstrate a strong graded relationships of the level of albuminuria, as well as the level of GFR, with risks of kidney disease progression, CVD, and mortality, this more detailed classification relates more closely to prognosis (see Table 52.1). The cause of disease is generally classified according to the presence or absence of systemic diseases (secondary or primary) and the presumed location of the pathologic-anatomic lesions (glomerular, tubulointerstitial, vascular, cystic, or disease in the kidney transplant; Table 52.3). Categories for GFR and albuminuria levels are shown in Tables 52.4 and 52.5. Fig. 52.2A shows the two-dimensional grid relating the risk of kidney outcomes and mortality to level of GFR and albuminuria. The green, yellow, orange, and red shaded categories represent patients at low, moderate, high, and very high risk of kidney outcomes and mortality, respectively.

Table 52.2   Definition of Chronic Kidney Disease

CKD is defined as abnormalities of kidney structure or function, present for >3 months, with implications for health.

Criteria for Chronic Kidney Disease[a]

Markers of kidney damage	• Albuminuria >30 mg/day • Urine sediment abnormalities • Electrolyte and other abnormalities caused by tubular disorders • Pathologic abnormalities • Imaging abnormalities • History of kidney transplantation
Decreased GFR	• GFR <60 mL/min per 1.73 m^2

[a]Either of the listed items for more than 3 months.
CKD, Chronic kidney disease; *GFR,* glomerular filtration rate.

Table 52.3   Classification of Cause of Chronic Kidney Disease Based on Presence or Absence of Systemic Disease and Location of Pathologic-Anatomic Findings

	Examples of Systemic Diseases Affecting the Kidney	Examples of Primary Kidney Diseases
Glomerular diseases	Diabetes, autoimmune diseases, systemic infections, drugs, neoplasia (including amyloidosis)	Diffuse, focal, or crescentric proliferative glomerulonephritis; focal and segmental glomerulosclerosis; idiopathic membranous nephropathy; minimal change disease
Tubulointerstitial diseases	Systemic infections, autoimmune diseases, sarcoidosis, drugs, urate, environmental toxins (lead, aristolochic acid), neoplasia (myeloma)	Urinary tract infections, stones, obstruction
Vascular diseases	Decreased perfusion (heart failure, liver disease, renal artery disease), atherosclerosis, hypertension, ischemia, cholesterol emboli, vasculitis, thrombotic microangiopathy, systemic sclerosis	ANCA-associated vasculitis; fibromuscular dysplasia
Cystic and congenital diseases	Polycystic kidney disease, Alport syndrome, Fabry disease, oxalosis	Renal dysplasia, medullary cystic disease
Diseases affecting the transplanted kidney	Recurrence of native kidney disease (diabetes, oxalosis, Fabry disease)	Chronic rejection; calcineurin inhibitor toxicity; BK virus nephropathy; recurrence of native kidney disease (glomerular disease)

ANCA, Antineutrophil cytoplasm antibody.
NOTE: Genetic diseases are not considered separately, because some diseases in each category are now recognized as having genetic determinants.

Table 52.4 Categories of Chronic Kidney Disease by the Level of Glomerular Filtration Rate and Corresponding Clinical Action Plan

Category	Glomerular Filtration Rate Levels (mL/min/1.73 m²)	Terms	Clinical Action Plan
G1[a]	>90	Normal or high	Diagnose and treat the cause Treat comorbid conditions Evaluate for CKD risk factors Start measures to slow CKD progression Start measures to reduce CVD risk
G2[a]	60–89	Mildly decreased[b]	Estimate progression
G3a	45–59	Mildly to moderately decreased	Adjust medication dosages as indicated
G3b	30–44	Moderately to severely decreased	Evaluate and treat complications
G4	15–29	Severely decreased	Prepare for kidney replacement therapy (transplantation and/or dialysis) if appropriate
G5	<15	Kidney failure (add D if treated by dialysis)	Start kidney replacement therapy (if uremia present) or continue conservative management

[a]GFR stages G1 or G2 without markers of kidney damage do not fulfill the criteria for CKD.
[b]Relative to young adult level.
CKD, Chronic kidney disease; *CVD,* cardiovascular disease; *GFR,* glomerular filtration rate.
NOTE: GFR in mL/min per 1.73 m² may be converted to mL/s per 1.73 m² by multiplying by 0.01667.

Table 52.5 Categories of Chronic Kidney Disease by the Level of Albuminuria and Corresponding Clinical Action Plan

Category	Albumin Excretion Rate (mg/day)	APPROXIMATELY EQUIVALENT ALBUMIN-TO-CREATININE RATIO (mg/mmol)	(mg/g)	Terms	Clinical Action Plan
A1	<30	<3	<30	Normal to mildly increased	Diagnose and treat the cause Treat comorbid conditions Evaluate for CKD risk factors Start measures to slow CKD progression Start measures to reduce CVD risk
A2	30–299	3–30	30–299	Moderately increased[a]	Treatment with renin-angiotensin system blockers and lower blood pressure goal if hypertensive
A3	>300	≥30	>300	Severely increased	Treat nephrotic syndrome (if present)

[a]Relative to young adult level.
CKD, Chronic kidney disease; *CVD,* cardiovascular disease.

PREVALENCE

Fig. 52.2 shows the prevalence estimates derived from measurements of serum creatinine to estimate GFR (eGFRcr) and albumin-to-creatinine ratio (ACR) during National Health and Nutrition Examination Surveys (NHANES) from 1999 to 2006. The prevalence of ACR greater than 30 mg/g or estimated GFR less than 60 mL/min per 1.73 m² is approximately 11.5% of the US adult population. The proportion of participants in the groups at moderate, high, and very high risk is about 73%, 18%, and 9%, respectively, representing a prevalence in the general population of about 8.5%, 2%, and 1%, respectively. This prevalence is more than 50 times greater than the prevalence of treated ESKD of approximately 0.2% reported by the US Renal Data System during this interval. Because kidney disease usually begins late in life and progresses slowly, most people in the earlier stages of CKD die before reaching kidney failure. In these patients, the burden of CKD is reflected in the complications of earlier stages, including increased mortality and morbidity, reduced quality of life, and high cost.

DETECTION, EVALUATION, PREDICTING PROGNOSIS, AND MANAGEMENT

Fig. 52.3 provides a five-step overview of the detection and evaluation of CKD. Care for patients with CKD requires multiple interventions and the coordinated, multidisciplinary effort of primary care physicians, allied health care workers, and other specialists, in addition to nephrologists. The KDIGO guidelines can provide a framework for care but cannot be a replacement of the physician's assessment of the needs of individual patients.

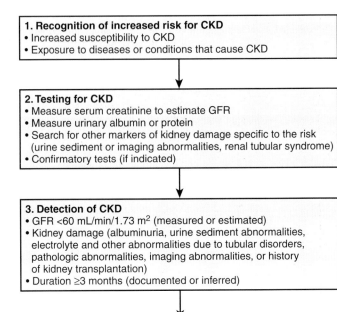

Percentage of US Population by eGFR and Albuminuria Category: KDIGO 2012 and NHANES 1999–2006			Persistent albuminuria categories Description and range			
			A1	A2	A3	
			Normal to mildly increased	Moderately increased	Severely increased	
			<30 mg/g <3 mg/mmol	30-300 mg/g 3-30 mg/mmol	>300 mg/g >30mg/mmol	
GFR categories (mL/min/ 1.73m²) Description and range	G1	Normal or high ≥90	55.6	1.9	0.4	57.9
	G2	Mildly decreased 60–89	32.9	2.2	0.3	35.4
	G3a	Mildly to moderately decreased 45–59	3.6	0.8	0.2	4.6
	G3b	Moderately to severely decreased 30–44	1.0	0.4	0.2	1.6
	G4	Severely decreased 15–29	0.2	0.1	0.1	0.4
	G5	Kidney failure <15	0.0	0.0	0.1	0.1
			93.2	5.4	1.3	100.0

Fig. 52.2 Prognosis and prevalence of chronic kidney disease in the United States by glomerular filtration rate and albuminuria category. Colors reflect the ranking of relative risk for kidney disease progression and cardiovascular risk. *Green,* low risk (if no other markers of kidney disease, no chronic kidney disease [CKD]); *Yellow,* moderately increased risk; *Orange,* high risk; *Red,* very high risk. Cells show the proportion of adult population in the United States. Data from the NHANES 1999 to 2006, *N* = 18,026. Glomerular filtration rate (GFR) is estimated from a single measurement of standardized serum creatinine with the CKD-EPI 2009 creatinine equation. Albuminuria is determined by one measurement of albumin-to-creatinine ratio, and persistence is estimated. Values in cells do not total to values in margins because of rounding. Category of very high albuminuria includes nephrotic range. *eGFR,* Estimated glomerular filtration rate; *KDIGO,* Kidney Disease: Improving Global Outcomes; *NHANES,* National Health and Nutrition Examination Survey. (Reproduced with permission from Kidney Disease: Improving Global Outcomes (KDIGO) CKD Work Group. KDIGO 2012 Clinical practice guideline for the evaluation and management of chronic kidney disease. *Kidney Int Suppl.* 2013;3:1–150.)

1. Recognition of increased risk for CKD
• Increased susceptibility to CKD
• Exposure to diseases or conditions that cause CKD

2. Testing for CKD
• Measure serum creatinine to estimate GFR
• Measure urinary albumin or protein
• Search for other markers of kidney damage specific to the risk (urine sediment or imaging abnormalities, renal tubular syndrome)
• Confirmatory tests (if indicated)

3. Detection of CKD
• GFR <60 mL/min/1.73 m² (measured or estimated)
• Kidney damage (albuminuria, urine sediment abnormalities, electrolyte and other abnormalities due to tubular disorders, pathologic abnormalities, imaging abnormalities, or history of kidney transplantation)
• Duration ≥3 months (documented or inferred)

4. Evaluation of clinical diagnosis for implementation of specific therapy
• Diabetic kidney disease (type 1 or type 2)
• Nondiabetic kidney disease (glomerular diseases other than diabetic kidney disease, vascular diseases, tubulointerstitial diseases, cystic diseases)
• Kidney disease in kidney transplant recipients

5. Evaluation of GFR and albuminuria categories for implementation of nonspecific therapy

Fig. 52.3 Five-step plan for detection and evaluation of chronic kidney disease. *CKD,* Chronic kidney disease; *GFR,* glomerular filtration rate. (Modified from Levey AS, Coresh J. Chronic kidney disease. *Lancet.* 2012;379:165–180.)

DETECTION

Screening for CKD in the general population is not recommended, but case finding is generally accepted in those deemed at high risk. As part of routine checkups, all patients should be evaluated to determine whether they are at increased risk for developing CKD. A reasonable approach to CKD testing in high-risk patients includes, at minimum, eGFRcr and urine ACR. Current guidelines suggest testing in patients with hypertension, diabetes, CVD, cancer, human immunodeficiency virus (HIV) infection, and before imaging procedures with iodine-based or gadolinium-based contrast. Clinical practice also includes measurement of serum creatinine with GFR estimation as part of the basic metabolic panel for patients with acute illness or before planned invasive procedures. The need for other measures (urinalysis or imaging) to ascertain other markers of kidney damage depends on the nature of the risk factors. eGFR less than 60 mL/min per 1.73 m² or urine ACR greater than 30 mg/g for more than 3 months meet the criteria for CKD. Values near these thresholds may arouse suspicion for CKD and prompt further testing. At present, there are few data regarding the optimal frequency of testing for CKD in high-risk individuals, although annual testing is recommended in patients with hypertension, diabetes, and HIV. Until evidence is available, it seems reasonable to suggest that others at increased risk be tested at least every 3 years.

EVALUATION

The goals of evaluation are to identify the duration and cause of CKD, to assess severity based on the levels of GFR and albuminuria, to identify the presence of complications, and to determine risk for progression of kidney disease and other outcomes. Evaluation includes a thorough history, including a review of past laboratory data, and physical examination to detect previous evidence of kidney disease, signs, and symptoms that may provide clues to the cause of kidney disease and, in particular, any reversible or treatable causes (e.g., uncontrolled hypertension, use of nonsteroidal antiinflammatory drugs). Medications should be reviewed to identify those that can cause kidney toxicity and others that must be adjusted based on level of GFR. The physical examination should include particular attention to details such as blood pressure, fundoscopy, and vascular examination. Laboratory tests should be performed to detect other markers of damage or functional disturbances (e.g., urine specific gravity, urine pH, urine sediment examination, serum electrolytes). Imaging studies should be performed if indicated based on clinical clues. Ultrasonography can be performed to detect anatomic abnormalities and to exclude obstruction of the urinary tract. It has been recommended that individuals with GFR less than 60 mL/min per 1.73 m² should have measurements of hemoglobin, as well as serum calcium, phosphate, albumin, and parathyroid hormone, but these measures are often not abnormal until GFR is less than 45 mL/min per 1.73 m². Laboratory evaluation should also include a search for traditional CVD risk factors, such as a lipid profile, and possibly tests for nontraditional risk factors such as insulin resistance and inflammation. Additional studies may be necessary to evaluate symptoms of CVD more fully or to detect asymptomatic CVD in patients with multiple risk factors.

Some elderly individuals meet the criteria for CKD solely because of eGFR less than 60 mL/min per 1.73 m². There is debate about the importance of a diagnosis of CKD in this setting. In the absence of risk factors for CKD, albuminuria, or other markers of kidney damage, patients with isolated decreased GFR may be at low risk for progression to kidney failure but remain at increased risk for CKD complications and for CVD. In such patients, clinicians may elect to defer some parts of the evaluation for CKD; however, a search for reversible causes of decreased GFR, adjustment of medication dosages for decreased GFR, appropriate attention to CVD risk factor management, and subsequent monitoring of GFR are appropriate.

EVALUATION OF DURATION

Kidney diseases and disorders may be acute or chronic depending on their duration. The distinction between acute and chronic is arbitrary but is useful in clinical practice. KDIGO defines chronicity as duration longer than 3 months (90 days), and the term *acute kidney diseases and disorders* (AKD) can be used to describe kidney disease with duration less than 3 months, including AKI. The duration of kidney disease may be documented or inferred based on the clinical context. For example, a patient with decreased kidney function or kidney damage in the midst of an acute illness, without previous documentation of kidney disease, may be inferred to have AKD. A patient with similar findings in the absence of an acute illness may be inferred to have CKD. In both cases, repeat ascertainment of kidney function and kidney damage is recommended for accurate diagnosis. The timing of the evaluation depends on clinical judgment, with earlier evaluation for patients suspected of having AKD and later evaluation for patients suspected of having CKD.

EVALUATION OF CAUSE

Identification of the cause of kidney disease, such as infection, drug toxicity, autoimmune disease, or obstruction of the urinary tract, enables specific directed treatments. In addition, the cause of kidney disease has implications for the rate of progression and the risk of complications. The cause of the disease is generally established by recognition of the clinical setting and the presence or absence of markers of kidney damage. A simplified system classifies kidney disease by anatomic location: glomerular, vascular, tubulointerstitial, and cystic kidney disorders (see Table 52.3). Clinical judgment is required to determine whether additional methods are necessary to characterize kidney disease, including imaging studies, other urine or serum markers, or biopsy

of the kidney. For many patients with CKD (especially older patients with hypertension or diabetes and no evidence of the other mentioned disorders), the cause will be unknown and presumed to be a result of vascular disease. In these cases, management will be based primarily on levels of GFR and albuminuria.

EVALUATION OF GLOMERULAR FILTRATION RATE

The KDIGO guideline recommends initial evaluation with eGFRcr, followed by confirmatory tests, if required. The guideline recommends using the Chronic Kidney Disease Epidemiology Collaboration (CKD-EPI) 2009 creatinine equation, or more accurate equations, if available. Confirmatory tests include measurement of clearances of exogenous filtration markers or creatinine clearance, or eGFR based on serum cystatin C with or without serum creatinine. GFR estimating equations are discussed in Chapter 3.

EVALUATION OF ALBUMINURIA

The KDIGO guidelines recommend initial evaluation with spot urine ACR, followed by confirmatory tests, if required. Alternative initial evaluation can include spot urine total protein-to-creatinine ratio (PCR), and urine dipstick with automated or manual reading. An early morning specimen is preferred, if possible. Confirmatory tests include a timed urine collection for measurement of albumin excretion rate. Table 52.6 provides a rough guide to measures of urine albumin and total protein in spot and timed urine collections that correspond to the KDIGO albuminuria stages. Further discussion of albuminuria and proteinuria is provided in Chapter 5.

PREDICTING PROGNOSIS

The KDIGO guideline recommends predicting risk for outcomes of CKD with the CGA classification and other risk factors and comorbid conditions specific for the outcome (see Table 52.1 and Fig. 52.2). Risk prediction instruments can be used to provide a numeric risk for specific outcomes. For example, the Kidney Failure Risk Equation (KFRE) has been validated in multiple cohorts worldwide. The KFRE is applicable for patients with eGFR less than 60 mL/min per 1.73 m² and uses age, sex, and current levels of eGFR and urine ACR to provide an estimate for the risk of developing kidney failure requiring treatment by dialysis or transplantation within 2 or 5 years. Change in eGFR and ACR can also be used to identify patients at higher risk for adverse outcomes. Recent data suggest a 30% decline in eGFR or a fourfold increase in urine ACR is associated with substantially increased risk for developing kidney failure, and a lesser increased risk for mortality, compared with patients with a stable eGFR or stable urine ACR. Quantitative risk predictions are not yet available based on changes in eGFR or urine ACR.

MANAGEMENT

CHRONIC KIDNEY DISEASE CARE

CKD care is directed by the CGA classification. For all patients, this includes treating specific causes of kidney disease, treating other reversible conditions causing kidney damage or decreased GFR, and prevention and treatment of complications. The action plan for each GFR and albuminuria stage is cumulative (see Tables 52.4 and 52.5). For patients

Table 52.6 Albuminuria and Proteinuria Measures

Measure	CATEGORIES		
	Normal to Mildly Increased	Moderately Increased	Severely Increased
AER (mg/24 hours)	<30	30–300	>300
PER (mg/24 hours)	<150	150–500	>500
Albumin-to-Creatinine Ratio			
(mg/mmol)	<3	3–30	>30
(mg/g)	<30	30–300	>300
Protein-to-Creatinine Ratio			
(mg/mmol)	<15	15–50	>50
(mg/g)	<150	150–500	>500
Protein reagent strip	Negative to trace	Negative to positive	Positive or greater

Urine albumin-to-creatinine ratio (ACR) may be divided into more than three categories. The normal urinary ACR in young adults is less than 10 mg/g; ACR 10 to 29 mg/g is high normal. Urine ACR greater than 2000 mg/g is accompanied by signs and symptoms of nephrotic syndrome (low serum albumin, edema, and high serum cholesterol).

Relationships between excretion rates and concentration ratios with urine creatinine are inexact. Excretion of urinary creatinine indicates muscle mass and varies with age, gender, race, diet, and nutritional status and generally exceeds 1.0 g/day in healthy adults; therefore the numeric value for urinary ACR (mg/g) is usually less than the rate of urinary albumin excretion (mg/day). Rates of 30 to 300 mg/day and greater than 300 mg/day correspond to microalbuminuria and macroalbuminuria, respectively.

Relationships between urinary albumin and total protein are inexact. Normal urine contains small amounts of albumin, low-molecular-weight serum proteins, and proteins that are from renal tubules and the lower urinary tract. In most kidney diseases, albumin is the main urine protein, comprising about 60% to 90% of total urinary protein when total protein is very high. Values corresponding to normal, high-normal, high, very high, and nephrotic-range total protein are approximately less than 50, 50 to 150, 150 to 500, greater than 500, and greater than 3500 mg/g, respectively.

Threshold values for standard international (mg/mol) and conventional units (mg/g) are not exact. Conversion factor for ACR: 1.0 mg/g = 0.113 mg/mmol.

AER, Albumin excretion rate; PER, protein excretion rate.

with albuminuria, key aspects include slowing progression of kidney disease by use of ACE inhibitors and ARBs and a lower blood pressure goal and preventing and treating complications of the nephrotic syndrome. For patients with decreased GFR, key aspects include assuring medication safety by avoiding drugs that are toxic to the kidney and adjusting doses of drugs that are excreted by the kidney, treating metabolic and endocrine complications of decreased GFR, and preparing for kidney replacement therapy or conservative care in patients with severely decreased GFR.

Patient education is central to the management strategy. CKD is often asymptomatic, and patients may not understand the importance of multidrug regimens and laboratory testing without explicit education. Complete management requires behavioral change by the patient, which may include lifestyle alterations, self-monitoring of blood pressure, and adherence to medication regimens and medical follow-up. Patient education is also important with respect to avoiding medications that are toxic to the kidneys. Patients must be aware that any drug or herbal remedy may be directly nephrotoxic or may require a dosage adjustment for the level of kidney function.

NEPHROLOGY REFERRAL

Nephrologists have multiple roles in the care of patients with CKD, including determining the cause of CKD, recommending specific therapy, suggesting treatments to slow progression in patients who have not responded to conventional therapies, identifying and treating kidney disease–related complications, and management in GFR stages 4 and 5 (GFR <30 mL/min per 1.73 m²).

Table 52.7 Recommendations for Referral to Specialists for Consultation and Comanagement of Chronic Kidney Disease

AKI or abrupt sustained fall in GFR
GFR <30 mL/min/1.73 m² (GFR categories G4–G5)
ACR ≥300 mg/g (albuminuria category A3)
Progression of CKD
Urinary red cell casts, RBC >20 per high-power field sustained and not readily explained
CKD and hypertension refractory to treatment with 4 or more antihypertensive agents
Persistent abnormalities of serum potassium
Recurrent or extensive nephrolithiasis
Hereditary kidney disease

ACR, Albumin-to-creatinine ratio; AKI, acute kidney injury; CKD, chronic kidney disease; GFR, glomerular filtration rate; RBC, red blood cells.
Adapted from Kidney Disease: Improving Global Outcomes (KDIGO) CKD Work Group. KDIGO 2012 Clinical practice guideline for the evaluation and management of chronic kidney disease. Kidney Int Suppl. 2013;3:1–150.

Recommendations for referral to a kidney disease specialist are not universal because specific practice patterns are dependent on health care systems and available resources in a geographic region. Table 52.7 lists clinical criteria for referral recommended by the KDIGO guideline. The strongest evidence regarding the importance of referral to a nephrologist is for management of GFR stages 4 and 5. Late referral to a nephrologist (i.e., <3 months before the start of dialysis therapy) has been associated with higher mortality after the initiation of dialysis. It is therefore recommended by many organizations, regardless of the health care system or geographic region, that all patients with GFR stages 4 and 5 be referred to a nephrologist. During GFR stage 4, it is important to prepare the patient for the possible onset of kidney failure (GFR stage 5). KDIGO recommends beginning preparations when the risk of kidney failure within 1 year is 10% to 20% or higher. Preparation involves estimating the risk of progression to kidney failure, holding discussions regarding kidney replacement therapy (dialysis and transplantation), and instituting conservative therapy for those who choose not to undergo kidney replacement therapy. In patients who elect replacement therapy, timely creation of vascular access for hemodialysis, home dialysis training, and donor evaluation for preemptive transplantation should occur during GFR stage 4. For patients with CKD in GFR stages 1 to 3 (GFR >30 mL/min per 1.73 m^2), only a subset is likely to require referral to a specialist.

KEY BIBLIOGRAPHY

Astor BC, Matsushita K, Gansevoort RT, et al. Lower estimated glomerular filtration rate and higher albuminuria are associated with mortality and end-stage renal disease. *Kidney Int.* 2011;79:1331-1340.

Carrero JJ, Grams ME, Sang Y, et al. Albuminuria changes are associated with subsequent risk of end-stage renal disease and mortality. *Kidney Int.* 2017;91:244-251.

Coresh J, Turin TC, Matsushita K, et al. Decline in estimated glomerular filtration rate and subsequent risk of end-stage renal disease and mortality. *JAMA.* 2014;311:2518-2531.

Eckardt KU, Berns JS, Rocco MV, et al. Definition and classification of CKD: the debate should be about patient prognosis—a position statement from KDOQI and KDIGO. *Am J Kidney Dis.* 2009;53:915-920.

Eckardt KU, Coresh J, Devuyst O, et al. Evolving importance of kidney disease: from subspecialty to global health burden. *Lancet.* 2013;382: 158-169.

Gansevoort RT, Matsushita K, van der Velde M, et al. Lower estimated GFR and higher albuminuria are associated with adverse kidney outcomes. *Kidney Int.* 2011;80:93-104.

Glassock RJ, Delanaye P, El-Nahas M. An age-calibrated classification of chronic kidney disease. *JAMA.* 2015;314:559-560.

Kidney Disease: Improving Global Outcomes (KDIGO) CKD Work Group. KDIGO 2012 clinical practice guideline for the evaluation and management of chronic kidney disease. *Kidney Int Suppl.* 2013;3:1-150.

Kovesdy CP, Coresh J, Ballew SH, et al. Past decline versus current eGFR and subsequent ESRD risk. *J Am Soc Nephrol.* 2016;27:2447-2455.

Levey AS, Becker C, Inker LA. Glomerular filtration rate and albuminuria for detection and staging of acute and chronic kidney disease in adults: a systematic review. *JAMA.* 2015;313:837-846.

Levey AS, Coresh J. Chronic kidney disease. *Lancet.* 2012;379:165-180.

Levey AS, Coresh J, Balk E, et al. National Kidney Foundation practice guidelines for chronic kidney disease: evaluation, classification, and stratification. *Ann Intern Med.* 2003;139:137-147.

Levey AS, de Jong PE, Coresh J, et al. The definition, classification and prognosis of chronic kidney disease: a KDIGO Controversies Conference report. *Kidney Int.* 2011;80:17-28.

Levey AS, Eckardt K, Tsukamoto Y, et al. Definition and classification of chronic kidney disease: a position statement from Kidney Disease: Improving Global Outcomes (KDIGO). *Kidney Int.* 2005;67:2089-2100.

Levey AS, Inker LA, Coresh J. Chronic kidney disease in older people. *JAMA.* 2015;314(6):557-558.

Levey AS, Stevens LA, Coresh J. Conceptual model of CKD: applications and implications. *Am J Kidney Dis.* 2009;53:S4-S16.

Matsushita K, van der Velde M, Astor BC, et al. Association of estimated glomerular filtration rate and albuminuria with all-cause and cardiovascular mortality in general population cohorts. *Lancet.* 2010;375: 2073-2081.

National Kidney Foundation. K/DOQI clinical practice guidelines for chronic kidney disease: evaluation, classification, and stratification. *Am J Kidney Dis.* 2002;39:S1-S266.

Tangri N, Grams ME, Levey AS, et al. Multinational assessment of accuracy of equations for predicting risk of kidney failure: a meta-analysis. *JAMA.* 2016;315:164-174.

van der Velde M, Matsushita K, Coresh J, et al. Lower estimated glomerular filtration rate and higher albuminuria are associated with all-cause and cardiovascular mortality. *Kidney Int.* 2011;79:1341-1352.

Full bibliography can be found on www.expertconsult.com.

T. Alp Ikizler

As chronic kidney disease (CKD) progresses, the requirements and utilization of different nutrients change significantly. Protein energy wasting (PEW), defined as a state of decreased body stores of protein and energy fuels, is common in individuals with CKD and has multifactorial causes. Changes in nutritional needs and utilization ultimately place kidney disease patients at high risk for nutritional abnormalities. Understanding the applicable nutritional principles and the available methods for improving nutritional status of these patients is essential. National Kidney Foundation Clinical Practice Guidelines for Chronic Kidney Disease and Nutrition in Chronic Kidney Disease provide in-depth information regarding these principles.

NUTRIENT METABOLISM IN KIDNEY DISEASE

PROTEIN METABOLISM AND REQUIREMENTS

AMINO ACID METABOLISM

CKD patients have well-defined abnormalities in their plasma and to a lesser extent in their muscle amino acid profiles. Commonly, essential amino acid concentrations are low and nonessential amino acid concentrations high. The etiology of this abnormal profile is multifactorial. The progressive loss of kidney tissue, where metabolism of several amino acids takes place, is an important factor. Specifically, glycine and phenylalanine concentrations are elevated, and serine, tyrosine, and histidine concentrations are decreased. Plasma and muscle concentrations of branched-chain amino acids (valine, leucine, and isoleucine) are reduced in CKD patients, especially in patients treated with maintenance dialysis. In contrast, plasma citrulline, cystine, aspartate, methionine, and both 1- and 3-methylhistidine levels are increased. Although inadequate dietary intake is a possible factor in abnormal essential amino acid profiles, certain abnormalities occur even in the presence of adequate dietary nutrient intake indicating that the uremic milieu has an additional effect. Indeed, it has been suggested that the metabolic acidosis commonly seen in uremic patients plays an important role in increased oxidation of branched-chain amino acids.

PROTEIN INTAKE IN NONDIALYSIS CKD PATIENTS

In general, the minimal daily protein requirement is one that maintains a neutral nitrogen balance and prevents protein wasting; this has been estimated to be a daily protein intake of approximately 0.6 g/kg in healthy individuals, with a safe level of protein intake equivalent to the minimal requirement plus 2 standard deviations, or approximately 0.75 g/kg per day. One of the most significant symptoms in advanced CKD is a decrease in appetite. Several studies have indicated that CKD patients spontaneously restrict their dietary protein intake, with levels often less than 0.6 g/kg per day among those with CKD stage 5, suggesting that anorexia predisposes CKD patients to malnutrition. Accumulation of uremic toxins may not be the sole cause of decreased dietary nutrient intake. Table 53.1 depicts factors that can cause decreased nutrient intake as well as other potential mechanisms of PEW in CKD patients. Individuals with CKD and coexisting diabetes mellitus are more prone to nutritional abnormalities because of additional dietary restrictions; gastrointestinal symptoms common in diabetes such as gastroparesis, nausea, and vomiting; and bacterial overgrowth in the gut and pancreatic insufficiency. Depression, which is common in CKD, is also associated with anorexia. CKD patients often are prescribed a large number of medications, particularly sedatives, phosphate binders, and iron supplements, all of which may have gastrointestinal complications. Finally, socioeconomic status, lack of mobility, and older age may all predispose to decreased dietary protein intake.

PROTEIN RESTRICTION IN NONDIALYSIS CKD PATIENTS

Dietary protein restriction, with or without supplementation of ketoanalogues of certain amino acids, has long been considered an attractive intervention to slow the progression of kidney disease. This is based on earlier studies indicating that excessive dietary protein intake causes hyperfiltration leading to progression of kidney disease, especially in high-risk populations such as individuals with coexisting diabetes mellitus and hypertension. As suggested by a number of meta-analyses, this dietary protein restriction effect is real, albeit relatively small in the context of progressive kidney disease (0.5 mL/min per year benefit). Several smaller studies suggest that the favorable effects of dietary protein restriction extend beyond slowing the progression. These include amelioration of metabolic acidosis and insulin resistance, antioxidant effects, and decreasing dietary phosphorus load. The optimal range of dietary protein restriction to exert the most beneficial outcome is not established, and the applicability of dietary protein restriction is limited by compliance.

In addition to protein restriction alone, a number of studies have also examined the effects of keto acid– or amino acid–supplemented low-protein diets (LPDs) or very low protein diets (VLPDs) on certain metabolic and kidney outcome parameters. Several studies indicate that protein-restricted diets supplemented with keto acids and amino acids result in a significant decrease in urea production and a beneficial effect on insulin resistance and oxidative stress in humans.

Table 53.1   Factors Leading to Nutritional and Metabolic Abnormalities in Chronic Kidney Disease Patients

Increased Protein and Energy Requirements

- Nephrotic syndrome
- Losses of nutrients (amino acids and/or proteins) during dialysis
- Increased resting energy expenditure
  - Acute or chronic inflammation
  - Hyperphosphatemia
  - Hemodialysis

Decreased Protein and Calorie Intake

- Anorexia (uremic toxins)
- Frequent hospitalizations
- Inadequate dialysis dose
- Comorbid conditions
  - Diabetes mellitus
  - Gastrointestinal diseases
  - Heart failure
  - Depression
- Multiple medications

Increased Catabolism/Decreased Anabolism

- Dialysis-induced catabolism
  - Amino acid losses
  - Induction of inflammatory cascade
- Metabolic acidosis
- Hormonal derangements
  - Hyperparathyroidism
  - Insulin resistance
  - Growth hormone resistance
  - Testosterone deficiency

An important consideration regarding dietary protein restriction in CKD is the potential to adversely affect nutritional status. These concerns have been mostly ameliorated by a number of studies showing that well-designed diets planned by skilled dietitians and followed by motivated and adherent patients are effective and do not have harmful effects on the nutritional condition. Long-term follow-up of several relatively large cohorts of CKD patients who received 0.47 g/kg per day protein with ketoacid supplementation showed no detrimental effect on clinical outcomes. Accordingly, one can conclude that prescribing LPD or VLPD with or without keto acid or amino acid supplementation with adequate caloric intake and close supervision does not seem to lead to PEW.

There are very limited data regarding the optimal level of dietary protein intake in patients with a kidney transplant. In general, these patients should also be considered as having CKD, and the same strategies for dietary protein intake and prescription should be applied. Table 53.2 depicts the most current recommendations for dietary protein and energy intake for patients with different stages of CKD.

MAINTENANCE DIALYSIS PATIENTS

Once CKD patients are initiated on maintenance dialysis, dietary restrictions are used to prevent hyperphosphatemia, hyperkalemia, or metabolic acidosis; however, these restrictions could predispose dialysis patients to an increased risk of PEW, primarily because of the increased metabolic stress associated with dialysis therapies. Nutrient losses through hemodialysis or peritoneal membranes, loss of residual kidney function due to long-term dialysis treatment, and increased inflammation due to indwelling catheters, bioincompatible hemodialysis membranes, and peritoneal dialysis (PD) solutions all may lead to an overly catabolic milieu and increase the minimal amount of nutrient intake needed to maintain a neutral nitrogen balance (see Table 53.2). In patients who cannot compensate for this increased need, a state of semistarvation ensues, resulting in the development or worsening of PEW. Although the current targets for acceptable dialysis

Table 53.2   Recommended Intakes of Protein, Energy, and Minerals in Kidney Disease

	Protein	Energy	Phosphorus	Sodium
Chronic Kidney Disease				
Stages 1–3	No restriction	No restriction	600–800 mg/day	<2 g/day[a]
Stages 4–5	0.60–0.75 g/kg/day[b]	30–35 kcal/kg/day[c]	600–800 mg/day[d]	<2 g/day
Dialysis				
Hemodialysis	>1.2 g/kg/day	30–35 kcal/kg/day[c]	600–800 mg/day[d]	<2 g/day
Peritoneal dialysis	>1.3 g/kg/day	30–35 kcal/kg/day[c]	600–800 mg/day[d]	<2 g/day
Acute Kidney Injury				
No dialysis	1.0–1.2 g/kg IBW/d	30–35 kcal/kg/day	600–800 mg/day[d]	<2 g/day
Dialysis	1.2–1.4 g/kg IBW/d	30–35 kcal/kg/day	600–800 mg/day[d,e]	<2 g/day

[a]If hypertensive.
[b]With close supervision and frequent dietary counseling.
[c]30 kcal/kg/day for individuals 60 years and older.
[d]Facilitated by phosphate binders, as needed.
[e]May need to replete if receiving continuous renal replacement therapy; check PO_4 levels daily.
IBW/d, Ideal body weight per day.

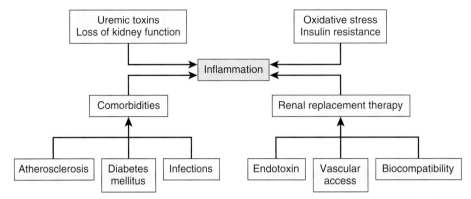

Fig. 53.1 Multiple factors can lead to systemic inflammation of patients with chronic kidney disease. Most of these factors are persistent, leading to a persistent inflamed state with short- and long-term adverse consequences.

dose should be adequate to prevent development of PEW in patients undergoing either hemodialysis or PD, there are limited data suggesting that a substantial increase in dose of dialysis could result in improvement in overall nutrition status in maintenance dialysis patients.

CHRONIC INFLAMMATION

Systemic inflammation is one of the major contributors to PEW in patients with CKD (Fig. 53.1). Increased levels of proinflammatory cytokines such as interleukin-1 (IL-1), interleukin-6 (IL-6), and tumor necrosis factor–α (TNF-α) play a crucial role in the exaggerated protein and energy catabolism present in individuals with CKD. Proinflammatory cytokines play integral roles in protein breakdown, resulting in muscle atrophy in chronic disease states such as advanced CKD. Recent data in maintenance hemodialysis patients clearly indicate exponentially increased protein catabolism, especially in the skeletal muscle compartment, in the setting of exaggerated systemic inflammation. In addition to increasing protein breakdown, chronic inflammation is associated with reduced physical activity and impairment in both insulin and growth hormone actions; it may also contribute to anorexia due to central effects. Small randomized studies suggest that certain antiinflammatory interventions such as IL1 receptor blockers, pentoxifylline, and fish oil could improve protein catabolism in maintenance dialysis patients.

METABOLIC ACIDOSIS

Metabolic acidosis is associated with increased muscle protein catabolism and promotes muscle wasting in patients with advanced CKD by stimulating the oxidation of essential amino acids. Multiple studies have shown improvements in nutrition status associated with oral bicarbonate supplementation in patients with advanced CKD, while some observational studies, but not all, and one randomized clinical trial suggest that the progression of CKD is slower among individuals treated with oral bicarbonate. This has led to a suggestion that attempts should be made to maintain a steady-state serum bicarbonate level of at least 24 mmol/L in nondialysis CKD patients. Data on bicarbonate supplementation in hemodialysis are mixed, although recent epidemiologic data suggest worse outcomes with very high predialysis serum bicarbonate levels,

potentially indicating a subset of the hemodialysis population with lower dietary protein intake. Dialysate base is covered in more detail in Chapter 57.

HORMONAL DERANGEMENTS

Resistance to the anabolic actions of insulin is a key endocrine abnormality implicated in the loss of muscle mass in chronic disease states including CKD. Enhanced protein catabolism applies to both insulin-deficient and insulin-resistant states. Maintenance hemodialysis patients with suboptimally controlled type 2 diabetes have a higher rate of muscle protein loss than hemodialysis patients without diabetes, a catabolic state that can be detected even in hemodialysis patients with insulin resistance.

Additional metabolic disorders such as increased parathyroid hormone concentration, low levels of testosterone, and several abnormalities in the thyroid hormone profile might also promote hypermetabolism and decrease protein anabolism, leading to excess net protein catabolism in patients with advanced CKD.

Acquired resistance to the anabolic actions of growth hormone is a potential cause of increased net protein catabolism in patients with advanced CKD. Growth hormone is the major promoter of growth in children and exerts anabolic actions even in adults, such as enhancement of protein synthesis, reduced protein degradation, increased fat mobilization, and increased gluconeogenesis, with insulin-like growth factor–1 (IGF-1) being the major mediator of these actions. Several studies showed that recombinant human growth hormone treatment over 6 months improves fat-free mass in maintenance hemodialysis patients.

Testosterone levels are also abnormally low among men and women with CKD, especially those treated with maintenance dialysis. Testosterone is an anabolic hormone that induces skeletal muscle hypertrophy by promoting nitrogen retention and stimulating fractional muscle protein synthesis. In dialysis and advanced CKD patients, low testosterone levels are associated with increased mortality risk. In one small clinical trial, nandrolone decanoate, an androgen analogue of testosterone, was associated with significant improvements in nutritional parameters, body composition, and physical functioning. However, its side effects, such as virilization, voice changes, hirsutism in women and abnormalities in prostate markers in men, and changes in liver enzymes limit its routine clinical use.

ENERGY METABOLISM AND REQUIREMENTS

The minimum energy requirement of patients with CKD is not well defined (see Table 53.2). An individual's energy requirement is dependent on resting energy expenditure, activity level, and effects of other ongoing illnesses. Resting energy expenditure is elevated in maintenance dialysis patients compared with age, sex, and body mass index matched normal controls and further increases during the hemodialysis procedure when catabolism is at a maximum due to amino acid losses into the dialysate. Several comorbid conditions also lead to hypermetabolism, including systemic inflammation, uncontrolled diabetes mellitus, and hyperparathyroidism, further increasing energy requirement in patients CKD. For earlier stages of CKD, energy requirements likely are similar to the general population. Among stage 4 and 5 CKD patients, the recommended energy intake is 35 kcal/kg body weight/day for those who are less than 60 years of age and 30 to 35 kcal/kg body weight/day for individuals 60 years and older.

LIPID METABOLISM AND REQUIREMENTS

Dyslipidemia is common in CKD patients, and abnormalities in lipid profiles can be detected once kidney function begins to deteriorate. The presence of nephrotic syndrome or other comorbid conditions such as diabetes mellitus and liver disease, as well as the use of medications altering lipid metabolism (e.g., thiazide diuretics, beta-blockers), further contribute to the dyslipidemia seen in patients with CKD.

In maintenance hemodialysis patients, the most common abnormalities are elevated serum triglycerides and very low-density lipoproteins and decreased low-density (LDL) and high-density (HDL) lipoproteins. The increased triglyceride component is thought to be related to increased levels of apoCIII, an inhibitor of lipoprotein lipase. A substantial number of chronic hemodialysis patients also have elevated lipoprotein (a) (Lp[a]) levels. Patients treated with PD exhibit higher concentrations of serum cholesterol, triglyceride, LDL cholesterol, and apoB, even though the mechanisms that alter the lipid metabolism are similar to maintenance hemodialysis patients. This may be related to increased protein losses through the peritoneum, possibly by mechanisms that are operative in the nephrotic syndrome and the glucose load supplied by dialysate causing increased triglyceride synthesis and hyperinsulinemia. PD patients also exhibit higher concentrations of Lp(a). Treatment of dyslipidemia is covered in detail in Chapter 55.

MINERAL, VITAMIN, AND TRACE ELEMENT REQUIREMENTS

Sodium intake should be restricted to less than 2 g/day in all CKD patients with hypertension and in dialysis patients regardless of blood pressure. Potassium intake should be less than 2 g/day in patients with stage 4 and 5 CKD and in maintenance hemodialysis patients; many PD patients require more liberal potassium intake. Foods containing high levels of potassium are listed in Table 53.3.

Table 53.3 Foods Containing High Levels of Potassium

Fruits	Vegetables	Other Foods
Apricots	Artichokes	Bran and bran products
Avocado	Beans, dried	Chocolate
Banana	Broccoli	Coconut
Cantaloupe	Brussels sprouts	Granola
Casaba melon	Escarole	Juices from high potassium fruits
Dried fruits (dates, figs, raisins, prunes)	Endive	and vegetables
Honeydew	Greens (Swiss chard, collard, beet,	Low-sodium baking powder or soda
Mango	dandelion, mustard)	Milk and milk products (ice cream,
Nectarine	Kale	yogurt—2 cups)
Orange	Kohlrabi	Molasses
Papaya	Lentils	Nuts/seeds
Rhubarb	Legumes	Peanut butter
Juice of fruits listed	Lima beans	Salt substitute or "lite" salt
Tangelo	Mushrooms	(containing potassium)
Watermelon	Parsnips	Snuff/chewing tobacco
	Potatoes (french fries, chips, baked,	
	mashed, boiled, sweet potatoes, yams)	
	Pumpkin	
	Rutabaga	
	Spinach, Swiss chard	
	Salt-free vegetable juice (ALL vegetable	
	juices)	
	Tomatoes	
	Winter squash (acorn, butternut, Hubbard)	

Table 53.4   Foods Containing High Levels of Phosphorus

Legumes, Nuts and Seeds, Whole Grains	Meat and Other Foods	Dairy and Beverages
Beans (navy, kidney, lima, pinto)	Chocolate	Beer
Soybeans	Dried fruit	Colas: Coke, Pepsi, Dr. Pepper
Black-eyed peas	Molasses	
Lentils	Beef liver, calf liver	Eggnog
Peanut butter	Liver sausage	Hot chocolate
Nuts	Liverwurst	Milk
Coconuts	Beef, bottom round	Casseroles
Pumpkin seeds	Pork, fresh	Cheese
Sunflower seeds	Veal, cubes, rib roast	Cream soups
Bran, bran flakes, bran muffins		Custard
Brown rice		Ice cream
Wheat germ		Pudding
Raisin bran, 100% bran		Yogurt
100% whole grain		

In early kidney disease (stages 2 to 3), restricting phosphorus intake to 600 to 800 mg/day is suggested. Because further restriction of dietary phosphorus in clinical settings is impractical, phosphate binders in addition to dietary phosphorus restriction are often necessary in very advanced CKD, particularly for patients treated with dialysis. High-phosphorus foods are listed in Table 53.4. Phosphorus is a "hidden" ingredient in most processed foods and often is not listed on nutritional labels; accordingly, nonprocessed food consumption should be emphasized if affordable. While use of calcium-containing binders can provide supplemental calcium that may be needed in advanced kidney disease, use of non-calcium-containing phosphate binders is generally preferred, especially in patients with higher burden of vascular calcification, including elderly patients and patients with underlying ischemic heart disease. A detailed review of calcium and phosphorus metabolism can be found in Chapter 54.

Vitamin A concentrations are usually elevated in maintenance dialysis patients, and intake of even small amounts leads to excessive accumulation. There have been several reports on the vitamin A toxicity in maintenance dialysis patients, and therefore it should not be supplemented. Vitamin E levels in patients with later stages of kidney disease are not well defined, and there have been reports of increased, decreased, or unchanged concentrations. Therefore it is not clear whether vitamin E supplementation is required in maintenance dialysis patients. Several randomized controlled studies suggested that the therapeutic use of pharmacologic doses of vitamin E as an antioxidant does not substantially alter the metabolic profile in advanced CKD patients. Vitamin K supplementation is usually not recommended in maintenance dialysis patients unless they are at high risk for developing vitamin K deficiency, as with prolonged hospitalization, with poor dietary intake, or antibiotic therapy, although

ongoing research is evaluating whether vitamin K has a role in preventing vascular calcification. Vitamin D (and calcium/phosphorus) metabolism is discussed in detail in Chapter 54.

Serum concentrations of the water-soluble vitamins may be low in maintenance dialysis patients mainly owing to decreased dietary intake and increased removal during hemodialysis. Multivitamin preparations specifically designed for CKD patients are available and useful for correcting these low concentrations without inducing toxicity.

The concentrations of most of the trace elements are primarily dependent on the stage of CKD. Although there is an extensive list of trace elements that may have altered concentrations in body fluids in maintenance dialysis patients, only a few are thought to be important. Serum aluminum is the most important trace element in maintenance hemodialysis patients because elevated levels are associated with dementia and bone disease. Aluminum intoxication can be caused either by use of inadequately processed hemodialysate water (mostly eliminated with the use of reverse osmosis for water purification) or by use of phosphate binders that contain aluminum hydroxide, which is also very limited currently. Aluminum levels are serially monitored in dialysis patients.

ASSESSMENT OF NUTRITIONAL STATUS IN CHRONIC KIDNEY DISEASE PATIENTS

A variety of parameters have been used to determine the nutrition status in CKD patients. Similar to the general population, an approach that incorporates continuous screening combined with more detailed assessment techniques is preferred (Table 53.5). Most screening tests are easy to perform, readily available, and inexpensive, rendering them clinically applicable. More sophisticated and expensive tools, such as dual-energy x-ray absorptiometry and magnetic resonance imaging, often are used for research purposes. Screening parameters can be collected routinely in clinical practice by any health professional and mostly provide a trigger to conduct more extensive assessment, confirm or establish the diagnosis, and determine the best course of treatment, if needed. Any of the screening tests are adequate to initiate a more thorough workup. On the other hand, nutritional assessment generally requires extensive training, provides comprehensive information to make a nutritional diagnosis, and aids in intervention and developing a monitoring plan. This should be performed by qualified individuals, preferably by dietitians. These tests should also be used for guiding nutritional therapies once the patient is deemed to be at risk or has overt PEW. A diagnosis of PEW necessitates confirmation by several tools and usually fits a strict criterion.

A number of considerations must be made on the unique situation of CKD patients for appropriate screening and assessment of their nutritional status. Some of these include fluid status, which could alter body composition and biochemical markers; the presence of systemic inflammation, which could change serum concentrations of acute-phase proteins; the presence and extent of proteinuria, a major determinant of serum albumin concentrations; and the level of residual kidney function, which could influence serum concentration of some biochemical markers, such as prealbumin, that are cleared by the kidneys.

Table 53.5   Suggestions for Monitoring Nutritional Status and Therapy in Kidney Failure

Simple Assessment (Monthly)	Findings	Possible Interventions
Body weight	Continuous decline or <85% IBW	Suspect PEW and perform more detailed nutritional assessment
Serum albumin	Below 4.0 g/dL	Consider preventive measures
Serum creatinine	Relatively low predialysis values	No specific intervention needed at this point

Detailed Assessment (as Indicated by Simple Assessment)	Findings	Possible Interventions (Simple)
Serum prealbumin	Below 30 mg/dL	Dietary counseling to increase DPI ≥1.2 g/kg/d and energy intake 30–35 kcal/d
Serum transferrin	Below 200 mg/dL	Consider timely initiation of maintenance dialysis
LBM and/or fat mass	Unexpected decrease	Assurance of optimal dialysis dose
SGA	Worsening	Upper GI motility enhancer in suitable patients

Repeat Detailed Assessment (2 to 3 Months From Previous)	Findings (Any of the Markers)	Possible Interventions (Moderate to Complex)
Serum prealbumin	Below 30 mg/dL	Nutritional supplements, including oral supplements, enteric tube feeding, IDPD, AAD
Serum transferrin	Below 200 mg/dL	Anabolic interventions, including anabolic steroids, rhGH (experimental)
Serum creatinine	Relatively low predialysis values	Appetite stimulants, including megestrol acetate, ghrelin (experimental)
LBM and/or fat mass	Unexpected decrease	Antiinflammatory interventions including IL-1ra (experimental), fish oil
C-reactive protein	Above 10 mg/L	

AAD, Amino acid dialysate; *DPI*, dietary protein intake; *IBW*, ideal body weight; *IDPN*, intradialytic parenteral nutrition; *IL1ra*, interleukin 1 receptor antagonist; *LBM*, lean body mass; *PEW*, protein-energy wasting; *rhGH*, recombinant human growth hormone; *SGA*, subjective global assessment.
Adapted with permission from Pupim LB, Cuppari L, Ikizler TA. Nutrition and metabolism in kidney disease. *Semin Nephrol.* 2006;26:134–157.

Estimation of dietary protein intake can also be used as a marker of overall nutritional status in the CKD patient. Although dietary recall is a direct and simple measure of dietary protein intake, several studies have shown that this method lacks accuracy in estimating the actual intake. Therefore other means of measuring dietary protein intake, such as 24-hour urine urea nitrogen excretion in CKD patients or urea nitrogen appearance (UNA) rate calculations derived from urea kinetic modeling in maintenance dialysis patients, have been suggested as useful methods to estimate protein intake. However, these indirect estimations of dietary protein intake are valid only in stable patients, and may easily overestimate the actual intake in catabolic patients where endogenous protein breakdown may lead to a high UNA.

In summary, there are many different methods available for assessing protein and energy nutritional status in CKD patients. Some are easy to perform, readily available, and inexpensive, while others are sophisticated, not available in many centers, and either expensive or carry an unfavorable cost-benefit ratio. For example, a monthly nutritional screening can be easily performed at nearly any clinic or hospital by measuring serum albumin, serum prealbumin, serum transferrin, and bioimpedance values. However, if the goal is to precisely and longitudinally follow changes in body composition, one may want to use anthropometry, dual-energy x-ray absorptiometry, and even more sophisticated methods,

if available. For all indirect methods, repeated measures and technical standardization are extremely important to reduce variability of results.

PREVENTION AND TREATMENT OF PROTEIN ENERGY WASTING

Given the importance of adequate nutritional status and the large number of factors that can result in PEW, especially in later stages of CKD, prevention and therapeutic strategies should involve a multidisciplinary approach to reduce protein and energy catabolism, prevent further losses, and restore negative balance (Fig. 53.2). Prescribing dietary nutrient intake appropriate for the stage of kidney disease (see Table 53.2) is critically important. Many maintenance dialysis patients will continue their predialysis diets while receiving kidney replacement therapy; this is inappropriate, and it is important that dietary protein and calorie intake increase to meet the requirements after dialysis initiation. Critical and often simple and straightforward steps to minimize the risk of the development or worsening of PEW include combating the catabolic effects of kidney replacement therapy, treating obvious causes of systemic inflammation, and managing comorbid conditions such as metabolic acidosis, diabetes, and depression. Managing food intake by either dietary counseling or positive reinforcement is crucial, particularly

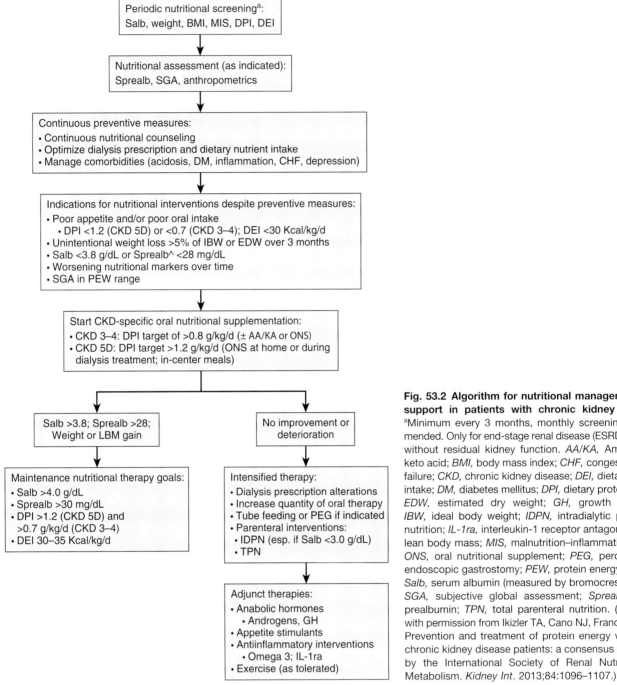

Fig. 53.2 Algorithm for nutritional management and support in patients with chronic kidney disease. [a]Minimum every 3 months, monthly screening recommended. Only for end-stage renal disease (ESRD) patients without residual kidney function. *AA/KA,* Amino acid/keto acid; *BMI,* body mass index; *CHF,* congestive heart failure; *CKD,* chronic kidney disease; *DEI,* dietary energy intake; *DM,* diabetes mellitus; *DPI,* dietary protein intake; *EDW,* estimated dry weight; *GH,* growth hormone; *IBW,* ideal body weight; *IDPN,* intradialytic parenteral nutrition; *IL-1ra,* interleukin-1 receptor antagonist; *LBM,* lean body mass; *MIS,* malnutrition–inflammation score; *ONS,* oral nutritional supplement; *PEG,* percutaneous endoscopic gastrostomy; *PEW,* protein energy wasting; *Salb,* serum albumin (measured by bromocresol green); *SGA,* subjective global assessment; *Sprealb,* serum prealbumin; *TPN,* total parenteral nutrition. (Reprinted with permission from Ikizler TA, Cano NJ, Franch H, et al. Prevention and treatment of protein energy wasting in chronic kidney disease patients: a consensus statement by the International Society of Renal Nutrition and Metabolism. *Kidney Int.* 2013;84:1096–1107.)

for patients treated with maintenance dialysis. Renal dietitians play a critical role in providing the majority of educational support and monitoring patient outcomes.

When dietary counseling to improve nutritional status is unsuccessful, other forms of supplementation such as enteral (including oral protein, amino acid, and energy supplementation, nasogastric feeding tubes, percutaneous endoscopic gastrostomy [PEG], or jejunostomy tubes) and intradialytic parenteral nutrition (IDPN) may be considered. Only a limited number of low-quality studies evaluating the effects of oral or enteral supplementation in CKD patients

not on maintenance dialysis are available. Furthermore, most of these studies demonstrate only a variable degree of success. It is usually a challenge to determine whether an oral or enteral form of supplementation is necessary and effective if administered in CKD patients not on maintenance dialysis. In these patients, recommendations that are developed for other comorbid conditions such as diabetes mellitus, frailty, and old age should be used while taking into account the implications of stage of kidney disease, especially in terms of mineral and electrolyte content of the supplementation.

In certain maintenance dialysis patients, where the standard measures are unable to prevent loss of protein and energy stores, nutritional supplementation is a suitable next step. In general practice, the gastrointestinal route is always preferred for nutritional supplementation. Oral supplementation should be given 2 to 3 times a day, preferably 2 hours before or after main meals and/or during hemodialysis. Oral supplementation can provide an additional 7 to 10 kcal/kg per day of energy and 0.3 to 0.4 g/kg per day of protein. This requires a minimum spontaneous dietary intake of 20 kcal/kg per day of energy and 0.4 to 0.8 g/kg per day of protein to meet the recommended dietary energy intake and dietary protein intake targets.

Although there are no well-designed, large sample size, prospective studies, the beneficial nutritional effects of these supplements have been reported primarily on serum biomarkers such as albumin, prealbumin, and transferrin, as well as gains in body weight and lean body mass. Improvements in markers of quality of life and physical functioning have also been reported. In prospective randomized studies examining hospitalizations and death, the statistical power to appropriately assess the efficacy of these interventions is mostly lacking. However, two recent large-scale observational studies reported significant survival benefit associated with oral nutritional supplement (ONS) administration during hemodialysis in hypoalbuminemic hemodialysis patients. The limitations of these studies include a retrospective design, convenience sampling, and residual confounding from unmeasured variables. A pragmatic cluster randomized clinical trial is under way to answer this question.

For patients who are unable to tolerate nutritional supplementation by mouth, nasogastric, PEG, or jejunostomy tubes can be considered. Although most of the studies reported beneficial nutritional effects of IDPN administration in maintenance hemodialysis patients with overt PEW, a relatively large sample sized, prospective, randomized, controlled study comparing IDPN plus ONS versus ONS alone showed similar improvements in nutritional parameters, with no additional benefit on hospitalization or death rates. Concerns regarding increased infectious complications, greater fluid volume requirement, and high cost remain as the barriers for the frequent use of IDPN. Hence, parenteral provision of nutrients should be reserved as an approach for individuals who cannot tolerate oral or enteral administration of nutrients. Studies using amino acid dialysate (AAD) in PD patients have provided conflicting results. In studies that suggested benefit from AAD, serum transferrin and total protein concentrations increased, and plasma amino acid profiles trended toward normal with one or two exchanges of AAD per day. On the other hand, exacerbations of uremic symptoms as well as metabolic acidosis are potential complications of AAD.

NUTRITION IN ACUTE KIDNEY INJURY

The nutritional hallmark of acute kidney injury (AKI), especially in the setting of critical illness, is excessive catabolism. Factors that have been postulated as the underlying mechanism for this high rate of protein and energy catabolism include concurrent illnesses leading to exaggerated proinflammatory cytokine release, inability to feed patients because of surgical and other reasons, and metabolic derangements predisposing patients to diminished utilization and incorporation of available nutrients. Whether uremic toxin accumulation further exacerbates these abnormalities is questionable because aggressive dialytic clearance does not substantially improve mortality in stage 3 AKI patients.

The nutritional markers that correlate best with efficacy of nutritional therapy and patient outcome are considerably different in AKI patients than in CKD patients. Blood levels of biochemical markers such as serum albumin and prealbumin are influenced by volume status and concurrent inflammatory state. Similarly, utilization of traditional measures of body composition such as anthropometry has limited application in AKI patients owing to major shifts in body water. The actual requirements for protein and energy supplementation in AKI patients are not well defined (see Table 53.2). In the presence of diminished utilization due to an altered metabolic state as well as diminished clearance due to decreased kidney function, excessive protein supplementation will result in increased accumulation of end products of protein and amino acid metabolism. Studies in the intensive care unit setting suggest that early enteral support is generally well tolerated in those without contraindication (e.g., anatomic, ongoing active resuscitation); this same recommendation should be applicable to AKI patients. Parenteral nutrition, in the short term, has a comparable safety profile to enteral nutrition in the overall intensive care unit population, although the risk of infectious complications increases over time and is higher in patients admitted with a diagnosis of sepsis. Parenteral nutrition can be considered as an adjunct if enteral goals are not being met, although it does remain more costly and may lack some nonnutritional benefits to the gut. Provision of large quantities of nutrients, especially intravenously, may result in more fluid administration and predispose patients to fluid overload, resulting in earlier initiation of dialytic support.

BIBLIOGRAPHY

Cano NJ, Fouque D, Roth H, et al. Intradialytic parenteral nutrition does not improve survival in malnourished hemodialysis patients: a 2-year multicenter, prospective, randomized study. *J Am Soc Nephrol.* 2007;18:2583-2591.

Carrero JJ, de Jager DJ, Verduijn M, et al. Cardiovascular and noncardiovascular mortality among men and women starting dialysis. *Clin J Am Soc Nephrol.* 2011;6:1722-1730.

Carrero JJ, Stenvinkel P, Cuppari L, et al. Etiology of the protein-energy wasting syndrome in chronic kidney disease: a consensus statement from the International Society of Renal Nutrition and Metabolism (ISRNM). *J Ren Nutr.* 2013;23:77-90.

Clinical practice guidelines for nutrition in chronic renal failure. K/DOQI, National Kidney Foundation [published erratum appears in Am J Kidney Dis 2001;38:917]. *Am J Kidney Dis.* 2000;35:S1-S140.

de Brito-Ashurst I, Varagunam M, Raftery MJ, Yaqoob MM. Bicarbonate supplementation slows progression of CKD and improves nutritional status. *J Am Soc Nephrol.* 2009;20:2075-2084.

Fouque D, Kalantar-Zadeh K, Kopple J, et al. A proposed nomenclature and diagnostic criteria for protein-energy wasting in acute and chronic kidney disease. *Kidney Int.* 2008;73:391-398.

Gould DW, Graham Brown MP, Watson EL, et al. Physiological benefits of exercise in pre-dialysis chronic kidney disease. *Nephrology (Carlton).* 2014;19:519-527.

Ikizler TA. A patient with CKD and poor nutritional status. *Clin J Am Soc Nephrol.* 2013;8:2174-2182.

Ikizler TA, Cano NJ, Franch H, et al. Prevention and treatment of protein energy wasting in chronic kidney disease patients: a consensus statement by the International Society of Renal Nutrition and Metabolism. *Kidney Int.* 2013;84:1096-1107.

Lacson E Jr, Wang W, Zebrowski B, et al. Outcomes associated with intradialytic oral nutritional supplements in patients undergoing maintenance hemodialysis: a quality improvement report. *Am J Kidney Dis.* 2012;60:591-600.

Naylor HL., Jackson H, Walker GH, et al. Renal Nutrition Group of the British Dietetic Association; British Dietetic Association. British Dietetic Association evidence-based guidelines for the protein requirements of adults undergoing maintenance haemodialysis or peritoneal dialysis. *J Hum Nutr Diet.* 2013;26:315-328.

Pupim LB, Ikizler TA. Assessment and monitoring of uremic malnutrition. *J Ren Nutr.* 2004;14:6-19.

Stenvinkel P. Can treating persistent inflammation limit protein energy wasting? *Semin Dialysis.* 2013;26:16-19.

Stratton RJ, Bircher G, Fouque D, et al. Multinutrient oral supplements and tube feeding in maintenance dialysis: a systematic review and meta-analysis. *Am J Kidney Dis.* 2005;46:387-405.

Bone and Mineral Disorders in Chronic Kidney Disease

54

L. Darryl Quarles; Pieter Evenepoel

Chronic kidney disease (CKD) alters the regulation of calcium, phosphate, and vitamin D homeostasis, leading to secondary hyperparathyroidism, elevations in serum fibroblast growth factor 23 (FGF23), metabolic bone disease, soft tissue calcifications, and other metabolic derangements that have a significant impact on morbidity and mortality. Although metabolic bone disease, reductions in circulating $1,25(OH)_2$ vitamin D, hyperphosphatemia, hypocalcemia, and abnormalities of parathyroid function are historically the main clinical manifestations of disordered mineral metabolism in CKD, elevated FGF23, α-Klotho deficiency, extraskeletal and vascular calcifications, and the impact of nontraditional risk factors on cardiovascular disease (CVD) and mortality are increasingly recognized as important aspects of CKD. Earlier interventions and stringent management guidelines to control serum parathyroid hormone (PTH), calcium, and phosphorus concentrations have been proposed for patients with CKD by several international foundations and initiatives, including the Kidney Disease: Improving Global Outcomes (KDIGO). An update of the 2009 KDIGO clinical practice guideline for chronic kidney disease–mineral and bone disorder (CKD-MBD) will be published before the release of this primer. Overall, there is lack of consensus regarding the best approach to treat abnormalities in mineral metabolism effectively and safely and to prevent the complications associated with these abnormalities.

Both active vitamin D analogues and calcimimetic drugs that target the calcium-sensing receptor (CaSR) in the parathyroid gland are available to suppress PTH, although the specific roles for each remain unspecified. There is similar lack of consensus on other issues, such as the clinical significance of low circulating 25(OH)D levels in people with CKD (which represents vitamin D deficiency in those without CKD); the optimal agent, dose, and route of active vitamin D analogue to treat secondary hyperparathyroidism; and the relative role of calcium- and noncalcium based binders to control serum phosphate. Most recommendations are graded as level 2 (weak), reflecting an important degree of remaining uncertainty.

The importance of vitamin D pathways in regulating innate immunity and cardiovascular function, in addition to its more traditional role in regulating mineral metabolism, is increasingly being recognized. However, although low vitamin D levels are associated with increased risk of CVD, infection, and mortality, there are only limited data that nutritional vitamin D supplementation (with cholecalciferol or ergocalciferol) improves clinical outcomes. In addition, treatment with active vitamin D or its analogues does not

appear to improve the severity of left ventricular hypertrophy (LVH) in CKD. Another word of caution against indiscriminate use of vitamin D supplements is that this treatment may exacerbate hyperphosphatemia, hypercalcemia, and hyperphosphatinonism (high FGF23).

Finally, emerging knowledge about the endocrine functions of bone (and specifically the role of the phosphaturic and vitamin D regulating hormone FGF23 in LVH, cardiovascular mortality, and glomerular filtration rate [GFR] loss) has led to a reexamination of the pathogenesis and treatment of disordered mineral metabolism in CKD.

PATHOGENESIS OF ABNORMAL MINERAL METABOLISM AND SECONDARY HYPERPARATHYROIDISM IN CHRONIC KIDNEY DISEASE

An increase in circulating PTH concentrations is the hallmark of secondary hyperparathyroidism. The major metabolic abnormalities leading to the increase in PTH are diminished production of $1,25-(OH)_2D_3$ (calcitriol, the activated form of vitamin D), decreased serum calcium, and increased serum phosphorus. In normal subjects, PTH is responsible for maintaining the serum calcium concentration within a narrow range through direct actions on the distal tubule of the kidney to increase calcium resorption and actions on bone to increase calcium and phosphate efflux (Fig. 54.1). In addition, some PTH effects are mediated by its effect on the production of calcitriol by the kidney via stimulation of Cyp27b1, the enzyme that converts inactive 25 hydroxyvitamin D to active $1,25(OH)_2D$. The net effects of PTH's bone and kidney actions are to create the positive calcium balance that is necessary to maintain calcium homeostasis. To prevent a concomitant positive phosphate balance due to the skeletal effects of PTH and the gastrointestinal actions of calcitriol, PTH acts secondarily to increase renal phosphorus excretion, mostly by decreasing activity of the sodium phosphate cotransporter in the proximal renal tubule.

Parathyroid disease in CKD is a progressive disorder characterized by both increased PTH secretion and expansion of the number of the PTH-secreting chief cells (hyperplasia). Elevations in serum PTH levels may first become evident when the GFR falls below 60 mL/min per 1.73 m². This occurs before hyperphosphatemia, reduction in calcitriol levels, or hypocalcemia is detectable by routine laboratory measurements. This delay in detectable serum chemistry abnormalities is presumably caused by the actions of increased

Parathyroid glands

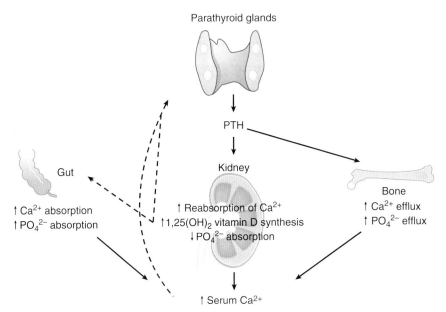

Fig. 54.1 Regulation of systemic calcium homeostasis. Parathyroid hormone (PTH) is a calcemic hormone that targets the kidney to promote renal calcium conservation and the bone to increase efflux of calcium and phosphorus. PTH-mediated production of 1,25(OH)$_2$D$_3$ (activated vitamin D) by the kidney increases gastrointestinal calcium and phosphate absorption. The phosphaturic actions of PTH on the kidney cause it to excrete the excess phosphate that accompanies calcium absorption by the intestines and calcium efflux from bone. Changes in calcium, 1,25(OH)$_2$D$_3$, and phosphate levels exert feedback on the parathyroid glands *(dotted line)*. In chronic kidney disease (CKD), elevation of serum fibroblast growth factor 23 (FGF23) is an early event leading to suppression of 1,25(OH)$_2$D production and possibly increased catabolism. FGF23-mediated suppression of 1,25(OH)$_2$D$_3$ may be the initiating event leading to secondary hyperparathyroidism. In advanced CKD, elevations of PTH appear to stimulate FGF23 further. Elevated levels of serum phosphate and FGF23 are associated with increased mortality in CKD.

PTH to restore homeostasis. PTH levels increase progressively as kidney function declines, such that all untreated subjects reaching stage 5 CKD (GFR <15 mL/min per 1.73 m^2 or dialysis) would be expected to have elevated PTH levels.

The initial event leading to an incremental rise in PTH has traditionally been attributed to primary reductions in 1,25(OH)$_2$D levels caused by decreased production by the diseased kidney. More recent data implicate an initial role of elevated FGF23 in the genesis of secondary hyperparathyroidism in CKD. In this scenario, increments in FGF23 reduce 1,25(OH)$_2$D production by suppressing Cyp27b1 activity in the proximal tubule and possibly enhance 1,25(OH)2D catabolism through increased Cyp24 activity. Cross-sectional studies in humans and serial studies of animal models with CKD suggest that increments in serum FGF23 precede elevations of PTH and correlate with reductions in circulating 1,25(OH)$_2$D concentrations. This sequence of events, however, is questioned by recent epidemiologic data. Given the multiple, complex, and often reciprocal interactions between the various players (calcium, phosphorus, FGF23, 1,25[OH]$_2$D), the exact role of each moiety in the pathogenesis of secondary hyperparathyroidism is hard to define.

FGF23, a key regulator of phosphate and vitamin D homeostasis, is perhaps the initial adaptive response in CKD and may also play a role in cardiovascular complications as well as progression of kidney disease. Gene transcription of FGF23 in mouse models is regulated both by systemic factors, such as hyperphosphatemia and elevated 1,25-(OH)$_2$D$_3$ levels, and by local bone-derived factors. FGF23 knockout mice are hyperphosphatemic and display soft tissue and vascular calcifications, growth retardation, and bone mineralization abnormalities. FGF23 is expressed mainly in osteocytes in bone and, to a much lesser extent, in the bone marrow, the ventrolateral thalamic nucleus, the thymus, and lymph nodes. FGF23 promotes phosphate excretion by inhibition of sodium-dependent phosphate resorption. It also suppresses renal and extrarenal calcitriol synthesis. FGF23 may also act in the heart through "off-target effects" to activate FGF receptors (FGFR) in the absence of its coreceptor α-Klotho, or on the kidney through "on-target" effects on FGFR: α-Klotho complexes to regulate genes, such as the suppression of angiotensin-converting enzyme 2 (ACE2). In addition, FGF23 may qualify both as a risk marker and mediator of (cardiovascular) disease. FGF23 production may be lowered by phosphate binders and/or dietary therapy. Whether FGF23 suppression translates to improved intermediate and hard outcomes remains to be proven.

Unless adequately treated, secondary hyperparathyroidism progresses inexorably, with the need for parathyroidectomy proportional to the number of years on dialysis. The difficulty in treating hyperparathyroidism in CKD partly reflects the massive hyperplasia and possibly adenomatous transformation of the parathyroid gland that occurs because of the chronic stimulation of PTH production. Enlarged, hyperplastic parathyroid glands retain some responsiveness to calcium-mediated

PTH suppression in secondary hyperparathyroidism. Because this responsiveness is lost with reductions in extracellular CaSR and vitamin D receptor (VDR) expression, as well as autonomous adenomatous transformation of the parathyroid gland, hypercalcemia develops in some patients. This is referred to as *tertiary hyperparathyroidism.*

Three molecular targets have been identified that regulate parathyroid gland function, including the G protein–coupled CaSR, the VDR, and the FGF23 receptor, which is constituted by the FGFR: α-Klotho complex. The molecular identity of the putative extracellular phosphate sensor remains undefined. Calcium, acting through the CaSR, is the major regulator of PTH transcription, secretion, and parathyroid gland hyperplasia. Calcitriol, which acts on the VDR in the parathyroid gland to suppress PTH transcription but not PTH secretion, has overlapping functions with the CaSR. It appears, however, that the physiologic role of the VDR in regulating parathyroid gland function may be subordinate to that of calcium. In this regard, secondary hyperparathyroidism and bone abnormalities in VDR-deficient mice can be corrected by normalizing the serum calcium concentration. Extracellular phosphate also has direct effects on parathyroid production, apparently through the regulation of PTH messenger RNA (mRNA) levels, possibly by stabilizing posttranscriptional PTH mRNA. Hyperphosphatemia may indirectly affect PTH production by lowering ionized calcium through chelation and suppressing 1α-hydroxylase and, hence, calcitriol production by the kidney. Finally, FGF23 has recently been shown to target the parathyroid gland via FGFR: α-Klotho complexes and to suppress PTH secretion. The actions of FGF23 on the parathyroid gland remain to be further elucidated, because most states of FGF23 excess are associated with elevations of PTH, and stimulation of FGFR pathways would be expected to lead to cell hyperplasia.

PATHOGENESIS OF BONE DISEASE ASSOCIATED WITH CHRONIC KIDNEY DISEASE

Bone is a dynamic tissue that undergoes repetitive cycles of removal and replacement. Osteoclasts, under the influence of paracrine and systemic factors, resorb bone, whereas osteoblasts fill in the resorptive cavities with new extracellular matrix that undergoes mineralization. This process is also regulated by physiochemical properties as well as proteins that either inhibit or promote the mineralization process. A subset of osteoblasts become embedded in the bone matrix to form an interconnected network of cells (osteocytes) that also respond to systemic and local stimuli to secrete factors regulating the bone remodeling process. During growth, new trabecular bone is added to the long bones beneath the growth plate, and factors that affect bone remodeling can also affect growth plate morphology, leading to rickets. In adults, bone disease can manifest as too little (osteopenia) or too much (osteosclerosis) bone, high or low states of bone turnover, and impaired mineralization.

PTH through PTH receptors, 1,25(OH)$_2$D through VDRs, and calcium and phosphate through effects on mineralization of bone extracellular matrix can all affect bone health. Osteoblast-mediated bone formation entails generation of a collagen matrix that undergoes mineralization controlled by a complex interplay among factors promoting and inhibiting mineralization. Bone formation is coupled to osteoclast-mediated bone resorption through osteoblastic paracrine pathways involving the secretion of a receptor activator of nuclear factor-κB ligand (RANKL), which stimulates osteoclast formation, function, and survival. Osteoblasts also secrete osteoprotegerin (OPG), which bind to RANKL to inhibit bone resorption. Denosumab, a monoclonal antibody that binds to RANKL and mimics the effects of OPG, is used to treat osteoporosis. Osteocytes also regulate bone formation through the production and secretion of sclerostin (SOST), an inhibitor of osteoanabolic Wnt signaling pathways.

The circulating level of PTH is the primary determinant of bone turnover in CKD and is a major determinant of bone disease type. PTH receptors are present in both osteoblasts and osteocytes. PTH suppresses SOST expression and stimulates cyclic adenosine monophosphate (cAMP) as well as other pathways leading to increased osteoblast-mediated bone formation. Long-term exposure to high circulating concentrations of PTH leads to increased bone resorption. In contrast, more short-term, intermittent exposure to PTH can result in increased bone formation in excess of bone resorption. Intermittent PTH administration is the basis for use of teriparatide to treat osteoporosis. In addition, 1,25(OH)$_2$D, at least in experimental settings, promotes mineralization and stimulates bone resorption. The specific types of histologic changes may also depend on patient age, the duration and cause of kidney failure, the type of dialysis therapy used, the presence of acidosis, vitamin D status, accumulation of metals such as aluminum, and other conditions affecting mineralization of the extracellular matrix.

HISTOLOGIC CLASSIFICATION OF BONE DISEASE IN CHRONIC KIDNEY DISEASE

Bone disease associated with CKD (Fig. 54.2) has traditionally been classified histologically according to the degrees of abnormal bone turnover and impaired mineralization of the extracellular matrix, although the current classification of bone histology adopted by KDIGO focuses on turnover, mineralization, and volume (TMV) (Fig. 54.3). These histologic changes in bone have been best studied in patients undergoing dialysis. Traditional categories are as follows:

1. Secondary hyperparathyroidism (high-turnover bone disease or osteitis fibrosa).
2. Osteomalacia (defective mineralization).
3. Mixed uremic bone disease (a mixture of high-turnover bone disease and osteomalacia).
4. Adynamic bone disease (decreased rates of bone formation without a mineralization defect).

The 2009 KDIGO initiative recommended the TMV classification. Especially if specific therapies that target each of these characteristics are developed, this classification could prove useful; however, treatments are at present directed toward maintaining serum PTH levels in a range that (1) prevents high-turnover osteitis fibrosa and increased cortical porosity on one end of the spectrum and (2)

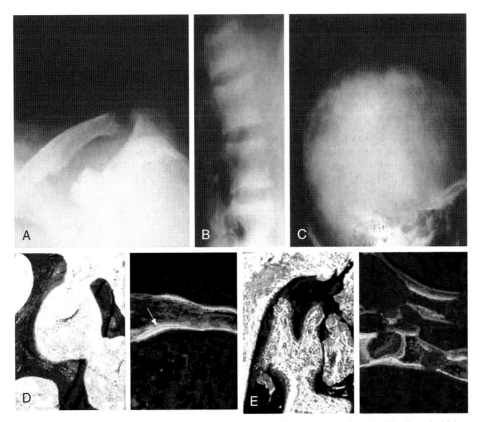

Fig. 54.2 Radiographic and histologic features of bone disease associated with chronic kidney disease (CKD). (A) Radiographic findings of severe erosion of the distal clavicle resulting from secondary hyperparathyroidism. (B) Example of "rugger-jersey spine" resulting from sclerosis of the end plates associated with hyperparathyroidism. (C) "Pepper-pot skull" with areas of erosion and patchy osteosclerosis associated with hyperparathyroidism. (D) Histologic appearance of normal bone. On the left, a section stained with Goldner Masson trichrome stain shows mineralized lamellar bone *(blue)* and adjacent nonmineralized osteoid surfaces *(red-brown)*. On the right, a Villanueva-stained section viewed under fluorescent light shows tetracycline labeling of freshly formed bone. Double staining *(arrow)* indicates amount of new bone laid down during the interval between the two periods of tetracycline administration. (E) Histologic appearance of osteitis fibrosa in a patient with stage 5 CKD and elevated parathyroid hormone levels. On the left, Goldner Masson trichrome stain shows increased numbers of multinucleated osteoclasts at resorptive surfaces *(white arrow)* and extensive bone-marrow fibrosis *(light blue staining of marrow)*. On the right, tetracycline labeling shows marked increases in the osteoid *(orange-red staining)* and in sites of new bone formation as measured by the yellow-green bands below the osteoid surfaces. (A–C from Martin KJ, Gonzalez EA, Slatopolsky E. Renal osteodystrophy. In: Brenner BM, ed. *Brenner and Rector's the Kidney.* 7th ed. Philadelphia: Saunders; 2004:2280, with permission.)

avoids low-turnover osteopenia (adynamic bone) at the other end.

HIGH-TURNOVER BONE DISEASE

High-turnover bone disease caused by excess PTH is characterized by greater number and size of osteoclasts and an increase in the number of resorption lacunae with scalloped trabeculae, as well as abnormally high numbers of osteoblasts. There is an increased amount of osteoid (unmineralized bone), which may have a woven appearance that reflects a disordered collagen arrangement under conditions of rapid matrix deposition. The excess in osteoid surfaces that accompanies increased bone turnover has been described as *mixed uremic bone disease*, but it may reflect a normal response to increased turnover rather than superimposed defective mineralization. Peritrabecular fibrosis (and even marrow fibrosis), reflecting PTH stimulation of osteoblastic precursors, is observed in severe disease.

OSTEOMALACIA

Osteomalacia is characterized by prolongation of the mineralization lag time as well as by increased thickness, surface area, and volume of osteoid. Osteomalacia was formerly linked to aluminum toxicity from both contamination of water in dialysates and the use of aluminum-based phosphate binders. Other causes of osteomalacia that may be present in CKD patients include 25-hydroxyvitamin D deficiency (secondary to poor dietary vitamin D and calcium intake, and lack of exposure to sunlight because of poor mobility and extended

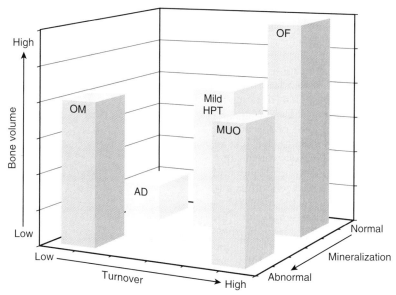

Fig. 54.3 The distribution of bone mineral disorders according to the Turnover, Mineralization, and Volume Classification System. *AD*, Adynamic bone disease; *HPT*, hyperparathyroidism; *MUO*, mixed uremic bone disease/osteomalacia; *OF*, osteitis fibrosa; *OM*, osteomalacia.

hospitalizations), metabolic acidosis (which inhibits both osteoblasts and osteoclasts), and hypophosphatemia (e.g., in Fanconi syndrome).

ADYNAMIC BONE DISEASE

Adynamic bone disease is a low-turnover bone state that has received increased attention. According to recent bone biopsy data, as many as 40% of patients on hemodialysis and 50% of patients on peritoneal dialysis have adynamic bone disease. In this disorder, the amount of osteoid thickness is normal or reduced, and there is no mineralization defect. The main findings are decreased numbers of osteoclasts and osteoblasts and very low rates of bone formation as measured by tetracycline labeling. High serum calcium levels sometimes seen in adynamic bone disease may in part be secondary to high oral calcium loads and suppression of PTH when calcium-based phosphate binders are used. There may also be a decreased ability of bone to buffer calcium loads. The main risk factors for adynamic bone disease are peritoneal dialysis, older age, corticosteroid use, and diabetes. It is thought that adynamic bone disease represents a state of relative hypoparathyroidism in CKD.

EPIDEMIOLOGY OF BONE DISEASE

Based on limited bone histologic data, approximately 40% of blacks and 20% of whites with end-stage kidney disease have high turnover disease, with the remainder having normal or low bone turnover in spite of elevated circulating PTH levels. Adynamic bone disease may not be a naturally occurring separate disease, but a consequence of overtreatment of hyperparathyroidism with calcium, calcitriol, and/or calcimimetics. CKD is a state of PTH hyporesponsiveness, most probably caused by downregulation of the PTH receptor and competing downstream signals.

CLINICAL MANIFESTATIONS OF BONE DISEASES ASSOCIATED WITH CHRONIC KIDNEY DISEASE

Most patients with CKD and mildly elevated circulating levels of PTH are asymptomatic. When clinical features of bone disease are present, they can be classified into musculoskeletal and extraskeletal manifestations.

MUSCULOSKELETAL MANIFESTATIONS

Fractures, tendon rupture, and bone pain resulting from metabolic bone disease, muscle pain and weakness, and periarticular pain are the major musculoskeletal manifestations associated with CKD. The most clinically significant effect of metabolic bone disease in CKD is hip fracture, which has a high incidence among stage 5 CKD patients and is associated with an increased risk for death. There is a roughly 4.4-fold increase in hip fracture risk in patients undergoing dialysis compared with the general population. Both high and low serum values of PTH are associated with increased fracture risks. Evidence from prospective cohort studies indicates that measurements of bone mineral density (BMD) may help in predicting fracture risk in CKD as in the general population.

EXTRASKELETAL MANIFESTATIONS

The most important advance in the understanding of the clinical significance of disordered bone and mineral metabolism in CKD has been the recognition that it is a systemic disorder affecting soft tissues, particularly blood vessels, heart valves, and skin. CVD accounts for approximately half of all deaths of patients on dialysis (see Chapter 55). Coronary and peripheral vascular calcifications occur frequently in stage 5 CKD and increase as a function of the number of years on dialysis. Gaining a better understanding of the etiology of increased vascular calcification and how it may influence clinical cardiovascular events is of critical importance.

Several patterns of vascular calcification have been described. The first occurs as focal calcification associated with lipid-laden foam cells that are seen in atherosclerotic plaques. These calcifications may increase both the fragility and the risk for rupture of plaques. Some have questioned the role of calcification in the pathogenesis of the athero sclerotic vascular lesions, raising the possibility that it is an epiphenomenon. The second pattern of vascular calcification is diffuse; it is not associated with atherosclerotic plaques and occurs in the media of vessels. This pattern is seen with aging, diabetes, and progressive kidney failure. This *Mönckeberg's sclerosis* was thought to be of little clinical significance for many years, but its effects of increasing blood vessel stiffness and reducing vascular compliance, which result in a widened pulse pressure, increased cardiac afterload, and LVH, are potential mechanisms that could contribute to cardiovascular morbidity (Fig. 54.4). Coronary calcium load as detected by electron-beam computed tomography (EBCT) has not been shown to correlate in dialysis patients with the degree of coronary vessel stenosis, suggesting that medial calcification is a disease entity separate from atherosclerosis in these patients.

The exact mechanisms of vascular medial calcification probably reflect the combined effects of decreased mineralization inhibitors, such as matrix Gla protein (a vitamin K–dependent calcification inhibitor known to be expressed by smooth muscle cells and macrophages in the artery wall) and increased mineralization inducers. Vascular calcification is an active, cell-mediated process. Accumulating evidence suggests that vascular smooth muscle cells undergo a phenotypic transition to an osteoblast-like cell that is important in driving the calcification process. Elevated serum phosphorus causes upregulation of a type III sodium-dependent phosphate cotransporter Pit-1 (POU1F1) in smooth muscle cells. The resulting increased intracellular phosphorus upregulates core binding factor alpha 1 (Cbfa1/RUNX2), a transcription factor believed to be critical in mediating this phenotypic switch to osteoblast-like cells. Concomitantly, bone matrix proteins, such as osteopontin and osteocalcin, are found only in calcified vessels.

An emerging area of study concerns how uremia may affect the vascular calcification process, independent of its effects on serum phosphorus. For example, the glycoprotein fetuin-A, which is downregulated during the acute-phase response, is an important inhibitor of calcification and may be associated with cardiovascular risk. Patients on dialysis have lower serum fetuin-A levels than do nondialysis patients.

The contribution of vitamin D to vascular calcification is controversial and debated. Some studies suggest that calcitriol can modulate vascular smooth muscle growth and influence vascular calcification by upregulation of the VDR and increased calcium uptake into smooth muscle cells. Vitamin D treatment enhances the extent of arterial calcification in animals that are also given warfarin to inhibit γ-carboxylation of the matrix Gla protein. On the other hand, low doses of both calcitriol and paricalcitol seem to be protective, probably through restoration of α-Klotho and osteopontin expression. A U-shaped dose response of active vitamin D can thus be

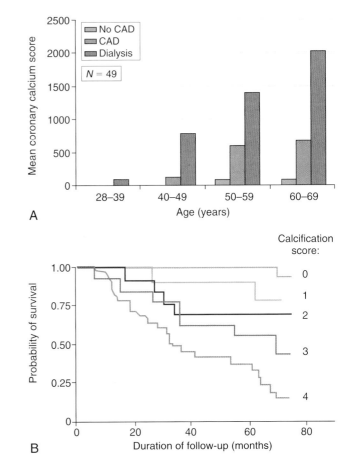

Fig. 54.4 Increased risk of death and cardiovascular calcification in dialysis patients. (A) Calcium score was determined by electron-beam computed tomography. The mean coronary artery calcium score was significantly higher in hemodialysis patients than in nondialysis patients with documented cardiovascular disease. (B) Risk of death in patients on hemodialysis increases as a function of a calcification score measured ultrasonographically (*P* < .0001 for comparisons among all curves). *CAD*, Calcium artery disease. (A from Braun J, Oldendorf M, Moshage W, et al. Electron beam computed tomography in the evaluation of cardiac calcifications in chronic dialysis patients. *Am J Kidney Dis.* 1996;27:394–401, with permission from the National Kidney Foundation. B from Blacher J, Guerin AP, Pannier B, et al. Arterial calcification, arterial stiffness, and cardiovascular risk in end-stage renal disease. *Hypertension.* 2001;38:938, with permission.)

postulated with regard to vascular calcification. A consistent survival benefit of treatment with active vitamin (analogues) in patients undergoing hemodialysis has been described in several retrospective studies and a recent meta-analysis, and the benefit seemed to be more pronounced in the low-dose range. It should be emphasized that, at present, no prospective randomized controlled trial (RCT) confirmed these results, leaving an important gap in the evidence.

CALCEMIC UREMIC ARTERIOLOPATHY

Calcemic uremic arteriolopathy (CUA), or calciphylaxis, is another form of vascular calcification that is observed primarily, although not exclusively, in stage 5 CKD. The prevalence is not well established, but it has been reported to occur in 1% to 4% of dialysis patients. CUA manifests with extensive calcifications of the skin, muscles, and subcutaneous tissues. Most often, skin lesions occur on the breast, abdomen, and thighs. Unusual presentations, such as necrosis of the tongue and of the penis, as well as visceral involvement of the lungs, pancreas, and intestines, have been described. Examination may not only show a violaceous rash, skin nodules, skin firmness, and eschars, but also livedo reticularis and painful hyperesthesia of the skin. Nonhealing ulcerations of the skin and gangrene resistant to medical therapy often lead to amputation, uncontrollable sepsis, and death. Histologically, there is extensive medial calcification of small arteries, arterioles, capillaries, and venules, as well as intimal proliferation, endovascular fibrosis, and sometimes thrombosis. Whether the molecular pathogenesis of CUA is similar to that of Mönckeberg sclerosis is not clear. Cases reported to be associated with very high PTH levels improved after parathyroidectomy. However, there are other cases in which the PTH levels were only mildly elevated. Interestingly, in the EVOLVE (Evaluation of Cinacalcet Therapy to Lower Cardiovascular Events) study, the use of cinacalcet in addition to standard therapy for secondary hyperparathyroidism reduced the incidence of CUA. Other risk factors for CUA are obesity, advancing age, female sex, diabetes mellitus, warfarin use, recent trauma, hypotension, and calcium ingestion. Anecdotal reports suggest that sodium thiosulfate, bisphosphonate therapy, daily hemodialysis, hyperbaric oxygen treatment, vitamin K, and normalization of serum phosphate levels may improve outcomes.

DISORDERED MINERAL METABOLISM AND MORTALITY IN CHRONIC KIDNEY DISEASE

Cardiovascular and all-cause mortality are high in CKD. In addition to traditional cardiovascular risk factors associated with underlying diseases leading to CKD and inflammation associated with CKD, abnormalities of bone and mineral metabolism are linked to increased mortality. In particular, hyperphosphatemia and elevated FGF23 concentrations show the most consistent and robust association with increased mortality.

Associative studies to date have shown that elevation of serum phosphorus is an independent risk factor for increased mortality in end-stage renal disease (ESRD) patients managed with hemodialysis, as well as CKD patients not yet on dialysis. Because increases in serum phosphorus greater than 3.5 mg/dL are independently associated with an incremental risk for mortality in nondialysis CKD, current recommendations emphasize keeping serum phosphate in the normal range. Some studies suggest that better control of serum phosphate, as well as use of noncalcium compared with calcium-based phosphate binders to control hyperphosphatemia, may be associated with improved outcomes. In addition, PTH in the 400- to 600-pg/mL range, hypercalcemia, and elevated alkaline phosphatase are associated with increased mortality in maintenance hemodialysis patients. However, the EVOLVE study, which compared the use of cinacalcet with standard therapy with active vitamin D analogues and phosphate binders, only showed a 7% nonsignificant survival benefit.

Elevated serum FGF23 is associated with increased LVH and mortality in CKD and ESRD. The increased mortality risk is independent of concomitant hyperphosphatemia in ESRD.

Of interest, in the EVOLVE study, treatment-induced reductions in serum FGF23 were found to be associated with lower rates of cardiovascular death and major cardiovascular events. Because high-dose active vitamin D analogues increase serum phosphate and FGF23 concentrations, associative studies indicating that treatment with active vitamin D analogues impart a survival advantage need to be reexamined. Indeed, the recently completed PRIMO and OPERA studies failed to show an effect of paracalcitol on left ventricular mass in CKD patients not yet on dialysis.

OTHER CONDITIONS AFFECTING MUSCULOSKELETAL HEALTH: AMYLOIDOSIS

Patients treated with dialysis for many years, particularly those treated with low-flux hemodialysis membranes, are at risk for developing osteoarticular amyloid depositions that consist of β_2-microglobulin (β_2M). This protein is normally released into the plasma with cell turnover and cleared by the kidney. Clinical manifestations of dialysis-related amyloidosis include destructive arthropathy, bone cysts, carpal tunnel syndrome, and fractures. Kidney transplant, high-flux hemodialysis, or hemofiltration, all of which provide increased clearance of β_2M, may be beneficial (see Chapter 57).

DIAGNOSIS OF BONE DISEASES ASSOCIATED WITH CHRONIC KIDNEY DISEASE

BIOCHEMICAL PARAMETERS

Abnormal parathyroid gland function is assessed by measurement of random circulating PTH levels. Full-length PTH has a half-life of 2 to 4 minutes. PTH is cleaved into an inactive C-terminal fragment, an active N-terminal fragment, and inactive midregion fragments in the peripheral tissues. These PTH fragments are normally excreted by the kidney and have a prolonged half-life in kidney failure. Circulating PTH thus is a heterogeneous mixture of full-length hormone and fragments, with (7-84)PTH accounting for up to 50% of overall PTH. The (7-84)PTH fragment may lack biologic activity or may potentially have distinct biologic actions. It may have hypocalcemic effects in vivo, and it has been shown to inhibit osteoclastic bone resorption in vitro.

Increasingly specific immunoreactive PTH assays have been developed over the years. Second-generation assays are currently most widely implemented. They use a capture antibody that binds near the N-terminus and a second solid phase-coupled antibody that binds to the C-terminus. Differences in antibody specificities and affinities of the assays translate into differing recovery of (1-84)PTH and differing cross-reactivity with (7-84)PTH and other fragments. This may explain, together with the lack of an agreed-upon common standard (calibrator), the large variability that exists among commercially available second-generation PTH assays. The third-generation assay uses the same capture antibody, but the detection antibody is more specific for the first four amino acids of PTH, thereby avoiding cross-reactivity with the N-terminal truncated PTH fragments. PTH levels using this bio-intact PTH assay are approximately 50% to 60% lower than those measured with the intact PTH assay.

Table 54.1   Kidney Disease: Improving Global Outcomes and Japanese Society of Dialysis Therapy Clinical Practice Guidelines for Bone Metabolism and Disease in Chronic Kidney Disease

	Phosphorus (mg/dL)	Calcium (Corrected, mg/dL)	Intact PTH (pg/mL)
KDIGO	Normal range	Normal range	150–600 (2–9 × normal)
JSDT	3.5–6	8.4–10	60–180

JSDT, Japanese Society of Dialysis Therapy; *KDIGO*, Kidney Disease: Improving Global Outcomes; *PTH*, parathyroid hormone.

Defining the target PTH level in the setting of CKD remains a challenge. Because of end-organ hyporesponsiveness (resistance) to PTH, the recommended target PTH levels are greater than the upper limit of the normal range in dialysis patients. The previously recommended target ranges for serum intact PTH are 35 to 70 pg/mL, 70 to 110 pg/mL, and 150 to 300 pg/mL for CKD stages 3, 4, and 5, respectively, reflect the progressive resistance to PTH as CKD progresses (Table 54.1). Because of the lack of standardization of PTH assays, KDIGO preferred to define the target in terms of times upper normal limit. In patients with ESRD, KDIGO recommends to maintain PTH levels between 2 and 9 times the upper limit of normal for the assay. The long-term impact of this more conservative management strategy still remains to be determined. This approach may minimize oversuppression of PTH and low-turnover bone disease, but it includes the risk of undersuppression of parathyroid gland hyperplasia leading to progression of secondary to tertiary hyperparathyroidism.

PTH levels are a direct measure of parathyroid gland function and an indirect measure of bone remodeling. PTH levels greater than 300 pg/mL correlate with the bony changes of secondary hyperparathyroidism and/or osteitis fibrosis. However, these observations are primarily derived from older studies in which patient demographics differed from those of today's dialysis population and before the widespread use of active vitamin D analogues. Patients with adynamic bone disease usually have intact PTH levels lower than 150 pg/mL, but these values also occur in subjects with normal bone.

PTH is only a crude indirect measure of bone turnover, because factors other than PTH can affect bone. The utility of PTH levels as an indicator of bone turnover can be increased by assessment of bone-specific alkaline phosphatase levels, which correlate with the degree of osteoblastic activity. Other biochemical markers of bone turnover are being developed that may provide a more accurate assessment of osteoblast and osteoclast activity in bone. For example, serum tartrate-resistant acid phosphatase 5b levels correlate well with histologic indices of osteoclasts and may serve as a specific marker for osteoclastic activity in CKD patients with bone disease. Efforts to correlate the different subtypes of bone disease with various markers of bone remodeling in both dialysis and predialysis patients are areas of ongoing research. Furthermore, prospective studies are required to determine whether evaluating trends in biomarker concentrations could guide therapeutic decisions.

BONE BIOPSY

The gold standard for assessing and diagnosing the various types of bone disease in patients with CKD is an iliac crest bone biopsy with double tetracycline labeling. Bone histomorphometric analysis of the biopsy specimen includes assessment of bone and fibrosis volumes, amount of osteoid and mineralization, and number of osteoblasts and osteoclasts seen on bony surfaces. Bone biopsies should be considered in the setting of atraumatic fracture with no other clear underlying cause, suspected aluminum toxicity (although rare today) to confirm the presence of osteomalacia before chelation therapy, before parathyroidectomy in patients with severe musculoskeletal symptoms and/or hypercalcemia with intermediate (100 to 500 pg/mL) intact PTH levels, and to exclude adynamic bone disease before the initiation of antiresorptive therapy.

IMAGING

In general, radiographic studies are not indicated in the diagnosis of the bone disorders associated with CKD, although certain radiographic changes can be seen (see Fig. 54.2A through C). Increased osteoblast function, especially in the setting of severe elevations of PTH, can lead to increased trabecular bone volume and accounts for the sclerotic changes that manifest as a "rugger-jersey spine" on radiography. Osteoclast-mediated bone resorption of secondary hyperparathyroidism results in cortical thinning and the classic radiographic evidence of subperiosteal, intracortical, and endosteal bone resorption. Subperiosteal erosions are best seen at the distal ends of the phalanges and clavicles and at the sacroiliac joints. Radiographically, expansile lytic lesions (brown tumors) can be seen in severe osteitis fibrosis. Pseudofractures, which appear as wide, radiolucent bands perpendicular to the bone long axis, can be seen in osteomalacia.

Osteoporosis is defined as a BMD that is at least 2.5 standard deviations lower than the mean BMD of a young adult of the same sex. Although patients with CKD typically have lower BMDs than the general population, the interpretations of dual-energy X-ray absorptiometry (DEXA) scans are complicated in secondary hyperparathyroidism because of focal areas of osteosclerosis, the presence of extraskeletal calcifications, and the variable presence of osteomalacia. Despite these limitations, DEXA BMD predicts fractures in CKD in the general population as evidenced by recent cohort studies. Current guidelines suggest BMD testing to assess fracture risk in patients with CKD stages 3a-5D with evidence of CKD-MBD and/or risk factors for osteoporosis if results will affect treatment decisions. Of note, there is no accurate correlation between BMD as measured by DEXA and the type of CKD-associated bone disease present.

TREATMENT OF MINERAL AND BONE DISORDER IN CHRONIC KIDNEY DISEASE

The treatment of disordered mineral metabolism in CKD is directed toward normalizing serum calcium, phosphate, PTH, and metabolic acidosis while minimizing the risks associated with the therapies. In the United States, the types of treatments chosen are influenced by the economic constraints of the health care system, which limits the frequency of hemodialysis in most patients to three treatments per week. Clinical practice guidelines for bone metabolism and disease in CKD have been developed by several organizations and are outlined in Table 54.1.

These recommendations are influenced by data linking an elevated serum phosphorus concentration or an elevated calcium concentration to increased mortality and by the growing concern that excessive calcium exposure may increase the risk of cardiovascular calcification. Of note, there are no clinical trial data demonstrating that any current treatments available for CKD-MBD reduce mortality, and achieving these targets with current treatment regimens is difficult. Nonetheless, these guidelines are a first step toward standardizing the approach to this difficult disorder.

The various tools for treating hyperphosphatemia and secondary hyperparathyroidism include dietary phosphorus restriction, calcium-based and non–calcium-based phosphate binders, calcitriol or other active vitamin D analogues, calcimimetics, daily or nocturnal hemodialysis, and parathyroidectomy.

CONTROLLING SERUM PHOSPHORUS

Dietary phosphorus restriction (800 to 1000 mg/day) is difficult to attain but should be initiated for all subjects with stage 5 CKD. There are actually three major sources of exogenous phosphorus to be considered: natural phosphate (as cellular and protein constituents) contained in raw or unprocessed foods, phosphate added to foods during processing (daily exposure may be as high as 1000 mg), and phosphate in dietary supplements/medications. Dairy products, nuts, beer, and chocolate all have a high content of phosphorus (see Chapter 53). For patients who are undergoing thrice-weekly dialysis and are receiving adequate nutrition, dietary phosphate restriction will be inadequate to correct the positive phosphate balance, especially in the presence of concurrent active vitamin D therapy, which increases phosphorus absorption from the gut. More frequent and prolonged hemodialysis (see Chapter 57) has been associated with lower serum phosphorus levels, but with thrice-weekly hemodialysis, phosphate binders are almost invariably required.

The choice of phosphate binder (i.e., calcium containing vs. nonaluminum, non–calcium containing) depends on many considerations, including the binder's efficacy, side effects, and cost. For many years, calcium-based phosphate binders were the mainstay of therapy to control serum phosphate levels. Commonly used calcium-based phosphate binders include calcium carbonate and calcium acetate. Calcium carbonate contains 500 mg of elemental calcium in a 1250-mg tablet (40%), whereas calcium acetate contains 169 mg of elemental calcium in one 667-mg tablet (25%). Calcium-based phosphate binders should be taken with meals to maximize binding of ingested phosphorus in the gut. When they are taken in the fasting state, more calcium is absorbed systemically and less phosphorus is bound. The concomitant use of active vitamin D sterols increases calcium absorption and the risk of hypercalcemia. The recent KDIGO update cautions against overzealous/excessive intake of calcium without defining a specific safe limit. Calcium acetate has greater

phosphorus-binding capacity than calcium carbonate, potentially allowing the use of lower doses of calcium binder. However, various small trials have not shown significant differences in the prevalence of hypercalcemia between these two compounds.

Vascular calcifications have been documented by EBCT in the coronary arteries of dialysis patients before 30 years of age. This, taken with growing concern about the possible clinical consequences of vascular calcifications, has led to the greater use of noncalcium binders. Sevelamer is a noncalcium phosphate binder containing cross-linked polyallylamine hydrochloride. It acts as an ion exchange polymer to bind phosphorus in the gut but is less effective than calcium on a weight basis. However, in human trials, sevelamer, when titrated to meet serum phosphorus goals, appeared equal in efficacy to the calcium-containing binders. Sevelamer has also been shown to decrease serum cholesterol and low-density lipoproteins and increase high-density lipoproteins in stage 5 CKD patients. Sevelamer has been associated with fewer arterial calcifications than calcium-based phosphate binders in dialysis patients. Sevelamer is more costly than calcium binders and may be associated with gastrointestinal side effects at higher doses that can limit its use in some individuals. Nevertheless, regimens with vitamin D analogues to raise calcium and suppress PTH, along with sevelamer to lower phosphorus, are effective in controlling both the skeletal and extraskeletal complications of stage 5 CKD.

The effect of sevelamer on cardiovascular mortality remains a critical question. Prospective trials comparing the effect of sevelamer versus calcium-containing phosphate binders on mortality produced equivocal results. One small, randomized trial with 127 incident hemodialysis patients monitored for a mean of 44 months demonstrated a significant overall survival advantage for sevelamer, although specific cardiovascular mortality was not assessed. The larger, open-labeled Dialysis Clinical Outcomes Revisited (DCOR) trial, which randomly assigned 2103 patients to either sevelamer or calcium-containing binders with a mean follow-up of 20.3 months, failed to show a difference in cardiovascular mortality between the two groups. In subgroup analysis of the DCOR results, patients older than 65 years who were treated with sevelamer had a lower all-cause mortality but not lower cardiovascular mortality. In addition, patients who remained in the study for longer than 2 years on treatment with sevelamer had a decrease in all-cause mortality. The short duration of follow-up, the high dropout rate, and the fact that the study was not powered statistically to detect differences in specific causes of death are limitations of this study. More recently, significant survival benefits were demonstrated for patients treated with sevelamer versus calcium-containing binders in a multicenter Italian study (INDEPENDENT Study). This study suffers, however, from a moderate risk of bias and therefore should be interpreted with caution. Together with data from formal calcium balance studies, this new evidence supported a more general recommendation to restrict calcium-based phosphate binders in hyperphosphatemic patients of all stages of CKD.

Although they are the most effective binders, aluminum-containing phosphate binders are not often used because of the potential for systemic aluminum absorption and subsequent neurologic, hematologic, and bone toxicity. Absorption of aluminum is increased by the concomitant use of sodium citrate for metabolic acidosis. Because of the potential for long-term toxicity, aluminum-containing antacids should be used only for a short period (<4 weeks) and only for severe hyperphosphatemia that is refractory to other treatments.

Another non–calcium-based phosphate binder is lanthanum carbonate. Lanthanum, like aluminum, is a trivalent cation with an ability to chelate dietary phosphate, but it has low systemic absorption. In a phase III trial over a 1-year period, lanthanum carbonate controlled serum phosphorus levels to an extent comparable to high-dose calcium carbonate. Mild gastrointestinal symptoms were the most common side effect in the lanthanum group. Lanthanum, unlike sevelamer, is an effective binder even in the acidic environment of the gut and does not bind bile acids. Adherence may be better than with calcium-based binders or sevelamer as a result of a lower pill burden. Because there is accumulation of small amounts of lanthanum over time, safety concerns have been raised. However, it is reassuring that, after more than 850,000 person-years of worldwide patient exposure, there is no evidence that lanthanum is associated with adverse safety outcomes in patients with ESRD. Sucroferric oxyhydroxide and ferric citrate have recently become available on the market. The added value of these iron-based phosphate binders as compared with established phosphate binders remains to be demonstrated. Also, data on patient-centered outcomes are not yet available.

ACTIVATING THE CALCIUM-SENSING AND VITAMIN D RECEPTORS TO SUPPRESS PARATHYROID HORMONE HYPERFUNCTION

Secondary hyperparathyroidism is a common complication of CKD that if left untreated may result in considerable morbidity and mortality. Current guidelines suggest to maintain PTH levels in the range of approximately 2 to 9 times the upper normal limit of the assay. Overall, there is no consensus on what should be the first-line treatment option to correct secondary hyperparathyroidism in CKD stage 5D patients: calcimimetics, calcitriol, or vitamin D analogues; a combination of calcimimetics and calcitriol; or vitamin D analogues. The individual choice should be guided by considerations about concomitant therapies and the present calcium and phosphate levels.

VITAMIN D ANALOGUES

Treatment with 1,25-$(OH_2)D_3$ (calcitriol) or an active vitamin D analogue (paricalcitol, doxercalciferol, alfacalcidol, or 22-oxacalcitrol) is a means of controlling secondary hyperparathyroidism. By binding to the VDR on parathyroid tissues, the vitamin D analogue suppresses PTH production. There is no uniform agreement about the route, dose, and type of active vitamin D analogue that should be given. Some of the available vitamin D analogues may cause less hypercalcemia than calcitriol, possibly because of decreased intestinal effect on calcium absorption. The "second-generation" analogue paricalcitol has generated interest because studies suggest that it leads to less elevation of serum calcium and phosphorus, as well as a greater PTH suppression, than calcitriol. When paricalcitol was compared with calcitriol in a large observational study of hemodialysis patients, its use was associated with significantly lower mortality. Although this study initially

raised questions about the extent to which efforts to control secondary hyperparathyroidism with vitamin D analogues might cause harm, subsequent retrospective studies suggested improved survival in dialysis patients treated with active vitamin D analogues compared with patients who did not receive vitamin D at all. However, a recent analysis of a large international dialysis database supported the possibility that the effect of vitamin D may represent a patient selection bias. Prospective clinical trials are needed to determine whether vitamin D therapy offers a survival advantage in dialysis patients.

Calcitriol and vitamin D analogues can be administered intravenously and orally. Equipotent intravenous doses of calcitriol, paricalcitol, and doxercalciferol for PTH suppression are 0.5, 2.5, and 5.0 μg, respectively, for PTH suppression. While it remains to be established which approach is most effective in lowering serum PTH and reducing toxicity, oral administration is gaining rapid popularity. Of note, in Europe, the oral route has been the preferential route of administration for years.

Stage 5 CKD patients whose PTH levels drop to less than 2 times the upper normal limit for the assay during treatment for secondary hyperparathyroidism require a reduction in their active vitamin D analogue or phosphate binders.

Current guidelines suggest to correct vitamin D deficiency and insufficiency, defined by 25(OH)D_3 levels below 20 and 30 ng/mL, respectively, with treatment strategies recommended for the general population. Clinical evidence in favor of vitamin D supplementation is limited. In a recent double-blind, placebo-controlled RCT, 6 months of supplementation with ergocalciferol increased serum 25(OH)D levels in patients on hemodialysis with vitamin D insufficiency or deficiency but had no effect on erythropoietin utilization or secondary biochemical and clinical outcomes. Nevertheless, the cost and risk of adverse side effects of nutritional vitamin D supplementation are small, and the potential effects of 25(OH)D on innate immunity and other cellular functions may still warrant hormonal replacement therapy in patients with low circulating 25(OH)D levels.

CALCIMIMETICS

Calcimimetics offer a novel approach for treating secondary hyperparathyroidism without using active vitamin D analogues or raising serum calcium levels. Calcimimetics are CaSR agonists that act on the parathyroid gland by allosterically increasing the sensitivity of the receptor to calcium. Cinacalcet, the first available drug of this group, was approved by the US Food and Drug Administration (FDA) in 2004 to treat secondary hyperparathyroidism in patients with stage 5 CKD. Treatment with cinacalcet causes significant decreases in PTH without elevating serum calcium or phosphorus concentrations (Fig. 54.5). In fact, there is usually a reduction in serum calcium and a tendency toward reduced serum phosphorus with calcimimetics. In one study, the use of cinacalcet resulted in approximately 41% of patients attaining the PTH and calcium-phosphorus product goals recommended by the K/DOQI guidelines, compared with fewer than 10% achieving these targets in the group treated with phosphate binders and vitamin D analogues alone. Additional studies are needed to evaluate the effect of cinacalcet in altering the natural history of parathyroid gland hyperplasia. Prospective trials examining the impact of lowering the calcium-phosphorus product with

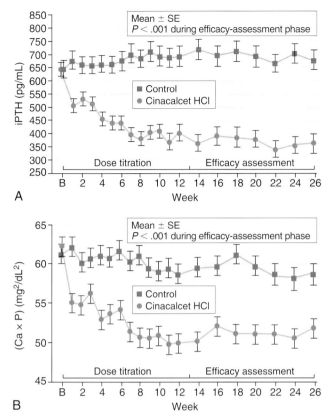

Fig. 54.5 Suppression of serum parathyroid hormone levels (A) by cinacalcet without elevation of the serum calcium-phosphorus product and (B) in patients on hemodialysis with secondary hyperparathyroidism not adequately controlled by treatment with phosphate binders and vitamin D analogues. *HCl,* Hydrochloride; *iPTH,* intact parathyroid hormone; *SE,* standard error. (From Block GA, Martin KJ, de Francisco AL, et al. Cinacalcet for secondary hyperparathyroidism in patients receiving hemodialysis. *N Engl J Med.* 2004;350:1516–1525, with permission.)

hypercalcemia and/or hyperphosphatemia despite medical management and for CUA or severe bone pain and fractures in the presence of elevated intact PTH levels. Either a subtotal parathyroidectomy or a total parathyroidectomy with forearm gland implantation can be performed. Some surgeons favor the latter procedure to avoid the need for repeated invasive neck surgery if hyperparathyroidism recurs. Glands can subsequently be removed from the forearm if necessary. Both subtotal and total parathyroidectomy with implantation are effective methods, and there are no studies comparing these approaches. Nonetheless, there is a 15% to 30% recurrence rate of hyperparathyroidism after complete or partial parathyroidectomy. Percutaneous ethanol injection into the gland as an ablation procedure for hyperparathyroidism refractory to medical management is performed in some centers in lieu of surgical parathyroidectomy. *Hungry bone syndrome* is a frequent complication of parathyroidectomy, especially when markedly elevated PTH values are acutely reduced. This syndrome is characterized by hypocalcemia, hypophosphatemia, and hypomagnesemia secondary to increased bone uptake of these three ions after removal of the resorptive influence of PTH. For unclear reasons, hyperkalemia is occasionally seen. If severe or symptomatic hypocalcemia develops, treatment with a continuous calcium infusion is necessary. Concomitant treatment with oral calcitriol before and after parathyroidectomy may mitigate the hungry bone syndrome.

PATIENTS WITH STAGE 3 AND STAGE 4 CHRONIC KIDNEY DISEASE

Treatment of patients with stage 3 and stage 4 CKD has not been well studied; however, the early development of parathyroid gland hyperplasia caused by chronic stimulation suggests that treatment should focus on prevention of parathyroid gland hyperplasia. Phosphate restriction, phosphate binders, and calcium supplementation are the mainstays of treatment in stages 3 and 4 CKD. Metabolic acidosis causes an efflux of calcium from bone as bone buffers hydrogen ions with carbonate release. Chronic metabolic acidosis should be corrected with sodium bicarbonate supplementation.

CKD patients are at increased risk for low levels of 25-hydroxyvitamin D for several potential reasons, including lack of sunlight if chronically ill or bedridden, poor oral intake of foods containing vitamin D, lower skin production of vitamin D_3 in elderly patients secondary to lower skin content of 7-dehydrocholesterol, and the presence of nephrotic syndrome causing loss of 25-hydroxyvitamin D and vitamin D–binding protein in the urine. Although the level of 25-hydroxyvitamin D in CKD that is diagnostic of hypovitaminosis D has not been firmly established, levels less than 30 ng/mL are associated with rising PTH levels. Stage 3 and 4 CKD patients with vitamin D levels lower than 30 ng/mL should be supplemented with ergocalciferol (vitamin D_2) or cholecalciferol (vitamin D_3). In patients without CKD, correction of vitamin D deficiency increases BMD and decreases the incidence of fractures.

The need for and timing of therapy with active vitamin D analogues in stages 3 and 4 CKD have not been firmly established. The demonstration of a significantly increased risk of hypercalcemia in patients treated with paricalcitol compared with placebo, in the absence of beneficial effects

calcimimetics in combination with active vitamin analogues, however, did not reduce vascular calcifications. The EVOLVE study also failed to meet its primary endpoint that cinacalcet reduces the risk of death or clinically important vascular events in CKD stage 5D patients. However, the results of secondary analyses suggest that cinacalcet may yet be beneficial in this population or a subset. These studies reflect the difficulty in demonstrating survival benefits from interventions directed at correcting the abnormalities of mineral metabolism in CKD.

Most recently, another calcimimetic, etelcalcetide, has been approved by FDA and European Medicines Agency (EMA). This intravenous calcimimetic proved to be superior to cinacalcet in reducing serum PTH concentration among patients receiving hemodialysis with moderate to severe secondary hyperparathyroidism. Intermediate or hard endpoint clinical trials with entelcalcetide are currently lacking.

PARATHYROIDECTOMY

As a remaining option for patients with uncontrolled hyperparathyroidism, parathyroidectomy should be considered for persistently elevated intact PTH levels associated with on surrogate cardiac endpoints (PRIMO and OPERA study), combined with the opinion that moderate PTH elevations may represent an appropriate adaptive response, urged KDIGO to recommend a more restricted use of active vitamin D (analogues) in the setting of predialysis CKD. In the revised guidelines, it is stated that the use of calcitriol or vitamin D analogs in patients with CKD stages 4 to 5 should be reserved for only severe and progressive secondary hyperparathyroidism.

Cinacalcet has not been well studied in patients with CKD stages 3 and 4 and is not approved by the FDA for these patients. Of note, the suppression of PTH in predialysis CKD patients goes along with an undesired increase of serum phosphate levels.

BISPHOSPHONATES

The use of bisphosphonates in patients with ESRD is poorly studied, and these agents are not widely prescribed in this setting because of concern that their use may exacerbate adynamic bone disease. In CKD, bisphosphonates may exacerbate kidney failure. In kidney transplant recipients, bisphosphonate may protect against immunosuppression-induced bone loss and prevent fracture. Limited data suggest that the bisphosphonates alendronate and risedronate are safe and effective for reducing fracture incidence in osteo-porotic patients with CKD.

KIDNEY TRANSPLANTATION

The bony changes of secondary hyperparathyroidism improve after transplantation; however, in patients with severe hyperparathyroidism before transplantation, elevated serum levels of PTH can persist for as long as 10 years. The incidence of parathyroidectomy remains high after kidney transplantation, probably reflecting the irreversible hyperplasia of parathyroid tissue that occurs during the course of CKD. It is not uncommon for patients to develop hypophosphatemia after kidney transplantation. This reduction in serum phosphorus may be mediated by persistent hyperparathyroidism and by other variables unrelated to PTH, such as increased levels of FGF23 that also reduce renal tubular reabsorption of phosphate. Typically, phosphate supplementation is reserved for severe hypophosphatemia (<1.5 mg/dL). More aggressive use of phosphate supplementation may exacerbate secondary hyperparathyroidism. Transplantation also prevents, but does not reverse, bone damage from amyloidosis caused by β_2M deposition. Symptoms of amyloidosis frequently abate after transplantation, perhaps because of concomitant steroid therapy.

Although successful kidney transplantation corrects many of the conditions that lead to disordered mineral metabolism associated with kidney failure, the glucocorticoids used to prevent rejection result in increased bone fragility, osteoporosis, and increased fracture rates. Other risk factors for fractures in this population include the presence of pretransplantation fracture, diabetes mellitus, and older age. In fact, the risk of fractures is greater in kidney transplant recipients than in patients on dialysis, at least in the first years after transplantation. While older studies demonstrated significant BMD loss, often exceeding 5% during the first year after transplantation, more recent cohort studies reported no or only minimal losses.

Steroid minimization most probably accounts to a large extent for this favorable trend. DEXA scans have been recommended in kidney transplant patients at the time of transplantation and then yearly, at least for the next several years. Mounting evidence indicates that low BMD by DEXA correlates with increased fracture risk in kidney transplant recipients, as in CKD patients and the general population. Calcium and vitamin D supplementation may be effective in counteracting the effects of glucocorticoids to reduce gastrointestinal calcium absorption. Studies have shown that calcium supplementation used with active vitamin D compounds preserves BMD at least early in the posttransplant period, but data showing that such treatment reduces fracture incidence are lacking. Bisphosphonates and denosumab appear to decrease the rate of bone loss as measured by BMD. However, given the concern for antiresorptive treatment-induced adynamic bone disease in this population and the lack of data on reduced facture incidence with this approach, there are currently no consensus recommendations on the use of this therapy in kidney recipients. Decisions should be individualized, and caution should be maintained.

Avascular necrosis is another complication of kidney transplantation. It most typically occurs in the femoral heads or other weight-bearing joints and is characterized by the collapse of surface bone and cartilage. The pathogenesis of this disorder is not clear, but it is probably related to prednisone therapy. Magnetic resonance imaging is the most sensitive technique to evaluate patients with hip pain after transplantation for the presence of avascular necrosis. Surgical therapies include core decompression and hip replacement.

KEY BIBLIOGRAPHY

Block GA, Klassen PS, Lazarus JM, et al. Mineral metabolism, mortality, and morbidity in maintenance hemodialysis. *J Am Soc Nephrol*. 2004;15:2208-2218.

Block GA, Martin KJ, de Francisco AL, et al. Cinacalcet for secondary hyperparathyroidism in patients receiving hemodialysis. *N Engl J Med*. 2004;350:1516-1525.

Block GA, Raggi P, Bellasi A, et al. Mortality effect of coronary calcification and phosphate binder choice in incident hemodialysis patients. *Kidney Int*. 2007;71:438-441.

Bricker NS, Fine LG. Uremia: formulations and expectations. The trade-off hypothesis: current status. *Kidney Int*. 1978;8:S5-S8.

Brown EM, Gamba G, Riccardi D, et al. Cloning and characterization of an extracellular Ca^{2+}-sensing receptor from bovine parathyroid. *Nature*. 1993;366:575-580.

Chertow GM, Burke SK, Raggi P, et al. Sevelamer attenuates the progression of coronary and aortic calcification in hemodialysis patients. *Kidney Int*. 2002;62:245-252.

D'Haese PC, Spasovski GB. A multicenter study on the effects of lanthanum carbonate (Fosrenol) and calcium carbonate on renal bone disease in dialysis patients. *Kidney Int*. 2003;85:S73-S78.

Faul C, Amaral AP, Oskouei B, et al. FGF23 induces left ventricular hypertrophy. *J Clin Invest*. 2011;121:4393-4408.

Gutierrez OM, Mannstadt M, Isakova T, et al. Fibroblastic growth factor 23 and mortality among patients undergoing hemodialysis. *N Engl J Med*. 2008;359:584-592.

Malluche HH, Mawad HW, Monier-Faugere MC. Renal osteodystrophy in the first decade of the new millennium: analysis of 630 bone biopsies in black and white patients. *J Bone Miner Res*. 2011;26:1368-1376.

Quarles LD, Lobaugh B, Murphy G. Intact parathyroid hormone overestimates the presence and severity of parathyroid-mediated osseous abnormalities in uremia. *J Clin Endocrinol Metab*. 1992;75:145-150.

Raggi P, Chertow GM, Torres PU, et al. The Advance study: a randomized study to evaluate the effects of cinacalcet plus low-dose vitamin D on vascular calcifications in patients on hemodialysis. *Nephrol Dial Transplant*. 2011;26:1327-1339.

Stehman-Breen CO, Sherrard DJ, Alem AM, et al. Risk factors fractures for hip fracture among patients with end-stage renal disease. *Kidney Int.* 2000;58:2200-2205.

Sugarman JR, Frederick PR, Frankenfield DL, et al. Developing clinical performance measures based on the Dialysis Outcomes Quality Initiative Clinical Practice Guidelines: process, outcomes and implications. *Am J Kidney Dis.* 2003;42:806-812.

Suki WN, Zabaneh R, Cangiano JL, et al. Effects of sevelamer and calcium-based phosphate binders on mortality in hemodialysis patients. *Kidney Int.* 2007;72:1130-1137.

Teng M, Wolf M, Lowrie E, et al. Survival of patients undergoing hemodialysis with paricalcitol or calcitriol therapy. *N Engl J Med.* 2003;349:446-456.

Teng M, Wolf M, Ofsthun MN, et al. Activated injectable vitamin D and hemodialysis survival: a historical cohort study. *J Am Soc Nephrol.* 2005;16:1115-1125.

Thadhani R, Appelbaum E, Pritchett Y, et al. Vitamin D therapy and cardiac structure and function in patients with chronic kidney disease: the PRIMO randomized controlled trial. *JAMA.* 2012;307:674-684.

The EVOLVE Trial Investigators. Effect of cinacalcet on cardiovascular disease in patients undergoing dialysis. *N Engl J Med.* 2012;367:2482-2494.

Weisinger JR, Carlini RG, Rojas E, et al. Bone disease after renal transplantation. *Clin J Am Soc Nephrol.* 2006;6:1300-1313.

Full bibliography can be found on www.expertconsult.com.

55

Cardiac Function and Cardiovascular Disease in Chronic Kidney Disease

Daniel E. Weiner; Mark J. Sarnak

Cardiovascular disease is the leading cause of mortality across the spectrum of chronic kidney disease (CKD), with increased risk seen in individuals with reduced glomerular filtration rate (GFR) and in those with even minimally elevated urine albumin excretion. Cardiovascular disease has many manifestations in individuals with CKD, including atherosclerotic and stiff vessels with resultant ischemic heart disease and heart failure and structural changes like left ventricular hypertrophy (LVH) and valvular diseases are common at all CKD stages. The risk of cardiovascular disease outcomes increases as kidney function declines, with the risk of cardiovascular death in patients undergoing dialysis 10 to 20 times that of the general population. This chapter focuses largely on individuals with reduced GFR, acknowledging that albuminuria identifies individuals with CKD and is a very strong predictor of cardiovascular disease risk at all levels of kidney function, including individuals with CKD stages 1 through 3a where metabolic sequelae of reduced GFR are not yet clinically apparent.

EPIDEMIOLOGY OF CARDIOVASCULAR DISEASE IN CHRONIC KIDNEY DISEASE

STAGES 3 TO 4 CHRONIC KIDNEY DISEASE

Manifesting with cardiac ischemia, heart failure, and arrhythmia, cardiovascular disease is overwhelmingly the leading cause of morbidity and mortality in individuals with CKD. Among individuals with reduced GFR, there is a progressive increase in the age-standardized incidence of cardiovascular disease events as kidney function declines, such that, compared with an age-standardized baseline rate of 21 cardiovascular events per 1000 person-years in individuals with estimated glomerular filtration rate (eGFR) greater than 60 mL/min per 1.73 m^2, rates increase to 37, 113, 218, and 366 events per 1000 person-years among people with eGFR of 45 to 59 (CKD stage 3a), 30 to 44 (CKD stage 3b), 15 to 29 (CKD stage 4), and less than 15 mL/min per 1.73 m^2 (CKD stage 5), respectively. Even in analyses that adjust for demographic factors as well as cardiovascular risk factors such as diabetes, hypertension, albuminuria, and dyslipidemia, the risk of cardiovascular death is dramatically increased at lower GFR (Fig. 55.1). The risk relationship between eGFR and cardiovascular disease events is independent of a person having preexisting cardiovascular disease (Fig. 55.2).

Prevalence of cardiovascular disease in people with CKD is similarly high. For example, in population screening programs administered by the National Kidney Foundation, 12% to 20% of individuals with eGFR of 30 to 60 mL/min per 1.73 m^2 (stage 3 CKD) state that they have had a previous "heart attack or stroke," versus 5% to 10% for those with eGFR of 60 mL/min per 1.73 m^2 or greater. In analyses adjusted for similar risk factors such as those mentioned earlier, both reduced eGFR and moderately increased albuminuria with preserved eGFR (urine albumin-to-creatinine ratio [UACR] 30 to 300 mg/g, indicating CKD stages 1 to 2) were independently associated with prevalent cardiovascular disease. Likewise, in pooled community cohorts, cardiovascular disease was prevalent in 31.3% of individuals with eGFR between 15 and 60 mL/min per 1.73 m^2 (stage 3 to 4 CKD) versus 14.4% with eGFR ≥60 mL/min per 1.73 m^2.

Cardiovascular disease may be subclinical in CKD populations; in Chronic Renal Insufficiency Cohort (CRIC) participants undergoing cardiac computed tomography, there was a graded increased risk of coronary calcification with both lower eGFR and higher levels of albuminuria, even in individuals with no known history of cardiovascular disease, although whether this suggests medial calcification or atheromatous disease is unknown. Similarly, in the elderly, the frequency of advanced atherosclerotic lesions on autopsy specimens increased as eGFR decreased (33.6% for eGFR ≥60 mL/min per 1.73 m^2, 41.7% for CKD stage 3a, 52.3% for CKD stage 3b, and 52.8% for CKD stage 4).

LVH is also highly prevalent in CKD stages 3 and 4, likely reflecting pressure and volume overload. In CRIC, the prevalence of LVH assessed by echocardiography was 32% for eGFR above 60 mL/min per 1.73 m^2, rising to 48%, 57%, and 75% for eGFR categories 45 to 59, 30 to 44, and less than 30 mL/min per 1.73 m^2, respectively. These findings contrast with a prevalence of LVH of less than 20% in older adults in the general population. Both incident and prevalent heart failure are common in people with CKD. Among adult members of a large group-model health maintenance organization in the northwestern United States, 6.0% of individuals with predominantly early stage 3 CKD had a diagnostic code for heart failure versus 1.8% in an age- and sex-matched population, while, in the Atherosclerosis Risk in Communities (ARIC) study, individuals with eGFR less than 60 mL/min per 1.73 m^2 at baseline were at twice the risk of incident heart failure hospitalization and death compared with those with

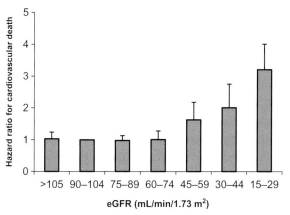

Fig. 55.1 Hazard ratios for cardiovascular events according to the baseline estimated glomerular filtration rate. Adjusted for age, sex, race, cardiovascular disease history, smoking status, diabetes mellitus, systolic blood pressure, serum total cholesterol, and urine albumin-to-creatinine ratio. (Plotted with data in van der Velde M, Matsushita K, Coresh J, et al. Lower estimated glomerular filtration rate and higher albuminuria are associated with all-cause and cardiovascular mortality. A collaborative meta-analysis of high-risk population cohorts. *Kidney Int.* 2011;79:1341–1352.)

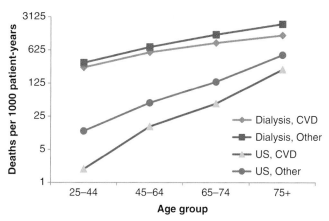

Fig. 55.3 Cardiovascular disease and noncardiovascular disease mortality in the general United States (US) population (2014) compared with patients with chronic kidney failure treated by dialysis (2012–2014). Cardiovascular disease (CVD) death in the US population includes "Diseases of the heart" (I00–I09, I11, I13, I20–I51) and "Cerebrovascular diseases" (I60–I69). CVD death in dialysis includes myocardial infarction, pericarditis, atherosclerotic heart disease, cardiomyopathy, arrhythmia, cardiac arrest, valvular heart disease, congestive heart failure, and cerebrovascular disease. The youngest general population group is 22 to 44 years old.

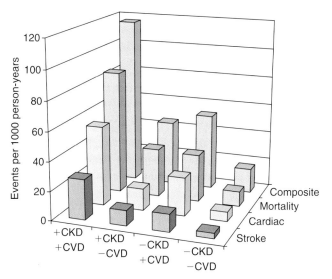

Fig. 55.2 Unadjusted event rates for individuals with and without baseline chronic kidney disease (estimated glomerular filtration rate of 15 to 59 mL/min per 1.73 m²) and cardiovascular disease. Cardiac events include myocardial infarction and fatal coronary disease. Stroke includes both fatal and nonfatal stroke events. Mortality includes all causes of death, and the composite outcome includes any cardiac, stroke, or mortality event. *CKD*, Chronic kidney disease; *CVD*, cardiovascular disease. (Reprinted with permission from Weiner DE, Tabatabai S, Tighiouart H, et al. Cardiovascular outcomes and all-cause mortality: exploring the interaction between CKD and cardiovascular disease. *Am J Kidney Dis.* 2006;48:392–401.)

of mitral annular calcification, with risk increased by 50%, 130%, 226%, and 278% for eGFR categories 50 to 60, 40 to 50, 30 to 40, and less than 30 mL/min per 1.73 m², respectively, when compared with eGFR ≥60 mL/min per 1.73 m². The Framingham Heart Study and other studies also have shown an increased prevalence of aortic valve calcification in individuals with CKD, with CRIC demonstrating a "dose-dependent" association between lower eGFR and greater aortic valve calcification that was independent of traditional cardiovascular risk factors.

STAGE 5 CHRONIC KIDNEY DISEASE/DIALYSIS

In patients undergoing dialysis, incident cardiovascular disease is common, with similar cardiovascular mortality rates in a 30-year-old patient undergoing dialysis and an 80-year-old individual from the general population (Fig. 55.3). This likely reflects a high prevalence of cardiovascular disease (~45% of prevalent dialysis patients in the United States in 2014 had known atherosclerotic heart disease and 40% had congestive heart failure) as well as a high case-fatality rate compared with the general population.

The incidence and prevalence of LVH and heart failure are also extremely high among patients undergoing dialysis. More than 30% of participants in the Frequent Hemodialysis Network studies (a group that overall was healthier than the general dialysis population) had LVH at study entry (defined with cardiac magnetic resonance imaging). Based on United States Renal Data System (USRDS) administrative data that rely on billing codes to identify heart failure events, for patients treated with dialysis in 2009 and followed for up to 3 years, incident heart failure rates were 464 events per 1000 patient-years for hemodialysis and 243 per 1000 patient-years for peritoneal dialysis.

Patients undergoing hemodialysis also have a high prevalence of valvular calcification; in one study, 45% of subjects

eGFR of ≥90 mL/min per 1.73 m², regardless of the presence of baseline coronary disease.

Other structural heart diseases seen commonly in CKD include aortic valve, mitral valve, and mitral annular calcification. Mitral valve or annular calcification was present in 20% of individuals with reduced kidney function (roughly stage 3 to 4 CKD) in the Framingham Offspring Study. In CRIC, lower eGFR was strongly associated with increased likelihood had calcification of the mitral valve, and 34% of subjects had calcification of the aortic valve, compared with expected prevalence of 3% to 5% in the general population. Studies have demonstrated rates of mitral annular calcification ranging from 30% to 50% in patients undergoing hemodialysis.

TYPES OF CARDIOVASCULAR DISEASES

Cardiovascular disease in individuals with CKD has a variety of manifestations, chiefly comprising atherosclerosis, arteriosclerosis, and cardiomyopathy/valvular disease (Table 55.1). In most cases, clinically apparent cardiovascular disease reflects the interplay among these manifestations. Although there is no consensus on terminology for arteriopathies, atherosclerosis can be defined as an occlusive disease of the vasculature that occurs because of the deposition of lipid-laden plaques, while arteriosclerosis is a nonocclusive remodeling of the vasculature accompanied by a loss of arterial elasticity. Both of these conditions may manifest with ischemic heart disease and heart failure, and clinical disease often reflects the concurrent presence of both atherosclerotic disease and vascular remodeling. Certain risk factors, including dyslipidemia, primarily predispose an individual to development and progression of atherosclerosis, whereas others, including elevated calcium-phosphorus product, may predispose to vascular stiffness. Volume overload and anemia may primarily predispose an individual to cardiac remodeling and LVH, whereas hypertension, which is common at all stages of CKD, is associated with all of these disease manifestations. Over time, the interplay among these manifestations may yield both segmental perfusion defects due to disease affecting larger coronary arteries and insufficient subendocardial perfusion secondary to cardiac hypertrophy (causing increased demand) and capillary dropout. The end result is myocyte death.

RISK FACTORS FOR CARDIOVASCULAR DISEASE

Much of the increased burden of cardiovascular disease in CKD is a result of increased prevalence of both traditional and nontraditional cardiovascular disease risk factors. Traditional risk factors were identified in the Framingham Heart Study as conferring increased risk of cardiovascular disease in the general population. Nontraditional risk factors were not defined in the initial reports of the Framingham Heart Study but increase in prevalence as kidney function declines, and they are hypothesized to be cardiovascular disease risk factors in patients with CKD (Table 55.2). All CKD stages, even stages 1 and 2 where GFR is preserved but albuminuria is at least moderately elevated, are independently associated with cardiovascular disease in epidemiologic studies. Although CKD, particularly late stage CKD, may directly cause cardiovascular disease through mechanisms that include fluid retention, anemia, abnormal mineral metabolism, and hypertension, it is likely that CKD also represents a risk state in which factors associated with the development of CKD (including diabetes, hypertension, and possibly dyslipidemia) account for the enhanced cardiac risk. In the latter hypothesis, the presence of CKD is a marker of the severity and duration of these other risk factors.

ISCHEMIC HEART DISEASE

PREDICTION OF ISCHEMIC HEART DISEASE

The Framingham coronary heart disease prediction equations use traditional risk factors including age, sex, diabetes, blood pressure, and lipid levels to estimate cardiac risk in the general US population. The 2013 American College of Cardiology/American Heart Association (ACC/AHA) Guideline on the Assessment of Cardiovascular Risk recommends use of a calculator based on these same variables plus race and smoking status to guide statin use, aspirin use, and blood pressure targets in the general population. In the general population, the addition of kidney measures, particularly albuminuria, to traditional risk factors appears to improve cardiovascular event prediction.

Use of these well-accepted prediction equations to assign cardiac risk to CKD patients (particularly those receiving dialysis) may be problematic, as risk factors that are at least in part dependent on intact nutrition (e.g., serum cholesterol) and cardiac health (e.g., systolic and diastolic blood pressure) appear to have different relationships with adverse outcomes. Accordingly, although many of the traditional risk factors that predict coronary heart disease in the general population are important risk factors in the late-stage CKD population, the relative importance of each risk factor may be different. In particular, diabetes in individuals with CKD is a more powerful marker of cardiac risk than it is in the general population, perhaps reflecting the fact that diabetes severe enough to cause kidney damage is also capable of causing systemic vascular disease.

In patients undergoing dialysis, the Framingham equations and other equations geared to the general population fail altogether, although older individuals and those with diabetes do have higher cardiovascular event rates. In patients undergoing hemodialysis, there is little increase in mortality risk at even markedly elevated systolic blood pressures, whereas lower systolic blood pressures (<120 mm Hg) are associated with the highest risk of mortality. These altered relationships do not speak to pathophysiology but rather likely reflect current health status and cardiac and nutritional reserve.

DIAGNOSIS OF ISCHEMIC HEART DISEASE

No single diagnostic test is optimal for identifying ischemic heart disease in patients with CKD, and each has pitfalls specific to CKD that may affect sensitivity and specificity. Currently, a functional assessment of perfusion that includes cardiac imaging is likely the best initial option to identify cardiac ischemia. These options include exercise or pharmacologic nuclear stress tests as well as exercise or pharmacologic stress echocardiography. Importantly, the ability to perform exercise stress testing is often limited by comorbid conditions in the CKD population. Overall, dobutamine stress echocardiography, assuming adequate institutional expertise and based on limited data, may have higher specificity and at least equivalent or higher sensitivity than pharmacologic nuclear stress tests for detecting angiographically apparent coronary lesions, while additionally providing information on valvular and other structural disease. Critically, there is no absolute contraindication to cardiac catheterization

Table 55.1   Types of Cardiac Diseases in Chronic Kidney Disease

Cardiovascular Disease Type	Pathologic or Structural Manifestation	Risk Factors	Indicators/Diagnostic Test	Clinical Sequelae
Arterial Disease	Atherosclerosis: Luminal narrowing of arteries because of plaques	Dyslipidemia Diabetes mellitus Hypertension Other traditional and nontraditional risk factors	Inducible ischemia on nuclear imaging Cardiac catheterization	Myocardial infarction Angina Sudden cardiac death Heart failure
	Arteriosclerosis: Diffuse dilatation and wall hypertrophy of larger arteries with loss of arterial elasticity	Hypertension Volume overload Hyperparathyroidism Hyperphosphatemia Other factors predisposing to medial calcification	Vascular calcification Increased pulse pressure Aortic pulse wave velocity Cardiac computed tomography Other arterial imaging	Myocardial infarction Angina Sudden cardiac death Heart failure LVH
Cardiomyopathy	LV Hypertrophy: Adaptive hypertrophy to compensate for increased cardiac demand	Pressure overload Increased afterload because of hypertension, valvular disease, and arteriosclerosis Volume overload Volume retention because of progressive kidney disease ± anemia	Echocardiography Cardiovascular magnetic resonance imaging	Myocardial infarction Angina Sudden cardiac death Heart failure
	Decreased LV contractility	Ischemic heart disease Hypertension LVH Other traditional and nontraditional risk factors	Echocardiography	Cardiorenal syndrome[a] Sudden cardiac death Heart failure Myocardial infarction Angina
	Impaired LV relaxation	Hypertension Anemia and volume overload Abnormal mineral metabolism Other arteriosclerosis risk factors Other traditional and nontraditional risk factors	Echocardiography	Heart failure Myocardial infarction Angina Sudden cardiac death
Structural Disease	Pericardial effusion	Delayed or insufficient dialysis	Echocardiography	Heart failure Hypotension
	Aortic and mitral valve disease	CKD stages 3 through 5 Abnormal calcium/phosphate/PTH metabolism Aging Dialysis vintage	Echocardiography	Aortic stenosis Endocarditis Heart failure
	Mitral annular calcification	CKD Stages 3 through 5 Abnormal calcium/phosphate/PTH metabolism	Echocardiography Uniform echodense rigid band located near the base of the posterior mitral leaflet	Arrhythmia Embolism Endocarditis Heart failure
	Endocarditis	Valvular disease Chronic venous catheters	Echocardiography	Arrhythmia Heart failure Embolism
Arrhythmia	Atrial fibrillation	Ischemic heart disease Cardiomyopathy	Electrocardiography	Hypotension Embolism
	Ventricular arrhythmia	Ischemic heart disease Cardiomyopathy Electrolyte abnormalities	Electrocardiography Electrophysiology study	Sudden cardiac death

[a]Cardiorenal syndrome is reviewed in Chapter 29.
CKD, Chronic kidney disease; *LV*, left ventricle; *LVH*, left ventricular hypertrophy; *PTH*, parathyroid hormone.

Table 55.2 Traditional and Nontraditional Cardiac Risk Factors in Chronic Kidney Disease

Traditional Risk Factors	Nontraditional Factors
Older age	Albuminuria
Male sex	Lipoprotein (a) and apo (a) isoforms
Hypertension	Lipoprotein remnants
Higher LDL cholesterol	Anemia
Lower HDL cholesterol	Abnormal mineral metabolism
Diabetes	Extracellular fluid volume overload
Smoking	Electrolyte abnormalities
Physical inactivity	Oxidative stress
Menopause	Inflammation
Family history of cardiovascular disease	Malnutrition
Left ventricular hypertrophy	Thrombogenic factors
	Sleep disturbances
	Altered nitric oxide/endothelin balance
	Sympathetic overactivity

HDL, High-density lipoprotein; *LDL*, low-density lipoprotein.
Revised from Sarnak MJ, Levey AS, Schoolwerth AC, et al. Kidney disease as a risk factor for development of cardiovascular disease: a statement from the American Heart Association Councils on Kidney in Cardiovascular Disease, High Blood Pressure Research, Clinical Cardiology, and Epidemiology and Prevention. *Circulation.* 2003;108:2154–2169.

in patients with CKD, including those already on dialysis, although preservation of existing kidney function is an important consideration in all stages of kidney disease, including those receiving hemodialysis and especially those treated with peritoneal dialysis. With careful management and conservative use of iodinated contrast (see Chapter 35), many individuals with advanced CKD can safely receive iodinated contrast.

PREVENTION AND TREATMENT OF ISCHEMIC HEART DISEASE

STAGES 3 TO 4 CHRONIC KIDNEY DISEASE

In the earlier stages of CKD, there is a moderate body of data, predominantly derived from subgroup analyses of larger clinical trials, demonstrating benefits with many interventions that are favorable in the general population. Therefore currently accepted treatment strategies for primary and secondary prevention of cardiac disease in individuals with CKD stages 3 to 4 mirror those seen in the general population, while exercising caution to minimize therapies with increased risk in patients with CKD.

In individuals with CKD stages 3 to 4, dyslipidemia (Table 55.3), hypertension, and diabetes likely should be treated similarly to current general population guidelines. Based on American Heart Association and American College of Cardiology joint guidelines, beta-blockers remain the first-line agent for stable symptomatic ischemic heart disease, for ischemic cardiomyopathy, and for immediate and up to 3 years postmyocardial infarction care, regardless of left ventricular function. There are limited data regarding benefits of longer-term beta-blocker use in ischemic heart disease, but they can

be considered for patients with coronary or other vascular disease. Specific indications for angiotensin-converting enzyme (ACE) inhibitors and angiotensin receptor blockers (ARBs) include ischemic cardiomyopathy, coexistent proteinuric kidney disease, and diabetes. Blood pressure management is discussed in detail in Chapter 65, and diabetes and diabetic nephropathy in Chapter 26.

Individualized care is important given the challenges associated with therapies. For example, there is an increased risk of hyperkalemia with blockade of the renin-angiotensin-aldosterone system that needs to be balanced against the benefits of this therapy in the individual patient. Hypotension and kidney perfusion may limit the ability to use multiple medications concurrently (such as ACE inhibitors, beta-blockers, and diuretics), although each may have reasonable clinical and evidence-based data supporting their use. Other concerns include an increased risk of rhabdomyolysis seen with dual statin and fibrate therapy, and this combination should be avoided in advanced CKD.

Most interventions for acute management as well as both primary and secondary prevention of coronary disease remain inadequately studied in advanced CKD, but, based on general population experience, many may be useful. Best studied are lipid lowering therapies, with the Study of Heart and Renal Protection (SHARP) demonstrating a significant benefit for primary prevention of cardiovascular disease events in individuals with CKD stage 3b to 4 (see Table 55.3). The 2013 Kidney Disease: Improving Global Outcomes (KDIGO) Clinical Practice Guideline for Lipid Management in CKD recommended statin or statin/ezetimibe treatment for all adults 50 years old or older with CKD stages 3a to 5 (nondialysis) and for all younger adults with CKD and diabetes, known coronary disease or stroke, or high cardiovascular disease risk. Critically, the KDIGO workgroup stressed a "fire-and-forget" approach to statin use in CKD rather than treating to a specific low-density lipoprotein (LDL)-cholesterol target. Recommended statin doses are in Table 55.4.

The benefits of other common interventions are less certain. For example, low-dose aspirin use in individuals with known cardiovascular disease or a high burden of cardiac risk factors is likely beneficial; however, data on more aggressive antiplatelet therapy with agents including glycoprotein IIb/IIIa inhibitors or clopidogrel following myocardial infarction or in the setting of acute coronary syndromes suggests that there may be a substantial risk of bleeding in individuals with advanced CKD, resulting in an overall equivocal benefit.

Choosing between medical management and invasive management of coronary disease in advanced CKD remains uncertain. Given existing data, an individualized approach appears optimal for CKD stage 3b and 4 patients with multivessel coronary artery disease, with options including intensive medical therapy as a first-line treatment. Percutaneous interventions and coronary artery bypass grafting may be deferred to a later time or used as part of a more aggressive first-line approach based on an individual patient's symptom burden, anatomic characteristics, longer-term prognosis, and lifestyle values, particularly if an intervention is likely to accelerate the need for dialysis or will facilitate kidney transplant.

STAGE 5 CHRONIC KIDNEY DISEASE/DIALYSIS

To date, clinical trial data demonstrating a significant survival benefit with accepted cardiovascular disease therapies in the

Table 55.3 **Randomized Controlled Studies of Statin Treatment Specifically in Chronic Kidney Disease**

Study	Intervention	Population	Median Follow-Up	Primary Outcome	Risk of Primary Outcome	Risk of All-Cause Mortality
4D	Atorvastatin 20 mg daily (vs. placebo)	1255 participants Age 18–80 years Type 2 diabetes Hemodialysis for <2 years LDL 80–190 mg/dL	4.0 years	Composite of death from cardiac causes,[a] fatal stroke, nonfatal MI, or nonfatal stroke	HR = 0.92 (0.77–1.10)	RR = 0.93 (0.79–1.08)
AURORA	Rosuvastatin 10 mg daily (vs. placebo)	2776 participants Age 50–80 years Hemofiltration or hemodialysis for more than 3 months	3.8 years	Composite of death from cardiovascular causes, nonfatal MI, or nonfatal stroke	HR = 0.96 (0.84–1.11)	HR = 0.96 (0.86–1.07)
ALERT	Fluvastatin 40 mg daily with dose increase permitted (vs. placebo)	2102 participants Age 30–75 years More than 6 months from transplant Stable kidney graft function No recent MI Total cholesterol 155–348 mg/dL	5.4 years	Major adverse cardiac event, defined as cardiac death, nonfatal MI, or coronary revascularization procedure	RR = 0.83 (0.64–1.06)	RR = 1.02 (0.81–1.30)
SHARP	Simvastatin 20 mg daily + ezetimibe 10 mg daily (vs. placebo)	9270 participants Age 40+ years No previous MI or coronary revascularization Creatinine more than 1.7 mg/dL (men) or more than 1.5 mg/dL (women)	4.9 years	Composite of coronary death,[b] nonfatal MI, ischemic stroke, or any revascularization procedure	RR = 0.83 (0.74–0.94)	RR = 1.02 (0.94–1.11)
	Subgroups within SHARP[c]	Nondialysis (n = 6247)	Not reported	As above	RR = 0.78 (0.67–0.91)	Not reported
		Hemodialysis (n = 2527)			RR = 0.95 (0.78–1.15)	
		Peritoneal dialysis (n = 496)			RR = 0.70 (0.46–1.08)	

Data in parentheses represents 95% confidence intervals. HR and RR report the relationship between treatment versus placebo, with values below 1 favoring treatment and above 1 favoring placebo.

[a]In 4D, death from cardiac causes comprised fatal myocardial infarction (death within 28 days after a myocardial infarction), sudden death, death due to congestive heart failure, death due to coronary heart disease during or within 28 days after an intervention, and all other deaths ascribed to coronary heart disease. Patients who died unexpectedly and had hyperkalemia before the start of the three most recent sessions of hemodialysis were considered to have had sudden death from cardiac causes.

[b]In SHARP, the original primary outcome included cardiac death, defined as death due to hypertensive heart disease, coronary heart disease, or other heart disease; the analytic plan was modified before data analysis to focus on death due to coronary heart disease rather than cardiac death.

[c]In SHARP, there was no statistically significant difference in the risk of the primary outcome between dialysis and nondialysis patients (P = 0.25) or between hemodialysis and peritoneal dialysis patients (P = 0.21).

4D, German Diabetes Dialysis Study; ALERT, assessment of Lescol in renal transplantation; AURORA, a study to evaluate the use of rosuvastatin in subjects in regular hemodialysis: an assessment of survival and cardiovascular events; HR, hazard ratio; LDL, low-density lipoprotein; MI, myocardial infarction; RR, risk ratio; SHARP, Study of Heart and Renal Protection.

dialysis population are lacking, although data from the United States and Australia do suggest that the rates of cardiovascular disease death in patients undergoing dialysis continue to decrease, although for reasons that remain uncertain. The overall failure to find specific interventions that significantly reduce the cardiovascular disease burden in individuals treated with maintenance dialysis most likely reflects the fact that there are numerous competing causes of death in these patients, and addressing single risk factors may be insufficient to reduce mortality.

Statin treatment has been best studied, with two large, adequately powered clinical trials both showing no benefit in patients undergoing hemodialysis, and a third trial, SHARP, showing no benefit in the subgroup receiving hemodialysis at trial initiation (see Table 55.3); patients on peritoneal dialysis remain inadequately studied. Based on these results, KDIGO did not recommend routinely initiating statin therapy in patients undergoing hemodialysis, although the guideline suggests continuing statins in those who were receiving them predialysis. In patients with longer life expectancies, such as patients expected to receive a kidney transplant, we suggest individualized decision making. Of note, KDIGO recommends statin therapy in transplant recipients.

Table 55.4   Recommended Doses of Statins in Adults With Chronic Kidney Disease

Agent	Intensity in General Population	Chronic Kidney Disease Stages 3–5 and Dialysis
Atorvastatin	High at 40–80 mg Moderate at 10–20 mg	20 mg
Rosuvastatin	High at 20–40 mg Moderate at 5–10 mg	10 mg
Simvastatin	Moderate 20–40 mg Low at 10 mg	20 mg
Pravastatin	Moderate at 40–80 mg Low at 10–20 mg	40 mg
Lovastatin	Moderate at 40 mg Low at 20 mg	Not evaluated
Fluvastatin	Moderate at 80 mg Low at 20–40 mg	80 mg
Pitavastatin	Moderate at 2–4 mg Low at 1 mg	2 mg

High-potency statins lower LDL cholesterol by at least 50% while lower potency statins lower LDL by 30% to 50% on average. Dosing recommendations are from the KDIGO guideline, and most are derived from medication doses safely used in trials. *KDIGO*, Kidney Disease: Improving Global Outcomes; *LDL*, low-density lipoprotein.

Current practice for other cardiovascular risk modifying therapy is chiefly based on observational data and extrapolations from the non-CKD population. In individuals receiving dialysis, interventions directed at blood pressure and diet are challenging given the difficulty of maintaining blood pressure in a narrow range as well as the catabolic nature of the dialysis milieu. In addition, some risk factors associated with adverse events in the general population appear to be protective in the dialysis population. For example, higher blood pressure and obesity both are associated with better survival in patients undergoing dialysis, probably because they reflect greater cardiac and nutritional reserves, respectively. Other challenges with risk-factor management include difficulty with ascertainment. For example, blood pressure measurements are often unreliable because of the presence of dialysis access and arterial calcification, home and ambulatory blood pressure measurements are infrequently used for clinical care, and glycated hemoglobin measurements may not accurately reflect glycemic control.

Despite a lack of definitive supporting evidence, the following targets could be reasonable, based predominantly on evidence from the nondialysis population. A predialysis blood pressure goal of less than 140 to 150/90 mm Hg should be targeted if achievable without hypotension-limiting ultrafiltration, optimally through appropriate dry weight before initiation of pharmacologic therapy. Modest glycemic control requires frequent glucose assessments, assuming that hypoglycemia can be avoided. In some patients, tighter control of cardiovascular disease risk factors, if achievable safely, may be advisable and cost effective, although tools to identify patients undergoing dialysis who are most likely to benefit from these interventions remain insufficient. Finally, smoking cessation efforts are essential in all stages of CKD. As with earlier stages of CKD, ischemic heart disease can be treated

successfully with invasive therapies in patients undergoing dialysis; however, the risk of complications is higher in patients with CKD. Accordingly, the optimal strategy remains unknown, and a policy of shared decision making is suggested.

LEFT VENTRICULAR HYPERTROPHY AND HEART FAILURE

DIAGNOSIS OF LEFT VENTRICULAR HYPERTROPHY AND HEART FAILURE

Diagnosis of LVH is readily accomplished with echocardiography, an inexpensive, noninvasive, and widely available test. Cardiac function should be assessed in the euvolemic state, as both significant volume depletion and overload may reduce left ventricular inotropy. Accordingly, in patients undergoing dialysis, two-dimensional echocardiography is likely to be most informative if performed on the interdialytic day. Although three-dimensional echocardiography may be useful to assess left ventricle (LV) structure because it avoids the use of geometric assumptions of LV shape that are required to estimate LV mass and volume, increasing availability likely makes cardiac magnetic resonance imaging the modality of choice if highly accurate assessment of LV structure is needed. Screening echocardiography is currently recommended for incident patients undergoing dialysis; however, there is no evidence that this improves clinical outcomes.

Heart failure and cardiorenal syndromes are extensively discussed in Chapter 29. Heart failure is a clinical syndrome characterized by specific symptoms, including dyspnea and fatigue, and signs, including edema and rales. Although this constellation of symptoms and signs may be consistent with heart failure, these symptoms also occur in many individuals with CKD and may simply reflect volume overload. Regardless of the specific cause, individuals with persistent or recurrent volume overload have poor clinical outcomes overall. Importantly in patients undergoing hemodialysis where preload is rapidly changing and fluid overload is managed with ultrafiltration, hypotension may be the only manifestation of heart failure.

TREATMENT OF LEFT VENTRICULAR HYPERTROPHY AND HEART FAILURE

Potentially modifiable risk factors for LVH include anemia, hypertension, extracellular volume overload, and abnormal mineral metabolism including hyperphosphatemia and secondary hyperparathyroidism, and, on rare occasions, arteriovenous fistulas cause high-output heart failure. Definitive clinical trials evaluating whether modifying these risk factors reduces mortality are not currently available, leading to reliance on surrogate outcomes. Some data suggest that ACE inhibitor and ARB therapy may result in favorable effects on a putative surrogate outcome (left ventricular mass reduction). In contrast, randomized trials in CKD patients targeting normalization of hemoglobin levels with recombinant human erythropoietin had no effect on the similar surrogate outcome of LVH or left ventricular mass. Critically, no trials in CKD stages 3 to 4 have demonstrated a reduction in cardiac outcomes or mortality with these interventions when they are used for the purpose of treating or preventing LVH. In patients undergoing hemodialysis enrolled in the Frequent Hemo-dialysis Network study, those who received more frequent hemodialysis experienced a significant improvement in LV mass, suggesting a critical role for consistent volume control.

Heart failure therapy differs by CKD stage because diuretics are a mainstay of therapy in advanced CKD, whereas fluid overload in patients undergoing dialysis is treated primarily with ultrafiltration. Chronic therapy for heart failure in CKD stages 3b through 5 has not been adequately studied; therefore recommendations are either extrapolated from the general population or based on small trials. As discussed previously, ACE inhibitors and ARBs may have cardiac benefits independent of their blood-pressure-lowering effects in systolic heart failure patients with CKD stages 1 to early stage 4, with limited data suggesting some improvement in LV geometry as well as cardiovascular outcomes. Potential further benefits associated with aldosterone blockade (e.g., spironolactone) are currently being studied, with a potential limitation of hyperkalemia, especially when used in conjunction with ACE inhibitors or ARBs. Beta-blocking agents, another mainstay of heart-failure therapy in the general population, are also likely beneficial in patients with nondialysis CKD, and evidence from one small trial supports carvedilol use to reduce mortality risk in patients undergoing dialysis with left ventricular dysfunction. Cardiac glycosides (e.g., digoxin) are occasionally used in heart failure in the general population where they decrease morbidity but not mortality. Although there are no specific studies of cardiac glycosides in CKD, they should be used judiciously if at all in these patients, with careful attention to dosage, drug levels, and potassium balance.

ARRHYTHMIA AND SUDDEN CARDIAC DEATH

Arrhythmias are extremely common in individuals with CKD, likely reflecting high prevalence of structural heart disease, ischemic heart disease, and electrolyte abnormalities. Atrial fibrillation is the most common arrhythmia, with prevalence estimates for paroxysmal and permanent atrial fibrillation as high as 30% in individuals with advanced CKD, including patients undergoing dialysis. Bradycardia, asystole, and ventricular arrhythmias are probably also exceedingly common, although true rates cannot be determined. Prevalent dialysis patients have cardiovascular disease mortality rates of more than 80 deaths per 1000 person-years, with cardiac arrest and arrhythmia accounting for 29% of all deaths and 39% of deaths with a known cause.

There are few data on prevention and treatment of arrhythmia and sudden cardiac death in the CKD or dialysis population, with most current treatment recommendations for individuals not treated with dialysis mirroring those seen in the general population. Although an increasing number of late-stage CKD and patients undergoing dialysis are receiving implantable cardioverter-defibrillators (ICDs) to prevent sudden cardiac death, there are no trial data that have shown a survival benefit or demonstrated cost effectiveness. Critically, ICD and other cardiac device wires typically traverse the left subclavian vein and may predispose to central stenosis, adversely affecting hemodialysis vascular access options. Newer, leadless devices may be particularly good options for the advanced CKD and dialysis populations, where vein preservation is paramount. Given the high incidence of sudden cardiac death, one sensible preventative strategy for ambulatory settings where CKD patients are treated, including clinics and dialysis facilities, is to ensure the presence of an automated external defibrillator (AED) and trained clinic personnel.

STROKE

Cerebrovascular disease is also common in individuals with CKD (see Fig. 55.2), with a higher incidence of both ischemic and hemorrhagic events than seen in the general population. Critically, even in the absence of clinically evident strokes, both silent lesions and substantial brain white matter disease may be present. Not surprisingly, the presence of cardiovascular disease is associated with cerebrovascular manifestations in individuals with CKD, including worse cognitive function.

Although not specifically studied, stroke prevention and treatment strategies for patients with earlier stages of CKD likely should follow general population guidelines, including management of traditional risk factors and the use of antithrombotic agents as indicated. For example, among individuals with CKD stage 3 participating in the Stroke Prevention in Atrial Fibrillation 3 trials, warfarin use based on general population recommendations was associated with a considerable reduction in the incidence of embolic stroke without a substantial increase in adverse events. Newer trials using direct oral anticoagulants (DOACs) rather than warfarin suggest that these agents are safe and effective in individuals with CKD stage 3. In contrast, clinical trial data examining either warfarin or DOACs are absent in patients undergoing dialysis, where the risk of bleeding complications and falls is substantially higher. Limited safety and efficacy data exist for DOACs in CKD stage 4, stage 5, or dialysis; all of these agents are at least in part cleared by the kidney, and there are no clinical trial data evaluating the safety of longer-term use of these agents in advanced CKD populations. Accordingly, until safety data are available, warfarin remains the oral anticoagulant of choice in advanced CKD.

In cohort data from dialysis populations, data on warfarin for primary thromboembolism prevention in atrial fibrillation is mixed, with some observational data suggesting an increased risk of death in patients treated with warfarin. If true, this may reflect the relationship between warfarin and increased vascular calcification, mediated by preventing vitamin K dependent carboxylation of matrix Gla protein, a calcification inhibitor. Given the frequency with which atrial fibrillation occurs in individuals with kidney failure, the lack of trial data on anticoagulation in patients undergoing dialysis, and the many competing risks of death in this population, optimal management of primary and secondary stroke prevention with anticoagulants urgently requires an adequately powered clinical trial to inform management decisions.

KEY BIBLIOGRAPHY

Baigent C, Landray MJ, Reith C, et al. The effects of lowering LDL cholesterol with simvastatin plus ezetimibe in patients with chronic kidney disease (Study of Heart and Renal Protection): a randomised placebo-controlled trial. *Lancet.* 2011;377:2181-2192.
Chronic Kidney Disease Prognosis Consortium. Association of estimated glomerular filtration rate and albuminuria with all-cause and

cardiovascular mortality in general population cohorts: a collaborative meta-analysis. *Lancet.* 2010;375:2073-2181.

Cice G, Ferrara L, D'Andrea A, et al. Carvedilol increases two-year survival in dialysis patients with dilated cardiomyopathy: a prospective, placebo-controlled trial. *J Am Coll Cardiol.* 2003;41:1438-1444.

deFilippi CWS, Rosanio S, Tiblier E, et al. Cardiac troponin T and C-reactive protein for predicting prognosis, coronary atherosclerosis, and cardiomyopathy in patients undergoing long-term hemodialysis. *JAMA.* 2003;290:353-359.

Fishbein GA, Fishbein MC. Arteriosclerosis: rethinking the current classification. *Arch Pathol Lab Med.* 2009;133:1309-1316.

Fox CS, Larson MG, Vasan RS, et al. Cross-sectional association of kidney function with valvular and annular calcification: the Framingham heart study. *J Am Soc Nephrol.* 2006;17:521-527.

Fox CS, Muntner P, Chen AY, et al. Use of evidence-based therapies in short-term outcomes of ST-segment elevation myocardial infarction and non-ST-segment elevation myocardial infarction in patients with chronic kidney disease: a report from the National Cardiovascular Data Acute Coronary Treatment and Intervention Outcomes Network registry. *Circulation.* 2010;121:357-365.

Go AS, Chertow GM, Fan D, et al. Chronic kidney disease and the risks of death, cardiovascular events, and hospitalization. *N Engl J Med.* 2004;351:1296-1305.

Hart RG, Pearce LA, Asinger RW, et al. Warfarin in atrial fibrillation patients with moderate chronic kidney disease. *Clin J Am Soc Nephrol.* 2011;6:2599-2604.

Kidney Disease: Improving Global Outcomes (KDIGO) Lipid Work Group. KDIGO clinical practice guideline for lipid management in chronic kidney disease. *Kidney Int Suppl.* 2013;3:259-305.

Lentine KL, Costa SP, Weir MR, et al. Cardiac disease evaluation and management among kidney and liver transplantation candidates: a scientific statement from the American Heart Association and the American College of Cardiology Foundation: endorsed by the American Society of Transplant Surgeons, American Society of Transplantation, and National Kidney Foundation. *Circulation.* 2012;126:617-663.

Matsushita K, Coresh J, Sang Y, et al. Estimated glomerular filtration rate and albuminuria for prediction of cardiovascular outcomes: a collaborative meta-analysis of individual participant data. *Lancet Diabetes Endocrinol.* 2015;3:514-525.

Ohtake T, Kobayashi S, Moriya H, et al. High prevalence of occult coronary artery stenosis in patients with chronic kidney disease at the initiation of renal replacement therapy: an angiographic examination. *J Am Soc Nephrol.* 2005;16:1141-1148.

Palmer SC, Di Micco L, Razavian M, et al. Effects of antiplatelet therapy on mortality and cardiovascular and bleeding outcomes in persons with chronic kidney disease: a systematic review and meta-analysis. *Ann Intern Med.* 2012;156:445-459.

Raggi P, Boulay A, Chasan-Taber S, et al. Cardiac calcification in adult hemodialysis patients: a link between end-stage renal disease and cardiovascular disease? *J Am Coll Cardiol.* 2002;39:695-701.

Roberts MA, Polkinghorne KR, McDonald SP, et al. Secular trends in cardiovascular mortality rates of patients receiving dialysis compared with the general population. *Am J Kidney Dis.* 2011;58:64-72.

Saran R, Li Y, Robinson B, et al. US Renal Data System 2015 Annual Data Report: epidemiology of kidney disease in the United States. *Am J Kidney Dis.* 2016;67:Svii, S1-S305.

Sarnak MJ. Cardiovascular complications in chronic kidney disease. *Am J Kidney Dis.* 2003;41:11-17.

Sarnak MJ, Levey AS, Schoolwerth AC, et al. Kidney disease as a risk factor for development of cardiovascular disease: a statement from the American Heart Association Councils on Kidney in Cardiovascular Disease, High Blood Pressure Research, Clinical Cardiology, and Epidemiology and Prevention. *Circulation.* 2003;108:2154-2169.

Umana E, Ahmed W, Alpert MA. Valvular and perivalvular abnormalities in end-stage renal disease. *Am J Med Sci.* 2003;325:237-242.

Full bibliography can be found on www.expertconsult.com.

Anemia and Other Hematologic Complications of Chronic Kidney Disease

56

Jay B. Wish

ANEMIA

EPIDEMIOLOGY AND PATHOGENESIS

Anemia is defined by the World Health Organization as hemoglobin (Hb) concentration of less than 13.0 g/L in adult men and nonmenstruating women and less than 12.0 g/dL in menstruating women. The incidence of anemia in patients with chronic kidney disease (CKD) increases as the glomerular filtration rate (GFR) declines. Population studies, including the United States National Health and Nutrition Examination Survey (NHANES) and the Prevalence of Anemia in Early Renal Insufficiency (PAERI) study, suggest that the incidence of anemia is less than 10% in CKD stages 1 and 2, 20% to 40% in CKD stage 3, 50% to 60% in CKD stage 4, and more than 70% in CKD stage 5.

The pathogenesis of anemia in patients with CKD is multifactorial (Box 56.1), but the contribution of erythropoietin (EPO) deficiency becomes greater as GFR declines. Hypoxia inducible factor (HIF), which is produced in the kidneys and other tissues, is a substance whose spontaneous degradation is retarded in the presence of decreased oxygen delivery because of anemia or hypoxemia. The sustained presence of HIF leads to signal transduction and the synthesis of EPO. In normal patients, plasma EPO levels increase dramatically in response to anemia. Because of their loss of functioning mass, the kidneys in patients with CKD fail to increase EPO production in response to anemia or other conditions that decrease oxygen delivery.

The kidneys produce about 90% of circulating EPO, and loss of EPO production in the setting of CKD is the primary cause of anemia in these patients. EPO binds to receptors on erythroid progenitor cells in the bone marrow, specifically the burst-forming units (BFU-E) and colony-forming units (CFU-E). The absence of EPO causes these cells to undergo programmed death or apoptosis, which is mediated by Fas ligand. In the presence of EPO, these erythroid progenitors differentiate into reticulocytes and red blood cells (RBCs).

Fig. 56.1 demonstrates the complex interactions among EPO, proinflammatory cytokines such as interleukin 1 (IL-1), tumor necrosis factor-α (TNF-α), IL-6, and interferon-γ (IFN-γ); hepcidin; and iron in the production of RBCs. Hepcidin is a peptide produced by the liver that interferes with RBC production by decreasing iron availability for incorporation into erythroblasts. Hepcidin gene expression is upregulated by IL-6 and iron overload and downregulated by TNF-α and iron deficiency. At the cell surface of macrophages and jejunal cells (and probably other cells), hepcidin binds to ferroportin, the membrane-embedded iron exporter, resulting in internalization and degradation of the complex. This inhibits iron transport across the cell membrane, trapping it in macrophages and preventing it from being absorbed from the intestine. Hepcidin activity is probably the basis for most "anemia of chronic disease" syndromes, and it contributes to the anemia in patients with CKD when inflammation and infection are present; however, in anemic CKD patients without inflammation or infection, EPO deficiency plays a much greater role than hepcidin.

The evidence for inhibition of RBC production by uremic toxins in patients with CKD is poor, as most CKD patients have an appropriate erythropoietic response to exogenously administered EPO if they are iron replete and free of inflammation or infection. It has been demonstrated that RBC survival is decreased from 120 days in normal individuals to 60 to 90 days in patients with CKD. This may be a result of RBC trauma from microvascular disease as well as decreased resistance to oxidative stress. The reduction of EPO in patients with CKD also contributes to neocytolysis, a physiologic process that leads to hemolysis of the youngest RBCs in the circulation.

CLINICAL MANIFESTATIONS

The major clinical manifestations of anemia in patients with or without CKD are fatigue (both with exercise and at rest), decreased cognitive function, loss of libido, and decreased sense of well-being. These symptoms tend to occur when the Hb is less than 10 g/dL, and they are more severe at lower Hb levels. More insidious are the cardiac complications of anemia, which may occur when the patient is otherwise asymptomatic and contribute to the adverse cardiovascular morbidity and mortality outcomes observed among patients with CKD. In patients with underlying coronary artery disease, anemia may lead to an exacerbation of angina because of decreased myocardial oxygen delivery. Decreased peripheral oxygen delivery because of anemia leads to peripheral vasodilation, increased sympathetic nervous system activity, increased heart rate and stroke volume, and, ultimately, left ventricular hypertrophy (LVH). LVH strongly correlates with adverse outcomes, including hospitalization and mortality, in patients with CKD. Each decrease in Hb of 0.5 g/dL is associated with a 32% increase in the likelihood that a patient has an increase in left ventricle (LV) mass over the course of a year; in contrast, each 5 mm Hg increase in systolic blood pressure correlates with only an 11% increase in LV

515

mass. Most anemic CKD patients treated with erythropoiesis-stimulating agents (ESAs) report a decrease in subjective symptoms and improved quality of life (QoL), but evidence supporting regression of LVH, fewer clinical cardiac events, or decreased mortality with ESA treatment is not compelling (see later discussion).

LABORATORY EVALUATION

Because anemia is common in CKD, the consequences of anemia are severe, and treatment is available, the 2012 Kidney Disease: Improving Global Outcomes (KDIGO) clinical practice guidelines for anemia in CKD recommended screening for all patients with CKD stage 3 at least annually and more frequently in those with more advanced CKD; in those with diagnosed anemia not receiving treatment, Hb concentration should be measured at least every 3 months in CKD stage 3 to 5 and monthly in dialysis. If anemia is present (defined as Hb <13.0 g/dL in adult men and Hb <12.0 g/dL in adult women), then further evaluation should be

undertaken to determine the cause. This evaluation should include a complete blood count including RBC indices, reticulocyte count, serum ferritin concentration, and transferrin saturation (TSAT) or reticulocyte Hb content (CHr). The anemia of EPO deficiency is normocytic (normal mean corpuscular volume, MCV) and normochromic (normal mean corpuscular Hb concentration, MCHC). A low MCV (microcytosis) is suggestive of iron deficiency but may be seen in hemoglobinopathies such as thalassemia. A high MCV (macrocytosis) is suggestive of vitamin B_{12} or folate deficiency. If the MCV is elevated, vitamin B_{12} and folate levels should be assessed.

The serum ferritin level correlates with iron bound to tissue ferritin in the reticuloendothelial (RE) system. Serum ferritin does not carry or bind to iron, and its function is unknown. Serum ferritin is also an acute phase reactant, and it increases in the setting of acute or chronic inflammation independent of tissue iron stores. TSAT is a measure of circulating iron available for delivery to the erythroid marrow and is calculated by dividing the serum iron concentration by the total iron binding capacity (TIBC). The TIBC correlates with the serum level of transferrin, which is the major iron-carrying protein in the blood. TSAT less than 16% in an anemic patient with CKD is consistent with absolute or functional iron deficiency, both of which are characterized by decreased delivery of iron to the erythroid marrow.

Absolute iron deficiency occurs in the setting of decreased total body iron stores and is accompanied by serum ferritin level less than 25 ng/mL in men and less than 12 ng/mL in women. Functional iron deficiency is seen in patients with low TSAT and normal or elevated serum ferritin. It may be a result of the pharmacologic stimulation of RBC production by ESAs, which causes iron demand by the erythroid marrow to outstrip the ability of the RE system to release iron to circulating transferrin. Functional iron deficiency may also result from the action of hepcidin in the setting of

> **Box 56.1 Factors That Cause or Contribute to Anemia in Patients With Chronic Kidney Disease**
>
> Insufficient production of endogenous EPO
> Iron deficiency
> Acute and chronic inflammatory conditions
> Severe hyperparathyroidism
> Aluminum toxicity
> Folate deficiency
> Decreased survival of RBCs and RBC loss
>
> *EPO*, Erythropoietin; *RBCs*, red blood cells.

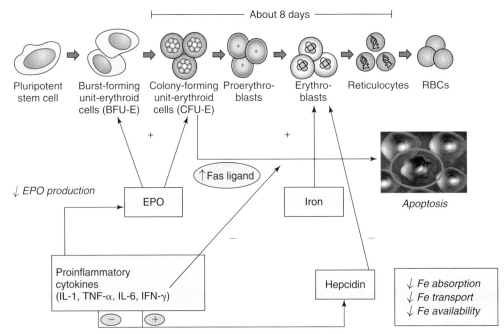

Fig. 56.1 Erythropoiesis in chronic kidney disease. *EPO*, Erythropoietin; *Fe*, iron; *IFN*, interferon; *IL*, interleukin; *RBCs*, red blood cells; *TNF*, tumor necrosis factor. (Courtesy Iain Macdougall, MD.)

inflammation or infection. The hallmark of functional iron deficiency anemia is that it responds to the administration of intravenous iron supplements, with increase in Hb level and/or decrease in ESA requirements despite the normal or elevated serum ferritin concentration. If the anemic patient with low TSAT and normal or high serum ferritin level does not respond to intravenous iron, the presumptive diagnosis is RE blockade, meaning that hepcidin has completely prevented the release of iron from macrophages to circulating transferrin. It should be noted that, although the diagnosis of iron depletion is based on serum ferritin concentration less than 25 ng/mL and that of iron-deficient erythropoiesis is based on TSAT less than 16%, anemic CKD patients with considerably higher serum ferritin and TSAT levels often respond to iron supplementation (see Iron Therapy, later).

The reticulocyte count is a useful and inexpensive test to distinguish anemia caused by underproduction of RBCs from that caused by RBC loss or destruction. In the setting of EPO deficiency, RBC production is decreased, and most anemic patients would be expected to have decreased absolute reticulocyte count (<40,000 to 50,000 cells per milliliter of whole blood). Elevated reticulocyte count is inconsistent with EPO deficiency, and an evaluation for hemolysis and blood loss should be undertaken.

Although it would seem that demonstration of decreased blood EPO level would secure the diagnosis of EPO deficiency, routine testing for EPO levels in anemic patients with CKD is not recommended. The reason is that patients who respond to exogenous ESAs may have normal or even elevated EPO concentration, which nevertheless may be inappropriately low for the severity of their anemia. Furthermore, the test is expensive. Therefore it is recommended that EPO deficiency be a diagnosis of exclusion (i.e., negative evaluation for other treatable causes of anemia) in the anemic CKD patient. However, a cause other than EPO deficiency should also be considered if anemia severity is disproportionate to the GFR or if leukopenia and/or thrombocytopenia are present.

ERYTHROPOIESIS-STIMULATING AGENTS

After other treatable causes of anemia have been excluded, and a diagnosis of EPO deficiency is inferred, the treatment of choice for many anemic patients with CKD is an ESA. Recombinant human erythropoietin (rHuEPO, or epoetin) has been available since 1989 and has revolutionized the treatment of anemia in patients with CKD who previously depended on blood transfusions and androgens. Although absorption of epoetin administered subcutaneously is incomplete with degradation of some of the protein before it reaches the circulation, the slower absorption and sustained serum epoetin levels may make this route of administration 20% to 30% more efficient than a comparable intravenously administered dose. Nonetheless, the vast majority of patients undergoing hemodialysis in the United States receive an ESA by the intravenous route because of convenience of administration. One possible additional motivation for intravenous administration is the association between cases of pure red cell aplasia (PRCA) in Europe and subcutaneous administration of the Eprex formulation of epoetin alfa (discussed later).

Patients with nondialysis dependent CKD and patients undergoing peritoneal dialysis usually receive ESAs subcutaneously. The package insert for epoetin recommends thrice-weekly dosing, because the clinical trials that were submitted for approval by the US Food and Drug Administration (FDA) involved patients undergoing hemodialysis who received the drug with each treatment. For CKD patients not on dialysis and patients on peritoneal dialysis, thrice-weekly dosing is not practical. It is more painful because of the subcutaneous route and not necessary because clinical trials in these patients have shown epoetin administered every 1 to 2 weeks equally effective. Epoetin is effective in maintaining target Hb levels in 76% of CKD patients not on dialysis when administered as infrequently as every 4 weeks.

Darbepoetin alfa is a bioengineered epoetin molecule with two additional N-linked carbohydrate side chains. It has a longer half-life and duration of action than epoetin. As with epoetin, studies have demonstrated that darbepoetin is effective in maintaining target Hb levels when administered as infrequently as every 4 weeks in selected patients. There appears to be no difference in subcutaneous versus intravenous administration in terms of efficacy. The side effect profile of darbepoetin is virtually identical to that of epoetin; both agents are associated with the development or exacerbation of hypertension in 20% to 30% of patients. The mechanism for hypertension is multifactorial and related to increased RBC mass, attenuation of the peripheral vasodilation associated with anemia, and, perhaps, a direct inhibitory effect on vascular endothelial vasodilatory mediators such as nitric oxide and prostaglandins. The existence or exacerbation of hypertension is not a contraindication to ESA therapy; rather, the hypertension should be treated with more aggressive pharmacologic therapy, increased ultrafiltration on dialysis, and/or a decrease in the ESA dose to slow the rate of Hb rise and to allow for physiologic vasomotor adaptation. There is no evidence that the rate of vascular access thrombosis is increased in patients undergoing hemodialysis when ESA treatment is used to maintain Hb levels within the currently recommended target range. All other side effects reported with ESA therapy are no greater than with placebo.

Mircera (methoxy polyethylene glycol-epoetin beta) has been extensively used in other parts of the world for a number of years and was introduced into the US market following the expiration of patents on epoetin in 2014. The pegylation of the molecule retards its metabolism and allows for once-monthly IV or SC dosing. Mircera carries the same FDA warnings as epoetin and darbepoietin. The pharmacologic properties of ESAs approved in the United States as of 2016 are summarized in Table 56.1.

PURE RED CELL APLASIA

PRCA is a form of aplastic anemia caused by the production of anti-EPO antibodies induced by administration of exogenous ESAs. The diagnosis of PRCA should be suspected in a patient with a sudden weekly drop in Hb of approximately 1 g/dL, or a weekly transfusion requirement and low reticulocyte count (<20,000 cells/μL), despite a high dose of ESA for several months. In contrast to classic aplastic anemia, the white blood cell and platelet counts are preserved in PRCA. A definitive diagnosis of PRCA is made by the demonstration of anti-EPO antibodies in the blood or a bone marrow examination showing normal cellularity and less than 4% erythroblasts. Treatment includes discontinuation of the ESA

Table 56.1 Erythropoiesis-Stimulating Agents Available in the United States, 2017

Generic Name	Brand Name	Dosing Frequency	Starting Dose
Epoetin	Epogen, Procrit	Three times weekly IV in HD patients; every 1–2 SC weeks in ND-CKD and PD patients	50 units/kg based on three times weekly dosing
Darbepoetin	Aranesp	Every 1–2 weeks IV or SC in ESRD patients; every 4 weeks SC in ND-CKD patients	0.45 µg/kg weekly or 0.75 mg/kg every 2 weeks in ESRD patients; 0.45 mg/kg every 4 weeks in ND-CKD patients
Methoxypolyethylene glycol epoetin beta	Mircera	Initiation: every 2 weeks; maintenance: monthly. IV in HD patients, SC in ND-CKD and PD patients	0.6 µg/kg every 2 weeks; monthly when Hb is stable at twice the every 2 weeks dose

CKD, Chronic kidney disease; *ESRD*, end-stage renal disease; *Hb*, hemoglobin; *HD*, hemodialysis; *IV*, intravenous; *ND*, nondialysis; *PD*, peritoneal dialysis; *SC*, subcutaneous.

and immunosuppressive therapy (e.g., cyclophosphamide); most patients respond after several months and do not relapse after the immunosuppressive therapy is discontinued. A cluster of PRCA cases in Europe was traced almost exclusively to subcutaneous administration of a form of epoetin alfa stabilized with Tween 80. This additive was never used in the United States where PRCA has always been rare. With removal of this preparation from the European market, the incidence of PRCA fell dramatically. An additional small cluster of PRCA cases was reported with one of the biosimilar ESAs (discussed below) approved in Europe. That cluster was traced to interaction of the agent with tungsten used in the manufacturing of the needles of prefilled syringes. Once the root cause was identified and eliminated, no further clusters of PRCA with that agent have been reported.

TARGET HEMOGLOBIN LEVEL

The target Hb level for anemic patients with CKD treated with ESAs has been controversial, because observational studies disagree with the results of interventional trials. Based on studies of epoetin efficacy in the early 1990s that compared outcomes in untreated patients with hematocrit (Hct) values in the mid-20s with those in treated patients with Hct values in the mid-30s, the first iteration of the NKF-DOQI anemia guidelines (1997) had an opinion-based recommendation that the target Hct for epoetin-treated patients should be 33% to 36%. However, observational studies from the United States Renal Data System (USRDS) and large dialysis chain databases suggested that the benefits of higher Hct or Hb levels extend to levels greater than 39% and 13 g/dL, respectively, with QoL increasing directly across the spectrum of Hct/Hb levels. In 1998, results from the Normal Hematocrit Study (NHS), which randomized 1223 patients undergoing hemodialysis with underlying cardiac disease receiving epoetin to target Hct 30% versus target Hct 42%, became available. The study was terminated early because of the low likelihood that the patients randomized to the higher Hct would show better outcomes. The patients in the higher target Hct group had a relative risk of 1.3 (confidence interval, 0.9 to 1.9) for the primary endpoints of death or myocardial infarction. Furthermore, patients in the higher target Hct group had a significantly greater incidence of vascular access thrombosis. Based on this study, the 2001 iteration of the NKF-K/DOQI

anemia guidelines recommended target Hb 11 to 12 g/dL in ESA-treated anemic patients with CKD.

The Cardiovascular Risk Reduction by Early Anemia Treatment with Epoetin Beta (CREATE) study randomly assigned 603 patients with GFRs between 15 and 35 mL/min per 1.73 m^2 and a baseline Hb of 11 to 12.5 g/dL to one of two groups. High target patients were immediately treated with epoetin beta to target Hb 13 to 15 g/dL, while low target patients were treated only when their Hb fell to less than 10.5 g/dL with target Hb 10.5 to 11.5 g/dL. There was no difference between the two groups in the primary endpoint (time to first cardiovascular event). Although there was no difference in the rate of decline in GFR between the two groups, more patients in the higher Hb target group required dialysis. Patients in the high target group had better general health and improved physical function, based on standard survey instruments. There was no difference between the two groups in combined adverse events.

The Correction of Hemoglobin and Outcomes in Renal Insufficiency (CHOIR) study randomized 1432 patients with stage 4 CKD to target Hb 11.3 g/dL versus 13.5 g/dL. The average follow-up period was 16 months, and the study was terminated early because of safety concerns in the higher target Hb group. The primary endpoint was a composite of death, myocardial infarction, hospitalization for congestive heart failure (without kidney replacement therapy), and stroke. The patients in the higher target Hb group had a significantly higher incidence of the composite endpoint, congestive heart failure, death, and hospitalization (cardiovascular and all-cause). There was no difference between the groups in rates of stroke, myocardial infarction, kidney replacement therapy, or QoL.

Based on the results of the CHOIR and CREATE studies, the FDA changed the product information for epoetin and darbepoetin to add a boxed warning regarding the risks for death and serious cardiovascular events when ESAs are administered to achieve target Hb levels 13.5 to 14.5 g/dL versus 10.0 to 11.3 g/dL. It was also stated that the physician should "individualize dosing to achieve and maintain Hb levels within the range of 10 to 12 g/dL" in patients with CKD. The FDA recommendations notwithstanding, in 2007 the NKF-K/DOQI anemia workgroup published an updated recommendation that the Hb target for ESA-treated CKD patients should be 11.0 to 12.0 g/dL and a guideline

Table 56.2 Large Randomized Studies of Erythropoiesis-Stimulating Agents in Chronic Kidney Disease Patients With Anemia

	NHS	CHOIR	CREATE	TREAT
Year published	1998	2006	2006	2009
Location	United States	United States	Europe	International
ESA	Epoetin alfa	Epoetin alfa	Epoetin beta	Darbepoetin alfa
CKD stage and comorbidity	Dialysis with cardiac disease	Nondialysis	Nondialysis	Nondialysis with type 2 diabetes
Number of patients	1223	1432	603	4038
High Hb target (g/dL)	14 (Hct 42)	13.5	13–15	13
Low Hb target (g/dL)	10 (Hct 30)	11.3	10.5–11.5	9
CV endpoints	RR 1.3 (CI 0.9–1.9)	Higher in high Hb group	No difference	No difference except higher stroke in high Hb group
Progression of CKD	Not applicable	No difference	More in high Hb group	No difference
Cancer deaths	Not noted	Not noted	Not noted	Higher in high Hb group among patients with previous cancer
QoL	Better in high Hb group	No difference	Better in high Hb group	No difference except less fatigue in high Hb group

CHOIR, Correction of Hemoglobin and Outcomes in Renal Insufficiency; *CI*, confidence interval; *CKD*, chronic kidney disease; *CREATE*, Cardiovascular Risk Reduction by Early Anemia Treatment with Epoetin; *CV*, cardiovascular; *ESA*, erythropoiesis-stimulating agent; *Hb*, hemoglobin; *Hct*, hematocrit; *NHS*, Normal Hematocrit Study; *QoL*, quality of life; *RR*, risk ratio; *TREAT*, Trial to Reduce Cardiovascular Events with Aranesp Therapy.

(moderately strong evidence) that the Hb target should not exceed 13 g/dL.

The Trial to Reduce Cardiovascular Events with Aranesp Therapy (TREAT) study was published in 2009. TREAT examined the use of darbepoetin in anemic patients with type 2 diabetes and nondialysis CKD. Unlike the CHOIR and CREATE studies, the TREAT study had a placebo arm. Important outcomes that were considered included death, cardiovascular events, progression of kidney disease, and QoL. One group received darbepoetin to target Hb of 13 g/dL, and the other was not administered any ESA unless the Hb level decreased to less than 9 g/dL. Other than a higher incidence of stroke in the higher target Hb group, cardiovascular events and deaths were similar in both arms. Fatigue scores were lower among patients in the higher target Hb arm, but the other QoL scores were similar in both groups. Unsurprisingly, there were more blood transfusions in the placebo group. A finding of some concern was that patients with a history of cancer were more likely to die of cancer if randomized to the higher Hb target. The findings of the NHS, CHOIR, CREATE, and TREAT studies are summarized in Table 56.2.

In 2011, the FDA substantially changed the product information for ESAs, eliminating the target Hb range of 10 to 12 g/dL and adding a new boxed warning regarding the risk of death, myocardial infarction, stroke, venous thromboembolism, thrombosis of vascular access, and tumor progression and recurrence. Other elements of the 2011 FDA guidelines are summarized in Box 56.2. The elimination of a target Hb range for ESA therapy, which had generally driven the development and use of standardized ESA dose titration protocols, and the substitution of a recommendation for "individualization" of ESA therapy with the goal of transfusion avoidance led to considerable confusion and controversy within the nephrology community. Especially challenging is the FDA recommendation that ESA therapy in CKD patients not on dialysis not be initiated until the Hb is less than

10 g/dL and that the dose be reduced or interrupted if Hb rises to greater than 10 g/dL. Given the stated goal of minimizing transfusions, perhaps the FDA should have simply recommended Hb target ranges of 9 to 10 g/dL and 9 to 11 g/dL in the nondialysis and dialysis CKD populations, respectively.

The concept of individualization in therapy is appropriate to properly balance the risk and benefit. Transfusion avoidance is a higher priority to avoid allosensitization in patients who are candidates for kidney transplantation. The QoL benefits of ESA therapy and higher Hb levels vary with patients' comorbidities, psychologic structures, functional levels, and expectations. Ideally, the goals of ESA therapy should incorporate the effect of treatment on patients' perception of their QoL with instruments that focus attention on the specific domains that are affected by anemia. The improvement in each of these domains, including fatigue, energy level, sense of vitality, and physical functioning, should be assessed on an individual basis to determine the Hb target range for each patient.

In 2012, the KDIGO Clinical Practice Guideline for Anemia in CKD was published. The KDIGO recommendations regarding target Hb level for patients receiving ESA therapy are summarized in Box 56.3. It should be noted that the KDIGO guideline acknowledges a QoL benefit from ESA therapy, which the FDA does not. The international 2012 KDIGO anemia guideline replaces the 2006 to 2007 K/DOQI anemia guidelines as the most current evidence basis for treatment of anemia in patients with CKD in the United States.

NEW AGENTS

Biosimilar ESAs, which are lower-cost versions of the originator or reference ESAs, are undergoing clinical trials in the United States and are already extensively used in other parts of the world. The FDA defines a biosimilar agent as one that is

Box 56.2   US Food and Drug Administration Guidelines on Use of Erythropoiesis-Stimulating Agents in Patients With Chronic Kidney Disease

General Guidance

In controlled trials, patients experienced greater risks for death, serious adverse cardiovascular reactions, and stroke when administered ESAs to target a Hb level of greater than 11 g/dL.

No trial has identified a Hb target level, ESA dose, or dosing strategy that does not increase these risks.

Use the lowest ESA dose sufficient to reduce the need for RBC transfusions.

Physicians and patients should weigh the possible benefits of decreasing transfusions against the increased risks of death and other serious cardiovascular adverse events.

For All Patients With CKD

When initiating or adjusting therapy, monitor Hb levels at least weekly until stable, then monitor at least monthly. When adjusting therapy consider Hb rate of rise, rate of decline, ESA responsiveness, and Hb variability. A single Hb excursion may not require a dosing change. Do not increase the dose more frequently than once every 4 weeks. Decreases in dose can occur more frequently. Avoid frequent dose adjustments.

If the Hb rises rapidly (e.g., more than 1 g/dL in any 2-week period), reduce the dose of ESA by 25% or more as needed to reduce rapid responses.

For patients who do not respond adequately (Hb increase <1 g/dL after 4 weeks of therapy), increase the dose by 25%.

For patients who do not respond adequately over a 12-week escalation period, increasing the ESA dose further is unlikely to improve response and may increase risks.

Use the lowest dose that will maintain a Hb level sufficient to reduce the need for RBC transfusions. Evaluate other causes of anemia. Discontinue ESA if responsiveness does not improve.

For Adult Patients Not on Dialysis

Consider initiating ESA treatment only when the Hb level is less than 10 g/dL, AND
   The rate of Hb decline indicates the likelihood of requiring RBC transfusion, AND
   Reducing the risk of allosensitization and/or other RBC transfusion related risks is a goal.

If the Hb level exceeds 10 g/dL, reduce or interrupt the dose of ESA.

For Adult Patients on Dialysis

Initiate ESA treatment when the Hb level is less than 10 g/dL.

If the Hb level approaches or exceeds 11 g/dL, reduce or interrupt the dose of ESA.

The intravenous route is recommended for patients on hemodialysis.

CKD, Chronic kidney disease; ESA, erythropoiesis-stimulating agent; Hb, hemoglobin; RBC, red blood cell.

Box 56.3   Key KDIGO Recommendations Regarding Target Hemoglobin Level in Patients Receiving ESA Therapy

For adult CKD nondialysis patients with Hb less than 10 g/dL, it is suggested that the decision to initiate ESA therapy is individualized based on the rate of fall of Hb, previous response to iron therapy, risk of needing transfusion, risks related to ESA therapy, and presence of symptoms attributable to anemia.

For adult CKD patients on dialysis, it is suggested that ESA therapy is used to avoid having the Hb concentration fall below 9 g/dL by starting ESA therapy when the Hb is 9 to 10 g/dL. Individualization of therapy is reasonable as some patients may have improvements in QoL at higher Hb concentration, and ESA therapy may be started above 10 g/dL.

In general, it is suggested that ESAs are not used to maintain Hb concentration above 11.5 g/dL in adult patients with CKD.

Individualization of therapy will be necessary as some patients experience improvements in QoL at Hb concentrations above 11.5 g/dL and will be prepared to accept the risks.

In all adult patients it is recommended that ESAs not be used intentionally to increase the Hb above 13 g/dL.

CKD, Chronic kidney disease; ESA, erythropoiesis-stimulating agent; Hb, hemoglobin; KDIGO, Kidney Disease Improving Global Outcomes; QoL, quality of life.

"highly similar to the reference product with no clinically meaningful differences in terms of the safety profile, purity or potency." Because of the molecular complexity of biologic drugs, biosimilars are not exact copies of the original product, unlike generic versions of small molecule drugs. Because the clinical safety and efficacy of an originator biologic molecule have already been demonstrated, the FDA does not require sponsors of biosimilar agents to repeat these studies. Instead, the FDA requires the sponsor of a biosimilar agent to demonstrate that it is not significantly different from the reference product using smaller-scale direct comparisons and extrapolation. The sponsor of the biosimilar agent must provide evidence demonstrating that its biological product is structurally and functionally similar to the reference product; that it uses the same mechanism of action for the proposed condition(s) of use; that the condition(s) of use proposed in labeling have been previously approved for the reference product; that it has the same route of administration, dosage form, and strength as the reference product; and that it is manufactured, processed, packed or held in a facility that meets standards designed to assure that the biological product continues to be safe, pure, and potent. It is anticipated that the first biosimilar ESA will be approved by the FDA in 2017.

Novel anemia treatments under development include agents that potentiate HIF activity by inhibiting the prolyl hydroxylase (PH) enzyme that normally degrades HIF. This stimulates the production of endogenous EPO, even in patients with end-stage renal disease (ESRD), suggesting that significant extrarenal EPO production can be induced.

These agents also down regulate hepcidin production, which may make them more effective than conventional ESAs for treating patients with underlying inflammation. Moreover, the HIF-PH inhibitors can be taken orally, which makes them potentially attractive to CKD patients not on dialysis and those on home dialysis who would otherwise have their ESA administered subcutaneously. As of this writing there are four HIF-PH inhibitor agents undergoing phase 2 and phase 3 studies in the United States, and it is anticipated that the first of these agents will be approved by the FDA in 2020.

IRON THERAPY

Iron deficiency frequently coexists with EPO deficiency as a cause of anemia in nondialysis CKD, and it almost universally develops in patients treated with hemodialysis because of blood losses in the extracorporeal circuit, frequent blood testing, oozing from vascular access sites after dialysis needles are withdrawn, and vascular access procedures. Nondialysis CKD patients may develop absolute iron deficiency because of inadequate oral iron intake resulting from dietary protein restriction or loss of a taste for red meat. Even if iron deficiency is not present at the time of initial anemia evaluation, it often develops after the initiation of ESA therapy, because the stimulation of new RBC production exhausts existing iron stores. Therefore it is important to regularly monitor iron status with serum ferritin and TSAT levels monthly during initiation of ESA therapy and every 3 months after stable Hb level has been achieved. As mentioned earlier, the target serum ferritin and TSAT levels for patients receiving ESAs are higher than those used to diagnose iron deficiency in the general population because of the phenomenon of functional iron deficiency.

Supplemental iron can be administered orally or intravenously. Oral iron may be sufficient to achieve target iron parameters in nonhemodialysis CKD patients because they do not have the ongoing blood losses of patients undergoing hemodialysis. However, even in nonhemodialysis CKD patients, oral iron may be ineffective because of incomplete adherence, side effects, and the magnitude of iron deficit. Commonly prescribed oral ferrous iron salts (sulfate, fumarate, gluconate) must be oxidized by stomach acid to the ferric form before they can be absorbed by the small intestine. This step may be impaired if stomach acid is buffered by food or an antacid or if the patient is taking a histamine-2 blocker or proton pump inhibitor. Therefore oral iron salts should be administered 1 hour before or 2 hours after a meal. The minimal effective oral iron dose to repair iron deficiency is 200 mg of elemental iron daily, but each 325-mg tablet of ferrous sulfate contains only 65 mg of elemental iron, requiring an iron-deficient patient to take at least three tablets daily in divided doses. A 325-mg tablet of ferrous fumarate contains approximately 100 mg of elemental iron, requiring an iron-deficient patient to take two tablets daily in divided doses. A 325-mg tablet of ferrous gluconate contains 39 mg of elemental iron, requiring 5 to 6 tablets daily in an iron-deficient patient. Oral polysaccharide-iron complex contains 150 mg of elemental iron in each 150-mg capsule, requiring 1 tablet twice daily to provide greater than 200 mg elemental iron. The bioavailability of oral iron salts is only 1% to 2% of the administered dose in patients with elevated serum ferritin, so even an adherent patient may be unable to repair an iron deficit with an oral agent. Finally, oral iron salts are associated with gastrointestinal side effects such as epigastric pain and constipation that may further limit compliance.

For nonhemodialysis patients with iron deficiency unresponsive to oral iron and for all patients undergoing hemodialysis receiving ESAs whose iron parameters are at or below target levels, intravenous iron therapy is recommended. Five forms of intravenous iron are available in the United States: iron dextran, iron sucrose, iron gluconate, ferumoxytol, and ferric carboxymaltose. Iron dextran is the least expensive, but it has been associated with fatal anaphylactic reactions leading to a "black box" warning by the FDA and the need for a test dose of 25 mg at the time of the first administration. The absence of a reaction to the test dose makes it less likely, but it does not guarantee that the patient will not have an anaphylactic reaction to a therapeutic dose of iron dextran. An advantage of iron dextran is that it can be administered in dosages as high as 1000 mg in a single session. This may be a consideration for nonhemodialysis patients with limited access to a healthcare facility to receive intravenous iron, and it preserves veins for future hemodialysis vascular access because fewer infusions are required. Iron sucrose and iron gluconate have never been associated with a fatal anaphylactic reaction and do not require a test dose. However, they can be administered to a maximum of only 250 to 300 mg per session, so a nonhemodialysis patient with severe iron deficiency will require several infusions to replete iron stores. Iron sucrose and iron gluconate are preferred in patients undergoing hemodialysis whose regular visits and access to the circulation through the extracorporeal circuit make smaller and more frequent dosing appropriate. Iron sucrose and iron gluconate have been associated with nonfatal anaphylactic reactions, hypotension, and nausea/vomiting. For iron dextran, sucrose, and gluconate, slower infusion rates and smaller doses in a single session are associated with a lower incidence of side effects.

There are two intravenous iron preparations, ferumoxytol and ferric carboxymaltose, that can be given in infusion doses of 510 and 750 mg, respectively. Ferumoxytol is approved by the FDA for administration of 510 mg over at least 15 minutes. A second dose can be administered 3 to 8 days later in a patient with TSAT less than 20%. Ferumoxytol has been associated with a small number of fatal anaphylactic reactions and received a strengthened warning from the FDA in 2015 due to anaphylaxis risk. Ferric carboxymaltose is given in a dose of 750 mg administered as an infusion over at least 15 minutes or a slow IV push over at least 7.5 minutes. A second 750-mg dose of ferric carboxymaltose can be administered at least 7 days later for a maximum cumulative dose of 1500 mg per course. These agents have potential appeal to nonhemodialysis CKD patients with iron deficiency because they allow decreased frequency and duration of clinic visits to receive intravenous iron therapy, and they preserve veins for future hemodialysis vascular access. The safety profiles of ferumoxytol and ferric carboxymaltose appear to be similar to those of iron sucrose and gluconate, with serious adverse events occurring in 0.4% to 0.6% of treatments. Characteristics of available intravenous iron preparations are summarized in Table 56.3. Iron isomaltoside is an IV iron preparation that is approved in Europe for administration of a single dose of 1000 mg. It is undergoing phase 3 trials in the United States

Table 56.3   Intravenous Iron Preparations Available in the United States

Generic Name	Brand Name	Labeled Dosing for Iron Deficiency	IV Administration Time	Test Dose Required?
Iron dextran	Dexferrum, INFeD	1000 mg in 10 divided doses or total dose as a single IV infusion	Infusion rate should not exceed 500 mL/hour	Yes
Iron sucrose	Venofer	1000 mg in 10 divided doses (hemodialysis)	5 min undiluted; 15 min if diluted in saline	No
		1000 mg in 5 divided doses (nondialysis)	Undiluted over 5 min or infused over 30–60 min	
		1000 mg in 2 doses of 300 mg and 1 dose of 400 mg (peritoneal dialysis)	300 mg infused over 1.5 hours 400 mg infused over 2.5 hours	
Iron gluconate	Ferrlecit, Nulecit	1000 mg in 8 divided doses (hemodialysis only)	60 min diluted in saline	No
Ferumoxytol	Feraheme	510 mg × 2 doses	Undiluted or infused over ≥15 min, 5–8 days apart	No
Ferric carboxymaltose	Injectafer (US), Ferinject	750 mg × 2 doses	Slow IV push over ≥7.5 min or infused over ≥15 min, ≥7 days apart	No

IV, Intravenous.

for a variety of iron deficiency anemia indications including dialysis dependent and nondialysis dependent CKD.

The Dialysis Patients' Response to IV Iron with Elevated Ferritin (DRIVE) study examined the efficacy of intravenous iron administration in patients undergoing hemodialysis who had Hb less than 11 g/dL on adequate ESA therapy, TSAT less than 25%, and serum ferritin 500 to 1200 ng/mL. The study showed that administration of eight 125-mg doses of iron gluconate resulted in more efficient erythropoiesis, a more rapid rise in Hb levels, a decrease in ESA requirements, and adverse events similar to those in a control group that received no intravenous iron. These findings suggest that there is a spectrum of responsiveness to intravenous iron that extends to patients with serum ferritin levels as high as 1200 ng/mL.

Concerns have been raised about the potential toxicity of intravenous iron supplements, including cellular and vascular damage from oxidative stress and impaired white blood cell function based on in vitro studies. There has been evidence of increased urinary excretion of markers of tubular injury, but not increased albuminuria, in CKD patients receiving intravenous iron sucrose. However, observational studies have not demonstrated increased hospitalizations or mortality in patients undergoing hemodialysis receiving an average of less than 400 mg of intravenous iron per month, and intravenous iron therapy was not identified as a risk factor for bacteremia in patients undergoing hemodialysis in a multivariate analysis. Liver magnetic resonance imaging studies of patients undergoing hemodialysis have shown abnormally high iron content, which correlates with serum ferritin level and cumulative iron dose. Because IV iron invariably exceeds the ability of the erythroid marrow to immediately assimilate it, most of the administered iron must be "parked" in the RE system for subsequent gradual release to transferrin. A significant portion of the RE system resides in the liver as Kupffer cells. Increased iron content in the liver on MRI may be a physiologic reflection of increased

storage iron and is of unclear significance because it is not known whether that liver iron is safely stored in RE cells or has "spilled over" to hepatocytes. Serial liver biopsies in patients with hemochromatosis showed no significant organ injury when the serum ferritin level was less than 2000 ng/mL. The 2012 KDIGO anemia guidelines recommend a trial of IV iron (or a 1- to 3-month trial of oral iron in nondialysis patients) for adult CKD patients with anemia not on iron or ESA therapy if an increase in Hb concentration without starting ESA therapy is desired, TSAT is ≤30%, and ferritin is ≤500 ng/mL. For those CKD patients receiving ESA therapy not receiving iron supplementation, a trial of IV iron (or a 1- to 3-month trial of oral iron in nondialysis patients) is recommended if an increase in Hb concentration or decrease in ESA dose is desired, TSAT is ≤30%, and ferritin is ≤500 ng/mL. The US commentary on the KDIGO anemia guideline considered the evidence to be insufficient to recommend a serum ferritin ceiling above which IV iron must be withheld but rather to weigh the risks and benefits of IV iron therapy including ESA responsiveness, Hb concentration, TSAT level, comorbid conditions, and health-related QoL in making decisions regarding iron administration in the setting of high serum ferritin.

Two new iron products have become available that provide lower doses of iron on a more continuous basis for patients undergoing dialysis and thereby may decrease the risk of excessive iron storage. Ferric citrate is an oral agent approved by the FDA as a phosphate binder for patients undergoing dialysis but which contains a form of iron that is more absorbable than conventional oral iron supplements. When ferric citrate is used in a dose to lower serum phosphorus to the target range, it leads to an increase in serum ferritin and TSAT while decreasing both IV iron and ESA requirements compared with conventional phosphate binder therapy. As of this writing, ferric citrate is seeking FDA approval as an oral iron supplement in patients with nondialysis CKD. Ferric pyrophosphate citrate (FFP) is added to the hemodialysate and provides the 5 to 7 mg of iron estimated to be lost during each dialysis treatment due to blood lost in the dialysate circuit, oozing from needle sites, and phlebotomy. Phase 3 studies with FFP demonstrated stable serum ferritin and TSAT levels with decreased IV iron and ESA requirements. FFP is added to the bicarbonate delivery system or to individual bicarbonate concentrate containers.

RESISTANCE TO ERYTHROPOIESIS-STIMULATING AGENTS AND ADJUVANT THERAPY

ESA resistance has been defined as failure to achieve Hb greater than 11 g/dL despite an epoetin dose of greater than 500 units/kg per week or the equivalent of another ESA. The causes of ESA resistance are the same as the causes of anemia in CKD (see Box 56.1), with the obvious exception of EPO deficiency and with the addition of PRCA. After iron deficiency, the most common cause of ESA resistance in patients with CKD is inflammation/infection. This is often associated with high levels of acute phase reactants such as serum ferritin, C-reactive protein, and erythrocyte sedimentation rate, but the source of the inflammation/infection may not be readily apparent. It has been demonstrated that patients undergoing hemodialysis who use catheters for vascular access have lower mean Hb levels and higher mean ESA doses, which probably reflects the inflammatory state induced by the presence of the catheter and its biofilm. Occult periodontal disease has been increasingly recognized as a cause of ESA resistance.

Although the intention-to-treat analyses of the CHOIR and TREAT studies conclude that higher target Hb levels are associated with increased cardiovascular events, secondary analyses of these studies implicate the higher ESA doses received by the patients in the higher Hb arms. The conclusion is that ESA doses should not be uptitrated indefinitely in patients who fail to achieve target Hb levels, because the risk of ESA therapy far exceeds the benefit in patients who do not respond readily to ESAs. For patients who have not responded adequately over a 12-week escalation period, the FDA recommends that increasing the dose further is unlikely to improve response and may increase risks. For CKD patients not on dialysis, an epoetin dose ceiling of 300 units/kg per week (or the equivalent of another ESA) should be considered, whereas the dose ceiling for patients undergoing dialysis should be 450 units/kg per week (or equivalent dose of another ESA).

There is insufficient evidence to support the use of adjuvants to ESA therapy, such as L-carnitine and vitamin C, in the management of anemia in patients with CKD. Although androgens were widely used to increase Hb levels in patients undergoing dialysis in the pre-ESA era, their use is not recommended because of insufficient evidence to support their efficacy in patients receiving adequate doses of ESAs and because of the potential for long-term toxicity.

Despite the use of adequate doses of ESA and iron therapy, transfusions with RBCs are sometimes required in the setting of ESA resistance or acute blood loss. Transfusions are considered a last resort because of the potential development of sensitization affecting future transplantation candidacy and the small risk of blood-borne infections. There is no single Hb concentration that necessitates transfusion, and the decision of whether and when to transfuse should be made based on the patient's individual situation, including comorbid illnesses, symptoms, acuity of Hb decrease, and potential for future transplantation, as well as the Hb level.

OTHER HEMATOLOGIC MANIFESTATIONS OF KIDNEY DISEASE

ABNORMALITIES OF HEMOSTASIS

Patients with advanced CKD typically have normal results on coagulation studies and normal platelet counts, but they exhibit an increased bleeding tendency because of defects in platelet function. This is manifested by prolonged bleeding time, abnormal studies of platelet aggregation and adhesiveness, and decreased release of platelet factor 3. There may also be an abnormal interaction between platelets and vascular endothelium, mediated by decreased activity of von Willebrand factor (vWF) as well as increased release of endothelial nitric oxide and prostacyclin in uremia. Thrombocytopenia has been reported to rarely occur in patients undergoing hemodialysis with polysulfone membranes sterilized by electron beam technology. The clinical manifestations of these abnormalities include an increased tendency to and increased duration of bleeding after trauma and in the setting of serosal inflammation. This often manifests as epistaxis, bleeding with tooth brushing, and easy bruisability, but it can result in life-threatening gastrointestinal hemorrhage or hemorrhagic pericarditis. The bleeding diathesis is only partially corrected by dialysis, and larger molecules that accumulate in the setting of kidney failure, such as parathyroid hormone, have also been implicated. Anemia may also contribute to the bleeding diathesis of uremia, as higher RBC counts push platelets closer to the vessel wall, making them more effective. Treatment of anemia with RBC transfusion and/or ESAs to Hb greater than 10 g/dL improves the bleeding diathesis. Platelet function improves after the initiation of ESA therapy but before the Hb rises, suggesting that ESAs may improve platelet function directly.

The treatment of choice for bleeding episodes in uremic patients is to provide adequate dialysis with minimal or no anticoagulation and to initiate ESA therapy. If bleeding continues or if the patient is at risk for bleeding from an invasive procedure, then treatment with desmopressin (DDAVP) should be considered. DDAVP is a synthetic form of antidiuretic hormone that has minimal vasopressor activity and is used in the treatment of diabetes insipidus. The mechanism of its action in the setting of uremic bleeding is thought to be related to the release of vWF from endothelial cells and platelets. The dose of DDAVP is 0.3 μg/kg intravenously or 3 μg/kg intranasally, and it can be repeated 1 to 2 times before tachyphylaxis develops. The onset of action is immediate, and the duration of action is 4 to 8 hours. More than half of patients treated with DDAVP respond with an improvement in bleeding time, and the reason for the lack of response in other patients is unknown. Because of tachyphylaxis, it is recommended that DDAVP be administered only once, immediately before an invasive procedure (and not the day before). DDAVP tachyphylaxis appears to abate after 48 hours, and twice-weekly therapy has been shown effective in some patients with chronic bleeding.

Conjugated estrogens (Premarin) act to reduce bleeding for up to 14 days, but the onset of action takes 6 hours. The dose is 0.6 mg/kg daily for 5 consecutive days, and this regimen has been effective in controlling gastrointestinal bleeding associated with arteriovenous malformations in uremic patients. The mechanism of action may be related to inhibition of vascular nitric oxide production.

Like DDAVP, cryoprecipitate provides vWF, but it is less convenient to use and carries the risk of blood-borne infections. The onset of action of cryoprecipitate is 1 hour, and its effect peaks at 12 hours. The dose is 10 units and can be repeated as necessary. The response to cryoprecipitate is highly variable, and it should be reserved for life-threatening hemorrhage.

The platelet hemostatic defect in uremia does not appear to protect against vascular access thrombosis, which is a common problem in patients on hemodialysis. The use of antiplatelet agents such as aspirin and clopidogrel to preserve vascular access may be associated with an unacceptably high rate of bleeding and is not recommended. Use of these agents for conventional indications, such as coronary artery and cerebrovascular disease, is not contraindicated in patients with CKD, although the benefit must be weighed against risk. Similarly, heparin and warfarin are frequently needed for conventional indications in patients with CKD, but the use of these agents superimposes a risk of bleeding on the underlying abnormalities of platelet function. It is estimated that the incidence of venous thrombotic and thromboembolic disease (exclusive of vascular access thrombosis) in patients with CKD is twice that of the general population. This is attributed to the complications of nephrotic syndrome with increased plasma fibrinogen and decreased plasma antithrombin III levels, the presence of systemic lupus with circulating "anticoagulants" such as antiphospholipid antibodies, elevated levels of homocysteine, venous injury from previous catheter placement, and the continued presence of intravascular "foreign bodies" such as dialysis catheters and arteriovenous grafts.

Increased experience with enoxaparin in patients with CKD has simplified anticoagulation in certain settings, because monitoring of the partial thromboplastin time is not required. The dose of enoxaparin for CKD patients with GFR less than 30 mL/min per 1.73 m^2 including those on dialysis is 1 mg/kg subcutaneous daily for deep venous thrombosis (DVT) and acute coronary syndromes or 30 mg daily subcutaneous for DVT prophylaxis. When given in prophylactic doses, enoxaparin has not been shown to increase the risk of bleeding complications irrespective of the degree of impairment of kidney function. In patients with CKD at high risk for bleeding receiving therapeutic doses of enoxaparin, anti-Xa monitoring is recommended with a target peak level to 1 to 2 IU/mL if enoxaparin is administered q24 hours and 0.6–1 IU/mL if enoxaparin is administered q12 hours. The novel oral anticoagulants have not been well studied in patients with advanced CKD.

ABNORMALITIES OF LEUKOCYTES

Except for a transient decrease in circulating granulocytes during the first 15 to 30 minutes of hemodialysis with older, unmodified cellulosic membranes, the white blood cell count of patients with uremia tends to be normal. The decrease in circulating granulocytes during unmodified cellulosic membrane hemodialysis is caused by alternative complement pathway activation, which leads to microleukoagglutination and margination of granulocytes in the pulmonary circulation. This may be responsible for the transient hypoxia that is sometimes observed during hemodialysis, and it is completely reversed by the end of the dialysis treatment. The function of granulocytes, including chemotaxis, adherence, phagocytosis, and production of reactive oxygen species, is altered in uremia; these changes may also be exacerbated by exposure to unmodified cellulosic membranes. Impaired granulocyte function is associated with increased susceptibility to infection with encapsulated bacteria, such as *Staphylococcus*, contributing to the high incidence of these infections in patients undergoing dialysis.

Monocyte and lymphocyte function are also impaired in uremia, leading to a decrease in cellular-type immunity. This may manifest as an increased susceptibility to viral infections such as influenza, decreased response to vaccinations, and anergy to immunologic skin testing. The activity of autoimmune diseases such as systemic lupus erythematosus may be attenuated after uremia supervenes. An impairment of cytokine release decreases the febrile response to pathogens in uremic patients so that infections may go unnoticed and may become more serious before diagnosis. The clinical implication is that symptoms suggestive of infection must trigger an aggressive diagnostic and therapeutic response in this vulnerable population.

BIBLIOGRAPHY

Besarab A, Bolton WK, Browne JK, et al. The effects of normal as compared with low hematocrit values in patients with cardiac disease who are receiving hemodialysis and erythropoietin. *N Engl J Med.* 1998;339:584-590.

Besarab A, Goodkin DA, Nissenson AR. The normal hematocrit study—follow-up. *N Engl J Med.* 2008;358:433-444.

Bonomini M, Del Vecchio L, Sirolli V, et al. New treatment approaches for the anemia of CKD. *Am J Kidney Dis.* 2016;67:133-142.

Coyne DW, Kapoian T, Suki W, et al; DRIVE Study Group. Ferric gluconate is highly efficacious in anemic hemodialysis patients with high serum ferritin and low transferrin saturation: results of the Dialysis Patients' Response to IV Iron with Elevated Ferritin (DRIVE) Study. *J Am Soc Nephrol.* 2007;18:975–984.

Drueke TB, Locatelli F, Clyne N, et al. Normalization of hemoglobin level in patients with chronic kidney disease and anemia. *N Engl J Med.* 2006;355:2071-2984.

Fishbane S, Nissenson AR. Anemia management in chronic kidney disease. *Kidney Int.* 2010;78:S3-S9.

Gupta A, Lin V, Guss C, et al. Ferric pyrophosphate citrate administered via dialysate reduces erythropoiesis-stimulating agent use and maintains hemoglobin in hemodialysis patients. *Kidney Int.* 2015;88:1187-1194.

Kidney Disease Improving Global Outcomes (KDIGO) Anemia Work Group. KDIGO clinical practice guideline for anemia in CKD. *Kidney Int Suppl.* 2012;2:1-335.

Kliger A, Fishbane S, Finkelstein FO. Erythropoietic stimulating agents and quality of a patient's life: individualizing anemia treatment. *Clin J Am Soc Nephrol.* 2012;7:354-357.

Lewis EF, Pfeffer MA, Feng A, et al. Darbepoetin alfa impact on health status in diabetes patient with kidney disease: a randomized trial. *Clin J Am Soc Nephrol.* 2011;6:845-855.

Lewis JB, Sika M, Koury MJ, et al. Ferric citrate controls phosphorus and delivers iron in patients on dialysis. *J Am Soc Nephrol.* 2015;26:493-503.

Macdougall IC, Bircher AJ, Eckardt K-U, et al. Iron management in chronic kidney disease: conclusions for a "kidney disease: improving global outcomes" (KDIGO) controversies conference. *Kidney Int.* 2016;89:28-39.

Manns BJ, Tonelli M. The new FDA labeling for ESA—implications for patients and providers. *Clin J Am Soc Nephrol.* 2012;7:348-353.

National Kidney Foundation. K/DOQI clinical practice guidelines and clinical practice recommendations for anemia in chronic kidney disease. *Am J Kidney Dis.* 2006;47:S1-S146.

Pfeffer M, Burdmann E, Chen C, et al. A trial of darbepoetinalfa in type 2 diabetes and chronic kidney disease. *N Engl J Med.* 2009;361: 2019-2032.

Saltiel M. Dosing low molecular weight heparins in kidney disease. *J Pharm Pract.* 2010;23:205-209.

Singh AK, Szczech L, Tang KL, et al. Correction of anemia with epoetin alfa in chronic kidney disease. *N Engl J Med.* 2006;355:2085-2098.

Szczech LA, Burnhart HXS, Inrig JK, et al. Secondary analysis of the CHOIR trial: epoetin-alfa dose and achieved hemoglobin outcomes. *Kidney Int.* 2008;74:791-798.

Vaziri ND, Kalantar-Zadeh K, Wish JB. New options for iron supplementation in hemodialysis patients. *Am J Kidney Dis.* 2016;67:367-375.

Wish JB. The approval process for biosimilar erythropoiesis-stimulating agents. *Clin J Am Soc Nephrol.* 2014;9:1645-1651.

DIALYSIS AND TRANSPLANTATION

57 Hemodialysis and Hemofiltration

Madhukar Misra

Hemodialysis (HD) is an extracorporeal therapy that is prescribed to reduce the signs and symptoms of uremia and to partially replace a number of the key functions of the kidneys when kidney function is no longer sufficient to maintain an individual's well-being or life. Although HD is one of several therapies (peritoneal dialysis, hemofiltration [HF]/hemodiafiltration [HDF], transplantation) that can be used for the treatment of acute or chronic end-stage kidney disease (ESKD), this chapter focuses primarily on HD. Peritoneal dialysis and transplantation are covered in detail elsewhere in the Primer.

PRINCIPAL FUNCTIONS OF HEMODIALYSIS

HD for the treatment of ESKD is effective in (1) reducing the concentration of uremic toxins, particularly small and medium-sized molecules, primarily by diffusion; (2) removing excess fluid volume by convection; and (3) correcting some of the metabolic abnormalities, such as acidosis and hyperkalemia, by the use of dialysate solutions with variable solute concentrations. The two major components of the HD procedure that will be discussed are the dialyzer and the dialysate.

DIALYZER

STRUCTURE

The most commonly used device for the performance of HD is the hollow fiber dialyzer, composed of several thousand hollow fibers made of thin, semipermeable membranes. These fibers are encased in a plastic tubing device that allows blood to be pumped from the patient through the hollow fibers while an aqueous solution, the dialysate, is pumped outside the fibers, typically in the opposite direction of the blood flow (countercurrent), to maximize the diffusion gradients across the membranes and along the length of the dialyzer.

There are generally two types of dialysis membranes (Fig. 57.1). The first are called "low-flux" membranes and are made up of fibers with small pore sizes, which allow the diffusion of small solutes such as urea and water but not the passage of larger molecules such as β2-microglobulin. "High-flux" membranes, the second type, have larger pore sizes that allow the passage of larger molecules such as β2-microglobulin. Because of these larger pores, the rate of water transfer (ultrafiltration coefficient) is much higher than that for low-flux membranes.

The manufacturing process of these membranes is such that, regardless of whether it is a low-flux or a high-flux membrane, the pore sizes are not uniform, and there is a distribution of pore sizes that allows the diffusion or removal of differently sized molecules at different rates (Fig. 57.2). It is important to note that the distribution of pore sizes for high-flux membranes is such that it does not allow for the passage of albumin.

PRINCIPAL FUNCTIONS OF THE DIALYZER

Diffusion

Diffusion describes the movement of solutes from a milieu with high concentrations across a semipermeable membrane into a milieu where it is in lower concentration. The rate and amount of solute that diffuses across the membrane in either direction depend on the difference in concentration between the blood and dialysate compartments; the molecular size of the solute; the characteristics of the membrane including its surface area, thickness, and porosity; and the conditions of flow (e.g., turbulent or smooth). These membrane characteristics are generally labeled *mass transfer characteristic* or *coefficient of diffusion* and are specific for the membrane used and the solute under consideration.

Using urea as an example of a small molecular solute, HD allows the movement of urea from the blood compartment, where it is in high concentration, to the dialysate compartment across the hollow fiber membranes. Thus, as blood is pumped and traverses through the dialyzer inside hollow fibers, the urea concentration of the blood is reduced; concurrently, the urea concentration of the dialysate increases as it flows outside the hollow fibers in the opposite direction. If the blood and dialysate were to flow in the same direction, then the urea concentration gradient between the blood and dialysate compartments would be considerably reduced at the exit site of the dialyzer, whereas a countercurrent flow ensures a maximum difference in concentration along the entire dialyzer length and therefore higher flux of solute from the blood compartment into the dialysate compartment.

The principles of diffusion apply not only to urea and other solutes that have a higher concentration in the blood than dialysate, but also to the diffusion of substances that have a higher concentration in the dialysate than blood. An example of the latter is the diffusion of bicarbonate from the dialysate into the blood compartment. The rate of diffusion (R) of a small blood solute like urea across the dialyzer membrane is proportional to the blood solute concentration (C) and is governed by laws of first-order kinetics. Based on this concept, R is proportional to C, or R = KC and therefore K = R/C, where K is a constant referred to as *clearance*. K of any solute across the dialyzer membrane is an

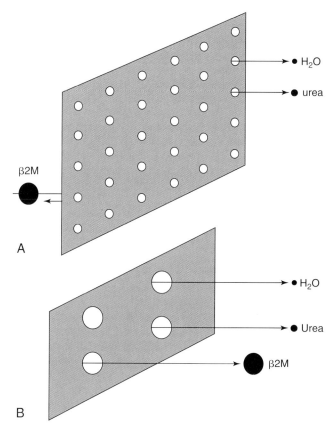

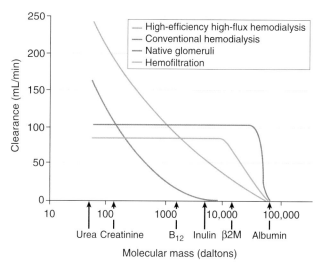

Fig. 57.1 Schematic diagrams of low-flux and high-flux membranes. (A) Low-flux membranes have small pores that are highly permeable to small solutes such as water and urea (60 Da) but restrict the transport of middle molecules such as β2-microglobulin (β2M). Because of their small pores, they also tend to have low ultrafiltration coefficients, although the ultrafiltration coefficient can be increased by increasing the surface area of the membrane. A low-flux membrane can be either high efficiency or low efficiency for urea transport, depending on its surface area and, to a lesser extent, its thickness. (B) High-flux membranes have large pores that facilitate the transport of middle molecules such as β2M in addition to small molecules. Their ultrafiltration coefficients are high. A high-flux membrane can be either high efficiency or low efficiency, depending on its surface area and, to a lesser extent, its thickness. (Reproduced with permission from Cheung A. Hemodialysis and hemofiltration. In: Greenberg A, ed. *Primer on Kidney Diseases*. 3rd ed. Philadelphia: National Kidney Foundation/Saunders; 2001:chap 47.)

Fig. 57.2 Solute clearance profile of various membranes. The curves are constructed based partially on data and partially on theoretical projection. The actual values may vary depending on the surface area of the membrane and operating conditions (e.g., blood flow rate). The curve for native glomeruli represents the summation of all the glomeruli in two normal kidneys. "Glomeruli" instead of "kidneys" are used because tubular reabsorption substantially lowers the kidney clearance of certain solutes, such as urea and glucose. Clearance of solutes by diffusion (via either conventional or high-efficiency/high-flux dialysis) deteriorates rapidly with increases in the molecular mass of the solute. In contrast, clearance by convection (hemofiltration or glomeruli) remains constant over a wide range of molecular mass. B_{12}, Vitamin B_{12}; *β2M*, β2-microglobulin. (Reproduced with permission from Cheung A. Hemodialysis and hemofiltration. In: Greenberg A, ed. *Primer on Kidney Diseases*. 4th ed. Philadelphia: National Kidney Foundation/Saunders; 2005:chap 90.)

Convection

The simple equation for solute clearance mentioned above does not take into account convective clearance of solutes. Convection refers to the mass transport of solutes along with the fluid it is dissolved in (plasma water) and is driven by the higher hydrostatic pressures in the blood compartment generated by the blood pump. The amount of solute removed by convection is not dependent on the concentration gradient of the solute, but rather on the difference in hydrostatic pressure between the blood and dialysate compartment and a specific membrane characteristic, termed the "sieving coefficient." The sieving coefficient (S) represents the ratio of the concentration of the solute in the ultrafiltrate and the concentration in plasma water, with values ranging from 0 (membrane impermeable to solute) to 1 (membrane freely permeable to the solute).

The relative contribution of convective transport to overall clearance depends on the pore size of the membrane as well as the size and charge of the solute. In general, the relative contribution of convective transport to the overall clearance for small molecules, such as urea, is minor, but it is more substantial for larger molecules (e.g., β2-microglobulin) because of the low diffusive clearance.

Therefore a more complete representation of solute clearance incorporating both diffusion and convection is:

$$K = \frac{Q_{Bi} \times C_A - Q_{Bo} \times C_V}{C_A} \approx \frac{Q_{Bo}(C_A - C_V)}{C_A} + Q_{uf}$$

expression of the effectiveness of dialysis. It remains constant during intermittent treatments as both blood concentrations of small solutes (C) and solute removal rates (R) decrease simultaneously. A useful way to express K is:

$$K = \frac{Q_B(C_A - C_V)}{C_A}$$

K of a solute from the blood compartment (in mL/min) is expressed as the difference in the amount of a solute at the inlet ($Q_B \times C_A$, where Q_B is the blood flow rate in mL/min and C_A is the concentration in mg/mL at the inlet or "arterial" side of the dialyzer) and the amount of solute at the outlet ($Q_B \times C_V$, where C_V is the concentration at the outlet or "venous" side of the dialyzer), divided by the concentration at the inlet (C_A).

where Q_{uf} is the difference between Q_{Bi} (inlet blood flow) and Q_{Bo} (outlet blood flow) and is termed the ultrafiltration rate (UFR) in mL/min.

Because any solute removed from the blood compartment appears in the dialysate, another expression of solute clearance (K) that includes both convective and diffusive removal is based on the measurement of the concentration of that solute at the outlet of the dialysate; this is true for all solutes that are not already present in dialysate and can be represented as:

$$K = \frac{Q_{DO} \times C_{DO}}{C_A}$$

where Q_{DO} is the dialysate flow rate at the outlet (mL/min), C_{DO} is the concentration of the solute in the dialysate (mg/mL) at the outlet, and C_A is the concentration (mg/mL) in the blood at the inlet. Because this represents the net loss of solute (both diffusive and convective) and does not depend on the partitioning of the solute between plasma water and red blood cells or on calculation of the sieving coefficient of the membrane, it is a more accurate measurement of solute clearance.

Hemofiltration and Hemodiafiltration

A technique that allows for the removal of solutes, as well as plasma water, primarily or solely by convection (i.e., without diffusion) is called *HF*. In this technique, there is no dialysate flow, and the ultrafiltrate has the same composition as plasma water. Conceptually, this technique mirrors the clearance mechanism that occurs across the native glomerulus (Fig. 57.3). However, in the absence of fluid reabsorption mediated by the renal tubules in the native kidney, the HF technique relies on infusion of large amounts of fluids to replace the large convective fluid losses. In convective removal techniques, the removal of small molecules is limited by their sieving coefficient "S" as well as the total volume of the ultrafiltrate. In contrast, diffusive removal is dependent on the concentration gradient and, therefore, is more efficient for the removal of small solutes. HF is particularly effective for removal of larger molecules that depend on convective removal.

HDF incorporates both diffusive and convective removal. Simply put, including the dialysate component in the HF circuit adds a diffusive component to the convective removal achieved by pure HF. A typical HDF procedure uses high-flux dialyzers, blood and dialysate flow rates of 300 and 500 mL/min, respectively, and a predefined amount of substitution fluid to achieve a minimum convection volume of 20% of total processed blood volume. Because of the requirement of large volumes of sterile substitution solutions to replace the ultrafiltrate, these techniques are not widely used for the treatment of chronic dialysis patients in the United States.

Net Clearance

Although the previous equations predict that the clearance of a substance will increase as blood flow (Q_B) and/or dialysate flow (Q_D) increase, in reality the clearance of solutes increases linearly with increases in blood and/or dialysate flow only up to a point before leveling off (Fig. 57.4). This plateau is reached at different clearance values depending on the size of the solute and the specific membrane characteristics

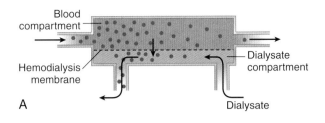

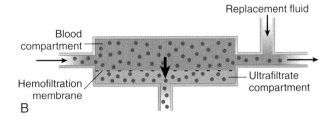

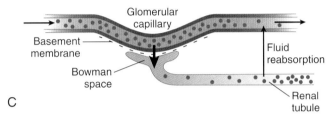

Fig. 57.3 Schematic representation of solute and fluid transport across the semipermeable artificial membranes and glomerular basement membrane. (A) Hemodialyzer. The plasma concentration of solutes *(solid circles)* in the blood inlet is high. Because of diffusive loss across the semipermeable hemodialysis membrane *(dotted line)*, the plasma concentration in the blood outlet is much lower. The thin arrow across the dialysis membrane represents a small amount of fluid loss (which is not necessary for solute removal). A high dialysate flow rate is used to maintain the concentration gradient across the dialysis membrane for solute removal. (B) Hemofilter. Plasma concentrations of solutes in the blood compartment remain unchanged as blood travels the length of the fiber and are similar to their concentrations in the ultrafiltrate. The hemofiltration membrane *(broken line)* has relatively large pores, which allow the necessary removal of a large volume of fluid *(heavy arrow)*. Replacement fluid is infused into the blood outlet to lower the plasma concentration of solutes and compensate for the fluid loss. (C) Glomerulus. Analogous to hemofiltration, plasma concentration of solutes remains unchanged throughout the length of the glomerular capillary and is similar to that in Bowman space. Fluid removal across the glomerular basement membrane *(broken curve)* is large *(heavy arrow)*. Reabsorption of fluid from the renal tubules lowers the plasma concentration of the solutes. (Reproduced with permission from Cheung A. Hemodialysis and hemofiltration. In: Greenberg A, ed. *Primer on Kidney Diseases.* 4th ed. Philadelphia, National Kidney Foundation, Saunders; 2005:chap 90.)

(porosity, thickness, surface charge, the chemical composition of the membrane, etc.). These summative membrane characteristics are called the mass transfer coefficient (Ko). The mass transfer coefficient is specific for the membrane used and the solute being considered; for dialyzers, this is usually represented as KoA, where A is the effective surface area of the specific dialyzer. Manufacturers generally provide the KoA of the different solutes for the specific dialyzer, and the clearance of specific solutes at different blood and dialysate concentrations can be calculated from such values. However, it is important to keep in mind that these KoA values are

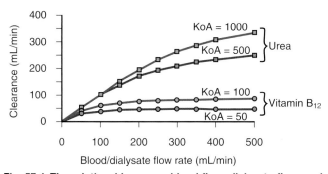

Fig. 57.4 The relationship among blood flow, dialysate flow, and membrane characteristics. The mass transfer coefficient is usually represented as KoA, where A is the effective surface area of the specific dialyzer.

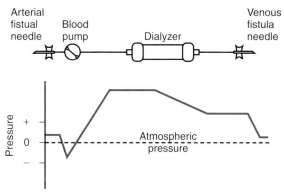

Fig. 57.5 The dialysis circuit, with positive and negative pressures at different points in the circuit.

determined by manufacturers in aqueous solutions, and the actual clearance obtained in vivo is typically lower than that supplied by the manufacturer.

Another important feature in the relationship between higher clearance and higher blood flow rate is the fact that, in the clinical setting, blood flow rate measured by the blood pump may not accurately represent the actual blood flow rate flowing through the hollow fibers of the dialyzer. For example, in cases where the size of the needle used in the inlet bloodline (arterial fistula needle) is too narrow or the HD vascular access is malfunctioning because of an inlet stenosis, it is possible that the volume of blood that is delivered by each rotation of the blood pump may be less than predicted, and therefore the blood flow rate noted on the dialysis machine, which is calculated from the number of rotations of the blood pump as well as the diameter of the intrapump segment of the dialysis tubing, may overestimate both the blood flow rate and the resultant solute clearance. Thus the use of higher blood flow rates can only improve clearance up to a certain point. In addition, at increasing blood flow rates, the prepump pressure (Fig. 57.5) may become excessively negative (greater than −250 mm Hg). This, in turn, leads to a higher risk of red blood cell lysis, presumably from the sudden change between the negative pressures in the blood tubing before the blood pump and the rapid rise in hydrostatic pressures after the pump.

Finally, there are practical limits to increasing the dialysate flow rate; not only is there cost associated with preparing water for dialysate preparation, but, because of the limitation of

the mass transfer coefficient for specific solutes and specific dialysis membranes, the optimal combination of dialysate flow is approximately 1.5 to 2.0 times the true blood flow rate inside the hollow fibers. Thus if the maximum blood flow rate (above which the negative arterial pressure prepump exceeds −250 mm Hg) is 350 mL/min, then the optimal dialysate flow rate is around 600 to 700 mL/min.

Assessing the Dialysis Dose

The total amount of solute removed during a dialysis procedure can be calculated from Kt (where K, the clearance in mL/min, is multiplied by the time [t] of the procedure in minutes); this assumes that the clearance (K) remains constant throughout the time of the procedure. The other variable that determines the net impact of solute removal from the patient by HD is the volume of distribution of the solute. Thus the dose of dialysis is usually defined as Kt/V, where V is the volume of distribution of that particular solute. Urea has been the index molecule used to define the dose of dialysis as it is easily measured, is small and therefore diffuses readily across a dialysis membrane, and, importantly, its volume of distribution (total body water) can be calculated from the weight of the patient. Thus the dose of dialysis traditionally is defined in terms of urea, rather than other solutes, and the K in the earlier equation typically refers to urea clearance.

A simpler but conventional measure of dialysis dose is the urea reduction ratio (URR). The URR is also based on urea but avoids the need to define or measure clearance or determine the volume of distribution. The URR usually is expressed as percent reduction, defined as:

$$URR = \frac{(C_{pre} - C_{post})}{C_{pre}} \times 100$$

where C_{post} is the urea concentration at the completion of dialysis, and C_{pre} is the urea concentration before the start of dialysis. The URR is traditionally expressed as a percentage.

Solute Clearance Other Than Urea

Although solute clearance by diffusion is dependent on the size of the solute molecule, other considerations, such as the electrical charge of the molecule and its *effective size*, also affect the net transfer of uremic solutes across the membrane. One example is the clearance of phosphate. Phosphate (PO_4) is a uremic toxin that accumulates as kidney failure progresses. Although phosphate has a low molecular weight and, based on its molecular size, would be expected to be easily cleared by high-flux dialysis membranes, in reality, phosphate is cleared rather poorly during dialysis because of its highly negative charge and the large number of water molecules that circulate with it; in addition, because of the large intracellular reservoirs of phosphate and slow transfer from the intracellular to the plasma compartment, net phosphate clearance by dialysis is poor. This results in a time-dependent slow clearance during conventional dialysis, with moderate clearance and declining removal during the first 2 hours of standard HD, and negligible removal afterward. However, as discussed later, the removal of phosphates is higher during longer dialysis treatments, such as occurs with nocturnal dialysis (~8 hours), since the longer sessions allow the time-dependent transfer of phosphate from the intracellular to the plasma compartment; accordingly, patients treated with nocturnal dialysis often require fewer or no phosphate binders.

Extracellular Volume Control (Ultrafiltration)

Another important function of HD is the removal of excess fluid that accumulates in the absence of effective kidney function. The major driving force that determines the rate of ultrafiltration or convective flow is the difference in hydrostatic pressure between the blood compartment and the dialysate compartments across the dialysis membrane; this is called the transmembrane pressure (TMP). Modern dialysis equipment adjusts these hydrostatic pressure gradients by varying the negative ("suction") pressure in the dialysate compartment rather than increasing the pressure in the blood compartment; this avoids the potential for increased lysis of red blood cells. Although the traditional low-flux dialysis membrane exhibited a linear relationship between the TMP and the amount of fluid removed, the commonly used high-flux membranes have much larger pore sizes allowing more rapid UFRs and more rapid transfer of plasma water. However, because this rapid transfer of plasma water occurs at the inlet of the dialyzer, the concentration of protein (oncotic pressure) rapidly rises in the blood compartment; because these proteins are also negatively charged, there is a corresponding development of a "concentration polarization" due to a rapid increase in negatively charged plasma protein concentration at the membrane surface (inside the blood compartment). This has the effect of disproportionately increasing the oncotic pressure at the interface between the blood compartment and the surface of the membrane. The high oncotic pressure at the surface of these high-flux membranes inhibits further ultrafiltration to the extent that, toward the blood outlet of high-flux dialysis membranes, "reverse filtration" may occur with dialysate solutions moving across the membrane into the blood compartment. This reverse filtration phenomenon is more likely to occur in membranes with large pore sizes (high-flux membranes) that allow more rapid ultrafiltration than in low-flux membranes, and it also results in a nonlinear relationship between the rate of ultrafiltration and TMP in dialysis with a high-flux membrane as shown in Fig. 57.6.

Because of this nonlinear relationship, the UFR is currently determined by accurately measuring the dialysate inflow and outflow rates in a closed-loop circuit rather than manually adjusting the TMP. An accurate fluid pump is used to remove fluid at the desired UFR; as fluid is removed from this closed-loop circuit, a negative pressure is generated in the dialysate loop that allows the ultrafiltration of exactly the same amount of fluid from the blood compartment. In this way, the rate of ultrafiltration is no longer dependent on the high-flux ultrafiltration characteristics of the membrane but rather the UFR set by the operator (Fig. 57.7).

DIALYSATE

In addition to removal of uremic solutes by diffusion and correction of extracellular volume by ultrafiltration, a third function of HD is to correct a number of metabolic abnormalities that result from the absence of kidney function. Although there are numerous abnormalities in the concentration of various metabolites that result from kidney failure, acid-base (bicarbonate) balance and potassium concentration are examples of the use of various dialysate solutions to correct such abnormalities.

BICARBONATE

In the absence of kidney function, the acidic moieties produced during metabolism accumulate in the blood and, after exhausting other available buffers, are neutralized by ambient serum bicarbonate molecules. This results in a metabolic acidosis with serum bicarbonate levels often ranging from 16 to 18 mEq/L in patients with chronic kidney disease (CKD) stage 5 before initiation of dialysis.

One of the functions of dialysis is to compensate for metabolic acidosis by replenishing blood bicarbonate. Most often, this is accomplished using formulations of dialysate solutions with bicarbonate concentrations generally above 30 mEq/L. This "higher than normal" bicarbonate concentration is needed to provide a concentration gradient from the dialysate to the blood compartment to replenish consumed bicarbonate and allow the patient to have an interdialysis bicarbonate "reserve." Thus the patient on dialysis cycles from a state of mild metabolic acidosis with respiratory

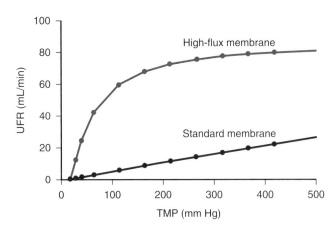

Fig. 57.6 The relationship between ultrafiltration rate (UFR) and transmembrane pressure (TMP) for different types of dialysis membranes.

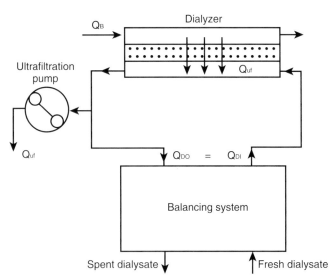

Fig. 57.7 Schematic diagram of the "closed-loop" ultrafiltration control used with high-flux membranes.

compensation at the beginning of dialysis to a state of mild metabolic alkalosis (and compensatory hypoventilation) at the end of dialysis.

Sodium bicarbonate is used as the source of bicarbonate in the dialysate. However, this product cannot simply be added as a component of dialysate as the presence of other electrolytes needed in the dialysate (specifically calcium and magnesium) would result in their precipitation as crystals, thereby reducing the concentration of all three components. Current dialysate delivery technology requires the preparation of two separate dialysate streams, one called "acid concentrate," which combines all the ingredients of dialysate except sodium bicarbonate, and a second stream that contains sodium bicarbonate and sodium chloride. These two concentrates are then separately diluted with treated water and combined just before reaching the dialysate inlet, resulting in a modestly alkaline (pH = 7.8) dialysate solution.

One important detail in the choice of dialysate bicarbonate levels is the presence of acetate in the formulation of the "acid concentrate" mentioned earlier. Depending on the manufacturer and whether the concentrate is liquid or powder, most "acid concentrates" contain organic acid (glacial acetic acid or citric acid) to maintain an acidic milieu and thus prevent precipitation of calcium and magnesium salts. The reaction between sodium bicarbonate and acetic acid or citric acid (in the acid concentrate) generates an equimolar amount of sodium acetate or sodium citrate ions that are metabolized to produce sodium bicarbonate in the body. The equimolar conversion does not change the total buffer base available to the patient.

The disodium acetate present in the acid concentrate (Granuflo) contains acetic acid and sodium acetate. The acetic acid reacts with sodium bicarbonate to generate 4 mmol of sodium acetate, while the sodium acetate component of sodium diacetate provides an additional 4 mmol of sodium bicarbonate in the body. If the dialysate sodium bicarbonate is 35 mEq/L to begin with based upon the prescribed sodium bicarbonate stream, the final buffer base available to the patient may reach 43 mEq/L ($35 + 4 + 4 = 43$), representing a significant contribution of alkali (8 mEq/L) from the acid concentrate. There are ongoing studies about the optimal concentration of total buffer, but most observational data suggest that a total buffer of around 35 to 37 mEq/L is optimal; ideally, such a concentration should be adjusted for each patient, depending on his or her dietary intake, protein catabolic rate, and the resulting predialysis and postdialysis bicarbonate level.

POTASSIUM

Similar therapeutic considerations apply to the prescription of dialysate potassium levels. In the absence of kidney function, potassium (and other electrolytes such as magnesium) accumulates in the blood; accordingly, an important function of dialysis is to reduce the potassium concentration during dialysis episodes to a level that prevents significant predialysis hyperkalemia during the interdialytic period while avoiding significant hypokalemia after dialysis.

As potassium removal depends on the difference in potassium concentration between the blood and the dialysate, the simplest way by which potassium removal can be maximized is to use a dialysate potassium concentration of 0 mEq/L. However, "0 Potassium" dialysate results in an early and very rapid decline in serum potassium concentrations, exceeding

the rate at which serum potassium can be replenished from intracellular stores and potentially predisposing to cardiac arrhythmias or cardiac arrest. In the opinion of the author, the optimal dialysate potassium for almost all patients is 2 or 3 mEq/L, and, for patients with a high predialysis potassium level, the safest option likely is to use a dialysate potassium of 2 or 3 mEq/L while extending the dialysis duration to remove more potassium but at a slower rate. The use of a low potassium diet and potentially enteric potassium binders are important adjuvants.

PREPARING PATIENTS FOR MAINTENANCE HEMODIALYSIS

PATIENT EDUCATION AND CHOICE OF THERAPY

It is important to emphasize that the selection of HD therapy should be a joint decision by the patient and the physician that follows a full discussion about other available kidney replacement therapy options (peritoneal dialysis, home HD, deceased- or living-donor transplantation), as well as the option of conservative management. Such a discussion provides the nephrology team with an opportunity to advise the patient about the medical aspects and the advantages and disadvantages of each modality, accounting for individual patient factors, including patient age, underlying kidney diagnosis and other medical conditions, and family and social conditions. Active management of patient's symptoms without dialytic support (comprehensive conservative care) is an option that may be recommended to appropriate patients, particularly the elderly and those with extensive comorbidity. Although the final decision should always take into account the patient's preferences, the nephrologist has the responsibility not only to discuss fully the therapeutic options available but also to offer advice and recommendations about the available choices.

If the patient is competent to make decisions, and the patient and physician are in agreement, there is little that should stand in the way of carrying out their choice, be it for or against the initiation of dialysis. Anecdotally, some patients refuse to consider dialysis treatment while in the office, but they seldom refuse it when confronting acute pulmonary edema or pericarditis; thus the relationship between the CKD patient and the nephrology team ideally should be longstanding to allow full discussion of the therapeutic options, the necessary time for the psychological acceptance of the therapy before dialysis is urgently needed, and sufficient time for the creation of a functional native arteriovenous (AV) fistula for repetitive blood access or placement of a peritoneal dialysis catheter.

30-20-10 Program for Dialysis Preparation

In the United States, more than 40% of patients who initiate dialysis do so without previous nephrology care, even though most patients have had some interaction with the healthcare system before kidney failure. Even for patients who are followed by nephrologists, there may be reluctance by the patient and even by the nephrologist to fully discuss the therapeutic options for treating kidney failure. Unless such discussion occurs, the patient will typically end up on HD ill prepared, resentful, and depressed.

A number of publications have highlighted the advantages of using the 30-20-10 "rule-of-thumb" for an orderly process of patient referral to a nephrologist and initiation of kidney replacement therapy. According to this rubric, at a glomerular filtration rate (GFR) of 30 mL/min, patients should be referred for active follow-up with a nephrologist, preferably jointly with the referring physician. When the patient's GFR is around 20 mL/min, an AV fistula should be placed in patients who have not already elected an alternative kidney replacement modality. Finally, at a GFR of around 10 mL/min, an informed choice of kidney replacement modality (including conservative care) should be in place for initiation when medically indicated.

Psychological Factors in Dialysis Initiations

Patients who are informed about the probable need to initiate dialysis often undergo the same reactions as those patients being informed about any life-threatening illness; most proceed through the stages of grief that have been described by Kübler-Ross—denial, anger, bargaining, depression, and finally acceptance of this lifelong chronic hardship.

It is essential to allay the anxiety and fear common in patients nearing kidney failure. Whenever possible, family members should be included in the decision-making process, and all members of the nephrology team, including the nephrologist, nurses, social workers, transplant coordinators, and dietitians, should participate in this process. If possible, patients and interested family members should visit the dialysis unit well before requiring treatment, as this simple exercise may help alleviate many of their fears and misconceptions. Because most patients also anticipate much pain during dialysis, it should be stressed that almost no pain is involved. This can be accomplished by introducing prospective patients to those already on dialysis. The need for adherence with diet, fluid intake, medications, and dialysis schedules should be stressed, and the patient should be empowered to participate in his or her own care, helping to ensure compliance and improve satisfaction. For patients presenting with an acute need to start dialysis, a trial can be presented, stressing that the decision to perform is not binding and can be reconsidered if individual goals are not met. This is especially relevant in older and frailer patients with multiple comorbidities.

Choice of Treatment Modalities

The cause of kidney failure and comorbid conditions are elements that should be integrated into the selection of treatment options; for example, patients with brittle diabetes or previous abdominal surgery may benefit from thrice weekly in-center HD, whereas those with cirrhosis or severe cardiomyopathy may be treated more successfully with peritoneal dialysis or daily HD regimens. When different dialysis modalities are equally possible from a medical standpoint, practical issues such as the presence of a supportive family environment, work habits, and economic factors (e.g., availability of transportation, housing issues, and distance from dialysis centers) often favor one modality over another.

VASCULAR ACCESS

Preparation and Timing of Vascular Access

Whichever option the patient chooses (except in cases of well-matched, living-related transplantation that can be preplanned), it is recommended that all patients approaching the need for HD initiation have an AV fistula created at a GFR around 20 mL/min.

Native AV fistulas have a significantly lower incidence of infection, and their half-life, if they are well developed before their use, is much longer than that of synthetic grafts. In some medical centers, access-related problems account for 30% to 40% of all nephrology admissions, representing a medical, emotional, and economic burden to the patient; thus the presence of either rapidly progressing or already advanced kidney disease should prompt AV fistula creation well before the expected date of dialysis initiation. Central vein catheters, even if placed for a short time, are associated with a high risk of infection and may adversely affect the longevity of any subsequent AV fistula or graft.

The following recommendations are useful guidelines:

1. A vascular access surgeon should evaluate patients with progressive GFR loss at the earliest opportunity to determine the best sites for vascular access (this should occur no later than at a GFR of around 20 mL/min, according to the 30-20-10 rubric). Early placement of AV fistulas not only allows for the development of the fistula (primary patency typically takes at least 6 to 8 weeks and perhaps longer) but also allows for needed interventions, including placement of a second fistula if the initial fistula does not mature. Studies show that in approximately 50% of cases of AV fistula creation, a second procedure is required before the fistula is usable for HD. This is often due to central venous stenoses, particularly in patients who previously had central venous catheters.
2. Although access should be planned first in the nondominant arm, sites also should be preserved in the other arm. The use of the nondominant arm is preferred, particularly for self-dialysis, as it facilitates self-cannulation. Radial arteries and cephalic veins should be preserved except in life-threatening situations. In particular, use of radial arteries for nonessential "arterial lines" as well as the use of peripherally inserted central catheter (PICC) lines should be discouraged. Whenever possible, phlebotomy should be limited to veins over the dorsum of the hand and the ulnar side of the forearm. If absolutely necessary, median antecubital veins may be punctured with small butterfly needles. Intravenous lines should spare the cephalic vein. If long-term outpatient infusions are required, consider using tunneled internal jugular catheters rather than PICC lines.
3. In hospitalized patients, sites being preserved should be marked with a black felt-tipped pen as a reminder to all. A notice on the wall above the patient's bed is also helpful.
4. Patients should be educated to preserve their own vasculature.

TYPES OF ARTERIOVENOUS FISTULAS

Radiocephalic Arteriovenous Fistulas

A standard vascular access now preferred by most access surgeons is a distal cephalic vein to radial artery end-to-side anastomosis near the wrist. Again, the preservation of both cephalic veins from the time of kidney disease diagnosis is critical, because the radiocephalic fistula is the optimal first option. This preserves upper-arm veins for later use (Fig. 57.8).

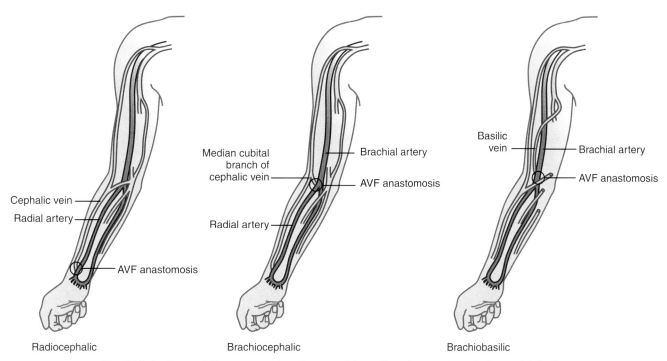

Fig. 57.8 Anatomy of the upper-extremity vasculature. Vessels named are instrumental for the creation of hemodialysis fistula and grafts for vascular access. *AVF*, Arteriovenous fistula. (Adapted with permission from Allon M, Robbin ML. Increasing arteriovenous fistulas in hemodialysis patients: problems and solutions. *Kidney Int.* 2002;62:1109–1124.)

Brachiocephalic and Brachiobasilic Fistulas

The next best approach is a more proximal fistula also using the patient's own vasculature, as described in Fig. 57.8. Upper-arm fistulas tend to have higher flow and therefore are more vulnerable to aneurysmal dilation; in addition, patients may have more difficulty self-cannulating an upper-arm access. Nevertheless, in patients without adequate forearm cephalic veins, brachiocephalic or brachiobasilic AV fistulas should still be placed approximately 6 months in advance of the time when dialysis is anticipated.

Access in Challenging Patients

Grafts. In patients who cannot receive either a forearm or an upper-arm fistula using their own vasculature, a synthetic graft may be placed in the forearm. Either a distal radial artery to basilic vein (straight) graft or a loop from the brachial artery to the basilic vein could be considered. Synthetic grafts are more prone to infection and clotting than fistulas with endogenous vessels. Therefore synthetic grafts should not be placed in anticipation of future dialysis need until generally 1 to 2 months before initiation of dialysis, with the understanding that optimal timing can be a challenge.

Catheters. Because kidney disease is often "silent," it is inevitable that some patients will present with clear indications for initiation of dialysis without a permanent access. In such cases, if HD is elected, dialysis initiation requires the placement of a catheter, preferably in the internal jugular vein. Because of the much higher propensity for infections, catheter malfunction, inadequate blood flow, and progressive vein stenosis along the path of the catheter, it is critical that a permanent access plan be developed and implemented as soon as it is determined that the patient has chronic (and not acute) kidney failure. Ideally, the placement of permanent access, preferably an AV fistula, should take place during the hospital admission for dialysis initiation.

INITIATION AND PRESCRIPTION OF HEMODIALYSIS

Assuming that HD is the modality of choice, what is the optimal dialysis prescription? This section briefly discusses different dialysis techniques, including short daily HD and nocturnal HD, with a focus on conventional, thrice weekly, in-center dialysis as this remains the most common HD strategy. The dialysis dose, the time needed to optimize kidney replacement therapy, and strategies for accomplishing this are reviewed. To place common HD strategies into context, current in-center HD regimens average approximately 3.5 hours per procedure and tend to provide less than 10 mL/min of creatinine clearance for the patient on an intermittent basis. Considering that this level is below the level at which HD is initiated, it is clear that the delivery of dialysis is inadequate and likely allows for shortened survival. It is therefore not surprising that the annual mortality rate of patients on such therapy approaches 15% to 20% and that the 5-year survival of ESKD patients is less than many forms of cancer. Several factors should be considered in the prescription of dialysis to optimize outcomes.

DIALYSIS TIME

It is possible to estimate the minimum dialysis time that a patient may need to achieve a specific target Kt/V or URR, taking into consideration the patient's residual kidney function (RKF). The first step is to calculate the volume of urea distribution, which is total body water. For the hypothetical 70-kg person, this is assumed to be 60% of body weight for men (42 L), whereas in women it is assumed to be 55% of body weight (38.5 L). The next step is to determine the clearance of the dialyzer at specific blood and dialysate flow rates. An in vitro evaluation of urea clearance is usually included in the package insert of the dialyzer, accounting for the surface area of the dialyzer, the dialysate flow rate, and other dialyzer factors. However, since this is an in vitro assessment based on an aqueous solution (rather than blood), it is reasonable to assume that the in vivo urea clearance is approximately 80% of the reported in vitro clearance. Accordingly, assuming the in vitro urea clearance at a "blood flow" of 300 mL/min and dialysate flow of 500 mL/min is 250 mL/min, then the presumed in vivo urea clearance is $250 \times 0.8 = 200$ mL/min.

If the goal of therapy is to achieve a minimum Kt/V of 1.2 as recommended by Kidney Disease Outcomes Quality Initiative (KDOQI) guidelines, then the minimum time needed for this hypothetical 70-kg man to achieve a Kt/V of 1.2 can be derived as below:

$$Kt/V = 1.2$$

$$t = 1.2 \times V/K = 1.2 \times (42,000 \text{ mL})/(200 \text{ mL/min}) = 252 \text{ min}$$

Although larger surface-area dialyzer and higher blood flow rates are means of reducing the dialysis duration, based on these data as well as observational data suggesting higher risk with high UFR, it is strongly recommended that, after the first several sessions, the maintenance dialysis time should be prescribed at no less than 4 hours thrice weekly.

Recently, retrospective analyses of large data sets from the United States and other countries have highlighted the impressive survival benefit of patients dialyzed for 4 or more hours. Possible explanations include theoretic benefits of an increase in the dose of dialysis as well as a decrease in the UFR to below 10 mL/kg per hour and resultant improved cardiovascular stability. A final important reason for starting patients at 4 hours is psychological; after a patient is initiated on dialysis for less than 4 hours, there is a strong reluctance on the part of many patients to increase the dialysis duration, regardless of the reason.

For stable CKD patients with progressive kidney failure who may have their initial HD in the outpatient setting, it would be reasonable to consider starting such patients for 2 hours in the first session, 3 hours in the second session, and 4 hours in the third session to avoid possible disequilibrium; however, in the author's opinion, the goal of at least a 4-hour treatment should be achieved as quickly as possible.

RESIDUAL KIDNEY FUNCTION

Almost all patients initiating dialysis have some RKF and urine output. RKF correlates strongly and consistently with patient survival. Although residual function provides additional (and continuous) clearance of solutes and water, the initiation of HD may lead to a more rapid loss of RKF, possibly reflecting dialysis-associated hypotension and ischemic kidney injury, progression of the underlying kidney disease, or the inflammatory burden associated with the dialysis procedure itself. Although it is important to preserve RKF, the mere presence of some RKF (native kidney urea

clearance greater than 2 mL/min) cannot justify shorter dialysis duration and/or reduced dialysis frequency. This is due to the fact that, after the initiation of dialysis, not only does RKF decline fairly rapidly, but there may also be strong resistance from patients to extend treatment time once RKF is lost.

TARGET OR "DRY" WEIGHT AND RATE OF ULTRAFILTRATION

A critical item for patients initiating dialysis is the establishment of a target weight, defined as the weight that the patient needs to achieve at the end of dialysis and at which the patient is close to euvolemia—the so-called "*dry weight.*" Although patients who present with dependent peripheral edema or pulmonary edema have excess fluid volume that can be easily targeted, often it is difficult to determine the target dry weight on clinical examination since fluid overload can be present even in the absence of edema.

For the rare patient not prescribed antihypertensive medications, the achievement of near-normal blood pressure may be one sign of achieving target weight; however, most CKD patients receive multiple blood pressure medications, complicating the use of blood pressure readings as an index of euvolemia. Blood pressure medications also complicate the achievement of the target weight, because these medications may predispose patients to hypotension during fluid removal. Accordingly, achievement of target weight based on clinical assessment is often a process of trial and error that subjects patients to frequent episodes of hypotension.

Several devices exist to help in determining target weight. The first, bioimpedance, can be used on the patient during dialysis by applying electrodes to the skin and estimating hydration status by measuring the resistance encountered by the electrical current passing through the body tissues. The use of a bioimpedance device for determining target weight has yet to receive US Food and Drug Administration (FDA) clearance in the United States. A second device monitors the relative blood volume (RBV) of the patient during HD. In overhydrated patients, the fluid removed during HD is replaced by transfer of fluid from the interstitial compartment, and the RBV does not change appreciably. However, as hydration status improves with time and the patients approach their target weight, the refill rate from the interstitium lags behind the UFR, and the RBV falls. This is accompanied by a drop in blood pressure ("critical" RBV). The blood volume monitor recognizes the "critical" RBV as the value around which hypotension can occur and, depending on the integration of the instrument, lowers the UFR to keep RBV above this value. This particular value of critical RBV varies from patient to patient. Clinical trial data supporting the use of either of these devices are mixed.

The attempt to determine target weight should not distract from another important consideration, namely the determination and prescription of UFRs, the rate at which fluid is removed from the total body water. Recent literature suggests that rates of ultrafiltration that exceed 13 mL/kg per hour are associated with higher morbidity and mortality. Strategies for fluid removal in excess of this amount should include extra dialysis sessions or increasing dialysis time. Additional measures in such situations may include an enhanced focus on dietary salt restriction and the use of diuretics to increase urine output in patients with significant RKF.

DOSE OF DELIVERED DIALYSIS

As discussed earlier, the dose of delivered dialysis is traditionally determined by changes in urea concentration before and after dialysis. Although urea is no longer considered the principal "uremic toxin," urea concentration in the blood and subsequent urea clearance with dialytic therapy correlate reasonably well with observed clinical changes. Furthermore, urea is easily measured in the blood and dialysate, is evenly distributed in total body water, and rapidly diffuses from intracellular to extracellular and vascular spaces. Therefore it is reasonable to assume that changes in urea concentration during dialysis represent a reasonable measure of the dose of dialysis.

Using urea as the accepted marker of the dose of dialysis, the KDOQI guidelines established by the National Kidney Foundation recommend that achievement of a urea single pool Kt/V of at least 1.2 represents the minimum accepted dose of thrice weekly HD. On the basis of limited long-term studies and no clinical trial data, the best patient outcomes appear associated with Kt/V values of 1.2 to 1.4, to be achieved in no less than 4 hours (as discussed previously) and at UFRs that do not exceed 13 mL/kg per hour. The determination of URR or Kt/V depends critically on the accurate measurement of pre- and postdialysis urea and the accurate determination of dialysis time. It is therefore important to be aware of the potential errors that could be introduced in determining each of these measures.

Potential Errors in Predialysis Urea Measurement

Blood for measurement of predialysis urea is generally collected after insertion of the needle in the patient's vascular access or is drawn directly from the catheter. If the blood sample is drawn from a catheter or a recently flushed bloodline, there is a strong likelihood that the blood sample will be diluted with residual saline solution. To address this, approximately 5 mL of blood should be drawn and discarded before the blood sample for urea measurement is obtained.

Potential Errors in Postdialysis Urea Measurement

The postdialysis urea blood sample must be drawn from the "arterial" (intake) needle at least 2 minutes after dialysis is terminated (preferred), the UFR is set to 0, and the blood pump has been stopped (after slowing it to 100 mL/min for at least 10 to 20 seconds before stopping) to avoid recirculation. *Recirculation* of blood not only refers to the possibility of mixing the inlet (arterial) blood with the outlet (venous) blood that occurs when access malfunction results in blood flow that is lower than the blood pump speed (access recirculation) but also to a phenomenon called *cardiopulmonary recirculation*. Cardiopulmonary recirculation occurs whenever the arterial blood feeds the dialyzer inlet (AV access). The dialyzed blood from the dialyzer outlet (relatively poor in urea) subsequently reaches the right heart (and mixes with urea-rich blood coming from other tissues) and passes through the lungs before finally reaching the aorta. The blood in the aorta (consisting of urea-"poor" and urea-"rich" components) is then pumped back to the AV access and to other tissues. The "urea-poor" component of the blood supply feeding the AV access lowers the overall concentration of blood urea in the AV access. This phenomenon does not occur when the access is fed via a venous catheter. This process occurs throughout a dialysis session and can be illustrated by the following observation: when tested, the urea concentration of the blood entering the dialyzer is often different from the urea concentration of the blood in distant peripheral tissues. Cardiopulmonary recirculation is more pronounced in patients dialyzed with high-efficiency dialysis (large dialyzer surface area or rapid blood flow) and in patients with low cardiac output. In many patients, the solute (urea) concentration at the arterial (inlet) bloodline rises by approximately 10% over a 3-minute period after dialysis is discontinued, and blood samples drawn immediately after termination of dialysis will have artificially lower urea concentration, resulting in overestimation of urea reduction and Kt/V compared with blood samples drawn after the urea concentration is uniformly distributed throughout the patient. It is therefore important to emphasize the need for prescribing exactly how the postdialysis urea sample needs to be drawn.

Potential Errors in Treatment Time

Although treatment time is generally considered to be the difference between the dialysis start time and termination time, actual treatment time may be significantly lower than "clock time," reflecting factors such as the time taken to reach maximum blood flow, alarm stoppages, and other interruptions, such as time for patients to use bathrooms. Modern dialysis machines report either actual dialysis time or blood volumes processed, the latter based on the rotation of the blood pump (with its attendant caveat mentioned earlier).

ANTICOAGULATION PRESCRIPTIONS

The contact of the blood with "foreign" surfaces such as the dialyzer membrane triggers the coagulation cascade. In the absence of anticoagulants, this results in blood clotting inside the dialyzer hollow fibers leading initially to loss of dialyzer surface area and eventually to possible loss of appreciable volumes of patient blood in the clotted dialyzer. Because the coagulation cascade is triggered as soon as blood is in contact with foreign surfaces, anticoagulation must be effective before such blood–membrane contact. The most commonly used anticoagulant is unfractionated heparin; initial dosing is most often weight based (approximately 50 units/kg), administered as a bolus immediately following needles insertion and establishment of access patency. Because it is important to allow the heparin to reach the systemic circulation, an interval of approximately 3 minutes following the administration of heparin should elapse before the blood is allowed to reach the extracorporeal circuit via the blood pump. If blood reaches the dialyzer membrane before full anticoagulation, it is likely that local clotting inside the fibers will occur, reducing the available dialyzer membrane surface area and therefore the clearance of uremic toxins.

Because of the steady decline in heparin concentration and level of anticoagulation during dialysis (via both heparin metabolism and adsorption on the extracorporeal surface), it is recommended that a continuous infusion of low doses of heparin be administered throughout most of the treatment at a rate of approximately 1000 units/h. For patients with permanent accesses (AV fistula or graft), it is also recommended that this continuous heparin be discontinued approximately 30 minutes before the end of dialysis to facilitate timely hemostasis of the vascular access after the withdrawal of the needles at the termination of dialysis. For patients dialyzed with a catheter, continuous heparin may be prescribed until the end of the treatment to reduce the risk of clotting of the catheter tips, because "hemostasis" of the catheter at the termination of dialysis is not required.

Although these recommendations are not based on extensive studies, they are clinically effective in most patients. In patients who may be using warfarin anticoagulation for other reasons, the dose of heparin should be reduced although not eliminated, as heparin and warfarin have different mechanisms of action on the coagulation cascade. In a small fraction of patients, heparin results in significant thrombocytopenia, and alternative methods of anticoagulation need to be considered. Very limited safety data exist supporting novel oral anticoagulant use in dialysis.

FREQUENCY OF DIALYSIS AND ALTERNATIVE MODALITIES

Thrice weekly dialysis, with each session lasting a few hours, was established as the standard for maintenance HD in the 1970s, primarily for practical reasons including patient and staff convenience. Because of technologic advances in the delivery of dialysis, the dialysis procedure has become much safer, with greater availability of equipment suitable for home use. Accordingly, regimens with different frequencies and different times of day are being explored. Nevertheless, thrice weekly, daytime, in-center HD remains by far the most common regimen.

Nocturnal Dialysis

Reflecting dialysis facility capacity issues, nephrologists who wanted to prescribe dialysis times of 6 to 8 hours implemented nocturnal dialysis. Patients begin their dialysis treatment in the evening, spending 6 to 8 hours receiving dialysis (generally while sleeping). This can be performed either in-center or at home. Such prolonged dialysis allows for an increase in the total dose of dialysis with much slower rates of ultrafiltration and diffusive clearance. Despite extensive observational data supporting the putative benefits of "more intensive dialysis" (extra session length/frequency or both), when tested in the Frequent Hemodialysis Network (FHN) Nocturnal trial, nocturnal dialysis did not show any benefits on prespecified outcomes of composite of mortality and either change in left ventricular mass or the physical component score of the Short Form (SF)-36. This trial, however, did demonstrate improvement in secondary outcomes of interdialytic weight gain, blood pressure, and predialysis phosphorous levels.

Although the concept of nocturnal dialysis is theoretically attractive, patient acceptance, nurse recruitment, and the need for physician visits at night are some of the barriers for this therapy. Nocturnal dialysis can be performed at home, but the fear of catastrophic events, such as severe hypotension and needle dislodgement while the patient is asleep, has limited this strategy. Of note, remote hemodynamic monitoring and devices that are activated by red blood cells and awaken the patient if there is a blood leak are now available; these may improve the safety of nocturnal dialysis procedure, both in-center and at home.

Short Daily Hemodialysis

An alternative to nocturnal dialysis that still increases the weekly number of dialysis hours is short daily HD, which is most often performed 5 or 6 times weekly for approximately 3 hours per session. The FHN Daily trial showed improvements in prespecified primary composite outcome of mortality and change in left ventricular mass. Secondary outcomes, specified above for nocturnal dialysis, also improved.

Regardless of the above discussion, it is clear that more attention needs to be paid to dialysis duration if patient outcomes are to continue to improve. Recent data clearly demonstrates that the adequacy of HD should not be solely based on small molecule clearance (which can be accomplished in shorter times with large surface-area dialyzers) but also consider the cumulative weekly dialysis time, as well as the rate of ultrafiltration.

BIBLIOGRAPHY

Chertow GM, Levin NW, Kliger AS, et al. In-center hemodialysis six times per week versus three times per week. *N Engl J Med.* 2010;363:2287-2300.

Culleton BF, Walsh M, Klarenbach SW, et al. Effect of frequent nocturnal hemodialysis vs conventional hemodialysis on left ventricular mass and quality of life: a randomized controlled trial. *JAMA.* 2007;298:1291-1299.

Eknoyan G, Beck GJ, Cheung AK, et al; Hemodialysis (HEMO) Study Group. Effect of dialysis dose and membrane flux in maintenance hemodialysis. *N Engl J Med.* 2002;347:2010-2019.

El Ters M, Schears GJ, Taler SJ, et al. Association between prior peripherally inserted central catheters and lack of functioning arteriovenous fistulas: a case-control study in hemodialysis patients. *Am J Kidney Dis.* 2012;60:601-608.

Finkelstein FO, Story K, Firenek C, et al. Perceived knowledge among patients cared for by a nephrologist about chronic kidney disease and end-stage renal disease therapies. *Kidney Int.* 2011;58:235-242.

Foley RN, Gilbertson DT, Murray T, et al. Long interdialytic interval and mortality among patients receiving hemodialysis. *N Engl J Med.* 2011;365:1099-1107.

Goldstein MB, Jindal KK, Levin A, et al. The adequacy of hemodialysis: assessment and achievement. In: Jacobson HR, Striker GE, Klahr S, eds. *The Principles and Practice of Nephrology.* St. Louis, MO: Mosby; 1995.

Grootman MP, Van den Dorpal MA, Bots ML, et al. Effect of online hemodiafiltration on all cause mortality and cardiovascular outcomes. *J Am Soc Nephrol.* 2012;23:1087-1096.

Lacson E Jr, Brunelli SM. Hemodialysis treatment time: a fresh perspective. *Clin J Am Soc Nephrol.* 2011;6:2523-2530.

Lacson E, Lazarus JM, Himmelfarb J, et al. Balancing fistula first with catheters last. *Am J Kidney Dis.* 2007;50:379-395.

Lacson E Jr, Wang W, DeVries C, et al. Effects of a nationwide predialysis educational program on modality choice, vascular access, and patient outcomes. *Am J Kidney Dis.* 2011;58:235-242.

Lacson E Jr, Wang W, Zebrowski B, et al. Outcomes associated with intradialytic oral nutritional supplements in patients undergoing maintenance hemodialysis: a quality improvement report. *Am J Kidney Dis.* 2012;60:591-600.

McIntyre CW, Rosensky SJ. Starting dialysis is dangerous. *Kidney Int.* 2012;82:382-387.

Mehrotra R, Agarwal R. *End stage renal disease and dialysis: nephrology re-assessment.* NephSAP, volume 11; November 2012. Available at: http://www.asn-online.org/education/nephsap/active.aspx. Accessed 24 May 2013.

Owen WF, Lew NL, Liu Y, et al. The urea reduction ratio and serum albumin concentration as predictors of mortality in patients undergoing hemodialysis. *N Engl J Med.* 1993;329:1001-1006.

Rocco MV, Lockridge RS Jr, Beck GJ, et al. The effects of frequent nocturnal home hemodialysis: the Frequent Hemodialysis Network Nocturnal Trial. *Kidney Int.* 2011;80:1080-1091.

Shen JI, Winklelmayer WC. Use and safety of unfractionated heparin for anticoagulation during maintenance hemodialysis. *Am J Kidney Dis.* 2012;60:463-486.

Spiegel DM. Avoiding harm and achieving optimal dialysis outcomes—the dialysate component. *Adv Chronic Kidney Dis.* 2012;19:166-170.

Suri RS, Nesrallah GE, Mainra R, et al. Daily hemodialysis: a systematic review. *Clin J Am Soc Nephrol.* 2006;1:33-42.

Peritoneal Dialysis 58

Anand Vardhan; Alastair J. Hutchison

Peritoneal dialysis (PD), hemodialysis (HD), and kidney transplantation are the cornerstones of kidney replacement therapy (KRT). These modalities are not mutually exclusive, and, during a lifetime of therapy, patients may transfer from one to the other. In the 1950s and 1960s, at its inception, PD was used predominantly to manage acute kidney injury, while patients with end-stage kidney failure were treated almost exclusively by HD. The introduction of continuous ambulatory peritoneal dialysis (CAPD) in 1976 transformed this situation, and there was a dramatic rise in the use of PD internationally during the 1980s and 1990s. PD use among incident patients in the United States declined steadily from the mid-1990s to 2007, when only approximately 6% of incident dialysis patients performed PD; these have rebounded somewhat since then, with PD utilization of approximately 10% in 2014 among incident US patients undergoing dialysis. On December 31, 2014, the prevalence of various KRT modalities in the United States was approximately 64% HD, 7% PD, and 29% functioning kidney transplant.

Although in the past many comparisons have been made between peritoneal and HD, focus has shifted more recently to the site of dialysis delivery, namely home-based or in-center. Home-based therapies have advantages for many patients and are particularly popular in Canada, the Netherlands, Iceland, Finland, Denmark, Australia, New Zealand, Mexico, and Hong Kong, where more than 20% of the dialysis population receive home therapies. Among these countries, PD accounts for almost 80% of dialysis in Hong Kong and about 65% in Mexico. In the United States, while home dialysis has increased in recent years, its use remains low, particularly for home HD. Contrary to prior concepts of self-care requiring a fully able patient, PD has expanded in some countries to become the therapy of choice for the elderly and those with multiple comorbidities. In many regions, this has largely been possible by the introduction of assisted PD, with patients given varying degrees of assistance by a trained health professional in carrying out dialysis in their home. It frees them from the tedium of hospital or center-based HD and the travel involved.

Acute or "urgent-start" PD is used in many parts of the world, especially for single-organ acute kidney injury requiring dialysis support and in "late-presenters" with chronic kidney failure. Most major kidney units around the world have developed pathways for rapid peritoneal access to facilitate an early start of PD.

PRINCIPLES OF PERITONEAL DIALYSIS

THE PERITONEAL MEMBRANE

In PD, the visceral peritoneum serves as the dialyzing membrane. The visceral peritoneal membrane tightly covers the intestine and mesentery, whereas the parietal peritoneum lines the insides of the abdominal cavity. The membrane consists of a single layer of mesothelial cells overlying an interstitium in which the blood and lymphatic vessels lie. The mesothelial cells are covered by microvilli that markedly increase the nominal surface area of the peritoneum, which is approximately 2 m^2. The effective peritoneal surface area available for dialysis, however, is estimated to be about one-third of this.

SOLUTE MOVEMENT

PD occurs across the peritoneal membrane with solute and water exchange between the peritoneal capillary blood and the dialysis solution that is instilled into the peritoneal cavity. There is also some net fluid and solute resorption via the intraperitoneal lymphatics. Solute movement occurs as a result of "diffusion" and "convective transport," whereas fluid shifts relate largely to "osmosis" created by the addition of osmotic agents to the dialysis solutions. During PD, solutes such as urea, creatinine, and potassium move from the peritoneal capillaries across the peritoneal membrane to the peritoneal cavity, while other solutes, such as lactate, bicarbonate, and potentially calcium, move in the opposite direction. Solute movement is mainly by diffusion and is therefore based on the concentration gradient between dialysate and blood. Solutes also move across the peritoneal membrane by convection, which is described as the movement of solutes as a result of fluid flux.

FLUID MOVEMENT

Standard PD fluids contain glucose in varying concentrations as the principal osmotic agent making the dialysate hyperosmolar in relation to plasma. When instilled in the peritoneal cavity this hyperosmolar solution causes net fluid removal (ultrafiltration) to occur. Dialysis fluid in the peritoneum is separated from capillary blood by three layers of tissue. These include the mesothelial cell layer, which offers little resistance to fluid and solute transport, the interstitium, which offers resistance mainly to large molecules, and the endothelium of the peritoneal capillaries, which is most active in restricting and regulating solute and fluid movement. The endothelial lining of the peritoneal capillaries has pores of three different sizes often referred to as the "three pore model." Small pores (radius 40 to 50 A°) located between the endothelial cells are responsible for transport of low-molecular-weight solutes. These account for most of the pore area available for solute transport and contribute significantly toward peritoneal ultrafiltration. The large pores (radius 250 A°), thought to correspond to interendothelial gaps, account for just 5% to 8% of the ultrafiltration coefficient and occupy less than 0.5% of the total pore area. The ultra-small pores (radius 3 to 5 A°), composed mainly of Aquaporin-1, are permeable only to water and are located within the endothelial cells. These account for up to 40% of the total ultrafiltration. The volume of ultrafiltration depends on the concentration of glucose in the solution used for each exchange, the length of time the fluid dwells in the peritoneal cavity, and the individual patient's peritoneal membrane characteristics (discussed later). With increasing dwell time, transperitoneal glucose absorption diminishes the dialysate glucose concentration and the osmotic gradient. Ultrafiltration is consequently decreased with longer dwell times, such as with the overnight exchange in CAPD or the long daytime dwell in automated peritoneal dialysis (APD), the most common form of which is referred to as continuous cycling peritoneal dialysis (CCPD).

The crucial physiologic components of the PD system are the magnitude of peritoneal blood flow and the permeability of the peritoneal membrane, neither of which is amenable to clinical manipulation. Also important are dialysate volume, dwell time, and number of exchanges per day, and these three variables can be manipulated to maximize solute and fluid removal. Various techniques and regimens have emerged as a consequence of increased understanding of peritoneal membrane transport characteristics or permeability in relation to the amount of solute and fluid to be removed.

ASSESSING PERITONEAL MEMBRANE CHARACTERISTICS

PD effectively removes substances with low molecular weights, such as creatinine, urea, and potassium, that are not in the infused dialysis fluid. With increasing dwell time, solutes move across the peritoneal membrane toward concentration equilibrium, and the ratio of dialysate to serum urea levels approaches 1.0. Because the peritoneal membrane has a net negative charge, negatively charged solutes, such as phosphate, move across it more slowly than positively charged solutes of similar size, such as potassium. Macromolecules such as albumin cross the peritoneum by mechanisms that are not completely understood, but probably via lymphatics and through large pores in the capillary membranes. During a dwell period, the osmotic gradient created by standard dialysate within the abdominal cavity declines as the glucose is absorbed. In time this can result in net fluid reabsorption back into the systemic circulation because of the added effects of intraperitoneal hydrostatic pressure and intravascular oncotic pressure. Continuous lymphatic absorption also diminishes net fluid removal.

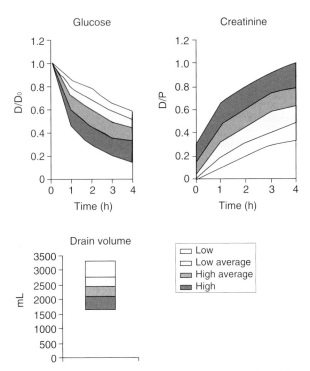

Fig. 58.1 The peritoneal equilibration test (PET) measures the peritoneal transport characteristics of glucose from the peritoneal fluid to plasma and of creatinine from plasma to the peritoneal fluid. The instilled peritoneal fluid volume for the PET is 2 L. D/D_0 represents the ratio of dialysate glucose concentration (D) at a given time point to the dialysate glucose concentration at time 0 (D_0). D/P represents the ratio of dialysate (D) to plasma (P) concentrations. The rate of transport of these molecules depends on the permeability of the membrane: the higher the permeability (high transporter), the more rapid the transport of glucose, with dissipation of the osmotic gradient and therefore less drain volume.

The rate of movement of small solutes between dialysate and blood differs from one patient to another. Peritoneal function characteristics are assessed by the peritoneal equilibration test (PET; Fig. 58.1). Classically, 2 L of dialysate containing 2.5 g/dL glucose is infused, and the ratio of dialysate to plasma creatinine (D/P_{Cr} ratio) at the end of a 4-hour dwell is calculated. With this test, each patient's peritoneal membrane can be categorized as having high (D/P_{Cr} >0.81), high-average (0.65 to 0.81), low-average (0.50 to 0.65), or low (<0.5) peritoneal transport characteristics. Use of 2 L of dialysate containing 4.25 g/dL glucose during the same dwell period as in the PET permits assessment of ultrafiltration failure; an effluent volume of less than 2.4 L is diagnostic of ultrafiltration failure; accordingly, 4.25% glucose dialysis is often substituted for 2.5% in the PET.

Removal of fluid and solutes is highly dependent on transport characteristics as described by the PET (Fig. 58.2). Patients with a high D/P_{Cr} ratio (high or fast transporters) have rapid clearance of small molecules but poor ultrafiltration because of rapid glucose absorption and dissipation of the osmotic gradient between dialysate and blood. These patients require short-dwell PD regimens to achieve adequate fluid removal. In addition, because the volume of fluid removed also contributes to the solute clearance of equilibrated dialysate via convection, fast transporters also have

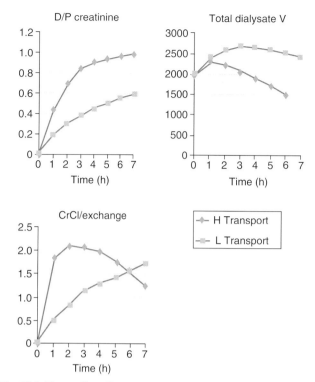

Fig. 58.2 The profiles of intraperitoneal dialysate volume (V) and solute transport (CrCl/exchange), in relation to dwell time in hours, vary in high transporters (H) and low transporters (L). These profiles are used in prescription setting of dwell times and fluid volumes. For long-dwell continuous ambulatory peritoneal dialysis, high transporters show both low fluid removal and low CrCl, compared with low transporters. *CrCl,* Creatinine clearance; *D/P creatinine,* dialysate-to-plasma creatinine ratio.

reduced solute clearance over long dwells because of low drain volumes. Patients with a low D/P_{Cr} ratio (low or slow transporters) have low clearance rates for solutes and usually require more dialysis exchanges or increased volume per exchange, or both, to avoid uremic symptoms once residual kidney function is lost. Ultrafiltration in this category of patient is relatively better. By virtue of the definition, most patients have high-average to low-average peritoneal transport, achieving adequate clearance and ultrafiltration on either CAPD or APD.

PERITONEAL CATHETERS

Access to the peritoneal cavity for dialysis is achieved by means of a self-retaining catheter inserted into the abdominal cavity, usually under local anesthetic with or without sedation. General anesthesia often is reserved for patients with previous abdominal surgery and complicated insertions, particularly those patients in whom laparoscopic insertion is planned. The catheter can be inserted under direct vision through a mini-laparotomy, percutaneously using the Seldinger technique with a guide-wire, or with peritoneoscopic or laparoscopic guidance. Although there are numerous catheter designs, such as the Swan-neck catheter (said to undergo less catheter tip migration and fewer exit-site infections) and curled catheters, none offers a significant proven advantage over the double-cuffed Silastic Tenckhoff catheter. This original and simple design is still the most commonly used catheter. The intraabdominal portion of the catheter has multiple perforations in addition to the hole at the end through which dialysate flows. The deep cuff placed at the rectus muscle in the mid-line or just laterally and the extraperitoneal portion of the catheter are tunneled through the subcutaneous tissue to exit the skin, pointing laterally and caudally. The superficial cuff is located inside the subcutaneous tunnel at least 2 to 3 cm from the exit site.

PD can be initiated immediately after catheter placement if it is urgently required; in this circumstance, exchange volumes are kept small, and the patient is kept recumbent to avoid dialysate leaks. Ideally, dialysis should be deferred for a few weeks after insertion to allow the surgical wound and exit site to heal properly. The surgical wound is secured in an occlusive dressing postoperatively and left untouched usually for 10 days, at which point patient training for exit-site care commences and training to perform CAPD or APD begins.

TECHNIQUES OF PERITONEAL DIALYSIS

CONTINUOUS AMBULATORY PERITONEAL DIALYSIS

CAPD is perhaps the simplest method for performing dialysis, involving the manual instillation of up to 3 L of dialysis fluid in the peritoneal cavity, through an indwelling abdominal catheter, three to five times a day. Typically this results in three to four shorter dwells during the day and a long dwell overnight. In adults the total volume of fluid exchanged in a day typically ranges from 8 to 10 L. Thus dialysis occurs continuously throughout the entire 24-hour period, and patients are free to go about their business in between exchanges. The prescription specifies the type of dialysis fluid, volume to be used, dwell time, and number of exchanges, and this prescription often varies according to patient size, peritoneal permeability, and residual kidney function.

PD fluid is instilled by gravity into the peritoneal cavity and drained out after a dwell period of several hours depending on the number of exchanges planned in the 24-hour period. The basic CAPD system, which has remained largely unchanged for almost 3 decades, consists of a plastic bag containing 0.5 to 3.0 L of dialysis fluid, a transfer set (tubing between the catheter and the plastic bag), and the permanent, indwelling Silastic catheter, which is implanted so that the tip of the intraperitoneal portion lies in the pelvis. Because the connection between the bag and the transfer set is interrupted three to five times a day to facilitate fluid exchange (approximately 1500 exchanges per year), the procedure must be carried out using a strict, aseptic, nontouch technique, which the patient or helper performs at home. The most common device in current use is based on a Y-shaped connection system. It comprises a filled bag and an empty bag of the same size with a Y-shaped junction, which can be connected to the PD catheter. Once the connection has been made, this device allows drainage of the effluent from the abdomen through the connection into the empty bag, before fresh dialysate is instilled. This ensures "flushing out" of any accidental "touch contamination" in the tubing before infusion of new fluid into the peritoneal cavity (Fig. 58.3). This

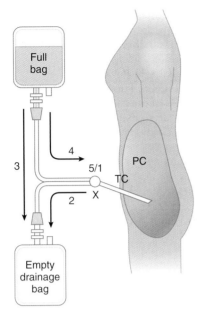

Fig. 58.3 Diagrammatic representation of a continuous ambulatory peritoneal dialysis exchange using a Y-set disconnect system. The Y-set consists of tubing with a full bag of dialysate at one end and an empty drainage bag at the other, placed on the floor. Fluid flow is by gravity, and the direction of flow is controlled by clamps on the tubing. Between exchanges, the peritoneal cavity (PC) contains dialysate and only a short, capped extension tubing attached to the peritoneal Tenckhoff catheter (TC). The exchange procedure comprises five steps: (1) To begin the exchange, the patient connects the Y tubing to the short extension tubing at X. (2) Keeping the clamp on the full bag closed, the patient or caregiver opens the clamp on the peritoneal catheter extension to allow the fluid in the PC to drain into the drainage bag by gravity. Time required: 10 to 15 minutes. (3) The patient then closes the clamp on the peritoneal catheter extension tubing and opens the clamp on the full bag, allowing fresh fluid to "flush" the tubing of air and any contamination into the drainage bag. Time required: a few seconds (count of 5). (4) Next, the patient closes the clamp on the drainage bag and opens the clamp on the peritoneal catheter extension tubing, allowing fresh dialysis fluid into the PC via the TC. Time required: 10 minutes. (5) The final step is to close the clamp on the peritoneal catheter extension tubing, disconnect the Y tubing, and cap the short extension tubing.

system reduces the risk of infection and also obviates the need for carrying an empty bag and transfer set, thus improving the psychologic aspects and quality of life of CAPD patients.

AUTOMATED PERITONEAL DIALYSIS

APD is a broad term that is used to refer to all forms of PD that use a mechanical device (called a *cycler*) for instillation and drainage of dialysis fluid. In its simplest form, APD was delivered in hospital, intermittently for prolonged periods of up to 24 hours, exchanging 20 to 60 L of dialysis fluid either in acute kidney failure or as a maintenance therapy in end-stage disease; this process was termed intermittent peritoneal dialysis (IPD). The technique is quite uncommon now, with most cycler-assisted exchanges carried out overnight by patients at home while asleep, thereby allowing freedom of movement during the day. APD regimens (illustrated in Table 58.1) can be tailored to individual need and include:

Table 58.1 Regimens Used in Peritoneal Dialysis

Type of Dialysis[a]	Typical Number of Daytime Exchanges	Typical Number of Nighttime Exchanges	Volume of Exchanges (L)
CAPD	2–3	1–2[b]	1.0–3.0
CCPD	1	3–4	1.0–3.0
NIPD	0	3–5	2.0–3.0
NIPD with "wet day"	1–2	3–5	2.0–3.0
TPD	0	4–20	1.0–2.0
IPD	5–10	5–10	1.0–2.0

[a]All regimens except continuous ambulatory peritoneal dialysis use a cycler machine and are therefore variants of automated peritoneal dialysis.
[b]If an additional exchange is needed during continuous ambulatory peritoneal dialysis to achieve adequate dialysis, a mechanical exchange device can be used to perform the exchange during the night while the patient is asleep.
CAPD, Continuous ambulatory peritoneal dialysis; *CCPD*, continuous cycling peritoneal dialysis; *IPD*, intermittent peritoneal dialysis; *NIPD*, nocturnal intermittent peritoneal dialysis; *TPD*, tidal peritoneal dialysis.

- CCPD, which provides three to four exchanges during the night and one during the day (a reversal of the CAPD regimen)
- Nocturnal intermittent peritoneal dialysis (NIPD), which provides rapid exchanges during the night, with no fluid in situ during the day (NIPD with "dry day")
- Nocturnal PD plus two exchanges during the day to allow for increased small-solute and fluid clearance (NIPD with "wet day")
- Tidal peritoneal dialysis (TPD), in which only a proportion of fluid in the abdomen is drained at the end of a cycle before it is filled again. The proportion of fluid removed can be set on the cycler and is usually between 50% and 85%. The lesser the proportion of fluid removed the more rapid is the cycling required and greater the total volume of dialysate used. The concept behind tidal PD is to allow continuous fluid-membrane contact to improve dialysis efficiency. In practice, however, tidal settings are often used with CCPD to relieve abdominal pain at the end of the drain cycle and to prevent catheter malfunction, rather than improve dialysis efficacy. When used for this purpose, 90% or more of the expected dialysate volume is typically removed.

APD regimens usually entail an increased number of short-dwell exchanges to enhance solute and fluid removal. The cycler delivers a set number of exchanges over 8 to 10 hours, with the last fill constituting the long day dwell, which may be necessary to provide additional dialysis to achieve solute and fluid removal targets. The most obvious advantage of APD is that it eliminates the need for intensive manual involvement, because most of the dialysis occurs at night during sleep. In essence, APD entails only two procedures daily: an initial connection of the catheter to the machine and a disconnection at the end of dialysis. APD is increasingly being used in the United States and Europe in lieu of CAPD and is gaining popularity in developing economies as well. This trend may be related to the convenience of performing the dialysis connections and to newer cycler models, which are smaller, lighter, and less expensive than previously, and more attractive to patients. In the past, APD tended to be offered only to patients who had been identified by PET as "high transporters" and who therefore required shorter dwell times. However, lifestyle issues and freedom from daytime exchanges are now major factors in patient modality choice.

ASSISTED PERITONEAL DIALYSIS

Although patients have been receiving assistance one way or another for as long as PD has been in existence, assisted peritoneal dialysis (aPD) is increasingly recognized as a distinct dialysis modality. Assistance may be provided by trained members of the family, paid nurses, or health care professionals, depending on the set-up of the health care system. Often, staff members at intermediate care facilities, assisted-living centers, and nursing homes are trained to carry out aPD for their residents. The advantages of aPD over in-center HD for the elderly include independence from hospital and slower removal of solute and fluid, reducing the likelihood of cardiovascular instability. In addition, older adult patients treated with aPD are less likely to suffer from malnutrition. Other patients who may be suitable for aPD include those with physical disabilities (e.g., rheumatoid arthritis), patients requiring terminal care (end-stage chronic disease, including malignancy and heart failure), those with learning disability, and others who are simply slow to learn because of other barriers.

Assistance can also be provided for CAPD, although this requires three or four visits daily. This model has been prevalent in France since the late 1970s. Assisted automated peritoneal dialysis (aAPD) is gaining in popularity as increased numbers of older patients are treated with dialysis. Varying degrees of assistance can be provided; one model includes one visit by the health care worker to the patient's home every day. During the visit, the health care worker will strip down and set up the cycler (each morning); review and dress the PD catheter exit site if required; check blood pressure, weight, and blood glucose if the patient has diabetes; document patient progress and communicate any variance to the dialysis unit; and maintain adequate stocks of dialysis fluids and consumables. This level of assistance greatly simplifies the patient role to connecting himself or herself to the machine before going to bed at night and then disconnecting in the morning.

PERITONEAL DIALYSIS SOLUTIONS

GLUCOSE-BASED SOLUTIONS

Standard PD solutions (Table 58.2) contain varying concentrations of glucose as the osmotic agent, electrolytes such as sodium, magnesium, calcium, and chloride and buffers like

Table 58.2 Composition and Properties of Standard Peritoneal Dialysis Fluids Including the Osmotic Agents Used

Type	Conventional	Low GDP[a]	Low GDP	Glucose Free	Glucose Free	Bicarbonate-Based	Bicarbonate-Based
Brand Name	Dianeal	Balance	Gambrosol Trio	Nutrineal	Extraneal	Physioneal	BicaVera
Solute	Glucose	Glucose	Glucose	Amino Acid[b]	Icodextrin	Glucose	Glucose
Solute Concentration[c]	1.5%, 2.5%, 4.25%	1.5%, 2.3%, 4.25%	1.5%, 2.5%, 3.9%	1.1%	7.5%	1.5%, 2.5%, 4.25%	1.5%, 2.3%, 4.25%
pH	5.2 (4–6.5)	7	5.5–6.5	6.6 (5.7–6.8)	5.0–6.0	7.4	7.4
Osmolarity (mosm/L)	345, 395, 483[d]	356, 399, 509[d]	357, 409, 483	365	282–286	344, 395, 483	358, 401, 511
Sodium (mmol/L)	132	134	131–133	132	132	132	134
Chloride (mmol/L)	96	100.5–101.5	96	105	96	95	104.5
Calcium (mmol/L)	1.25–1.75	1.25–1.75	1.70–1.79	1.25	1.75	1.25	1.75
Magnesium (mmol/L)	0.25	0.5	0.24–0.26	0.25	0.25	0.25	0.5
Lactate (mmol/L)	40	35	39–41	40	40	15	0
Bicarbonate (mmol/L)	0	0	0	0	0	25	34

[a]Newer glucose-based solutions with low levels of glucose degradation products and physiologic pH are now available and are being used increasingly.
[b]Amino acid solutions are used infrequently in practice because evidence for definite nutritional benefit is equivocal, but they do serve to reduce the glucose exposure of the peritoneal membrane.
[c]1.5% indicates 15 g per liter of glucose monohydrate, 2.5% is 25 g/L, and 4.25% is 42.5 g/L; the equivalent anhydrous glucose is 13.6 g/L, 22.7 g/L, and 3.86 g/L, respectively.
[d]Osmolarity listed above reflects lower calcium dialysate and is 1 to 2 mosm/L higher with higher dialysate calcium concentrations. Lower dialysate calcium is more common in the United States.

lactate. Lactate was initially used as the buffer in preference to the more physiologic bicarbonate for technical reasons, specifically that the low pH of lactate prevents caramelization of the glucose while autoclaving for sterilization during the manufacturing process. The biocompatibility of these solutions has been intensively studied. There is no doubt that their unphysiologically low pH, high osmolarity, and presence of glucose degradation products (GDPs) generated during manufacture and autoclaving are harmful to peritoneal cells in vitro and are implicated in peritoneal neovascularization, collagen production, and peritoneal thickening, all of which may contribute to loss of function.

Other dialysate buffer options exist. One relatively newer, more physiologic dialysate, also described in Table 58.2, uses bicarbonate as the buffer and is dispensed in twin bags, one of which contains the glucose solution and the other the bicarbonate solution. At the point of use, the two solutions are mixed by breaking a protective seal to produce a dialysate with a neutral pH and low GDP content. Alternative osmotic agents such as "icodextrin" and a mixture of amino acids have also been developed and are in routine use worldwide. While there is no conclusive clinical trial evidence to demonstrate that the newer more physiologic solutions preserve the peritoneal membrane and result in longer technique and patient survival, there is little doubt about their more physiologic constitution; hence increased utilization of these novel solutions appears limited only by higher costs. They may also be used in patients in whom standard solutions cause abdominal pain, as this is less of a problem with the newer solutions possibly because of the more physiologic pH and osmolarity.

NONGLUCOSE-BASED SOLUTIONS

ICODEXTRIN DIALYSATE

While glucose remains the most common osmotic agent in use because of its relatively low immediate toxicity, low cost, and ease of manufacture, two alternative osmotic agents have interesting and attractive properties. Icodextrin is a starch-derived glucose polymer that produces ultrafiltration by exerting colloid oncotic pressure when administered intraperitoneally. A 7.5% icodextrin solution is almost isosmolar to serum but produces sustained ultrafiltration over a period of up to 12 hours, with minimal absorption into the circulation. The volume of ultrafiltrate is comparable to that produced by a hyperosmolar 4.25% glucose dialysate without the accompanying calorie load or glucose exposure to the peritoneal membrane. It can improve fluid balance as it can be left for the long overnight dwell in CAPD and long daytime dwell in APD (CCPD). It serves to achieve sustained ultrafiltration irrespective of transporter status and even in situations where there is peritoneal inflammation (during an episode of peritonitis). The current license limits the amount of icodextrin used to one exchange per day, with the volume used ranging from 1 L to 2.5 L, depending on patient size and need for ultrafiltration, although studies are in progress investigating the safety and benefits of two dwells per day.

Small amounts of complex carbohydrate do get absorbed into the circulation via the lymphatic system and, with regular daily use, reach a steady-state plasma level in 7 to 10 days. This carbohydrate polymer is hydrolyzed in part to maltose by circulating amylase, and maltose levels of around 1.4 mg/mL are observed with no significant impact on plasma osmolality. The long-term adverse effects of this are not known but are not thought to be harmful. Critically, the maltose in the circulation interferes with blood glucose estimation in patients with diabetes using home blood glucose monitoring equipment. Blood glucose measurement therefore must be done with a glucose-specific method to prevent maltose interference. Glucose dehydrogenase pyrroloquinolinequinone (GDH-PQQ) or glucose-dye-oxidoreductase (GDO)-based methods should not be used. Similarly, the use of some glucose monitors and test strips using glucose dehydrogenase flavinadenine dinucleotide (GDH-FAD) methodology have resulted in falsely elevated glucose readings because of the presence of maltose. In case of any doubts, the manufacturer(s) of the monitor and test strips should be contacted to seek clarification. Falsely high readings can result in insulin overdose with ensuing hypoglycemia or cause an apparently normal glucose reading when the patient is actually hypoglycemic. Multiple deaths have been reported because of the failure to appreciate maltose cross-reactivity with glucose measures.

Most antibiotics are compatible with icodextrin and can be administered dissolved in this solution during the long dwell in the event of peritonitis. While antibiotic combinations are well studied and reported in glucose-based solutions, there is less evidence of their safety and efficacy in icodextrin-based dialysate.

AMINO ACID–BASED DIALYSATE

Amino acid–based solutions intend to provide nutritional supplementation while enabling reduced glucose PD. The commercially available solution is a mixture of 15 amino acids in a concentration of 1.1%. The solution also contains standard concentrations of sodium, calcium, magnesium, chloride, and lactate. The amino acids act as the osmotic agent and are variably absorbed across the peritoneal membrane during the dwell. The evidence to support improvement in nutrition as well as overall outcome is not compelling, but this dialysate can be considered in malnourished patients both for nutritional supplementation and for reduction of glucose exposure. Used in combination with icodextrin, amino acid–based solutions have the potential to preserve peritoneal membrane integrity and reduce excessive glucose absorption. A 2-L bag contains approximately 25% of the daily protein requirement of a 70-kg adult. Successful utilization of the amino acids is dependent on an adequate calorie load, and amino acid dialysate (Nutrineal) should be instilled after the patient has had a meal. In CAPD regimens Nutrineal is usually administered after the midday meal and, in APD regimens, can be the first exchange on the cycler. One exchange per day of 2 to 2.5 L is recommended, and a maximum of two exchanges may be used. Amino acid–based dialysate should be avoided in severe uremia, disorders of amino acid metabolism, severe liver disease, acidosis, hypokalemia, and hypersensitivity.

MANAGEMENT OF PERITONEAL DIALYSIS

PERITONEAL DIALYSIS PRESCRIPTION

In determining the appropriate prescription for an individual patient, one needs to account for the fixed components

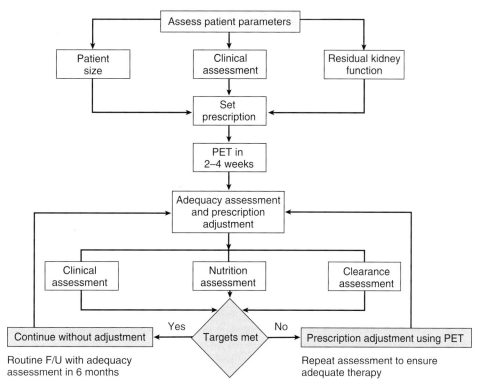

Fig. 58.4 Algorithm for prescription setting. After the initial peritoneal equilibration test (PET) at 2 to 4 weeks, the prescription is altered according to the membrane permeability results. For high transporters, short-dwell automated peritoneal dialysis is appropriate; for high-average and low-average transporters, continuous ambulatory peritoneal dialysis would suffice. *F/U*, Follow-up.

at the time, including residual kidney function, peritoneal membrane permeability, and patient size, as well as the variable components of dialysate volume, dwell times, concentration of glucose, and number of exchanges. A prescription entails modifications of the variable components to arrive at a regimen that provides for adequate solute and fluid removal to meet clinical needs and maintain reasonable quality of life. Setting a PD prescription is outlined in Fig. 58.4. Dialysis adequacy regarding solute removal, fluid status, nutritional status, and clinical well-being are monitored regularly as discussed below, and the prescription is modified accordingly.

The overall clearance capacity of the peritoneum for small solutes is limited by the volume of dialysis fluid that can be provided daily. Many CAPD patients are prescribed four exchanges of 2 L of dialysate per day. Four 2-L CAPD exchanges per day with 2 L daily net ultrafiltration represents a drain volume of 70 L/week, which is inadequate for most patients in the absence of significant residual kidney function, especially those who weigh more than 80 kg. Initially, most patients will have residual kidney function that contributes to the total solute clearance. As kidney function is gradually lost, patients will require larger exchange volumes (2.5 or 3.0 L) and may also need five daily exchanges to avoid uremic symptoms and reach target values of urea Kt/V and creatinine clearance (CrCl) described below. In a CAPD regimen, the fifth exchange may be provided by use of an automated device that performs an extra exchange during the night. However, this technique is in decline, because it effectively introduces a mini-APD machine, and most patients and physicians would opt to switch completely at this point from CAPD to APD. Larger patients should be started on

exchange volumes of 2.5 to 3.0 L. APD can achieve higher clearance of small solutes, but it may necessitate 1 or 2 day dwells ("wet day") in addition to three or four nocturnal exchange volumes of 2.5 to 3.0 L each.

PERITONEAL DIALYSIS ADEQUACY

Adequacy of PD is determined by clinical assessment, solute clearance measurements, nutritional status, and fluid removal. The well-dialyzed patient has a good appetite, no nausea, and minimal fatigue; is well nourished; and feels well. In addition to these clinical parameters, two biochemical measures are used to assess adequacy of solute removal:

1. An index of peritoneal urea removal, expressed as Kt/V, which is urea clearance (K) multiplied by time (t) and related to total body water volume, which is assumed to be the urea distribution volume (V). Kt is obtained by multiplying the ratio of effluent dialysate to plasma urea nitrogen concentration (D/P_{urea}) by the 24-hour effluent drain volume. Kidney urea clearance is added to this value to yield the total daily body clearance. The daily value is multiplied by 7 to provide a weekly value. V can be estimated as 60% of weight in males or 55% of weight in females although the Watson formula is more often used. A typical calculation is given in Table 58.3.

2. CrCl, which is provided by both peritoneal clearance and that contributed by residual kidney function. Peritoneal CrCl is also obtained from the 24-hour collection of dialysate, but to this is added an estimate of the glomerular filtration rate (GFR) achieved by the residual kidney

Table 58.3 An Example of Urea Kt/V Calculation for a 70-kg Adult Woman Receiving Continuous Ambulatory Peritoneal Dialysis With Four 2-L Exchanges Per Day and 1-L Residual Urine Output Per Day

Data to Be Obtained	Calculations/Assumptions
24-hour dialysate volume (4 × 2 L infusion) + 1 L net ultrafiltrate = 9 L	Requires measuring the total effluent, which consists of spent dialysate plus the net ultrafiltrate
D/P ratio for urea (0.9)	Determined by collecting the total drained dialysate for 24 hours and measuring the dialysate and concurrent blood urea nitrogen (UN)
Residual kidney urea clearance Using the formula (U × V)/P, where U = 24-hour urine urea nitrogen, V = urine volume, and P = BUN	In this example $U_{UN}/P_{UN} = 2.9$ V = 1 L/24 hours (or 0.7 mL/min) Clearance = 2.9 × 0.7 = 2 mL/min 2 mL/min = 20.2 L/week ~ 20 L/week
Formulas	
Peritoneal urea clearance/day (Durea/Purea × Volume)	= 0.9 × 9 L = 8.1 L
Weekly peritoneal urea clearance	= 8.1 L/day × 7 days/week = 56.7 L/week
Residual kidney urea clearance	= 20 L/week (from above)
Total urea clearance (Kt)	= 56.7 L/week + 20 L/week = 76.7 L/week
Volume of urea distribution (V)[a]	= (0.55 × weight in kg) = 38.5 L
Weekly Kt/V	= 76.7 L ÷ 38.5 L = 1.99

[a]Volume of urea distribution (V) can be estimated as 0.60 (male) or 0.55 (female) times the body weight in kilograms. However, it is more accurate to use the formula of Watson and Watson, which takes into account weight (in kilograms), height (in centimeters), gender, and age (in years). For males, V(L) = 2.477 + (0.3362 × Weight) + (0.1074 × Height) − (0.09516 × Age). For females, V(L) = −2.097 + (0.2466 × Weight) + (0.1069 × Height). The data collection for creatinine clearance (CrCl) is similar to that for Kt/V. However, the urinary component of CrCl is usually corrected for creatinine secretion by averaging it with the urinary urea clearance. The peritoneal CrCl is simply calculated by dividing the creatinine content of the 24-hour dialysate by the serum creatinine concentration. The total CrCl (peritoneal + kidney) is normalized to 1.73 m[2] body surface area.
BUN, Blood urea nitrogen; *CAPD*, continuous ambulatory peritoneal dialysis; *D/P ratio*, Dialysate-to-plasma creatinine ratio.

function. By tradition, residual kidney clearance is determined by averaging CrCl and urea nitrogen clearance as an estimate of the GFR. This is performed to correct for tubular secretion of creatinine, which substantially overestimates GFR at low levels of kidney function. An adjustment for body surface area is also usually applied.

Although the validity of these measurements and calculations continues to cause some controversy, they are the accepted methods of estimating dialysis adequacy, and various national and international organizations have set minimum targets for both CrCl and urea clearance based on them. However, it is sometimes difficult for patients to achieve one or both targets, and doubt remains about the precise level at which the targets should be set. The National Kidney Foundation Kidney Disease Outcomes Quality Initiative (K/DOQI) Practice Guidelines for Peritoneal Dialysis were first published in 1997 and were last updated in 2006. In 2006, the target minimum Kt/V for urea was reduced from 2.0 to 1.7, and the target total weekly CrCl from 60 L to 50 L, largely as a result of one large, well-conducted and randomized prospective study (ADEMEX), which showed no survival advantage with the higher dialysis dose. Several other guidelines have similar conclusions, including the United Kingdom Renal Association Guidelines, the European Renal Best Practice, and the International Society for Peritoneal Dialysis Guidelines. It is thought that failure to achieve these clearance thresholds will result in a higher risk of uremic symptoms, decreased nutritional status, and mortality, but conclusive evidence is lacking as investigators are naturally reluctant to test the point at which reducing the dialysis "dose" produces clinical symptoms.

Although current guidelines suggest the minimum solute clearance targets required to achieve an acceptable long-term clinical outcome, some patients may need more dialysis to overcome uremic symptoms. In addition, it must always be remembered that the term *dialysis adequacy* is restricted to the description of solute removal and does not cover other aspects of care. Control of hypertension, correction of dyslipidemia, maintenance of fluid balance, maximal cardiovascular risk reduction, and management of comorbidities can hugely influence outcomes in any dialysis patient. Critically, anuric patients can usually be successfully managed with PD by appropriate prescription adjustments, including the use of APD regimens and icodextrin.

It is well recognized that residual kidney function is extremely important in providing adequate solute and fluid clearance. Most studies show that residual kidney function correlates with improved survival and less morbidity, and its preservation forms an important part of PD patient management. To preserve residual kidney function, nephrotoxic drugs such as aminoglycosides and nonsteroidal antiinflammatory agents should be avoided whenever possible, and episodes of hypotension from any cause should be corrected as rapidly as possible. Residual kidney function is better preserved in patients receiving PD than in those receiving HD, so PD could be a better initial therapy option for both acute and chronic kidney failure.

FLUID REMOVAL

Although PD patients benefit from continuous daily fluid removal, most patients are at least mildly fluid overloaded. There are multiple reasons for this, potentially including less frequent medical assessments. Whether this state of continuous mild overload is more or less harmful than the thrice-weekly rapid variation in fluid status experienced by a HD patient is unknown, but volume management may become more troublesome in the longer term, when residual kidney function is lost and PD ultrafiltration capacity is reduced, particularly as adequate fluid removal appears to have a more significant impact on outcomes than solute clearance. Net ultrafiltration of at least 750 mL/day is associated with better survival in anuric patients, although the exact reason for this association is unclear. Greater emphasis is now placed on optimizing fluid status, and algorithms are available that help the physician manage fluid overload in PD patients (Fig. 58.5). The use of icodextrin for the longest dwell may achieve better fluid balance and result in improved left ventricular indices.

NUTRITION IN PERITONEAL DIALYSIS

Up to 40% of PD patients are protein malnourished as defined by anthropometric studies, in part reflecting losses of amino acids and protein in the dialysate, with protein loss approximating 8 to 12 g/day. In addition to factors common in kidney failure, PD-specific factors include peritonitis, which markedly increases dialysate protein losses and appetite suppression by the absorbed dialysate glucose. Both the Kt/V and the weekly CrCl correlate, albeit weakly, with dietary protein intake, suggesting that a certain minimum dose of dialysis is required for adequate protein intake. While lower serum albumin level is associated with both mortality and hospitalization in PD patients, albumin is greatly influenced by inflammation and is a poor marker of nutritional status when used alone. Protein intake of at least 1.2 g/kg per day is recommended for PD patients, but many ingest only 0.8 to 1.0 g/kg per day. The KDOQI recommendations are that such patients should first receive dietary counseling and education; then, if protein intake remains inadequate, oral supplements should be prescribed. The use of amino acid dialysate (in which amino acids replace the glucose) has been tried on a limited basis as a means of correcting protein malnutrition, but proof of its long-term nutritional benefit is lacking. It is especially difficult to correct malnutrition related to inflammation and comorbidity. This "type II" malnutrition may well be cytokine mediated, and its correction necessitates establishing an underlying cause for inflammation.

The number of calories absorbed from dialysate glucose depends on the dextrose concentration used (1.5, 2.5, or 4.25 g/dL) and on the membrane permeability of the patient. The development of obesity is not unusual in patients undergoing PD, especially in those who were already overweight at the start of dialysis. In addition, glucose absorption frequently results in hyperlipidemia, which may contribute to atherosclerotic cardiovascular disease.

COMPLICATIONS OF PERITONEAL DIALYSIS

PERITONITIS

Peritonitis remains a major complication of PD despite advances in connectology and aseptic technique. Peritonitis accounts for 15% to 35% of hospital admissions and is the major cause of catheter loss and technique failure resulting

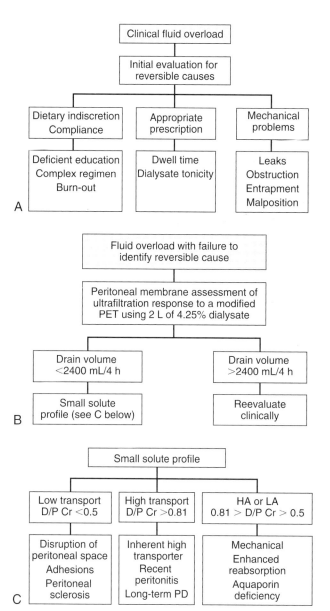

Fig. 58.5 (A) Evaluation of the clinical syndrome of fluid overload. This initially entails the evaluation and search for reversible causes. (B) After reversible causes are excluded, it is appropriate to evaluate peritoneal membrane function using the modified peritoneal equilibration test (PET) with 2 L of 4.25% glucose. (C) Algorithm for further evaluation and treatment based on the small solute profile. For high-transport patients, the therapy is outlined. For low-transport patients peritoneal dialysis may not be possible and peritoneal sclerosis should be excluded, especially encapsulating peritoneal sclerosis. *D/P Cr*, Ratio of dialysate to plasma creatinine; *HA*, high-average transport; *LA*, low-average transport; *PD*, peritoneal dialysis.

in transfer to HD. Entry of bacteria into the catheter during an exchange procedure (touch contamination) is the most common source, but organisms can also track along the external surface of the catheter or migrate into the peritoneum from another abdominal viscus.

Diagnosis of peritonitis requires the presence of any two of the following:

- Organisms identified on Gram staining or subsequent culture

Table 58.4 Microorganisms Causing Peritonitis

Microorganisms	Frequency (%)
Gram Positive	
Staphylococcus epidermidis	30–40
Staphylococcus aureus	15–20
Streptococcus	10–15
Other gram positive	2–5
Gram Negative	
Pseudomonas	5–10
Enterobacter	5–20
Other gram negative	5–7
Fungi	2–10
Other organisms	2–5
Culture negative	10–30

- Cloudy fluid (white cell count $>100/mm^3$; $>50\%$ neutrophils)
- Symptoms and signs of peritoneal inflammation

Cloudy dialysate effluent is almost invariably present, and abdominal pain is present in about 80% to 95% of peritonitis cases. Gastrointestinal symptoms, chills, and fever are present in as many as 25% of the cases, and abdominal tenderness in 75%. Bacteremia is rare. Gram staining of the effluent is seldom helpful, except with fungal peritonitis, but cultures are usually positive. In many centers up to 20% of peritonitis episodes result in a "no growth" culture result, predominantly because of suboptimal sample collection, transportation, and inadequate culture techniques or a combination of these.

Causes of peritonitis are summarized in Table 58.4, together with the frequency of infection with these organisms. The rate of peritonitis with *Staphylococcus epidermidis* has decreased since the introduction of the Y-set and the "flush-before-fill" technique; accordingly *Staphylococcus aureus* and enteric organisms now account for a larger proportion of peritonitis episodes than in the past. Because patients infected with these organisms are more symptomatic than those with *S. epidermidis* peritonitis, peritonitis has become a less frequent but more severe complication, often requiring hospital admission. Peritonitis rates, originally very high in the late 1970s and early 1980s, have decreased to less than one episode every 2 to 3 dialysis years, owing to improvements in connectology and resultant decreases in touch contamination.

Catheter removal for peritonitis depends on the infecting microorganism. Peritonitis due to *S. epidermidis* is less likely to result in catheter loss than peritonitis due to *S. aureus* or *Pseudomonas aeruginosa*. If these more virulent organisms are associated with a catheter tunnel or exit-site infection, the catheter loss rate can be as high as 90%. Fungal peritonitis almost invariably requires catheter removal, because a medical cure can only rarely be achieved. There is no apparent difference in rates of peritonitis between CAPD and APD; however, detection of peritonitis on APD can be delayed because the effluent is less readily available for inspection after each drain, and the volume of fluid dilutes the cells so that the patient may not notice any clouding.

The initial treatment of peritonitis is empiric and designed to cover both gram-positive cocci and gram-negative bacilli. The International Society for Peritoneal Dialysis Guidelines published in *Peritoneal Dialysis International* in 2016 recommend a center-specific empiric therapy based on the local history of sensitivities of organisms causing peritonitis. Gram-positive organisms may be covered by vancomycin or a first-generation cephalosporin if methicillin resistance is rare and gram-negative organisms by a third- or fourth-generation cephalosporin or aminoglycoside while dialysate effluent culture report is awaited; subsequent therapy is tailored to the sensitivity results. As mentioned, first-generation cephalosporins may not adequately cover methicillin-resistant staphylococci and do not cover most coagulase negative staphylococci, whereas widespread empiric use of vancomycin raises concerns about the promotion of resistance in staphylococci and the development of vancomycin-resistant enterococci (VRE). However, the long half-life of vancomycin in PD patients makes it very simple to administer, and it is widely used as a result. When used, aminoglycoside levels should be monitored to avoid accelerated loss of residual kidney function and vestibulo-ototoxicity; however, because these antibiotics also have a relatively long half-life in PD, the traditional advice regarding peak and trough levels is invalid, and serum values may not be informative of intraperitoneal levels.

A listing of antibiotics and suggested dosing schedules is given in Table 58.5. Antibiotics are usually administered intraperitoneally in the long-dwell exchange (overnight in CAPD and during the daytime long dwell in APD). They can also be given continuously in every exchange. The dosage may need adjustment if residual kidney function is significant. Duration of therapy depends on the organisms and the severity of the peritonitis; it is usually 14 days for *S. epidermidis* infections and 3 weeks for most other infections.

It is possible in most cases to achieve complete cure without having to resort to catheter removal. Persistent symptoms beyond 96 hours occur in 10% to 30% of episodes, suggesting that the catheter should be removed. Occasionally, cure may be obtained if antibiotics alone are continued beyond 96 hours without catheter removal, but there is a high risk of damage to the peritoneum, and neither the short-term bacterial outcome nor the long-term peritoneal membrane effect is good. Therefore if there is not clear evidence of improvement (i.e., reduction in abdominal pain, falling dialysis fluid cell count, visual clearing of the PD effluent) after 96 hours of treatment with appropriate antibiotic therapy, the catheter should be removed as soon as possible. In a study in which antibiotics were continued for 10 days for "resistant" peritonitis without clearing of the fluid and without catheter removal, one-third of the patients died; another third lost ultrafiltration necessitating discontinuation of PD; and only one-third were able to continue with PD. Two or more episodes of peritonitis can be characterized as relapsing, recurrent, or repeat. An episode that occurs within 4 weeks of completion of therapy of a previous episode with the same organism or a sterile episode is defined as relapsing peritonitis. An episode that occurs within 4 weeks of completion of therapy of a previous episode but with a different organism is defined as recurrent peritonitis. Finally, peritonitis that occurs more than 30 days after completion of therapy of a previous episode, but with the same organism that caused the previous episode, is defined as repeat peritonitis, whereas

Table 58.5   Common Antibiotics and Dosing Schedules (Intraperitoneal Use Unless Otherwise Stated)

Antibiotic	Intermittent Dosing (One Exchange Daily)	Continuous Dosing (All Exchanges)
Vancomycin	15–30 mg/kg every 5–7 days	LD 30 mg/kg MD 1.5 mg/kg/bag
Gentamicin	0.6 mg/kg daily	LD 8 mg/L MD 4 mg/L
Cefazolin	15–20 mg/kg daily	LD 500 mg/L MD 125 mg/L
Ceftazidime	1–1.5 g daily	LD 500 mg/L MD 125 mg/L
Amikacin	2 mg/kg daily	LD 25 mg/L MD 12 mg/L
Aztreonam	2 g daily	LD 1000 mg/L MD 250 mg/L
Ciprofloxacin	No data	MD 50 mg/L
Meropenem	1 g daily	No data
Teicoplanin	15 mg/kg every 5 days	LD 400 mg/bag MD 20 mg/bag
Fluconazole	200 mg every 24–48 hours	No data

Once-daily antibiotic dosing with the long dwell is preferred to the addition of antibiotic to each exchange. Patients receiving automated peritoneal dialysis (APD) may be changed to a continuous ambulatory peritoneal dialysis schedule; if they remain on an APD schedule, antibiotics are added to each exchange.
LD, Loading dose; *MD*, maintenance dose.

if the organism is different, it is defined as a reinfection. Relapsing peritonitis is a feature in about 10% to 15% of episodes. Catheter removal is necessary in as many as 15% of these cases, and death has been reported in 1% to 3%. For fungal peritonitis, it is now standard practice to remove PD catheters in addition to giving antifungal treatment for a minimum of 3 weeks and modality transfer to HD.

Peritonitis results in a marked increase in acute peritoneal protein losses and a transient decrease in ultrafiltration due to the increased permeability to the dialysate dextrose. Although peritoneal membrane changes are usually transient and related to acute peritonitis, peritoneal fibrosis (often referred to as sclerosis) may be involved in severe episodes or as a cumulative effect of multiple episodes of peritonitis (see later discussion).

PERITONEAL CATHETER EXIT-SITE AND TUNNEL INFECTION

Peritoneal catheter infections can involve the exit site (erythema or purulent drainage), the tunnel (edema, erythema, or tenderness and collections along the subcutaneous pathway), or both simultaneously. *S. aureus* is the most common cause of exit-site and tunnel infections, with *Pseudomonas* being the next most frequent organism. *S. aureus* exit-site infections are difficult to treat and frequently progress to tunnel infections and peritonitis, in which case catheter removal is required for resolution. *S. aureus* nasal carriage is associated with an increased risk of *S. aureus* catheter infection. Treatment of nasal carriers with intranasal mupirocin twice daily for 5 days each month, mupirocin applied daily to the exit site regardless of carrier status, or oral rifampin 600 mg/day for 5 days every 12 weeks has been shown to be effective in reducing *S. aureus* catheter infections.

The application of mupirocin at the exit site as part of routine exit-site care has resulted in a dramatic reduction in exit-site infections and peritonitis related to *S. aureus*. Bacteriologic monitoring of the PD population for *S. aureus* carriage is unnecessary when this approach is adopted. Concerns about development of resistance to mupirocin have not proved true in clinical practice over the past decade, but it may in the future encourage growth of resistant organisms. *P. aeruginosa* catheter exit-site infections are very difficult to resolve and frequently relapse. Ciprofloxacin is often used to treat such catheter infections, but if the infection does not resolve within a couple of weeks or if *P. aeruginosa* peritonitis develops, the catheter must be removed.

CATHETER MALFUNCTION, HERNIAS, AND FLUID LEAKS

The most important noninfectious complications during PD are abdominal wall hernias, leakages of dialysis fluid, and inflow and outflow malfunctions. Before PD treatment is started, all significant abdominal wall hernias should be corrected. With the presence of 2 to 3 L of dialysate in the abdominal cavity, there is an increased intraabdominal pressure, and preexisting hernias will worsen during PD treatment. The most frequently occurring hernias after commencement of PD are incisional, umbilical, and inguinal hernias. Significant hernias should be repaired surgically, and IPD may be continued postoperatively using low dwell volumes in a supine position.

Leakage of peritoneal fluid is related to catheter implantation technique, trauma, or patient-related anatomic abnormalities. It can occur early (<30 days) or late (>30 days) after implantation and can have various clinical manifestations depending on whether the leak is external or subcutaneous. Early leakage is usually external, appearing as fluid through the incision site or the catheter exit site. Late leakage may develop at the site of any incision and entry into the peritoneal cavity. The exact site of the leakage can be determined by computed tomography after infusion of 2 L of dialysis fluid containing radiocontrast material. Scrotal or labial edema can be a sign of an early or late fluid leak, usually through a patent processus vaginalis. Therapy usually entails a period off PD, during which the patient is maintained on HD or on limited, small-volume PD in the supine position as necessary. For recurrent leaks, surgical repair is essential. Leakage of fluid into the subcutaneous tissue is sometimes occult and difficult to diagnose. It may manifest as diminished drainage, which might be mistaken for ultrafiltration failure. Computed tomography and abdominal scintigraphy may identify the leak.

Outflow-inflow obstruction is the most frequently observed early event, occurring within 2 weeks after implantation of the catheter, although it may also be seen later in association with other problems such as peritonitis. One-way outflow obstruction is the most frequent problem and is characterized by poor flow and failure to drain the peritoneal cavity.

Common causes include both intraluminal factors (blood clot, fibrin) and extraluminal factors (constipation, occlusion of catheter holes by adjacent organs or omental wrapping, catheter tip dislocation out of the true pelvis, incorrect catheter placement at implantation). A kidney, ureter, and bladder (KUB) radiographic study is useful in localizing the PD catheter tip for malposition. Depending on the cause, appropriate therapy may entail laxatives to clear the bowels, heparinized saline flushes, urokinase or tissue plasminogen activator (TPA) instillation into the catheter to relieve blockages, manipulation under fluoroscopy guidance (using a stiff wire or stylet with a "whiplash" technique), and laparoscopic revision or open replacement of the catheter in cases of catheter displacement.

PERITONEAL MEMBRANE CHANGES

ENCAPSULATING PERITONEAL SCLEROSIS

The peritoneum undergoing dialysis reacts in response to the new environment. Over time there is thickening of the interstitium and basement membrane reduplication, both in the mesothelium and in the capillaries. These changes likely occur in response to the nonphysiologic composition of standard dialysis solutions and from the direct actions of glucose and GDPs, which result in the formation of advanced glycation end products (AGEs) and consequent changes in the peritoneal membrane. Changes in peritoneal microvessels and neovascularization occur, analogous to those seen in diabetic retinopathy, with deposition of type IV collagen. Other conditions that are important in the pathogenesis of peritoneal thickening are recurrent acute peritonitis and chronic inflammatory reactions mediated by uremic or low-level bacterial activation of peritoneal macrophages and intraperitoneal production of proinflammatory and profibrotic cytokines such as vascular endothelial growth factor, interleukin 6, and transforming growth factor-β.

Data from an international biopsy registry showed that thickening of the membrane usually occurs over a period of 4 to 5 years of PD and is associated with increasing severity of vasculopathy, although there is considerable interpatient variability, and some patients show only relatively minor changes even after more than 5 years on dialysis. For patients who have been undergoing PD for more than 5 years, it is prudent to be vigilant for signs of a sudden increase in peritoneal permeability, particularly in association with raised inflammatory markers or gastrointestinal symptoms of intermittent obstruction. These signs may indicate development of the rare condition known as *encapsulating peritoneal sclerosis* (EPS), which is characterized by dense fibrosis and thickening of the peritoneum with bowel adhesions and encapsulation.

The pathogenesis of EPS is complex, and no single etiologic factor has been identified; factors such as multiple episodes of peritonitis, use of high-glucose dialysis solutions, and genetic predisposition have been proposed, with little substantiating evidence. Although EPS is rare, its incidence rises significantly after 5 years of PD therapy. EPS is a serious, life-threatening condition with variable reported mortality, which probably depends on severity at the time of diagnosis. One series reported a 60% death rate within 4 months after presentation with intestinal obstruction. Progressive loss of ultrafiltration and sudden development of high-transporter status may be early warning signs in some patients. However, the designation "EPS" should be reserved for the point at which *encapsulation* has clearly occurred. Clinically, the features are those of ileus or frank intestinal obstruction. Diarrhea is also observed when partial obstruction spontaneously resolves. Gut motility is compromised as a result of binding of the intestinal loops to the parietal peritoneum and abdominal wall by an aggressive fibrotic process. Treatment consists of resting the bowel with total parenteral nutrition and surgical enterolysis for obstructive symptoms, which is best undertaken at specialist centers. Some advocate cessation of PD and conversion to HD, but others suspect that such a change may exacerbate the fibrotic process. There are anecdotal reports of use of antifibrotic agents such as tamoxifen or immunosuppressive agents, but with limited success.

ULTRAFILTRATION FAILURE

Net ultrafiltration failure is the most important transport abnormality in patients undergoing long-term PD. On the basis of clinical symptoms, its prevalence has been reported to increase from 3% after 1 year on CAPD to about 30% after 6 years. *Ultrafiltration failure* is defined as net ultrafiltration of less than 400 mL after a 4-hour dwell using 2 L of 4.25% glucose-containing dialysate. This condition is associated with a large peritoneal vascular surface area and impaired aquaporin channel–mediated water transport. It is best managed with frequent, short dwells and elimination of long dwells, such as with nocturnal APD, combined with daytime icodextrin. Because icodextrin is such a large molecule, its reabsorption is relatively unaffected by membrane permeability. It exerts colloid oncotic pressure and is able to maintain gradual but sustained ultrafiltration for 12 hours or longer. Improvement of peritoneal function can be brought about by minimizing glucose exposure (i.e., using glucose-free dialysate), providing peritoneal rest (being "dry" during the day on APD), using solutions that are low in GDPs, and using icodextrin, which has been shown to extend PD therapy time in patients with loss of ultrafiltration. Mortality in this group is higher than for other patients on PD, probably because of poor fluid control, which adds to the overall cardiovascular risk, as well as increased protein loss in the dialysate, which compromises nutrition.

DIABETES AND PERITONEAL DIALYSIS

Diabetic glomerulosclerosis is the most common cause of kidney failure worldwide. Most diabetic patients require insulin while they are on PD, even if they did not require it before the initiation of dialysis, in part the result of glucose absorption from the dialysate and associated weight gain. Insulin can be given to PD patients via the intraperitoneal route, the subcutaneous route, or a combination of both. If given intraperitoneally, the total daily dose of insulin required must be increased because insulin adsorbs onto the polyvinylchloride bags. Patients undergoing APD usually require long-acting subcutaneous insulin (with or without intraperitoneal regular insulin) for adequate glucose control. Injection of insulin into dialysis fluid bags confers a theoretical risk of bacterial contamination and subsequent peritonitis and is not widely used at present.

OUTCOMES IN PERITONEAL DIALYSIS

Patient survival on PD is similar to that on HD and is probably slightly better during the initial years of dialysis therapy. Underlying comorbidities very much dictate outcome, although several observational studies from Canada and Europe have suggested that there is a survival advantage in commencing dialysis therapy with PD and then changing to HD when therapy fails, rather than initiating with HD. Beginning with PD maximizes the advantages that it confers during the first few years of dialysis, in terms of preservation of residual kidney function and better fluid control, plus preservation of sites for future vascular access.

Patient and technique survival with PD continue to improve. According to the latest United States Renal Data System (USRDS) Report 2016 adjusted survival for incident HD patients in 2009 was only 56% at 3 years after the onset of end-stage renal disease (ESRD) while for PD the figure was 67% at 3 years. Between the years 2001 and 2009 5-year survival rose from 36% to 42% among HD patients and from 39% to 51% among PD patients.

Patients transfer from PD to HD for a multitude of reasons, including peritonitis or exit-site infection, catheter malfunction, inability to perform the dialysis procedure, and inadequate clearance or ultrafiltration (particularly with loss of residual kidney function). Patients who lose a catheter because of peritonitis or a catheter infection often elect to switch to HD permanently. The use of the Y-set and "flush-before-fill" systems is associated with improved technique survival on CAPD that is primarily due to lower peritonitis rates. It is hoped that long-term outcomes will improve with greater emphasis on maintenance of residual kidney function, greater use of more physiologic PD solutions, and the use of PD in an integrated kidney replacement treatment program as an equally important modality to HD and perhaps as the first dialytic treatment for most patients with ESRD.

Transplantation is the goal for many patients undergoing dialysis. The allograft and patient survival rates of transplanted PD patients are similar to those of transplanted HD patients, but there is reduced delayed graft function in the former group. Delayed graft function, in combination with graft rejection, is a strong predictor of graft survival. If the transplant does not initially function, PD may be continued, provided that the peritoneal cavity was not breached during surgery. The PD catheter is usually left in place for several weeks until the kidney graft is functioning well.

PERITONEAL DIALYSIS FOR ACUTE KIDNEY INJURY

Intermittent PD can be successfully used to manage acute kidney injury. In the past "acute PD" was performed using a rigid peritoneal catheter that was inserted percutaneously using a stylet without a subcutaneous tunnel. PD exchanges would be commenced immediately to provide solute clearance and ultrafiltration; however an increased risk of fluid leakage and peritonitis led to its disuse. Bedside insertion of a Tenckhoff catheter using the Seldinger technique under local anesthesia is equally straightforward and carries a much lower risk of infection. Rapid exchanges are performed to maximize

clearance of small solutes at a frequency of up to one exchange per hour, ideally using a cycler. Exchanges more frequent than once per hour are unlikely to improve solute clearance and may result in more "down time," when the peritoneum is mostly empty in between dwells, than dialysis time. After acute solute and volume issues are under control, any of the PD regimens discussed above can be adopted. Of note, although these PD procedures are extremely effective for volume control and are better tolerated by hemodynamically unstable patients than intermittent HD, clearance of small solutes may be inadequate in catabolic patients or patients receiving total parenteral nutrition with large protein loads. Although several publications, largely from Europe, describe positive outcomes in single organ system failure treated with "acute PD," PD has been largely replaced by HD and by continuous venovenous hemofiltration or hemodiafiltration for the management of acute kidney injury.

URGENT-START PERITONEAL DIALYSIS

Conventionally there is a gap of several weeks after the insertion of a PD catheter before initiating PD exchanges, allowing for the incision and exit site to heal and for the patient to be taught exit-site care before commencing training to carry out manual or cycler-assisted exchanges. This delay may be particularly important in patients who have undergone complicated PD catheter insertion procedures, where an early start is more likely to cause fluid leak from the incision or exit site. Urgent-start PD is the term used to describe initiation of exchanges immediately or soon after catheter insertion.

Despite improvements in patient pathways for commencing PD, many PD units do not have the staffing and infrastructure to offer this form of therapy to the late presenting kidney failure patients. One key requirement for running an urgent-start PD program is to have operators who can place a PD catheter within 24 to 48 hours of referral. These could be interventional nephrologists, radiologists, or surgeons who use a minimally invasive technique of insertion allowing for early use for dialysis exchanges with a lower risk of pericatheter leaks. Often a low volume (1 L) rapid cycling regimen in the supine position is the treatment of choice in the initial week before moving on to ambulatory PD. Other key team members are dialysis education nurses who can provide information to the patients at short notice on what to expect with PD as well as other personnel, including social workers who can carry out a rapid assessment of the patient's social circumstances and address any potential barriers to home dialysis, PD nurses who can train patients in carrying out the exchanges and assist with exchanges during the first weeks of therapy (often in-center but perhaps at home), and administrative support to arrange for rapid delivery of dialysis cyclers and consumables to the patient's home.

Urgent-start PD gives the choice of long-term PD to patients who need to start therapy at short notice, avoiding the use of temporary HD catheters, which are not without complications. Patients are usually reluctant to move from HD to PD; accordingly, an urgent-start PD program may increase the overall utilization of PD.

Contraindications to urgent-start PD include severe illness and comorbidity that would preclude patient involvement or be poorly responsive to acute PD and anatomic issues that would preclude successful exchanges.

KEY BIBLIOGRAPHY

Abu-Alfa AK, Burkart J, Piraino B, Pulliam J, Mujais S. Approach to fluid management in peritoneal dialysis: a practical algorithm. *Kidney Int Suppl.* 2002;S8-S16.

Brown EA, Davies SJ, Rutherford P, et al. Survival of functionally anuric patients on automated peritoneal dialysis: the European APD Outcome Study. *J Am Soc Nephrol.* 2003;14:2948-2957.

Brown EA, Johansson L, Farrington K, et al. Broadening options for long-term dialysis in the elderly (BOLDE): differences in quality of life on peritoneal dialysis compared to haemodialysis for older patients. *Nephrol Dial Transplant.* 2010;25:3755-3763.

Brown N, Vardhan A. Developing an assisted automated peritoneal dialysis (aAPD) service—a single centre experience. *NDT Plus.* 2011;4:16-18.

Burkart JM, Piraino B, Bargman J, et al. NKF KDOQI clinical practice recommendations for peritoneal dialysis adequacy. *Am J Kidney Dis.* 2006;48:S130-S158.

Devuyst O, Rippe B. Water transport across the peritoneal membrane. *Kidney Int.* 2014;85(4):750-758.

Garcia-Lopez E, Lindholm B, Davies S. An update on peritoneal dialysis solutions. *Nat Rev Nephrol.* 2012.

Gokal R. Peritoneal dialysis in the 21st century: an analysis of current problems and future developments. *J Am Soc Nephrol.* 2002;13:S104-S116.

Li PK, Szeto CC, Piriaino B, et al. ISPD Peritonitis Recommendations: 2016 update on prevention and treatment. *Perit Dial Int.* 2016;36:481-508.

Lo WK, Ho YW, Li CS, et al. Effect of Kt/V on survival and clinical outcome in CAPD patients in a randomized prospective study. *Kidney Int.* 2003;64:649-656.

Lobbedez T, Moldovan R, Lecame M, Hurault dL, El Haggan W, Ryckelynck JP. Assisted peritoneal dialysis. Experience in a French renal department. *Perit Dial Int.* 2006;26:671-676.

Mujais S, Nolph K, Gokal R, et al. Evaluation and management of ultrafiltration problems in peritoneal dialysis. International Society for Peritoneal Dialysis Ad Hoc Committee on Ultrafiltration Management in Peritoneal Dialysis. *Perit Dial Int.* 2000;20:S5-S21.

Pajek J, Hutchison AJ, Bhutani S, Brenchley PE, Hurst H, Perme MP, Summers AM, Vardhan A. Outcomes of peritoneal dialysis patients and switching to hemodialysis: a competing risks analysis. *Perit Dial Int.* 2014;34:289-298.

Paniagua R, Amato D, Vonesh E, et al. Effects of increased peritoneal clearances on mortality rates in peritoneal dialysis: ADEMEX, a prospective, randomized, controlled trial. *J Am Soc Nephrol.* 2002;13:1307-1320.

Piraino B, Bernardini J, Brown E, Figueiredo A, Johnson DW, Lye WC, Price V, Ramalakshmi S, Szeto CC. ISPD position statement on reducing the risks of peritoneal dialysis-related infections. *Perit Dial Int.* 2011;31:614-630.

Povlsen JV, Ivarsen P. Assisted automated peritoneal dialysis (AAPD) for the functionally dependent and elderly patient. *Perit Dial Int.* 2005;25:S60-S63.

Qi H, Xu C, Yan H, Ma J. Comparison of icodextrin and glucose solutions for long dwell exchange in peritoneal dialysis: a meta-analysis of randomized controlled trials. *Perit Dial Int.* 2011;31:179-188.

Saran R, Li Y, Robinson B, et al. US Renal Data System 2015 Annual Data Report of Kidney Disease in the United States. *Am J Kidney Dis.* 2016;67:S1-S305.

Summers AM, Abrahams AC, Alscher MD, et al. A collaborative approach to understanding EPS: the European perspective. *Perit Dial Int.* 2011;31:245-248.

Szeto CC. Peritoneal dialysis-related infection in the older population. *Perit Dial Int.* 2015;35:659-662.

Full bibliography can be found on www.expertconsult.com.

59

Outcomes of Kidney Replacement Therapies

Rajnish Mehrotra; Kamyar Kalantar-Zadeh

Patients with chronic kidney disease (CKD) stage 5 often require either kidney transplantation or maintenance dialysis to sustain life. In general, the paucity of living and deceased donors and the medical ineligibility of many end-stage renal disease (ESRD) patients for transplantation substantially limit the number of patients who can receive a kidney transplant. In contrast, many countries and states around the world have made a social compact to make maintenance dialysis therapy available to every kidney failure patient in whom this treatment is indicated. Thus maintenance dialysis is the dominant method of treatment for chronic kidney failure.

It is estimated that there are some 2 million patients treated with maintenance dialysis worldwide including almost half a million alone in the United States. The global census of patients undergoing dialysis continues to increase, in part reflecting exponential growth in patient populations undergoing dialysis in such emerging economies as China and India. It is believed that currently over 80% of patients undergoing dialysis worldwide are treated with in-center hemodialysis (HD), generally delivered thrice weekly in most industrialized nations, while once- to twice-weekly HD may be common in some other countries either as incremental transition to thrice weekly dialysis or as palliative dialysis, although resource constraints may also lead to less frequent treatment; most of the rest are treated with home peritoneal dialysis (PD).

In the last 10 years, variations in the conventional method of delivery of different therapies, but particularly HD, are increasingly being used, creating a veritable menu of kidney replacement therapies from which patients can choose (Table 59.1). In recent years, there also has been heightened interest in better understanding the implications of transition from advanced CKD (estimated glomerular filtration rate [eGFR] <30 mL/min/1.73 m^2) to kidney replacement therapy as well as transitions within kidney replacement modalities (Fig. 59.1).

Notwithstanding the myriad options and different transitions, the median life expectancy of ESRD patients starting dialysis therapy still remains short, ranging from 3 to 5 years, prompting increased interest in determining if the method of delivery of kidney replacement therapy affects the survival of ESRD patients. More important, for reasons that remain uncertain, mortality of patients on dialysis is the highest in the first several months following dialysis initiation (Fig. 59.2). Although it has been speculated that the excessively high mortality associated with transition to dialysis may be related to the rapid loss of residual kidney function in the first several months following dialysis initiation, other factors may also contribute, including loss of functionality and worsening quality of life in the setting of a dialysis-dependent lifestyle. Finally, acute kidney injury (AKI) as the cause of dialysis

initiation, potentially mislabeled as transition to ESRD, may contribute, as AKI is associated with high death rates.

There are ongoing discussions as to whether very old persons with advanced CKD or those with more severe comorbid states and shorter life expectancy would have similar or even better survival and quality of life if they receive conservative management without dialysis or transplantation. This chapter reviews the contemporary studies comparing the survival of patients treated with different kidney replacement therapy modalities; more focused discussion of comprehensive conservative care occurs in Chapter 50.

MAINTENANCE DIALYSIS VERSUS KIDNEY TRANSPLANTATION

For many patients, a functioning kidney transplant is less intrusive in their daily lives than maintenance dialysis and, hence, offers a substantial lifestyle advantage. However, these advantages are partially counterbalanced by the short-term surgical risks and longer term medical risks from lifelong immunosuppression. Studies suggest that, despite these short- and longer term risks, ESRD patients who receive a kidney transplant have a longer life expectancy when compared with individuals with equivalent health status who remain on the waiting list for a deceased donor organ while undergoing maintenance dialysis. The survival advantage with a successful transplant extends even to transplants where the kidney is harvested from marginal or expanded criteria deceased donors and in individuals whose age or coexisting medical conditions would have precluded them from being considered as donors over a decade ago. Furthermore, the earlier in the course of kidney failure that a patient receives a kidney transplant, the longer the allograft functions.

These observational reports are limited given systematic differences among individuals who receive a kidney transplant versus those who remain on the waiting list or those who receive an organ transplant earlier during the disease that cannot be fully accounted for in statistical models. While it is important to recognize these limitations, it is equally important to acknowledge that a clinical trial comparing kidney transplantation with maintenance dialysis in general, or the various dialysis modalities separately, is unlikely to be undertaken. Accordingly, the substantial lifestyle advantages along with the possibility of increased longevity make a compelling case for ensuring that every eligible kidney failure patient can undergo a kidney transplant as early as feasible within the constraints imposed by the availability of living donors and waiting time for a deceased donor transplant.

Table 59.1   Various Forms of Kidney Replacement Therapies Used in End-Stage Kidney Disease

In-Center Hemodialysis

Thrice Weekly

Standard duration (3–4 hours)
Diurnal, long duration
Nocturnal, long duration

Frequent (four times weekly to daily hemodialysis)

Infrequent (once to twice weekly)

Incremental (upon transition to dialysis)
Palliative

Hemodiafiltration

On-line hemodiafiltration

Home Hemodialysis

Diurnal, twice to thrice weekly with conventional machines
Frequent with conventional or low-flow machines
Frequent long-duration nocturnal

Peritoneal Dialysis

Continuous ambulatory peritoneal dialysis
Automated peritoneal dialysis

Kidney Transplantation

Living related or unrelated donor
Deceased donor

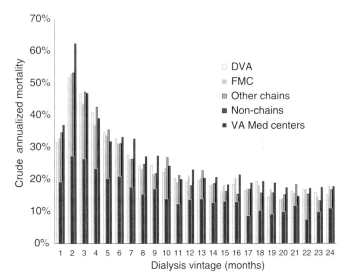

Fig. 59.2 High mortality rate during the first 12 months of hemodialysis therapy in more than 52,000 incident ESRD Veterans in the United States over 4 years (10/2007 to 9/2011). *DVA,* DaVita; *FMC,* Fresenius Medical Center; *VA,* Veterans Affairs. (Adapted from the Transition of Care in Chronic Kidney Disease Chapter of the United States Renal Data System Annual Data Report.)

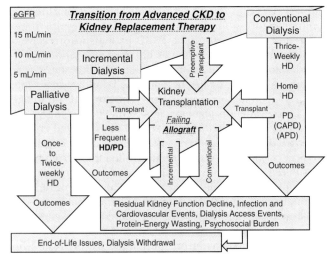

Fig. 59.1 Transition from advanced chronic kidney disease (eGFR <30 mL/min/1.73 m²) to kidney replacement therapy with different modalities, also highlighting intermodality transitions and impact on clinical outcomes. *APD,* Automated peritoneal dialysis; *CAPD,* continuous ambulatory peritoneal dialysis; *CKD,* chronic kidney disease; *HD,* hemodialysis; *PD,* peritoneal dialysis.

HEMODIALYSIS OR PERITONEAL DIALYSIS

Both HD and PD require significant but different adaptations to patients' lifestyles. First, HD requires high flow access to the bloodstream. Second, except for some recent trends,

virtually all patients treated with HD are treated in a dialysis facility (referred to as in-center HD), and, throughout the developed world, HD is most commonly provided thrice weekly for 3 to 4 hours per session. Given transportation needs and time to achieve vascular access hemostasis posttreatment, HD requires a minimum total commitment of 4 to 5 hours thrice weekly. Variations from this general approach are increasingly being used and include differences in length and/or frequency of each treatment session (e.g., short daily HD of 2.5 to 4.0 hours, long thrice-weekly HD sessions of 5 to 7 hours each) as well as the site where dialysis is performed (home vs. in-center including conventional vs. nocturnal).

PD, in contrast, is almost exclusively performed at home. While traditionally patients performed four exchanges every day with continuous ambulatory peritoneal dialysis (CAPD), PD is increasingly performed with the use of a cycler at night, referred to as automated peritoneal dialysis (APD) or continuous cycling peritoneal dialysis (CCPD). APD usually requires patients to be connected to the machine for 8 to 10 hours with or without a daytime manual exchange. Thus the flexibility of dialyzing at home with PD is counterbalanced by the need to perform dialysis daily.

The necessary lifestyle adjustments for either dialysis modality are extremely important when considering the studies that have compared the outcomes of HD and PD patients. It is widely accepted that randomized, controlled clinical trials are the gold standard when comparing the outcomes of patients treated with two different therapies. However, the disparate effects of each treatment on patients' lifestyles have stymied efforts to undertake randomized, controlled comparisons of HD and PD. For example, one clinical trial comparing these two modalities in the Netherlands was abandoned for futility as over 90% of eligible patients, when explained about the two treatment modalities, had a preference for one modality over the other and refused to be randomized (Table 59.2).

Table 59.2 Summary of Randomized, Controlled Trials Undertaken to Compare Various Kidney Replacement Therapies

First Author (Publication Year)[a]	Control Group	Intervention Group	Sample Size	Primary Outcome Measures	Key Results
Thrice-Weekly In-Center Hemodialysis Versus Peritoneal Dialysis					
Korevaar (2003)	Thrice-weekly hemodialysis	Peritoneal dialysis	38	Quality-adjusted life year score	95% of eligible subjects refused to be randomized, limiting external validity; in first 2 years, hemodialysis associated with slightly better quality-adjusted life year score
Thrice-Weekly In-Center Hemodialysis Versus Frequent In-Center Hemodialysis					
Chertow (2010)	2.9 treatments/week, mean duration, 213 min	5.2 treatments/week, mean duration, 154 min	245	Death or 12-month change in left ventricular mass; death or 12-month change in physical health score	Frequent hemodialysis associated with significant benefits with respect to both coprimary outcomes and improved control of blood pressure and serum phosphorus but higher incidence of vascular access procedures
Thrice-Weekly Hemodialysis Versus Frequent Nocturnal Home Hemodialysis					
Culleton (2007)	3 treatments/week, in-center	5–6 treatments/week, at least 6 hours per treatment	51	6-month change in left ventricular mass	Nocturnal hemodialysis associated with significant improvement in primary outcome, as well as kidney-specific domains of quality of life, blood pressure, and mineral metabolism
Rocco (2011)	2.9 treatments/week, mean duration, 256 min, home	5.1 treatments/week, mean duration, 379 min	87	Death or 12-month change in left ventricular mass; death or 12-month change in physical health score	No significant effect of nocturnal home hemodialysis or either of the two coprimary outcomes, but associated with improved control of hypertension and hyperphosphatemia; trend toward increased vascular access events
Thrice-Weekly Low Flux Hemodialysis Versus Post-Dilution On-Line Hemodiafiltration					
Grooteman (2012)	Low flux in-center hemodialysis	Post-dilution online hemodiafiltration with 6 L/hour convective clearances with high-flux dialyzers	714	All-cause mortality	No significant difference in all-cause mortality or cardiovascular events; post-hoc analyses showed that patients with higher convective clearances had lower all-cause mortality
Continuous Ambulatory Versus Automated Peritoneal Dialysis					
De Fijter (1994)	Continuous ambulatory peritoneal dialysis	Automated peritoneal dialysis	82	Patient and technique survival, time to first peritonitis, and hospital admission and catheter removal rates	Significantly fewer hospitalizations, and peritonitis rate with automated peritoneal dialysis; no difference in patient, or technique survival, or time to first peritonitis
Bro (1999)	Continuous ambulatory peritoneal dialysis	Automated peritoneal dialysis	34	Health-related quality of life	No difference in quality of life; too few events to assess the effect on clinical outcomes; automated peritoneal dialysis patients reported more time for work, family, and social activities

[a]Please see the full bibliography on www.expertconsult.com for a list of these studies.

In this clinical trial, patients randomized to HD had a slightly better health-related quality of life, but these findings have substantially limited external validity. A more recent effort to conduct a randomized, controlled comparison of HD and PD in China (Clinicaltrials.gov identifier: NCT01413074) that aimed to randomize 1370 patients with all-cause mortality as the primary outcome measure was terminated in December 2013 after 416 patients were enrolled. As of February 2017, results from this study remain unreported. Until then, one has to depend upon observational studies to compare the survival of HD and PD patients.

Over the 35 years since the advent of widespread use of PD for treatment of kidney failure, numerous single- and multicenter observational studies have compared the outcomes of patients treated with PD to those treated with HD. Despite differences among individual studies, analyses of survival data from national registries of patients who started treatment through the 1990s reveal a few common themes: overall, patients who started treatment with PD had a lower death risk for the first 1 to 2 years but a higher long-term risk. The apparent "early survival advantage" with PD was greater and of longer duration for younger and healthier patients, particularly among nondiabetics with no additional comorbidity. In contrast, there was little if any apparent "early survival advantage" with PD among older and sicker patients, and there appeared to be a higher long-term death risk.

In addition, since the mid-1990s, there has been a differential change in outcome of patients treated with the two dialysis therapies such that improvements in survival of patients treated with PD appear to outpace those seen for patients treated with HD, whereas the outcome of any types of kidney transplantations remains superior to both HD and PD (Fig. 59.3). This differential improvement in outcomes appears worldwide, with data emerging from the United States, France, Australia, New Zealand, Canada, Denmark, and Taiwan. The reasons for these differential changes over time are unclear but highlight the importance of considering an "era effect," or secular trend, in addition to the complexities in comparing the HD and PD outcomes mentioned earlier.

The results of observational studies that have compared the outcomes of HD and PD patients who started treatment after 2000 are summarized in Table 59.3. These contemporary studies, even though nonrandomized, have been more diligent in attempting to account for potential bias when comparing two therapies as different as HD and PD, with some applying advanced statistical tools like propensity scores and/or marginal structural models. Notwithstanding the sophistication of statistical models used, the risk for residual confounding persists. Stated differently, it remains uncertain if differences in outcomes of patients treated with the two therapies are a result of the dialysis modality or simply reflect the differences in outcomes of patients treated with HD and PD. With this caveat, these studies suggest that the "early survival advantage" with PD described in studies of earlier cohorts may be attributable to the high risk of death for patients who start HD with central venous catheters and disproportionate representation of late-referred patients in the HD cohort. In other words, the "early survival advantage" with PD may not be a direct benefit of PD but rather a result of differences in patients who were treated with PD compared with HD. More important, these studies demonstrate that the 4-, 5-, and 10-year survival of patients treated with HD and PD in different parts of the world with different PD utilization rates are similar. In addition, there are studies that demonstrate equivalent outcomes with HD and PD in subgroups of patients like those infected with hepatitis C, those with atheroembolic disease, or those returning to dialysis after a failed kidney transplant. Two studies seem to be the exception to the theme of equivalency of outcomes with HD and PD. One study, with data from the European registry, showed a robust survival advantage for patients who started treatment with PD, while a study from France showed a higher death risk among kidney failure patients with congestive heart failure treated with PD.

ALTERNATIVE HEMODIALYSIS REGIMENS

The length and frequency of hemodialysis sessions are primarily based upon feasibility and convenience, with thrice-weekly treatment regimens necessarily entailing one 3-day interval between HD treatments. Several observational studies have indicated that the death risk of patients is highest immediately after this long interdialytic interval—that is, on Monday for Monday-Wednesday-Friday and on Tuesday for Tuesday-Thursday-Saturday patients. Similarly, several studies have demonstrated an inverse association between length of each HD session and patient survival. This has led to an increasing use of HD with a frequency higher than thrice weekly and/or treatment duration longer than 3 to 4 hours per session (see Table 59.1).

Over the past 5 years, three randomized, controlled clinical trials have tested two of these alternative regimens (see Table 59.2). Patients treated with both short-daily in-center and nocturnal home HD achieved significant reductions in blood

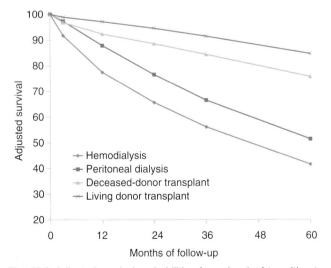

Fig. 59.3 Adjusted survival probabilities from day 1 of transition to kidney replacement therapy to compare 5-year survival of end-stage renal disease patients in the United States across hemodialysis, peritoneal dialysis, deceased donor transplantation, and living donor transplantation. The probabilities are adjusted for age, sex, race, Hispanic ethnicity, and primary diagnosis. (Adapted from the United States Renal Data System Annual Data Report.)

Continued

Table 59.3 Observational Studies That Compared Mortality in Entire Regional Populations of Incident In-Center Hemodialysis and Peritoneal Dialysis Patients Since 2000

First Author (Publication Year)[a]	Cohort Period/ Country	Sample Size	Statistical Approach	Follow-up Duration	Key Results
Liem (2007)	1987–2002 Netherlands	16,643 (HD 10,841; PD 5802)	Cox proportional hazards model	Up to 16 years	In younger diabetic and nondiabetic patients, lower risk for PD patients for the first 15 months; no difference thereafter. In older nondiabetics, lower risk for PD patients in the first 6 months, but higher risk after the first 15 months. In older diabetics, no difference in early death but higher risk for PD patients after the first 15 months
Huang (2008)	1995–2002 Taiwan	48,629 (HD 45,820; PD 2809)	Cox proportional hazards model	Up to 6 years	Overall similar 5-year (HD, 54%; PD, 56%) and 10-year survival (HD, 34%; PD, 35%); subgroup analysis showed higher risk for death among all diabetics, and older nondiabetics (>55 years age)
Sanabria (2008)	2001–2003 Colombia	923 (HD 437; PD 486)	Cox proportional hazards model	Up to December 2005	No difference in overall adjusted mortality rates between HD and PD; lower death risk for young, nondiabetic patients treated with PD but similar outcomes in all other groups
McDonald (2009)	1991–2005 Australia and New Zealand	25,287 (HD 14,733; PD 10,554)	Cox proportional hazards model, including analyses in propensity-score quartiles	Up to December 31, 2005	Overall 11% lower risk for death for PD patients in the first year, but 33% higher risk after the first 12 months; early survival advantage with PD seen only in young patients without comorbidities; in the most recent cohort (2004), no difference in long-term mortality of HD and PD patients
Weinhandl (2010)	20C3 USA	6337 pairs (HD 6337; PD 6337)	Propensity-score matched cohort	Up to 4 years	Overall mortality risk was 8% lower for PD patients. Similar adjusted 4-year-survival (HD, 48%; PD, 47%)
Mehrotra (2011)	1996–2004 USA	684,426 (HD 620,020; PD 64,406)	Marginal structural model	Up to 5 years	In 2002–2004, no significant difference in the 5-year adjusted survival of HD and PD patients (35% and 33%, respectively); lower risk for death for younger, nondiabetic PD patients; higher death risk for older diabetics—particularly those with additional comorbidity—treated with PD
Perl (2011)	2001–2008 Canada	38,512 (HD, 31,100; PD, 7412)	Proportional and nonproportional piecewise exponential survival model	Up to 5 years	First-year mortality of HD patients who started dialysis with a fistula or graft was similar to that with PD but significantly higher for those HD patients who started with central venous catheters; during entire follow-up period, HD patients with fistula/graft had lower and those with central venous catheters higher death risk than PD patients
Quinn (2011)	1998–2006 Ontario, Canada	6573 (HD, 4538; PD, 2035)	Cox proportional hazards model	—	No significant difference in early or late mortality of HD and PD patients who started dialysis electively as outpatients and had at least 4 months of predialysis nephrology care
Tranyor (2011)	1982–2006 Scotland	3197 (HD, 2107; PD, 1090)	Cox proportional hazards model	Through December 31, 2006	No significant difference in survival of nondiabetic transplant-listed patients treated with either hemodialysis or peritoneal dialysis

Table 59.3 Observational Studies That Compared Mortality in Entire Regional Populations of Incident In-Center Hemodialysis and Peritoneal Dialysis Patients Since 2000—cont'd

First Author (Publication Year)[a]	Cohort Period/ Country	Sample Size	Statistical Approach	Follow-up Duration	Key Results
Van de Luijtgaarden (2011)	1998–2006 ERA-EDTA Registry	15,828 (HD, 12,731; PD, 3097)	Cox proportional hazards model	Up to 3 years	18% lower 3-year death risk in patients starting treatment with PD; survival benefit greater in those with no underlying comorbidity and no difference in death risk in those with comorbidity
Yeates (2012)	1991–2004 Canada	46,839 (HD, 32,531; PD, 14,308)	Cox proportional hazards model	Up to December 31, 2007	For the 2001–2004 cohort, PD patients had a lower death risk than HD patients for the first 2 years, but there was no difference in death risk thereafter
Happio (2013)	2000–2009 Finland	4463 (HD, 3246; PD, 1217)	Cox proportional hazards model	Up to December 31, 2009	No significant difference in adjusted survival of patients treated with peritoneal dialysis or in-center hemodialysis
Choi (2013)	2008–2011 South Korea	1060 (HD, 736; PD, 324)	Cox proportional hazards model	Up to December 30, 2011	Overall, patients treated with PD had a 51% lower risk for death compared with those treated with in-center hemodialysis
Heaf (2014)	1990–2010 Denmark	12,095 (HD: 8273; PD, 3822)	Piecewise Cox regression	—	Significantly greater improvement in risk for death for patients treated with peritoneal dialysis than hemodialysis; starting 1995, significantly lower risk for death for patients treated with peritoneal dialysis, compared with hemodialysis; for the 2005–2010 cohort, 20% lower death risk
Kumar (2014)	2001–2013 Kaiser Permanente, Southern California	1003 propensity-score matched pairs	Stratified proportional hazards model	Up to June 30, 2013	There was a significantly higher risk for death for patients treated with in-center hemodialysis compared with peritoneal dialysis; the cumulative hazard ratio for death for patients treated with hemodialysis was 2.38 (1.68–3.40) and 2.10 (1.50–2.94), compared with peritoneal dialysis, in the as-treated and intent-to-treat analyses, respectively
Waldum-Grevbo (2015)	2005–2012 Norway	692 propensity-matched pairs	Cox proportional hazards model	Up to December 3, 2012	No significant difference in 2- or 5-year mortality of patients treated with hemodialysis or peritoneal dialysis or in subgroups by gender, diabetic status, or patients >65 years of age; significantly lower risk for death for patients ≤65 years age treated with PD compared with in-center hemodialysis
Van de Luijtgaarden (2016)	1993–2012 ERA-EDTA Registry	140,527 (HD, 112,258; PD, 28,269)	Cox proportional hazards model	Up to 5 years	No significant difference in 5-year survival of patients treated with hemodialysis or peritoneal dialysis for 1993–2002; 9% lower 5-year mortality for patients treated with peritoneal dialysis in 2003–2007, compared with hemodialysis. Generally lower risk for death with peritoneal dialysis in patients <65 years and without diabetes and higher risk for patients >65 years and with diabetes

[a]Please see the full bibliography on www.expertconsult.com for a list of these studies.

ERA-EDTA, European Renal Association, European Dialysis and Transplant Association; *HD,* hemodialysis; *PD,* peritoneal dialysis.

pressure, antihypertensive medications, serum phosphorus levels, and use of phosphate binders. Furthermore, patients randomized to short daily in-center HD had significant improvements in each of the two coprimary composite outcomes in these trials—death or change in left ventricular mass and death or change in physical health composite on a quality of life measure. In contrast, the results of the two clinical trials of nocturnal home HD have been inconsistent. While the smaller clinical trial from Canada showed a salutary effect of the treatment on left ventricular mass, there was no significant improvement in either of the two coprimary composite outcomes in the trial undertaken by the Frequent Hemodialysis Network (death or change in left ventricular mass; death or change in physical health composite). More important, the latter study illustrated yet again the challenges in randomizing patients to two therapies, with the investigators achieving only one-third of their enrollment goal. These data support the notion that intensive HD regimens are superior in improving a variety of intermediate outcomes, but whether they will lower death risk remains to be determined in larger studies.

At least 14 recent observational studies have evaluated the survival of patients treated with alternative HD regimens of varying combinations of increased length of each session and/or frequency compared with either conventional in-center HD or PD (Table 59.4). Four of five studies demonstrate a lower death risk with nocturnal HD, whether performed thrice weekly in-center or at home, when compared with patients treated with thrice-weekly, conventional duration in-center HD. Furthermore, the results of two studies comparing outcomes for patients treated with nocturnal home HD compared with those undergoing kidney transplantation are inconsistent: while one shows a no significant difference in risk for death, the more recent study demonstrates a significantly better survival rate for patients who undergo transplant compared with those treated with nocturnal HD. The only study that has compared outcomes of nocturnal HD with PD shows lower risk for death for patients treated with the former. A small but consistent survival advantage has also been reported for patients treated with short daily home HD, whether using the low-flow NxStage system or conventional machines, compared with conventional in-center HD or PD. Yet, the survival of elderly patients who undergo kidney transplantation is significantly better than those undergoing daily home HD.

These data are quite encouraging, but, as discussed above, caution needs to be exercised when interpreting observational studies comparing treatments with disparate effects on patients' lifestyle. Furthermore, the overall health and functional status of patients starting treatment with these alternative HD regimens is considerably better than even those treated with PD, and these differences cannot readily be accounted for by matching or other statistical adjustments. Thus there is substantial uncertainty as to whether the survival benefit seen in observational studies is attributable to the dialysis modality or reflects other characteristics of patients treated with these alternative HD regimens.

In summary, it is highly unlikely that a randomized trial testing the efficacy of any of these alternative HD regimens, adequately powered for mortality, will be undertaken in the near future. Thus providers should be aware of the proven benefits of these alternative HD regimens on important

intermediate measures and ensure patients are offered the wide range of HD treatment options.

INCREMENTAL AND INFREQUENT HEMODIALYSIS

Although the prevailing dialysis modality paradigm has been to initiate "full-dose" thrice-weekly HD treatment schedules irrespective of native kidney function in most industrialized nations, recent data suggest that a more gradual approach with less than thrice-weekly HD may preserve residual kidney function longer in those who have substantial native kidney function at initiation. Given consistent data that suggest a strong association between higher residual kidney function and better clinical outcomes in both HD and PD patients, a renewed interest in incremental transition has emerged. Registry and large national dialysis data suggest that a sizeable proportion of patients on dialysis have substantial levels of residual kidney function at the start of dialysis therapy.

Recognizing the benefits of residual kidney function on health-related quality of life and survival of patients treated with dialysis, as well as other relevant outcomes such as less burden of dialysis vascular access, there has been growing interest in incremental HD in recent years, in which HD frequency and dose are tailored to patients' residual native kidney function. Infrequent (once- to twice-weekly) HD can also be offered as an alternative to those who prefer a more conservative approach in managing uremia including palliative dialysis. Clinical practice guidelines support the use of once- to twice-weekly HD among patients with adequate residual kidney function including a renal urea clearance greater than 3 mL/min per 1.73 m^2 and urine output greater than 600 mL/min per day, while other criteria should also be considered (Table 59.5). These criteria can also be used to make recommendations or the decision to transition the patient from twice- to thrice-weekly HD. Recent data suggest that incremental HD is associated with longer preservation of residual kidney function, while survival is comparable in those with substantial native kidney function. Currently, incremental HD remains an underutilized approach in North America and Europe.

ON-LINE HEMODIAFILTRATION

Hemodiafiltration (HDF) combines both hemofiltration (HF) and HD in a single procedure. Whereas in the United States HDF is mostly performed in intensive care units, many other countries have adapted this modality for outpatient therapy, mostly known as "on-line" HDF. On-line HDF, where replacement fluid is prepared from ultrapure dialysate, can be performed safely because of recent technologic advances; however, in some countries, including the United States, government restrictions prohibit the use of on-line HDF. HDF was initially performed in adults in 1977, and later used in children in the early 1980s. The use of HDF allows significantly higher convective clearances to be combined with the diffusive dialysis clearances, resulting in a better tolerated treatment session. Although at least six randomized trials have compared HDF to either low-flux (three trials) or high-flux HD (three trials), HDF was associated with a lower risk for all-cause and cardiovascular mortality in only one of these six trials.

Table 59.4 Observational Studies of Mortality With Alternative Hemodialysis Regimens

First Author (Publication Year)[a]	Treatment Group	Comparator Group	Key Results
Nocturnal In-Center Hemodialysis			
Lacson (2010)	655 patients, 3 HD sessions/week, mean duration 470 min	15,334 patients, 3 HD sessions/week, mean duration 222 min	No significant difference in adjusted death risk but lower hospitalizations in patients treated with nocturnal in-center hemodialysis
Lacson (2012)	746 patients, 3 HD sessions/week, mean duration 471 min	2062 propensity-score matched conventional HD patients	Nocturnal in-center hemodialysis associated with 25% lower death risk
Rivara (2016)	1206 patients, on average 2.8 sessions/week, treatment duration of 399 min	111,707 patients undergoing conventional hemodialysis, on average 2.9 sessions/week, treatment duration 211 min	33% lower adjusted risk for death in patients undergoing extended hours nocturnal in-center hemodialysis
Frequent, Diurnal Home Hemodialysis			
Johansen (2009)	43 patients, median 5 HD sessions/week, 2.8 hours/session, majority with Aksys machine	Propensity-score matched in-center hemodialysis patients from the United States Renal Data System	No difference in death risk or composite outcome of death, acute myocardial infarction, or stroke, with frequent, diurnal home hemodialysis
Weinhandl (2012)	1873 patients treated with NxStage One HD system	9365 propensity-score matched in-center hemodialysis patients from the United States Renal Data System	Home hemodialysis with NxStage One system associated with 13% lower risk for all-cause mortality and 8% lower risk of cardiovascular mortality
Marshall (2016)	1763 patients with quasi-intensive home HD (longer and more/or more frequent HD but <5/week) and 375 patients treated with intensive home HD (≥5×/week, any hours per session)	32,283 patients treated with conventional facility HD	44% lower mortality with quasi-intensive home HD; lower risk with intensive home HD seen in some but not all statistical models
Molnar (2016)	480 patients ≥65 years of age starting frequent home HD between 2007 and 2011	480 propensity-score matched patients undergoing kidney transplant between 2007 and 2011	The adjusted risk for death in patients undergoing home HD was almost fivefold higher than those who underwent kidney transplantation
Nesrallah (2016)	2688 consecutive adults starting daily home hemodialysis (≥5 days/week for ≥1.5 hours/day)	2688 propensity-score matched patients starting peritoneal dialysis	25% lower death risk in patients starting treatment with home hemodialysis compared with peritoneal dialysis
Weinhandl (2016)	4201 patients treated with NxStage One HD system	4201 propensity-score matched patients treated with peritoneal dialysis	Home HD associated with 20% lower all-cause mortality, 8% lower hospitalizations, and 37% lower risk for transfer to in-center hemodialysis; no significant difference in outcomes in patients that started home HD within 6 months of ESRD onset, compared with those treated with peritoneal dialysis
Nocturnal or Long-Duration Home Hemodialysis			
Johansen (2009)	94 patients, median 6 sessions/week, 8 hours/session	Propensity-score matched in-center hemodialysis patients from the United States Renal Data System	Significantly lower death risk with nocturnal home hemodialysis; no difference in hospitalizations
Pauly (2009)	177 patients, 3–7 sessions/week, 6–8 hours/session	533 matched deceased donor and 533 matched living donor kidney transplant recipients	Survival of nocturnal home hemodialysis patients similar to that of deceased donor transplant recipients but inferior to that of living donor transplant recipients
Nesrallah (2012)	338 patients, 4.8 sessions/week, mean duration, 441 min	1388 matched patients from Dialysis Outcomes and Practice Patterns study participants, 3 sessions/week, mean duration 236 min	45% lower death risk in patients treated with intensive home hemodialysis
Tennankore (2014)	173 patients undergoing ≥16 hours of home HD/week; 165 with 5–7 sessions/week, ≥5.5 hours/session; 8 patients 3–4 sessions/week, ≥5.5 hours/session	673 living donor recipients, 642 standard criteria deceased donor recipients, and 202 expanded criteria deceased donor recipients	Patients with a kidney transplant, without regard to the donor type, had lower risk for composite outcome of time to treatment failure or death
Nadeau-Fredette (2015)	706 incident patients, included conventional, long, frequent, or long/frequent sessions	10,710 incident patients starting treatment with peritoneal dialysis	53% lower adjusted death risk and 66% lower adjusted risk for death or transfer to in-center dialysis in patients treated with home hemodialysis compared with peritoneal dialysis

aPlease see the full bibliography on www.expertconsult.com for a list of these studies.

ESRD, End-stage renal disease; HD, hemodialysis.

Table 59.5   Proposed Decision Support System With 11 Criteria for Initiating and Maintaining Incremental (Twice-Weekly) Hemodialysis Treatment Upon Transition to End-Stage Renal Disease and for Incremental Transition to Thrice-Weekly Hemodialysis

Incremental (Twice-Weekly) Hemodialysis Treatment Criteria

1. Adequate residual kidney function with a urine output >600 mL/day (transition to thrice-weekly if urine output drops to <500 mL/day)[a]
2. Limited fluid retention between two consecutive hemodialysis treatments with a fluid gain <2.5 kg (or <5% of the ideal dry weight) without hemodialysis for 3 to 4 days
3. Limited or readily manageable cardiovascular or pulmonary symptoms without clinically significant fluid overload[b]
4. Suitable body size relative to residual renal function; patients with larger body size may be suitable for twice-weekly hemodialysis if not hypercatabolic
5. Hyperkalemia (K > 5.5 mEq/L) infrequent or readily manageable
6. Hyperphosphatemia (P > 5.5 mg/dL) infrequent or readily manageable
7. Good nutritional status without florid hypercatabolic state
8. Lack of profound anemia (hemoglobin >8 g/dL) and appropriate responsiveness to anemia therapy
9. Infrequent hospitalization and easily manageable comorbid conditions
10. Satisfactory health-related quality of life and functional status
11. Residual urea clearance (KRU) >3 mL/min/1.73 m^2 (transition to thrice-weekly if KRU <2 mL/min/1.73 m^2)¶

Implementation Strategies

1. To initiate twice-weekly hemodialysis, the patient should meet the first (urine output >600 mL/day) *and* the last criteria (KRU > 3 mL/min/1.73 m^2),[c] *plus* most (five out of nine) other criteria.
2. Examine these criteria every 1–3 months in all twice-weekly hemodialysis patients and compare outcome measures between twice-weekly and thrice-weekly hemodialysis patients to assure outcome noninferiority for continuation of twice-weekly hemodialysis.
3. Consider transition from a twice-weekly to thrice-weekly hemodialysis regimen if patient's urine output drops <500 mL/day, if KRU declines <2 mL/min/1.73 m^2, or if patient's nutritional status or general health condition shows a deteriorating trend over time.

[a]The minimum required urine output to initiate twice-weekly hemodialysis has been changed to 600 mL/day in this adaptation, while >500 mL/day is needed to maintain twice-weekly regimen.
[b]Lack of systolic dysfunction (ejection fraction > 40%) and no major coronary intervention over the past 3 months.
[c]Added criterion in this adaptation.
Adapted from Kalantar-Zadeh K, Unruh M, Zager PG, Kovesdy CP, Bargman JM, Chen J, Sankarasubbaiyan S, Shah G, Golper T, Sherman RA, Goldfarb DS. Twice-weekly and incremental hemodialysis treatment for initiation of kidney replacement therapy. *Am J Kidney Dis.* 2014;64:181–186.

VARIATIONS IN PERITONEAL DIALYSIS REGIMENS

As indicated earlier, PD can be performed either as CAPD or APD. In addition to the different lifestyle implications, APD is more expensive than CAPD. In most of the developed world, APD has become the dominant PD modality, driven largely by lifestyle considerations associated with PD with a cycler performed overnight. On the other hand, PD patients in the developing world, including the emerging economies, are almost exclusively treated with CAPD primarily for economic reasons. There are potential medical differences between the two PD modalities that have been considered, with several studies suggesting that APD is associated with a more rapid decline in residual kidney function. Moreover, there is concern that frequent nighttime exchanges with APD may lead to inadequate volume removal compared with that achieved with CAPD. However, evidence for these potential adverse effects of APD is, at best, inconsistent. Nevertheless, it is important to determine if the medical outcomes with CAPD and APD are equivalent.

Two randomized, controlled trials that have compared CAPD and APD were unable to demonstrate any significant differences in any medical outcomes (see Table 59.2).

However, because of small sample sizes, these studies were inadequately powered to determine relevant differences in outcomes by modality. In recent years, at least eight large observational studies have examined the relative outcomes with CAPD and APD (Table 59.6). The preponderance of evidence suggests that there is no overall difference in either all-cause mortality or technique survival in patients treated with CAPD and APD (Fig. 59.4), although APD may offer a survival advantage in the high/fast transporter subgroup of patients. Thus as the available data seems to support no significant differences in the medical outcomes of patients treated with CAPD and APD, it follows that lifestyle and economic considerations will continue to drive the differential utilization of the two PD modalities in different parts of the world.

DIALYSIS MODALITY IN CHILDREN

Most children with ESRD who need dialysis before receiving a kidney transplant undergo PD, although a significant proportion is treated with in-center and home HD therapies. Despite interest and feasibility of on-line HDF in children, the majority of pediatric dialysis units across the world still

Table 59.6 Multicenter Observational Studies of Continuous Ambulatory Peritoneal Dialysis and Automated Peritoneal Dialysis

First Author et al. (Publication Year)[a]	Cohort Period/ Country	Data Source	Sample Size (CAPD vs. APD)	Follow-Up Duration	OUTCOME COMPARISON BETWEEN CAPD AND APD	
					Patient Survival	Technique Survival
Mujais (2006)	2000–2003 USA	Baxter Healthcare Corporation On-Call system	Total 40,869	Through June 2005	No difference	Better in APD group
Badve (2008)	1999–2004 Australia and New Zealand	Australia and New Zealand Dialysis and Transplant (ANZDATA) Registry	2393 vs. 1735	Through March 2004	No difference	No difference
Mehrotra (2009)	1996–2004 USA	United States Renal Disease System (USRDS)	42,942 vs. 23,439	Through September 2006	No difference	No difference
Michels (2009)	1997–2006 Netherlands	The Netherlands Cooperative Study on the Adequacy of Dialysis (NECOSAD)	562 vs. 87	Through August 2007	No difference	No difference
Johnson (2010)	1999–2004 Australia and New Zealand	Australia and New Zealand Dialysis and Transplant (ANZDATA) Registry	High transporters (142 vs. 486) Low transporters (n = 196)	—	Lower death risk with APD for high transporters and higher for low transporters	No difference
Cnossen (2011)	2001–2008 USA	Renal Research Institute	179 vs. 441	—	No difference	No difference
Sun (2011)	1997–2008 Taiwan	University-affiliated hospitals in Northern Taiwan	121 vs. 161	Through December 2008	Lower risk with APD in patients <65 years of age	Lower risk with APD in patients <65 years of age
Beduschi (2015)	2004–2011 Brazil	BRAZPD II	1445 propensity-score matched pairs	Through December 2011	Higher risk for death with CAPD	No difference

[a]Please see the full bibliography on www.expertconsult.com for a list of these studies.
APD, Automated peritoneal dialysis; *CAPD*, continuous ambulatory peritoneal dialysis.

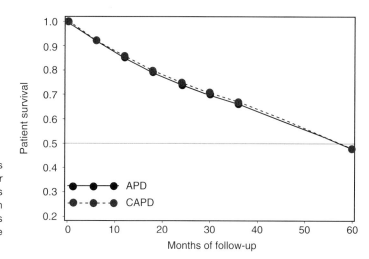

Fig. 59.4 Comparison of survival of patients treated with continuous ambulatory and automated peritoneal dialysis in the United States for 1996 to 2004. *APD*, Automated peritoneal dialysis; *CAPD*, continuous ambulatory peritoneal dialysis. (Figure reproduced with permission from Mehrotra R, Chiu YW, Kalantar-Zadeh K, et al. Similar outcomes with hemodialysis and peritoneal dialysis in patients with end-stage renal disease. *Arch Intern Med*. 2011;171:110–118.)

perform HD using highly permeable membranes, allowing back filtration in the filter and therefore a degree of convective flow (i.e., internal HDF). Notwithstanding the general assumption that transplant is the best option for children, there are currently no convincing data as to which of the dialysis modalities offers better outcome in children who are awaiting a kidney transplant.

IMPLICATIONS FOR DIALYSIS MODALITY SELECTION

Understanding the differences in outcomes with the various kidney replacement therapies will help guide individual patients as they weigh their choices for the treatment of kidney failure. A diagnosis of advanced CKD (eGFR <30 mL/ min/1.73 m^2) and the imminent need to transition to dialysis is stress provoking and sometimes devastating, with approximately 10% of patients having a constellation of symptoms consistent with posttraumatic stress disorder. Structured interviews and focus groups of ESRD patients indicate that, when considering dialysis modalities, many are confronting their mortality and worrying about being a burden on others; patients and their families seek knowledge about treatment options, are concerned about actual or perceived lack of choice, and weigh alternatives to determine what effect the treatment will have on their lifestyles.

It is unclear whether very old persons with advanced CKD or those with more severe comorbid states and shorter life expectancy will benefit from transition to dialysis. It has been argued, although not unequivocally proven, that some of these patients may have similar or even better quality of life and longevity if they continue with a conservative management of kidney failure without dialysis or kidney transplantation. Some others may prefer to choose palliative and infrequent dialysis regimen to mitigate the level of dialysis-associated anxiety and reduce personal and family burden. It is against this background of emotional turmoil that practitioners should juxtapose the paucity of adequately powered randomized, controlled trials to determine the effect of any given dialysis therapy versus none on hard outcomes, and the uncertainty of attribution from observational studies. It appears reasonable

to conclude that, for most ESRD patients, there are no compelling medical reasons to choose one dialysis therapy over another. Instead, the primary goal of the health care provider should be to provide iterative education about different treatment options and allow the patient to choose the kidney replacement therapy that best allows him or her to lead a fulfilling and productive life.

KEY BIBLIOGRAPHY

Chertow GM, Levin NW, Beck GJ, et al. In-center hemodialysis six times per week versus three times per week. *N Engl J Med*. 2010;363: 2287-2300.

Culleton BF, Walsh M, Klarenbach SW, et al. Effect of frequent nocturnal hemodialysis vs conventional hemodialysis on left ventricular mass and quality of life: a randomized controlled trial. *JAMA*. 2007;298: 1291-1299.

Foley RN, Gilbertson DT, Murray T, et al. Long interdialytic interval and mortality among patients receiving hemodialysis. *N Engl J Med*. 2011;365:1099-1107.

Grooteman MP, van den Dorpel MA, Bots ML, et al. Effect of online hemodiafiltration on all-cause mortality and cardiovascular outcomes. *J Am Soc Nephrol*. 2012;23:1087-1096.

Johansen KL, Zhang R, Huang Y, et al. Survival and hospitalization among patients using nocturnal and short daily compared to conventional hemodialysis: a USRDS study. *Kidney Int*. 2009;76:984-990.

Kalantar-Zadeh K, Unruh M, Zager PG, Kovesdy CP, Bargman JM, Chen J, Sankarasubbaiyan S, Shah G, Golper T, Sherman RA, Goldfarb DS. Twice-weekly and incremental hemodialysis treatment for initiation of kidney replacement therapy. *Am J Kidney Dis*. 2014;64: 181-186.

Korevaar JC, Feith GW, Dekker FW, et al. Effect of starting hemodialysis compared with peritoneal dialysis in patients new on dialysis treatment: a randomized controlled trial. *Kidney Int*. 2003;64:2222-2228.

Lacson E Jr, Xu J, Suri R, et al. Survival with three-times weekly in-center nocturnal versus conventional hemodialysis. *J Am Soc Nephrol*. 2012;23:687-695.

McDonald SP, Marshall MR, Johnson DW, et al. Relationship between dialysis modality and mortality. *J Am Soc Nephrol*. 2009;20: 155-163.

Mehrotra R, Chiu YW, Kalantar-Zadeh K, et al. Similar outcomes with hemodialysis and peritoneal dialysis in patients with end-stage renal disease. *Arch Intern Med*. 2011;171:110-118.

Mehrotra R, Chiu YW, Kalantar-Zadeh K, et al. The outcomes of continuous ambulatory and automated peritoneal dialysis are similar. *Kidney Int*. 2009;76:97-107.

Mehrotra R, Kermah D, Fried L, et al. Chronic peritoneal dialysis in the United States: declining utilization despite improving outcomes. *J Am Soc Nephrol*. 2007;18:2781-2788.

Morton RL, Tong A, Howard K, et al. The views of patients and carers in treatment decision making for chronic kidney disease: systematic review and thematic synthesis of qualitative studies. *BMJ.* 2010;340:c112.

Nesrallah GE, Lindsay RM, Cuerden MS, et al. Intensive hemodialysis associates with improved survival compared with conventional hemodialysis. *J Am Soc Nephrol.* 2012;23:696-705.

Obi Y, Streja E, Rhee CM, Ravel V, Amin AN, Cupisti A, Chen J, Mathew AT, Kovesdy CP, Mehrotra R, Kalantar-Zadeh K. Incremental hemodialysis, residual kidney function, and mortality risk in incident dialysis patients: a cohort study. *Am J Kidney Dis.* 2016;68:256-265.

Rocco MV, Lockridge RS Jr, Beck GJ, et al. The effects of frequent nocturnal home hemodialysis: the frequent hemodialysis network nocturnal trial. *Kidney Int.* 2011;80:1080-1091.

Vonesh EF, Snyder JJ, Foley RN, et al. The differential impact of risk factors on mortality in hemodialysis and peritoneal dialysis. *Kidney Int.* 2004;66:2389-2401.

Weinhandl ED, Foley RN, Gilbertson DT, et al. Propensity-matched mortality comparison of incident hemodialysis and peritoneal dialysis patients. *J Am Soc Nephrol.* 2010;21:499-506.

Weinhandl ED, Liu J, Gilbertson DT, et al. Survival in daily home hemodialysis and matched thrice-weekly in-center hemodialysis patients. *J Am Soc Nephrol.* 2012;23:895-904.

Wolfe RA, Ashby VB, Milford EL, et al. Comparison of mortality in all patients on dialysis, patients on dialysis awaiting transplantation, and recipients of a first cadaveric transplant. *N Engl J Med.* 1999;341:1725-1730.

Full bibliography can be found on www.expertconsult.com.

Selection of Prospective Kidney Transplant Recipients and Donors

60

Greg Knoll; Todd Fairhead

Kidney transplantation is the treatment of choice for most patients with end-stage kidney disease (ESKD) because it prolongs survival, improves quality of life, and is less costly than the alternative therapy of dialysis. However, less than 20% of ESKD patients actually receive a transplant. Many patients are not suitable candidates because of coexisting illness that may affect perioperative risk and survival after transplantation, but for those patients who are eligible, there are simply not enough organs available. As the primary contact for patients with advanced chronic kidney disease (CKD), as well as for those already on dialysis, nephrologists are in a unique position to counsel and guide patients through the transplantation process. A thorough understanding of who is suitable for transplantation and the required evaluation will facilitate this process.

WHO SHOULD BE CONSIDERED FOR KIDNEY TRANSPLANTATION?

There are very few absolute contraindications for kidney transplantation. In most populations studied, including the elderly and patients with diabetes with ESKD, kidney transplantation confers a survival advantage. All patients should be evaluated by their nephrologist for transplant suitability and potentially referred to a transplant center for further evaluation. Eligibility should not be based on age, sex, race, or socioeconomic status. Given that donor kidneys are a rare and limited resource, a patient must be expected to survive beyond current waiting times for transplantation. Careful evaluation of physiologic age, medical comorbidities, and functional status will help determine whether a patient may be eligible for transplantation. Box 60.1 lists the contraindications for transplantation.

TIMING OF REFERRAL

Both mortality and graft outcomes are improved with early transplantation. Patients who receive a preemptive kidney transplant have a superior outcome compared with patients who undergo dialysis treatments before receiving a transplant. Similarly, the length of exposure to dialysis affects transplant outcomes and mortality. Improved outcomes are inversely related to the duration of dialysis. Thus to allow adequate time to complete the required medical tests before transplantation and to facilitate potential preemptive transplantation, patients with CKD should be referred to a kidney transplant center early in their disease course. Many potential transplant recipients are medically complex. Determining their suitability for transplantation may require multiple specialist visits and medical tests. This process may take 6 to 12 months to complete and should be factored into the overall referral time. For patients with potential living donors, appropriate time should be allocated for donor workup as well.

In the United States, the United Network for Organ Sharing (UNOS) allows listing for transplantation when a patient's estimated glomerular filtration rate (eGFR) falls below 20 mL/min, whereas organizations in other countries have established stage 5 CKD (eGFR below 15 mL/min) as the upper limit for listing. Thus patients should be referred for transplantation evaluation when they have stage 4 CKD (eGFR below 30 mL/min) that is progressing. In many programs, transplantation assessment is initiated with referral to a multidisciplinary kidney replacement therapy planning clinic. In these clinics, transplant eligibility is considered, and teaching is provided alongside planning for dialysis initiation. Education and identification of potential living kidney donors should be prioritized. It is important to recognize that certain barriers to transplant referral have been identified. Access to transplantation may be decreased for patients of certain ethnicities, those with lower socioeconomic status and/or education level, or those living a greater distance from a transplant referral center.

MEDICAL EVALUATION FOR TRANSPLANTATION

A complete medical, surgical, and psychosocial history is required upon consideration for transplantation. A thorough physical examination may identify underlying systemic diseases that may affect transplant suitability, such as poor dentition or diminished arterial pulses. Table 60.1 lists the minimum investigations required before transplantation. Additional testing based on medical comorbidities may be necessary. Each coexisting illness should be evaluated for its potential effect on transplant outcome. In addition, total disease burden and functional capacity must be factored into a final decision. The American Society of Transplantation (2001), the Canadian Society of Transplantation (2005), and the European Renal Best Practice group (2015) have published clinical practice guidelines for the eligibility of kidney transplant recipients. The international guideline group, Kidney Disease: Improving Global Outcomes (KDIGO) has begun work on a clinical

Box 60.1 Contraindications to Kidney Transplantation

Chronic illness with life expectancy <1 year
Active malignancy with short life expectancy
Active infection
Poorly controlled psychosis
Medical nonadherence or active substance abuse

Table 60.1 Proposed Workup for Potential Kidney Transplant Candidates

Test	Comments
Physical examination	Attention to dentition, arterial pulses
Tissue typing	ABO blood type, HLA identification, PRA
Viral serology	CMV, EBV, VZV, HSV, HCV, HBV, HIV, HTLV, VDRL
Cardiac testing	ECG
	Echocardiogram
	Risk stratification if high risk
Imaging	Chest radiograph
	Abdominal ultrasound or imaging equivalent
	Arterial vascular imaging if high risk (Doppler ultrasound, CT scan, angiogram)
Female specific	Breast examination and mammogram
	Pap smear
Male specific	Prostate examination
Consultations	Transplant surgeon
	Cardiologist (if high risk)
	Social worker

CMV, Cytomegalovirus; *CT*, computerized tomography; *EBV*, Epstein-Barr virus; *ECG*, electrocardiogram; *HBV*, hepatitis B virus; *HCV*, hepatitis C virus; *HIV*, human immunodeficiency virus; *HLA*, human leukocyte antigen; *HSV*, herpes simplex virus; *HTLV*, human T-lymphotropic virus; *PRA*, panel-reactive antibody; *VDRL*, Venereal Disease Research Laboratory (test); *VZV*, varicella-zoster virus.

practice guideline for the evaluation and management of candidates for kidney transplantation. This guideline will update existing literature and provide detailed guidance on the assessment of complex patients. The guideline scope is no longer appearing on the KDIGO website.

GENERAL CONSIDERATIONS

Advanced age is not a contraindication to transplantation. At present, patients over 65 years of age are the fastest growing group of wait-listed potential recipients. Death-censored graft outcomes are similar or better in these older adult recipients. With advanced age, special attention should be paid to pretransplant medical comorbidities, functional status, and quality of life. The cost of maintaining a proposed recipient on the waiting list is not insignificant. A patient's capacity to survive beyond current waiting list times to transplantation

and beyond must be considered. The technical aspects of the transplant surgery limit transplantation in extremely young children. However, this should not delay transplant workup, and preemptive transplantation should be considered when possible.

OBESITY

Patients with extreme obesity are susceptible to an increased risk for transplant-related complications, including delayed graft function, wound complications, and infections, as well as an increased risk for new-onset diabetes after transplantation. In some studies, long-term graft failure rates and mortality are higher among obese recipients when compared with otherwise comparable recipients. As such, many transplant programs avoid transplanting patients with extreme obesity. Individual programs limit transplantation to individuals under a certain body mass index (BMI), usually 40 kg/m^2. In patients with a BMI between 30 and 39 kg/m^2, weight-loss counseling should be provided. Bariatric surgery may be considered in individuals with a BMI greater than 40 kg/m^2.

KIDNEY DISEASE

Many kidney diseases recur after transplantation. Recent analyses suggest that allograft failure secondary to recurrent disease is now the third most common reason for graft failure, behind rejection and death with a functioning graft. In an analysis of the Australia and New Zealand Dialysis and Transplant Registry (ANZDATA), allograft loss due to recurrent disease occurred in 8.4% of patients with biopsy-proven glomerulonephritis who received a kidney transplant. Similarly, when the Mayo Clinic retrospectively analyzed specific causes of kidney allograft loss, recurrent disease was diagnosed in 14.3% of all lost allografts. An additional 6.5% of graft loss was due to glomerular pathology that could not be classified as recurrent because of incomplete clinical information. Despite this, the risk for recurrence rarely precludes transplantation, and allograft failure from recurrence is rare in the first 5 years posttransplant. In the ANZDATA analysis, the overall 10-year incidence of allograft loss was similar among transplant recipients with glomerulonephritis versus those with other causes of kidney failure, and no risks were identified that would preclude transplantation. It is important to counsel prospective transplant recipients about the risk for recurrent disease. Table 60.2 shows the incidence of recurrence of different forms of kidney disease.

Immunoglobulin A (IgA) nephropathy may recur in up to 60% of allograft biopsies; however, clinically significant recurrence (with elevated creatinine or proteinuria) develops in only 30% of kidney transplants. Furthermore, clinical recurrence tends to be late, and graft loss due to IgA nephropathy occurs in only 10% of patients. Focal segmental glomerulosclerosis (FSGS) can recur in up to 30% of transplant recipients and is more common in those with primary FSGS. In patients with a previously failed allograft due to recurrent FSGS, the risk for recurrence rises to as high as 50%–80%. In many cases, recurrence appears to be secondary to a circulating permeability factor that affects podocyte foot process and glomerular slit diaphragm integrity. Plasma exchange may reduce proteinuria and prolong the life of the allograft. Recently, the circulating permeability factor was proposed

Table 60.2 Risk for Recurrence and Graft Loss After Transplantation

Type of Glomerulonephritis	Risk for Clinically Relevant Recurrence (% of patients)	Risk for Graft Failure 5–10 Years Posttransplant (% of patients)
IgA nephropathy	15–50	10
FSGS	30	20
Membranous nephropathy	40	15
MPGN (immune complex)	30–50	15
MPGN (dense deposit disease)	80	50
ANCA glomerulonephritis	10–15	5
SLE	5	3
Anti-GBM	<5	Rare
Fibrillary/immunotactoid glomerulopathy	>50	Unknown

ANCA, Antineutrophil cytoplasmic antigen; *FSGS,* focal segmental glomerulosclerosis; *GBM,* glomerular basement membrane; *MPGN,* membranoproliferative glomerulonephritis; *SLE,* systemic lupus erythematosus.

to be soluble urokinase-type plasminogen activator receptor (suPAR); although this is unproven, this line of research gives hope for more definitive treatments for recurrent FSGS in the future. Membranous nephropathy can recur in up to 40% of cases posttransplant. Unlike in the nontransplanted kidney, spontaneous remission is rare, and graft failure can occur in as many as 50% of cases by 10 years. Rituximab may limit proteinuria and allograft damage after recurrence.

Membranoproliferative glomerulonephritis (MPGN) has a high rate of recurrence posttransplantation, with immune complex-mediated MPGN recurring in 30% to 50% of patients and dense deposit disease recurring in over 80% of patients. The presence of serum monoclonal proteins and low complement levels at the time of transplantation are risks for MPGN recurrence. Recurrence of MPGN is usually early in the transplant course and is associated with proteinuria. The risk for graft loss from immune complex-mediated MPGN is approximately 15% at 10 years, whereas it is as high as 50% after 5 years in dense deposit disease. Recurrence of rapidly progressive glomerulonephritis is rare if disease is quiescent at the time of transplantation. In patients with antiglomerular basement membrane (anti-GBM) disease, the absence of circulating anti-GBM antibodies should be confirmed before considering transplantation. Although the presence of antineutrophil cytoplasmic antibodies (ANCA) does not preclude transplantation, patients should achieve a clinical remission period in which they are not taking immunosuppressive medications before transplantation. Similarly, a positive serostatus in patients with systemic lupus erythematosus (SLE) does not preclude transplantation; however, disease should be quiescent. Recurrence of lupus nephritis is rare (<20%), possibly because of protection from immunosuppressive transplant medications. Glomerular

diseases with organizing deposits, such as amyloidosis, fibrillary, and immunotactoid glomerulonephritis, can all recur with rates greater than 50%. With both primary and secondary forms of amyloidosis, transplantation is often limited by severe cardiac disease; early death from cardiovascular disease or infection is quite high. The total burden of amyloidosis needs to be considered before transplantation.

Genetic forms of kidney disease may affect the transplanted allograft. Rarely, patients with Alport disease can develop antibodies against type IV collagen leading to a condition similar to anti-GBM disease. Patients with primary oxalosis are highly susceptible to rapid oxalate deposition in the transplanted kidney without treatment. These patients are best managed with concurrent liver transplantation and supplementation with orthophosphate and pyridoxine. Patients with atypical hemolytic uremic syndrome (HUS) due to complement mutations have a rate of recurrent disease and graft failure of up to 60% to 70% at 2 years' posttransplantation. Treatment with the complement C5 inhibitor, eculizumab, should strongly be considered. Patients with kidney failure secondary to sickle cell nephropathy can be safely transplanted with good results, providing their overall health allows transplantation.

INFECTION

The presence of an active infection—bacterial, fungal, or viral—is a contraindication for transplantation. All potential recipients should be screened for chronic infections during the transplant evaluation and assessed for acute infection at the time of transplantation. Clinical and occult dialysis access-related infections in indwelling peritoneal dialysis catheters and tunneled hemodialysis catheters need to be fully treated before transplantation.

Efforts to protect immunosuppressed recipients should occur before transplantation. Transplant candidates should be immunized against seasonal influenza, hepatitis B virus (HBV), and pneumococcal pneumonia. In addition, vaccination against human papillomavirus and primary (chickenpox) and secondary (shingles) varicella-zoster infection should be considered in high-risk recipients. Although efficacy of immunization is notably poor in the ESKD population, risk for infection posttransplant is high.

Cytomegalovirus (CMV) can be transmitted via kidney transplant, and it commonly leads to disease if untreated. Measuring a potential recipient's CMV serostatus is important before transplantation, but a negative serostatus does not preclude receipt of a kidney transplant from a CMV-positive donor. In addition, potential recipients and donors should be screened for Epstein-Barr virus (EBV) and herpes simplex virus (HSV) before transplant. Those recipients with an EBV-mismatched kidney transplant should undergo EBV virus surveillance for posttransplant lymphoproliferative disorder (PTLD), whereas HSV-mismatched patients may be offered acyclovir for prophylaxis.

Tuberculosis (TB) infection is common in immunosuppressed kidney transplant patients, and it may approach 15% in TB-endemic areas. Risk factors for developing TB after transplant include a positive tuberculin skin test reaction before transplant, prior residence in a TB-endemic area, a chest radiograph suggestive of prior TB, and older age. Before transplantation, all potential recipients should undergo tuberculin skin testing and a chest radiograph. High-risk patients should undergo prophylactic TB treatment for 6 to 12 months in the absence of documented prior treatment. It is probably safe to proceed with transplantation after beginning prophylactic TB treatment, but evidence is lacking.

Although once considered an absolute contraindication, kidney transplantation in human immunodeficiency virus (HIV)–positive recipients has become possible in the current era of highly active antiretroviral therapy (HAART). Patient and allograft survival in this population is acceptable, and no worse than other high-risk groups (e.g., older recipients), although the incidence of acute rejection is increased. Patients with HIV should be referred to a transplant center with experience managing this infection. In general, patients should be compliant with HAART therapy, HIV RNA should be undetectable, and the CD4 count should be greater than 200 mm^3 before consideration for transplant.

In the modern era of immunosuppression, allograft loss due to BK (polyoma) virus has emerged as an important threat to graft survival. Polyoma virus infection is ubiquitous in the general population, with overimmunosuppression thought to be responsible for clinically evident disease. Limited evidence suggests that retransplantation in patients who have suffered a previous allograft failure from the BK virus may be successful; thus the BK virus should not preclude retransplantation.

MALIGNANCY

Immunosuppression likely promotes tumor growth and increases the risk for cancer recurrence. As allograft survival lengthens, death from malignancy increases. Thus active malignancy is an absolute contraindication to transplantation, with the exception of superficial squamous cell and basal cell skin cancers. In patients with a history of malignancy, a waiting period between successful treatment of cancer and transplantation is recommended. The length of this waiting period depends on the type of malignancy and the risk of recurrence. In general, a waiting period of 2 years is recommended for most types of cancers. In high-risk malignancies, such as breast cancer, colon cancer, melanoma, and invasive and/or symptomatic renal cell cancer, a waiting period of 5 years is recommended. However, with improved knowledge of cancer biology, it has become apparent that different molecular subtypes of certain malignancies have very different outcomes. Genomic profiling assays can now be used to provide a more individualized granular assessment of cancer recurrence risk. In cases with very low risk profiles, a wait of 2 years may not be necessary, but further work in transplant candidates is needed before this becomes routine practice. Small, incidentally discovered renal cell cancers and cervical cancer in situ do not require any waiting period. Multiple myeloma is a contraindication for transplantation unless considered concurrently with an allogeneic bone marrow transplant.

Although life expectancy is shortened in dialysis-dependent prospective kidney transplant recipients, most programs perform pretransplant malignancy screening. This screening should be based on clinical practice guidelines for the general population as part of a periodic health examination. All patients should receive a chest radiograph, abdominal ultrasound, and age-appropriate colon cancer screening

as part of their workup. Women should undergo breast examination, pelvic examination, and Pap smear as dictated by their age. Men should receive a prostate examination and prostate-specific antigen (PSA) screening as dictated by their age, or if symptomatic. In addition, patients who have received cyclophosphamide in the past should be considered for urine cytology and cystoscopy to rule out bladder malignancy.

Prospective transplant recipients should be counseled about the risk of malignancy posttransplant. The risk of nonmelanoma skin cancer and lymphoma is much higher than similarly matched dialysis controls. The risk of squamous cell cancer increases with increased age, lighter skin tones, a prior history of skin cancer, and cumulative lifetime sun exposure. Recipients should be counseled to avoid prolonged direct sun exposure and should wear ultraviolet A (UVA) and ultraviolet B (UVB) sunscreens and protective clothing. The posttransplant lymphoma risk is much higher in EBV-naïve recipients.

CARDIOVASCULAR DISEASE

Cardiovascular disease is the leading cause of death in patients on dialysis and in kidney transplant recipients, with diabetics at particular risk. Therefore all potential transplant recipients should be carefully evaluated for the presence of heart disease before listing. At a minimum, patients should be assessed for signs and symptoms of cardiovascular disease and undergo an electrocardiogram (ECG) and an echocardiogram. Patients with progressive angina symptoms or a myocardial infarction within 6 months should not be offered transplantation. In patients with severe and irreversible coronary artery disease, projected life expectancy must be balanced against the risks of transplant surgery. It is worth noting that left ventricular dysfunction due to uremic cardiomyopathy is not a contraindication to transplantation and frequently improves after surgery. In patients at high risk for underlying coronary disease (including men over age 40, women over age 50, patients with diabetes, patients with multiple traditional cardiovascular risk factors), noninvasive testing may be performed to identify underlying disease. Patients with positive noninvasive stress test results may be referred for angiography and potential revascularization before transplantation.

At present, cardiac risk stratification of potential kidney transplant candidates is guided by little supporting evidence. Although data demonstrate that noninvasive testing can accurately diagnose coronary artery disease in patients with diabetes and in CKD patients without diabetes, subsequent management varies widely from center to center. Current guidelines from the American College of Cardiology (ACC)/American Heart Association (AHA) recommend revascularization only in symptomatic patients with high-risk cardiac lesions. In two clinical trials that examined preoperative revascularization versus medical management in moderate- to high-risk individuals, perioperative event rates and mortality did not differ. It should be noted that patients with advanced CKD have not been studied in this context, nor has the question of life expectancy after organ transplant in individuals with a significant burden of coronary artery disease been directly addressed. With prolonged waiting times, cardiovascular disease in high-risk individuals may progress. Many programs perform periodic noninvasive rescreening in wait-listed patients; however, the value of this practice is unknown, and newly detected disease is only variably acted upon.

Modifiable risk factors for cardiovascular disease should be managed appropriately in prospective kidney transplant recipients. Blood pressure should be treated to a target of at least 140/90 mm Hg, and smoking cessation should be encouraged. The utility of treating dyslipidemia in patients undergoing dialysis has recently come into question (see Chapter 55); however, control of low-density lipoprotein (LDL) cholesterol should be considered in high-risk individuals.

CEREBROVASCULAR DISEASE

After transplantation, recipients are at an increased risk for cerebrovascular disease when compared with pretransplant patients or the general population. Patients with symptomatic transient ischemic attacks or a recent stroke should be symptom free for 6 months before transplantation. Consideration of carotid endarterectomy should be given to those individuals with known carotid stenosis. The screening of asymptomatic patients is unclear. Again, modifiable risk factors, including smoking and blood pressure, should be addressed before transplant.

LIVER DISEASE

Because progressive liver disease causes significant morbidity and mortality in transplant patients, all prospective recipients should be screened. In patients with liver disease not caused by viral hepatitis, liver function testing and a liver biopsy should be considered to assess the severity of disease. The patient's immunosuppressed state in the posttransplantation period permits viral replication that can accelerate chronic viral hepatitis. Therefore all patients should be screened for HBV and hepatitis C virus (HCV) infection. In patients with significant liver disease and/or cirrhosis, consideration of combined liver-kidney transplant may be an option.

Patients with positive hepatitis B surface antigen (HBsAg) should undergo testing for hepatitis B viral load by protein-creatinine ratio (PCR), hepatitis B early antigen (HBeAg), and hepatitis D virus (HDV). Patients with evidence of active viral replication (HBeAg-positive, or hepatitis B viral load–positive) should forgo transplantation until HBV is effectively treated. Those with both HBV and HDV should not be considered for transplantation because of the risk of severe liver disease. In patients with chronic active hepatitis and elevated liver enzymes, liver biopsy should be performed, and posttransplant antiviral therapy (e.g., lamivudine) should be considered. Transplant outcomes are generally worse in patients who are HBsAg-positive compared with those who are not. The decision whether to transplant can be difficult, and specialist assistance will usually be required.

HCV infection can lead to accelerated liver disease after transplantation. All prospective transplant recipients who have serologic evidence of HCV exposure should undergo HCV load testing by PCR and liver biopsy. Although patients with HCV have worse outcomes after transplantation when compared with those without infection, the outcomes are improved over remaining on dialysis. Treatment outcomes of HCV infection in ESKD patients, including posttransplantation, have significantly improved after the introduction of direct-acting antivirals (DAAs). Treatment of HCV with DAAs can occur before or after kidney transplantation. Physicians should be aware of drug interactions with calcineurin inhibitors posttransplantation. Patients with HCV may be able to accept a kidney from an HCV-positive donor, especially given improved treatment outcomes.

PULMONARY DISEASE

Patients with pulmonary disease are at increased risk for perioperative respiratory complications. Thus patients with severe, irreversible lung disease, including severe chronic obstructive pulmonary disease (COPD), cor pulmonale, and those needing supplemental oxygen, should not be offered kidney transplantation. Current smokers and patients with known lung disease should undergo pulmonary function testing for risk stratification before transplantation. Smokers who undergo transplantation are at risk for increased perioperative events and have poor long-term outcomes compared with nonsmokers. All smokers should be offered smoking cessation aids and counseling as necessary to encourage smoking cessation.

THROMBOTIC RISK

Patients with a history of venous or arterial thromboembolic disease may be at risk for perioperative graft loss due to thrombosis. Screening for genetic risks of thrombosis should be considered in those individuals with a positive medical history, and a plan for perioperative anticoagulation should be constructed. Patients with a history of SLE should be screened for antiphospholipid antibodies. Inherited disorders of complement may lead to atypical HUS, with recurrent disease occurring in up to 25% to 50% of allografts. Screening for genetic abnormalities may allow for an individualized perioperative plan, including plasma exchange and/or calcineurin inhibitor avoidance, which may lessen recurrence risk.

UROLOGIC EVALUATION

Patients with a history of lower urinary tract abnormalities, bladder dysfunction, or recurrent urinary tract infections (UTIs) require urologic investigation and voiding cystourethrogram. In addition, high-risk patients, such as those with diabetes, should be screened with a postvoid residual. Efforts should be made to preserve the native bladder, and self-intermittent catheterization is preferable to urinary diversion with ureteroileostomy. Patients with significant exposure to cyclophosphamide should be screened with cystoscopy to rule out malignancy. Pretransplant nephrectomy should be considered in patients with severe reflux or recurrent nephrolithiasis with infection, difficult-to-control hypertension, severe nephrotic syndrome, and symptomatic polycystic kidneys.

PSYCHOLOGICAL EVALUATION

All prospective transplant recipients should undergo screening to identify cognitive or psychological impairments that may alter their ability to provide informed consent or their ability to follow medical protocols after transplantation. Medication nonadherence remains a major cause of graft loss. However, identification of individuals at risk is difficult and not often apparent during the transplant workup. In general, one should be cautious in restricting access to transplantation in those at risk for nonadherence. Patients with addiction or a history of chemical dependency should be offered counseling and rehabilitation. Many programs require a period of abstinence before a patient is put on the waiting list. Those individuals with major psychiatric illness should receive appropriate psychiatric care with the recognition of potential medication interactions and side effects.

IMMUNOLOGIC CONSIDERATIONS BEFORE TRANSPLANTATION

Tissue compatibility between donor and recipient is determined by matching ABO blood type, human leukocyte antigen (HLA), and/or major histocompatibility complex (MHC). Blood and HLA tissue typing is performed on all suitable transplant candidates at the time of wait-listing. For the most part, the donor kidney must be ABO compatible with the recipient. In North America, ABO B blood type recipients have a longer waiting period as compared with other blood types. Many programs now allocated ABO A2 kidneys to ABO B recipients to improve equity.

Although HLA matching is desired, it is rarely achieved because of the tremendous allelic polymorphisms present in the MHC genes. In kidney transplantation, HLA A, B, and DR are thought to be most important in histocompatibility. Both early rejection and long-term allograft survival are affected by HLA matching, with a zero-antigen mismatched kidney having a decreased risk for rejection and better long-term survival as compared with a six-antigen mismatched kidney.

A major barrier to transplantation is the development of antibodies against HLA epitopes, called sensitization. Anti-HLA antibodies are formed during exposure to foreign HLA through blood transfusions, pregnancy, and prior transplantation. The presence of anti-HLA antibodies against a donor HLA type precludes transplantation in most circumstances because of the extreme risk for hyperacute rejection and graft failure. Thus all candidates on the waiting list are screened for the presence of anti-HLA antibodies at least every 3 months.

Screening for anti-HLA antibodies is performed through serologic testing (by mixing donor lymphocytes with recipient serum) or, now more routinely, through solid-phase assays, such as flow cytometry or the Luminex platform. An estimate of a recipient's anti-HLA antibody burden can be assessed by mixing recipient serum with a panel of lymphocytes representing random donors from the general population. The percentage of lymphocytes that react to recipient antibodies is called panel-reactive antibody (PRA) and provides an estimate of the likelihood of finding a suitable donor within the population. A high PRA means it will be more difficult to find a compatible donor. In addition, a high PRA is associated with worse graft survival, even if the final cross-match against the donor is negative. Using solid-phase assays, most transplant centers are now able to determine the specificity of a recipient's anti-HLA antibodies. A list of unacceptable HLA antigens can then be compiled for a recipient. Comparing this profile to the donor's HLA type to assess tissue histocompatibility is termed a *virtual cross-match*. Solid-phase assays to detect anti-HLA antibodies are much more sensitive than serologic detection and can often identify low-titer antibodies that were previously undetectable. Even with a negative cross-match, presence of low-titer antibodies against donor HLA is associated with antibody-mediated rejection and higher rates of graft loss.

At the time of transplantation, a final cross-match is completed to ensure tissue compatibility. Recipient serum is mixed with donor tissue. A positive cross-match indicates the presence of donor-specific anti-HLA antibodies (DSAs) and predicts hyperacute rejection. Because not all positive cross-match results are due to antibodies that cause hyperacute rejection, further laboratory tests may be necessary before transplantation. In patients with a high PRA, the cross-match is often performed with historical sera that have the highest PRA value. Recipients with a current negative cross-match but a historical positive cross-match may undergo transplantation, but they are at a higher risk for antibody-mediated rejection.

Patients with a high PRA are disadvantaged and often have prolonged waiting times because of the limited number of compatible donors. Strategies to lower a patient's PRA to increase the probability of finding a suitable donor are constantly evolving. Noninvasive strategies, such as enrollment in a living donor–paired exchange program, have increased access for mismatched living donor pairs (see later). Strategies to decrease or eliminate anti-HLA or anti-ABO antibodies may include targeting of either the antibodies or the B cell/plasma cell clones that produce the antibodies. Plasmapheresis and high-dose intravenous immunoglobulin (IVIG) have been used successfully to greatly reduce or eliminate anti-HLA antibodies. Rituximab and bortezomib (and, rarely, splenectomy) target B cells and plasma cells. Although these strategies have allowed successful transplantation with ABO-incompatible or positive cross-match donors, the risk for antibody-mediated rejection and graft loss remains increased.

DECEASED DONOR ORGANS

Because of the shortage of deceased donor organs, novel sources of kidneys for transplantation continue to be explored. In North America, the majority of organs are removed from deceased donors following the neurologic determination of death (NDD). More recently, organs have been removed from donors not meeting the criteria for brain death but whose death is determined by cardiac criteria (donation after cardiocirculatory death, or DCD). Organ procurement in DCD donors can be controlled or uncontrolled. In controlled DCD donation, consent for donation is obtained before death, and life support is withdrawn in a controlled fashion. An uncontrolled donor dies before consent for organ donation, and attempts are made to preserve the organs until consent can be obtained. DCD kidneys have a higher rate of delayed graft function; however, long-term outcomes are similar to recipients who received a kidney from an NDD donor. In the United Kingdom, DCD donors now account for approximately 40% of all deceased organ donors.

There is substantial variability in the quality of donor kidneys. Most obviously, a kidney from a donor with a decreased glomerular filtration rate (GFR), older age, or significant medical comorbidities might be expected to have a shorter graft survival as compared with a kidney from a young healthy donor. Attempts have been made to evaluate donor organ quality and allocate donor kidneys based on expected outcomes. The concept of marginal donor kidneys affecting transplant outcome was formalized in 2002 with the definition of expanded criteria donors (ECDs). ECD kidneys include those from donors over the age of 60 or from donors between 50 and 59 years old with two of the following: cerebrovascular accident as the cause of death, hypertension, or terminal serum creatinine greater than 1.5 mg/dL. ECD kidneys have a 1.7-fold higher probability of graft failure 2 years after transplantation as compared with standard criteria donor (SCD) kidneys; however, early access to transplantation may benefit potential transplant recipients. In patients over the age of 65 or patients over the age of 40 with diabetes and prolonged deceased donor transplant wait times, receipt of an ECD kidney confers a survival advantage over waiting for an SCD kidney. Younger, healthier kidney transplant candidates may be better served by waiting for an SCD kidney.

In the United States, donor kidney quality is now assessed and quantified on a continuous scale by calculating the Kidney Donor Risk Index (KDRI), which estimates donor kidney quality based on 10 donor characteristics including age, ethnicity, creatinine, and specific donor health comorbidities. The Kidney Donor Profile Index (KDPI) converts the KDRI into a percentile used to express the quality of the donor kidney relative to other kidneys. A higher KDRI or KDPI indicates a lower expected graft survival. By using the KDPI, healthy donor kidneys (<20%) can be allocated to recipients with the longest life expectancy, while higher KDPI kidneys can be allocated to older recipients, similar to ECD recipients. Fig. 60.1 shows the expected half-life of donor kidneys based on KDPI.

ALLOCATION OF DECEASED DONOR ORGANS IN THE UNITED STATES

UNOS and the Organ Procurement and Transplant Network (OPTN) allocate donated kidneys in the United States. Patients who are medically ready for transplantation may be placed on the UNOS waiting list for a deceased donor kidney. Kidneys are allocated by policies designed to balance equity and efficacy. Only a brief overview of this process will be provided; policies can be viewed in more detail online (https://optn.transplant.hrsa.gov/learn/professional-education/kidney-allocation-system/).

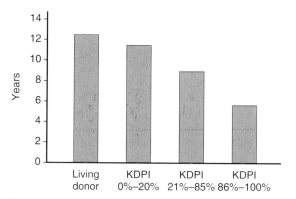

Fig. 60.1 Estimated graft half-lives (years). *KDPI*, Kidney donor profile index. (Data accessed on August 26, 2016, from https://optn.transplant. hrsa.gov/.)

Deceased donor kidneys are generally allocated by ABO blood type—thus blood type O donor kidneys are available only to O recipients. This allocation is followed for A, B, and AB kidneys also. Donor kidneys are first offered locally, then regionally, and then nationally. All potential recipients on the UNOS waiting list are allocated points, which determine their priority for transplantation. Patients with more points receive higher priority. Points are awarded for length of waiting time, quality of DR antigen match, degree of sensitization and PRA, medical urgency, and pediatric recipient status. Details of the point system for kidney allocation can be reviewed at the OPTN website (see earlier).

In 2015, a new kidney allocation policy was introduced, which attempts to account for factors associated with allograft and recipient survival to increase the efficiency of organ utilization and to increase access for certain underrepresented recipient candidates. Policy changes attempt to increase access to patients with a high PRA, those of ABO blood type B, and those who are referred late for transplant assessment. An estimated posttransplant survival score (EPTS) is calculated for all adult candidates on the waiting list and is based on recipient age, time on dialysis, presence or absence of diabetes, and history of a prior transplant. Those candidates with a high probability of long-term survival (EPTS <20%) are eligible to receive kidneys from donors with a KDPI of <20%. In this manner, kidneys are matched to the recipient based on the expected survival of the kidney and the recipient. With the new policy, concern remains that certain groups may be disproportionately disadvantaged. An analysis of outcomes over time will allow adjustments to the current allocation system.

LIVING KIDNEY DONATION

Although the number of deceased donors has increased significantly since 1990 (Fig. 60.2), this has not kept pace with the increased number of patients being added to the kidney transplant waiting list. As of 2015, approximately 99,000 patients were wait-listed for kidney transplantation in the United States. As such, wait times have increased dramatically, to the point where the median waiting time for a deceased donor kidney nationwide is over 6 years. Looking at it another way, only 30% of candidates will receive a kidney transplant within 3 years of being placed on the wait-list. The lack of access to deceased donor organs, as well as the superior outcomes with live donors, has resulted in the increased usage of living kidney donors for transplantation. In the 15 years from 1990 to 2005, the number of living kidney donors used in the United States increased dramatically (see Fig. 60.2). Unfortunately, since 2005, the number of living donors has fallen, but there were still more than 5500 living kidney donors used for transplantation in 2015 alone.

Living kidney donation offers several potential advantages over deceased donor transplantation. First, the procedure is elective and scheduled, thus ensuring that both donor and recipient are in optimal medical condition. The planned nature of the operation also facilitates the use of preemptive transplantation (i.e., kidney transplantation without prior dialysis), which has been associated with both improved patient and allograft survival. Second, the incidence of delayed graft function (the need for dialysis in the first week

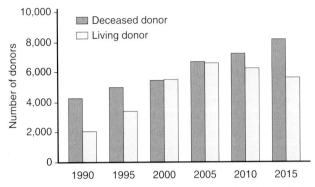

Fig. 60.2 Living and deceased organ donors in the United States. (Data accessed on August 26, 2016, from https://optn.transplant.hrsa.gov/.)

Box 60.2   Key Points of Informed Consent Process for Living Kidney Donors

Living kidney donors should understand the following items as part of the informed consent process:

- Consent may be withdrawn at any time.
- The evaluation process and operation both involve risk.
- Abnormalities discovered during the evaluation might affect future insurability or may require reporting to another agency (e.g., positive HIV test).
- There is a small but real risk for death with live donor nephrectomy (3.1 per 10,000 donors).
- All donors will lose kidney function postoperatively, but the actual amount is difficult to predict.
- The risk of ESKD in living donors is no greater than the general population but is higher than comparatively healthy nondonors (attributable risk 26.9 per 10,000 donors).
- There is an increased risk of hypertension, gestational hypertension, preeclampsia, and gout among kidney donors.

ESKD, end-stage kidney disease; *HIV*, human immunodeficiency virus.

---

posttransplantation) is much lower for recipients of living donor kidneys. In 2016, only 3% to 5% of living donor kidney recipients had delayed graft function, compared with 25% of deceased donor transplant patients. Finally, patient and allograft survival rates are superior for living donor kidneys compared with deceased donors. In the most recently available data, patients who received a living donor kidney transplant in 2014 had a 1-year allograft survival of 97%, compared with 92% for deceased donor recipients. For patients who received a living donor kidney transplant in 2008, the 5-year patient survival was 92%, compared with only 84% for deceased donor recipients. Similarly, for those who received a living donor transplant in 2008, the 5-year allograft survival was 85%, compared with only 73% for recipients of deceased donor kidney transplant.

Prospective recipients with a willing living donor who is ABO-incompatible or possesses an incompatible HLA antigen may consider registering in a local, regional, or national paired exchange program. Incompatible donor pairs are entered into a computer registry that compares the medical information on all registered pairs and identifies pairs that might be able to exchange donors. Proposed matches can identify a single matching pair or may identify a series of pairs that may exchange donors in a chain-like or domino fashion. Living donor paired exchange increases access to transplantation and offers the benefits of living donor transplantation to those recipients with an incompatible living donor.

LIVING DONOR EVALUATION PROCESS

Living donation is a unique medical situation in which the patient (donor) undergoes an operation with risk, yet receives no direct medical benefit from the procedure. Living kidney donation carries small but measurable risks of perioperative complications and adverse long-term health outcomes including ESKD. However, many donors do report benefits, such as an improved sense of well-being from seeing a friend or relative thrive after transplantation. Given the exceptional circumstances surrounding living donation, it is crucial that informed consent be obtained in an open and thoughtful manner. Consent should be obtained for both the evaluation process and the surgical procedure itself. The potential donor needs to understand that the evaluation process requires a

series of tests—and that the results of some of these tests may be abnormal. Certain test results may prompt disclosure to another agency (e.g., HIV-positive test results reported to public health) or may affect future insurability (e.g., significant proteinuria). Donors need to be counseled on the lifetime risk of kidney failure. This can be estimated at http://www.transplantmodels.com/esrdrisk/. Other points that should be fully discussed as part of the informed consent process are outlined in Box 60.2.

After informed consent, the evaluation consists of a psychosocial and medical assessment. The psychosocial assessment must be conducted by an appropriate professional with experience in living kidney donation. This person will vary from site to site but is most often a social worker, clinical psychologist, or psychiatrist. Important components of the psychosocial assessment are outlined in Box 60.3. Significant concerns with any of these factors may preclude donation or require further assessment by other health care professionals (e.g., psychiatrist).

The medical assessment should be conducted by a surgeon or physician (ideally both) with expertise in living kidney donation. The goal of the medical evaluation is to determine (1) the overall health of the potential donor and whether he or she is fit for surgery; (2) the current kidney health of the potential donor and his or her risk for kidney disease or medical complications in the future; (3) the presence of any conditions that may result in disease transmission (e.g., infection) to the recipient; and (4) the immunologic compatibility of the potential donor with the intended recipient. The tests required to address these components of the medical evaluation are listed in Box 60.4. In 2017, KDIGO published clinical practice guidelines on the evaluation and care follow-up care of living kidney donors. The guidelines can be found at http://kdigo.org/home/guidelines/.

Before proceeding with specific testing, a medical history and physical examination is required for all living donors.

The history should focus on conditions related to overall health and fitness for surgery, such as the presence of cardiovascular disease, liver disease, pulmonary disease, or hematologic conditions (bleeding disorders or thrombosis). Significant abnormalities in any of these areas may preclude donation or require more specialized testing and/or referral to another consultant.

AGE OF THE LIVING KIDNEY DONOR

Age is an important consideration when assessing living kidney donors. Most programs will not allow living donors younger than 18 years of age, and 15% of transplant centers require donors to be at least 21 years old. On the opposite end of the age spectrum, wide variation exists in practice. The most common upper age limit for living donors is 65 years old, and this cutoff was reported at 21% of American transplant centers in a 2007 survey. Notably, 59% of programs reported

that no upper age limit was in effect at their center. Despite these survey results, between 1992 and 2011, there were only 1200 living kidney donors 65 years of age or older in the United States, with approximately 100 per year in the past few years.

The age of the living donor is important for three main reasons. The first reason is that advanced age may lead to inferior graft outcomes in the recipient. This question has been addressed in a few recent analyses, and fortunately, the results are encouraging. A large analysis using the United States Renal Data System (USRDS) registry showed that transplant patients who received a kidney from a living donor older than 55 years of age had a risk for graft loss similar to those who received a kidney from a living donor 55 years of age or younger (adjusted relative risk 1.00; 95% confidence interval [CI] 0.47 to 2.13). It is important to note that graft survival from these older living donors was actually superior to younger standard criteria *deceased* donors. A subsequent analysis showed that recipients of live kidneys from donors above the age of 70 had similar graft survival to those who received standard criteria allografts from 50- to 59-year-old deceased donors (hazard ratio 1.19; 95% CI 0.87 to 1.63).

A second reason for the importance of the age of living donors is related to comorbidity. Advanced age is often associated with increased comorbidity, which may lead to more perioperative complications at the time of the donor nephrectomy. Other than a longer hospital stay (median difference, 1 day), living donors older than 60 years of age do not have a significant difference in minor complications (e.g., UTI), major complications (e.g., reoperation), or even death following nephrectomy. In an analysis of 80,347 live donors, the 90-day mortality rate was 3.1 per 10,000 donors, and this rate was not significantly different for donors above or below 60 years of age. In addition, the long-term survival

---

Box 60.3 Key Points to Be Addressed in the Psychosocial Assessment of Living Kidney Donors

Capacity suitable for informed consent

No evidence of coercion to donate

Social support network adequate to assist with recovery from surgery

Financial stability to take time off from work and cover expenses

High-risk behavior (e.g., IV drug use) that might increase risk for disease transmission to the recipient

Current or previous psychiatric disorders that might influence decision making or response to adverse outcomes

---

Box 60.4 Medical Assessment of Living Kidney Donors

1. General donor health and immediate surgical risk
   - Complete blood count, prothrombin time or INR, partial thromboplastin time
   - HCG for women of childbearing potential
   - Electrolytes, transaminases, bilirubin, calcium, phosphorus, albumin
   - Chest radiograph and electrocardiogram
2. Current kidney health and future disease risk
   - Serum creatinine
   - Fasting blood glucose, total cholesterol, HDL-cholesterol, LDL-cholesterol, triglycerides
   - Urinalysis, urine culture
   - Proteinuria measurement: ACR, PCR, or 24-hour urine collection for total protein and/or albumin
   - Kidney function measurement: 24-h urine collection for creatinine clearance or measured GFR using an exogenous marker (inulin; radioactive or cold iothalamate, iohexol, DTPA, or EDTA)
   - CT or MR angiogram
3. Potential disease transmission to recipient
   - CMV, HSV, and EBV antibody
   - HIV
   - HTLV
   - HBV surface antigen, core antibody, and surface antibody
   - HCV virus antibody
   - Rapid plasma reagin test for syphilis
   - Emerging/geographic-specific infections (e.g., West Nile virus, Zika virus)
   - Papanicolaou test for women
   - Mammogram for women over 40 years
   - Prostate-specific antigen for men over 50 years (40 years if black or positive family history)
   - Colon cancer screen for donors over 50 years (fecal occult blood testing or visualization with colonoscopy, virtual colonoscopy, or flexible sigmoidoscopy)
4. Immunologic compatibility with recipient
   - ABO blood type
   - HLA typing

ACR, Albumin-creatinine ratio; *CMV,* cytomegalovirus; *DTPA,* diethylenetriaminepentaacetic acid; *EDTA,* ethylenediaminetetraacetic acid; *EBV,* Epstein-Barr virus; *GFR,* glomerular filtration rate; *HBV,* hepatitis B virus; *HCV,* hepatitis C virus; *HCG,* human chorionic gonadotropin; *HIV,* human immunodeficiency virus; *HLA,* human leukocyte antigen; *HSV,* herpes simplex virus; *HTLV,* human T lymphotropic virus; *INR,* international normalized ratio; *PCR,* protein-creatinine ratio.

to 12 years was actually greater for donors older than 60 years compared with an age-matched cohort of nondonors who did not have contraindications to live donation.

The third reason is that age is important when considering live donors because it influences the amount of time that the donor is at risk to develop ESKD or other complications that might negatively affect someone with a solitary kidney. For example, a 22-year-old overweight black man with pre-diabetes has a significant risk for developing overt diabetes and ESKD given the many potential years of life ahead of him. Although being overweight and having prediabetes are not absolute contraindications to donation on their own, this young man may not be an appropriate donor because of his future risk for disease. In contrast, a 63-year-old white woman with well-controlled hypertension on one medication might be a suitable donor given that her lifetime risk for kidney failure is much lower than that for a younger patient without risk factors.

KIDNEY FUNCTION

Ninety percent of programs in the United States use a 24-hour urine collection for creatinine clearance as the measure of kidney function, with the remainder using a direct measure of GFR, such as a radioisotopic clearance. The threshold for declining donors based on GFR or creatinine clearance is somewhat controversial with varied practice. Approximately two-thirds of American centers exclude donors with a creatinine clearance less than 80 mL/min per 1.73 m^2, whereas 25% require the value to be within two standard deviations of the mean creatinine clearance for the donor's age. See Table 60.3 for creatinine clearance values in the normal population.

From the perspective of the transplant recipient, it is crucial to ensure that kidney mass and function are adequate to prevent premature graft loss. On average, a kidney donor will lose 25% of kidney function after donation. When the donor's creatinine clearance is above 80 mL/min per 1.73 m^2, postnephrectomy kidney mass is usually adequate. Lower values can provide adequate kidney mass and may be appropriate for certain recipients (e.g., older adults). However, from the perspective of the living donor, the appropriate clearance threshold might be somewhat different. It is well known that

GFR declines with age, and thus a creatinine clearance of 80 mL/min per 1.73 m^2 in a 20-year-old is very different from a clearance of 80 mL/min per 1.73 m^2 in a 65-year-old donor. For 20-year-olds, this cutoff is well below two standard deviations of the mean for their age, and nephrectomy (with a further loss of GFR) may put them at increased risk for ESKD given their long potential lifetime. For 65-year-old donors, a clearance of 80 mL/min per 1.73 m^2 is within the normal range for their age, and the risk for ESKD is much less given that they have fewer years of life remaining. For these reasons, it is preferred to individualize donor acceptance with age-based creatinine clearance or GFR values, with consideration also given to the intended recipient, rather than with rigid cutoffs.

BLOOD PRESSURE

Sitting blood pressure should be measured at least 2 times in any potential living donor. Ambulatory blood pressure monitoring should be considered if isolated office hypertension is suspected. Hypertension was previously considered a contraindication to donation, but practice is now quite varied. Only 47% of programs exclude donors with normal blood pressure on one antihypertensive medication; 36% continue to exclude only those with persistently borderline blood pressure values. The increased acceptance of hypertensive donors is based on favorable data from select, mostly white, patients with well-controlled hypertension who have undergone living donation. Limited outcome data are available from hypertensive donors in other populations who may be at higher risk (e.g., blacks). The Amsterdam forum and the KDIGO guideline on the care of the live kidney donor suggest that patients with easily controlled blood pressure who meet other criteria (i.e., age >50 years, GFR >80 mL/min, no proteinuria) may be acceptable as live kidney donors. Until further data are available, the use of living donors with hypertension should be restricted to white donors.

PROTEINURIA

The 24-hour urine collection is still used by most programs (75%) to assess for proteinuria, but spot urine protein or albumin (PCR or albumin-creatinine ratio) measurements are becoming more commonly used. Mildly abnormal values should be repeated, especially if patients were acutely ill with fever or were exercising before testing. The threshold for excluding donors based on proteinuria is not consistent among centers. Whereas 36% of programs exclude donors with greater than 150 mg/day of total protein, 44% require proteinuria to be greater than 300 mg/day before exclusion. The KDIGO guideline recommends using albuminuria (albumin excretion rate, AER), rather than proteinuria. Albuminuria more closely reflects glomerular disease and is a better predictor of cardiovascular events. Given the strong link with proteinuria and kidney disease, it seems prudent to exclude any donor with abnormal albuminuria (>30 mg/day) or total proteinuria greater than 300 mg/day. A lower threshold may be needed in cases of familial kidney disease, borderline blood pressure, or other abnormalities, such as microscopic hematuria.

HEMATURIA

Isolated microscopic hematuria should be confirmed with repeat urinalysis including microscopy to verify the presence

---

Table 60.3 Measured Creatinine Clearance According to Age

Age (Year)	Mean Creatinine Clearance (mL/min/1.73 m^2)	SD	Mean—SD	Mean—2 SD
17–24	140	12	128	116
25–34	140	21	119	98
35–44	133	20	113	93
45–54	127	17	110	93
55–64	120	16	104	88
65–74	110	16	94	78
75–84	97	16	81	65

Used with permission of the American Society of Nephrology; previously published in Kher A, Mandelbrot DA. The living kidney donor evaluation: focus on renal issues. *Clin J Am Soc Nephrol.* 2012;7:366–371.

of red blood cells as the cause of dipstick hematuria. Infection, nephrolithiasis, malignancy, and glomerulonephritis need to be ruled out in potential donors with hematuria. Urine culture should be performed to rule out infection, and menstrual contamination should always be considered in premenopausal women. Imaging will rule out a structural kidney cause, but most donors must undergo cystoscopy to rule out local bladder causes. Finally, glomerular hematuria from IgA nephropathy, hereditary nephritis, or thin basement membrane nephropathy must be considered in an otherwise healthy donor. These conditions can only be diagnosed by kidney biopsy, and this test should be considered if the donor understands the risks and is motivated to continue the evaluation. The most common practice (43% of programs) is to accept donors with hematuria only if urologic evaluation and kidney biopsy are both normal. However, 21% of programs would exclude patients with hematuria (>10 red blood cells/high-power field) regardless of these investigations.

DIABETES

Given the risk for diabetic nephropathy, established diabetes is a contraindication to donation. All donors should have a fasting blood glucose performed to rule out undiagnosed diabetes, impaired fasting glucose, or prediabetes. Patients at increased risk for diabetes (e.g., history of gestational diabetes, first-degree relative with diabetes, BMI >30) should have an oral glucose tolerance test or glycated hemoglobin test. Potential donors with impaired fasting glucose need to be assessed on a case-by-case basis; young patients or those with other risk factors, such as obesity, hypertension, or dyslipidemia, should be excluded from donation.

OBESITY

Obesity (BMI >30) is associated with short-term surgical complications following nephrectomy, as well as an increased risk for future medical conditions, such as diabetes, hypertension, and dyslipidemia. Fifty-two percent of programs exclude donors with a BMI greater than 35, whereas 20% exclude those with BMI above 40. A recent study found that obesity was associated with more hypertension and dyslipidemia after a mean follow-up of 11 years but was not significantly different from an obese control group who did not donate. In addition, obese donors had a GFR that was similar to nonobese donors and were not at increased risk for long-term deterioration in kidney function. Not all patients with an elevated BMI have central obesity, and potential donors should be examined for body habitus and muscle mass before exclusion based on BMI alone. Obese donors may also lose weight to a certain target before proceeding with surgery, with appropriate support and counseling to prevent immediate weight gain postnephrectomy.

NEPHROLITHIASIS

Kidney stones are a very common occurrence, with as many as 19% of men and 9% of women having a symptomatic kidney stone in their lifetime. The majority of these stones are composed of calcium oxalate. Improved imaging techniques have increased the ability to detect small, asymptomatic kidney stones as well. As such, nephrolithiasis is not an uncommon problem in potential living donors. The major concern for the living donor is recurrence postnephrectomy, leading to obstruction of the single remaining kidney. The majority

of programs (53%) accept donors with a history of kidney stones as long as the metabolic workup is normal. Another consideration is age at onset and time since symptomatic episode. Younger patients are at an increased risk for recurrence, given their long projected lifespan. Patients whose stone episode was remote (>10 years) are at decreased risk for recurrence. Patients with a history of stone disease or stones on imaging should have a metabolic workup done, including serum calcium and bicarbonate to rule out metabolic acidosis. A 24-hour urine collection (preferably on two occasions) should be performed to assess calcium, oxalate, uric acid, and citrate excretion. Patients who should be excluded as donors include those with recurrent stones and those at high risk for recurrence, such as those with metabolic abnormalities (e.g., hypercalciuria), chronic diarrhea/malabsorption, gout, cysteine, uric acid, or struvite stones.

CONCLUSION

Limited data are available to guide the selection of living kidney donors. Most studies to date have been single-center or small in sample size, have had a relatively short duration of follow-up, and, notably, may have been biased by not including all donors in follow-up. As such, donor selection is often made with personal opinion or center-based protocols. Contraindications to living donation have been published and are presented in Table 60.4. It is important to assess potential donors individually and to use the information available as a guide. Younger donors have a much higher lifetime risk for developing complications, such as diabetes or ESKD, and the evaluation should be conducted with this

Table 60.4	**Absolute and Relative Contraindications to Living Kidney Donation**
Absolute Contraindications	**Relative Contraindications**
Age <18 years	Age 18–21 years
Mentally incapable of making informed decision	Creatinine clearance <2 SD below mean for age
Uncontrolled hypertension, or hypertension with end-organ damage	Albuminuria or proteinuria
	Hypertension in non-white race
Diabetes	Hypertension in young donor
BMI >35 kg/m²	Prediabetes in young donor
Untreated psychiatric conditions	BMI >30 kg/m²
	Bleeding disorder
Nephrolithiasis with high likelihood of recurrence	History of thrombosis or embolism
Evidence of donor coercion	Nephrolithiasis
Active malignancy or incompletely treated malignancy	History of malignancy, especially if metastatic
	Significant cardiovascular
Persistent infection	disease

BMI, Body mass index.
Used with permission of the American Society of Nephrology; previously published in Kher A, Mandelbrot DA. The living kidney donor evaluation: focus on renal issues. *Clin J Am Soc Nephrol.* 2012;7:366–371.

in mind. Similarly, older donors have a much lower lifetime risk for complications and may be appropriate for donation with certain conditions (e.g., hypertension). Further research focusing on complete and long-term follow-up, especially involving those with medical abnormalities, is needed to enrich the data available to make evidence-based decisions in living kidney donation.

KEY BIBLIOGRAPHY

Abramowicz D, Cochat P, Claas FH, Heemann U, Pascual J, Dudley C, Harden P, Hourmant M, Maggiore U, Salvadori M, Spasovski G, Squifflet JP, Steiger J, Torres A, Viklicky O, Zeier M, Vanholder R, Van Biesen W, Nagler E. European Renal Best Practice Guideline on kidney donor and recipient evaluation and perioperative care. *Nephrol Dial Transplant.* 2015;30:1790-1797.

Briganti EM, Russ GR, McNeil JJ, et al. Risk of renal allograft loss from recurrent glomerulonephritis. *N Engl J Med.* 2002;11:103-109.

De Vriese AS, De Bacquer DA, Verbeke FH, et al. Comparison of the prognostic value of dipyridamole and dobutamine myocardial perfusion scintigraphy in hemodialysis patients. *Kidney Int.* 2009;76:428-436.

Dew MA, Jacobs CL, Jowsey SG, et al. Guidelines for the psychosocial evaluation of living unrelated kidney donors in the United States. *Am J Transplant.* 2007;7:1047-1054.

Fairhead T, Knoll G. Recurrent glomerular disease after kidney transplantation. *Curr Opin Nephrol Hypertens.* 2010;19:578-585.

Frassetto LA, Tan-Tam C, Stock PG. Renal transplantation in patients with HIV. *Nat Rev Nephrol.* 2009;5:582-589.

Gill J, Bunnapradist S, Danovitch GM, et al. Outcomes of kidney transplantation from older living donors to older recipients. *Am J Kidney Dis.* 2008;52:541-552.

Hart A, Smith JM, et al. OPTN/SRTR annual data report 2014: kidney. *Am J Transplant.* 2016;16:11-46.

Kasiske BL, Cangro CB, Hariharan S, et al. The evaluation of renal transplant candidates: clinical practice guidelines. *Am J Transplant.* 2001;1:3-95.

Kher A, Mandelbrot DA. The living kidney donor evaluation: focus on renal issues. *Clin J Am Soc Nephrol.* 2012;7:366-371.

Kidney Disease: Improving Global Outcomes (KDIGO) Living Kidney DonorWork Group. KDIGO Clinical Practice Guideline on the Evaluation and Care of Living Kidney Donors. *Transplantation.* 2017;101(suppl 8S):S1-S109.

Knoll G, Cockfield S, Blydt-Hansen T, et al. Canadian Society of Transplantation: consensus guidelines on eligibility for kidney transplantation. *CMAJ.* 2005;8:S1-S25.

Lefaucheur C, Suberbielle-Boissel C, Hill GS, et al. Clinical relevance of preformed HLA donor-specific antibodies in kidney transplantation. *Am J Transplant.* 2008;8:324-331.

Lentine KL, Costa SP, Weir MR, et al. Cardiac disease evaluation and management among kidney and liver transplantation candidates: a scientific statement from the American Heart Association and the American College of Cardiology Foundation: endorsed by the American Society of Transplant Surgeons, American Society of Transplantation, and National Kidney Foundation. *Circulation.* 2012;126:617-663.

Mukhtar RA, Piper ML, Freise C, Van't Veer LJ, Baehner FL, Esserman LJ. The novel application of genomic profiling assays to shorten inactive status for potential kidney transplant recipients with breast cancer. *Am J Transplant.* 2017;17:292-295. doi:10.1111/ajt.14003.

Muzaale AD, Massie AB, Wang MC, et al. Risk of end-stage renal disease following live kidney donation. *JAMA.* 2014;311:579-586.

Rule AD, Larson TS, Bergstralh EJ, et al. Using serum creatinine to estimate glomerular filtration rate: accuracy in good health and in chronic kidney disease. *Ann Intern Med.* 2004;141:929-937.

Saran R, Li Y, Robinson B, et al. United States renal data system 2015 annual data report: epidemiology of kidney disease in the United States. *Am J Kidney Dis.* 2016;67:S1-S305. Svii.

Segev DL, Muzaale AD, Caffo BS, et al. Perioperative mortality and long-term survival following live kidney donation. *JAMA.* 2010;303:959-966.

Tavakol MM, Vincenti FG, Assadi H, et al. Long-term renal function and cardiovascular disease risk in obese kidney donors. *Clin J Am Soc Nephrol.* 2009;4:1230-1238.

Full bibliography can be found on www.expertconsult.com.

Posttransplantation Monitoring and Outcomes

61

Jagbir S. Gill; James Lan

The management of kidney transplant recipients is complex and spans a wide range of clinical scenarios. Posttransplant care begins in the immediate postsurgical period and continues through the various phases that make up the natural history of kidney transplantation. Whereas the early phases of care focus primarily on postsurgical management, monitoring of allograft function, and optimization of immunosuppression, later phases extend this focus to include ongoing assessment and management of factors that contribute to chronic allograft dysfunction, allograft loss, and death with a functioning graft. The nuances of posttransplant care have changed significantly over time as our understanding of the natural history of transplantation has evolved. The case-mix of transplant recipients has become more complex, and new technologies to monitor transplant recipients have emerged. In this chapter, we will review the major aspects of posttransplant care through this continuum in the current era of transplantation.

RECIPIENT AND DONOR CHARACTERISTICS

With changes in the demographics of the population with end-stage renal disease (ESRD) and improvements in technologies and immunosuppression, kidney transplantation may benefit many patients who previously would not have been eligible. With these successes come increased challenges and complexities in posttransplant care, along with a greater need to individualize care for various subgroups of kidney transplant recipients. For instance, transplantation in older adult patients has increased significantly in the past decade, with patients 65 years of age and older accounting for 18.5% of all transplant recipients in the United States in 2016. The complexities of pre- and posttransplant care are unique in older adult recipients, because they are more likely to have a greater burden of comorbid disease and a higher risk for death with a functioning allograft. However, the risk for acute allograft rejection is lower in older transplant recipients as a result of immunosenescence, which may allow for decreased use of immunosuppression. Therefore posttransplant care must be tailored to risks and outcomes within individual populations. Also, with the advent of desensitization strategies, both human leukocyte antigen (HLA)- and ABO-incompatible transplantation are realities in our current era, but these cases require more intense follow-up, given their higher risk for rejection and allograft loss. Other high-risk recipient groups include human immunodeficiency virus (HIV)-positive recipients, repeat transplant recipients, and multiorgan

transplant recipients, each of which brings unique challenges to posttransplant care.

Similarly, the characteristics of deceased donors have changed over time, further complicating early posttransplant care. In the face of increasing demand for transplantation, organs from higher risk deceased donors are routinely transplanted in selected recipients. The Kidney Donor Profile Index (KDPI) is a continuous measure (percentile) of deceased donor quality that characterizes donors according to 10 characteristics that are associated with posttransplant allograft survival. The KDPI provides a relative estimation of posttransplant allograft survival relative to the kidneys transplanted in the United States within the previous year. For example, a kidney with a KDPI of 20% is anticipated to last longer than 80% of kidneys that were transplanted (i.e., it is among the top 20% of donor kidneys in terms of expected longevity). Conversely, a kidney with a KDPI of 85% is anticipated to last longer than only 15% of kidneys that were transplanted (i.e., it is among the bottom 15% of donor kidneys in terms of expected longevity). In 2015 nearly 10% of transplant recipients received a kidney with a KDPI of 85% or greater. In addition to having an increased risk of allograft loss, recipients who receive these kidneys also have an increased risk for delayed graft function (DGF) compared with recipients who receive kidneys with lower KDPIs. These high KDPI kidneys should typically be allocated only to recipient populations that continue to derive a significant survival benefit from transplantation, such as older adult and diabetic transplant candidates.

THE FIRST WEEK

Most kidney transplant recipients have a hospital duration of 4 to 7 days following surgery. In the acute postoperative phase, transplant recipient care involves assessment for immediate graft function, management of potential surgical complications, and treatment of postoperative fluid and electrolyte shifts.

The details of kidney transplantation surgery vary depending on whether the kidney comes from a living donor or a deceased donor, as well as the specific anatomy of a given recipient. In general, the surgery involves engraftment in the iliac fossa with vascular anastomoses of the donor renal artery to the recipient external iliac artery and of the donor vein to the external iliac vein. Perioperative complications that may require surgical exploration and management include bleeding and thrombosis of the renal artery or vein.

Assessment of graft function involves quantifying urine output (keeping the preoperative urine output of the recipient in mind) and following serum chemistries every 12 to 24 hours. Immediate graft function is denoted by a rapid drop in serum creatinine levels and urine output in excess of 100 mL/hour; this is expected in all living donor kidney transplant recipients and in most recipients of deceased donor kidneys. Immediate graft function is less likely in recipients of higher KDPI kidneys and in cases with prolonged cold ischemic times (>24 hours).

DGF is typically denoted as the requirement for dialysis within the first week posttransplant and occurs in less than 5% of living donor transplant recipients. Conversely, DGF is seen in more than 30% of recipients of deceased donor kidneys with a KDPI ≥85%. In addition to donor factors, the duration of cold ischemic time and warm ischemic time is an important predictor of DGF. Dialysis is performed based on volume status and metabolic parameters, and either hemodialysis or peritoneal dialysis may be used, depending on the patient's baseline dialysis modality. In the case of peritoneal dialysis, it is important to confirm that the peritoneum was not breached during the surgery before resumption of dialysis.

Although the cause of DGF is usually acute ischemia-reperfusion injury, alternate causes (including vascular thrombosis and early acute rejection) need to be considered. Therefore a Doppler kidney ultrasound to assess for blood flow in the allograft is recommended within hours of a clinical change in allograft function. Elevated resistive indices may suggest either tubular injury or rejection; thus the baseline risk for rejection and duration of DGF should be considered in assessing the cause of early graft dysfunction. If rejection is suspected or DGF persists beyond 1 week, an allograft biopsy should be performed. In cases of prolonged DGF, serial biopsies should be considered to rule out immune-mediated injury.

Reduced exposure to calcineurin inhibitors (CNIs) in the setting of DGF is recommended to avoid further tubular injury associated with CNI nephrotoxicity, but this must be balanced with the risk for rejection. The use of induction immunosuppressive agents is recommended if CNIs are to be reduced or avoided in the setting of DGF. There are few data to support a uniform approach to immunosuppression in the setting of DGF, but some centers prefer to use T lymphocyte–depleting antibodies (thymoglobulin) for induction, along with immediate initiation of an antimetabolite (mycophenolate) and corticosteroids, with delayed introduction of CNI only once there is evidence of graft function. A number of novel therapeutic agents are currently being studied to minimize the risk of DGF in kidney transplantation. QPI-1002 (formerly I5NP) is an intravenously administered synthetic small interfering ribonucleic acid (siRNA) that is currently in a phase 3 clinical trial to prevent DGF. The agent is designed to temporarily inhibit the expression of the proapoptotic gene p53 in order to allow proximal tubular cells the opportunity to repair ischemia reperfusion-associated cellular damage.

The majority of DGF cases recover within the first 2 to 3 weeks, but numerous studies have demonstrated inferior allograft survival in patients who have developed DGF, although it remains unclear how much of this is directly attributable to cold ischemia–induced DGF versus baseline donor and recipient factors that may independently contribute to both

an increased risk of DGF and allograft loss. Importantly, although DGF appears to be associated with an increased risk of allograft loss, the survival benefit of transplantation is retained even among recipients who develop DGF and largely irrespective of the KDPI of the transplanted kidney.

Fluid and electrolyte management is a key component of early postoperative care. Hemodynamic extremes of hypotension and volume overload should be avoided in all patients and, particularly, in older adult patients and in those with compromised cardiac function. Electrolyte shifts, including hypercalcemia and hypophosphatemia associated with secondary hyperparathyroidism and hypomagnesemia associated with diuretic use, may be seen early posttransplantation and should be managed accordingly.

OUTPATIENT CARE

Following discharge from the hospital, transplant recipients are closely followed by the transplant center. The frequency of monitoring is greatest during the first 3 months, as the risk for rejection is highest during this period. Many centers follow patients twice weekly during the first month posttransplant and then weekly for the remainder of the first 3 months, with the frequency of visits gradually reduced to every 4 to 8 weeks by the end of the first year.

Routine posttransplant monitoring includes a follow-up history and physical examination, along with measurement of serum chemistries, a complete blood count, liver enzymes, whole blood CNI levels, and urinalysis. Spot albumin-to-creatinine ratios are also periodically monitored. Preemptive viral screening and monitoring are indicated at a high frequency (weekly) for the first 3 to 6 months, depending on the patient's risk for infection, and should continue at a lower frequency for the duration of the first year posttransplantation. Testing beyond the first year should be tailored to each patient's risk.

IMMUNOSUPPRESSION

Immunosuppression after transplantation consists of induction therapy followed by lifelong maintenance immunotherapy. Chapter 62 provides greater details on specific induction and maintenance agents, including their side-effect profiles. Induction therapy is administered at the time of transplantation and includes intravenous methylprednisolone, along with either an anti-CD25 antibody (basiliximab) or a T lymphocyte–depleting antibody (the polyclonal antibody thymoglobulin). Alemtuzumab is a monoclonal antibody used in the management of chronic lymphocytic leukemia that results in potent lymphocyte depletion and is increasingly used as an induction agent in kidney transplantation.

Maintenance immunosuppression typically consists of triple immunosuppressive therapy with a CNI, an antimetabolite, and low-dose corticosteroids. Until the early 2000s, azathioprine was the preferred posttransplantation antimetabolite; however, mycophenolic acid (MPA) agents more selectively target lymphocytes, resulting in superior efficacy in preventing acute rejection and increased patient tolerability. Rapamycin has been studied as an alternative to CNIs or for use in combination with CNIs. Although concerns regarding wound healing and nephrotoxicity have minimized the use of rapamycin as a primary de novo immunosuppressant agent after transplantation, data suggesting a reduced risk for malignancies with the use of rapamycin have renewed interest in this agent, particularly for patients with recurrent skin cancers posttransplant. Belatacept is an intravenously administered costimulatory blocker that binds CD80 and CD86 on the surface of antigen-presenting cells to inhibit T-cell activation and promote anergy and apoptosis. While long-term outcomes comparing this agent with cyclosporine have been very promising, the optimal indication and immunosuppressive cocktail within which this agent should be used still remains uncertain and will likely be refined in the coming years.

IMMUNOSUPPRESSIVE PROTOCOLS

The majority of transplant recipients are maintained on triple immunosuppressive therapy, including CNI, MPA, and corticosteroids. Low rates of acute rejection and growing concern with the adverse effects of these agents, including chronic CNI nephrotoxicity, have led to strategies to minimize immunosuppressive exposure. Minimization of CNI and corticosteroid exposure has been most frequently studied, but the merits of immunosuppression minimization with the increasingly recognized importance of chronic immune-mediated injury are debatable in the current era.

Posttransplant corticosteroid exposure has been reduced significantly, with prednisone doses rapidly tapered to 5 to 10 mg daily within the first 4 to 6 weeks after surgery. Late withdrawal of corticosteroids has been largely abandoned in the face of numerous studies demonstrating an increased risk for rejection when corticosteroids are withdrawn beyond 3 to 6 months posttransplant. Early corticosteroid withdrawal or avoidance strategies, however, are associated with largely favorable outcomes. A meta-analysis of 34 studies, including 5637 patients receiving steroid withdrawal or avoidance regimens, found that steroid avoidance reduced the risk for hyperlipidemia, hypertension, and new-onset diabetes after transplantation (NODAT). Woodle and colleagues conducted a multicenter randomized controlled trial of early corticosteroid withdrawal (within 7 days) compared with low-dose maintenance corticosteroids in a CNI- and MPA-based regimen. The early steroid withdrawal group had an increased rate of biopsy-proven acute rejection and chronic allograft nephropathy, but no difference was found in the composite primary endpoint of death, graft loss, or severe acute rejection through 5 years. When examined separately, graft and patient survival also did not differ. Although steroid exposure should be minimized whenever possible, corticosteroid avoidance or early withdrawal should be reserved for patients at low risk for rejection and only with careful and frequent posttransplant monitoring.

LONG-TERM DRUG DOSING AND MONITORING

Because of inter- and intrapatient variability in the bioavailability and absorption of CNI, routine whole-blood drug-level monitoring is essential. Trough levels of CNI correlate well with drug exposure and clinical events, particularly for tacrolimus. However, evidence exists that peak drug levels (2 hours after dose) of cyclosporine correlate better with drug exposure and clinical events, including acute rejection. As a result, certain centers have adopted peak level, or "C2" monitoring, for cyclosporine. Although specific therapeutic targets may vary depending on concomitant immunosuppression, levels are typically kept highest in the first month after transplant, with a gradual reduction over the next 6 months. In interpreting drug levels, it is important to remember that different labs may use different assays, resulting in different results.

Routine therapeutic drug level monitoring is not recommended for MPA, because trough levels do not correlate well with clinical efficacy, and the repeat measurements required to appropriately calculate the area under the curve are labor intensive and not feasible for routine measurement. Target doses (2 g daily for mycophenolate mofetil and 1440 mg daily for mycophenolate sodium, typically in divided doses) are based on clinical trials demonstrating efficacy at these doses. Transient dose reduction or temporary discontinuation of MPA is recommended in cases of significant diarrheal symptoms or profound leukopenia. However, full doses should be resumed after resolution of symptoms, if tolerated, because prolonged dose reductions or discontinuations are associated with inferior allograft survival.

Nonadherence to immunosuppressive medications after kidney transplantation significantly increases the risk of acute and chronic immune-mediated allograft dysfunction and allograft loss. Therefore assessment and management of nonadherence are important aspects of immunosuppressive management. An assessment of patient-level risk factors for nonadherence (including young age, a history of nonadherence to other therapies, psychiatric/psychological disorders, substance abuse, cognitive impairment) should be completed, and mechanisms to monitor adherence should be implemented before transplantation. Tools to optimize adherence should be explored, including increased education and support to promote adherence, tailoring the immunosuppressive regimen, or consideration of once-daily formulations of medications when available, blister packaging of medications, and increased frequency of follow-up. Importantly, these interventions require frequent reassessment and evaluation in the early and late posttransplant setting.

ADVERSE EFFECTS AND DRUG INTERACTIONS

Adverse effects of immunosuppressant medications should be assessed during each follow-up visit. Significant effects of corticosteroids include cataracts, bone loss and fractures, avascular necrosis, hypertension, weight gain, dyslipidemia, glucose intolerance, mood lability, and acne. MPAs may confer bone marrow toxicity (leukopenia, anemia), gastric reflux, diarrhea, and pancreatitis. Calcineurin inhibitors may cause acute and chronic nephrotoxicity, although the impact of CNIs on chronic graft function is being increasingly questioned. Other significant effects of CNIs include hypomagnesemia, hyperkalemia, hyperuricemia, neurotoxicity (e.g., tremor), and, rarely, thrombotic microangiopathy. Tacrolimus is more strongly associated with NODAT than cyclosporine, whereas cyclosporine is more commonly associated with cosmetic changes, including gingival hyperplasia and hirsutism.

The narrow therapeutic and toxic window for CNIs, in addition to the high potential for altered metabolism from

Table 61.1 Selected Common Drug Interactions With Calcineurin Inhibitors

Increase CNI Level (Inhibits Enzyme)[a]	Decrease CNI Level (Stimulates Enzyme)[a]
Calcium channel blockers	Antibiotics
• Diltiazem	• Rifabutin
• Verapamil	• Rifampin
Antiarrhythmics	Antiepileptics
• Amiodarone	• Phenobarbital
HIV protease inhibitors	• Phenytoin
• Ritonavir	• Carbamazepine
• Saquinavir	Herbal substances
• Indinavir	• St. John wort
Azole antifungal agents	
• Ketoconazole	
• Clotrimazole	
• Itraconazole	
• Voriconazole	
Antibiotics	
• Erythromycin base	
• Synercid (quinupristin and dalfopristin)	
Antidepressants	
• Fluvoxamine	
Other agents	
• Grapefruit juice	

[a]Listed drugs interact with the calcineurin inhibitors, cyclosporine, and tacrolimus because they are metabolized by the cytochrome P450 CYP3A4 isoenzyme.
CNI, Calcineurin inhibitors; *HIV,* human immunodeficiency virus.

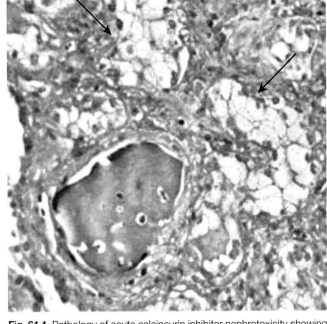

Fig. 61.1 Pathology of acute calcineurin inhibitor nephrotoxicity showing isometric tubular vacuolization *(arrows).*

interference of the cytochrome 450 (CYP450) mechanism, mandates careful examination and recognition of potential drug interactions. Common CYP450 drug inhibitors (which will increase CNI levels) and inducers (which will lower CNI levels) are outlined in Table 61.1. New drugs should be introduced with care, and drug levels should be carefully monitored, when indicated. MPA is not metabolized via the CYP450 enzyme pathway, and there are fewer drug interactions compared with CNI; however, any drugs that may potentiate leukopenia should not be used in conjunction with these agents.

ALLOGRAFT DYSFUNCTION

The immune response to an allograft involves (1) recognition of foreign antigens, (2) activation of recipient lymphocytes, and (3) effector mechanisms leading to rejection of the allograft. The human major histocompatibility complex (MHC) is a cluster of genes on chromosome 6 that encodes HLA, in addition to other agents critical in controlling the immune response; MHC is the key factor in the initiation of the immune response to an allograft. The HLA antigens are the major barriers to transplantation, and allogeneic donor HLA antigens are the main targets of the immune system in rejection of the graft. However, the role of non-HLA antigens in inciting an immune response and subsequent rejection is increasingly being realized.

ACUTE ALLOGRAFT DYSFUNCTION

A 15% to 20% increase in serum creatinine from baseline suggests graft dysfunction and warrants a thorough evaluation, including an assessment of risk factors for acute kidney injury, an ultrasound of the allograft, and often an allograft biopsy. Nonimmune causes of allograft dysfunction should be ruled out, including CNI nephrotoxicity, acute interstitial nephritis, pyelonephritis, ischemic injury, recurrent native kidney disease, and BK nephropathy. Supratherapeutic CNI levels and the presence of isometric tubular vacuolization or arteriolar hyalinosis on biopsy (Fig. 61.1) strongly suggest acute CNI nephrotoxicity, although an allograft biopsy is not usually required for diagnosis because a reduction in CNI dose will quickly improve kidney function. Recurrent native kidney disease rates vary, depending on the original cause of ESRD, and require allograft biopsy for diagnosis. BK polyomavirus nephropathy may cause graft injury with a high risk for subsequent graft loss, but a histologic diagnosis is often difficult.

The Banff classification, originally published in 1993 and subsequently revised in multiple iterations, was instrumental in standardizing criteria for allograft pathology, including those for acute rejection (Box 61.1). The glomeruli, tubules, interstitium, and vessels should be examined for the presence of inflammation and lymphocyte infiltration. Interstitial inflammation with lymphocytes is scored from absent (i0) to severe (i3). Tubulitis is the definitive aspect of acute cellular rejection and is quantified from mild (t1) to severe (t3). Vessel wall infiltration, or arteritis, represents a greater severity of rejection (grade II) and ranges from mild/moderate (v1) to severe (v2). Although lymphocyte infiltration in the glomeruli may accompany acute rejection, it is not a criterion of rejection.

Box 61.1   Banff 2007 Criteria for Allograft Pathology With Banff 2013 Revision (Simplified)

1. **Normal**
2. **Antibody-mediated changes** (may coincide with categories 3, 4, and 5)
   Acute/active AMR: all three features must be present
   1. Histologic evidence of tissue injury (one or more): microvascular inflammation (g >0 and/or ptc >0); intimal or transmural arteritis (v >0); acute thrombotic microangiopathy; ATN without other cause
   2. Evidence of antibody interaction with vascular endothelium (one or more): C4d staining in peritubular capillaries; moderate-severe microvascular inflammation (g + ptc ≥2); validated molecular markers for AMR
   3. Serologic evidence for donor-specific antibodies (HLA or non-HLA)
   Chronic active AMR: all three features must be present
   1. Chronic tissue injury (one or more): transplant glomerulopathy (by light microscopy or by EM alone); severe peritubular capillary basement membrane multilayering; unexplained new arterial intimal fibrosis
   2. Evidence of antibody interaction with vascular endothelium (one or more): C4d staining in peritubular capillaries; moderate-severe microvascular inflammation (g + ptc ≥2); validated molecular markers for AMR
   3. Serologic evidence for DSAs (HLA or non-HLA)
   C4d staining without evidence of rejection (require all three):
   1. C4d staining in peritubular capillaries
   2. No acute or chronic microvascular inflammation, intimal or transmural arteritis, thrombotic microangiopathy, or unexplained ATN
   3. No acute T-cell mediated rejection or borderline changes
3. **Borderline changes**
   Suspicious for acute T-cell–mediated rejection. No intimal arteritis, but foci of tubulitis (t1, t2, or t3) with minor interstitial inflammation (i0 or i1) or interstitial infiltration (i2, i3) with mild (t1) tubulitis (t1, i1, or greater)
4. **T-cell–mediated rejection** (TCMR; may coincide with 2, 5, and 6)
   Acute T-cell–mediated rejection (type/grade)
   1. Significant interstitial infiltration (i2; >25% of parenchyma affected) and foci of moderate tubulitis (t2; >4 mononuclear cells/tubular cross section or group of 10 tubular cells)
   2. Significant interstitial infiltration (i2; >25% of parenchyma affected) and foci of severe tubulitis (t3; >10 mononuclear cells/tubular cross section or group of 10 tubular cells)
   3. Mild to moderate intimal arteritis (v1)
   4. Severe intimal arteritis comprising >25% of the luminal area (v2)
   5. Transmural arteritis and/or arterial fibrinoid change and necrosis of medial smooth muscle
   Chronic active T-cell–mediated rejection
   Chronic allograft arteriopathy (arterial intimal fibrosis with mononuclear cell infiltration)
5. **Interstitial fibrosis and tubular atrophy,** no evidence of any specific etiology (grade)
   1. Mild interstitial fibrosis (ci1) and tubular atrophy (ct1); <25% of cortical area affected
   2. Moderate interstitial fibrosis (ci2) and tubular atrophy (ct2); 26%–50% of cortical area affected
   3. Severe interstitial fibrosis (ci3) and tubular atrophy (ct3); >50% of cortical area affected
6. **Other:** changes not considered to be due to rejection—acute and/or chronic (may coincide with categories 2, 3, 4, and 5)

AMR, Antibody-mediated rejection; *ATN*, acute tubular necrosis; *C4d+*, activated complement component C4d; *cg*, glomerulopathy; *ci*, interstitial fibrosis; *ct*, tubular atrophy; *EM*, electron microscopy; *g*, glomerulitis; *i*, interstitial infiltration; *ptc*, peritubular capillaritis; *t*, tubulitis; *v*, vessel wall infiltration or arteritis.

Treatment of acute cellular rejection includes intravenous pulse corticosteroids, intensification of maintenance immunosuppression, and polyclonal antilymphocyte antibodies (thymoglobulin) in more severe cases. Although recovery from acute rejection has improved dramatically over time, an episode of acute rejection (even if successfully treated) significantly increases the risk for early graft loss.

Antibody-mediated rejection (AMR) involves the production of antidonor antibodies by plasma cells, either from memory or naive B cells. These donor-specific antibodies (DSAs) may be directed against both HLA and non-HLA targets on allograft vascular endothelium, resulting in complement activation, cell death, loss of vascular integrity, and subsequent ischemic injury. In addition to the presence of circulating DSA, the revised 2013 Banff diagnosis of AMR also requires demonstration of antibody interaction with vascular endothelium, which may be indicated by (1) complement component C4d deposition in peritubular capillaries, (2) a significant burden of microvascular injury, or (3) validated molecular markers for AMR. Bolstered by evidence from molecular studies and protocol biopsies, the previous

requirement for C4d positivity is no longer absolute under the current Banff criteria, as numerous groups have independently confirmed the existence and significance of C4d-negative AMR, particularly in patients presenting with late antibody-mediated allograft dysfunction. Finally, histologic evidence of acute or chronic tissue injury must be present. These findings may include acute tubular injury, vasculitis, and peritubular capillary inflammation.

The importance of DSA appears to extend beyond the acute rejection episode; chronic exposure to low levels of DSA (even in the absence of a clinical episode of AMR) may lead to chronic AMR and inferior graft survival. As a result, the treatment of AMR primarily targets DSA reduction either through elimination of B cells that secrete alloantibodies and/or removal of circulating DSA. Plasmapheresis and high-dose intravenous immune globulin (IVIG) aim to lower DSA levels through removal or inactivation, respectively. Anti-CD20 agents (rituximab) aim to reduce antibody levels by depleting B lymphocytes and preventing the maturation of new DSA-producing plasma cells. The proteasome inhibitor bortezomib causes apoptosis of normal plasma cells and had favorable results in the treatment of AMR in small single-center uncontrolled studies. Although its benefit is largely unproven, bortezomib may be considered in refractory cases of AMR. Recently, eculizumab, a novel anti-C5 complement inhibitor, showed promise in reducing the rate of acute AMR in recipients transplanted with a positive crossmatch, although patients with persistently strong DSA still progressed to chronic AMR on longer follow-up. The optimal use of this new class of therapeutics will require further study.

CHRONIC ALLOGRAFT DYSFUNCTION

A gradual decline in kidney function manifested by a slowly rising creatinine, increasing levels of proteinuria, and worsening hypertension denotes chronic allograft dysfunction and typically precedes chronic allograft loss. Chronic allograft loss is defined as allograft failure that occurs after 1 year posttransplant. For years, the term *chronic allograft nephropathy* was cited as the most common cause of chronic allograft loss, without a clear understanding of its underlying etiology. In the 2005 Banff reclassification, this term was abandoned and replaced with the term *interstitial fibrosis and tubular atrophy (IF/TA)* to more accurately represent the histologic findings associated with chronic allograft loss, without ascribing any specific cause to the histologic changes. A number of histologic changes may be seen in chronic failing allografts, including vascular changes (endothelial inflammation and intimal thickening), glomerular changes (glomerular capillary wall thickening, often with a double contour appearance, termed transplant glomerulopathy), and interstitial fibrosis with tubular atrophy. Many of these histologic changes are associated with inferior allograft survival. For instance, transplant glomerulopathy carries one of the worse prognoses, with 5-year graft survival rates of less than 50% from the time of diagnosis. The Banff classification grades the degree of IF/TA (I, II, III) according to the severity of interstitial fibrosis (mild, moderate, severe) and tubular atrophy (mild to severe), but these grades have not been precisely correlated with allograft outcomes.

It is clear from long-term protocol biopsy studies that the underlying causes of these histologic changes are multifactorial and include both immune-mediated and nonimmune-mediated processes, such as chronic CNI nephrotoxicity, recurrent disease, and subclinical and overt chronic AMR.

Chronic CNI nephrotoxicity was first described in the 1970s and is attributed to the renal vasoconstrictive effects of CNI and direct tubular toxicity. The histologic hallmarks of chronic CNI nephrotoxicity are largely nonspecific and include stripped interstitial fibrosis, glomerular sclerosis, and arteriolar hyalinosis (the only specific finding of CNI nephrotoxicity). Calcineurin inhibitor nephrotoxicity has been touted as a key contributor to chronic allograft dysfunction, but recent studies have suggested a more prominent role for immune-mediated injury in chronic allograft dysfunction, bringing into question the safety of CNI minimization posttransplantation. Therefore the relative importance of CNI nephrotoxicity and chronic rejection remains an active source of debate.

Chronic active AMR is a subset of AMR and is characterized by the presence of circulating DSA and histologic evidence of chronic allograft injury, including transplant glomerulopathy, peritubular capillary basement membrane multilayering, and interstitial fibrosis and tubular atrophy. After binding

of antibody on target antigens, activation of the complement cascade, direct endothelial cell activation, and recruitment of inflammatory cells have all been shown to take part in this complex process. Consequently, the treatment of chronic antibody-mediated damage is not precisely defined, but it is recognized as a key therapeutic target in reducing the risk for chronic allograft loss.

ASSESSMENT OF ALLOGRAFT DYSFUNCTION

Current strategies to monitor allograft function are limited to serum creatinine, proteinuria, and surveillance allograft biopsies in some programs. Unfortunately, aside from the invasive procedure of an allograft biopsy, these are late markers of allograft dysfunction and are inadequate to detect early immune injury, subclinical rejection, and chronic allograft inflammation, all of which are increasingly recognized as important contributors of chronic allograft function.

Allograft biopsy remains the gold standard for early detection of allograft changes because histologic rejection can be seen before changes in serum creatinine. However, the impact of interventions that are guided solely by biopsy findings remains unclear, with a recent randomized study demonstrating no effect with treatment. Ultimately, the invasive nature of a biopsy and patient reluctance limit the widespread use of surveillance biopsies. Therefore novel noninvasive markers of immune-mediated injury and chronic inflammation are needed.

DSAs are routinely monitored *before* transplantation because they correlate with increased rates of subclinical and clinical AMR in the early posttransplant period. In the setting of AMR, DSA levels may be monitored to guide the duration and choice of treatment regimens, although it is recognized that the output of solid-phase immunoassays only provides a semiquantitative assessment of antibody strength and should be interpreted in the context of the platform's known limitations. De novo DSAs posttransplant have also been associated with higher transplant failure rates and may occur before proteinuria or changes in serum creatinine. Consensus guidelines have advocated for routine monitoring of DSAs posttransplant. However, the cost-effectiveness of routine DSA monitoring, particularly in stable low-risk and intermediate-risk patients, remains unclear. More recently, the advent of modified single-antigen bead assays (C1q, C3d, IgG subtypes) permits discrimination of the pathogenicity of DSA by interrogating their complement-activating potential. While many studies associate complement-fixing DSA with inferior graft outcomes, it remains controversial whether these tests provide prognostic value beyond conventional clinical data and antibody characteristics. Thus more research and studies are required to define the utility of these diagnostics before implementation into clinical care.

A number of candidate biomarkers have been studied to predict and detect acute rejection and early allograft injury, including urinary markers related to cytotoxic T lymphocytes (granzyme A/B, perforin, Fas ligand, serpin B9), regulatory T cells (FOXP3), CD4 T cells (chemokines, TIM-3), and markers of renal tubular injury (NGAL, A1M, cleaved B2M). Functional assays such as IFN-γ ELISPOT can detect donor-reactive memory T cells that correlate with an increased risk of cellular rejection posttransplant. With the evolution and cost reduction of high-throughput technologies, transcriptome profiling of tissue biopsy allows characterization of unique gene signatures that improve the diagnostic accuracy and prognostication of cellular and AMR events. Similarly, peripheral blood mRNA analysis has been shown to predict subclinical and acute rejection and has the advantage to serve as a noninvasive method of immune monitoring posttransplant. On the horizon, quantitation and tracking the dynamics of donor-derived cell-free DNA in recipient blood is a novel method of allograft surveillance without the associated shortcomings of allograft biopsy. Although a number of promising observations have been made, most of these markers still require further validation and controlled trials to document their clinical applicability and ability to improve clinical outcomes.

INFECTIOUS COMPLICATIONS

PROPHYLAXIS AND MONITORING

The risk for infection is related to the overall level of immunosuppression, recipient factors, donor factors, and community exposures. Strategies to minimize infection after transplantation include pretransplant vaccination and a combination of universal posttransplant prophylaxis (e.g., perioperative antibiotic prophylaxis) and preemptive therapy (e.g., monitoring and treating for viremic states).

Universal prophylaxis is given to all patients for a defined time period and includes the administration of perioperative antibiotics and low-dose trimethoprim-sulfamethoxazole (TMP-SMX) for 6 months to a lifetime after transplant to prevent *Pneumocystis jirovecii* pneumonia (formerly known as PCP), *Toxoplasma gondii*, many *Nocardia* and *Listeria* species, and common urinary and respiratory pathogens. Patients intolerant to TMP-SMX may receive either atovaquone or dapsone instead.

Preemptive therapy uses quantitative assays at predetermined intervals to detect early infection, with initiation of therapy when there is a positive assay. Preemptive therapy is often used in monitoring for cytomegalovirus (CMV), Epstein-Barr virus (EBV), BK polyomavirus, and viral hepatitis, depending on donor and recipient factors.

APPROACH TO POSTTRANSPLANT INFECTIONS

Clinical presentations of infectious disease may be variable and atypical in immunosuppressed patients. Therefore workup for a suspected infection should be broad and may include blood and urine cultures, a chest radiograph, and bronchoscopic evaluation when investigating pulmonary infiltrates. In cases where the source of infection is unclear, the threshold for initiation of broad-spectrum antibiotics should be low. Consideration of donor-derived infections, latent viral infections, and new opportunistic infections, factoring in the timing posttransplant, is important in developing a differential diagnosis.

A detailed approach to and management of infectious complications posttransplant are outlined in Chapter 63 and will not be discussed in this chapter, with the exception of human BK polyomaviruses. The human polyomavirus BK (BKV) causes BK nephropathy in up to 10% of kidney transplant recipients. BKV may be harbored within the recipient or in the uroepithelium of the donor, with reactivation and replication upon immunosuppression. Renal tubular epithelial invasion produces an inflammatory response similar to acute rejection, with resultant atrophy and fibrosis. A creeping increase of serum creatinine, along with BKV viruria and viremia, is often the only clinical sign of BK nephropathy. Therefore preemptive screening is essential. BKV polymerase chain reaction (PCR) should be performed once every 3 months for the first 2 years posttransplant, and then annually until the fifth year. Viremic patients should have immunosuppressive doses reduced and undergo an allograft biopsy if there is evidence of kidney dysfunction. In patients with sustained viremia despite a reduction in immunosuppression, adjunctive therapy with cidofovir, leflunomide, IVIG, and fluoroquinolones may be considered, although these treatments remain largely unproven. The role of fluoroquinolones in preventing BK viruria was recently examined in a double-blinded, placebo-controlled trial of 154 Canadian living or deceased donor kidney transplant recipients who were randomized to receive levofloxacin or placebo for the first 3 months post transplantation. There was no difference in the time to occurrence of BK viruria between groups, and there was an increased risk of adverse events with levofloxacin, including bacterial resistance.

HEMATOLOGIC COMPLICATIONS

Common hematologic complications and their causes are outlined in Table 61.2. Nearly half of kidney transplant recipients will be anemic within the first 6 months post transplant, with 10% to 40% remaining anemic at 1 year, irrespective of graft function. Within days of kidney transplantation, erythropoietin (EPO) levels increase as a result of the functioning allograft, with an early surge to supraphysiologic levels in the first 2 to 3 weeks. Despite this, anemia may persist because of a number of factors, including baseline anemia, surgical blood loss, iron deficiency, allograft dysfunction, and viral illness. In addition, a number of drugs introduced posttransplant may cause anemia, including antimetabolites (MPA, azathioprine), antiviral agents, antibiotics (e.g., TMP-SMX), and angiotensin-converting enzyme (ACE) inhibitors. Although some agents, such as ACE inhibitors, may result in isolated anemia, most of these drugs typically affect other cell lines as well.

Workup of posttransplant anemia should include iron studies, a reticulocyte count, and an assessment of other cell lines. If the etiology remains unclear or involves more than one cell line, a hematologist should be consulted. Parvovirus B19 should also be considered with unexplained isolated anemia.

Leukopenia, with or without anemia, is most often associated with immunosuppressive or antiviral medications. Dose reductions or discontinuation usually improves medication-related cytopenias within a matter of days to weeks. If cytopenias persist, alternate etiologies should be explored. Anemia and thrombocytopenia, with or without allograft dysfunction, may indicate hemolytic uremic syndrome. This may be secondary to CNI or recurrent hemolytic uremic syndrome–thrombotic thrombocytopenic purpura (HUS-TTP) and generally portends a poor prognosis, warranting therapy with plasmapheresis.

Table 61.2 Hematologic Complications Post Kidney Transplantation

Hematologic Complication	Cause(s)
Anemia	Allograft dysfunction (early or late posttransplant)
	Iron deficiency
	Blood loss
	EPO resistance
	Immunosuppressive medications (mycophenolic acid agents, azathioprine, rapamycin)
	Other medications (TMP-SMX, valganciclovir, ganciclovir, ACE inhibitors)
	Infections (parvovirus B19, CMV, BK polyomavirus, tuberculosis, varicella-zoster virus)
	Comorbid conditions (e.g., cardiovascular disease, peripheral vascular disease)
	Hemolytic anemia (minor ABO incompatibility, rhesus D unmatching, autoimmune anemia)
Leukopenia	Immunosuppressive medications (mycophenolic acid agents, azathioprine, rapamycin, thymoglobulin, alemtuzumab)
	Other medications (valganciclovir, ganciclovir, TMP-SMZ)
	Infections (cytomegalovirus, tuberculosis, and overwhelming bacterial infections)
Thrombocytopenia	Immunosuppressive medications (thymoglobulin, alemtuzumab, azathioprine, rapamycin)
	Other medications (antibiotics, antiviral agents, heparin)
	Infection
	HUS-TTP (CNI use)
	Autoimmune thrombocytopenia

ACE, Angiotensin-converting enzyme; *CMV,* cytomegalovirus; *CNI,* calcineurin inhibitor; *EPO,* erythropoietin; *HUS-TTP,* hemolytic uremic syndrome–thrombotic thrombocytopenic purpura; *TMP-SMX,* trimethoprim-sulfamethoxazole.

METABOLIC COMPLICATIONS

Many of the metabolic abnormalities that contribute to renal osteodystrophy in ESRD patients, such as phosphate retention, secondary hyperparathyroidism, decreased calcitriol synthesis, and β_2-microglobulin (β_2M) accumulation, are reversed with transplantation; however, a degree of hyperparathyroidism may persist. Persistent uncontrolled hyperparathyroidism-associated hypercalcemia increases the risk for posttransplant bone disease and contributes to vascular calcification. In cases of severe, symptomatic, or persistent hypercalcemia, parathyroidectomy may be indicated. The use of calcimimetics posttransplant is not well established, with trials ongoing to examine their use in this setting. To date, cinacalcet therapy has been shown to effectively normalize serum calcium levels, but the impact on parathyroid hormone (PTH) and serum phosphorous levels appears variable.

Hypophosphatemia after transplantation is induced by phosphate wasting in the urine as a result of hyperparathyroidism and PTH-independent pathways, such as persistent elevations of FGF-23. Plasma phosphate levels below 1.0 mg/dL can cause muscle weakness and possibly osteomalacia, and should be reversed with supplementation. Osteopenia and osteonecrosis posttransplant are caused by multiple factors, including persistent uremia-induced abnormalities in calcium homeostasis and acquired defects in mineral metabolism induced by immunosuppressive medications. Measures to prevent and treat posttransplant bone disease include minimizing corticosteroid exposure, providing supplemental calcium, treating vitamin D deficiency, and encouraging weight-bearing exercise. Antiresorptive agents may be considered, but data on their benefits in kidney transplant recipients are lacking.

POSTTRANSPLANT MALIGNANCY

Incidence rates of malignancies at 1 and 3 years post transplant compared with the general population are outlined in Table 61.3. Kidney transplant recipients have a higher incidence of most cancers post transplant, but the risks are particularly high for certain viral-mediated malignancies, including EBV-related posttransplant lymphoproliferative disease (PTLD), skin and lip cancers, and human herpesvirus 8 (HHV-8)–associated Kaposi sarcoma. In addition, certain malignancies are more common in patients with kidney disease, such as kidney and urinary tract malignancies. Risk factors for cancer after transplant include advanced recipient age, white race, male sex, and a history of cancer. Recipients with previous cancers must be disease-free for an established time before transplantation and should be monitored more intensively after transplantation.

Successful treatment of malignancy relies on regular screening and early detection. Typically, malignancy-screening guidelines from the general population are applicable in the posttransplant setting and should be coordinated annually after transplant. Cancers of the skin are the most common malignancies in adult kidney transplant recipients and include squamous and basal cell carcinomas, malignant melanomas, and Merkel cell tumors. Kidney transplant recipients have a 250-fold and 10-fold increased incidence of squamous cell carcinoma and basal cell carcinoma, respectively, compared with the general population. Patients should be counseled to minimize sun exposure, use protective clothing and sunscreen regularly, and perform annual self-examinations for skin lesions. Suspicious lesions should be biopsied, and patients with recurrent lesions should be routinely followed by a dermatologist.

EBV-associated PTLD is characterized by lymphoproliferation, and it includes clinical syndromes ranging from infectious mononucleosis to life-threatening malignancies. Of note, PTLD remains relatively uncommon in kidney transplant recipients (1% to 2%), typically occurring in the context of primary EBV infection within the first year posttransplant. Additional risk factors for PTLD include young recipient age, CMV mismatch or disease, and the use of T lymphocyte–depleting antibody. Universal prophylaxis for EBV is not recommended. However, antiviral prophylaxis (acyclovir or ganciclovir) may be considered for EBV-negative

Table 61.3   Age-Adjusted Cancer Rates[a] in Male and Female Transplant Recipients Compared With the US Population

Type of Cancer	CANCER RATES IN MEN			CANCER RATES IN WOMEN		
	US Population	1 Year Posttransplant	3 Years Posttransplant	US Population	1 Year Posttransplant	3 Years Posttransplant
Skin Cancers						
Melanoma	19.0	60.4	131.3	12.1	99.9	63.5
Nonmelanoma skin	24.0	2017.1	2160.2	14.3	851.6	1320.5
Lymphomas						
Hodgkin lymphoma	3.2	37.9	98.6	2.5	11.5	93.5
NHL	22	882	150.7	15.7	667.5	456.7
Gastrointestinal						
Colon	66.4	137.2	107.7	48.5	91.1	137.0
Esophagus	8.8	17.4	21.3	2.2	3.6	6.2
Hepatobiliary	9.4	33.5	39.2	5.4	83.2	24.3
Pancreas	12.3	19.8	12.4	9.6	25.1	44.1
Small intestine	2.0	3.8	4.1	1.4	25.1	0
Stomach	11.0	38.9	4.1	5.1	23.7	21.4
Genitourinary						
Bladder	38.3	148.9	60.9	10.0	69.0	36.3
Kidney	16.0	671.0	226.1	8.4	767.7	122.9
Prostate	162.0	477.4	265.8	—	—	—
Testes	5.5	21.3	20.4	—	—	—
Cervix	—	—	—	9.4	9.4	53.7
Ovary	—	—	—	16.2	29.5	42.4
Uterus	—	—	—	0.7	51.7	21.5
Vulvovaginal	—	—	—	3.0	14.6	26.5
Other						
Breast	1.5	6.8	6.0	134.1	343.4	144.3
Lung	89.1	149.4	202.8	53.4	141.8	194.1
CNS	7.9	15.1	36.3	1.7	8.9	21.0
Kaposi sarcoma	1.5	55.0	26.1	0.1	56.0	6.2

[a]Rates per 100,000 for US population and for transplant recipients. All rates standardized to the 2000 US census population.

CNS, Central nervous system; *NHL*, non-Hodgkin lymphoma.

Modified from table 3 in Kasiske BL, Snyder J, Gilbertson DT, Wang C. Cancer after kidney transplantation in the United States. *Am J Transplant*. 2004;4:905–913.

recipients with EBV-positive donors, because it may result in a reduced rate of PTLD. Prophylaxis with IVIG has been shown to reduce the incidence of non-Hodgkin lymphoma posttransplant in retrospective studies, but prospective randomized controlled trials in pediatric patients have been inconclusive. High viral loads often predate the clinical presentation of PTLD; therefore frequent EBV viral load monitoring is recommended in high-risk populations. If viremia occurs in the absence of other clinical signs of PTLD, reduction of immunosuppression and initiation of antiviral therapy may be indicated. Most PTLD cases are non-Hodgkin lymphomas of B-cell origin and are CD20-positive. Mortality rates with PTLD are greater than 50%, with increased age, elevated lactate dehydrogenase levels, multiorgan involvement, and the presence of constitutional symptoms predicting a higher risk for death. The importance of clonality in PTLD is often debated, with monoclonal B-cell lymphomas considered more malignant and resistant to treatment compared with

polyclonal lymphomas. Treatment involves reduction of immunosuppression and typically includes administration of an anti-CD20 agent (rituximab), with or without additional cytotoxic therapies.

Immunosuppressive reduction should be considered in all patients with malignancy posttransplant, but it should be reviewed in each case to balance the risks for rejection and recurrent malignancy. The role of the mammalian target of rapamycin (mTOR) in malignancies has been the subject of increased study in the last decade. Indeed, rapamycin has been shown to suppress the growth and proliferation of certain tumors in various animal models. Small studies in humans have suggested that rapamycin may confer a reduced risk for malignancy compared with CNIs, particularly in skin and kidney cancers. However, in an analysis of Medicare claims data for transplant recipients in the United States, de novo use of rapamycin was associated with an increased risk for PTLD. Although further studies are clearly needed to delineate the benefits of rapamycin in reducing the risk for posttransplant malignancy, many centers currently consider converting patients with recurrent malignancies to a rapamycin-based immunosuppressive regimen.

CARDIOVASCULAR RISK FACTORS

Cardiovascular death is the leading cause of allograft loss and accounts for nearly 60% of posttransplant mortality. Risk factors for coronary disease after transplantation include the traditional markers of increased age, diabetes mellitus, hypertension, cigarette smoking, and hyperlipidemia, as well as proteinuria, reduced kidney function, elevated lipoprotein(a) levels, elevated CRP and IL6 levels, and obesity, particularly in the context of the metabolic syndrome (Table 61.4).

Table 61.4   Cardiovascular Risk Factors Post Kidney Transplantation

Cardiovascular Risk Factor	Contributing Factors Posttransplant
Hypertension	Volume overload
	Calcineurin inhibitors
	Corticosteroids
	Allograft dysfunction
	Renal artery stenosis
Obesity	Liberalization of dietary restrictions
	Persistent physical inactivity
	Chronic corticosteroid use
Dyslipidemia	Corticosteroids may cause elevations in LDL and total cholesterol but are associated most strongly with hypertriglyceridemia posttransplant
	Calcineurin inhibitors are associated with elevated total cholesterol and LDL levels and reductions in HDL levels independent of corticosteroid use
	Rapamycin is mostly associated with hypertriglyceridemia
Diabetes	Calcineurin inhibitors (especially tacrolimus) are associated with hyperglycemia and NODAT
	Corticosteroids are associated with hyperglycemia and NODAT
	Rapamycin is associated with hyperglycemia and NODAT
	Chronic hepatitis C infection is associated with pretransplant and posttransplant diabetes possibly due to HCV-induced islet cell dysfunction and liver dysfunction associated with insulin resistance
Reduced kidney function	Immune- and non–immune-mediated allograft injury with resultant chronic kidney disease
Elevated homocysteine	Homocysteine levels continue to rise post kidney transplantation and may be associated with cyclosporine use

HCV, Hepatitis C virus; *HDL,* high-density lipoprotein; *LDL,* low-density lipoprotein; *NODAT,* new-onset diabetes after transplantation.

METABOLIC SYNDROME

The constellation of central obesity, dyslipidemia, hypertension, and fasting hyperglycemia is called metabolic syndrome and is associated with an increased risk for diabetes mellitus, proteinuria, reduced kidney function, and cardiovascular disease in the general population. Numerous studies have reported a high prevalence of metabolic syndrome both before and after transplantation. In one US study, the pretransplant prevalence of metabolic syndrome was 57.2% in nondiabetic recipients, and metabolic syndrome pretransplant was an independent risk factor for NODAT in 31.4% of recipients. After transplantation, metabolic syndrome has been reported in up to 63% of recipients and is associated with worse kidney function and allograft survival. Among the various components of metabolic syndrome, systolic hypertension and hypertriglyceridemia have been reported to have the greatest negative impact on long-term allograft function.

OBESITY

Pretransplant obesity (body mass index [BMI] >30) increases the risk for surgical wound infections, allograft loss, and cardiovascular disease posttransplant. Weight gain is common posttransplant, particularly in women, blacks, low-income patients, and recipients with pretransplant obesity. All transplant recipients should receive counseling on the importance on diet and exercise. Pharmacologic agents and surgical options for weight loss may be considered in morbidly obese patients both before and after transplantation.

HYPERTENSION

Hypertension is seen in 60% to 80% of all transplant recipients and is associated with worse allograft survival. In the early posttransplant period, volume management, allograft function, and changes to baseline antihypertensive therapy may contribute to hypertension. Immunosuppressive agents, including CNIs and corticosteroids, may further exacerbate hypertensive states. For instance, cyclosporine increases both systemic and renal vascular resistance and induces renal vasoconstriction via increased release of vasoconstrictors, such as endothelin.

The presence of atherosclerotic disease and complications during organ procurement and transplantation increase the risk for transplant renal artery stenosis. In addition, CMV infection and DGF have been found to be associated with renal artery stenosis. Therefore in cases of refractory hypertension posttransplant, particularly when associated with unexplained allograft dysfunction, transplant renal artery stenosis should be considered. As in the nontransplant setting, ACE inhibitor–induced reversible decline in kidney function may be suggestive of renal artery stenosis. Blood pressure targets are variable and depend on comorbid disease, including diabetic status and presence of proteinuria. The Kidney Disease: Improving Global Outcomes (KDIGO) guideline for care of the kidney transplant recipient suggests maintaining blood pressure at less than 130/80 mm Hg.

Calcium channel blockers, ACE inhibitors, and beta-blockers may all be considered first-line antihypertensive agents posttransplant, with selection of a specific agent dependent on other patient-specific factors. A recent Cochrane Group meta-analysis of randomized trials found that only calcium channel blockers reduced graft loss and improved glomerular filtration rate (GFR) compared with placebo, whereas ACE inhibitors more effectively reduced proteinuria. Importantly, the renoprotective benefits of ACE inhibitors have not been proven in transplant recipients. In a double-blind, placebo-controlled trial conducted at 14 centers in Canada and New Zealand, 213 adult kidney transplant recipients with an estimated GFR of 20 mL/min per 1.73 m^2 or greater and proteinuria of 0.2 g/day or greater were randomized to receive ramipril versus placebo for up to 4 years. Treatment with ramipril was not associated with a significant reduction in doubling of serum creatinine, ESRD, or death.

DYSLIPIDEMIA

The Assessment of Lescol in Renal Transplantation (ALERT) trial was a large multicenter study of stable transplant recipients who received either fluvastatin (Lescol) or placebo with the outcome of lowering LDL cholesterol and reducing the risk for cardiac events. After 5 years of follow-up, the fluvastatin group had lower total and LDL cholesterol and fewer cardiac deaths and nonfatal myocardial infarctions, but there was no difference in major adverse cardiac events. It is important to note that despite concerns regarding increased risks for statin-induced rhabdomyolysis due to CNI coadministration, no increased risk for rhabdomyolysis was noted in the statin arm of the trial. Therefore, although the mortality benefit of statins posttransplant remains unproven, statins remain the drug of choice for the treatment of dyslipidemia in transplant recipients.

NEW-ONSET DIABETES AFTER TRANSPLANTATION

The incidence of NODAT has been variably reported, but recent studies note a prevalence of 16% at 1 year posttransplant. The development of NODAT confers a 46% increased risk for graft loss and an 87% increased risk for death posttransplant, with a tripling of the risk for cardiovascular death. The reason for an increased risk for graft loss remains unclear, but it may be due to a combination of diabetic nephropathy and the implications of reduced immunosuppression to avoid NODAT.

In addition to traditional risk factors for diabetes (older age, obesity, preexisting glucose intolerance, and a family history of diabetes mellitus), risk factors for NODAT include the type and degree of immunosuppression, black race, level of HLA matching, chronic hepatitis C infection, and the cause of ESRD, with some reports suggesting a higher risk associated with polycystic kidney disease. Calcineurin inhibitors, particularly tacrolimus, may cause pancreatic beta-cell dysfunction and contribute to insulin resistance. Cyclosporine is less diabetogenic than tacrolimus, and some centers have advocated the use of cyclosporine in patients at high risk for developing NODAT. Alternatively, reduced doses of CNI are recommended to minimize the risk for NODAT. However, no comparative studies have been conducted to demonstrate the benefit and safety of cyclosporine-based immunosuppression or low-dose CNI in patients at high risk for NODAT. Rapamycin is also diabetogenic and has

been shown to worsen glycemic control after conversion from a CNI.

Corticosteroids cause hyperglycemia through a number of mechanisms in a dose-dependent manner. Therefore rapid reduction of prednisone to maintenance doses (5 to 10 mg/day) significantly improves hyperglycemia. However, the relative benefit of complete steroid withdrawal versus maintenance with low-dose prednisone has not been consistently demonstrated.

All transplant recipients should have fasting blood glucose levels checked weekly for the first month, and then at 3, 6, and 12 months thereafter. Impaired fasting blood glucose results should be further evaluated with an oral glucose tolerance test. Hemoglobin A1c (HbA1c) assessment should be used to direct therapy in patients with NODAT. Hyperglycemic patients should receive counseling on diet and lifestyle modification and be initiated on therapy if hyperglycemia persists. All oral hypoglycemic agents have been found to be safe and effective posttransplant; however, the metabolism and adverse effects of each drug should be considered in relation to immunosuppressant medications and the level of allograft function.

KEY BIBLIOGRAPHY

Engels EA, Pfeiffer RM, Fraumeni JF, et al. Spectrum of cancer risk among US solid organ transplant recipients. *JAMA*. 2011;306:1891-1901.

Fishman JA. Infection in solid-organ transplant recipients. *N Engl J Med*. 2007;357:2601-2614.

Gloor J, Cosio F, Lager DJ, et al. The spectrum of antibody-mediated renal allograft injury: implications for treatment. *Am J Transplant*. 2008;8:1367-1373.

Haas M. The Revised (2013) Banff classification for antibody mediated rejection of renal allografts: update, difficulties, and future considerations. *Am J Transplant*. 2016;16:1352-1357.

Hart A, Smith JM, Skeans MA, et al. OPTN/SRTR 2015 Annual Data Report: kidney. *Am J Transplant*. 2017;17:21-116.

Ho J, Wiebe C, Gibson IW, et al. Immune monitoring of kidney allografts. *Am J Kidney Dis*. 2012;60:629-640.

Holdaas H, Fellstrom B, Jardine AG, et al. Effect of fluvastatin on cardiac outcomes in renal transplant recipients: a multicentre, randomised, placebo-controlled trial. *Lancet*. 2003;361:2024-2031.

Hricik DE. Metabolic syndrome in kidney transplantation: management of risk factors. *Clin J Am Soc Nephrol*. 2011;6:1781-1785.

Humar A, Michaels M. AST ID Working Group on Infectious Disease Monitoring. American Society of Transplantation recommendations for screening, monitoring and reporting of infectious complications in immunosuppression trials in recipients of organ transplantation. *Am J Transplant*. 2006;6:262-274.

Kasiske B, Cosio FG, Beto J, et al. Clinical practice guidelines for managing dyslipidemias in kidney transplant patients: a report from the Managing Dyslipidemias in Chronic Kidney Disease Work Group of the National Kidney Foundation Kidney Disease Outcomes Quality Initiative. *Am J Transplant*. 2004;4:13-53.

Kidney Disease. Improving global outcomes (KDIGO) transplant work group. KDIGO clinical practice guideline for the care of kidney transplant recipients. *Am J Transplant*. 2009;9:S1-S157.

Lo DJ, Kaplan B, Kirk AD. Biomarkers for kidney transplant rejection. *Nat Rev Nephrol*. 2014;10:215-225.

Mannon RB. Immune monitoring and biomarkers to predict chronic allograft dysfunction. *Kidney IntSuppl*. 2010;S59-S65. doi:10.1038/ki.2010.425.

Mennon MC, Murphy B, Heeger PS. Moving biomarkers toward clinical implementation in kidney transplantation. *J Am SocNephrol*. 2017.

Merion RM, Ashby VB, Wolfe RA, et al. Deceased-donor characteristics and the survival benefit of kidney transplantation. *JAMA*. 2005;294:2726-2733.

Nankivell BJ, Borrows RJ, Fung CL, et al. The natural history of chronic allograft nephropathy. *N Engl J Med*. 2003;349:2326-2333.

Nickerson P. Post-transplant monitoring of renal allografts: are we there yet? *CurrOpinImmunol.* 2009;21:563-568.

Stegall MD, Gloor JM. Deciphering antibody-mediated rejection: new insights into mechanisms and treatment. *CurrOpin Organ Transplant.* 2010;15:8-10.

Tait BD, Susal C, Gebel HM, et al. Consensus guidelines on the testing and clinical management issues associated with HLA and non-HLA antibodies in transplantation. *Transplantation.* 2013;95:19-47.

Woodle ES, First MR, Pirsch J, et al. A prospective, randomized, double-blind, placebo-controlled multicenter trial comparing early (7 day) corticosteroid cessation versus long-term, low-dose corticosteroid therapy. *Ann Surg.* 2008;248:564-577.

Full bibliography can be found on www.expertconsult.com.

Immunosuppression in Transplantation

62

Sindhu Chandran; Flavio G. Vincenti

The central issue in organ transplantation remains the suppression of allograft rejection. Understanding the physiology of the immune response to a transplanted organ, developing targeted immunosuppressive drugs, and devising the best combinations to maintain safety and improve efficacy are keys for successful graft function and long-term graft survival.

PHYSIOLOGY OF IMMUNORECOGNITION

The immune system evolved to discriminate self from nonself, and this response against nonself consists of an array of receptor-mediated sensing and effector mechanisms broadly described as innate and adaptive. *Innate immunity* is primitive, does not require priming, and is of relatively low affinity but broadly reactive. *Adaptive immunity* is antigen-specific, depends on antigen exposure or priming, and can be of very high affinity. The major effectors of innate immunity are complement, granulocytes, monocytes/macrophages, natural killer (NK) cells, mast cells, and basophils. The major effectors of adaptive immunity are B and T lymphocytes.

A transplant between genetically distinct individuals of the same species is called an allogeneic graft, or an allograft. The immune response to an allograft requires three elements: recognition of foreign antigens, activation of antigen-specific lymphocytes, and the effector phase of graft rejection. The recognition of antigens as peptide fragments bound to major histocompatibility complex (MHC) molecules, known as human leukocyte antigens (HLAs), is the central event in the initiation of an alloresponse. HLA molecules (Fig. 62.1) are highly polymorphic, follow Mendelian codominant inheritance, and constitute the principal antigenic barrier to transplantation. The degree of HLA matching between the donor and the recipient plays an important role in graft survival, and HLA matching has been incorporated into kidney allocation. In addition, non-HLA molecules, such as MHC class I–related chain A (MICA), are recognized as playing a significant role in rejection, particularly in recipients of well–HLA-matched kidneys.

There are two types of HLA molecules: class I and class II. Class I HLA molecules are expressed on all nucleated cells, whereas class II molecules are usually expressed only on antigen-presenting cells (APCs), which include dendritic cells, B lymphocytes, and macrophages. Cytokines such as interferon-γ (IFN-γ) induce, upregulate, and broaden HLA expression, so that all cells in a graft can become potential targets of the immune response. Ischemia-reperfusion injury in the graft leads to the production of inflammatory cytokines and recruitment of macrophages, and acute rejection episodes are more common in grafts with prolonged ischemia times. Recipient T cells may respond directly to peptides/HLA complexes presented by donor APCs in the graft or to donor HLA peptides presented on the recipient's own APCs (Fig. 62.2). Acute rejection of an allograft is believed to be primarily dependent on direct allorecognition, whereas the indirect pathway may play a larger role in chronic rejection.

T cells are critically important in the rejection of allogeneic grafts. CD4 T cells (helper T cells) are thought to mediate the initial recognition of an allograft and to help amplify and coordinate the subsequent immune response, including providing help to CD8 (effector) T cells. T cell recognition of the alloantigen occurs via binding of the T cell receptor (TCR)/CD3 complex on the T cell's surface to the peptide/MHC complex on APCs. This is referred to as *signal 1* and leads to phosphorylation of TCR-associated proteins and downstream activation of several pathways, including calcineurin, protein kinase C, and mitogen-activated protein (MAP) kinase pathways. The calcineurin pathway has been best characterized, and it involves the activation of calcineurin (a phosphatase) by an increase in cytosolic calcium. Calcineurin dephosphorylates nuclear factor of activated T cells (NFAT), allowing NFAT to translocate from the cytoplasm to the nucleus. The NFAT binds to regulatory sequences and increases gene transcription of several cytokines, including interleukin (IL)-2, a T cell growth factor, as well as IL-4, IFN-γ, and tumor necrosis factor-α (TNF-α).

Although the specificity of the immune response is determined by *signal 1*, a costimulatory signal, *signal 2*, which occurs though accessory molecules, is essential for T cell activation. The most potent of these signals regulating T cell clonal expansion and differentiation is provided by the B7/CD28 family of molecules (Fig. 62.3). B7-1 (CD80) and B7-2 (CD86) are ligands on APCs that bind to CD28, expressed on most T cells. Engagement of CD28 increases the production of IL-2 and other cytokines, resulting in T cell proliferation. CD80 and CD86 also regulate T cells by binding another antigen on T cells called cytotoxic T-lymphocyte antigen-4 (CTLA-4), which inhibits T cell proliferation. A costimulatory interaction between CD40 on APCs and CD40 ligand (CD154, CD40L) on T cells is also critical for activation of APCs and upregulation of B7 expression on T cells. One way to induce T cell anergy in vitro is to provide the T cell with an antigen-specific signal through the TCR (signal 1) in the absence of CD28 engagement (signal 2). However, in most in vivo models of B7 blockade, anergy has been difficult to demonstrate, which is possibly due to the complexity of costimulation that involves multiple stimulatory and inhibitory signals.

589

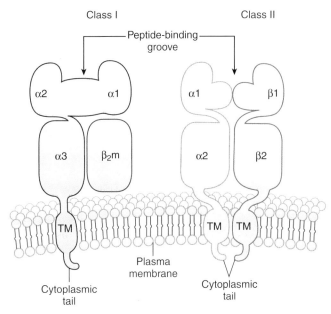

Fig. 62.1 Structure of human leukocyte antigens class I and class II molecules. Beta$_2$-microglobulin (β_2m) is the light chain of the class I molecule. The α chain of the class I molecule has two peptide-binding domains (α1 and α2), an immunoglobulin-like domain (α3), the transmembrane (TM) region, and the cytoplasmic tail. Each of the class II α and β chains has four domains: the peptide-binding domain (α1 or β1), the immunoglobulin-like domain (α2 or β2), the transmembrane region, and the cytoplasmic tail. (From Klein J, Sato A. The HLA system. *N Engl J Med.* 2000;343:702–709.)

Antigen-specific activation of T cells, particularly CD4 T cells, leads to the production of cytokines, the recruitment of monocytes, and the proliferation of CD8 T cells, NK cells, and B cells. CD8 T cells cause cell death in the graft through the release of soluble cytotoxic factors (granzymes and perforin) as well as upregulated Fas ligand on T cells that bind to Fas (CD95) on target cells and trigger apoptosis.

In addition to T cells, B cells and the humoral arm of the immune system play a major role in acute and chronic graft injury. Antibodies produced by the differentiation of B cells into plasma cells cause cell injury through complement fixation or antibody-dependent cellular cytotoxicity. Hyperacute

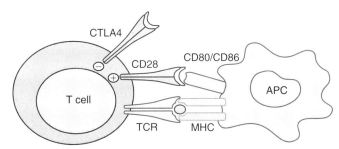

Fig. 62.3 Signal 1 and signal 2. *APC,* Antigen-presenting cell; *MHC,* major histocompatibility complex; *TCR,* T-cell receptor. (From Vincenti F. Costimulation blockade in autoimmunity and transplantation. *J Allergy Clin Immunol.* 2008;121:299–306.)

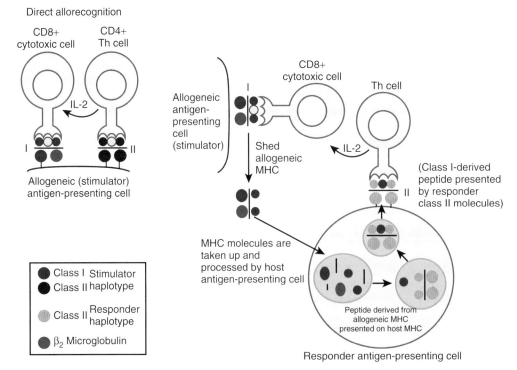

Fig. 62.2 Diagrammatic representation of the direct and indirect pathways of allorecognition. *IL,* Interleukin; *MHC,* major histocompatibility complex. (From Rogers NJ, Lechler RI. Allorecognition. *Am J Transplant.* 2001;1:97–102.)

rejection occurs when preformed recipient antibodies to donor HLA antigens or ABO blood group antigens result in complement activation, intravascular coagulation, and graft necrosis within 24 hours of transplantation. Although cross-matching and ABO blood typing have virtually eliminated hyperacute rejection, B cells and plasma cells continue to play an important role in subsequent antibody-mediated rejection (AMR) and may be important mediators of chronic graft injury and late graft loss.

STRATEGIES FOR IMMUNOSUPPRESSION

The first attempts at immunosuppression used total-body irradiation. Subsequently, azathioprine was introduced in the early 1960s, and soon thereafter was routinely accompanied by prednisolone in an immunosuppressive regimen. The polyclonal antilymphocyte antibody preparations became available in the mid-1970s. The introduction of cyclosporine in the early 1980s dramatically improved 1-year graft survival rates from 50% to over 80%, and, in 1985, OKT3, a monoclonal antibody to CD3, was introduced for the treatment of acute rejection. In the 1990s, tacrolimus and mycophenolate mofetil (MMF) emerged as alternatives to cyclosporine and azathioprine, anti–IL-2 receptor antibodies were approved for induction, and sirolimus became available. In 2011, belatacept was approved as the first biologic agent for use in maintenance immunotherapy. Commonly used immunosuppressants and their mechanisms of action are listed in Table 62.1.

Transplant immunosuppression is guided by three key principles. First, multiple agents directed at different molecular targets within the alloimmune response are used simultaneously to maximize synergy and efficacy while minimizing toxicity. Second, greater immunosuppression (induction) is needed for early engraftment or to treat established rejection rather than for long-term graft maintenance. And third, continuous vigilance is essential to identify rejection, drug toxicity, and infection so that the immunosuppressive regimen can be modified appropriately.

Table 62.1 Commonly Used Induction and Maintenance Immunosuppressive Agents

Drug	Phase of Use	Mechanism of Action	Side Effects
Glucocorticoids: methylprednisolone (Solu-Medrol), prednisone (Deltasone)	Induction and maintenance	Binds cytosolic receptors and heat shock proteins, and blocks transcription of IL-1, IL-2, IL-3, IL-6, TNF-α, and IFN-γ	Hypertension, hyperglycemia, dyslipidemia, osteoporosis, impaired wound healing, cosmetic effects
Calcineurin inhibitors: cyclosporine (Sandimmune, Neoral, Gengraf), tacrolimus (Prograf)	Maintenance	Forms a complex with cyclophilin or FK-binding protein, which binds to calcineurin, preventing dephosphorylation of regulatory proteins and decreasing transcription of IL-2, IL-4, IFN-γ, and TNF-α; also increases TGF-β, which inhibits IL-2	Tremor, nephrotoxicity, hypertension, hyperglycemia, hyperuricemia, hyperlipidemia (CsA), hirsutism (CsA), gingival hyperplasia (CsA), hair loss (tacrolimus)
Antiproliferative Agents			
Azathioprine (Imuran, Azasan)	Maintenance	Purine analog that blocks DNA, RNA, and protein synthesis	Marrow suppression, pancreatitis
Mycophenolate mofetil (Cellcept), mycophenolic acid (Myfortic)	Maintenance	Inhibits IMPDH, preventing de novo guanosine nucleotide synthesis	Diarrhea, marrow suppression, teratogenic
mTOR inhibitors: sirolimus (Rapamune), everolimus (Zortress)	Maintenance	Forms a complex with FK-binding protein-12, which blocks p70 S6 kinase, causing G1 cell cycle arrest	Hyperlipidemia, hyperglycemia, thrombocytopenia, impaired wound healing, interstitial pneumonitis, embryotoxic
Biologics			
Basiliximab (Simulect)	Induction	Monoclonal antibody to CD25 (IL-2 receptor α chain), which blocks IL-2 engagement	Rare infusion reactions
Rabbit antithymocyte globulin (Thymoglobulin)	Induction	Polyclonal antithymocyte antibody, which depletes T cells	Cytokine release syndrome, serum sickness, thrombocytopenia, prolonged lymphopenia
Alemtuzumab (Campath)	Induction	Monoclonal antibody to CD52, which depletes T cells, B cells, and NK cells	Cytokine release syndrome, prolonged lymphopenia
Belatacept (Nulojix)	Maintenance	CTLA-4-Ig fusion protein, which competes with CD28 for CD80/86 binding, inhibiting T-cell costimulation	Rare infusion reactions

CSA, Cyclosporine A; *IFN*, interferon; *IL*, interleukin; *IMPDH*, inosine monophosphate dehydrogenase; *mTOR*, mammlian target of rapamycin; *NK*, natural killer; *TGF-β*, transforming growth factor-β; *TNF-α*, tumor necrosis factor-α.

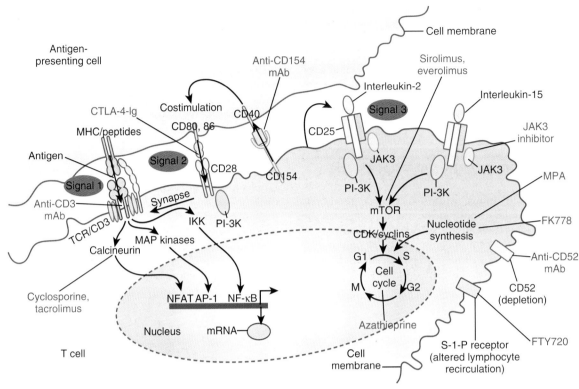

Fig. 62.4 Individual immunosuppressive drugs and sites of action in the three-signal model. *CDK,* Cyclin-dependent kinase; *IKK,* IκB kinase; *MAP,* mitogen-activated protein; *MHC,* major histocompatibility complex; *MPA,* mycophenolic acid; *NFAT,* nuclear factor of activated T cells; TCR/CD3, T-cell receptor. (From Halloran PF. Immunosuppressive drugs for kidney transplantation. *N Engl J Med.* 2004;351:2715–2729.)

MECHANISMS OF ACTION OF IMMUNOSUPPRESSIVE DRUGS

T cells have historically been the major target of immunosuppression. The three-signal model of T cell activation and subsequent cellular proliferation provides a useful guide to the sites of action of the major immunosuppressive agents (Fig. 62.4). Signal 1 is the antigen-specific signal provided by the interaction of the MHC/peptide complex on APCs with the TCR/CD3 complex. Signal 2 is a non-antigen-specific costimulatory signal provided by the engagement of B7 on APCs with CD28 on the T cell. These two signals activate intracellular pathways leading to the production of IL-2 and other cytokines. Stimulation of the IL-2 receptor (CD25) leads to activation of mammalian target of rapamycin (mTOR), a protein kinase, and provides signal 3, which triggers cell proliferation. Therapies targeting antibody-mediated injury are directed against B cells, plasma cells, and complement activation. In general, all drugs in current clinical use have been more effective at suppressing primary rather than memory immune responses.

INDUCTION THERAPY

High intravenous doses of corticosteroids are used as part of nearly all induction immunosuppression protocols. Induction therapy with biologic agents is used to delay the use of nephrotoxic calcineurin inhibitors (CNIs) and/or to intensify the initial immunosuppressive therapy in patients at high immunologic risk (i.e., broadly sensitized, black individuals, children, or individuals with a prior transplant). Biologic agents for induction therapy are currently used in over 80% of kidney transplant recipients and are divided into two groups: depleting agents and immune modulators.

Depleting agents diminish the recipient's lymphocyte population at the time of transplantation, and induction with these agents has been shown to improve graft survival. Antithymocyte globulin (ATG), a polyclonal antilymphocyte preparation directed against T cells and approved for the reversal of acute rejection (usually rabbit-derived thymoglobulin), is used off-label as the most common induction agent in kidney transplantation. It is interesting to note that ATG also causes sustained and rapid expansion of regulatory T cells, which play an important part in maintaining immune homeostasis and limiting antigraft immunity. The standard dose of rabbit-derived thymoglobulin is 1.5 mg/kg daily for 4 to 10 days. Alemtuzumab (Campath-1H) is a humanized anti-CD52 monoclonal antibody that targets lymphocytes, monocytes, macrophages, and NK cells and causes prolonged B and T cell depletion. Alemtuzumab is also used off-label as induction therapy in about 10% of kidney transplants, particularly as part of steroid-sparing protocols. It is usually given as a single dose of 30 mg intraoperatively when infusion-related events are often masked by general anesthesia. ATGAM, an equine ATG, is rarely used in the United States because of its poorer efficacy. OKT3, a murine monoclonal antibody to CD3, was associated with significant acute side effects, such as cytokine release syndrome, and was withdrawn from the market.

Depleting agents can elicit major side effects, including fever, chills, and hypotension. The polyclonal agents are xenogeneic proteins. Cell death and cytokine release peak with the first infusion and diminish substantially with subsequent doses. Premedication with corticosteroids, acetaminophen, and an antihistamine along with slow infusion (over 4 to 6 hours) through a large-diameter vessel minimize reactions. Other side effects include leukopenia, thrombocytopenia, serum sickness, glomerulonephritis, and, rarely, anaphylaxis. In the long term, depleting agents have been associated with a higher incidence of infections and malignancy, particularly posttransplant lymphoproliferative disorders (PTLDs).

Immune-modulating induction agents do not deplete T cells, with the possible exception of T regulatory cells, but rather they block IL-2–mediated T cell activation. Daclizumab (Zenapax) and basiliximab (Simulect) are chimeric and humanized monoclonal antibodies, respectively, that bind to the α chain of the IL-2 receptor, thus blocking IL-2–mediated responses. Daclizumab has a longer half-life ($T_{1/2}$) than basiliximab (20 days vs. 7 days), and the typical dosing schedule results in longer saturation of the IL-2Rα on circulating T cells (120 days vs. 30 to 45 days). However, saturation of the IL-2Rα may not prevent rejection and was noted to be similar in patients with or without an acute rejection episode. Rejection in patients despite IL-2R blockade may occur through a mechanism that bypasses the IL-2 pathway as a result of cytokine-cytokine receptor redundancy (i.e., IL-7, IL-15). Both drugs are fairly well tolerated, and no cytokine release syndrome has been observed, although anaphylaxis may occur rarely. Since the manufacturer's withdrawal of daclizumab from the market in October 2008, basiliximab is the only anti-IL2R antibody currently available for use as induction therapy.

More aggressive approaches to induction therapy have been used in patients with high levels of anti-HLA antibodies, donor-specific antibodies, or previous humoral rejection. These include plasmapheresis and intravenous immune globulin (IVIG) to reduce the levels of preformed antibodies, and rituximab, a chimeric anti-CD20 monoclonal antibody, to selectively deplete B cells.

MAINTENANCE IMMUNOTHERAPY

The basic immunosuppressive protocols use multiple drugs simultaneously. Therapy typically involves a CNI, glucocorticoids, and MMF, each directed at a discrete site in T cell activation. Protocols using rapid steroid withdrawal (within 1 week) are being used in over one-third of kidney transplant recipients with good short-term results, although the effects on long-term graft function are unknown. Azathioprine has mostly fallen out of favor, but it is still used during pregnancy and sometimes as part of lower cost regimens. Sirolimus and everolimus have been used mostly in de novo or conversion regimens that spare/minimize CNI exposure. Maintenance biologic therapy with belatacept, in combination with a steroid and an antiproliferative agent, permits complete avoidance of calcineurin inhibition and has been associated with superior kidney function, improved metabolic parameters, and improved graft survival in recipients with low immunologic risk.

GLUCOCORTICOIDS

Glucocorticoids are used in high doses both as part of induction protocols and for the treatment of acute rejection episodes and in low doses for maintenance immunosuppression. Steroids exert broad antiinflammatory effects on multiple components of cellular immunity but have little effect on humoral immunity. They lyse (in some species) and redistribute lymphocytes, causing a rapid transient lymphopenia. To effect long-term responses, steroids bind to intracellular receptors and downregulate the transcription of numerous genes such as IL-1, IL-2, IL-3, IL-6, TNF-α, and IFN-γ, thereby inhibiting T cell activation. Neutrophils and monocytes display poor chemotaxis and decreased lysosomal enzyme release. In addition, steroids curtail the activation of NF-κB, thus increasing the apoptosis of activated cells.

The long-term use of steroids is associated with several adverse effects, including growth retardation in children, avascular osteonecrosis, osteopenia, increased risk for infection, poor wound healing, cataracts, hyperglycemia, and hypertension. Steroid minimization (avoidance and withdrawal) protocols are associated with improved metabolic parameters at the cost of higher acute rejection rates and unknown long-term effects on the graft.

CALCINEURIN INHIBITORS

Cyclosporine A (CsA) ushered in the modern era of organ transplantation, increasing the rates of early engraftment, extending kidney graft survival, and making cardiac and liver transplantation possible. Cyclosporine and tacrolimus are structurally unrelated agents that bind to distinct molecular targets (cyclophilin and FK-binding protein [FKBP] 12, respectively), blocking calcineurin and selectively inhibiting signal transduction in activated T cells. Cyclosporine also increases the expression of transforming growth factor-β (TGF-β), which inhibits IL-2 and the generation of cytotoxic T cells.

CsA, a lipophilic and highly hydrophobic cyclic polypeptide of 11 amino acids, is produced by the fungus *Beauveria nivea*. CsA, as supplied in the original soft gelatin capsule (Sandimmune), is absorbed slowly, with 20% to 50% bioavailability. A modified microemulsion formulation (Neoral) with improved bioavailability has become the most widely used preparation. Generic preparations of both are available and are bioequivalent to the original formulation but not to each other. The initial dose is usually 10 to 15 mg/kg per day, divided into two doses. The administration of CsA with food delays and decreases its absorption, and it can lower the peak concentration by 33% and the area under the drug concentration curve (AUC) by 13%. The elimination of cyclosporine from the blood is generally biphasic, with a terminal $T_{1/2}$ of 5 to 18 hours. It is metabolized extensively in the gut and the liver by CYP3A and P-glycoprotein. CsA and its metabolites are excreted principally through the bile into the feces, with 6% being excreted in urine. Dosage adjustments are required for hepatic dysfunction but not for reduced glomerular filtration rate. Despite being the most commonly used monitoring tool, 12-hour trough CsA levels (C0 level) are poorly reflective of the AUC and thus are not an accurate indication of CsA exposure in individual patients. Drug levels 2 hours after Neoral dose administration (C2 levels) have shown better correlation with the AUC but are difficult to obtain in routine clinical practice.

The principal adverse reactions to CsA therapy are kidney dysfunction and hypertension. Tremor, hirsutism, hyperlipidemia, hyperuricemia, and gingival hyperplasia are also frequently encountered. Nephrotoxicity occurs in the majority of patients and is the major reason for the cessation or modification of therapy. It initially causes a dose-related, reversible renal vasoconstriction that particularly affects the afferent arteriole. In the long term, fibrosis occurs as a consequence of both chronic ischemia and CsA-enhanced TGF-β expression. The increased production of TGF-β also promotes cancer progression through its effect on the proliferation of tumor cells. Thrombotic microangiopathy (TMA) is an uncommon but distinct form of CNI-induced endothelial toxicity. It can be systemic or limited to the kidney, and it usually responds to withdrawal of the CNI.

Tacrolimus (FK506; Prograf) is a macrolide antibiotic produced by *Streptomyces tsukubaensis*. Because of perceived slightly greater efficacy and ease of blood level monitoring, tacrolimus has become the preferred CNI in most transplant centers. It is indicated for the prophylaxis of solid-organ allograft rejection and is also used as rescue therapy in patients who develop rejection episodes despite maintaining therapeutic levels of CsA. Oral bioavailability is about 25%, and $T_{1/2}$ of tacrolimus is 8 to 12 hours. Similar to CsA, it is extensively metabolized in the gut and liver by CYP3A, and the majority is excreted in the feces. The recommended initial oral dose is 0.2 mg/kg per day in two divided doses. Trough tacrolimus levels seem to correlate better with the drug AUC and with clinical events than they do for CsA. The first generic tacrolimus product gained US Food and Drug Administration (FDA) approval in August 2009. Dose requirements and trough levels are similar between brand and generic tacrolimus, but postconversion monitoring is prudent because patients may require dose titration. Care should also be taken when switching from one generic version to another. Two extended release formulations of tacrolimus, which allow once-daily dosing, have been approved by the FDA for use in kidney transplant recipients: Astagraf XL in 2013 and Envarsus XR in 2015. Compared with both immediate release tacrolimus and Astagraf XL, Envarsus XL demonstrates greater bioavailability (higher AUC_{24}) and a flatter pharmacokinetic profile (lower C_{max} and more prolonged time to peak of 6 hours). Similar to CsA, nephrotoxicity is a limiting factor with tacrolimus. Neurotoxicity (e.g., tremor, headache, paresthesias, seizures), hyperglycemia, hypomagnesemia, and gastrointestinal (GI) complaints tend to occur more commonly in patients on tacrolimus as compared with CsA, whereas elevations in uric acid and low-density lipoprotein (LDL) cholesterol are less common. Diarrhea and alopecia are common in patients on both tacrolimus and mycophenolate. Unlike CsA, tacrolimus does not cause hirsutism or gingival hyperplasia.

Both CsA and tacrolimus are extensively metabolized by hepatic microsomal enzymes, especially CYP3A, as well as through P-glycoprotein, and interact with a wide variety of commonly used drugs. These interactions are better characterized for CsA but usually apply to both drugs. CYP3A inhibitors can decrease CsA metabolism and increase blood CsA concentrations (Table 62.2). These include calcium channel blockers (e.g., verapamil, diltiazem), antifungal agents (e.g., fluconazole, ketoconazole), antibiotics (e.g., erythromycin), human immunodeficiency virus protease inhibitors (e.g., ritonavir), and other drugs (e.g., amiodarone). Grapefruit juice inhibits CYP3A and the P-glycoprotein multidrug efflux pump and can increase the blood concentrations of both CNIs. In contrast, hepatic microsomal inducers, such as some antibiotics (e.g., nafcillin, rifampin), anticonvulsants (e.g., phenobarbital, phenytoin), and St. John wort, can decrease CsA and tacrolimus blood levels. CsA and tacrolimus also affect the concentration of other drugs by competing for the hepatic microsomal system and plasma protein binding, and they decrease the clearance of drugs, such as statins, digoxin, and methotrexate. Close monitoring of drug levels and attention to dosage are required when such combinations are used. CNI nephrotoxicity can also be exaggerated by the combination with amphotericin, aminoglycosides, and nonsteroidal antiinflammatory drugs.

Table 62.2 Notable Drug Interactions With Cyclosporine

Drug Class	Agents	Effect on Cyclosporine Level
Anticonvulsants	Barbiturates, phenytoin, carbamazepine, oxcarbazepine	↓
Antibiotics	Nafcillin, IV trimethoprim, imipenem, cephalosporins, terbinafine	↓
	Clarithromycin, erythromycin, telithromycin	↑
Antifungals	Terbinafine	↓
	Ketoconazole, fluconazole, itraconazole, voriconazole	↑
Antimycobacterials	Rifampin, rifabutin (to a lesser extent)	↓
	Pyrazinamide	↑
Antiretrovirals	Efavirenz, etravirine, nevirapine	↓
	Atazanavir, boceprevir, darunavir, delavirdine, fosamprenavir, indinavir, ritonavir, saquinavir, telaprevir	↑
Antiarrhythmics	Amiodarone, dronedarone, quinidine	↑
Calcium channel blockers	Diltiazem, nicardipine, verapamil	↑
Food and herbs	St. John wort	↓
	Grapefruit juice	↑
Glucocorticoids	Methylprednisolone, prednisone	May ↓ or ↑ via CYP3A4 induction or competitive inhibition
Miscellaneous	Bosentan, octreotide, orlistat	↓
	Carvedilol, bromocriptine, metoclopramide, cimetidine	↑

ANTIPROLIFERATIVE AGENTS

Azathioprine (Imuran) is an imidazolyl derivative of 6-mercaptopurine, which inhibits de novo purine synthesis. Cell proliferation is thereby blocked, impairing a variety of lymphocyte functions. Azathioprine was the first chemical immunosuppressive agent used in organ transplantation, but it has been mostly superseded by mycophenolate in current clinical practice. Oral bioavailability of azathioprine is about 50%, and it is metabolized by oxidation and methylation in the liver and/or erythrocytes. The major side effect is myelosuppression, which can be severe if it is used in combination with allopurinol. Allopurinol inhibits the enzyme xanthine oxidase, which converts azathioprine to inactive 6-thiouric acid. Other adverse effects of azathioprine include hepatotoxicity, alopecia, GI toxicity, pancreatitis, and increased risk for neoplasia.

MMF (Cellcept) is a prodrug that is rapidly hydrolyzed to the active drug mycophenolic acid (MPA), a selective, noncompetitive, reversible inhibitor of inosine monophosphate dehydrogenase (IMPDH). B and T cells lack nucleotide salvage pathways, are highly dependent on de novo purine synthesis for cell proliferation, and are therefore selectively inhibited by this drug. MMF is indicated for the prophylaxis of transplant rejection and is typically used in combination with a CNI and glucocorticoids. In addition, it has benefits in the treatment of acute and chronic rejection, which arise from its ability to inhibit the recruitment and interaction of mononuclear cells and to prevent the development and progression of proliferative arteriolopathy, respectively. The typical starting dose is 1 g twice daily, although a higher dose (1.5 g twice daily) may be recommended for black recipients. The parent drug is cleared from the blood within a few minutes, and MPA in turn is conjugated to glucuronide (MPAG) before excretion in bile. Enterohepatic cycling of MPAG occurs, producing a second peak at 5 to 6 hours, after which MPAG is excreted in the urine. Although oral bioavailability is about 90% with a $T_{1/2}$ of 12 hours, plasma concentrations of MPA after a single dose in kidney transplant patients within the first month are about half of those found in healthy volunteers or long-term transplant recipients. A generic version of MMF was approved in 2009 and can be safely substituted for Cellcept. As with the use of tacrolimus and cyclosporine generics, it is important to ensure that patients consistently receive the same generic product, that patients and clinicians are aware when substitutions occur, and that enhanced vigilance is provided during the transition.

The principal toxicities of MMF are GI and hematologic. These include leukopenia, anemia, diarrhea, abdominal pain, and vomiting. An enteric-coated form of MPA (Myfortic) is also available, which anecdotally has superior GI tolerability, although this has not been convincingly demonstrated in controlled studies. There is also an increased incidence of certain infections with MMF, especially sepsis associated with cytomegalovirus (CMV) and an association with progressive multifocal leukoencephalopathy (PML) caused by John Cunningham (JC) virus. Because of the higher potency of CsA in interrupting enterohepatic circulation, the combination of MMF with tacrolimus leads to higher AUC for MPA and is more immunosuppressive than when it is used in combination with CsA. The use of MMF in pregnancy is associated with congenital malformations and increased risk for pregnancy loss. Women of childbearing potential must adhere to a Risk Evaluation and Mitigation Strategy (REMS) and use effective contraception while taking MMF.

Sirolimus (Rapamycin; Rapamune) is a macrocyclic lactone produced by *Streptomyces hygroscopicus*. It also forms a complex with FKBP-12, but unlike with tacrolimus, this complex binds to and inhibits the protein kinase mTOR leading to a cell-cycle arrest in the G1 phase. Sirolimus is indicated for the prophylaxis of kidney transplant rejection, usually in combination with a reduced dose of a CNI and glucocorticoids. Particular attention has focused on its use in protocols using early or late CNI withdrawal or minimization, although enthusiasm has dampened for early use because of higher rates of acute rejection, possibly due to the expansion of CD8 memory T cells. However, sirolimus has also been associated with the expansion of CD4 regulatory T cells and therefore may find utility as part of regimens that promote transplant tolerance. One unique advantage is its antitumor effect, which arises from its inhibition of angiogenesis and G1 to S cell cycle transition. mTOR inhibition has shown clinical benefit in both primary and metastatic Kaposi sarcoma and renal cell carcinoma, and it shows promise in the treatment of other solid and hematologic malignancies. A clinical trial of conversion from a CNI-based regimen to sirolimus-based regimen in kidney transplant recipients showed a reduction in the incidence of repeat skin cancers without any increase in the risk of acute rejection or graft dysfunction.

Sirolimus is absorbed rapidly after an oral dose, and bioavailability is about 15%. It is extensively metabolized in the liver by CYP3A4 and P-glycoprotein. The blood $T_{1/2}$ after multiple doses in stable kidney transplant patients is 62 hours. It is usually dosed once daily, with target trough blood levels of 5 to 15 ng/mL. Interactions of sirolimus are common with drugs that are metabolized or transported by CYP3A4 and P-glycoprotein (see Table 63.2). In healthy volunteers, concomitant administration of sirolimus and CsA (as Neoral) increased the AUC for sirolimus by 230% compared with sirolimus alone. Therefore it is recommended that sirolimus be administered 4 hours after the morning CsA dose. Everolimus is closely related chemically and clinically to sirolimus but has a shorter $T_{1/2}$ (23 hours) and therefore a shorter time to achieve steady-state drug concentrations. The toxicities and reported drug interactions appear to be the same.

The major adverse effects of sirolimus in the early posttransplant period arise from its antiproliferative actions, including impaired wound healing and wound dehiscence, prolonged delayed kidney graft function, and a higher incidence of lymphoceles. Hypercholesterolemia and hypertriglyceridemia, hyperglycemia, bone marrow suppression, oral ulcers, and GI side effects are well known. Rarely, it can cause localized limb edema, angioedema, and interstitial pneumonitis. Sirolimus given alone does not produce acute or chronic decreases in kidney function; however, it can cause direct tubular and podocyte toxicity resulting in hypokalemia, de novo proteinuria, and nephrotic syndrome. In combination with standard doses of CNI, there is a potentiation of nephrotoxicity that is not completely explained by their pharmacokinetic interaction. For this reason, it is recommended that the CNI dose be reduced when sirolimus is added. Sirolimus is embryotoxic, and its use is contraindicated in pregnancy. Women must use effective contraception while on sirolimus. Reversible oligospermia and reduced testosterone levels have also been described.

BIOLOGICS FOR MAINTENANCE IMMUNOSUPPRESSION

Abatacept (CTLA4-Ig) contains the binding region of CTLA4 and the constant region of human IgG₁, and it competitively inhibits CD28 (Fig. 62.5). However, CTLA4-Ig was less effective when used in nonhuman primate models of kidney transplantation. Belatacept (LEA29Y; Nulojix) is a second-generation CTLA4-Ig with two amino acid substitutions, which has higher affinity for CD80 (twofold) and CD86 (fourfold), yielding a 10-fold increase in potency. Preclinical studies showed that belatacept did not induce tolerance but did prolong graft survival. BENEFIT and BENEFIT-EXT were two randomized, multicenter trials in which adult patients receiving a kidney transplant were randomized to one of three regimens for maintenance immunosuppression: a more intensive (MI) regimen of belatacept, a less intensive (LI) regimen of belatacept, or cyclosporine (Fig. 62.6). Patients

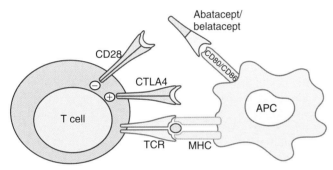

Fig. 62.5 Abatacept and belatacept bind to CD80 and CD86 and block costimulation. *APC*, Antigen-presenting cell; *MHC*, major histocompatibility complex; *TCR*, T cell receptor. (From Vincenti F. Costimulation blockade in autoimmunity and transplantation. *J Allergy Clin Immunol.* 2008;121:299–306.)

in all treatment arms received basiliximab induction and were maintained on MMF and corticosteroids. The demonstration of comparable efficacy to CsA associated with superior kidney function and metabolic parameters led to the LI belatacept regimen receiving FDA approval in 2011 for maintenance immunotherapy in kidney transplantation. The more intense regimen was associated with more infections and PTLD, and therefore belatacept is not approved for use in Epstein-Barr virus (EBV)-negative patients. Although belatacept was associated with more rejections, which were also histologically more severe when compared with those in cyclosporine-treated patients, these rejections lacked other characteristics that are usually associated with poor outcomes, such as the development of donor-specific antibodies. Interestingly, graft function in patients with acute rejection was nevertheless superior to cyclosporine-treated patients without rejection, again underscoring the contribution of CNI-nephrotoxicity to graft dysfunction. A preexisting repertoire of memory T cells, which are resistant to costimulation blockade and may not be affected by anti-IL2-receptor antibodies, may be responsible for the difference in acute rejection rates.

Despite the increased risk of early acute rejection, an analysis of the 7-year safety and efficacy data from the belatacept clinical trials published in 2016 showed a significantly lower rate of death or graft loss with both the MI and the LI regimens of belatacept compared with cyclosporine (12.7% and 12.8% vs. 21.7%). The risk of early acute rejection can be abrogated using belatacept in combination with a depletional induction agent and an mTOR inhibitor, and this strategy could further improve long-term graft outcomes. Belatacept has also been used as part of a CNI-free conversion strategy in stable kidney transplant recipients and has demonstrated superior improvement in GFR with conversion versus CNI continuation.

A second costimulatory pathway involves the interaction of CD40 on activated T cells with CD40 ligand (CD154) on

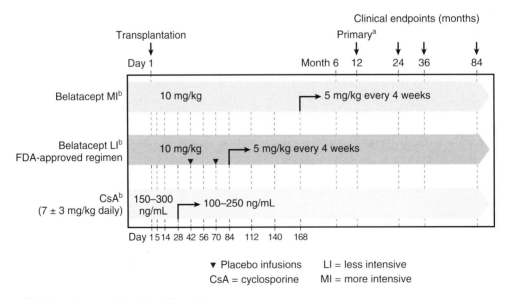

ᵃBelatacept arms unblinded at 12 months.
ᵇAll patients received basiliximab induction, mycophenolate mofetil, and corticosteroid taper.

Fig. 62.6 BENEFIT and BENEFIT-EXT study design and medication dosing.

APCs. Two humanized anti-CD154 monoclonal antibodies have been used in clinical trials in kidney transplantation and autoimmune diseases but were associated with thromboembolic events. An alternative approach with monoclonal antibodies to CD40 is more attractive. Although clinical trials of ASKP1240 or 4D11 (Astellas Pharma US, Inc.)—a fully human anti-CD40 monoclonal IgG4 antibody—provided evidence of efficacy with reduced dose tacrolimus and steroids, there was an unacceptably high rate of acute rejection, and additional studies in transplantation were placed on hold. Other anti-CD40 antibodies are in development.

SMALL MOLECULES

Cytokine receptors are enticing targets for modulation by new small molecules. Janus kinases (JAK) are important cytoplasmic tyrosine kinases involved in cell signaling. Tofacitinib (CP-690550) inhibits JAK3, which is expressed on NK cells, activated T cells, B cells, and myeloid cells. In clinical trials, it was noninferior to tacrolimus in terms of rejection rates and graft survival. It also showed a lower rate of hyperglycemia but a trend toward more infections, including CMV and polyomavirus. Sotrastaurin (AEB071) inhibits multiple protein kinase C isoforms, leading to decreased T cell activation, but it showed poor efficacy in preventing rejection after CNI withdrawal in clinical trials.

TARGETING B CELLS AND HUMAN LEUKOCYTE ANTIGEN ANTIBODY

Most of the advances in transplantation can be attributed to drugs designed to inhibit T cell responses. As a result, T cell–mediated acute rejection became much less of a problem. Disappointingly, long-term graft loss rates did not change substantially even with the reduction in 1-year acute cellular rejection rates to <10% with newer protocols. The development of newer methods to identify donor-specific anti-HLA antibodies (DSA, using single antigen beads), recognize histologic features of antibody-mediated injury (C4d staining), and characterize the gene expression profiles associated with rejection has led to the understanding that a chronic injury mediated by preexisting or de novo alloantibody is the major cause of late graft loss. Therefore, therapies that address B cell responses and the humoral response to the graft are critical not only for the treatment of acute AMR, which is rare, but also to address the larger problem of late graft attrition. Current strategies include B cell depletion, modulation of B cell activation and survival, plasma cell depletion, antibody removal, and inhibition of antibody effector function (Fig. 62.7).

Rituximab (Rituxan), a chimeric monoclonal antibody directed against CD20 on B cells, causes rapid sustained depletion of circulating and lymphoid B cells for more than 6 months. Because CD20 is not found on pro-B cells or plasma cells, rituximab does not prevent the regeneration of B cells from precursors and does not directly affect immunoglobulin levels, although some studies have reported a reduction in DSA. It has been used pretransplant to reduce high levels of preformed anti-HLA or ABO antibodies, as well as posttransplant to treat acute AMR. It has not yet been rigorously tested in clinical trials. Infusion reactions can occur and are usually prevented by premedication. Rare cases of PML have been associated with its use. Newer fully human

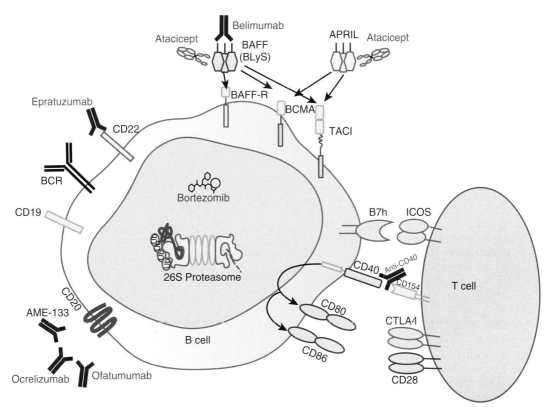

Fig. 62.7 Novel strategies targeting humoral alloimmunity. (From Webber A, Hirose R, Vincenti F. Novel strategies in immunosuppression: issues in perspective. *Transplantation*. 2011;91:1057–1064.)

and humanized monoclonal anti-CD20 antibodies are less immunogenic, more efficacious, and can overcome rituximab resistance. Obinutuzumab (Gazyva, Genentech), also known as afutuzumab until 2009, is a fully humanized monoclonal antibody to CD20 on mature B cells that is currently approved by the FDA for the treatment of chronic lymphocytic leukemia in combination with chlorambucil. An early phase trial is currently under way to test preliminary efficacy as a desensitization strategy in kidney transplant recipients.

IVIG is a preparation of human polyclonal IgG (95%) derived from the pooled plasma of adults. The mechanism of action of high-dose IVIG in immune modulation is complex and involves multiple pathways. It provides antiidiotypic antibodies, reduces the expression and function of Fc receptors on leukocytes and endothelial cells, increases IgG clearance, downregulates the activation and effector function of T and B cells, and inhibits complement activation and cytokine production. IVIG causes a rapid reduction in DSA and has shown efficacy in clinical trials as part of the desensitization strategies. The standard dose is 2 g/kg up to a maximum of 140 g in a single administration infused over 4 to 8 hours. Minor reactions, such as flushing, chills, headache, nausea, myalgia, and arthralgia, are common; these are reduced with premedication and by slowing the infusion rate. Hemolytic anemia, aseptic meningitis, and thrombotic complications are rare. Acute kidney injury, due to osmotic nephrosis from the sucrose or sorbitol vehicle, is usually self-limited.

Bortezomib (Velcade) is a 26S proteasome inhibitor that is approved for the treatment of multiple myeloma. Proteasomal inhibition results in the accumulation of misfolded IgG and causes apoptosis of plasma cells. Bortezomib also reduces NF-κB activity by inhibiting the degradation of IκB, which then leads to the reduced transcription of IL-6, a potent plasma cell survival factor. Bortezomib has been used for desensitization, the treatment of acute AMR, and in the experimental protocols of transplant tolerance. It has been shown to significantly reduce anti-HLA antibody levels. The main toxicity of bortezomib is neurologic, with de novo or worsened peripheral neuropathy being common. Hematologic and GI toxicity can also occur. Carfilzomib (Kyprolis) is a second-generation proteasome inhibitor that irreversibly binds to and inhibits the chymotrypsin-like activity of the 20S proteasome. An advantage of carfilzomib over bortezomib is the reduced risk of neuropathy. A phase I clinical trial of carfilzomib as part of a desensitization strategy in kidney transplant candidates is currently under way.

Eculizumab (Soliris) is a monoclonal antibody to the complement protein C5, which blocks C5 cleavage and halts the formation of the membrane attack complex. It is approved for the treatment of paroxysmal nocturnal hemoglobinuria and is emerging as a novel therapy for the treatment of acute AMR due to its ability to arrest complement-mediated injury. This creates a window of opportunity for other therapies to clear DSA. Because eculizumab diminishes the defense against encapsulated bacteria, especially meningococci, patients should ideally undergo meningococcal vaccination before receiving the first eculizumab treatment. Plasma-derived C1 esterase inhibitor (Cinryze) has shown some promise in the treatment of acute AMR, and clinical trials are under way.

BAFF (B cell–activating factor, also known as BLys, TALL-1, and THANK) belongs to the TNF family and is an important stimulator of B cell survival and expansion.

Belimumab (Benlysta) is a humanized monoclonal antibody that specifically inhibits BAFF, is approved for the treatment of systemic lupus, and may be useful for B cell depletion and to decrease antibody production. Atacicept is a fusion protein formed from TACI, the extracellular domain of one of the receptors for BAFF. It binds BAFF and APRIL (a proliferation-inducing ligand), which also promotes B cell and plasma cell survival. Atacicept may be useful in sensitized patients with established plasma cells.

TREATMENT OF REJECTION

Maintenance immunosuppression is effective in preventing acute cellular rejection; however, it is less effective in blocking activated T cells and thus in treating established acute rejection or preventing chronic rejection. After the acute rejection episode has been treated, intensification of the maintenance regimen and closer monitoring are often indicated.

Treatment of acute cellular rejection requires the use of agents directed against activated T cells. These include glucocorticoids in high doses (pulse therapy), polyclonal antilymphocyte antibodies, or muromonab-CD3. Steroids reverse about 75% of first acute rejections and are typically tapered down over a few weeks to maintenance doses of 5 to 10 mg/day. Thymoglobulin has largely replaced OKT3, and it reverses about 90% of severe acute rejections. The treatment of acute AMR consists of strategies to remove DSA (plasmapheresis), decrease antibody production (IVIG, rituximab, and bortezomib), and inhibit complement activation (eculizumab).

The management of chronic allograft rejection is difficult because the histologic changes seen are often irreversible and lead to the progression of kidney disease, regardless of the original injury. Intensification of calcineurin inhibition is generally not effective, and some studies have shown benefit with reduction/elimination of the CNI while maintaining or increasing adjunctive therapy. Most of the experience has been with MMF in these situations, although sirolimus may be an appropriate alternative in the absence of proteinuria. C4d positivity in patients with chronic rejection is a marker for ongoing humoral injury, and these patients may benefit from intensification of immunosuppression and IVIG. The risks and benefits of immunosuppression must be weighed carefully at every stage. If graft function continues to deteriorate, immunosuppression should be withdrawn in a stepwise fashion to avoid precipitating acute rejection, and the patient should be prepared for dialysis, preemptive transplant, or comprehensive conservative care.

TOLERANCE

Operational transplant *tolerance* is defined as prolonged survival of a transplanted organ in the absence of immunosuppression, without evidence of a destructive response. In addition, the recipient should be able to respond normally to immune stimuli, such as infection and tumors. Transplant tolerance is therefore an active state of antigen-specific nonresponsiveness, rather than a failure to respond to the allograft.

Chimerism (coexistence of cells from two genetic lineages in a single individual) can be induced by first dampening or eliminating immune function in the recipient and then providing a new source of immune function by adoptive transfer (transfusion) of bone marrow or hematopoietic stem cells. Upon reconstitution of immune function, the recipient no longer recognizes new antigens provided during a critical period as nonself. Early animal studies showed that fetal/neonatal exposure to donor blood cells led to hematopoietic chimerism and specific transplant tolerance. In the precyclosporine era, improved kidney transplant outcomes were seen with donor-specific blood transfusions. These disappeared after the introduction of CsA, presumably due to the efficacy of this drug in blocking T cell activation. It is possible that the effect may have been from cell surface or soluble HLA molecules. Soluble HLA and peptides corresponding to linear sequences of HLA molecules have been shown to induce immunologic tolerance in animal models.

The creation of bone marrow chimeras as a tool for transplant tolerance was first demonstrated when patients who had undergone bone marrow transplantation (BMT) for the treatment of hematologic malignancies subsequently underwent successful kidney transplantation for kidney failure from their original BMT donor, without the requirement for maintenance immunosuppression. However, the toxicity of the myeloablative therapy and the risk of lethal graft-versus-host disease (GVHD) precludes this protocol for routine transplantation. Two approaches to reduce toxicity involve the creation of a mixed allogeneic chimera using (a) cytotoxic drugs and thymic irradiation in combination with a limited course of immunosuppression or (b) total lymphoid irradiation (TLI), which targets the thymus, the spleen, and the supradiaphragmatic lymph nodes. TLI, compared with total body irradiation, resulted in a markedly reduced incidence of GVHD by sparing recipient NK cells, but neither approach has been reliable in achieving durable operational tolerance in HLA-mismatched patients.

Several combinations of biologics can be envisioned as potentially inducing tolerance. Although preclinical trials of a monoclonal antibody to CD40 ligand (CD40L) with CTLA4Ig were promising, clinical trials were halted due to increased thromboembolic events. The combination of belatacept and anti-CD40 antibody may be useful.

Regulatory T cells (T_{regs}) were found to suppress the rejection response of naive T cells in adoptive transfer assays. T_{regs} express the transcription factor FOXP3 that is responsible for their suppressive functions, whereas activated effector T cells do not stably express FOXP3. Several studies involving the use of T_{regs} in kidney transplant recipients as either tolerogenic agents or immunotherapy for graft inflammation are currently under way.

Operational tolerance in transplantation has not yet been routinely achieved. The development of new agents and improved understanding of transplant immunology are now allowing us to create simplified immunosuppressive regimens with low toxicities that have the potential to improve long-term patient and graft survival.

IMMUNE MONITORING

Current monitoring of kidney transplant recipients consists primarily of serial measurements of kidney function and of immunosuppressive drug levels. These methods have limited sensitivity and specificity for the diagnosis of rejection, which is usually made by kidney biopsy. However, a kidney biopsy is invasive, cannot be used for frequent monitoring, and only identifies an established rejection process.

Biomarkers may serve not only as diagnostic parameters but also as predictive tools that anticipate the subsequent development of subclinical and clinical acute rejection. The identification of biomarkers of immune alloreactivity in blood, urine, and tissue would allow the early identification of patients at risk for rejection, the optimization of drug regimens, and the monitoring of responses to changes in therapy and would guide the development of novel therapies. Studies in human kidney recipients suggest unique protein and genetic signatures that may identify biomarkers of injury as well as potential targets of therapy.

Preformed and de novo anti-HLA antibodies are associated with both acute and chronic AMR and graft loss. Anti-HLA antibodies developed in one-third of recipients at 5 years, and about 30% are donor-specific. Serial monitoring of DSA is used mostly in highly sensitized patients, and further studies are needed to identify their cost-effectiveness and clinical utility in broader populations, especially given the limited effect of current therapies on decreasing DSA.

Cell-based assays aim to measure recipient T cell reactivity. The cell-mediated lympholysis (CML) assay primarily measures class I alloreactivity through the direct pathway, whereas the mixed lymphocyte culture (MLC) test recognizes class II differences between the recipient and the donor by both direct and indirect recognition pathways. Alloreactive T cells can be measured with flow cytometry-based assays, as well as with HLA class I and class II tetramers. An enzyme-linked immunosorbent spot assay (ELISPOT) can measure the secretion of cytokines, such as IFN-γ from T cells after alloantigen stimulation and provides a useful means of assessing the indirect pathway. ELISPOT may identify recipients at risk for acute rejection posttransplant, and further testing is under way to establish its role. The ImmuKnow assay (Cylex) quantifies the amount of intracellular ATP that is released from CD4 T cells in response to a nonspecific mitogenic stimulus. It is less specific, and changes in test values may be more predictive than single time point assessments. The kidney solid organ response test (kSORT) is a recently identified 17-gene set that is able to predict acute rejection up to 3 months in advance using quantitative polymerase chain reaction (PCR) on peripheral blood samples; it is currently being developed for commercial use.

Urine proteomics, as well as messenger RNA (mRNA) isolation, have been proposed as another means of identifying acute rejection, graft IF/TA, and drug toxicity. Urinary mRNA levels of several cytolytic proteins, such as granzyme B and perforin, have been demonstrated to significantly discriminate acute rejection from stable allograft function or tubular necrosis and are currently undergoing development in commercial assays.

Microarray analysis and real-time PCR of candidate transcripts in allograft tissue obtained from kidney biopsy have demonstrated unique findings in clinical settings, such as ischemia-reperfusion injury, stable graft function, acute rejection, subclinical rejection, and polyomavirus infection. A common rejection module consisting of 11 genes that are significantly overexpressed in acute rejection was initially identified in four different types of transplanted organs. It is now being developed as a urinary biomarker to identify kidney transplant recipients with subclinical rejection.

The development of reliable biomarkers is crucial for individualizing therapy aimed at extending allograft survival and improving patient health, particularly when incorporating novel immunosuppressive agents, implementing drug minimization protocols, and selecting patients for transplant tolerance trials.

KEY BIBLIOGRAPHY

Boffa DJ, Luan F, Thomas D, et al. Rapamycin inhibits the growth and metastatic progression of non-small cell lung cancer. *Clin Cancer Res.* 2004;10:293-300.

Brennan D, Daller J, Lake K, et al. Rabbit antithymocyte globulin versus basiliximab in renal transplantation. *N Engl J Med.* 2006;355:1967-1977.

Ekberg H, Grinyo J, Nashan B, et al. Cyclosporine sparing with mycophenolate mofetil, daclizumab and corticosteroids in renal allograft recipients: the CAESAR study. *Am J Transplant.* 2007;7:560-570.

Ekberg H, Tedesco-Silva H, Demirbas A, et al; for ELITE-Symphony Study. Reduced exposure to calcineurin inhibitors in renal transplantation. *N Engl J Med.* 2007;357:2562-2575.

Gloor JM, Sethi S, Stegall MD, et al. Transplant glomerulopathy: subclinical incidence and association with alloantibody. *Am J Transplant.* 2007;7:2124-2132.

Halloran PF. Immunosuppressive drugs for kidney transplantation. *N Engl J Med.* 2004;351:2715-2729.

Hanaway MJ, Woodle ES, Mulgaonkar S, et al; for INTAC Study Group. Alemtuzumab induction in renal transplantation. *N Engl J Med.* 2011;364:1909-1919.

Jordan SC, Vo AA, Peng A, et al. IVIG: a novel approach to improve transplant rates and outcomes in highly HLA-sensitized patients. *Am J Transplant.* 2006;6:459-466.

Knight S, Russell N, Barcena L, et al. Mycophenolate mofetil decreases acute rejection and may improve graft survival in renal transplant recipients when compared with azathioprine: a systematic review. *Transplantation.* 2009;87:785-794.

Li L, Khatri P, Sigdel TK, et al. A peripheral blood diagnostic test for acute rejection in renal transplantation. *Am J Transplant.* 2012;12(10):2710-2718.

Maluccio M, Sharma V, Lagman M, et al. Tacrolimus enhances transforming growth factor-beta1 expression and promotes tumor progression. *Transplantation.* 2003;76:597-602.

Patel R, Terasaki PI. Significance of the positive crossmatch test in kidney transplantation. *N Engl J Med.* 1969;280:735-739.

Scehna F, Pascoe M, Albaru J, et al. Conversion from calcineurin inhibitors to sirolimus maintenance therapy in renal allograft recipients: 24-month efficacy and safety results from the CONVERT trial. *Transplantation.* 2009;87:233-242.

Starzl TE. Immunosuppressive therapy and tolerance of organ allografts. *N Engl J Med.* 2008;358:407-411.

Vincenti F, Kirkman R, Light S, et al. Interleukin-2-receptor blockade with daclizumab to prevent acute rejection in renal transplantation. Daclizumab Triple Therapy Study Group. *N Engl J Med.* 1998;338:161-165.

Vincenti F, Larsen C, Durrbach A, et al. Costimulation blockade with belatacept in renal transplantation. *N Engl J Med.* 2005;353:770-781.

Vincenti F, Rostaing L, Grinyo J, et al. Belatacept and long-term outcomes in kidney transplantation. *N Engl J Med.* 2016;374:333-343.

Vincenti F, Schena F, Paraskevas S, et al; For the FREEDOM Study Group. A randomized, multicenter study of steroid avoidance, early steroid withdrawal or standard steroid therapy in kidney transplant recipients. *Am J Transplant.* 2008;8:307-316.

Zachary AA, Montgomery RA, Ratner LE, et al. Specific and durable elimination of antibody to donor HLA antigens in renal transplant patients. *Transplantation.* 2003;76:1519-1525.

Full bibliography can be found on www.expertconsult.com.

Infectious Complications of Solid Organ Transplantation

63

Michael G. Ison

Infections remain among the most common complications following kidney transplantation. While advances in surgical techniques and modern induction and maintenance immunosuppression regimens have improved the outcomes of the allograft, they have also resulted in an alteration in the risk of posttransplant infections over time. For example, lymphocyte depletion induction combined with tacrolimus–mycophenolate–based maintenance has resulted in an increase in the frequency of BK virus nephropathy (BKVN). To counter the enhanced risk of infection, broader use of modern antimicrobial prophylaxis has been deployed in an attempt to delay and reduce the incidence of posttransplant infections. This chapter will summarize the timing of infectious complications, discuss key issues related to donor-derived disease transmission and methods to mitigate the risk of these events, review key strategies to minimize the risk of infectious complications of kidney transplantation, and finish with focused reviews of common infections complicating kidney transplantation, including BKVN, cytomegalovirus (CMV), infectious diarrhea, and urinary tract infections (UTI).

TIMING OF INFECTIOUS COMPLICATIONS IN KIDNEY TRANSPLANTATION

Infectious complications typically occur in one of three time periods posttransplant: early posttransplant infections, infections during peak immunosuppression, and late-onset infections. A number of factors affect the timing of the infections, including specific donor and recipient factors, such as preexisting infection or immunity, the use of antimicrobial prophylaxis, and the net state of immunosuppression. Of these, the net state of immunosuppression requires the closest consideration as there are no direct measures to assess the impact of various factors on risk of rejection or infectious complications. Instead, the clinician must assess a variety of factors including current and past immunosuppression; underlying immunodeficiency; neutropenia; lymphopenia; a variety of complex metabolic conditions, such as presence of uremia, malnutrition, poorly controlled diabetes mellitus, cirrhosis; and replication of immunomodulatory viruses, including human immunodeficiency virus (HIV), CMV, Epstein-Barr virus (EBV), hepatitis B (HBV), and hepatitis C (HCV). Reviews of immunosuppression must keep in mind both medications that may not be readily apparent on the patient's medication list (i.e., alemtuzumab for induction, or rituximab for prior treatment of antibody-mediated rejection as such antibody-based immunosuppression may have long-standing impacts of components of the immune system), as

well as the impact of recent immunosuppression, such as recent rejection treatment, high plasma levels of tacrolimus, or recent conversion from one immunosuppression to another. For example, with many immunosuppression conversions, the patient is effectively exposed to multiple agents with effective immunosuppression as one agent is titrated off and another is titrated on. Taken together, these inform the net state of immunosuppression for an individual patient.

Early posttransplant infections occur in the first 30 days posttransplant. The majority of such infections (~98%) are typical of any surgical patient, but they may be more severe or more common. The most common postsurgical infections include deep and superficial surgical site infections at the operative site, hospital-acquired pneumonia as a consequence of intubation during transplant surgery, UTI as a consequence of bladder catheterization, bacteremia secondary to use of intravenous (IV) catheters, and *Clostridium difficile* colitis as a complication of perioperative antimicrobial utilization. Management approaches for such infections are consistent with the local epidemiology and susceptibility of predicted pathogens and published guidelines. Rarely, donor-derived infections may present during the first 30 days posttransplant, as discussed in greater detail below. Finally, recipient-origin infections may manifest in the first 30 days. Examples of recipient-origin infections include respiratory viral infections, such as influenza, or occult bacteremias that were incubating in the candidate at the time they present for their transplant procedures.

Infections during peak immunosuppression are typically opportunistic infections or pathogens that reactivate from latent infection in the recipient and generally occur between 30 days and 6 months posttransplant or within 3 months of treatment of rejection. Use of prophylactic antimicrobials may delay the onset of such infections, resulting in later than typical onset. For example, high-risk CMV donor seropositive, recipient seronegative (D+/R−) patients frequently will be given 6 months of anti-CMV prophylaxis, and as a result, CMV incidence peaks 1 to 3 months after such prophylaxis is discontinued. Examples of infections that typically occur during the period of peak immunosuppression include BK virus, CMV, herpes simplex virus (HSV), varicella-zoster virus (VZV), HBV, HCV, tuberculosis, *Listeria*, *Strongyloides*, and Chagas.

Late-onset infections typically present greater than 6 months posttransplant or greater than 3 months after treatment for a rejection episode. Most late-onset infections are community-acquired infections, such as community-acquired pneumonia, respiratory viral infections including influenza, and UTI. Such infections may lead to hospitalization or require aggressive antimicrobial therapy to resolve the infections. Patients may acquire infections from exposure to the environment or travel, which increases over time as the patient returns to normal function. Examples of environmental exposures include endemic mycoses (histoplasmosis, blastomycosis, and coccidioidomycosis), West Nile virus, and travel-associated malaria. Some opportunistic infections notoriously present late, including nocardiosis, mucormycosis, and JC virus–mediated progressive multifocal leukoencephalopathy (PML). Lastly, some infections such as CMV, EBV-positive and EBV-negative posttransplant lymphoproliferative disorder (PTLD), hepatitis, and TB may present in this late period. *Pneumocystis jirovecii* (PCP) historically was an infection complicating the period of peak immunosuppression, although with universal prophylaxis, most cases of PCP occur late posttransplant in the current era.

DONOR-DERIVED INFECTIONS AND RISK MITIGATION STRATEGIES

Donor-derived infections are defined as any infection present in the donor that is transmitted to the recipient with the transplanted organ or vessels. Such infections can be categorized as either expected disease transmissions, where the pathogen is known to be present in the donor at the time of procurement and steps are taken to mitigate the disease transmission, or unexpected disease transmissions, when the donor is not recognized to have an infection that is identified after resulting in clinical disease in one or more of the transplant recipients. Examples of expected disease transmissions include CMV or EBV in which the donor is recognized to have an infection and the recipient is either monitored for evidence of disease or given prophylactic medications to prevent clinical diseases. Examples of unexpected disease transmissions include bacteria (*Escherichia coli*, *Mycobacteria tuberculosis*, and *S. aureus*), fungi (Candida, Cryptococcus, and Histoplasmosis), parasites (Chagas, Strongyloides, and Acanthamoeba), and viruses (lymphocytic choriomeningitis virus [LCMV], rabies, HIV, and HCV). In the United States, any documented or suspected unexpected donor-derived disease transmissions need to be reported to the Organ Procurement and Transplantation Network (OPTN) as soon as possible but not greater than 24 hours after initially suspecting transmission (OPTN Policy 15.4); the report is made through the Patient Safety Portal. Timely reporting of suspected transmissions is essential to facilitate communication and rapidly allow screening and treatment of recipients of other organs from the same donor. Data on such disease transmissions have been collected and categorized based on standardized methodologies and have been summarized in detail elsewhere.

There are several ways in which potential living and deceased donors can be screened to mitigate the risk of disease transmission. All donors should have a thorough review of their medical and social history, receive a complete physical examination and assessment of the potential organs, and undergo thorough testing of blood. The donor medical and social history should be reviewed for history of documented infection or exclusion from blood donation. The donor's social history should be reviewed for residence or travel to regions of endemicity for potentially transmissible infections, including Chagas, and Coccidioidomycosis, *M. tuberculosis*,

strongyloidosis, toxoplasmosis, and West Nile virus. Patients with evidence of prior exposures to such potentially transmissible diseases should be screened for latent infection, as is required for living donors (OPTN Policy 15.3). The social history should also be reviewed for risk factors that place the donor at increased risk of transmission of HIV, HBV, and HCV as defined by the US Public Health Service (PHS) as summarized in Table 63.1. Current US policy (OPTN Policy 15.3) requires transplant centers to be informed if a potential donor meets any of the US PHS Increased Risk criteria and that the centers must obtain special informed consent from potential recipients of organs from such donors. Further, policy requires that the recipients of organs of such donors

---

Table 63.1   US Public Health Service Definitions of Donors at Increased Risk of HIV, Hepatitis B Virus, and Hepatitis C Virus Transmission

All Age Groups

- People who have had sex with a person known or suspected to have HIV, HBV, or HCV infections in the preceding 12 months
- Men who have sex with men (MSM) in the preceding 12 months
- Women who have had sex with a man with a history of MSM behavior in the preceding 12 months
- People who have had sex in exchange for money or drugs in the preceding 12 months
- People who have had sex with a person who had sex in exchange for money or drugs in the preceding 12 months
- People who have had sex with a person who has injected drugs by IV, IM, or subcutaneous routes for nonmedical reasons in the preceding 12 months
- People who have injected drugs by IV, IM, or subcutaneous routes for nonmedical reasons in the preceding 12 months
- People who have been in lockup, jail, prison, or a juvenile correctional facility for ≥72 hours in the preceding 12 months
- People who have been newly diagnosed with or have been treated for syphilis, gonorrhea, Chlamydia, or genital ulcers in the preceding 12 months
- People who have been on hemodialysis in the preceding 12 months (RISK FOR HCV ONLY)

Pediatric Donors

- A child who is ≤18 months of age and born to a mother known to be infected with, or at increased risk for, HIV, HBV, or HCV infections
- A child who has been breastfed within the preceding 12 months and the mother is known to be infected with, or at increased risk for, HIV

Laboratory Criteria

- Any evidence of hemodilution

HBV, Hepatitis B virus; *HCV*, hepatitis C virus; *HIV*, human immunodeficiency virus; *IM*, intramuscular; *IV*, intravenous.
From Seem DL, Lee I, Umscheid CA, Kuehnert MJ, United States Public Health Service. PHS guideline for reducing human immunodeficiency virus, hepatitis B virus, and hepatitis C virus transmission through organ transplantation. *Public Health Rep.* 2013;128:247–343.

be screened for development of potential donor-derived disease after transplantation. Because serology may miss transmission, early screening, optimally within the first 1 to 3 months posttransplant, for HIV, HBV, and HCV should include both serologic and direct detection of the virus (i.e., polymerase chain reaction [PCR]) unless the recipient had infection documented pretransplant. Because transmission of HBV may be missed with early posttransplant screening, repeat screening for HBV should be considered around 1 year posttransplant.

One unique category of donors are the US PHS Increased Risk Donors who have engaged in behaviors that place them at increased, albeit low, risk of transmission of HIV, HBV, and HCV. Despite current screening practices (Table 63.2), these donors harbor a residual risk of unrecognized disease transmission because of the fact that the donors may be within either the eclipse period (the period between infection and detection of infection by PCR or nucleic acid test [NAT])

or the serologic window period (the period between infection and detection of antibodies in the blood); the specific eclipse and window periods are summarized in Table 63.3. Because specific informed consent is required from potential recipients before the use of organs from US PHS Increased Risk Donors, the residual risk of disease transmission needs to be known to the consenting clinician to accurately estimate the risk of disease transmission (Table 63.4). Given the recent rise in donors who die of acute drug overdoses, even negative nucleic acid testing of donors will not fully rule out the risk of transmission, and the higher estimated residual risk should be made clear to the recipient (see Table 63.4); there have been documented examples of disease transmission, particularly HCV, from such drug overdose donors with negative testing within the eclipse period.

Donors with recognized infections require additional attention. While full discussion of relevant risk and prevention strategies are available elsewhere, three unique situations warrant review here: HBV infection in the donor, bacteremic donors, and donors with meningitis or encephalitis. Required screening of donors includes hepatitis B surface antigen (HBsAg) and hepatitis B core antibody (HBcAb); many donors may also have HBV NAT available. Donors with detectable virus by positive HBV NAT or HBsAg have active infection and can transmit infection effectively to kidney transplant recipients. As such, these organs are typically reserved for recipients with preexisting HBV infection with the use of HBV-active antivirals to prevent replication. Use of HBV-infected donor kidneys in select hepatitis B surface antibody (HBsAb)-positive recipients has rarely been described, typically with excellent outcomes, but in the setting of careful monitoring, antiviral medication, and informed consent. Donors with HBcAb positivity alone have a history of infection with HBV that remains latent in the donor. Because these donors account for up to 15% of the donor population, there is a greater body of evidence for the outcomes of recipients of such donors. Typically, HBcAb-positive donors are used in recipients with prior HBV vaccination and positive HBsAb titers of greater than 10 IU/L (although optimal protection is with ≥100 IU/L). Outcomes of such transplants are generally excellent without the need of antivirals with a low rate of HBV transmission, typically

---

Table 63.2   Screening Assays for Living and Deceased Organ Donors

Required Screening for All Living and Deceased Donors

- FDA licensed anti-HIV I, II or combined HIV antibody-antigen assay
- Hepatitis B: HBsAg, HBcAb
- Hepatitis C: anti-HCV, HCV NAT
- Syphilis screening
- Anti-CMV
- EBV serologic testing
- Blood and urine cultures (deceased donors only)
- Toxoplasmosis (for heart donors only)

Screening for Endemic Infections (Required for Living Donors With Relevant Risks)

- Strongyloides
- Tuberculosis
- *Trypanosoma cruzi* (Chagas disease)
- West Nile virus

Screening of US PHS Increased Risk Donors

- Combined HIV antibody-antigen assay or HIV NAT
- Hepatitis B NAT

Optional Screening Test

- HSV (herpes simplex) IgG antibody
- Varicella-zoster virus antibody
- Measles antibody
- Mumps antibody
- Rubella antibody
- HHV8 serology

CMV, Cytomegalovirus; *EBV*, Epstein-Barr virus; *FDA*, US Food and Drug Administration; *HBcAb*, hepatitis B core antibody; *HBsAg*, hepatitis B surface antigen; *HCV*, hepatitis C virus; *HHV*, human herpesvirus; *HIV*, human immunodeficiency virus; *HSV*, herpes simplex virus; *IgG*, immunoglobulin G; *NAT*, nucleic acid testing; *US PHS*, US Public Health Service.
From Fischer SA, Lu K, AST Infectious Diseases Community of Practice. Screening of donor and recipient in solid organ transplantation. *Am J Transplant.* 2013;13:9–21; and Rosen A, Ison MG. Screening of living organ donors for endemic infections: understanding the challenges and benefits of enhanced screening. *Transpl Infect Dis.* 2016. doi: 10.1111/tid.12633. [Epub ahead of print].

Table 63.3   Eclipse and Serologic Window Period for Human Immunodeficiency Virus, Hepatitis B Virus, and Hepatitis C Virus

Virus	Eclipse Period	Serologic Window Period
HIV	5–9 days	22 days
HBV	22 days	44 days
HCV	5–7 days	66 days

Eclipse period is the period between initial infection and first detection of virus by direct detection methods, such as polymerase chain reaction, nucleic acid testing, or antigen detection. The serologic window period is the time between initial infection and first detection of virus-specific antibodies.
HBV, Hepatitis B virus; *HCV*, hepatitis C virus; *HIV*, human immunodeficiency virus.
From Ison MG, Grossi P, AST Infectious Diseases Community of Practice. Donor-derived infections in solid organ transplantation. *Am J Transplant.* 2013;13:22–30.

Table 63.4 Residual Risk of Human Immunodeficiency Virus and Hepatitis C Virus for Screen Negative US Public Health Service Increased Risk Donors by Risk Factor

Risk Factor	Residual Risk of Human Immunodeficiency Virus	Residual Risk of Hepatitis C Virus	Risk Relative to Remaining on Hemodialysis for 1 year[a]
Injection drug user (nonwindow period)	0.05%	0.32%	Same risk as HD
Injection drug user (window period)	0.12%	3.0%	Higher risk than HD
Prostitute	0.03%	0.12%	3 times higher risk with HD
Sex partner with any of the above	0.01%	0.14%	3 times higher risk with HD
Men who have sex with men	0.04%	0.04%	10 times higher risk with HD
Exposed to HIV through blood	0.006%	0.004%	15 times higher risk with HD
Incarceration	0.009%	0.008%	5 times higher risk with HD

[a]The residual risk of human immunodeficiency virus and hepatitis C virus transmission for remaining on hemodialysis for 1 year are approximately 0.05% and 0.34%, respectively, according to USRDS data.
HIV, Human immunodeficiency virus; *HD*, hemodialysis.
From Kucirka LM, Sarathy H, Govindan P, et al. Risk of window period hepatitis-C infection in high infectious risk donors: systematic review and meta-analysis. *Am J Transplant.* 2011;11:1188–1200; and Kucirka LM, Sarathy H, Govindan P, et al. Risk of window period HIV infection in high infectious risk donors: systematic review and meta-analysis. *Am J Transplant.* 2011;11:1176–1187.

4% or lower. Such patients should be monitored for HBV replication posttransplant. If HBcAb-positive donors are used in HBsAb-negative recipients, antivirals can be considered until vaccination is given to the recipient.

Donors with bacteremia are another group requiring careful consideration as they comprise up to 5% of organ donors. Donors with active bacteremia pose a clear risk of disease transmission, and use requires careful review of the donor, informed consent of the recipient, and posttransplant antibacterial therapy. Most cases of transmission have involved resistant bacteria or recipients who receive inadequate therapy. Generally, it is recommended that the bacteremic donor receives antimicrobial treatment targeted at the causative bacteria with known susceptibility patterns for at least 24 to 48 hours and that the donor optimally has some degree of clinical response (improved white blood cell count, improved hemodynamics, defervescence). The donor should be carefully assessed for the presence of metastatic infection, particularly to the organ to be transplanted, and for endocarditis in cases of more than transient bacteremia or risk factors (i.e., IV drug use, recent dental work). Use of donors with gram-negative bacteria producing carbapenemases, which usually exhibit extended drug-resistant phenotypes and remain susceptible to only a few antibiotics, must be done with caution and with active engagement of transplant infectious disease experts, as these pose the highest rates of disease transmission and active agents may be associated with nephrotoxicity. Recipients are typically treated for at least 14 days of active antibiotic posttransplant and then monitored closely for evidence of recrudescent bacteremia.

Donors with documented bacterial meningitis, with or without bacteremia, can generally be safely used with little risk of disease transmission. Generally, donors are treated for 24 to 48 hours with antibiotics directed at the identified bacteria before procurement, optimally with evidence of clinical improvement. The recipient is typically treated for 7 to 14 days posttransplant with antibiotics directed at the cultured bacteria. Meningitis caused by highly virulent or intracellular organisms, such as *Listeria* species or *Mycobacteria*, are considered a contraindication. Donors with a presumptive diagnosis of bacterial meningitis but with negative bacterial cultures, may transmit infections and malignancies, and these donors generally should be avoided. Donors with encephalitis, particularly with fever, without a documented cause are frequently associated with disease transmission. Transmission of rabies, parasitic infections, lymphomas, and leukemias has occurred when donors with encephalitis without a proven cause were accepted as organ donors. As such, donors dying of encephalitis without a proven cause should likely be avoided. The one exception is a donor with documented *Naegleria fowleri* meningitis/meningoencephalitis; as the risk of disease transmission is low, such donors generally can be safely used.

INFECTIOUS DISEASE PREVENTION STRATEGIES

While available therapies have improved the outcome of infectious disease complications of solid organ transplantation, prevention remains the key to optimize patient care. Prevention strategies include thorough recipient screening, optimization of vaccination of recipients and their contacts, and use of selected antimicrobial prophylaxis. All recipients should be screened pretransplant for HIV; HBV; HCV; CMV; EBV; VZV; measles, mumps, rubella (MMR); tuberculosis (with either a purified protein derivative [PPD] or interferon-gamma release assay); and relevant latent endemic infections, including Chagas disease, Coccidiomycosis, and Strongyloides. Patients who plan to travel to underdeveloped regions of the world posttransplant should be seen by travel medicine experts for consideration of protective vaccines before transplant and at least 30 days before any such travel. Candidates should have a thorough screening to ensure their vaccine status is up to date before transplant. Special attention should be paid to candidates with negative VZV serology who should receive pretransplant varicella vaccine, patients with negative MMR titers who should receive the MMR vaccine, and patients with negative HBsAb who should receive the three-dose HBV vaccine series. Pretransplant and posttransplant, candidates and their family members should have up-to-date influenza (annually), tetanus-diphtheria-acellular

Table 63.5   Vaccines for Transplant Candidates, Recipients, and Contacts

Vaccine	Type	Recommended Pretransplant	Recommended Posttransplant	Safe for Contacts of Transplant Recipients
Influenza–injectable	I	YES	YES	YES
Influenza–intranasal	LA	YES	NO[a]	NO[a]
Hepatitis A	I	YES	YES	YES
Hepatitis B	I	YES	YES	YES
TDaP	I	YES	YES	YES
Haemophilus influenzae	I	YES	YES	YES
Conjugated Streptococcus pneumoniae	I	YES	YES	YES
Polysaccharide S. pneumoniae	I	YES	YES	YES
Neisseria meningitidis	I	YES	YES	YES
HPV	I	YES	YES	YES
Rabies	I	YES	YES	YES
Varicella	LA	YES	NO	YES
Rotavirus	LA	YES	NO	YES
MMR	LA	YES	NO	YES
BCG	LA	YES[b]	NO	YES
Anthrax	I	NO	NO	YES
Smallpox	LA	NO	NO	NO

For all vaccines, follow recommended dose and frequency consistent with national guidelines.

[a]Can use if no other alternative vaccine available but monitor for clinical disease.

[b]Use only if recommended by national guidelines.

HPV, Human papillomavirus; I, inactivated; LA, live attenuated; MMR, measles, mumps, rubella; TDaP, tetanus, diphtheria, acellular pertussis.

From Danziger-Isakov L, Kumar D, ASwT Infectious Diseases Community of Practice. Vaccination in solid organ transplantation. Am J Transplant. 2013;13:311–317.

pertussis (TDaP, once every 10 years), and pneumonia vaccines (Table 63.5). In general, use of live attenuated vaccines (see Table 63.5) should be avoided on patients receiving immunosuppressive medications.

Selected antimicrobial prophylaxis should be given to patients beginning with the transplant procedures. Published guidelines recommend cefazolin or vancomycin plus either aztreonam or a fluoroquinolone given no more than 60 minutes before the skin incision as a single dose. *P. jirovecii* prophylaxis consists of trimethoprim-sulfamethoxazole (TMP-SMX) single or double strength daily to three times per week for the first 6 to 12 months posttransplant; for sulfa-allergic patients, atovaquone 1500 mg daily, dapsone 50 to 100 mg daily (must not be used with G6PD deficiency), or pentamidine 300 mg nebulized every 4 weeks are alternatives. Prophylaxis for CMV is discussed below, although CMV D–/R– recipients need prevention of VZV and HSV with acyclovir, valacyclovir, or famciclovir for 3 to 6 months posttransplant. Kidney transplant recipients benefit from UTI prophylaxis while ureteral stents are in place; TMP-SMX daily or cephalexin 500 mg daily are adequate.

COMMON INFECTIOUS COMPLICATIONS OF KIDNEY TRANSPLANTATION

BK VIRUS NEPHROPATHY

BK virus is a polyomavirus that infects most children by 3 to 4 years of age and remains latent in the uroepithelium for the remainder of the individual's life. Immunosuppression results in increased frequency of replication, and in some patients a lack of control of the viral replication can lead to damage to the kidney and graft loss. Such BKVN occurs in 4% to 8% of kidney transplant recipients. Rarely, a related polyoma virus, JC virus, can cause a similar disease that is clinically indistinguishable from BKVN, other than JC virus being detected in the blood and urine instead of BK virus. Replication begins in the uroepithelium with initial detection of virus or shed infected cells (decoy cells). This typically precedes spillover of the virus in the blood compartment by 3 to 6 months. Viremia, without intervention, leads to subsequent development of BKVN 1 to 3 months after initial detection. As a result of these replication characteristics, routine screening of kidney transplant recipients can identify those at risk. Screening of blood and, less commonly, urine should be performed every 1 to 3 months for the first 2 years posttransplant; screening may be continued beyond 2 years, although new infections are uncommon unless there is enhancement of immunosuppression. Screening should also be performed with any rise in creatinine and at the timing of any biopsy performed either based on protocol or for cause. While the gold standard to diagnose BKNV is biopsy with immunohistochemical stains for the large T antigen, plasma viral loads greater than 10,000 are used by many to diagnose BKVN. Detection of replication should typically prompt reduction of immunosuppression, which reduces progression to BKVN. Optimal strategies for immunosuppression reduction have not been defined in prospective studies, but the overall goal is to reduce the net state of immunosuppression. If viuria or viremia persists despite reduction of immunosuppression, further reduction of immunosuppression and use of systemic cidofovir (typically 0.25 to 1 mg/kg every other week) or leflunomide can be considered; prospective studies have not documented superiority of any specific interventions. Fluoroquinolones have been tried in the past, but two prospective, randomized studies failed to demonstrate clinical success so they are not recommended currently for the prevention or management of BK viremia.

CYTOMEGALOVIRUS

CMV remains the most common viral infection complicating kidney transplantation. The risk is highest among seronegative recipients of seropositive donor organs (CMV D+/R−). Intermediate risk of CMV is present in the seropositive recipient with slightly higher risk in donor seropositive than donor seronegative. The lowest risk is among D−/R−, which still have an incidence of ~2% because of false-negative serology or posttransplant acquisition of infection. Given the high prevalence of CMV in the general population and the efficacy of antiviral therapy, serologic matching is typically not used. Instead, prevention of CMV is achieved with one of three approaches: universal prophylaxis, preemptive monitoring, or a hybrid approach. With universal prophylaxis, all at-risk patients receive prophylaxis with ganciclovir, valganciclovir, or valacyclovir for a fixed period of time. For preemptive monitoring, patients have regular (weekly or twice weekly) CMV viral load measurements and only receive antivirals when there is documented replication. The hybrid approach applies universal prophylaxis for a period of time and follows it with preemptive monitoring. Universal prophylaxis is frequently the easiest to implement in most settings, is associated with the greatest graft outcomes but has the high cost of the drug and complications of prophylaxis, including neutropenia, late-onset CMV replication, and development of resistance. Preemptive monitoring requires logistic systems to optimize testing but is associated with high rates of rejection and graft loss and can result in resistance emergence. The hybrid approach intuitively would be the optimal approach, although prospective studies have failed to document consistent superiority to clinical monitoring.

While valacyclovir is effective in preventing CMV, it requires high doses with high rates of neurologic side effects. Given the ease and efficacy, most centers use valganciclovir. While approved at 900 mg daily (or an equivalent dose adjusted for kidney function), some centers use a lower dose of 450 mg daily or the kidney function adjusted equivalent. This is associated with less neutropenia but may result in high rates of clinical failure. Among high-risk patients, 6 months of valganciclovir is associated with 16% of patients developing CMV. Current guidelines recommend CMV D+/R− pairs, and patients given lymphodepleting induction receive 6 months of prophylaxis, while lower risk patients receive 3 to 6 months of prophylaxis.

In patients that develop CMV viremia or tissue invasive disease, treatment is with full-dose valganciclovir or IV ganciclovir. A randomized controlled trial demonstrated similar outcomes with either approach except in patients with severe CMV, defined as CMV pneumonitis, high-level CMV replication (>50,000 to 100,000 copies/mL), or CMV colitis. As a result, oral valganciclovir 900 mg twice daily (or equivalent dose adjusted for kidney function) is preferred for most patients. IV therapy is generally reserved for patients with severe disease or CMV colitis. Treatment is generally continued until patients have no evidence of CMV end-organ disease and undetectable CMV viral loads on two sequential measurements. Treatment is typically followed by a period, from 1 to 3 months, of secondary prophylaxis. Full details on diagnostics and treatment are available in published guidelines. Patients who fail to have clinical or virologic response should be tested for resistance. Management of resistance is complex and is best done by an experienced Transplant Infectious Diseases expert.

DIARRHEA

Diarrhea is a frequent complication of solid organ transplantation and can be the result of drug side effects, infection, or other causes, including graft-versus-host disease or malignancy, especially PTLD. The optimal approach to diarrhea begins with an initial evaluation of stool for C. difficile, norovirus PCR, stool cultures, Giardia and Cryptosporidium enzyme immunoassay (EIA), and serum CMV viral load. If diarrhea persists with negative studies, reduction of mycophenolic acid can be attempted; if diarrhea still persists, colonoscopy with random biopsies assessed with immunohistochemical stains for CMV should be performed. C. difficile is the most common infectious cause of diarrhea among transplant patients and can occur in the context of recent antibiotics or without obvious inciting events. Treatment is consistent with published guidelines, which typically includes metronidazole, vancomycin, or fidaxomicin. Norovirus is the second most common infectious cause of diarrhea in solid organ transplant patients and can result in chronic diarrhea that may be relapsing and remitting in nature. Reduction of immunosuppression typically does not have a significant impact of shedding or diarrhea. Although intravenous immunoglobulin (IVIG), oral immunoglobulin, breast milk, and nitazoxanide have been tried to treat chronic norovirus, superiority or efficacy has not been clearly demonstrated for any one intervention. The focus of therapy should be aggressive hydration and antimotility agents to control diarrhea. The third most common infectious cause of diarrhea is CMV colitis. Approximately 15% of cases of CMV colitis may be demonstrated in the absence of systemic viremia, highlighting the need for colonoscopy for diagnosis. Treatment is with IV ganciclovir as outlined above.

URINARY TRACT INFECTIONS

UTIs are common among kidney transplant recipients, particularly in patients with frequent pretransplant UTIs, women, and patients with foreign material, including stents and drains, in the urinary tract. Asymptomatic bacteriuria is a frequent occurrence in transplant patients but does not warrant treatment. Only patients with abnormal urine analysis, symptoms, and greater than 100,000 CFUs of bacteria or Candida on urine culture should be treated with antibiotics. Given rising resistance to fluoroquinolones among enteric gram-negative bacteria, the preferred first-line therapy is cephalexin dosed to kidney function. Definitive therapy is dictated by the specific susceptibility patterns of the cultured bacteria. Patients with limited cystitis likely can be treated with 3 to 7 days of antibiotics, while patients with bacteremia or signs or symptoms of pyelonephritis, which is more frequent among transplant patients, require a longer course of 14 to 21 days of therapy. Patients with recurrent UTIs should undergo urologic evaluation for correctable issues in the urinary tract. While antibiotic-based suppression can be considered, this frequently leads to resistance and challenges in managing subsequent infections. Nonantibiotic preventative strategies, including methenamine hippurate, can be tried.

KEY BIBLIOGRAPHY

Danziger-Isakov L, Kumar D, AST Infectious Diseases Community of Practice. Vaccination in solid organ transplantation. *Am J Transplant.* 2013;13:311-317.

Dorschner P, McElroy LM, Ison MG. Nosocomial infections within the first month of solid organ transplantation. *Transpl Infect Dis.* 2014;16:171-187.

Echenique IA, Penugonda S, Stosor V, Ison MG, Angarone MP. Diagnostic yields in solid organ transplant recipients admitted with diarrhea. *Clin Infect Dis.* 2015;60:729-737.

Fischer SA, Lu K, AST Infectious Diseases Community of Practice. Screening of donor and recipient in solid organ transplantation. *Am J Transplant.* 2013;13:9-21.

Fishman JA. Infection in solid-organ transplant recipients. *N Engl J Med.* 2007;357:2601-2614.

Garzoni C, Ison MG. Uniform definitions for donor-derived infectious disease transmissions in solid organ transplantation. *Transplantation.* 2011;92:1297-1300.

Hirsch HH, Randhawa P, AST Infectious Diseases Community of Practice. BK polyomavirus in solid organ transplantation. *Am J Transplant.* 2013;13:179-188.

Huprikar S, Danziger-Isakov L, Ahn J, et al. Solid organ transplantation from hepatitis B virus-positive donors: consensus guidelines for recipient management. *Am J Transplant.* 2015;15:1162-1172.

Ison MG, Nalesnik MA. An update on donor-derived disease transmission in organ transplantation. *Am J Transplant.* 2011;11:1123-1130.

Ison MG, Grossi P, AST Infectious Diseases Community of Practice. Donor-derived infections in solid organ transplantation. *Am J Transplant.* 2013;13:22-30.

Kotton CN, Kumar D, Caliendo AM, et al. Updated international consensus guidelines on the management of cytomegalovirus in solid-organ transplantation. *Transplantation.* 2013;96:333-360.

Kucirka LM, Sarathy H, Govindan P, et al. Risk of window period hepatitis-C infection in high infectious risk donors: systematic review and meta-analysis. *Am J Transplant.* 2011;11:1188-1200.

Kucirka LM, Sarathy H, Govindan P, et al. Risk of window period HIV infection in high infectious risk donors: systematic review and meta-analysis. *Am J Transplant.* 2011;11:1176-1187.

Martin SI, Fishman JA, AST Infectious Diseases Community of Practice. Pneumocystis pneumonia in solid organ transplantation. *Am J Transplant.* 2013;13:272-279.

Parasuraman R, Julian K, AST Infectious Diseases Community of Practice. Urinary tract infections in solid organ transplantation. *Am J Transplant.* 2013;13:327-336.

Razonable RR, Humar A, AST Infectious Diseases Community of Practice. Cytomegalovirus in solid organ transplantation. *Am J Transplant.* 2013;13:93-106.

Seem DL, Lee I, Umscheid CA, Kuehnert MJ, United States Public Health S. PHS guideline for reducing human immunodeficiency virus, hepatitis B virus, and hepatitis C virus transmission through organ transplantation. *Public Health Rep.* 2013;128:247-343.

Suryaprasad A, Basavaraju SV, Hocevar SN, et al. Transmission of Hepatitis C virus from organ donors despite nucleic acid test screening. *Am J Transplant.* 2015;15:1827-1835.

Full bibliography can be found on www.expertconsult.com.

HYPERTENSION

64

Pathogenesis of Hypertension

Christopher S. Wilcox

Hypertension implies an increase in either cardiac output or total peripheral resistance (TPR). Essential hypertension developing in young adults may be initiated by an increase in cardiac output, associated with signs of overactivity of the sympathetic nervous system; the blood pressure (BP) is labile, and the heart rate is increased. Later, the BP increases further because of a rise in TPR, with return to a normal cardiac output. Most patients in clinical practice with sustained hypertension have an elevated TPR accompanied by constriction of resistance vessels. Over time, vascular remodeling contributes a structural component to vasoconstriction.

The abrupt left ventricular systole creates a shock wave that is reflected back from the peripheral resistance vessels and reaches the ascending aorta during early diastole. It is often visible in tracings of aortic pressure in younger subjects as the dicrotic notch. With aging, there is loss of elasticity, an increase in the tone of the resistance vessels, and often a reduced aortic diameter. Thus the pressure wave is transmitted more rapidly within the arterial tree. Eventually, this shock wave in the aorta coincides with the upstroke of the aortic systolic pressure wave, leading to an abrupt increase in the height of the systolic BP. This largely accounts for the frequent finding of isolated, or predominant, systolic hypertension in the elderly. In contrast, systolic hypertension in the young usually reflects an enhanced cardiac contractility and output.

PATHOPHYSIOLOGY OF HYPERTENSION

INTEGRATION OF CARDIORENAL FUNCTION

The integration of cardiorenal function is illustrated by the response of a normal person to standing. Upon standing, there is an abrupt fall in venous return and hence in cardiac output; this elicits a baroreflex response, as resistance vessels contract to buffer the immediate fall in BP, and capacitance vessels contract to restore venous return. The end result is only a small drop in the systolic BP, with a modest rise in diastolic BP and heart rate. During prolonged standing, increased renal sympathetic nerve activity enhances the reabsorption of sodium chloride (NaCl) by the renal tubules, as well as the release of renin from the juxtaglomerular apparatus. Renin release results in the subsequent generation of angiotensin II and aldosterone, which maintain systemic BP and circulating volume. In contrast, the BP of patients with autonomic insufficiency declines progressively upon standing, sometimes to the point of syncope. Patients with autonomic failure vividly

illustrate the crucial importance of a stable BP for efficient function of the brain, heart, and kidneys. Therefore it is no surprise that evolution has provided multiple, coordinated BP-regulatory processes. The understanding of the cause of a sustained change in BP, such as hypertension, requires knowledge of a number of interrelated pathophysiologic processes. The most important and best understood of these are discussed in this chapter.

KIDNEY MECHANISMS AND SALT BALANCE

The kidney has a unique role in BP regulation. Renal salt and water retention sufficient to increase the extracellular fluid (ECF) volume, blood volume, and mean circulatory filling pressure enhances venous return, cardiac output, and BP. The kidney is so effective in excreting excess fluid during periods of surfeit, or retaining fluid and electrolytes during periods of deficit, that the ECF volume and, specifically, the blood volume normally vary less than 10% with changes in salt intake. Consequently, the role of body fluids in hypertension is subtle. For example, a 10-fold increase in daily NaCl intake in normal subjects increases ECF volume by only about 1 L (about 6%) and normally produces no change, or only a small increase, in BP. Conversely, a diet with no salt content leads to the loss of approximately 1 L of body fluid over 3 to 5 days and only a trivial fall in BP. Different effects can be seen in patients with chronic kidney disease (CKD), whose BP often increases with the level of salt intake. This "salt-sensitive" component to BP increases progressively with loss of kidney function. Among normotensive subjects, a salt-sensitive component to BP is apparent in about 30% and appears to have a genetic component. Salt sensitivity is almost twice as frequent in patients with hypertension and is particularly common among blacks, the elderly, and those with CKD. It is generally associated with a lower level of plasma renin activity (PRA).

What underlies salt sensitivity? Normal kidneys are exquisitely sensitive to BP. A rise in mean arterial pressure (MAP) of as little as 1 to 3 mm Hg elicits a subtle increase in renal NaCl and fluid elimination. This "pressure natriuresis" also works in reverse and conserves NaCl and fluid during decreases in BP. It is rapid, quantitative, and fundamental for normal homeostasis. It is primarily a result of changes in tubular NaCl reabsorption rather than total renal blood flow (RBF) or glomerular filtration rate (GFR). Indeed, renal autoregulation maintains RBF and GFR remarkably constant during modest changes in BP. The pressure natriuresis mechanism accurately adjusts salt excretion and body fluids in persons with healthy kidneys across a range of BPs.

Two primary mechanisms of pressure natriuresis have been identified.

First, a rise in kidney perfusion pressure increases blood flow selectively through the medulla, based on data in salt-loaded rats. Medullary blood flow is not as tightly autoregulated as cortical blood flow. These increases in pressure and flow enhance renal interstitial hydrostatic pressure throughout the kidney, which is an encapsulated organ. This rise in interstitial pressure reduces proximal tubule reabsorption and impairs fluid return to the bloodstream. Therefore net NaCl and fluid reabsorption is diminished. Second, the degree of stretch of the afferent arteriole regulates the secretion of renin into the bloodstream and hence the generation of angiotensin II. Thus an increase in BP that is transmitted to this site reduces renin secretion. Angiotensin II coordinates the body's salt and fluid retention mechanisms by stimulating thirst and enhancing NaCl and fluid reabsorption in the proximal and distal nephron segments. By stimulating secretion of aldosterone and arginine vasopressin, and inhibiting atrial natriuretic peptide (ANP), angiotensin II further enhances reabsorption in the distal tubules and collecting ducts. Thus, during normal homeostasis, an increase in BP is matched by a decrease in PRA. It follows that a normal or elevated value for PRA in hypertension is effectively "inappropriate" for the level of BP, and is thereby contributing to the maintenance of hypertension.

The relationships among long-term changes in salt intake, the renin-angiotensin-aldosterone system (RAAS), and BP are shown in Fig. 64.1. Healthy people regulate the RAAS closely with changes in salt intake. An increase in salt intake brings about only a modest and transient rise in MAP, because the RAAS is suppressed and the highly effective pressure natriuresis mechanism rapidly increases renal NaCl and fluid elimination sufficiently to restore a near-normal blood volume and BP. Expressed quantitatively in Fig. 64.1, the slope of

the long-term increase in NaCl excretion with BP is normally almost vertical. One factor contributing to the steepness of this slope, or the gain of the pressure natriuresis relationship, is the reciprocal changes in the RAAS with BP that dictate appropriate alterations in salt handling by the kidney. Therefore, when the RAAS is artificially fixed, the slope of the pressure natriuresis relationship flattens, resulting in salt sensitivity, displacement of the set point, and a change in ambient BP. For example, an infusion of angiotensin II into a normal subject raises the BP. Because angiotensin II is being infused, the kidney cannot suppress angiotensin II levels appropriately by reducing renin secretion. Therefore the pressure natriuresis mechanism is prevented, and the BP elevation is sustained without an effective and complete kidney compensation. In contrast, normal individuals treated with an angiotensin-converting enzyme (ACE) inhibitor to block angiotensin II generation or an angiotensin receptor blocker (ARB) to block AT_1 receptors have a fall in BP. Again, the kidney cannot stimulate an appropriate effect of angiotensin II and aldosterone that would be required to retain sufficient NaCl and fluid to buffer the fall in BP. Therefore when the RAAS is fixed, the BP changes as a function of salt intake and becomes highly "salt sensitive" (see Fig. 64.1). These studies demonstrate the unique role of the RAAS in long-term BP regulation and its importance in isolating BP from NaCl intake.

Some recent findings add complexity to these simple relationships. Renin is also generated within the connecting tubule and collecting ducts. This renal renin may contribute to the very high level of angiotensin within the kidney that does not share the same relationship with dietary salt. Animal models of diabetes mellitus demonstrate an increase in local angiotensin generation and action in the kidneys that may contribute to the beneficial effects of ACE inhibitor and ARB therapy, despite low circulating renin levels. Other studies

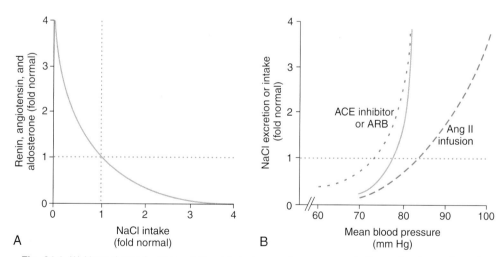

Fig. 64.1 (A) Normal steady-state relationship between plasma concentrations of renin, angiotensin II (Ang II), and aldosterone and dietary salt intake. (B) Relationships between sodium excretion relative to intake and mean arterial blood pressure in normal subjects (*solid line*), in subjects given an angiotensin-converting enzyme (ACE) inhibitor or angiotensin receptor blocker (ARB; *short dashes*), and in subjects given an infusion of Ang II (*long dashes*) to prevent adaptive changes in Ang II levels. *NaCl*, Sodium chloride. (Modified from Guyton AC, Hall JE, Coleman TG, et al. The dominant role of the kidneys in the long-term regulation of arterial pressure in normal and hypertensive states. In: Laragh JH, Brenner BM, eds. *Hypertension, Pathophysiology, Diagnosis and Management.* New York: Raven; 1995:1311–1326, with permission.)

have shown that prorenin, although not itself active, becomes activated after binding to a renin receptor in the tissues, notably the kidneys, where novel signaling adds another component to the effects of the RAAS. This is important because conventional RAAS antagonists may not block these actions, nor do the novel renin inhibitors block this renin receptor.

Four compelling lines of evidence implicate the kidney and RAAS in long-term BP regulation. First, kidney transplant studies in rats showed that a normotensive animal that received a kidney from a hypertensive animal becomes hypertensive, and vice versa. Similarly, human kidney transplant recipients frequently become hypertensive if they receive a kidney from a hypertensive donor. Apparently, the kidney in hypertension is programmed to retain salt and water inappropriately for a normal level of BP, thereby resetting the pressure natriuresis to a higher level of BP and dictating the appearance of hypertension in the recipient, even if the neurohumoral environment is that of normotension. Nevertheless, recent studies in gene-deleted or transgenic mice subjected to kidney transplantation concluded that the increase in BP during prolonged infusion of angiotensin II was mediated by the combined effects within the kidney and the systemic circulation, most likely involving the renal afferent arterioles and the brain. A second observation was that the BP was normally reduced 5% to 20% by an ACE inhibitor, an ARB, an aldosterone receptor antagonist, or a renin inhibitor. The fall in BP was greatest in those with elevated PRA values, and it was enhanced by dietary salt restriction or concurrent use of diuretic drugs (see Fig. 64.1). Third, almost 90% of patients approaching end-stage renal disease (ESRD) have hypertension. Fourth, the major monogenetic causes of human hypertension involve genes that activate RAAS signaling (such as glucocorticoid-remediable hypertension) or renal sodium transport (such as Liddle syndrome).

TOTAL-BODY AUTOREGULATION

An increase in cardiac output necessarily increases peripheral blood flow. However, each organ has intrinsic mechanisms that adapt its blood flow to its metabolic needs. Therefore, over time, an increase in cardiac output is translated into an increase in TPR. The outcome is that organ blood flow is maintained, but hypertension becomes sustained. This total-body autoregulation is demonstrated in human subjects who are given salt-retaining mineralocorticosteroid hormones. An initial rise in cardiac output is translated in most individuals into sustained hypertension and an elevated TPR over 5 to 15 days.

STRUCTURAL COMPONENTS TO HYPERTENSION

Hypertension causes not only hypertrophic or eutrophic remodeling in the distributing and resistance vessels and the heart, but also fibrotic and sclerotic changes in the glomeruli and interstitium of the kidney. Hypertrophy of resistance vessels limits the ratio of lumen to wall and dictates a fixed component to TPR. This is evidenced by a higher TPR in hypertensive versus normotensive individuals during maximal vasodilatation. Moreover, thickened and hypertrophied resistance vessels have greater reductions in vessel diameter during vasoconstrictor stimulation. This is apparent as an increase in

vascular reactivity to pressor agents. Remodeling of resistance arterioles diminishes their response to changes in perfusion pressure. This manifests as a blunted myogenic response contributing to incomplete autoregulation of RBF, thereby adding a component of barotrauma to hypertensive kidney damage. Sclerotic and fibrotic changes in the glomeruli and kidney interstitium, combined with hypertrophy of the afferent arterioles, limit the sensing of BP in the juxtaglomerular apparatus and kidney parenchyma. This blunts renin release and pressure natriuresis, thereby contributing to salt sensitivity and sustained hypertension. Rats receiving intermittent weak electrical stimulation of the hypothalamus initially had an abrupt increase in BP followed by a sudden fall after the cessation of the stimulus. However, eventually the baseline BP increased in parallel with the appearance of hypertrophy of the resistance vessels. These structural components may explain why it often takes weeks or months to achieve maximal antihypertensive action from a drug, a reduction in salt intake, or correction of a renal artery stenosis or hyperaldosteronism. Vascular and left ventricular hypertrophy is largely, but usually not completely, reversible during treatment of hypertension, whereas fibrotic and sclerotic changes are not.

SYMPATHETIC NERVOUS SYSTEM, BRAIN, AND BAROREFLEXES

A rise in BP diminishes the baroreflex, thereby reducing the tone of the sympathetic nervous system and increasing the tone of the parasympathetic nervous system. Paradoxically, human hypertension is often associated with an increase in heart rate, maintained or increased plasma catecholamine levels, and an increase in directly measured sympathetic nerve discharge despite the stimulus to the baroreceptors. What is the cause of this inappropriate activation of the sympathetic nervous system in hypertension? Studies in animals show that the baroreflex "resets" to the ambient level of BP after 2 to 5 days. Thereafter, the baroreflex no longer continues to "fight" the elevated BP but defends it at the new higher level. Much of this adaptation occurs within the baroreceptors themselves. With aging and atherosclerosis, the walls of the carotid sinus and other baroreflex sensing sites become less distensible. Therefore the BP is less effective in stretching the afferent nerve endings, and the sensitivity of the baroreflex is diminished. This may contribute to the enhanced sympathetic nerve activity and increased plasma catecholamines that are characteristic of elderly hypertensive subjects. Additionally, animal models have identified central mechanisms that alter the gain of the baroreflex process, and therefore the sympathetic tone, in hypertension. The importance of central mechanisms in human hypertension is apparent from the effectiveness of drugs, such as clonidine, that act within the brain to decrease the sympathetic tone. The kidneys themselves contain barosensitive and chemosensitive nerves that can regulate the sympathetic nervous system. In one study, hemodialysis patients experienced an increased sympathetic nervous system discharge and increased BP that were not apparent after bilateral nephrectomy. This suggests that the renal nerves were maintaining enhanced sympathetic tone. Based on this pathophysiology, radiofrequency ablation of the renal nerves has successfully improved BP control in some, but not all, studies of patients with drug-resistant hypertension, further illustrating the importance of the renal nerves in setting the long-term level of BP in human subjects.

ENDOTHELIUM AND OXIDATIVE STRESS

Calcium-mobilizing agonists, such as bradykinin or acetylcholine, as well as shear forces produced by the flow of blood result in the release of endothelium-dependent relaxing factors, predominantly nitric oxide (NO). NO has a half-life of only a few seconds because of inactivation by oxyhemoglobin or reactive oxygen species (ROS), such as superoxide anion (O_2^-). People with essential hypertension have defects in endothelium-dependent relaxation of peripheral vessels and also diminished NO generation. One underlying mechanism is oxidative stress, with excessive O_2^- formation inactivating NO and leading to functional NO deficiency. Another mechanism is the appearance of inhibitors of nitric oxide synthase (NOS), including asymmetric dimethyl arginine (ADMA). Finally, atherosclerosis, prolonged hypertension, or the development of malignant hypertension causes structural changes in the endothelium that limit endothelial function further. NO inhibits renal NaCl reabsorption in the loop of Henle and collecting ducts of the kidney. Therefore NO deficiency not only induces endothelial dysfunction and vasoconstriction but also reduces renal pressure natriuresis. Functional NO deficiency in large blood vessels contributes to vascular inflammation and atherosclerosis.

GENETIC CONTRIBUTIONS

The heritability of human hypertension can be assessed from differences in the concordance of hypertension between identical twins (who share all genes and a similar environment) versus nonidentical twins (who share only a similar environment). These studies suggest that genetic factors contribute less than half of the risk for developing hypertension in modern humans. Studies in mice with targeted disruption of individual genes or insertions of extra copies of genes provided direct evidence of the critical regulatory roles for certain gene products in hypertension. Deletions of the gene in mice for endothelial NOS lead to salt-dependent hypertension, and the BP of mice decreases with the number of copies of the gene encoding ACE. While these are compelling examples of circumstances in which a single gene can sustain hypertension, there is increasing recognition of the complexity and importance of gene–gene interactions and the crucial effects of the genetic background on the changes in BP that accompany insertion or deletion of a gene.

Currently there is evidence that certain individual gene defects can contribute to human essential hypertension. However, the net effect on BP is small. Certain rare forms of hereditary hypertension are caused by single-gene defects. For example, dexamethasone-suppressible hyperaldosteronism is caused by a chimeric rearrangement of the gene encoding aldosterone synthase that renders the enzyme responsive to adrenocorticotropic hormone. Liddle syndrome is caused by a mutation in the gene encoding one component of the endothelial sodium channel that is expressed in the distal convoluted tubule. The mutated form has lost its normal regulation, leading to a permanent "open state" of the sodium channel that dictates inappropriate renal NaCl retention and salt-sensitive, low-renin hypertension (see Chapters 9, 38, and 66).

IMPLICATED MEDIATORS OF HYPERTENSION

Alterations in the synthesis, secretion, degradation, or action of numerous substances are implicated in hypertension. Some of the most important mediators are described in the following paragraphs.

RENIN, ANGIOTENSIN II, AND ALDOSTERONE

The PRA is not appropriately suppressed in most patients with essential hypertension and is above normal values in approximately 15%. Individuals with normal or high PRA have a greater antihypertensive response to single-agent therapy with an ACE inhibitor, an ARB, or a beta-blocker than patients with low-renin hypertension, who respond notably to salt restriction and diuretic therapy. The RAAS is particularly important in the maintenance of BP in patients with renovascular hypertension, although its importance wanes during the chronic phase when structural alterations in blood vessels or damage in the kidney dictate an RAAS-independent component to the hypertension.

SYMPATHETIC NERVOUS SYSTEM AND CATECHOLAMINES

Pheochromocytoma is a catecholamine-secreting tumor, often occurring in the adrenal medulla, that increases plasma catecholamines 10- to 1000-fold. However, even such extraordinary increases in pressor amines are rarely fatal, because there is downregulation of the catecholamine receptors. Moreover, an intact renal pressure natriuresis mechanism reduces the blood volume, thereby limiting the rise in BP. Indeed, such patients can have orthostatic hypotension between episodes of catecholamine secretion (see Chapter 66).

Increased sympathetic nerve tone of resistance vessels in human essential hypertension causes α_1-receptor-mediated vasoconstriction of the blood vessels and β_1-receptor-mediated increases in contractility and cardiac output; these are incompletely offset by β_2-receptor–mediated vasorelaxation of peripheral blood vessels. Increased sympathetic nerve discharge to the kidney leads to α_1-mediated enhancement of NaCl reabsorption and β_1-mediated renin release.

DOPAMINE

Dopamine is synthesized in the brain and renal tubular epithelial cells independent of sympathetic nerves. Dopamine synthesis in the kidney is enhanced during volume expansion and contributes to decreased reabsorption of NaCl in the proximal tubule. Defects in tubular dopamine responsiveness are apparent in genetic models of hypertension. Recent evidence relates single-nucleotide polymorphisms of genes that regulate dopamine receptors to human salt-sensitive hypertension.

ARACHIDONATE METABOLITES

Arachidonate is esterified as a phospholipid in cell membranes. It is released by phospholipases that are activated by agents such as angiotensin II. Three enzymes principally metabolize arachidonate. Cyclooxygenase (COX) generates unstable intermediates whose subsequent metabolism by specific enzymes yields prostaglandins that are either generally vasodilative (e.g., prostaglandin I_2 [PGI_2]), vasoconstrictive (e.g., thromboxane), or of mixed effect (e.g., PGE_2). COX-1 is expressed in many tissues, including platelets, resistance vessels, glomeruli, and cortical collecting ducts. Inflammatory mediators induce COX-2. However, the normal kidney is unusual in expressing substantial COX-2, which is located in macula densa cells, tubules, renal medullary interstitial cells, and arterioles. The net effect of blocking COX-1 generally is to retain NaCl and fluid while raising BP and dropping PRA. Blockade of COX-2 has little effect on normal BP, but it can increase BP in those with essential hypertension. Nonsteroidal antiinflammatory agents exacerbate essential hypertension, blunt the antihypertensive actions of most commonly used agents, predispose to acute kidney injury during periods of volume depletion or hypotension, and blunt the natriuretic action of loop diuretics. In contrast, aspirin reduces BP in patients with renovascular hypertension, testifying to the prohypertensive actions of thromboxane and other prostanoids that activate the thromboxane-prostanoid receptor in this condition. Metabolism of arachidonate by cytochrome P-450 monooxygenase yields 19,20-hydroxyeicosatetraenoic acid (HETE), which is a vasoconstrictor of blood vessels but inhibits tubular NaCl reabsorption. Metabolism by epoxygenase leads to epoxy-eicosatrienoic acids (EETs), which are powerful vasodilators and natriuretic agents. Arachidonate metabolites act primarily as modulating agents in normal physiology. Their role in human essential hypertension remains elusive.

L-ARGININE–NITRIC OXIDE PATHWAY

NO is generated by three isoforms of NOS that are widely expressed in the body. NO interacts with many heme-centered enzymes. Activation of guanylyl cyclase generates cyclic guanosine monophosphate, which is a powerful vasorelaxant and inhibits NaCl reabsorption in the kidney. Defects in NO generation in the endothelium of blood vessels in human essential hypertension may contribute to increased peripheral resistance, vascular remodeling, and atherosclerosis, whereas defects in renal NO generation may contribute to inappropriate renal NaCl retention and salt sensitivity. NOS activity is reduced in hypertensive human subjects and in those with CKD.

REACTIVE OXYGEN SPECIES

The incomplete reduction of molecular oxygen, either by the respiratory chain during cellular respiration or by oxidases such as nicotinamide adenine dinucleotide phosphate (NADPH) oxidase, yields ROS like O_2^- and generates peroxynitrite ($ONOO^-$). $ONOO^-$ has long-lasting effects through oxidizing and nitrosylating reactions. Reaction of ROS with lipids yields oxidized low-density lipoprotein (LDL) that promotes atherosclerosis and isoprostanes that cause

vasoconstriction, salt retention, and platelet aggregation. O_2^- can be quantitated by eight-isoprostane $F_{2\alpha}$. Hypertension, especially in the setting of CKD, is a state of oxidative stress. Drugs that effectively reduce O_2^- lower BP in animal models of hypertension, but they are largely unexamined in human hypertension.

ENDOTHELINS

Endothelins are produced primarily by cells of the vascular endothelium and collecting tubules. Discrete receptors mediate either increased vascular resistance (type A) or the release of NO and inhibition of NaCl reabsorption in the collecting ducts (type B). Endothelin type A receptors potentiate the vasoconstriction accompanying angiotensin II infusion or blockade of NOS. Endothelin is released by hypoxia, specific agonists such as angiotensin II, salt loading, and cytokines. Nonspecific blockade of endothelin receptors lowers BP in models of volume-expanded hypertension, whereas collecting duct specific deletion of endothelin B (ETB) receptors increases BP. The role of endothelin in human essential hypertension is unclear.

ATRIAL NATRIURETIC PEPTIDE

ANP is released from the heart during atrial stretch. It acts on receptors that increase GFR, decrease NaCl reabsorption in the distal nephron, and inhibit renin secretion. ANP is released during volume expansion and contributes to the natriuretic response. Its role in essential hypertension is unclear. Endopeptidase inhibitors that block ANP degradation are natriuretic and antihypertensive but also inhibit the metabolism of kinins. Although an increase in kinins may contribute to the fall in BP with endopeptidase or ACE inhibitors, kinins can cause an irritant cough or a more serious anaphylactoid reaction.

PATHOGENESIS OF HYPERTENSION IN CHRONIC KIDNEY DISEASE

With progression of CKD, the prevalence of salt-sensitive hypertension increases in proportion to the fall in GFR. Hypertension is almost universal in patients with CKD caused by primary glomerular or vascular disease, whereas those with primary tubulointerstitial disease may be normotensive or, occasionally, salt losing.

With declining nephron number, CKD limits the ability to adjust NaCl excretion rapidly and quantitatively during changes in intake. The role of ECF volume expansion is apparent from the ability of hemodialysis to lower BP in patients with ESRD.

Additional mechanisms besides primary renal fluid retention contribute to the increased TPR and hypertension in patients with CKD. The ESRD kidney generates abnormal renal afferent nerve impulses, which entrain an increased sympathetic nerve discharge that is reversed by bilateral nephrectomy. Plasma levels of endothelin increase with kidney failure. CKD induces oxidative stress, which contributes to vascular disease and impaired endothelium-dependent relaxation. A decreased generation of NO from L-arginine follows the accumulation of ADMA, which inhibits NOS. The thromboxane-prostanoid receptor is activated and contributes to vasoconstriction and structural damage.

Clearly, hypertension in CKD is multifactorial, but volume expansion and salt sensitivity are predominant. Pressor mechanisms mediated by angiotensin II, catecholamines, endothelin, or thromboxane-prostanoid receptors become more potent during volume expansion. This fact may underlie the importance of these systems in the ESRD patients. Finally, many of the pathways that contribute to hypertension in ESRD (such as impaired NO generation and excessive production of endothelin, ROS, and ADMA) also contribute to atherosclerosis, cardiac hypertrophy, and progressive kidney fibrosis and sclerosis. Indeed, kidney damage in poorly treated hypertension further enhances hypertension, which itself engenders further kidney damage, generating a vicious spiral culminating in accelerated hypertension, progressively diminishing kidney function, and the requirement for kidney replacement therapy. Therefore rational management of hypertension in CKD first entails salt-depleting therapy with a salt-restricted diet

and diuretic therapy. Patients frequently require additional therapy to combat the enhanced vasoconstriction and to attempt to slow the rate of CKD progression.

BIBLIOGRAPHY

Carlestrom M, Wilcox CS, Arendshorst W. Renal autoregulation in health and disease. *Physiol Rev.* 2015;95:405-511.

DiBona GF. Sympathetic nervous system and the kidney in hypertension. *Curr Opin Nephrol Hypertens.* 2002;11:197-200.

Guyton AC, Hall JE, Coleman TG, et al. The dominant role of the kidneys in the long-term regulation of arterial pressure in normal and hypertensive states. In: Laragh JH, Brenner BM, eds. *Hypertension: Pathophysiology, Diagnosis and Management.* New York: Raven; 1989: 1029-1052.

Navar LG. The role of the kidneys in hypertension. *J Clin Hypertens.* 2005;7:542-549.

Wilcox CS. Oxidative stress and nitric oxide deficiency in the kidney: a critical link to hypertension? *Am J Physiol Regul Integr Comp Physiol.* 2005;289:R913-R935.

Wilcox CS. *Therapy in Nephrology and Hypertension.* 3rd ed. Philadelphia: WB Saunders; 2008.

65

Evaluation and Management of Hypertension

Raven Voora; Debbie L. Cohen; Raymond R. Townsend

Hypertension remains the leading cause of cardiovascular (CV) morbidity and mortality including stroke, heart disease, kidney disease, and other vascular disease. The relationship between blood pressure (BP) and CV risk is linear, continuous, and additive to other well-known risk factors including diabetes, dyslipidemia, obesity, and cigarette smoking. For individuals aged 40 to 69 years, each increment of either 20 mm Hg in systolic BP or 10 mm Hg in diastolic BP doubles the mortality risk related to stroke, ischemic heart disease, and other vascular causes across the entire BP range from 115/75 to 185/115 mm Hg.

Hypertension affects nearly a third of the US adult population, and the prevalence continues to increase steadily because of aging and increasing obesity in the US population. The lifetime risk of developing hypertension is about 90%. In 2003, the Joint National Committee (JNC 7) on Prevention, Detection, Evaluation, and Treatment of High Blood Pressure classified BP into four categories as listed in Table 65.1; this classification system remained unchanged in JNC 8, published in 2014. In JNC 7, a "prehypertension" category was created to reflect its association with higher CV risk compared with normal BP; prehypertension affects, on average, about a quarter of the US adult population.

Correctly assessing BP status and overall CV risk is key to optimizing therapy to reduce CV morbidity and mortality. At first diagnosis, a comprehensive evaluation is usually undertaken in those with a consistent systolic BP greater than 140 mm Hg and/or diastolic BP greater than 90 mm Hg.

EVALUATION OF HYPERTENSION

Three key questions are addressed when assessing each hypertensive patient. The first question is whether the BP increase is essential (primary) or represents a secondary form of hypertension. Most hypertensive patients have primary or essential hypertension and are likely to remain hypertensive for life. However, some patients have identifiable, or secondary, causes, for their elevated BP that may warrant specific therapy in addition to antihypertensive medications to address the underlying specific or dominant pathology and offer possible cure. The clinical clues suggesting the possible presence and cause of secondary hypertension are discussed later in this chapter.

The second question assesses the presence of other CV risk factors as summarized in Table 65.2. Defining overall CV risk is important in the choice of antihypertensive medications, BP target, and management of other treatable factors such as dyslipidemia.

The third question evaluates the presence of end-organ damage, defined as clinically evident cardiovascular diseases (CVDs) related to hypertension as summarized in Table 65.3. The presence of end-organ damage redirects the goal of treating BP from primary prevention of target-organ integrity to the more challenging realm of secondary prevention.

MEASURING BLOOD PRESSURE

Measuring BP correctly is the key to proper BP classification. Fig. 65.1 lists steps recommended to obtain reliable BP readings, and Table 65.4 lists common mistakes leading to inaccurate BP measurements. During the initial visit, BP should be measured in both arms (and in the leg if aortic coarctation is suspected). For proper BP assessment, it is important to take the BP in the correct way at least twice on any occasion and on at least two, and preferably three, separate days for the initial diagnosis of hypertension. The 2015 US Preventive Services Task Force (USPSTF) guidelines on hypertension recommend that all individuals 18 years or older be screened for elevated BP.

Pseudohypertension is a problem occasionally encountered in examining patients with very stiff and difficult to compress blood vessels due to arterial wall calcification. The pressure required to compress the stiff brachial artery and to stop the audible blood flow with a standard BP cuff can be much greater than the actual intraluminal BP obtained invasively. Osler's maneuver can be used to identify this condition by inflating the BP cuff at least 30 mm Hg above the palpable systolic pressure and then trying to "roll" the brachial or radial artery underneath the fingertips. Pseudohypertension may be present when something resembling a stiff tube is felt underneath the skin because a normal artery should not be palpable when empty. It is important to identify pseudohypertension as it tends to occur in the elderly and chronically ill who are also more prone to orthostatic and postprandial hypotension, which can be aggravated by the unwarranted intensification of BP treatment.

Electronic devices are increasingly used to measure BP at home and in the office setting. Most of these devices work on oscillometric principles. The cuff is inflated until the disappearance of the brachial pulses is detected. Upon deflation, sensors detect the increasing amplitude in the brachial pulsation and measure the mean arterial pressure. The systolic and diastolic BP readings are then derived from the mean arterial BP. Typically, systolic BP is slightly lower and diastolic BP is slightly higher when measured with electronic devices when compared to invasively measured arterial pressure.

Also available are specialized electronic devices to perform automated office blood pressure monitoring (AOBP) in the office setting. With AOBP, multiple BP readings are recorded using a fully automated sphygmomanometer with the patient resting quietly and sitting alone. Proper timing, patient positioning, cuff size, and placement are still necessary to be certain that the readings are accurate. There are currently three validated devices available for performing AOBP, and each can be programmed to take multiple consecutive BP measurements in intervals of typically 1 to 2 minutes. The devices differ in the number of readings taken and the number of minutes before the first BP measurement is recorded. AOBP has the same cut-point as home BP and awake ambulatory BP (135/85 mm Hg) for defining hypertension, because systolic pressure readings are 5 to 10 mm Hg lower with AOBP than with auscultatory measurement. In 2011, the Canadian Hypertension Education Program recommended AOBP for the diagnosis of hypertension, and, in 2013, the European Society of Hypertension recommended using AOBP if feasible.

AOBP has some specific advantages, including that AOBP is not associated with the white-coat effect (the response in some patients in which BP readings taken by doctors and nurses tend to be higher because of increased patient anxiety), multiple readings are obtained, and readings more significantly correlate with awake ambulatory BP readings when compared with manual office readings as demonstrated in the Conventional Versus Automated Measurement of BP in the Office (CAMBO) study.

ASSESSING CARDIOVASCULAR RISK AND END-ORGAN DAMAGE

The evaluation of each hypertensive patient should include a detailed personal and family history, thorough physical examination, and selected tests focused on addressing the above three key questions. Key components of the history and physical examination are listed in Table 65.5.

A detailed personal history of hypertension includes its onset, duration, severity and related symptoms, presence of other CV risk factors, and target-organ complications. The medication history should include the prior and current use of any prescription and over-the-counter agents. Special attention should be paid to antihypertensive medications with their related clinical responses and adverse effects, as well as common offending agents, such as nonsteroidal antiinflammatory drugs (NSAIDs), oral contraceptives, and cold/cough remedies. NSAIDs can increase BP directly and can decrease the efficacy of antihypertensive medications by inhibiting the vasodilatory and natriuretic effects of

Table 65.1 Classification of Blood Pressure Status

BP Classification	Systolic BP (mm Hg)		Diastolic BP (mm Hg)
Normal	<120	and	<80
Prehypertension	120–139	or	80–89
Stage 1 hypertension	140–159	or	90–99
Stage 2 hypertension	≥160	or	≥100

BP, Blood pressure.

Table 65.2 Other Cardiovascular Risk Factors in Individuals with Hypertension

Risk Factors	Level Considered Abnormal	Approximate Frequency (%)
Obesity	BMI >30 kg/m²	40
Increased total cholesterol	Total cholesterol >240 mg/dL	40
Reduced HDL	HDL cholesterol <35 mg/dL	25
Albuminuria[a]	≥30 mg/g	16
Diabetes	Type 1 and type 2 diabetes mellitus; fasting glucose >126 mg/dL	15
Insulin resistance	Elevated fasting insulin and/or impaired glucose tolerance	50
LVH[a]	Defined by various ECG or echocardiogram criteria	~30[b]
Sedentary	Arbitrary	~30

[a]Albuminuria and left ventricular hypertrophy are both risk factors and markers of target-organ damage.
[b]Based on echocardiogram definition.
BMI, Body mass index; *HDL,* high-density lipoprotein; *LVH,* left ventricular hypertrophy.

Table 65.3 Target-Organ Effect of Hypertension

Organ	History/Symptom(s)	Physical Examination	Laboratory
Retina	Blurry vision, headache, disorientation	Retinopathy	—
Brain	Stroke, TIA, confusion/disorientation	Signs of stroke, carotid bruits	MRI, CT, or ultrasound
Heart	Angina, MI, heart failure, cardiac arrest, atrial fibrillation	Cardiomegaly, S4, rales, irregular heartbeats	ECG may show LVH and/or prior MI
Kidney	Chronic kidney disease, polyuria, nocturia, anorexia, nausea, weight loss, peripheral edema	Palpable kidneys, epigastric bruits	Elevated creatinine, proteinuria, hematuria; ultrasound may show small kidneys with increased echogenicity
Circulation	Peripheral arterial disease, claudication, ischemic digits	Femoral bruits, diminished or absent pedal pulses	Ankle-brachial index <0.9

CT, Computed tomography; *ECG,* electrocardiogram; *LVH,* left ventricular hypertrophy; *MI,* myocardial infarction; *MRI,* magnetic resonance image; *TIA,* transient ischemic attack.

1. Have patient relax for at least 5 minutes before taking blood pressure. Feet should be on the floor, with the back supported.

2. The patient's arm should be supported (i.e., resting on a desk) for the measurement.

3. The stethoscope bell, not the diaphragm, should be used for auscultation.

4. Blood pressure should first be checked in both arms with the patient sitting.
   Note which arm gives the higher reading. This arm (with the higher reading) should then be used for all other (standing, lying down) and future readings.

5. All measurements should be separated by 2 minutes.

6. Measure the blood pressure in the sitting, standing, and lying positions.

7. Use the correct cuff size, and note if a larger or smaller than normal cuff size is used.

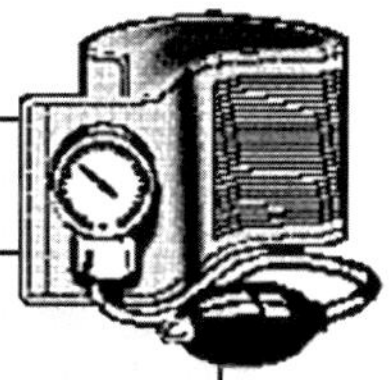

Blood Pressure Cuff Size Criteria			
	Weight		
Arm Circumference	Female	Male	Cuff Size to Use
24–32 cm	<150	<200	REGULAR
33–42 cm*	>150	>200	LARGE
38–50 cm*	–	–	THIGH
Either cuff is acceptable in the overlap diameter zone			

8. Record systolic (onset of first sound) and diastolic (disappearance of sound) pressures.

9. Do not round off results to zeros or fives. Record exact results to nearest even number.

Fig. 65.1 Instructions for taking blood pressure. Steps in obtaining accurate blood pressure measurements by aneroid sphygmomanometry.

Table 65.4 Common Causes Contributing to Inaccurate Blood Pressure Readings

Failure to sit quietly for 5 min before a reading is taken
Lack of arm and foot support
Too small a cuff size relative to the arm (cuff bladder should encircle ≥80% of upper arm circumference)
Too rapid cuff deflation (i.e., more than 2 mm Hg per second)
On-going conversation
Recent caffeine intake or cigarette smoking

---

prostaglandins and potentiating vasoconstrictive effects of angiotensin-II. Dietary salt intake, alcohol consumption, tobacco use, physical activity, and weight changes should be recorded. With the increasing prevalence of obesity, essential hypertension manifests at a younger age, often in the 30s. In addition, more elderly patients are expected to develop essential hypertension as systolic BP increases throughout life. Family history of hypertension, diabetes, and related CV complications should also be noted, as a positive family history further increases the individual's CV risk. Excluding monogenic causes of hypertension, available data suggest that the heritability of essential hypertension ranges from 20% to 40%.

Physical examination should start with measurement of height, weight, and waist circumference. BP is usually measured in supine, sitting, and standing positions on the initial evaluation, and at least once in both arms (and at least one leg if aortic coarctation is suspected). Subsequent BP measurements are obtained in the seated position from the arm with the higher initial BP reading.

The optic fundi are the only place where blood vessels can be directly examined. The fundoscopic examination looks for arteriolar narrowing (grade 1), arteriovenous compression (grade 2), hemorrhages and/or exudates (grade 3), and papilledema (grade 4), which not only provide information on the degree of target-organ damage related to BP but also provide important prognostic information on overall CV outcomes.

Bruits in the neck, abdomen, and groin should be noted. Bruits may simply result from vascular tortuosity, particularly with high-flow vessels. However, they may be a sign of vascular

Table 65.5   Key Elements of History and Physical in Evaluating Hypertensive Patients

Key Elements	Evaluation
History	
Age of onset, duration, and severity	Onset at younger age (<30 years) or older age (>55 years) suggests secondary causes; new onset of severe hypertension also suggests a secondary cause
Contributing factors	Dietary salt intake, physical inactivity, psychosocial stress, symptoms of sleep apnea
Concomitant medications	Common offenders include NSAIDs, oral contraceptives, corticosteroids, licorice, cough/cold/weight-loss sympathomimetic agents (pseudoephedrine, ma huang, ephedrine)
Risk factors for cardiovascular disease	Diabetes, smoking, family history of premature cardiovascular disease particularly in a first-degree relative (parent or sibling)
Symptoms suggestive of secondary causes	Palpitations or tachycardia, spontaneous sweating, migraine-like headaches in paroxysms (catecholamine excess); muscle weakness, polyuria (decreased potassium from aldosterone excess); personal or family history of kidney disease or findings (proteinuria, hematuria), or symptoms like ankle swelling (edema); thinning of skin and stigmata of cortical excess; snoring and daytime somnolence (sleep apnea); heat intolerance and weight loss (hyperthyroidism)
Target-organ damage	Chest pain or chest discomfort (possible coronary artery disease); neurologic symptoms consistent with stroke or transient ischemic attack; dyspnea and easy fatigue (possible heart failure); claudication (peripheral arterial disease)
Physical Examination	
General appearance, skin lesions, distribution of body fat	Patient may fit criteria for metabolic syndrome (increased cardiovascular risk); evidence of prior stroke from gain/station; rarely secondary forms as striae (Cushing syndrome) or mucosal fibromas (MEN II)
Fundoscopy	See text for lesion grades; retinal changes reflect severity of hypertension (target-organ damage to the eyes) and future cardiovascular risk
Neck	Diffuse multinodular goiter indicating Graves' disease; presence of carotid bruits suggests potential stroke risk
Cardiopulmonary examination	Rales and cardiac gallops consistent with target-organ damage (heart enlargement or heart failure), interscapular murmur during auscultation of the back for aortic coarctation
Abdominal examination	Palpable kidneys suggest polycystic kidney disease; mid-epigastric bruits indicate renal artery disease
Neurologic examination	Signs of previous stroke (reduced grip, hyperreflexia, spasticity, Babinski sign, muscle atrophy, and gait disturbances) reflect target-organ damage
Pulse examination	Delayed or absent femoral pulses may reflect coarctation of the aorta or atherosclerosis

MEN, Multiple endocrine neoplasia; *NSAIDs,* nonsteroidal antiinflammatory drugs.

stenosis and irregularity and be a clue to vascular damage leading to future loss of target-organ function. The radial artery is similarly distant from the heart as the femoral artery, and the pulse should arrive at approximately the same moment when palpating both sites simultaneously. In aortic coarctation, a palpable delay in the arrival of the femoral pulse compared with the radial pulse supports this diagnosis, as does an interscapular murmur heard during auscultation over the back of the patient. A systolic BP in the leg behind the knee (popliteal) lower than the brachial value suggests the presence of aortic or iliac obstruction, but it may also reflect more peripheral arterial disease in certain patients such as smokers and those with target-organ damage. Patients should be advised that measuring leg BP may be uncomfortable given the large cuff and the amount of pressure required to occlude the femoral artery.

Cardiac examination by palpation may reveal a displaced apical impulse, indicative of left ventricular enlargement. A sustained apical impulse may suggest left ventricular hypertrophy (LVH). Auscultation should focus on listening for an S4 that is heard with left ventricular stiffness. An S3 indicates impairment in left ventricular function and usually underlying heart disease when rales are present on lung examination, although the presence of S3 and rales is uncommon on initial office evaluation of new hypertensive patients. The lower extremities should also be examined for peripheral arterial pulses and edema. The loss of pedal pulses is a sign of peripheral vascular disease (target-organ damage) and is associated with higher CV risk.

Finally, a brief neurologic examination for evidence of remote stroke should assess gait, bilateral grip strength, speech, memory, and mental acuity. Given the link between hypertension and future loss of cognitive function, it is useful to establish the cognitive function status before starting antihypertensive medications, as some patients may complain of memory loss after starting pharmacotherapy.

Several laboratory studies are recommended in the routine evaluation of the hypertensive patient. Testing should include hemoglobin or hematocrit, urinalysis with microscopic examination, serum potassium, bicarbonate, creatinine, fasting glucose, lipid profile, and 12-lead electrocardiogram (ECG). Assessing albuminuria is important as albuminuria has been associated with increased CV risk and may warrant more aggressive BP reduction. Assessing kidney function is also an important part of evaluation as chronic kidney disease (CDK) is not only a sign of target-organ damage but also a common cause of hypertension. Depending on the degree of glomerular filtration rate (GFR) loss, up to 90% of patients with advanced CKD or end-stage kidney disease have hypertension. Uric acid may be checked in those with a history of gout as diuretics can increase uric acid level and lead to gouty flares. In some cases, checking calcium, thyroid-stimulating hormone (TSH), or other thyroid studies may be reasonable when clinically indicated.

Plasma renin activity and serum aldosterone levels are useful in screening for aldosterone excess and salt sensitivity. However, these measurements are usually reserved for patients with hypokalemia, metabolic alkalosis, or those who fail to achieve BP control on a three-drug regimen (which includes a diuretic). A suppressed renin activity level with increased aldosterone-to-renin ratio supports a contribution of dietary sodium excess to hypertension; this scenario should respond well to dietary salt restriction and diuretics. It is worth noting that primary hyperaldosteronism is more common than previously thought. In patients referred to one hypertension center in Italy, 11% had primary hyperaldosteronism, with 5% having a potentially curable aldosterone-secreting adenoma and 6% having idiopathic hyperaldosteronism. In the same study, only 50% of patients with a confirmed aldosterone-producing adenoma had hypokalemia, underscoring the importance of considering this diagnosis in patients with normal levels of potassium.

Additional testing may be indicated in some patients depending on the clinical situation. Limited echocardiography is more sensitive than an ECG for detection of LVH. The presence of LVH, a sign of target-organ damage, can help establish or reinforce the need of antihypertensive therapy, especially in those who have borderline BP and/or are reluctant to start antihypertensive medications.

AMBULATORY AND HOME BP MONITORING

Since BP can be influenced by an environment such as an office or hospital, ambulatory BP monitoring (ABPM) or self-monitored BP (SMBP) in the home is useful in establishing or excluding the diagnosis of hypertension in those with white-coat hypertension or masked hypertension (Fig. 65.2). ABPM and SMBP are also useful in assessing the adequacy of BP control in outpatients and helping identify those with morning surges in BP (i.e., >55 mm Hg increase in systolic BP during the early waking hours compared with sleeping). The morning surge has been associated with increased risk of cerebrovascular diseases, including brain white matter lesions and stroke. In addition, ABPM is helpful in screening for nocturnal hypertension or nondipper status (i.e., <10% reduction in nighttime BP compared with daytime). Data from large ABPM cohorts suggests that nighttime BP provides the greatest information regarding CV risk. CV risks associated with elevated nighttime BP levels outweigh the risks associated with elevated routine office BP measurements and those of the cumulative daytime hours. In addition, the BP variability data from ABPM suggests that a greater degree of BP variability during the 24 hours of monitoring is associated with a greater risk of CV target-organ damage. ABPM is typically programmed to take BP measurements every 15 to 30 minutes during awake hours and every 30 to 60 minutes during sleep hours. It is important for patients to complete the diary correctly so that the hours

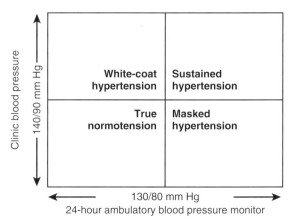

Fig. 65.2 **Use of ambulatory blood pressure monitoring in diagnosing hypertension.** This grid helps to integrate ambulatory blood pressure (BP) monitor data with office BP results. Sustained hypertension is diagnosed if office BP is ≥140/90 mm Hg and 24-hour average of ambulatory BP is ≥130/80 mm Hg. White-coat hypertension is diagnosed when office BP is ≥140/90 mm Hg but 24-hour average of ambulatory BP is <130/80 mm Hg. Masked hypertension is diagnosed when office BP is <140/90 mm Hg but 24-hour average of ambulatory BP is ≥130/80 mm Hg.

of sleep (including naps) can be incorporated into the ABPM report.

Current estimates suggest that more than half of hypertensive patients measure their BP at home. Although not reimbursed by most insurers in the United States, home BP monitors are relatively inexpensive and reasonably accurate. Specific recommendations have been published on how to incorporate home blood pressure monitoring (HBPM) into overall BP assessment. For the diagnosis of hypertension, it is recommended to take two BP readings in the morning between 7 am and 10 am and two measurements in the evening between 7 pm and 10 pm for 7 consecutive days. Values from the first day are discarded, and the subsequent 6 days' values are averaged. For the diagnosis of hypertension in untreated patients, hypertension is not present if the average is less than 125/80 mm Hg, but hypertension is likely present if the value is greater than 135/85 mm Hg. For values in between, ABPM is recommended and hypertension is considered present when the ABPM 24-hour average is greater than 130/80 mm Hg. Cutoff values for ABPM and HBPM are listed in Table 65.6.

ABPM and HBPM have important similarities, but they also have meaningful differences. They are viewed as complementary rather than alternative techniques because they provide different information regarding BP. Table 65.7 compares similarities and differences among the various techniques available for BP measurement.

The National Center for Health and Clinical Excellence (NICE) in the United Kingdom recommended using ABPM or HBPM to confirm all new diagnoses of hypertension. Similarly, the 2015 USPSTF guidelines recommended that the diagnosis of hypertension be confirmed with ABPM. However, the USPSTF recognized that ABPM is not widely available because of equipment cost and lack of widespread insurance coverage and stated that HBPM is an acceptable alternative to ABPM if not available. Because all the data for treating hypertension have been based on standard office

Table 65.6 Ambulatory and Home Blood Pressure Values

Category	Interval	Optimal, mm Hg	Normal, mm Hg	Elevated, mm Hg
ABPM	Daytime	<120/80	<130/85	≥135/85
HBPM	Daytime	<120/75	<125/80	≥135/85
ABPM	Nighttime	<100/65	<110/70	≥120/70
ABPM	24-hour	<115/75	<125/75	≥130/80

ABPM, Ambulatory blood pressure monitoring; *HBPM*, home blood pressure monitoring.

Table 65.7 Comparison of Ambulatory, Home, and Office Blood Pressure Monitoring

	ABPM	Home	Office
Detects WCH and masked HTN	Yes	Yes	No
Multiple measurements	Yes	Yes	Yes
Evaluates circadian rhythm of BP	Yes	No	No
Predicts events	Yes	Yes	Yes
Evaluates BP variability	Yes	No	No
Improves compliance and BP control	?	Yes	Yes
Cost	High	Low	Low
Reimbursement	Partial	No	Yes

ABPM, Ambulatory blood pressure monitoring; *HTN*, hypertension; *WCH*, white-coat hypertension.

Table 65.8 2015 USPSTF Recommendations for High Blood Pressure Screening in Adults

Recommendation

Screening: Screen for hypertension in adults aged ≥18 years old without known hypertension; obtain measurements outside of the clinical setting for diagnostic confirmation.

Risk assessment: Persons at increased risk for hypertension are those who have high-normal blood pressure (130–139/85–89 mm Hg), overweight or obese individuals, and African Americans.

Screening tests: Using proper protocol, average 2 office measurements while patient is seated using a manual or automated sphygmomanometer. Ambulatory and home blood pressure monitoring can be used to confirm a diagnosis of hypertension after initial screening.

Screening interval: Adults aged ≥40 years old and persons at increased risk for hypertension should be screened annually. Adults 18–39 years old with normal blood pressure (<130/85 mm Hg) who do not have other risk factors should be rescreened every 3–5 years.

Treatment and interventions: For nonblack patients, initial treatment consists of a thiazide diuretic, calcium channel blocker, angiotensin-converting enzyme inhibitor, or angiotensin-receptor blocker. For black patients, initiate treatment with a thiazide or a calcium channel blocker. Initial or add-on treatment for patients with chronic kidney disease consists of either an angiotensin-converting enzyme inhibitor or an angiotensin-receptor blocker (not both).

USPSTF, U.S. Preventive Services Task Force.
From Siu A. Screening for high blood pressure in adults: U.S. preventive services task force recommendation statement. *Ann Intern Med.* 2015;163:1–9.

BP measurement and because ABPM is currently only reimbursed by the Center for Medicare and Medicaid Services (CMS) for suspected untreated white-coat hypertension, it remains uncertain whether ABPM and HBPM will be used more widely to help diagnose and manage hypertension in the United States as recommended by the USPSTF. A summary of the 2015 USPSTF recommendations is listed in Table 65.8.

MANAGEMENT OF HYPERTENSION

LIFESTYLE MODIFICATIONS

Several nonpharmacologic approaches are used in lowering BP. In obese patients, the most effective measure to reduce BP is weight loss. For all patients, reducing dietary sodium intake to less than 100 mmol/day (2300 mg of sodium) and increasing physical activity to at least 30 minutes daily on most days of the week are high-yield lifestyle modifications. Finally, limiting alcohol intake to two drinks a day for men (one drink a day for women) helps reduce BP. Other approaches, including modification of intake of fish oil, garlic, and green tea and supplementation of potassium, magnesium, and calcium, have had variable success in managing BP. Although they do not appear harmful, these approaches lack robust data to support their widespread use in the management of prehypertension and hypertension. Table 65.9 summarizes the effects of various lifestyle modifications on BP.

There is evidence for the benefit of lifestyle measures in hypertension management. The Dietary Approaches to Stop Hypertension (DASH) Study showed that a diet low in sodium and high in fruits, vegetables, and calcium is effective in lowering BP. In addition, the Trials of Hypertension Prevention (TOHP2) and Trials of Non-Pharmacological Interventions in the Elderly (TONE) reported that in middle-aged (TOHP2) and elderly (TONE) subjects with mild to moderate hypertension, diet, exercise-induced weight loss, and sodium restriction can be sustained and are associated with significant BP reductions. A recent meta-analysis of 24 randomized controlled trials showed that dietary modifications are associated with significant incremental reductions in BP. The authors found that the net reduction in systolic and diastolic BP was 3.1 mm Hg and 1.8 mm Hg, respectively. From this same analysis, it appears that some dietary patterns are more effective than others, as the DASH diet was associated with the greatest overall reduction in BP with a net reduction in systolic and diastolic BP of 7.6 mm Hg and 4.2 mm Hg, respectively.

The effect of aerobic exercise was evaluated in a meta-analysis of 54 randomized controlled trials and demonstrated that aerobic exercise reduces systolic and diastolic BP by 3.8 mm Hg and 2.6 mm Hg, respectively. This BP reduction was noted in both overweight and normal-weight participants, as well as in normotensive individuals.

Viewed in sum, these studies demonstrate the importance of individually evaluating the various lifestyle factors associated

Table 65.9   Lifestyle Modification to Manage Hypertension

Modification	Recommendation	Approximate SBP Reduction
Weight reduction	Maintain normal body weight (BMI 18.5–24.9)	5–20 mm Hg/10-kg weight loss
Adopt DASH eating plan	Consume a diet rich in fruits, vegetables, and low-fat dairy products with a reduced content of saturated and total fat	8–14 mm Hg
Dietary sodium reduction	Reduced dietary sodium intake to no more than 100 mmol/L (2.3 g sodium or 6 g sodium chloride)	2–8 mm Hg
Physical activity	Engage in regular aerobic physical activity such as brisk walking (at least 30 min per day, most days of the week)	4–9 mm Hg
Moderation of alcohol consumption	Limited consumption to no more than two drinks per day for most men and no more than one drink per day for most women and lighter-weight persons	2–4 mm Hg

For overall cardiovascular risk reduction, stop smoking. The effects of implementation of these modifications are dose and time dependent and could be higher for some individuals.
BMI, Body mass index, *DASH*, Dietary Approaches to Stop Hypertension.

with hypertension in all patients as part of the initial management of hypertension.

PHARMACOLOGIC AGENTS

Many patients with hypertension find it difficult to make necessary lifestyle modifications to effectively lower BP. Treatment with antihypertensive medications is recommended when BP remains above the goal despite lifestyle modifications.

Major classes of antihypertensive medications with their mechanism of actions, common side effects, and compelling indications are listed in Table 65.10. Heart failure and stroke are the target-organ damage that is prevented to the greatest extent by long-term antihypertensive therapy. A recent large meta-analysis suggests that all five major classes of antihypertensive agents (angiotensin-converting enzyme [ACE] inhibitor, angiotensin II receptor blocker [ARB], beta-blocker, calcium channel blocker [CCB], and diuretic) can reduce target-organ damage when used to control BP effectively. Choosing an agent involves a decision-making process that takes into account demographics (age and ethnicity), drug cost, and the anticipated side-effect profile. The usual response to a single antihypertensive agent is a reduction in systolic BP of 12 to 15 mm Hg and diastolic BP of 8 to 10 mm Hg. Follow-up visits for BP assessment and dose titration are often scheduled in 2 to 4 weeks for single-agent therapy as most agents will exert their antihypertensive effects at that dose by then.

In patients with systolic BP greater than 20 mm Hg and/or diastolic BP greater than 10 mm Hg above the goal, beginning treatment with combination drug therapy can shorten the time to achieve BP goal, require less dose titration of antihypertensive agent, and increase the likelihood of achieving BP goal. Combination therapy is often more desirable than a stepwise approach of maximizing one agent before adding another agent because of the better efficacy in BP control and side-effect profile.

A useful approach in building an effective combination therapy is based on a convenient model shown in Fig. 65.3. This approach is similar to the popular "Birmingham Square" used in the United Kingdom to develop combination regimens. The art in building or adjusting a combination antihypertensive regimen is to use medications with complementary, and not overlapping, mechanisms of action and to try to minimize side effects by leveraging known pharmacology. Examples include adding an ACE inhibitor to a diuretic to reduce occurrence of hypokalemia or adding an ACE inhibitor (or an ARB) to a CCB to reduce CCB-dependent edema.

MAJOR CLASSES OF ANTIHYPERTENSIVE AGENTS AND ASSOCIATED CARDIOVASCULAR BENEFITS

DIURETICS

Diuretics are proven antihypertensive agents and play a key role in building a successful combination regimen. They work mostly by inhibiting renal sodium absorption. There is abundant evidence to support the benefit of diuretics compared with placebo in reducing CV morbidity and mortality, including ischemic heart disease, heart failure, stroke, other vascular disease, and death. Data from the Antihypertensive and Lipid Lowering Treatment to Prevent Heart Attack Trial (ALLHAT) suggest that thiazide diuretics are as effective as CCBs and ACE inhibitors in lowering BP and reducing coronary events. Despite the concern of higher incidence of new onset of diabetes with diuretics, secondary analyses from ALLHAT found a diuretic to be equally effective as an ACE inhibitor and a CCB in reducing CV risk, including ischemic heart disease, heart failure, stroke, kidney disease, and death in both diabetic and nondiabetic patients. The published data on long-term outcomes of the Systolic Hypertension in the Elderly Program (SHEP) further affirm the benefits of diuretic therapy in reducing CV endpoints.

Hydrochlorothiazide (HCTZ) is the most commonly prescribed diuretic for hypertension. Chlorthalidone is a thiazide-like diuretic that is not as commonly prescribed. HCTZ and chlorthalidone are pharmacologically different. Chlorthalidone has a duration of action of 48 to 72 hours versus 16 to 24 hours for HCTZ. The longer duration of action may explain the observation of improved mean 24-hour ambulatory BPs (including daytime and nighttime) with chlorthalidone versus HCTZ and the superiority of chlorthalidone in preventing CV events when compared with HCTZ in one meta-analysis.

Table 65.10   Major Classes of Available Antihypertensive Medications With Their Mechanisms and Side Effects

Class	Mechanisms	Side Effects	Compelling Indications
Diuretics	Reduce renal sodium absorption	—	Heart failure, high CAD risk diabetes, stroke
Thiazide diuretics	Inhibit sodium and chloride cotransporter in the distal convoluted tubule; more effective in BP control than loop diuretics	Hypokalemia, hyponatremia, hypomagnesemia, hyperuricemia, photosensitivity, and metabolic effects including dyslipidemia and impaired glucose tolerance	
Loop diuretics	Inhibit sodium, potassium, and chloride cotransporter in the thick ascending limb of the loop of Henle	Hypokalemia but less other metabolic side effects	
Potassium-sparing diuretics	Inhibit the epithelial sodium channel in the distal tubule	Hyperkalemia	
Renin Angiotensin System Blockers	Dampen arterial wave reflections, increasing aortic distensibility and venodilation	—	Heart failure, post MI, high CAD risk, diabetes, CKD, stroke
ACE inhibitors	Block the conversion of angiotensin I to angiotensin II	Cough, hyperkalemia, elevated creatinine and angioedema, fetal toxicity, angioedema	
ARB	Block binding of angiotensin-II to the type 1 angiotensin receptor	Similar to ACE inhibitors except no cough	
Direct renin inhibitor (aliskiren)	Block conversion of angiotensinogen to angiotensin I	Similar to ARB; diarrhea at high doses	
Calcium Channel Blockers	Inhibit the L-type voltage-gated plasma membrane channel	—	High CAD risk, diabetes
Dihydropyridine	Vasodilatation	Dependent edema, gingival hyperplasia	
Diltiazem	Vasodilation and AV nodal blockade	Bradycardia	
Verapamil	Vasodilation and AV nodal blockade	Bradycardia, constipation	
Beta-Blockers	Inhibit adrenergic receptors	Reduced exercise tolerance, depression, bronchospasm	Heart failure, post MI, high CAD risk, diabetes, stroke
Nonselective beta-blockers	Inhibit both beta 1 and 2 receptors	More bronchospasm	
Selective beta-blockers	Block beta 1 receptors	Less bronchospasm	
Combined alpha- and beta-blockers	Block both beta and alpha receptors	—	
Aldosterone Blocker	Block aldosterone receptor	—	Heart failure, post MI
Spironolactone	—	Androgen-blocking effect including irregular menses, gynecomastia, impotence	
Eplerenone	—	Less potent but fewer side effects related to androgen blocking	
Direct Vasodilators	Smooth muscle relaxant	Peripheral edema	
Alpha-1 Blockers	Vasodilatation	Postural hypotension	
Central Adrenergic Agonists	Inhibit central adrenergic tone	Drowsiness, fatigue, and dry mouth	

ACE, Angiotensin-converting enzyme; *ARB,* angiotensin II receptor type I blocker; *AV,* atrioventricular; *BP,* blood pressure; *CAD,* coronary artery disease; *CKD,* chronic kidney disease; *MI,* myocardial infarction.

RENIN-ANGIOTENSIN-ALDOSTERONE SYSTEM BLOCKADE

ACE inhibitors, ARBs, direct renin inhibitors, and spironolactone/eplerenone block the conversion of angiotensin I to II, the binding of angiotensin II to its receptor, the conversion of angiotensinogen to angiotensin I, and the binding of aldosterone to the mineralocorticoid receptor, respectively. ACE inhibitors and ARBs have been shown in many studies to reduce CV events, prevent stroke, improve kidney outcomes, and lower the incidence of new-onset diabetes. Aliskiren, a direct renin inhibitor, is an effective antihypertensive agent with a side-effect profile that appears similar to ARBs, but it

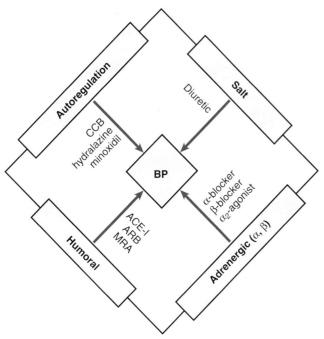

Fig. 65.3 Building successful combination antihypertensive therapy. The diagram emphasizes four basic physiologic processes that regulate blood pressure and places the major classes of antihypertensive medications along the side, corresponding to the process responsible for the primary antihypertensive effect of the class. Combining agents to control hypertension is usually more effective when drugs are chosen from different sides (e.g., diuretic plus ARB) as opposed to the same side (e.g., beta-blocker plus alpha$_2$-agonist) of the diagram. *ACE-I,* Angiotensin-converting enzyme inhibitor; *ARB,* angiotensin receptor blocker; *CCB,* calcium channel blocker; *MRA,* mineralocorticoid antagonist.

lacks evidence of benefit in hard endpoint outcome trials. Although spironolactone and eplerenone both have potential benefits in congestive heart failure, they are currently used as third- or fourth-line antihypertensive agents. The recently published PATHWAY-2 Study found that spironolactone, when compared with bisoprolol and doxazosin, was more effective for BP lowering among patients with resistant hypertension already on a three-drug regimen, indicating that spironolactone is an effective fourth-line agent.

CALCIUM CHANNEL BLOCKERS

CCBs inhibit the L-type voltage-gated channels resulting in vasodilatation (and decreased cardiac output with non-dihydropyridine CCBs). Data from ALLHAT suggests that dihydropyridine CCBs are as effective as thiazide diuretics and ACE inhibitors in lowering BP and reducing CV events, including myocardial infarction (MI), stroke, and overall mortality. In addition, data from the Anglo-Scandinavian Cardiac Outcomes Trial (ASCOT) showed that a combination of CCB with ACE inhibitor was superior in reducing stroke than a combination of beta-blocker with ACE inhibitor. Data from the Avoiding Cardiovascular Events through Combination Therapy in Patients Living with Systolic Hypertension (ACCOMPLISH) trial demonstrated that, despite identical BP control, combination therapy with an ACE inhibitor and a CCB seemed superior to the combination of an ACE inhibitor and a diuretic in hypertensive patients with high CV risk.

BETA-BLOCKERS

Beta-blockers generally decrease cardiac output, but several beta-blockers also show vasodilatory effects, either from a combined alpha blockade (labetalol and carvedilol) or through nitric oxide potentiation (nebivolol). Beta-blockade is useful in treating ischemic heart disease and congestive heart failure. However, in older patients, beta-blockers have been increasingly replaced by other classes of agent because of concerns that beta-blockade does not prevent stroke as effectively as other agents. Although the ASCOT trial suggests the combination of dihydropyridine CCB plus ACE inhibitor is better than the selective beta-blocker atenolol plus diuretic, the newer generation of beta-blockers with combined alpha- and beta-blocking activities or nitric oxide potentiating effect may provide benefit in lowering CV events, although this remains speculative at present.

OTHER AGENTS

Alpha$_1$-blockers and other direct vasodilators are used as add-on therapy in resistant hypertension. However, as previously mentioned, the PATHWAY-2 study found that spironolactone is more effective than doxazosin (an alpha$_1$-blocker) for BP lowering in patients with resistant hypertension. In addition, the doxazosin arm in ALLHAT was terminated early because of its inferior CV outcomes, particularly for the risk of new heart failure, compared with the diuretic, ACE inhibitor, and CCB arms. Because of these studies, alpha$_1$-blockers are not commonly prescribed for BP lowering as the initial or even the second agent.

NOVEL ANTIHYPERTENSIVE THERAPIES

Several device-based interventions are under investigation to treat hypertension either alone or as a complement to standard antihypertensive medications. One approach uses the known effects of carotid baroreceptor activation therapy (BAT) to reduce sympathetic output and lower BP. This requires surgical implantation of a pacemaker-like device that has an electrode placed on the carotid body in the neck. When the signal generator is activated, it stimulates the carotid baroreceptors to reduce signals to the brain stem, resulting in lower BP and heart rate. Initial experience showed significant and sustained mean reduction in BP of 21/12 mm Hg at 3 months and 33/22 mm Hg at 2 years; however, a recent pivotal study of 265 patients with drug-resistant hypertension failed to achieve two of its five primary endpoints. This study observed that 35% of patients had a serious procedure-related adverse event, including nerve injury. The device is not approved currently in the United States, but it remains in use in Europe.

Another approach uses either radiofrequency energy from an intravascular signal source or focused external ultrasound or a delivery of an ablative chemical such as alcohol into the perivascular renal nerve supply. The procedure usually takes less than an hour to complete and reduces sympathetic flow into (efferent) and out of (afferent) the kidneys. Initial studies suggested that renal denervation could substantially lower BP in patients with drug-resistant hypertension. However, a large randomized controlled trial failed to demonstrate superiority of renal denervation over sham procedure. Multiple reasons emerged to explain these results, and there are still several trials under way evaluating the utility of this approach in hypertensive individuals. No denervation device or procedure is currently approved in the United States.

Lastly, another device approach to hypertension management has been the creation of a 4-mm fistula between the iliac artery and the iliac vein with a vascular coupler device. Initial studies in patients with resistant hypertension treated with this device showed reductions in office systolic BP of 27 mm Hg compared with a fall of 4 mm Hg in the normal care group, corroborated by ABPM. The principal adverse effect noted with this procedure is unilateral leg edema due to venous stenosis occurring in about one in four patients. Although usually managed successfully with stenting and venoplasty, it is currently the largest drawback to this approach. This technology is not currently approved in the United States, although a US trial is scheduled to begin in late 2016.

GOAL BLOOD PRESSURE LEVELS

In 2003, JNC 7 recommended a BP goal of less than 140/90 for patients less than 80 years of age in the absence of comorbidities or compelling indications. A revised recommendation, published in 2014 by members of the Joint National Committee (JNC 8), suggested a goal of less than 140/90 mm Hg for the general population under 60 years of age and a goal less than 150/90 mm Hg for those aged 60 years and older. In addition, they recommended a goal of less than 140/90 mm Hg in diabetics and those with CKD, representing a change from prior recommendations. The JNC 8 members based their recommendations for raising the BP goal among patients aged greater than 60 years on several studies including the Principal Results of the Japanese Trial to Assess Optimal Systolic Blood Pressure in Elderly Hypertensive Patients (JATOS) Study, the Target Blood Pressure for Treatment of Isolated Systolic Hypertension in the Elderly: Valsartan in Elderly Isolated Systolic Hypertension (VALISH) Study, the Treatment of Hypertension in Patients 80 Years of Age or Older (HYVET) Study, the Randomised Double-Blind Comparison of Placebo and Active Treatment for Older Patients with Isolated Systolic Hypertension (SYST-EUR) Study, and SHEP. The recommendation for raising the goal systolic BP in this group was not unanimous and remains controversial.

In 2015, the Systolic Blood Pressure Intervention Trial (SPRINT) was published. SPRINT was a large, multicenter, randomized controlled trial that enrolled 9361 patients aged 50 years or older who had a systolic BP of 130 to 180 mm Hg plus one or more of the following additional risks factors for CVD: age 75 years or older; clinically evident CVD; an estimated GFR (eGFR) of 20 to 59 mL/min; or a 10-year Framingham Risk Score greater than or equal to 15%. SPRINT excluded patients with diabetes, prior stroke, polycystic kidney disease (PKD), greater than 1 g of proteinuria, or an eGFR of less than 20 mL/min. Automated oscillometric BP was used to measure BP in the study.

SPRINT tested whether a systolic BP goal of less than 120 mm Hg compared with less than 140 mm Hg would reduce the occurrence of CVD and CKD events in a moderately high CV risk population. The SPRINT study was terminated early when it was observed that the patients in the lower SBP target group had significantly lower rates of heart failure and death. However, there were more acute kidney injury events

and electrolyte disturbances in the lower SBP goal group, suggesting that patients who were targeted more aggressively require closer monitoring.

The findings from the SPRINT study are expected to have important implications for BP guidelines relevant to the population included in the study, and new guidance regarding BP goals is anticipated from the American Heart Association (AHA) and American College of Cardiology.

SPECIAL POPULATIONS

WOMEN

Women show similar BP response to antihypertensive agents as men. Before menopause, women have lower BP than men of a similar age. This trend reverses after menopause, and black women tend to have the highest BP. In women of childbearing age, ACE inhibitors and ARBs are usually avoided because of the risk of fetal malformation. Women tend to have a higher risk of hypokalemia when treated with diuretics and a greater risk of hyponatremia when treated with thiazide diuretics but in general show similar benefits from antihypertensive agents as men.

BLACKS

Hypertension is more prevalent in blacks, tends to be more salt sensitive, and responds better to diuretics and CCB than ACE inhibitors, ARBs, or beta-blockers when used as monotherapy. In addition, blacks tend to experience higher rates of target-organ damage than whites at any level of BP. The reason is not entirely clear, but recent advances in genetic predisposition, particularly the presence of APOL1 risk alleles, explain part of this enhanced predisposition. Compared with whites, blacks have more frequent CV complications, such as heart failure, and about a fourfold higher risk of end-stage kidney disease. In 2010, the International Society of Hypertension in Blacks (ISHIB) released a consensus statement on the recommendations for managing hypertension in black patients. It recommended a goal BP of less than 135/85 mm Hg in black patients without target-organ damage and goal BP less than 130/80 mm Hg in patients with evidence of target-organ damage, although robust evidence is lacking for this recommendation. Most expert panels still recommend similar BP goals for black patients as compared with other patient groups.

ELDERLY

The pattern of BP elevation in older patients is characterized predominantly by systolic hypertension. This relates in large part to the significant role of vascular stiffness, which also contributes to a decline in diastolic BP and, therefore, an increase in the pulse pressure. With low diastolic pressure, concern exists with further therapeutic lowering of diastolic BP while targeting SBP, especially in those with existing coronary artery disease due to increasing CV events below a certain threshold of BP. Current recommendations are to avoid lowering diastolic BP less than 70 mm Hg in those with active coronary artery disease at any age.

As previously mentioned, current guidelines are controversial and inconsistent with respect to the optimal SBP treatment goal in the elderly. Among patients 75 years of age and older who participated in SPRINT, targeting intensive BP control reduced mortality and CV events even among those who were frail or had decreased gait speed. In addition, there was no increase in serious adverse events, falls, or orthostatic hypotension with intensive BP control. The results suggest that older patients with similar characteristics as those included in SPRINT can benefit from intensive BP lowering.

DIABETES MELLITUS

The presence of both diabetes mellitus (DM) and hypertension represents a substantial CV risk. Treating hypertension is an effective way of reducing this risk. An ACE inhibitor or ARB is preferred as initial therapy in a hypertensive diabetic patient with albuminuria to slow progression of kidney disease. Several studies have indicated that a combination of ACE inhibitor *and* ARB is *not* superior to monotherapy with one of these agents and is associated with more side effects.

Major guidelines suggest that the goal BP in patients with DM is less than 140/90 mm Hg, although prior guidelines had suggested more intensive lowering to less than 130/80 mm Hg. The American Diabetic Association (ADA) does recommend a lower target of less than 130 mm Hg systolic in patients with albuminuria and in younger patients if tolerated. The Action to Control Cardiovascular Risk in Diabetes (ACCORD) trial greatly influenced current recommendations about target goals in diabetics. In ACCORD, the intensive group with SBP goal less than 120 mm Hg did not experience an improvement in the primary outcome of a composite fatal and nonfatal CV events despite an SBP that was 14 mm Hg lower than the standard group. Stroke, a prespecified secondary outcome, however, was significantly reduced in the lower BP goal group. As in SPRINT, the increased medication requirement in the lower BP group resulted in more side effects, including reduced kidney function.

Follow-up data from the ACCORD BP trial were recently published in the Action to Control Cardiovascular Risk in Diabetes Follow-Up Study (ACCORDION). The ACCORDION trial looked at 3957 participants from the ACCORD BP trial who were followed up for an additional 5 years. Results showed that during a median follow-up of 8.8 years, there remained a nonsignificant reduction in the primary outcome of CVD with intensive lowering of BP. In addition, the stroke benefit that was observed in ACCORD did not persist after BP differences waned.

There are theories as to why the SPRINT study demonstrated lower CV and mortality rates with an SBP target under 120 mm Hg, whereas the ACCORD trial failed with intensive treatment to the same target in diabetes. The factorial design of ACCORD and differences in patient population may have contributed to the discrepant results.

CHRONIC KIDNEY DISEASE

Hypertension is a frequent finding in both acute and CKD. Mortality and morbidity from CVD are high among those with CKD, and CKD is an independent risk factor for coronary heart disease. The risk of death, particularly due to CVD, is typically higher than the risk of eventually requiring kidney replacement therapy. Risk factor modification, including BP lowering, can reduce the CV complications associated with CKD. Abundant evidence supports the current recommendation of using ACE inhibitors and ARBs in patients with CKD, especially those with proteinuria.

Findings from SPRINT indicate that patients with an eGFR of 20 to 59 mL/min and less than 1 g of proteinuria had a lower rate of fatal and nonfatal CV events and death when targeted to a lower SBP goal of less than 120 mm Hg. However, as in the ACCORD trial, the increased medication requirement in the lower BP group resulted in an increased risk of reduced kidney function. Because the trial was stopped early, long-term outcomes for CKD events (doubling of serum creatinine or development of end-stage kidney disease) were not significant, in part, because of the low event rates of the CKD endpoint in both the standard and intense BP lowering groups. Further analysis of the CKD subgroup will offer more insight as to how best to manage patients with CKD.

As the SPRINT study excluded patients with PKD, eGFR less than 20 mL/min, kidney transplants, and proteinuria greater than 1 g per 24 hours, findings cannot be applied to these patient groups. There are no randomized trials examining the optimal BP targets in kidney transplant recipients. Patients with PKD were studied in the Halt Progression of Polycystic Kidney Disease (HALT-PKD) Study which showed that rigorous BP control was associated with a slower increase in total kidney volume, no overall change in the estimated GFR, a greater decline in left ventricular mass index, and greater reduction in albuminuria.

With respect to proteinuria, some guidelines have recommended a lower BP goal in this population. Some of the data that support this recommendation in patients with nondiabetic CKD comes from the Modification of Diet in Renal Disease (MDRD) trial that assessed the effect of more aggressive BP lowering in patients with CKD. The study suggested that with increasing degrees of proteinuria at baseline, more aggressive BP lowering was associated with a slower rate of GFR loss, compared with less aggressive BP lowering.

HEART DISEASE

Hypertension is a major risk factor for ischemic heart disease and heart failure. Beta-blockers and renin-angiotensin system blockers have been shown to reduce morbidity and mortality associated with acute MI and high-risk ischemic heart disease. Although beta-blockers may worsen acute congestive heart failure, beta blockade remains a key agent in managing chronic congestive heart failure. Diuretics also play an essential role in managing patients with congestive heart failure.

The 2015 guidelines from the AHA recommend a BP target of less than 140/90 mm Hg for the majority of patients with hypertension and coronary artery disease. However, the guidelines do suggest that a lower BP target of less than 130/80 mm Hg is reasonable in some patients with coronary artery disease (CAD), such as those who have had a prior MI, stroke, transient ischemic attack (TIA), peripheral arterial disease, or abdominal aortic aneurysm.

STROKE

Hypertension is the most common and most important risk factor for ischemic stroke, the incidence of which can be markedly reduced by effective antihypertensive therapy. Hypertension is also an important risk factor for hemorrhagic stroke. The approach to BP management of a stroke patient differs in the acute and chronic phases of stroke and depends on whether a patient has an acute ischemic versus acute hemorrhagic stroke. Many patients are hypertensive in the setting of an acute stroke.

In 2015, the America Heart Association/American Stroke Association (AHA/ASA) published guidelines regarding BP targets in the acute phase of ischemic stroke. The targets depend on whether thrombolysis is indicated. The guidelines recommend a goal BP less than 185/110 mm Hg in the setting of an acute ischemic stroke and thrombolysis. There does not appear to be a benefit to BP lowering without thrombolytic therapy.

Persons who survive a stroke or TIA are at increased risk of experiencing another stroke. Treatment of hypertension with diuretics, renin-angiotensin blockers, CCBs, and beta-blockers are all beneficial for reducing risk of recurrent stroke. As mentioned previously, beta blockade may not provide *as much* benefit in stroke reduction as other forms of antihypertensive drug therapy.

The optimal SBP targets to prevent recurrent stroke was tested in the Secondary Prevention of Small Subcortical Strokes (SPS3) trial, which studied 3020 patients with recent lacunar infarctions. Patients were randomized to an SBP target of 130 to 149 mm Hg versus a lower target of less than 130 mm Hg. There was a nonsignificant reduction in recurrent stroke in the group randomized to the lower SBP goal. The AHA/ASA recommends a target BP level less than 140/90 mm Hg for secondary prevention of stroke/TIA, but it suggests that a target systolic BP less than 130 mm Hg is not unreasonable given the SPS3 trial findings.

RESISTANT HYPERTENSION

Resistant hypertension is defined as a BP that remains above goal in spite of concurrent use of three antihypertensive agents of different classes, with one of the three agents a diuretic (if tolerated) and all agents prescribed at optimal doses (50% or more of the maximum recommended antihypertensive dose). The true prevalence of resistant hypertension is not known, but it is estimated that about 7% to 14% of treated hypertensives have resistant hypertension. These patients are more likely to have target-organ damage and are at greater risk of stroke, MI, heart failure, and CKD compared with patients who have more easily controlled hypertension.

Pseudoresistance refers to poorly controlled hypertension that appears resistant to treatment but is actually attributable to other factors, including inaccurate BP measurement, poor adherence, and white-coat effect. Out-of-office BP monitoring is a valuable tool to determine the presence of true drug resistance, including both ABPM and SMBP.

Medication adherence (taking medication as prescribed) and persistence (refilling prescriptions) data increasingly indicate that patients prescribed antihypertensive regimens with multiple drugs take either no drug or fewer than the prescribed number of drugs in about half of the cases of drug-resistant hypertension. These are important factors to consider before making a diagnosis of resistant hypertension.

Mineralocorticoid receptor antagonists like spironolactone and eplerenone are evidence-based treatment options for patients with resistant hypertension. The antihypertensive effect of spironolactone was evaluated in the ASCOT in which the addition of spironolactone (median dose of 25 mg daily) as a fourth drug was associated with a mean 22/10 mm Hg reduction in BP at 1-year follow-up. In addition, the previously mentioned PATHWAY-2 study was the first randomized controlled trial comparing multiple agents with placebo for resistant hypertension. The mineralocorticoid antagonist spironolactone was the most effective agent.

OBSTRUCTIVE SLEEP APNEA

Obstructive sleep apnea (OSA) is common among patients with hypertension, especially in resistant hypertension. Both of these highly prevalent conditions contribute to an increased CV risk. Patients with more severe OSA are also more likely to have abnormal nocturnal BP patterns. Although OSA increases the risk of CV disease through a number of mechanisms, repetitive cycles of hypoxemia and reoxygenation probably play a central role in increasing CV risk by augmenting sympathetic nervous system activity, systemic inflammation, and oxidative stress. The effects of continuous positive airway pressure (CPAP) on BP reduction are modest, and use of supplemental nocturnal oxygen as salvage therapy has been shown to be ineffective for BP reduction in patients with OSA for whom CPAP is problematic. Combining weight loss with CPAP has been shown to be more effective in reducing SBP than either intervention alone. CPAP has also been shown to restore nocturnal dipping in resistant hypertensive patients, and the number of hours of CPAP use is correlated with the degree of BP improvement. Patients with OSA and either resistant hypertension or frequent apneic episodes are also more likely to have a greater reduction in BP from use of CPAP.

OBESITY

Obesity (body mass index greater than 30 kg/m^2) is a global pandemic. As the prevalence of obesity increases, so does its associated comorbidities, including hypertension. Resistant hypertension and OSA are common in obese patients. The mechanism by which obesity raises BP is not completely understood. Theories implicate insulin resistance and hyperinsulinemia, adipokines that are secreted by adipose tissue, and elevated plasma aldosterone levels that are often found in obese patients. All of these factors contribute to impaired sodium excretion, increased sympathetic nervous system activity, reduced vascular compliance, and activation of the renin-angiotensin-aldosterone system (RAAS).

The approach to lowering BP in obese patients includes treating sleep apnea if present, weight loss, lower sodium diet, and pharmacologic therapy. In addition, bariatric surgery may be helpful. Bariatric surgery (e.g., Roux-en-Y gastric bypass [RYGB], sleeve gastrectomy [SG], and adjustable gastric band [AGB]) is increasingly being used as a therapeutic option for controlling obesity. In a meta-analysis of 136 studies, average weight loss and improvement in hypertension control with several bariatric procedures were significant, with 78.5% of patients categorized as having resolved or improved BPs. In a prospective study comparing the various bariatric surgery approaches, resolution or remission of hypertension at 1 year after the procedure occurred in 79% of patients managed with an RYGB, 68% undergoing a SG, and 44% undergoing an AGB.

CONCLUSION

Hypertension is common, and the prevalence continues to rise with an increasingly older and obese population. Adequate treatment of hypertension remains the key to lowering CV morbidity and mortality. Correctly assessing BP status, CV risk, and the presence of target-organ damage is important in optimizing therapy to reduce CV morbidity and mortality. The optimal BP level to reduce the risk associated with hypertension is still debatable and varies across patient populations. The most effective approach to BP lowering is addressing lifestyle factors, secondary causes of hypertension, and medications that are complementary in action. Novel therapies with devices may provide additional options in managing the truly resistant hypertension, but they are not currently available.

BIBLIOGRAPHY

ALLHAT Officers and Coordinators for the ALLHAT Collaborative Research Group. Major outcomes in high-risk hypertensive patients randomized to angiotensin-converting enzyme inhibitor or calcium channel blocker vs diuretic: the antihypertensive and lipid-lowering treatment to prevent heart attack trial (ALLHAT). *J Am Med Assoc.* 2002;288:2981-2997.

Calhoun DA, et al. Resistant hypertension: diagnosis, evaluation, and treatment: a scientific statement from the American Heart Association Professional Education Committee of the Council for High Blood Pressure Research. *Circulation.* 2008;117:e510-e526.

Chobanian AV, et al. Seventh report of the Joint National Committee on the Prevention, Detection, Evaluation, and Treatment of High Blood Pressure (JNC 7): resetting the hypertension sails. *Hypertension.* 2003;41:1178-1179.

Cushman WC, Evans GW, et al. Effects of intensive blood-pressure control in type 2 diabetes mellitus. *N Engl J Med.* 2010;362:1575-1585.

DASH Collaborative Research Group. A clinical trial of the effects of dietary patterns on blood pressure. *N Engl J Med.* 1997;336:1117-1124.

Flack JM, Sica DA, et al. Management of high blood pressure in Blacks: an update of the International Society on Hypertension in Blacks consensus statement. *Hypertension.* 2010;56:780-800.

Gay H, et al. Effects of different dietary interventions on blood pressure: systemic review and meta-analysis of randomized controlled trials. *Hypertension.* 2016;67:733-739.

Jamerson K, Weber MA, et al. Benazepril plus amlodipine or hydrochlorothiazide for hypertension in high-risk patients. *N Engl J Med.* 2008;359:2417-2428.

James PA, et al. Evidence-based guidelines for the management of high blood pressure in adults (JNC 8). *J Am Med Assoc.* 2014;311:507-520.

Kernan WN, et al. Guidelines for the prevention of stroke in patients with stroke and transient ischemic attack: a guideline for healthcare professionals from the American Heart Association/American Stroke Association. *Stroke.* 2014;45:2160-2236.

McCormack T, et al. Management of hypertension in adults in primary care: NICE guideline. *Br J Gen Pract.* 2012;62:163-164.

Myers MG, et al. Conventional versus automated measurement of blood pressure in the office (CAMBO) trial. *Fam Pract.* 2012;29:376-382.

Pareek AK, et al. Efficacy of low-dose chlorthalidone and hydrochlorothiazide as assessed by 24-h ambulatory blood pressure monitoring. *J Am Coll Cardiol.* 2016;67:379-389.

Rosendorf C, et al. Treatment of hypertension in patients with coronary artery disease: a scientific statement from the American Heart Association, American College of Cardiology, and American Society of Hypertension. *Circulation.* 2015;131:e435-e470.

Rossi GP, et al. A prospective study of the prevalence of primary aldosteronism in 1,125 hypertensive patients. *J Am Coll Cardiol.* 2006;48:2293-2300.

Rousch GC, et al. Chlorthalidone compared with hydrochlorothiazide in reducing cardiovascular events: systemic review and network meta-analyses. *Hypertension.* 2012;59:1110-1117.

Siu A. Screening for high blood pressure in adults: U.S. preventive services task force recommendation statement. *Ann Intern Med.* 2015;163:1-9.

The Sprint Research Group. A randomized trial of intensive versus standard blood-pressure control. *N Engl J Med.* 2015;373:2103-2116.

Whelton SP, et al. Effect of aerobic exercise on blood pressure: a meta-analysis of randomized, controlled trials. *Ann Intern Med.* 2002;136:493-503.

Williams B, et al. Spironolactone versus placebo, bisoprolol, and doxazosin to determine the optimal treatment for drug-resistant hypertension (PATHWAY-2): a randomised, double-blind, crossover trial. *Lancet.* 2015;386:2059-2068.

Secondary Hypertension

Aldo J. Peixoto

66

DEFINITION AND PREVALENCE OF SECONDARY HYPERTENSION

Secondary hypertension is generally defined as hypertension associated with a specific cause and therefore is potentially curable if that cause is removed. The use of this definition generates two separate lines of diseases. The first are considered "classic" causes of secondary hypertension, which, if diagnosed in a timely manner, can be effectively cured. Examples include acute glomerulonephritis, primary aldosteronism, some cases of renal artery stenosis (RAS), pheochromocytoma, Cushing syndrome, hypothyroidism and hyperthyroidism, and coarctation of the aorta. Other conditions may be associated with higher blood pressure (BP) levels; however, given their complex pathophysiologic mechanisms and association with multiple other cardiovascular risk factors, their correction does not necessarily result in the resolution of hypertension. Examples in this category include chronic kidney disease (CKD), sleep apnea, and obesity.

The prevalence of secondary hypertension is estimated around 10% of all cases of hypertension in adults. Absent from most prevalence studies, all of which were conducted from the 1970s to the 1990s, is the recognition that primary aldosteronism was underdiagnosed, that the definitions of kidney disease were too conservative, and that sleep apnea was not considered as a diagnosis. Therefore it is likely that an updated survey of the prevalence of secondary hypertension would result in higher prevalence estimates.

The relationship between age and prevalence of secondary causes must be acknowledged. Among hypertensive children, secondary causes are the rule rather than the exception, with up to 90% of young children having an identifiable secondary cause, most commonly structural kidney disease. The prevalence of "classic" causes of secondary hypertension among hypertensive adolescents had been about 65% in older observations, although the obesity epidemic has somewhat masked this relationship. While obesity is associated with a higher prevalence of primary hypertension in children and adolescents, its presence does not exclude the presence of a typical secondary cause (~40%). Therefore the coexistence of obesity should not prevent the clinician from investigating secondary hypertension in children and adolescents.

The transition point of prevalence rates from childhood/adolescence numbers to more typical adult numbers is unknown. The only study that investigated the effect of age on the prevalence of secondary hypertension was unable to show a higher prevalence among patients aged 18 to 29 years (5.6%) compared with any other age bracket; in fact, because of the high rate of renovascular disease and primary aldosteronism in older patients, the prevalence of secondary hypertension was lowest among the youngest group. Mindful of these somewhat unexpected data, it must be recognized that there is a transition period and that ignoring it would inevitably lead to frequently missing the diagnosis of a secondary cause. Accordingly, our search for secondary hypertension in younger adults, especially those under the age of 30 years, is always more "aggressive" than in older patients. In this chapter, we will restrict discussion of secondary hypertension to adults.

CLINICAL OPPORTUNITIES TO DIAGNOSE SECONDARY HYPERTENSION

There are two critical opportunities to identify secondary hypertension during the evaluation and management of hypertensive patients. First, and most important, is during the initial evaluation of a patient diagnosed with hypertension. It is important to consider the breadth of possibilities at this time, especially as diagnostic tests often perform at their best when patients are not on treatment. Table 66.1 lists clinical features suggestive of each of the major causes of secondary hypertension. The clinician should explore the presence of these different clinical signs and symptoms in every patient. The list of general diagnostic tests recommended as part of the initial evaluation of hypertensive individuals (see Table 66.1) broadly addresses the identification of secondary causes. It should be reviewed carefully for every patient, and further investigations should be pursued if suggested by this initial review.

The second occasion to explore secondary causes is when patients are noted to be resistant to therapy. Resistant hypertension, identified in approximately 12% of treated patients with hypertension, is defined as BP that remains above target (in general, above 140/90 mm Hg) despite the use of three adequately dosed drugs, of synergistic drug classes, preferably including a diuretic. Patients with resistant hypertension have higher rates of secondary hypertension, in particular primary aldosteronism (~20%), renovascular disease (~25%), and obstructive sleep apnea (>50%). Therefore every patient with resistant hypertension should be reconsidered for secondary causes, and, if not previously screened, objective testing for these conditions should be considered.

Table 66.1 Clues That Suggest Secondary Hypertension Based on Simple Diagnostic Tests That Are Routinely Recommended for the Initial Evaluation of Hypertensive Patients

Test	Possible Causes of Secondary Hypertension
Basic Metabolic Panel	
eGFR (based on creatinine)	Low: CKD (any etiology), RAS
Potassium	Low: aldosterone excess (primary or secondary), hypercortisolism, apparent mineralocorticoid excess syndromes, primary reninism
	High: Gordon syndrome, CKD
Bicarbonate	High: aldosterone excess (primary or secondary), apparent mineralocorticoid excess syndromes, primary reninism
	Low: Gordon syndrome, CKD (any etiology)
Calcium	High: Hyperparathyroidism
Urinalysis	
Hematuria	Glomerulonephritis, interstitial nephritis
Proteinuria	Glomerulonephritis
Complete Blood Count	
Hematocrit/ Hemoglobin	High: sleep apnea, any polycythemic disorder (e.g., polycythemia vera)

CKD, Chronic kidney disease; *eGFR,* estimated glomerular filtration rate; *RAS,* renal artery stenosis.

CLINICAL SYNDROMES SUGGESTIVE OF SECONDARY HYPERTENSION

HYPERTENSION AND HYPOKALEMIA

The coexistence of hypertension and spontaneous hypokalemia should always raise the possibility of secondary causes of hypertension. The approach should start with a clinical evaluation that confirms that the kidney is the source of potassium wasting. This can be achieved with measurement of the transtubular potassium gradient (TTKG) ([urine potassium/plasma potassium]:[urine osmolality/plasma osmolality]) or the urine potassium/creatinine ratio. In the presence of hypokalemia, a TTKG greater than 2 or a urine potassium/creatinine ratio greater than 13 mEq/g is diagnostic of renal potassium wasting. Once renal potassium wasting is confirmed, paired measurement of plasma renin activity (PRA; in ng/mL per hour) and plasma aldosterone (in ng/dL) allows a thoughtful differential diagnosis according to three different diagnostic patterns:

1. *High aldosterone* (>15 ng/mL) *with high PRA* (>1.5 ng/mL per hour). This combination results in a variable aldosterone-to-renin ratio, but it is usually less than 20. These patients have secondary hyperaldosteronism, commonly caused by diuretic therapy (thiazides, loop diuretics), RAS (particularly unilateral), malignant hypertension (of

any etiology), or the rare syndrome of primary reninism, which is usually caused by a benign renin-producing tumor of the juxtaglomerular cells, though several extrarenal tumors have been reported (teratomas, adenocarcinomas of the adrenal, lung, pancreas, or ovary, or hepatocellular carcinoma).

2. *High aldosterone with suppressed renin activity* (<0.6 ng/mL per hour), leading to an aldosterone-to-renin ratio greater than 30. This is diagnostic of primary aldosteronism and should lead to further subtype differentiation (see specific section below).

3. *Low aldosterone* (often suppressed to undetectable levels) *and low renin activity.* These patients behave clinically as if they had hyperaldosteronism but have undetectable aldosterone levels. This implicates one of three possibilities: (1) an alternative source of mineralocorticoid activity (e.g., deoxycorticosterone or cortisol from a tumor, or congenital adrenal hyperplasia due to 11β-hydroxylase or 21-hydroxylase deficiency); (2) a disorder of impaired degradation of cortisol, thus leaving it available to activate the mineralocorticoid receptor (e.g., licorice ingestion or primary 11β-hydroxysteroid dehydrogenase type 2 deficiency); or (3) mutations in the epithelial sodium channel (Liddle syndrome) or the mineralocorticoid receptor (Geller syndrome). Some of these conditions are briefly presented in Table 66.2.

HYPERTENSION WITH A STRONG FAMILY HISTORY OF HYPERTENSION EARLY IN LIFE

Hypertension has a significant genetic component, with multiple genes associated with small effects on BP. However, patients who have a strong family history of hypertension early in life should be approached more carefully, as they may have a genetic disorder responsible for the hypertension. The most common of these conditions is autosomal-dominant polycystic kidney disease (1:500 to 1:1000 live births), which can result in hypertension several years before producing symptoms or causing loss of kidney function. There are several rare monogenic causes of hypertension that the clinician should entertain in the right clinical setting; Table 66.2 summarizes their key clinical and genetic features.

HYPERTENSION AND OBESITY

Obesity is strongly associated with hypertension. It is mediated by increased activity of the renin-angiotensin system and the sympathetic nervous system, increased production of aldosterone by adipocytes, and impaired production of natriuretic peptides. Localized fat accumulation in the liver (as in nonalcoholic steatohepatitis) or kidney (renal sinus fat) is also associated with an increased prevalence of hypertension.

Weight gain often results in loss of BP control, and weight loss, when significant, can lead to resolution of hypertension. This can be achieved with lifestyle changes (dietary caloric restriction, exercise, behavioral modification to adjust caloric intake patterns), with or without the addition of drugs (orlistat, lorcaserin, phentermine/topiramate) or bariatric surgery. It is important to remember that some drugs used to treat obesity, such as lorcaserin (a serotonin 5-HT2 receptor

Table 66.2   Clinical Clues to Guide the Investigation in Young Hypertensive Patients With a Potential Hereditary Cause

Possible Causes of Familial Hypertension		Clinical Clues
Catecholamine-Producing Tumors		
PPGL	Familial cases are responsible for up to 40% of cases	Paroxysmal palpitations, headaches, diaphoresis, pale flushing. Syndromic features of any of the associated disorders (see PPGL section for details)
Neuroblastomas (adrenal)	1%–2% of neuroblastomas are familial	Symptoms of the abdominal tumor (pain, mass) or catecholamine release (same as PPGL)
Parenchymal Kidney Disease		
Glomerulonephritis	Alport disease (X-linked, AR or AD), familial IgA nephropathy (AD with incomplete penetrance)	Proteinuria, hematuria, low eGFR
Polycystic kidney disease	ADPKD type 1 or 2, ARPKD	Multiple kidney cysts (as few as 3 in patients under the age of 30)
Adrenocortical Disease		
Glucocorticoid-remediable aldosteronism (familial hyperaldosteronism type 1)	AD chimeric fusion of the 11β-hydroxylase and aldosterone synthase genes	Cerebral hemorrhages at young age, cerebral aneurysms. Mild hypokalemia. High plasma aldosterone, low renin
Familial hyperaldosteronism type 2	AD. Unknown defect	Severe hypertension in early adulthood. High plasma aldosterone, low renin. No response to glucocorticoid treatment
Familial hyperaldosteronism type 3	AD mutation in the KCJN5 potassium channel	Severe hypertension in childhood with extensive target-organ damage. High plasma aldosterone, low renin. Marked bilateral adrenal enlargement
Congenital adrenal hyperplasia	AR mutations in 11β-hydroxylase or 21-hydroxylase	Hirsutism, virilization. Hypokalemia and metabolic alkalosis. Low plasma aldosterone and renin
Monogenic Primary Renal Tubular Defects		
Gordon syndrome	AD mutations of KLHL3, CUL3, WNK1, WNK4. AR mutations of KLHL3	Hyperkalemia and metabolic acidosis with normal renal function
Liddle syndrome	AD mutations of the epithelial sodium channel	Hypokalemia and metabolic alkalosis. Low plasma aldosterone and renin
Apparent mineralocorticoid excess	AD mutation in 11β-hydroxysteroid dehydrogenase type 2	Hypokalemia and metabolic alkalosis. Low plasma aldosterone and renin
Geller syndrome	AD mutation in the mineralocorticoid receptor	Hypokalemia and metabolic alkalosis. Low plasma aldosterone and renin. Increased BP during pregnancy or exposure to spironolactone
Unknown Mechanisms		
Hypertension-brachydactyly syndrome	AD mutation in the phosphodi-esterase 3 (PDE3) gene	Short fingers (small phalanges) and short stature. Brainstem compression from vascular tortuosity in the posterior fossa

AD, Autosomal dominant; *ADPDK,* autosomal-dominant polycystic kidney disease; *aldo,* aldosterone; *AR,* autosomal recessive; *ARPKD,* autosomal-recessive polycystic kidney disease; *PKD,* polycystic kidney disease; *PPGL,* pheochromocytoma/paraganglioma.
Modified from Peixoto AJ. Attending rounds: a young patient with a family history of hypertension. *Clin J Am Soc Nephrol.* 2014;9: 2164–2172.

agonist) and phentermine (a sympathomimetic amine) can induce significant hypertension in some patients.

The impact of bariatric surgery on hypertension control in obese patients is now well established. A meta-analysis of 57 studies in over 50,000 patients showed that 64% of patients had improved BP levels, and up to 50% were able to fully come off medications. In general, the amount of weight loss is greater with a Roux-en-Y gastric bypass than with other techniques that are purely restrictive (gastric banding, gastric sleeve), and in many studies, this is also associated with greater BP reduction.

DRUG-INDUCED HYPERTENSION

Patients presenting with hypertension or whose BP control suddenly worsens should always be evaluated for exposure to hypertensogenic substances (Table 66.3). These include substances of abuse and over-the-counter and prescription drugs. Oral contraceptive pills (OCP), especially earlier generation pills that had higher estrogen and progesterone content, can cause hypertension. Modern low-estrogen pills can also produce hypertension, though at rates much lower than with older preparations. Stopping the OCP

Table 66.3   Drugs Commonly Associated With Hypertension

Oral contraceptives
NSAIDs (selective and nonselective)
Sympathomimetics: pseudoephedrine, phenylpropanolamine, phentermine, cocaine, amphetamines (prescription or illegal), yohimbine (α_2-anatagonist)
SSRIs and SNRIs
MAOIs
Cyclosporine and tacrolimus
Erythropoietin and darbepoietin
Corticosteroids, mineralocorticoids (fludrocortisone)
Anti-VEGF antibodies (bevacizumab, ramucirumab) and certain tyrosine kinase inhibitors with anti-VEGF activity (e.g., sorafenib, sunitinib)
Licorice
Ethanol

MAOIs, Monoamine oxidase inhibitors; *NSAIDs,* nonsteroidal antiinflammatory drugs; *SNRIs,* serotonin-norepinephrine reuptake inhibitors; *SSRIs,* selective serotonin reuptake inhibitors; *VEGF,* vascular endothelial growth factor.

cures the hypertension after several weeks to months in most, but not all, women. Nonsteroidal antiinflammatory drugs (NSAIDs) result in a modest average hypertensive effect (up to ~5 mm Hg), but some patients can have very large BP responses. In addition, NSAID-induced hypertension often presents as loss of BP control in patients taking a diuretic or a blocker of the renin-angiotensin system, whereas calcium channel blockers tend to be less affected in NSAID users.

Sympathomimetic amines (legal or illegal) usually cause hypertension acutely, close to the time of ingestion. Alcohol has an acute hypotensive effect, but chronic use in large amounts (>4 to 5 drink-equivalents per day) is associated with increased BP. Glucocorticoids and mineralocorticoids can produce a dose-dependent rise in BP. Although generally seen only with systemic treatment, there are isolated reports of hypertension resulting from high-exposure topical therapy. Glucocorticoids with low mineralocorticoid activity (dexamethasone, budesonide) induce lesser pressor responses. Selective serotonin reuptake inhibitors (SSRIs) and serotonin-norepinephrine reuptake inhibitors (SNRIs) can produce a modest increase in BP. SNRIs are more commonly culprits, and the hypertensive response in some patients can be severe. Interestingly, when used for hypertensive patients with depression, BP often improves as depressive symptoms improve.

Angiogenesis inhibitors, such as anti–vascular endothelial growth factor (VEGF) antibodies (bevacizumab, ramucirumab) and tyrosine kinase inhibitors (sorafenib, sunitinib), can produce hypertension that often persists despite discontinuation. Most cases are related to systemic therapy, although there are isolated reports following intravitreal administration of bevacizumab. Because hypertension during the use of these drugs correlates with better tumor responses (likely a reflection of successful antiangiogenesis), treatment is usually continued unless BP control to acceptable levels is not achievable or if severe kidney injury develops.

LABILE HYPERTENSION OR HYPERTENSION WITH SYMPTOMS OF CATECHOLAMINE EXCESS

Some patients present with paroxysmal hypertension (isolated episodes interspersed with normotension), labile hypertension (wide fluctuations in BP during any given time interval), or hypertension accompanied by stereotypical spells suggestive of catecholamine excess (headaches, palpitations, diaphoresis, pallor). In these situations, ruling out pheochromocytoma/paraganglioma (PPGL) is the first initial step. However, because these symptoms are nonspecific and PPGL is rare, most patients turn out to have an alternative diagnosis, and often no specific etiology can be identified. Important considerations to be entertained in patients presenting as "pseudopheochromocytoma" include sympathomimetic drug use, alcohol withdrawal, hyperthyroidism, RAS, carcinoid, intracranial hypertension, neurovascular brainstem compression, panic disorder, and baroreflex failure (as in patients with bilateral carotid sinus injury due to trauma, surgery, or irradiation). Further testing is based on specific symptoms and signs associated with each of these conditions.

SPECIFIC CAUSES OF SECONDARY HYPERTENSION

PARENCHYMAL KIDNEY DISEASE

Chronic kidney disease (CKD) of any etiology can lead to hypertension. Approximately 75% of patients with glomerular filtration rate (GFR) less than 45 mL/min are hypertensive. Patients with polycystic kidney disease and glomerulopathies tend to be hypertensive earlier in the course of the disease (at higher GFR) than patients with interstitial diseases. However, with progressive decline in kidney function, the prevalence of hypertension is relatively similar across all causes of CKD. Proteinuria is linked to increased sodium retention and hypertension. This relationship starts at relatively low levels of proteinuria and progressively strengthens with higher degrees of protein excretion. Low GFR and proteinuria have a synergistic association with higher BP.

The pathogenesis, diagnosis, and management of CKD (including hypertension), glomerular and interstitial diseases, and polycystic kidney disease are discussed elsewhere in this book.

RENOVASCULAR DISEASE

Renovascular hypertension due to RAS is present in 1% to 5% of hypertensive patients. There are two main types of RAS that can lead to hypertension: atherosclerotic RAS (ARAS, >90% of cases) and fibromuscular dysplasia (FMD, <10%). ARAS is an atherosclerotic process indistinct from atherosclerosis in any other vascular bed, with similar pathobiologic mechanisms. Conversely, FMD is a nonatherosclerotic, noninflammatory disease of the arterial wall that results in stenosis of the arterial lumen.

Many hypertensive patients may have renovascular atherosclerotic lesions without a role in the pathogenesis of hypertension. Renovascular atherosclerosis is associated with increased cardiovascular risk but should be differentiated from renovascular hypertension. In this chapter, I refer solely to RAS (atherosclerotic or fibromuscular) that leads to hypertension through ischemia-induced activation of the renin-angiotensin-aldosterone system (RAAS) as well as progressive endothelial dysfunction, capillary rarefaction, and kidney injury. In animal models of arterial flow restriction, unilateral RAS results in ipsilateral ischemia and renin production, which leads to increased angiotensin II levels that produce a systemic pressor response. Because the other kidney is normal, there is pressure-induced natriuresis and the animals do not become volume overloaded. In contrast, in bilateral disease natriuresis is impaired so hypertension is initially driven by angiotensin II–stimulated vasoconstriction but is maintained by sodium retention, which ultimately leads to decreased renin production. However, in humans, perhaps reflecting the chronicity of this process, there is wide variability in plasma renin levels in bilateral disease, although it is generally accepted that kidney tissue renin levels are high.

Recent animal models have provided new insights, especially on atherosclerotic disease, demonstrating that renal artery flow restriction induces a proinflammatory and profibrotic environment that results in endothelial dysfunction, microvascular rarefaction, and interstitial fibrosis. The degree of flow restriction to trigger these responses in humans is a matter of debate. Available evidence from a study testing ipsilateral renin generation during balloon inflation indicates that a 20% drop in perfusion pressure is required and that renin generation progressively increases with greater degrees of hypoperfusion (Fig. 66.1). The degree of luminal stenosis necessary to produce this pressure gradient typically exceeds 70%, although it may occur with lesions in the 50% to 70% range.

DIAGNOSIS OF RENAL ARTERY STENOSIS

Renovascular hypertension should be suspected in patients with hypertension and an unexplained decrease in GFR, hypokalemia due to secondary hyperaldosteronism (seen in unilateral RAS), worsening of kidney function with use of angiotensin-converting enzyme (ACE) inhibitors or angiotensin receptor blockers (ARBs) (this suggests bilateral disease, unilateral stenosis in a single kidney, or unilateral stenosis accompanied by underlying parenchymal disease), kidney asymmetry (difference in kidney length of 1.5 cm or more), abdominal and/or flank bruits, generalized atherosclerosis, or unexplained acute pulmonary edema (particularly if recurrent).

Once suspected, the diagnosis of RAS is based on imaging tests. Renal angiography is the gold standard for the diagnosis of RAS; however, most patients are evaluated noninvasively before angiography. The three accepted noninvasive diagnostic modalities are computed tomography angiography (CTA), magnetic resonance angiography, and duplex renal ultrasound (DRU). All other tests, including renal scintigraphy and several previously used biochemical tests, should no longer be used for screening because of poor sensitivity and specificity.

CTA and magnetic resonance angiography are preferred because they are easy to perform, are operator independent, and provide good anatomic detail, including visualization of plaque burden in ARAS, morphology of the renal artery in FMD, detailed information on degree of stenosis, and assessment of the typical poststenotic dilatation. Despite the fact that many in the past have used 50% stenosis as the cutoff for diagnosis, and that the presence of any atherosclerotic

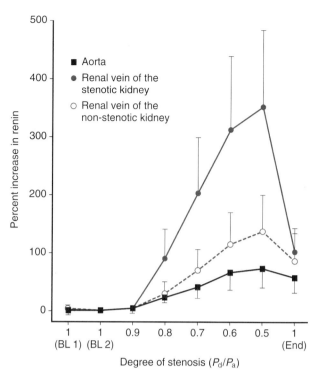

Fig. 66.1 Transstenotic pressure thresholds for renin secretion after graded renal artery occlusion in patients with unilateral renal artery stenosis. The experiment was performed after the lesion was treated with stenting. The pressure gradient was induced by progressive inflation of an angioplasty balloon. P_d/P_a indicates the systolic blood pressure (BP) ratio between the renal artery (distal to the balloon) and the aorta. A ratio of 1.0 indicates no difference in BP (i.e., no stenosis). The graph shows significant increases in ipsilateral renin secretion with transstenotic systolic BP gradients greater than 20% (i.e., ratio of 0.8 or lower). Renin data are presented for the aorta (*squares*), renal vein of the stenotic kidney (*closed circles*), and renal vein of the nonstenotic kidney (*open circles*). BL 1 is the baseline before stenting; BL 2 is the baseline after stenting. (From De Bruyne B, et al. Assessment of renal artery stenosis severity by pressure gradient measurements. *J Am Coll Cardiol.* 2006;48:1851–1855, with permission.)

renal artery lesion (of any severity) is associated with increased cardiovascular mortality, current guidelines call for luminal occlusion greater than 70% to be considered hemodynamically significant. The quality of the images with CTA (Fig. 66.2) is generally better than magnetic resonance angiography, but its use may be precluded by the coexistence of impaired kidney function and the attendant risk of contrast-induced nephropathy. Magnetic resonance angiography has the caveats of requiring breath holding; accordingly, motion artifacts are common. In addition, if gadolinium is used, there may be a risk of nephrogenic systemic fibrosis in patients with GFR less than 30 mL/min, although imaging can be done without gadolinium. Both CTA and magnetic resonance angiography are limited by a tendency to overestimate lesions and the inability to provide any functional information.

DRU, in experienced hands, is approximately 90% accurate for the diagnosis of RAS. The diagnosis is not made through visualization of the stenosis but by the detection of increased flow velocity at the site of stenosis compared with the adjacent aorta. A renal-to-aortic ratio greater than 3.5 (peak systolic velocity within the renal artery divided by the peak systolic

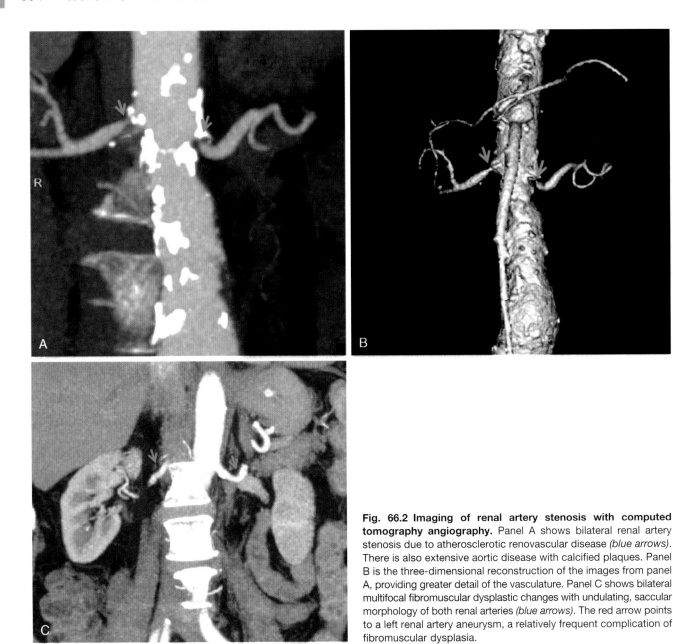

Fig. 66.2 Imaging of renal artery stenosis with computed tomography angiography. Panel A shows bilateral renal artery stenosis due to atherosclerotic renovascular disease *(blue arrows)*. There is also extensive aortic disease with calcified plaques. Panel B is the three-dimensional reconstruction of the images from panel A, providing greater detail of the vasculature. Panel C shows bilateral multifocal fibromuscular dysplastic changes with undulating, saccular morphology of both renal arteries *(blue arrows)*. The red arrow points to a left renal artery aneurysm, a relatively frequent complication of fibromuscular dysplasia.

velocity in the aorta) accompanied by a peak systolic velocity greater than 280 m/s is suggestive of greater than 60% RAS on angiography (this was the cutoff used by the seminal validating studies). In addition, functional information on the RAS can be derived from Doppler tracings obtained from the renal parenchyma. Acceleration times reflect the time needed for the incident pulse wave to reach its peak. In conditions of restricted flow, the acceleration time is increased (>100 ms), which results in a pulse wave of decreased amplitude and late peak (i.e., a "pulsus parvus et tardus"). While this abnormality is insensitive for the diagnosis of severe RAS, it is quite specific for hemodynamically significant lesions, and the tracings should always be inspected to try to identify it. The resistive index [(peak systolic velocity − diastolic velocity)/peak systolic velocity] is a marker of increased parenchymal resistance to blood flow due to increased renovascular resistance but is also influenced by systemic factors, such as heart rate, peripheral vascular resistance, and arterial stiffness. It can be increased

(>0.8) in the setting of acute kidney injury or CKD of any cause. The resistive index is low in a kidney with a hemodynamically significant inflow restriction, and a low resistive index (<0.6) in a kidney with a visualized RAS suggests that the lesion is hemodynamically significant. If the contralateral kidney has a resistive index greater than 0.8, the likelihood of clinical response to revascularization is lower, as the high resistive index in the contralateral kidney suggests systemic microvascular disease and parenchymal kidney damage. Because it does not involve contrast administration, DRU is often used in patients with advanced kidney disease. However, it is time consuming and dependent on both operator skill and patient body habitus, resulting in unreliable results in up to 25% of patients.

Novel techniques are under development to provide functional data in RAS. The most promising appears to be blood-oxygen-level-dependent magnetic resonance imaging (BOLD-MRI), a technique that detects areas of ischemia (based on deoxyhemoglobin levels) in the kidney. This modality is being perfected to identify kidneys that remain viable despite underlying ischemia, allowing clinicians to identify good candidates for revascularization. Unfortunately, difficulties with protocol validation and lack of studies demonstrating its value are still restricted to small case series, and thus its use in clinical practice cannot yet be recommended.

MANAGEMENT OF ATHEROSCLEROTIC RENAL ARTERY STENOSIS

All patients with ARAS should receive maximal medical therapy including smoking cessation (if applicable), antiplatelet therapy, statins, and a blocker of the RAAS. Even though there are no data demonstrating a benefit from smoking cessation and antiplatelet therapy, there is general agreement based on the management of vascular disease in other arterial beds that smoking cessation, antiplatelet therapy (aspirin or clopidogrel), and statins should be offered to all patients.

Observational studies support the use RAAS blockers (ACE inhibitors or ARBs) to improve cardiovascular and kidney outcomes in ARAS. This is important to recognize because clinicians are often fearful of using these agents in ARAS. In fact, ACE inhibitors are associated with decreased risk of death and kidney failure in this population, even among patients with bilateral disease. The inability to tolerate a RAAS blocker (i.e., a drop in GFR >20%) in such patients is an indication of hemodynamic significance of the lesions and should lead the clinician to strongly consider revascularization.

There is little evidence from clinical trials to support an advantage of revascularization over medical therapy in patients with disease of mild severity (<70% stenosis), in those incidentally discovered without accompanying hypertension or kidney dysfunction, or in those with well-controlled hypertension and stable kidney function during follow-up. Although meta-analyses indicate that BP is approximately 7/3 mm Hg lower in patients randomized to revascularization compared with medical therapy, two randomized clinical trials, STAR (STent placement and blood pressure and lipid-lowering for the prevention of progression of renal dysfunction caused by Atherosclerotic ostial stenosis of the Renal artery) and Angioplasty and Stenting for Renal Artery Lesions (ASTRAL), studied patients with relatively mild degrees of stenosis, stable clinical course, and reasonable BP control, and demonstrated no significant BP reduction, kidney function improvement, or effect on the occurrence cardiovascular events, end-stage kidney disease, or death associated with renal artery stenting.

The Cardiovascular Outcomes in Renal Atherosclerotic Lesions (CORAL) trial was the most detailed trial comparing renal artery stenting with medical therapy in patients with hypertension and significant stenosis (>80% or 60% to 80% with a transstenotic systolic BP gradient >20 mm Hg). In CORAL, renal artery stenting resulted in minimally lower systolic BP than medical therapy (2.3 mm Hg, $P = .03$), but there was no difference in the occurrence of the composite primary endpoint of cardiovascular or kidney death, myocardial infarction, hospitalization for congestive heart failure, stroke, progressive kidney disease, and the need for kidney replacement therapy (35.1% in the stent group, 35.8% in the medical group, $P = .58$), any of the components of this composite outcome, or any secondary endpoints. The results did not differ between patients with unilateral or bilateral

disease. Lastly, a meta-analysis of five randomized clinical trials revealed no role for intervention to reduce the occurrence of nonfatal myocardial infarction in ARAS (the risk ratio compared with medical therapy was 0.86 [0.51–1.43], $P = .55$), a finding that was independent of follow-up kidney function or duration of follow-up.

It is important to recognize that the available clinical trials excluded a large number of patients. For example, ASTRAL included only patients whose clinicians were "uncertain that patients would definitely benefit from revascularization." None of the studies included patients with rapid loss of kidney function or patients presenting with recurrent unexplained pulmonary edema. Because of this, I believe that rapid loss of kidney function, resistant hypertension in the hands of a hypertension specialist, and unexplained recurrent pulmonary edema are acceptable indications for intervention in ARAS. I often recommend intervention in patients who have bilateral disease and develop kidney hypoperfusion and loss of kidney function upon achievement of adequate BP control and/or initiation of RAAS blockade. A 2014 expert consensus from the Society for Cardiovascular Angiography and Interventions suggests these indications and also considers it justified when ARAS is identified in the setting of acute coronary syndrome complicated by severe hypertension.

Revascularization is currently accomplished via percutaneous transluminal angioplasty and stenting (PTRAS) in 98% of patients who require an intervention. Angioplasty alone (without stenting) is not an adequate technique in ARAS because of the extensive amount of arterial recoiling following the procedure. This is due to the proximal nature of the lesions and shared plaque with the aorta. In addition, stent use results in significantly lower rates of restenosis compared with angioplasty alone. Surgical intervention is rarely needed and is left for patients with extensive aortic disease that would require simultaneous open correction.

Approximately one-third of patients undergoing intervention experience worsening kidney function. This may be the result of contrast nephropathy or atheroembolic kidney disease, which often goes unsuspected and undiagnosed.

Monitoring patients closely is extremely important. Patients with ARAS who are followed without intervention are at risk of occlusion and atrophy of the ipsilateral kidney (~10% and 22% over 3 years, respectively). However, studies of incidental ARAS suggest a stable kidney course over time, although patients with ARAS have a high risk of cardiovascular events, which is likely a reflection of overall atherosclerotic disease burden. Current recommendations suggest yearly ultrasounds to monitor kidney size. My practice is to do so for 2 to 3 years, but if patients have stable BP and kidney function, I typically stop and reserve re-imaging to cases of loss of clinical stability.

FIBROMUSCULAR DYSPLASIA

FMD predominantly affects younger women, most often diagnosed between 40 and 50 years old. The renal arteries are the vessels most commonly affected (80% to 100% of patients, up to 60% bilateral), although many other sites can be involved, including the carotid and vertebral arteries (up to ~70% in some series, 20% to 30% in most). Most cases are sporadic, although ~10% are familial, and rare cases can be associated with specific genetic diseases, such as neurofibromatosis, tuberous sclerosis, Ehlers-Danlos syndrome, Alagille syndrome, Williams syndrome, and Turner syndrome. Renal FMD is associated with smoking in about 30% of patients.

Renal FMD is subdivided according to its radiographic appearance as multifocal (~80% of cases, usually representing involvement of the media) or unifocal (~20%, usually due to intimal or perimedial disease). The radiographic appearance does not seem to affect the clinical presentation, which is one of hypertension, usually with preserved kidney function. However, data from the most comprehensive series indicates that, although the median BP response to angioplasty is similar for both FMD subtypes (~30 mm Hg), the cure of hypertension is not the norm, occurring in 54% of patients with unifocal disease and 26% with multifocal disease.

The goal in FMD is early identification and treatment with percutaneous angioplasty, which is indicated in patients with hypertension as long as there is no significant atrophy of the affected kidney (e.g., kidney length <8 cm on ultrasound). Stenting is rarely necessary, and surgical correction is reserved for patients with complex anatomic lesions. Despite the absence of comparative trials, most believe that medical management is a less preferred option in FMD. In patients who opt against angioplasty, treatment is a drug regimen that includes an ACE inhibitor (or an ARB). Antiplatelet therapy (beyond a few weeks postangioplasty) and statins are not necessary, but smoking cessation should be strongly encouraged.

PRIMARY ALDOSTERONISM

Primary aldosteronism is a common cause of secondary hypertension, with an estimated prevalence of 5% to 10% among hypertensive patients. In patients with resistant hypertension, that number approaches 20%. Most cases are due to adrenal hyperplasia (~60%), which is typically bilateral, or aldosterone-producing adrenal adenomas (~40%). Uncommon causes include adrenal carcinoma, unilateral adrenal hyperplasia, and glucocorticoid-remediable aldosteronism.

Recent advances have significantly improved the understanding of the pathobiology of adrenal proliferation and aldosterone excess in primary aldosteronism. Somatic mutations in the *KCJN5* gene coding for an inward rectifying potassium channel in adrenal adenomas are present in about one-third of adenomas. These mutant channels expressed in the adrenal glomerulosa lose their specificity for potassium and allow inward flow (i.e., into the cell) of sodium, resulting in chronic cell depolarization and calcium inflow, which, in turn, stimulates cell proliferation and aldosterone production. The same mutation has been identified as a germline mutation in patients with a rare form of adrenal hyperplasia (familial aldosteronism type 3) and results in massive adrenal hyperplasia, aldosterone production, and severe hypertension with cardiovascular complications. Similar effects on cell depolarization and inward calcium inflow have been demonstrated with other somatic mutations in adenomas, such as in the *CACNA1D* gene coding a voltage-gated calcium channel, the *ATP1A1* gene coding the α1 subunit of the Na/K ATPase, and the *ATP2B3* gene encoding the plasma membrane Ca-ATPase 3. In addition, mutations in other pathways for adrenal adenoma formation have been recently described, such as those in the β-catenin gene *CTNNB1*, leading to tumor growth and aldosterone secretion through mechanisms that are not yet fully understood but seem to involve overexpression of β-catenin, and, therefore, overactivity of the WNT signaling pathway.

While hypokalemia is the most common clue to the diagnosis, the prevalence of primary hyperaldosteronism is quite variable and usually restricted to a minority of patients (only 9% to 37% have serum potassium <3.5 mEq/L). It is more common in patients with adenomas (~50%) than bilateral hyperplasia, likely reflecting the generally higher aldosterone levels in adenomas. Therefore clinicians must be attuned to the possibility of primary aldosteronism in many other situations. Recognizing this, the Endocrine Society recommends screening for primary aldosteronism when hypertension is associated with one of seven specific circumstances: (1) BP consistently greater than 150/100 mm Hg; (2) resistant hypertension (>140/90 mm Hg on >3 drugs); (3) spontaneous or diuretic-induced hypokalemia; (4) adrenal incidentaloma; (5) sleep apnea; (6) family history of early-onset hypertension or stroke at age younger than 40 years; or (7) family history of primary aldosteronism (of any type).

BIOCHEMICAL DIAGNOSIS

Screening is performed with simultaneous measurement of plasma aldosterone and PRA and calculation of the aldosterone/renin ratio (ARR). There are numerous factors that impact on this ratio, and it is particularly sensitive to the PRA, as small changes in value can result in significant changes in the ARR. To maximize the accuracy of the test, it is best to obtain it in the morning, after the patient has been out of bed for at least 2 hours, after 5 to 15 minutes in the seated position, and preferably under liberal salt intake and appropriate potassium repletion. While many drugs can affect the ARR (Table 66.4), most patients are screened while taking antihypertensive medications, with the exception of mineralocorticoid receptor antagonists (MRA) and other potassium-sparing diuretics, and renin inhibitors. Long-acting drugs, such as spironolactone must be stopped for at least 4 weeks before testing.

If the ARR results (see later) obtained while the patient is receiving medications are counter to the clinical suspicion, patients should come off all drugs that can affect the ARR (see Table 66.4) for at least 2 weeks and undergo retesting. Medications with minimal or no effects on the ARR, such as nondihydropyridine calcium channel blockers (diltiazem, verapamil), alpha-blockers (doxazosin, terazosin), and hydralazine, should be used as needed to control BP during this washout period.

An ARR greater than 30 (with aldosterone measured in ng/dL and PRA measured in ng/mL per hour) is suggestive of primary aldosteronism, especially if accompanied by plasma aldosterone levels greater than 15 ng/dL. However, one must keep in mind that using higher aldosterone cutoff levels decreases the sensitivity of the approach, while improving specificity. Lowering the cutoff has the opposite effect, but may be worth considering, especially in high-risk patients. For example, 30% to 40% with high ARR and plasma aldosterone between 10 and 15 ng/dL have positive confirmatory tests that assess aldosterone production; this number is approximately 4% if the aldosterone is less than 10 ng/dL. Therefore it is plausible to consider a confirmatory test in patients with a high ARR and plasma aldosterone greater than 10 ng/dL, especially in those with a high a priori probability of the diagnosis. In

Table 66.4   Factors Affecting the Interpretation of the Aldosterone/Renin Ratio

	False Positives	False Negatives
Aldosterone relatively high	Potassium loading	—
Renin relatively low	β-Blockers Central antiadrenergics Direct renin inhibitors NSAIDs CKD Sodium loading	—
Aldosterone relatively low	—	Hypokalemia
Renin relatively high	—	Diuretics (any type) ACE inhibitors Angiotensin receptor blockers Dihydropyridine calcium blockers Serotonin reuptake inhibitors Acute sodium depletion Estrogens, oral contraceptives Pregnancy

Direct renin inhibitors uniformly lower aldosterone levels. However, their effect on renin differs if measured plasma renin activity (PRA) falls or plasma renin concentration (PRC) increases.
ACE, Angiotensin-converting enzyme; *CKD,* chronic kidney disease; *NSAIDs,* nonsteroidal antiinflammatory drugs.

patients with a high ARR, low PRA (<0.2 ng/mL per hour), and aldosterone greater than 20 ng/dL, confirmatory testing is not necessary; these patients are virtually certain to have primary aldosteronism.

Confirmatory tests are designed to document persistent autonomous production of aldosterone despite the use of a physiologic factor that strongly suppresses aldosterone secretion (i.e., sodium loading). There are several accepted confirmatory tests, the most important being the oral sodium loading test (OSLT), the saline infusion test (SIT), and the fludrocortisone suppression test. I prefer either the OSLT or the SIT, both for ease of performance and overall safety. In the OSLT, sodium intake is liberalized to achieve greater than 200 mEq/day sodium intake for 3 days. Potassium should be effectively replaced during the collection to avoid hypokalemia. A 24-hour urine collection is performed starting in the morning of the third day. We measure urine creatinine (to assess the completeness of the collection), sodium (to confirm >200 mEq/day intake), and aldosterone. Urine aldosterone excretion greater than 12 to 14 µg/day is confirmatory, while levels less than 10 µg/day convincingly exclude the diagnosis. In case of intermediate values, repeating the collection is necessary. In the SIT, the patient lies supine for 1 hour before administration of 2 L of normal saline over 4 hours with the patient remaining in the supine position. Both presaline and postsaline plasma aldosterone are measured. A postinfusion aldosterone greater than 10 ng/dL

confirms the diagnosis, while aldosterone less than 5 ng/dL rules it out. Levels between 5 and 10 ng/dL are considered indeterminate and require either repeat testing or an alternative confirmatory test. Prepotassium and postpotassium and corotisol are also measured to exclude an effect of potassium or adrenocorticotropic hormone (ACTH) on the changes in aldosterone concentration. Because both tests involve the administration of substantial amounts of sodium, they are contraindicated in patients with congestive heart failure, severe hypertension, or severe hypokalemia. In such cases, a pragmatic decision is made regarding the likelihood of the diagnosis simply using the screening aldosterone and PRA.

SUBTYPE DIFFERENTIATION

Once the biochemical diagnosis of autonomous aldosterone excess is confirmed, the next step is subtype differentiation. The two most common subtypes are bilateral hyperplasia (~60% of cases) and adrenal adenomas (~40% of cases). Rare causes include adrenal carcinoma, unilateral adrenal hyperplasia, and glucocorticoid-remediable aldosteronism.

The differential diagnosis starts with a thin-cut adrenal CT. The major role of the CT is to rule out an adrenal carcinoma, which is typically a large mass (rarely <4 cm). Visualization of a small (<3 cm), hypodense (<10 Hounsfield units) adrenal nodule is virtually diagnostic of an adenoma. However, evidence based on adrenal venous sampling (AVS) studies suggests that nodules are nonfunctional in 20% to 25% of cases. Moreover, a meta-analysis showed that imaging (CT and MRI) and AVS data are discordant in almost 40% of cases. This includes the occurrence of not only nonfunctional adenomas but also cases when no adenoma was visualized, but there was lateralization on AVS (microadenomas or unilateral adrenal hyperplasia). Therefore the most appropriate method to distinguish between the clinical subtypes is AVS, and indeed, current recommendations call for AVS in almost all patients in whom surgical treatment of a possible functioning adenoma is being entertained. The only possible exception refers to patients who are younger than 35 years, have hypertension with hypokalemia and high aldosterone levels (>20 ng/dL), and have an adenoma on CT. This is justified by the very low rate of incidental adrenal masses in this age range. Patients who are not interested in or are high risk for surgery do not require AVS and should be treated medically.

AVS should be performed by an experienced interventional radiologist who is familiar with the protocol and is skilled in the procedure, especially because of the angle of the right adrenal vein, which precludes successful catheterization in up to 25% of cases. The test starts with the administration of cosyntropin, which is used to produce maximal cortisol secretion from both adrenal glands to provide a good means for "adjustment" of the aldosterone results. I use a continuous infusion of 50 µg/h intravenously starting 30 minutes before the catheterization and continuing until the end of the procedure. Blood is sampled from each of the adrenal glands and a peripheral site (can be the inferior vena cava or an upper extremity vein) and is sent for both aldosterone and cortisol.

Interpretation of Adrenal Venous Sampling Results

First, each aldosterone and cortisol level should be analyzed as ratios of aldosterone-to-cortisol from each of the three sampling sites. Second, the aldosterone/cortisol ratio for the right adrenal vein is compared with the left adrenal vein, and both are compared with the peripheral ratio. If the aldosterone/cortisol ratio on one of the adrenal veins is greater than or equal to 4 times higher than the contralateral side, the diagnosis of lateralization is made, indicating the presence of an aldosterone-producing adenoma or, rarely, unilateral adrenal hyperplasia. Most adenomas have lateralizing ratios greater than 10 to 20 times. In addition, patients with adenomas typically have suppressed secretion from the contralateral side (defined as aldosterone/cortisol ratio from the contralateral side lower than that from the periphery).

Other Testing

In the past, several biochemical tests and nuclear medicine imaging (iodocholesterol) were used to help in subtype differentiation. The accuracy of these tests is low, and they are no longer recommended. In patients suspected of having glucocorticoid-remediable aldosteronism (early hypertension, personal or family history of hemorrhagic strokes or brain aneurysms), the diagnosis should be made through formal genetic testing to identify the chimeric gene mutation (between the aldosterone synthase and 11β-hydroxylase genes). Indirect physiologic tests, such as the dexamethasone suppression test or the measurement of urinary hybrid steroids, are no longer recommended, although they may still be used in resource-poor areas where genetic testing is not available.

TREATMENT OF PRIMARY ALDOSTERONISM

Primary aldosteronism is associated with cardiovascular and kidney damage, which is likely related to aldosterone excess. The removal or blockade of this excess results in improved clinical outcomes. Patients with an aldosterone-producing adenoma or unilateral adrenal hyperplasia should be offered laparoscopic unilateral adrenalectomy. All adrenalectomized patients experience normalization of serum potassium levels. On the other hand, BP improvement occurs primarily in younger patients who are lean (body mass index <26 kg/m^2), more often female, have a relatively recent history of hypertension (<5 to 6 years), require less than two drugs for treatment of their hypertension, and have normal kidney function. Patients who have few or none of these characteristics have poor BP response to adrenalectomy; accordingly, an initial attempt at medical therapy may be a more reasonable choice in the group.

Bilateral hyperplasia is managed medically, with an MRA as the backbone of therapy. A recent clinical trial showed that spironolactone was slightly better than eplerenone, although the doses may not have been precisely exchangeable. I typically start with spironolactone 25 mg once daily and escalate the dose as needed (typically 50 to 150 mg/day) to achieve BP and potassium control. For those patients who develop intolerable side effects to spironolactone, especially those related to its antiandrogenic effects, I substitute eplerenone using a 2:1 dosing ratio and twice-daily dosing. The Endocrine Society guidelines recommend against the use of MRAs in patients with estimated GFR (eGFR) less than 30 mL/min. I disagree with this recommendation because MRAs are effective antihypertensive agents even in anephric patients. The risk of hyperkalemia obviously exists but can be mitigated with the use of smaller doses (e.g., starting at 12.5 mg daily) and closely monitoring serum potassium levels.

Aldosterone synthase inhibitors are under development and have been tested in patients with primary aldosteronism. The early experience indicates that, while successful in suppressing aldosterone levels, the efficacy of managing BP is significantly less than eplerenone. At the present time, they are not yet marketed and their role in treatment remains uncertain, although one could envision a situation in which they are used in combination with an MRA or other BP agents, especially as patients often need additional agents to reach BP control despite the use of an MRA. Thiazide diuretics are often helpful, although potassium levels must be monitored closely as they may drop precipitously with the thiazide. Calcium channel blockers are also effective for BP control in primary aldosteronism.

PHEOCHROMOCYTOMA-PARAGANGLIOMA

Pheochromocytoma is a tumor arising from the adrenomedullary chromaffin cells. Paraganglioma is a tumor derived from extraadrenal chromaffin cells of the sympathetic paravertebral and neck ganglia. Pheochromocytomas are almost always biochemically active, producing epinephrine, norepinephrine, or dopamine, alone or in combination. Paragangliomas may be biochemically silent, especially when originating in the neck and base of the skull. Overall, pheochromocytomas represent approximately 80% to 85% of these tumors, whereas paragangliomas account for approximately 15% to 20%.

PPGLs are rare tumors, with an incidence of two to eight cases per million per year. However, knowledge about their clinical presentation and the appropriate approach to diagnosis and management are important because of the cardiovascular risk they pose through severe hypertension. Most PPGL patients are hypertensive (~90%), particularly those with pheochromocytoma. Approximately one-third of patients have only paroxysmal BP elevations, and, of the two-thirds with sustained hypertension, about half also have episodic peaks. These paroxysms are associated with catecholamine release and are clinically characterized by the classic triad of headaches, palpitations, and diaphoresis. This diagnostic triad is present in the majority of patients but has limited specificity (positive predictive value 6%), so that most patients with the triad actually do not have PPGL. Other common symptoms are anxiety, tremulousness, pallor, pale flushing, and orthostatic hypotension. There is growing acknowledgment of the fact that PPGL may be asymptomatic more often than previously considered and needs to be entertained in the diagnostic approach to adrenal masses and other masses of the neck, abdomen, and pelvis with the right location and radiographic appearance.

Overall, 5% to 10% of PPGL are extraabdominal, 10% to 15% are multifocal (including bilateral adrenal lesions), and approximately 10% are malignant. Recent advances in genetic testing have significantly increased the percentage of patients with PPGL associated with a specific syndrome or germline mutations. In the past, genetic causes of PPGL had been restricted to syndromic forms of PPGL, such as multiple endocrine neoplasia type 2 (MEN2), hereditary retinoblastoma (RET), neurofibromatosis type 1 (NF1), and von Hippel-Lindau disease (VHL). However, recent data estimate that up to 40% of PPGL patients have a germline mutation, even in patients with sporadic PPGL, a number that is likely to increase as novel mutations continue to be identified. One dozen germline mutations have already been described and have contributed to the understanding of the pathobiology of PPGL. For example, one cluster of germline mutations involving the VHL gene and the genes for the different succinate dehydrogenase (SDX) subunits and somatic mutations of the hypoxia-induced factor 2A (HIF2A) gene are characterized by an impact on abnormal transcription in response to hypoxia. Another cluster of mutations that involve *RET* and *NF1* among other genes is characterized by activation of kinase-mediated cell proliferation pathways, such as the PI3/AKT/mTOR. These developments not only have diagnostic and genetic counseling relevance but also may have treatment implications in the future.

PPGL should be suspected in every hypertensive patient with symptoms suggestive of catecholamine excess. While there are several reports of hypertensive PPGL presenting without any symptoms, these are unusual (probably ~1%), and, as a rule, I do not screen patients referred to us for the evaluation of nonparoxysmal hypertension who are fully asymptomatic. The exceptions are very young patients or those who have the sudden development of hypertension that is not explained by other more common secondary causes. It should also be suspected in patients with one of the syndromic forms of PPGL, such as MEN2, hereditary RET, NF1, and VHL, and in adult patients with chronic congenital cyanotic heart disease, an association that has been based on the role of chronic hypoxia as a mediator of tumor development.

BIOCHEMICAL DIAGNOSIS AND IMAGING OF PHEOCHROMOCYTOMA-PARAGANGLIOMA

Biochemical documentation of catecholamine excess is essential during the evaluation of PPGL. No other tests (e.g., localizing imaging tests) should be performed until there is laboratory evidence of excessive catecholamine production and/or metabolism. The measurement of free metanephrines in serum or urine is the preferred diagnostic test. Metanephrines are produced continuously within chromaffin cells (or chromaffin-derived PPGL); this is different and independent from the pattern of catecholamine release, which can be intermittent.

Plasma or urine free metanephrines are acceptable screening measurements, both having an accuracy in the 96% to 99% range. Sensitivity is very high, although there are shortcomings in specificity due to substances that may cause falsely elevated levels. In the case of plasma metanephrines, false-positive normetanephrine can be observed with acetaminophen (only certain assays), tricyclic antidepressants, methyldopa, phenoxybenzamine, and sulfasalazine, whereas buspirone may elevate plasma metanephrines. Monoamine oxidase (MAO) inhibitors, cocaine and other sympathomimetics, and levodopa can provoke false elevations of both plasma metanephrine and normetanephrine. Similar patterns are observed for urine metanephrine and normetanephrine levels. In addition, labetalol and sotalol can increase both urinary levels (but have no effect on plasma measurements).

Measurement of plasma free metanephrines requires cautious attention to position. When levels are obtained in the seated position, there is almost a threefold increase in false positives compared with supine measurements. The Endocrine Society recommends supine measurements; however, it recognizes the practical limitations of this recommendation, as most laboratories are unable to accommodate this request. Accordingly, it is acceptable to obtain samples in the seated position and, in case results are high, have them repeated in the supine position or corroborated by a 24-hour urine collection.

Most PPGLs result in metanephrine levels more than 3 times above the normal range. In such cases, anatomic localization is indicated. In patients with repeatedly borderline levels, the clonidine suppression test can be performed to distinguish between a normal variant (suppressible plasma metanephrines) and PPGL (nonsuppressible levels). In this test, clonidine 0.3 mg is given orally immediately after measurement of plasma metanephrines, which are measured again 3 hours later. Normally, clonidine lowers catecholamine and metanephrine levels by more than 40%; however, no such effect occurs in PPGL.

When convincing biochemical evidence of PPGL is available, radiographic localization is indicated. The screening method of choice is a contrast-enhanced CT of the abdomen and pelvis, as 85% of PPGL are intraabdominal. If negative, imaging extension to the chest (CT) and neck (MRI) should be performed. In patients in whom a tumor cannot be identified despite the above approach, ^{123}I-metaiodobenzylguanidine (MIBG) scintigraphy is indicated as another method to locate the tumor. Other techniques, including ^{123}I-MIBG positron emission tomography (PET) and 5-fluorodopamine-PET, are not easily available outside of research institutions.

GENETIC TESTING IN PHEOCHROMOCYTOMA-PARAGANGLIOMA

The Endocrine Society recommends the use of shared decision making with the patient regarding genetic testing. The guidelines suggest individual screening for mutations based on the familial distribution, the presence of a defined syndrome, and the guided choice of genes to be tested based on location and biochemical profile of the tumor. Because of the continued rise in identification of mutations in PPGL, many clinicians from several referral centers do not follow this approach and instead screen all patients (including those with sporadic PPGL) using a next-generation sequencing package that covers all known mutations. As the field evolves, more uniformity in the practice is likely to emerge.

TREATMENT OF PHEOCHROMOCYTOMA-PARAGANGLIOMA

The treatment of choice for PPGLs is surgical excision and should take place in referral centers with large experience with neuroendocrine tumors. Pheochromocytomas can be managed laparoscopically, whereas paragangliomas are usually resected with an open approach. All patients should be treated medically for at least 1 to 2 weeks in anticipation of surgery. The cornerstone of therapy is an alpha-blocker (either the nonselective phenoxybenzamine or a selective alpha$_1$-blocker, such as doxazosin or terazosin). Calcium channel blockers (amlodipine or nifedipine) are the first option as add-on treatment if BP is not adequately controlled with an alpha-blocker, followed by the addition of a beta-blocker (propranolol or atenolol). Many clinicians also routinely use metyrosine (a tyrosine hydroxylase inhibitor that blocks the first step in catecholamine synthesis) to improve BP control and intraoperative stability in these patients.

The evaluation and management of metastatic disease are nuanced and beyond the scope of this chapter. Follow-up is planned based on individual clinical and genetic characteristics. In most cases, biochemical screening is repeated 6 months following resection and then yearly. In high-risk patients, such as those with large pheochromocytomas, multifocal paragangliomas, or biochemically silent disease, yearly imaging is indicated.

OTHER ENDOCRINE CAUSES OF HYPERTENSION

CUSHING SYNDROME

Approximately 80% of patients with glucocorticoid excess due to Cushing syndrome have hypertension. However, they typically come to medical attention due to other features of the syndrome (weight gain, fatigue, muscle weakness, skin changes, anxiety, glucose intolerance, hyperlipidemia, osteopenia) rather than hypertension. Patients with ectopic ACTH production tend to have more severe hypertension. In many cases, hypokalemia can be significant. It is important to always consider the possibility of glucocorticoid excess in patients with hypertension accompanied by low aldosterone and suppressed PRA.

THYROID DISEASE

Hypertension may be observed in both hypothyroidism and hyperthyroidism, although the hemodynamic profile of each condition is quite distinct. Hypertension is seen in ~40% of patients with hypothyroidism and has a predominantly diastolic phenotype associated with increased systemic vascular resistance and decreased arterial compliance. Because of low cardiac output, patients may have a narrow pulse pressure despite stiff vessels. Hypertension in hyperthyroidism is primarily systolic and is related to increased cardiac output. Because vascular resistance is decreased, pulse pressure is often wide. Hyperthyroid patients may present with spells and paroxysmal features that at times resemble pheochromocytoma. Specific treatments for each thyroid disturbance are sufficient to normalize BP in most patients.

PRIMARY HYPERPARATHYROIDISM

Up to 70% of patients with primary hyperparathyroidism due to a parathyroid adenoma are hypertensive. Despite the absence of a direct correlation between serum calcium or parathyroid hormone levels and BP in these patients, it is presumed that it is the increase in cytosolic calcium that results in hypertension due to increased vascular resistance and cardiac output. Hypercalcemia-induced renal vasoconstriction and kidney damage due to hypercalciuria are additional mechanisms that may mediate hypertension. Removal of the adenomatous gland cures or improves BP in most hyperparathyroid patients with a new diagnosis of hypertension.

ACROMEGALY

Hypertension is common in acromegaly, although much of its prevalence may be explained by age and sex. Despite this, BP decreases following successful treatment in many patients, thus raising the possibility that growth hormone and insulin-like growth factor 1 are indeed related to hypertension in this condition. BP elevations are seldom severe.

OBSTRUCTIVE SLEEP APNEA

Obstructive sleep apnea (OSA) is a common disorder in the general population, and it is associated with hypertension, in particular due to the shared common occurrence of obesity. OSA results in not only nocturnal but also diurnal elevations in BP, and there is a direct relationship between the severity of OSA and the frequency and severity of hypertension. In patients with resistant hypertension, the prevalence of OSA is approximately 60%.

OSA should be suspected in obese patients (men more so than women) who report severe snoring, daytime somnolence, witnessed nocturnal choking or gasping, and have a "crowded oropharynx" (limited or no visualization of the soft palate) on physical examination. The diagnosis of OSA is based on an ambulatory sleep study or in-center polysomnography (the gold standard).

OSA can be considered a "nonclassic" cause of secondary hypertension because its treatment with continuous positive airway pressure ventilation (CPAP) does not necessarily result in the cure of hypertension. In fact, the overall BP-lowering effect of CPAP is low (~3/2 mm Hg). However, patients who have more severe hypertension (resistant hypertension with BP >145/85 mm Hg despite the use of three or more drugs), more severe OSA (apnea/hypopnea index >30), higher daytime sleepiness score (Epworth Sleepiness Score >10), and greater adherence to CPAP (average use >4 hours per night) tend to have greater responses.

Despite the limited magnitude of the BP-lowering effect of CPAP, I still believe there is value in asking about and screening for OSA in hypertensive patients and referring those with high sleepiness scores for formal sleep testing. In nonsleepy OSA patients, the strength of the evidence for benefit on BP lowering is weak, and a recent trial failed to demonstrate improvements in cardiovascular outcomes. Therefore I tend to pursue the diagnosis and treatment of OSA in nonsleepy patients only in the setting of resistant hypertension.

Aside from CPAP, patients with sleep apnea can benefit from medical therapy. Hypertension of OSA is associated with both sympathetic activation and aldosterone excess. While there is no definitive trial demonstrating the superiority of one drug class over another in OSA, there is some evidence that beta-blockers are particularly effective, and some recent data demonstrate the value of spironolactone, either alone or in combination with a loop diuretic. It is interesting that spironolactone can improve not only the BP but also the OSA. This may be due to an improvement in extracellular volume and a decrease in rostral fluid accumulation during recumbence/sleep.

COARCTATION OF THE AORTA AND OTHER AORTOPATHIES

Coarctation of the aorta (CoA) is a constriction of the descending thoracic aorta, most commonly distal to the left subclavian artery, but should be interpreted as a diffuse large vessel arteriopathy. It is an unusual cause of hypertension in adults and should be suspected in patients with hypertension in the arms but normal or low BP in the thigh/leg. A bicuspid aortic valve is a common accompaniment, present in 50% of CoA patients. Conversely, approximately 6% of patients with a bicuspid aortic valve have CoA. Therefore in patients with a known bicuspid aortic valve who develop hypertension at a young age or have new, otherwise unexplained, hypertension should have the possibility of CoA entertained, especially as bicuspid aortic valves are relatively common (1% to 2% of the population). Hypertension is noted in the upper extremities due to mechanical obstruction to blood flow, which in turn results in renal ischemia and activation of the RAAS. The diagnosis is made with magnetic resonance angiography or CT angiography to locate and define the severity of the coarctation. Echocardiography is an alternative method, although it is not as accurate. Once diagnosed, patients should undergo angiography to define the translesional gradient and, if it is elevated (>20 mm Hg), they should undergo repair either surgically or with balloon angioplasty with or without stenting. In recent years, percutaneous angioplasty has been increasingly used in lieu of open surgical techniques for the successful treatment of localized CoA in adults. Surgery is preferred for complex lesions not suitable for percutaneous management.

Stenotic lesions of the aorta due to other forms of aortic disease can be seen at any level and may result in hypertension through similar mechanisms as CoA. Although rare, the most common such aortopathy is Takayasu arteritis, which should be considered in patients with evidence of a systemic inflammatory disease with progressive involvement of the aorta and large branches, in particular among women (~90%) of East Asian descent, although the disease has been identified with increasing frequency in the Indian subcontinent, the Middle East, and both Central and South America.

KEY BIBLIOGRAPHY

Anderson GH Jr, Blakeman N, Streeten DH. The effect of age on prevalence of secondary forms of hypertension in 4429 consecutively referred patients. *J Hypertens.* 1994;12:609-615.

Caielli P, Frigo AC, Pengo MF, et al. Treatment of atherosclerotic renovascular hypertension: review of observational studies and a meta-analysis of randomized clinical trials. *Nephrol Dial Transplant.* 2015;30:541-553.

Cano-Pumarega I, Duran-Cantolla J, Aizpuru F, et al. Obstructive sleep apnea and systemic hypertension: longitudinal study in the general population. *Am J Respir Crit Care Med.* 2011;184:1299-1304.

Dorresteijn JA, Visseren FL, Spiering W. Mechanisms linking obesity to hypertension. *Obes Rev.* 2012;13:17-26.

Elliot WE, Peixoto AJ, Bakris GB. Primary and secondary hypertension. In: Skorecki K, Chertow GM, Marsden PA, Yu ASL, Taal MW, eds. *Brenner and Rector's the Kidney.* Philadelphia: Elsevier; 2016: 1522-1566.

Funder JW, Carey RM, Mantero F, et al. The management of primary aldosteronism: case detection, diagnosis, and treatment: an endocrine society clinical practice guideline. *J Clin Endocrinol Metab.* 2016;101:1889-1916.

Grossman A, Messerli FH, Grossman E. Drug induced hypertension—an unappreciated cause of secondary hypertension. *Eur J Pharmacol.* 2015;763:15-22.

Hannemann A, Wallaschofski H. Prevalence of primary aldosteronism in patient's cohorts and in population-based studies—a review of the current literature. *Horm Metab Res.* 2012;44:157-162.

Iftikhar IH, Valentine CW, Bittencourt LR, et al. Effects of continuous positive airway pressure on blood pressure in patients with resistant hypertension and obstructive sleep apnea: a meta-analysis. *J Hypertens.* 2014;32:2341-2350, discussion 2350.

Japanese Society of Hypertension Committee for Guidelines for the Management of Hypertension. Secondary Hypertension. *Hypertens Res.* 2014;37:349-361.

Kempers MJ, Lenders JW, van Outheusden L, et al. Systematic review: diagnostic procedures to differentiate unilateral from bilateral adrenal abnormality in primary aldosteronism. *Ann Intern Med.* 2009;151: 329-337.

Lenders JW, Duh QY, Eisenhofer G, et al. Pheochromocytoma and paraganglioma: an endocrine society clinical practice guideline. *J Clin Endocrinol Metab.* 2014;99:1915-1942.

Montesi SB, Edwards BA, Malhotra A, et al. The effect of continuous positive airway pressure treatment on blood pressure: a systematic review and meta-analysis of randomized controlled trials. *J Clin Sleep Med.* 2012;8:587-596.

Omura M, Saito J, Yamaguchi K, et al. Prospective study on the prevalence of secondary hypertension among hypertensive patients visiting a general outpatient clinic in Japan. *Hypertens Res.* 2004;27:193-202.

Parikh SA, Shishehbor MH, Gray BH, et al. SCAI expert consensus statement for renal artery stenting appropriate use. *Catheter Cardiovasc Interv.* 2014;84:1163-1171.

Parthasarathy HK, Menard J, White WB, et al. A double-blind, randomized study comparing the antihypertensive effect of eplerenone and spironolactone in patients with hypertension and evidence of primary aldosteronism. *J Hypertens.* 2011;29:980-990.

Persu A, Giavarini A, Touze E, et al. European consensus on the diagnosis and management of fibromuscular dysplasia. *J Hypertens.* 2014;32:1367-1378.

Rossi GP, Auchus RJ, Brown M, et al. An expert consensus statement on use of adrenal vein sampling for the subtyping of primary aldosteronism. *Hypertension.* 2014;63:151-160.

Wachtel H, Cerullo I, Bartlett EK, et al. Long-term blood pressure control in patients undergoing adrenalectomy for primary hyperaldosteronism. *Surgery.* 2014;156:1394-1402, discussion 402-403.

Wilhelm SM, Young J, Kale-Pradhan PB. Effect of bariatric surgery on hypertension: a meta-analysis. *Ann Pharmacother.* 2014;48:674-682.

Full bibliography can be found on www.expertconsult.com.

Index